Embryo and Fetal Pathology

COLOR ATLAS WITH ULTRASOUND CORRELATION

Exhaustively illustrated in color with more than 1000 photographs, figures, histopathology slides, and sonograms, this uniquely authoritative atlas provides the clinician with a visual guide to diagnosing congenital anomalies, both common and rare, in every organ system in the human fetus. It covers the full range of embryo and fetal pathology, from point of death, autopsy and ultrasound, through specific syndromes, intrauterine problems, organ and system defects to multiple births and conjoined twins. Gross pathologic findings are correlated with sonographic features in order that the reader may confirm visually the diagnosis of congenital abnormalities for all organ systems. Obstetricians, perinatologists, neonatologists, geneticists, anatomic pathologists, and all practitioners of maternal-fetal medicine will find this atlas an invaluable resource.

Enid Gilbert-Barness is Professor of Pathology, Laboratory Medicine, Pediatrics and Obstetrics and Gynecology at the University of South Florida and Professor Emeritus of Pathology and Laboratory Medicine and Distinguished Medical Alumni Professor Emeritus at the University of Wisconsin-Madison. She is a leading authority in pediatric pathology with an international reputation for her contributions to the areas of congenital abnormalities, tumor biology, abnormal skeletal growth, sudden infant death syndrome, and many genetic and hereditary disorders.

Diane Debich-Spicer is a pathologists' assistant and highly accomplished medical illustrator. She has had more than twenty years of experience in pediatric pathology.

Embryo and Fetal Pathology

COLOR ATLAS WITH ULTRASOUND CORRELATION

Enid Gilbert-Barness, MD, MBBS, FRCPA, FRCPath, DSci(hc), MD(hc)
Tampa General Hospital, University of South Florida
University of Wisconsin School of Medicine

Diane Debich-Spicer, BS
Tampa General Hospital, University of South Florida

Ultrasound contributions from:
Mark Williams, MD
Kathy B. Porter, MD
Susan Guidi, MS, RDMS

FOREWORD BY JOHN M. OPITZ, MD, MD(hc), DSci(hc), MD(hc)
Pediatrics (Medical Genetics), Human Genetics, Obstetrics and Gynecology, and Pathology
University of Utah Medical School

CAMBRIDGE
UNIVERSITY PRESS

PUBLISHED BY THE PRESS SYNDICATE OF THE UNIVERSITY OF CAMBRIDGE
The Pitt Building, Trumpington Street, Cambridge, United Kingdom

CAMBRIDGE UNIVERSITY PRESS
The Edinburgh Building, Cambridge CB2 2RU, UK
40 West 20th Street, New York, NY 10011-4211, USA
477 Williamstown Road, Port Melbourne, VIC 3207, Australia
Ruiz de Alarcón 13, 28014 Madrid, Spain
Dock House, The Waterfront, Cape Town 8001, South Africa

http://www.cambridge.org

First published 2004

Printed in Singapore

Typefaces Minion 10.5/14 pt. and ITC Symbol *System* LATEX 2_ε [TB]

A catalog record for this book is available from the British Library.

Library of Congress Cataloging in Publication Data

Gilbert-Barness, Enid, 1927–

Embryo and fetal pathology : color atlas with ultrasound correlation / Enid Gilbert-Barness, Diane Debich-Spicer ; with a foreword by John M. Opitz.

p. cm.

Includes bibliographical references and index.

ISBN 0-521-82529-6

1. Fetus – Diseases – Diagnosis – Atlases. 2. Human embryo – Diseases – Diagnosis – Atlases. 3. Fetus – Abnormalities – Atlases. 4. Ultrasonics in obstetrics – Atlases. 5. Embryology – Atlases. I. Spicer, Diane Debich. II. Title.

RG626.G34 2003
618.3′2′00222 – dc22 2003055422

ISBN 0 521 82529 6 hardback

To Lew, Mary, Elizabeth, Jennifer, Rebecca and grandchildren Alexandra,
Louis, Christian, James, Thomas, Blake, Spencer, Curtis,
Kiara and Rebecca

and

To Scott and Andrew

Contents

Foreword

With the publication of ***Embryo and Fetal Pathology***, developmental pathology has come full circle. It is no coincidence that the development of this branch of biology was almost exactly congruent with that of morphology. And while morphology, since its founding by Goethe and Burdach, respectively, in 1796 and 1800, continued to grow slowly but steadily, especially after shedding its neo-Platonic philosophical trappings, developmental pathology matured in fits and spurts with some astonishing *hiatus*, which to date remain unexplained by the historians of biology. And while the description of the malformed *fetus*, some of them with remarkable accuracy, antedated the 19th century, it was not until 1802–1805 that we can date a modern (i.e., scientific) analysis of malformations. It was on the 8th of April 1802 that Joannes Fridericus Meckel, *Halensis*, at the age of 21, *publice defendet* his *dissertatio inauguralis "de cordis conditionibus abnormibus"* (on congenital heart defects, published in *Reil's Archive* three years later).

What happened between 1802 and 1805 in Meckel's life was of the utmost importance for the subsequent development of the field, for it was during that time that the prodigiously gifted, young Meckel – working with Cuvier in Paris – became master of comparative anatomy but with the difference that, while Cuvier ignored embryonic and fetal stages and considered malformations irrelevant, Meckel did not. Indeed, it was Meckel's attention to prenatal stages of life, whether normal or abnormal, that led to the formulation of the concepts of vestigia (persistence of embryonic/fetal stages) and atavisms (recurrence of an ancestral stage) and an initial recapitalulationist attempt to relate evolution and development.

And while, in the words of Virchow, Meckel, during his short life of 52 years, accomplished the best and most in what was in Virchow's days called the science of Teratology, the oblivion that befell his work after his death was so complete that the science was independently reinvented several times in the subsequent century, beginning with Rokitansky, Isidore Geoffroy St.-Hilaire, Taruffi, Dareste, and, finally, Ballantyne. Ernst Schwalbe began his *Morphologie der Missbildungen des Menschen und der Tiere* (Morphology of malformations of humans and animals) in 1906 and finished Parts I (on the science of malformations or Teratology) and II (conjoined twinning, 1907) himself before enlisting the collaboration of coworkers who completed the work after Schwalbe's death; lastly, under Georg Gruber's editorship, the last fascicle (on the malformation of the male genitalia) appeared in 1958. John W. Ballantyne of Edinburgh completed the second part of his *Manual of Antenatal Pathology and Hygiene* (The Embryo) in 1904.

Thereafter, virtually no text for the medical profession comprehensively addressed the science, that is, the causes and pathogenesis of human malformations. I for one received no instruction on the subject in medical school; the somewhat idiosyncratic text by Willis (*The Borderland of Embryology and Pathology*, 1958) with its denunciation of atavisms did not appear until the year before my medical school graduation. After Lejeune's discovery of trisomy "21" in Down syndrome in 1959, there was a sudden and highly productive renaissance of the study of human developmental anomalies – in my case, facilitated by a marvelous undergraduate education in embryology and the evolutionary aspects of development (under Emil Witschi). I had met Josef Warkany in Dr. Witschi's office and, during my first year of residency, was struggling with a decision of whether to continue my training as a teratologist in Cincinnati under Warkany, or as a clinical geneticist in Madison with David Smith and Klaus Patau. I applied to both institutions; a few minutes after I accepted the position in Madison, late at night shortly before the first of July 1961, the chair of Pediatrics in Cincinnati called and was disappointed at my unreasonable decision. In retrospect, it was a fortunate decision because my training placed heavy emphasis on genetics and cytogenetics at a time when medical morphology was barely beginning a rebirth and was not considered a science fit for a respectable geneticist. Nevertheless, after David Smith's departure for the University of Washington in Seattle, pediatric/clinical genetics continued to grow in Madison complemented by a supportive and productive anatomical genetics program where we were privileged to dissect the first few 18- and 13-trisomy infants previously studied by Drs. Smith, Patau, and Pallister (in far-off Montana). The field was stimulated by continuing discoveries in cytogenetics, biochemical genetics, and animal genetics (e.g., Hans Grüneberg in the mouse, Curt Stern and Ernst Hadorn in *Drosophilia*).

And then in 1970, *mirabile cum dictu*, Enid Gilbert was appointed Professor of Pediatric Pathology at the University of Wisconsin, and my life has not been the same since then. Now it was finally possible for me, under the guidance of this enormously experienced, wise, and gentle colleague, to complete my training in developmental pathology and for us to develop together a research, service, and training program combining anatomy, genetics, embryology, and experimental approaches. It must be remembered that Enid was not only the consummate pediatric and fetal pathologist, but also a marvelous teratologist who conducted pioneering studies on the production of cardiovascular malformations in chicks with a successful and well-funded research team. Enid's knowledge in all of these fields was then already so legendary that her future husband, Lew Barness, stumped when asked to come up with a (correct) diagnosis in a CPC exercise, thought to be really clever in reading through Enid's bibliography for her favorite subject in the field to which he had narrowed his nosology (a storage disorder), at which point, he threw his hands up in wonder saying: "... why she has written on *all* of them."

Embryo and Fetal Pathology could not have been published at a more propitious time. At the beginning of this year the National Institute of Child Health and Human Development of the United States will support five centers to conduct exemplary, multidisciplinary studies to determine the causes of stillbirth. Surely, ***Embryo and Fetal Pathology*** will be the resource *par excellence* to guide those of us in the five centers, and *all* other pediatric/fetal pathologists throughout the world, to do the analyses most likely to yield the data needed to inform parents on pathogenesis, cause and recurrence risk pertaining to the death of their infant.

Meckel apologized that his "Beyträge" – contributions to pathologic anatomy of 1811 – were not illustrated, probably *the* crucial factor for that work's oblivion. He tried to amend in 1817 with the publication of his *Tabulae Anatomico-Pathologicae* which covered only the heart. Probably there is no more visually aesthetic science in biology than development and developmental pathology and the Gilbert-Barness text ***Embryo and Fetal Pathology*** is superbly illustrated (with the assistance of Diane Debich-Spicer) with more than 1000 images. Meckel could not have imagined the means available to us now to visually assess the structural and functional status of the embryo and fetus. But ***Embryo and Fetal Pathology*** is a model of coordinating information from ultrasonography, indeed, all means of prenatal diagnosis (with the expert collaboration of Mark Williams, Kathy Porter, and Susan Guidi), anatomy, embryology, radiology, molecular biology, and genetics to assist in our goal of assessing the fetus.

The stepchild of the 19th- and early 20th-century fetal pathology was the placenta and its relationship to fetal pathology; even now, we do not routinely give the placentas the same meticulous attention we pay to the fetus. Thus, Chapter 5 in ***Embryo and Fetal Pathology*** is called to particular attention of all students of human development for its detailed analysis of placental ontogeny, structure, and function.

There are two books Meckel would have considered fundamental in the progress of developmental history and pathology – he was ready, far, far ahead of his contemporaries for the *Origin of Species*... and he would have considered ***Embryo and Fetal Pathology*** the fulfillment of all of his efforts to unite comparative anatomy, embryology, "heredity," pathology, and the relationship of all animals on this earth, whether normal or abnormal. I feel humbly and profoundly gratified to greet and introduce this *opus maximus* of my friend and most distinguished collaborator, Dr. Enid Gilbert-Barness.

John M. Opitz
Lacosalensis, Utah
December 2003

Preface

This Atlas represents almost 50 years of study of embryos, fetuses, and perinatally dead infants. It includes more than 200 ultrasound images essential to modern diagnosis and important in the correlation with pathologic examination and for genetic counseling. In the past, products of conception frequently have been discarded or given only a cursory pathologic examination; however, in recent years it has become important to carefully examine these specimens and study embryonic tissue to accurately determine the nature and cause of prenatal death.

The Atlas includes more than 2000 illustrations in color, with a brief text of essential concepts and comments. Generous use of tables is made to replace more extensive text and important references are given at the end of each chapter.

A catalog of genetic syndromes with updated references is available through OnLine Mendelian Inheritance in Man OMIM (http://www3.ncbi.nlm.nih.gov/omim/). In general, OMIM does not provide specific testing sites but often discusses the potential for molecular testing and gives references that can be used to contact experts in the field.

It is our hope that this volume will be a useful reference for obstetricians engaged in fetal–maternal and reproductive medicine, geneticists, pediatricians – neonatologists, in particular, and pathologists who have an interest in pediatric and genetic pathology.

Enid Gilbert-Barness, MD
Diane Debich-Spicer, BS

Acknowledgments

The authors wish to express their thanks and deep gratitude to their many friends and colleagues who have been so generous with their time, encouragement, and support of this work, and to those who have contributed illustrations. In particular, we especially thank Carlos Abramowsky, Jeanne Ackerman, Jeff Angel, Sonja Arnold, John Balis, Lewis Barness, Stephen Brantley, Irwin Browarsky, M. Michael Cohen Jr., John Curran, Monica Drut, Philip Farrell, Jamie Frias, Americo Gonzalvo, Robert Gorlin, Susan Guidi, Silvaselvi Gunasekaran, James Huhta, Stanley Inhorn, Craig Kalter, Judith Krammer, Atilano Lacson, Renata Laxova, Jane Messina, Santo Nicosia, William O'Brien, John M. Opitz, Kathy Porter, Helga Rehder, Allen Root, Karen Schmidt, David Shields, Jürgen Spranger, George Tiller, Mark Williams, and Gabriele ZuRhein. We most sincerely appreciate the untiring dedication of Kathleen Lonkey in the preparation of the manuscript – without her expertise this book would not have been possible. We also thank Margaret Petro and Gerda Anderson, Tampa General Hospital librarians, whose help has been inestimable. To the editors Catherine Felgar and Eleanor Umali, we are profoundly indebted.

ONE

The Human Embryo and Embryonic Growth Disorganization

STAGES OF EMBRYONIC DEVELOPMENT

Carnegie staging in the development of the human embryo categorizes 23 stages.

Fertilization and Implantation (Stages 1–3)

Embryonic development commences with fertilization between a sperm and a secondary oocyte (Tables 1.1 to 1.5). The fertilization process requires about 24 hours and results in the formation of a **zygote** – a diploid cell with 46 chromosomes containing genetic material from both parents. This takes place in the ampulla of the uterine tube.

The embryo's sex is determined at fertilization. An X chromosome-bearing sperm produces an XX zygote, which normally develops into a female, whereas fertilization by a Y chromosome-bearing sperm produces an XY zygote, which normally develops into a male.

The zygote passes down the uterine tube and undergoes rapid mitotic cell divisions, termed cleavage. These divisions result in smaller cells – the **blastomeres.** Three days later, after the developing embryo enters the uterine cavity, compaction occurs, resulting in a solid sphere of 12–16 cells to form the **morula**.

At 4 days, hollow spaces appear inside the compact morula and fluid soon passes into these cavities, allowing one large space to form and thus converting the morula into the **blastocyst** (blastocyst hatching). The blastocyst cavity

Table 1.1 Human embryonic development and growth

Period	Conception* (d)	Gestational age** (d)	CR length (mm)	External characterizations	Carnegie staging
Blastogenesis					
First 2 weeks	0–14	0–28	0–0.4	Unicellular to bilaminar plate	1–6b
Days 14–28	15–28	29–35	0.4–4.6	Trilaminar embryo to open neural groove	7–10
Organogenesis					
Second 4 weeks	22–35	36–49	4.6–8	Neural tube closure to limb buds	11–13
Days 32–56	36–60	50–75	8–30	Limb growth to fused eyelids	14–22
Fetal	61–266	75–280	35–350	Fetal maturation	

* Embryonic development is dated from fertilization.
** Prenatal growth evaluation by ultrasound is dated from day of last menstrual period. This is termed "gestational age."
Adaped from Wilson RD: Prenatal evaluation of growth by ultrasound, *Growth Genetics & Hormones*, v.9(1), 1993.

separates the cells into an outer cell layer, the trophoblast, which gives rise to the placenta, and a group of centrally located cells, the **inner cell mass**, which gives rise to both embryo and extraembryonic tissue.

The **zona pellucida** hatches on day 5 and the blastocyst attaches to the endometrial epithelium. The trophoblastic cells then start to invade the endometrium.

Implantation of the blastocyst usually takes place on day 7 in the midportion of the body of the uterus, slightly more frequently on the posterior than on the anterior wall.

Gastrulation

Changes occur in the developing embryo as the bilaminar embryonic disc is converted into a trilaminar embryonic disc composed of three germ layers.

Table 1.2 Measurements of gestation age by ultrasound

Mean gestational age (wk)*	Mean gestational sac diameter (mm)†	Embryo CR length (mm)	BPD (mm)	Femur length (mm)
5 + 0	2	–	–	–
6 + 0	10	6	–	–
7 + 0	18	10	–	–
8 + 0	26	17	–	–
9 + 0	–	25	–	–
10 + 0	–	33	–	–
11 + 0	–	43	–	6
12 + 0	–	55	17	9
13 + 0	–	68	20	12
14 + 0	–	85	25	15

* From 1st day of last menstrual period †Daya et al., 1991 ‡Jeanty, 1983
Adaped from Wilson RD: Prenatal evaluation of growth by ultrasound, *Growth Genetics & Hormones*, v.9(1), 1993.

The process of germ layer formation, called gastrulation, is the beginning of embryogenesis (formation of the embryo).

Gastrulation begins at the end of the 1st week with the appearance of the hypoblast; it continues during the 2nd week with the formation of the epiblast and is completed during the 3rd week with the formation of intraembryonic mesoderm by the primitive streak. The three primary germ layers are called ectoderm, mesoderm, and endoderm. As the embryo develops, these layers give rise to the tissues and organs of the embryo.

The blastocyst begins to become attached to the uterine lining (the endometrium).

Table 1.3 Number of somites correlated to approximate age in days

Approximate age (days)	No. of somites
20	1–4
21	4–7
22	7–10
23	10–13
24	13–17
25	17–20
26	20–23
27	23–26
28	26–29
30	34–35

Implantation

Implantation includes dissolution of the zona pellucida and adhesion between the blastocyst and the endometrium, trophoblastic penetration, and migration

Table 1.4 Summary of embryonic development highlights

CR length (mm)	Days after ovulation	Carnegie stage	Main external features
0.1	0–2	1	Fertilized oocyte
	4–6	3	Blastocyst
0.2–0.4	6–15	5	Trilaminar embryo with primitive streak
1.5–2.0	20–22	9	Heart tubes begin to fuse
2.0–3.0	22–24	10	Neural folds begin to fuse; heart begins to beat
3.0–4.0	24–26	11	Rostral neuropore closing
4.0–5.0	26–30	12	Upper limb buds appear
5.0–6.0	28–32	13	Four pairs of branchial arches
6.0–7.0	31–35	14	Lens pits and nasal pits visible
Highlights 35–56 days, organogenesis			
7.0–10.0	35–38	15	Hand plates formed; retinal pigment visible
10.0–12.0	37–42	16	Foot plates formed
12.0–14.0	42–44	17	Finger rays appear; auricular hillocks developed
14.0–17.0	44–48	18	Toe rays appear
16.0–20.0	48–51	19	Trunk elongating; midgut herniation to umbilical cord
20.0–22.0	51–53	20	Fingers distinct but webbed
22.0–24.0	53–54	21	Fingers free and longer
24.0–28.0	54–56	22	Toes free and longer
28.0–30.0	56–60	23	Head more rounded; fusing eyelids

Table 1.5 Major landmarks for early development

Retinal pigment 35–37 days
Separation of common aorticopulmonary trunk (A & PA separate) 42 days
Distinct elbow and/or developing eyelids 44 days
Scalp vascular plexus 49 days
Intestines into umbilical cord 7–10 weeks
Perforation of anal membrane 51 days
Lack of tail 56 days
Fingernails and a well-defined neck 10–12 weeks (a fetus not embryo)

of the blastocyst through the endometrium. Implantation occurs by the intrusion of trophoblastic extensions, which penetrate between apparently intact endometrial cells.

Second Week of Development (Stages 4 and 5)

During the 2nd week, a bilaminar **embryonic disc** forms, **amniotic and primary yolk sac** cavities develop, and there are two layers of trophoblast (Figure 1.1).

The two-layered disc separates the blastocyst cavity into two unequal parts (a smaller amniotic cavity and a larger primary yolk cavity). The thick layer of embryonic cells bordering the amniotic cavity is called the **epiblast** and a thin layer bordering the primary yolk cavity is called the **hypoblast**.

The trophoblast differentiates into two layers, an inner **cytotrophoblast** and an outer **syncytiotrophoblast**. The trophoblast continues to penetrate deeper into the endometrium. At the end of the 2nd week, the site of implantation is recognized as a small elevated area of endometrium having a central pore filled with a blood clot.

Third Week of Development (Stages 6–9)

Formation of the primitive streak and three germ layers (ectoderm, mesoderm, and endoderm) (Figure 1.2) occurs during the 3rd week.

The **primitive streak** results from a proliferation of ectodermal cells at the caudal end of the embryonal disc. Cells at the primitive streak proliferate to form the embryonic endoderm and mesoderm. The cephalic end of

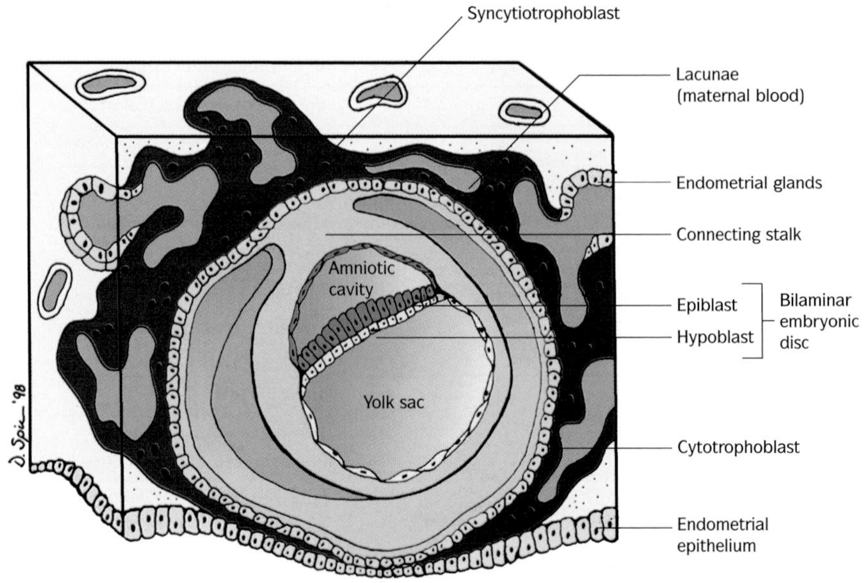

1.1. Bilaminar embryonic disc in the 2nd week of development (stage 5), with amniotic and primary yolk sac cavities.

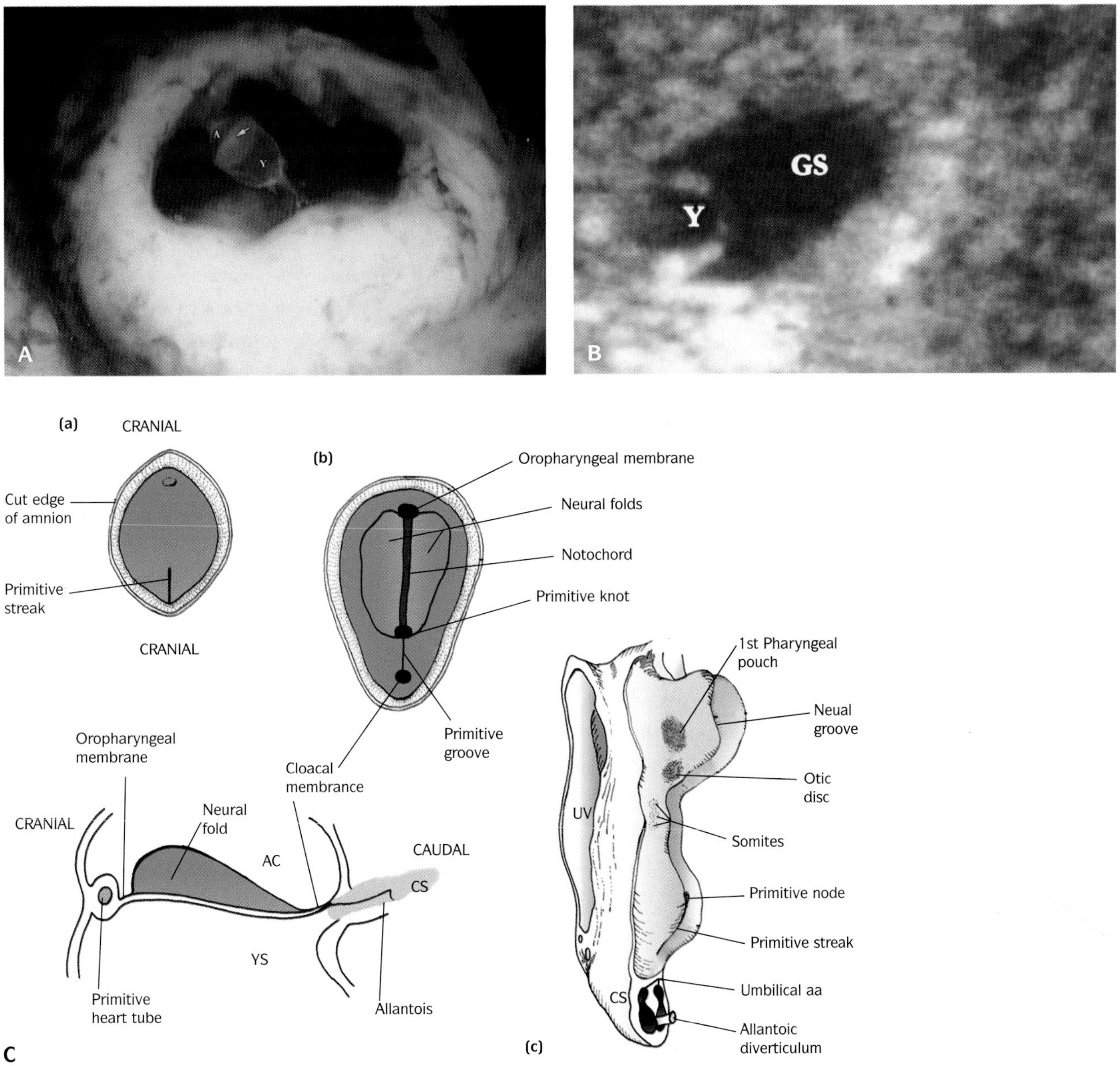

1.2. (A) Ectopic pregnancy at day 17 showing an embryonic disc with opacity (arrow) representing the primitive streak. The amniotic cavity (A) and the primary yolk sac cavity (Y) are present. **(B)** Ultrasound of a human embryo at the same stage of development as A (GS, gestational sac; Y, yolk sac). **(C)** Diagram of development of the primitive streak (a), notochord (b), and neural folds (c) in a trilaminar embryo (stages 6–9).

the primitive streak is the primitive node, and this cord of cells is the **notochord.**

Thickening of ectodermal cells gives rise to the **neural plate**, the first appearance of the nervous system, which becomes depressed below the surface along the long axis of the embryo to form the neural groove. The **neural groove** deepens and its margins elevate to form the **neural folds**. The fusion is completed during the 4th week of development. The neural tube ultimately will give rise to the central nervous system. The cephalic end will dilate to form the forebrain, midbrain, and hindbrain. The remainder of the neural tube will become the spinal cord.

The mesoderm on either side of the midline of the embryo (the paraxial mesoderm) undergoes segmentation, forming **somites**. The first pair of somites arises in the cervical region of the embryo at approximately day 20 of development. From there new somites appear in craniocaudal sequence, approximately three per day, until 42–44 pairs are present at the end of week 5. There are 4 occipital, 8 cervical, 12 thoracic, 5 lumbar, 5 sacral, and 8–10 coccygeal pairs. The first occipital and the last 5–7 coccygeal somites later disappear, while the remainder form the axial skeleton. During this period of development, the age of the embryo is expressed in the number of somites. Each somite differentiates into bones, cartilage, and ligaments of the vertebral column as well as into skeletal voluntary muscles, dermis, and subcutaneous tissue of the skin. The intermediate mesoderm and the lateral mesoderm give rise to portions of the urogenital system. The lateral plate mesoderm is involved in the development of pericardial, pleural, and peritoneal cavities as well as the muscle of the diaphragm.

Mesoderm also forms a primitive cardiovascular system during the 3rd week of development. Blood vessel formation begins in the extraembryonic mesoderm of the yolk sac, the connecting stalk, and the chorion. Embryonic vessels develop 2 days later. The linkage of the primitive heart tube with blood vessels takes place toward the end of week 3, after which blood circulation begins. The beating heart tube begins at 17–19 days.

The embryo changes shape from a disc to a tube with a cranial and a caudal end and the third germ layer, the endoderm, becomes incorporated into the interior of the embryo.

The formation of **chorionic villi** takes place in the 3rd week. The cytotrophoblast cells of the chorionic villi penetrate the layer of syncytiotrophoblast to form a cytotrophoblastic shell, which attaches the chorionic sac to the endometrial tissues.

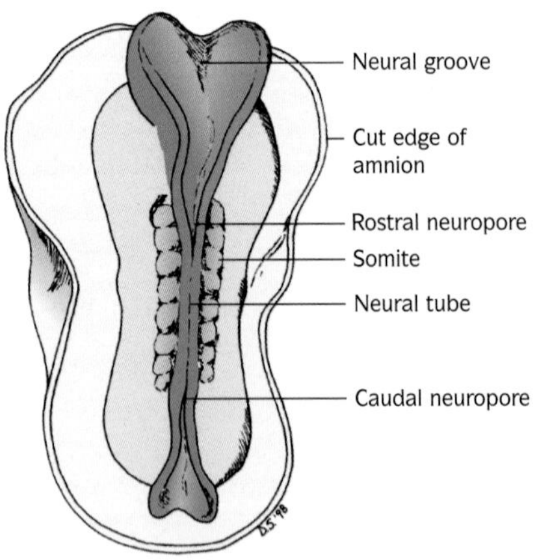

1.3. Diagram of human embryo at stage 10. Neural folds are partially fused with the neural tube open at the rostral and caudal neuropore.

Fourth Week of Development (Stages 10–12: Up to Day 28, End of Blastogenesis)

At this stage, the embryo measures 2–5 mm (Figures 1.3 to 1.6). At *stage 10*, the embryo (at 22–24 days) is almost straight and has between 4 and 12 somites that produce conspicuous surface elevations. The neural tube is closed between the somites but is widely open at the rostral and caudal neuropore. The first and second pairs of branchial arches become visible.

During *stage 11*, a slight curve is produced by folding of the head and tail. The heart produces a large ventral prominence. The rostral neuropore continues to close and optic vesicles are formed.

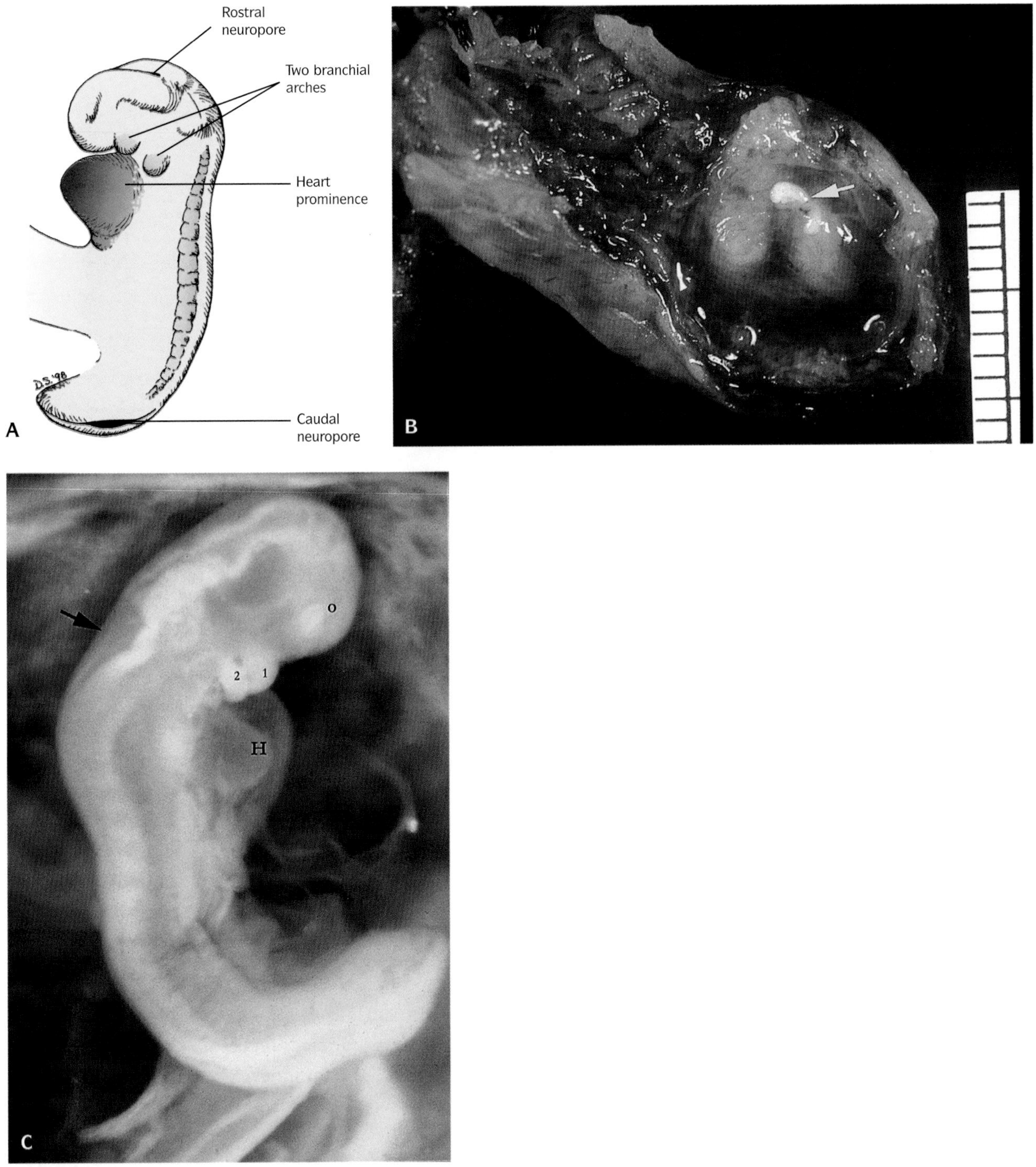

1.4. (A) Diagram of a human embryo at stage 11. **(B)** A human embryo at stage 11 (arrow) showing a slight curve. The size should range from 2 to 5 mm. **(C)** Human embryo at stage 11 with a slight curve, two pairs of branchial arches, heart prominence (H), and optic vesicle (O). Rostral neuropore (arrow) continues to close.

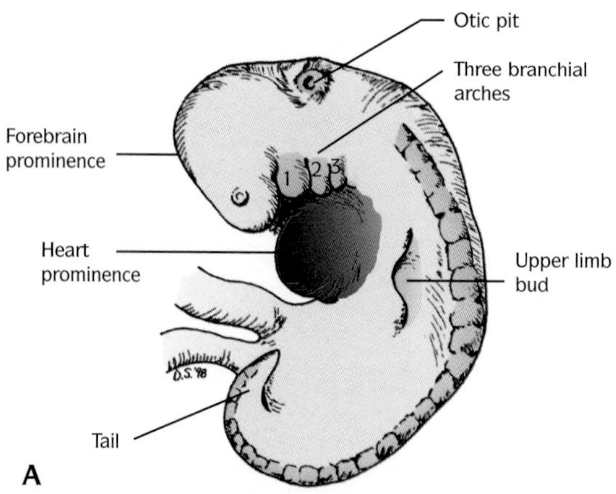

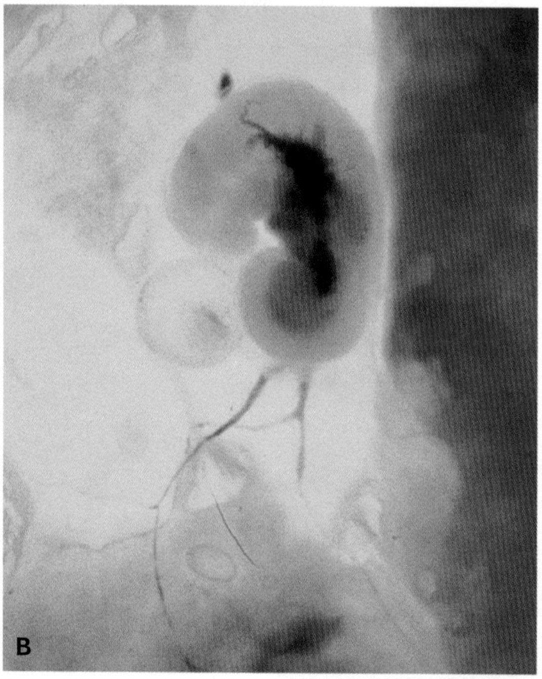

1.5. **(A)** Drawing of a human embryo at stage 12. **(B)** Embryo at stage 10–12 (4th week of development) with early vascular development.

In *stage 12*, three pairs of **branchial arches** complete closure of the rostral hemisphere and recognizable upper-limb buds on the ventral lateral body wall appear. The **otic pits** and the primordia of the inner ears become visible. Growth of the forebrain produces an enlargement of the head, and further folding of the embryo in the longitudinal plane results in a C-shaped curvature. Narrowing of the connection between the embryo and the yolk sac produces a **body stalk** containing one umbilical vein and two umbilical arteries.

Fifth Week of Development (Stages 13–15)

At this stage, the embryo measures 5–10 mm in length. Rapid head growth occurs, caused mainly by rapid development of the brain. The upper limbs

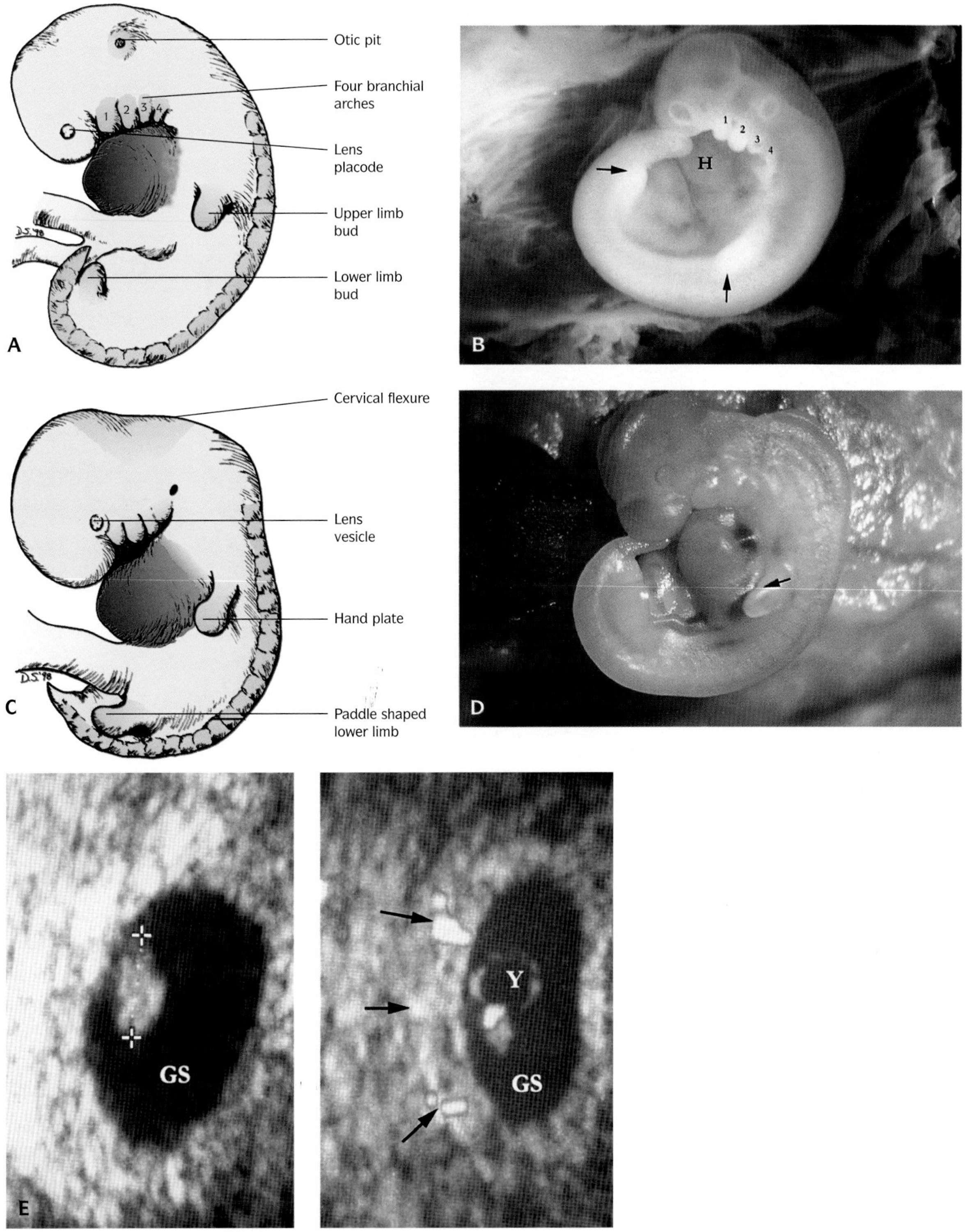

1.6. (A) Drawing of a human embryo at stage 13. **(B)** Human embryo at stage 13. Note body curvature, four pairs of branchial arches, heart prominence (H), and upper and lower limb buds (arrows). The lens placode and otic pit are identifiable and the neural tube is closed. **(C)** Drawing of a human embryo at stage 15. **(D)** Human embryo at stage 15 with well-defined lens vesicle and an area representing hand plate formation (arrow). The cervical flexure is prominent. **(E)** Ultrasound at stages 13–15: (Right) CR length of embryo in the gestational sac. (Left) Doppler imaging showing blood flow (arrows) surrounding the gestational sac (GS) and in the embryo (transverse plane at the level of the heart). Yolk sac (Y) is also indicated.

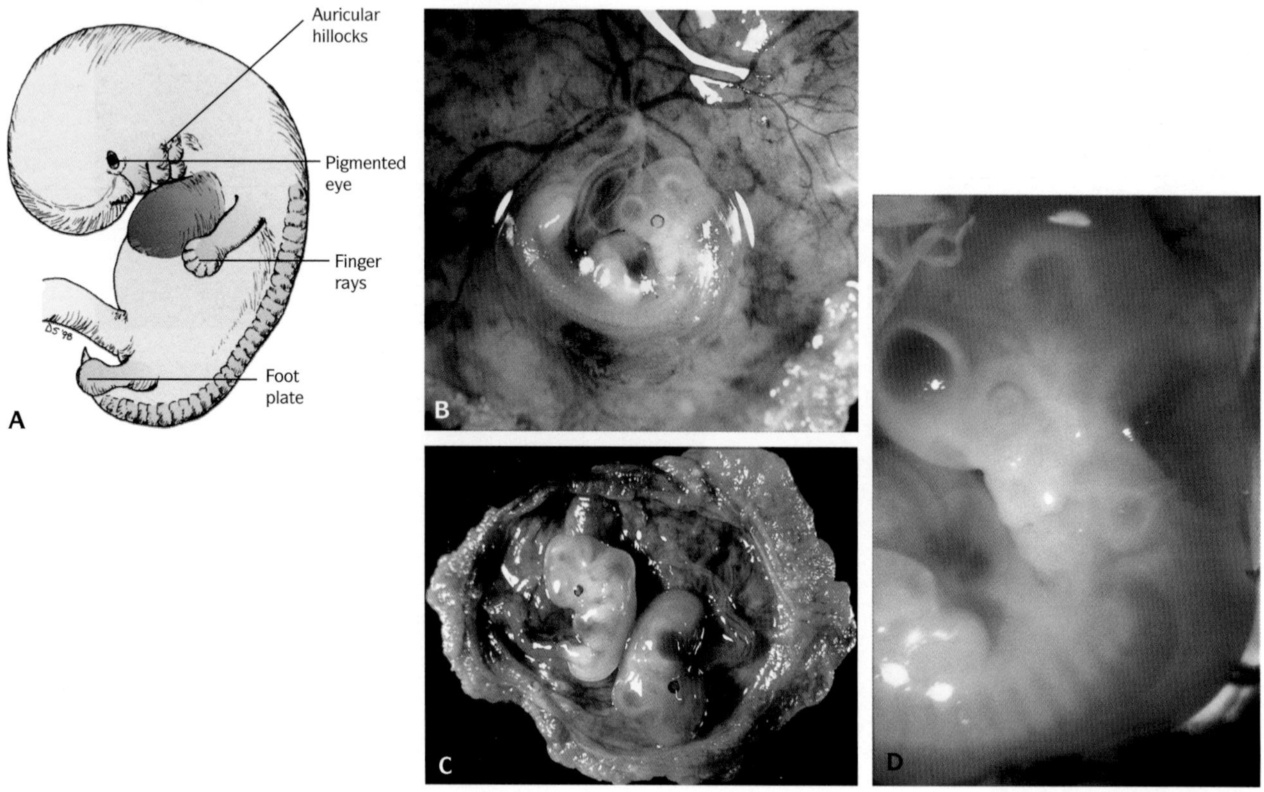

1.7. **(A)** Drawing of a human embryo at stage 17, lateral view. **(B)** Human embryo with early formation of retinal pigment, finger rays and foot plate. **(C)** Monochorionic monoamniotic twin embryos with well-developed retinal pigment. **(D)** Embryo at 12 weeks fertilization age showing auricular hillocks.

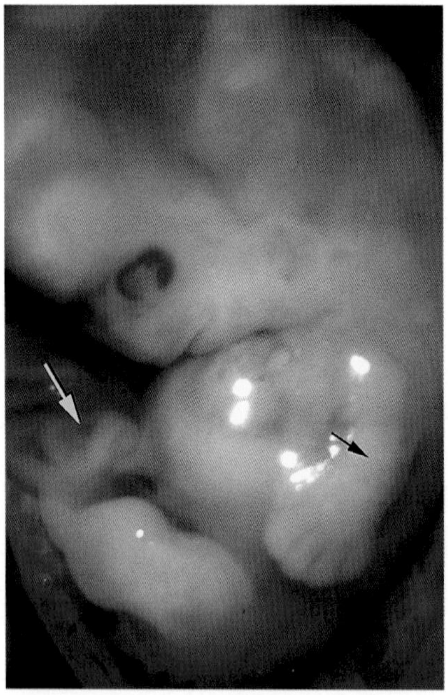

1.8. Human embryo at stage 18 and 19 showing elbow region (black arrow), toe rays, and herniation of intestinal loops into the umbilical cord (yellow arrow).

begin to show differentiation as the **hand plates** develop toward the end of this week. The fourth pair of **branchial arches** and the **lower-limb buds** are present by 28–32 days of development. Lens placodes of the eyes are visible on the sides of the head. The attenuated tail with its somites is a characteristic feature at the beginning of week 5.

Sixth Week of Development (Stages 16 and 17)

The crown–rump (CR) length of the embryo in this time period is 10–14 mm. At *stage 16*, **nasal pits** face ventrally, **retinal pigment** becomes visible, **auricular hillocks** appear, and the **foot plate** is formed. In *stage 17*, the C-shape of the embryo is still present. Development of **finger rays** and basic facial-structure formation advances (Figure 1.7). The **upper lip** appears when medial nasal prominences and maxillary prominences merge. The nostrils become clearly defined and the eyes are directed more anteriorly.

1.9. **(A)** Human embryo at stage 20 showing webbed fingers and notches between the toe rays. The vascular plexus becomes visible (arrows). **(B)** Human embryo at stage 21 and 22 with free fingers. The hands and feet approach each other. Note the intestine in the umbilical cord (arrow). **(C)** Human embryo at stage 23 with more typical human characteristics

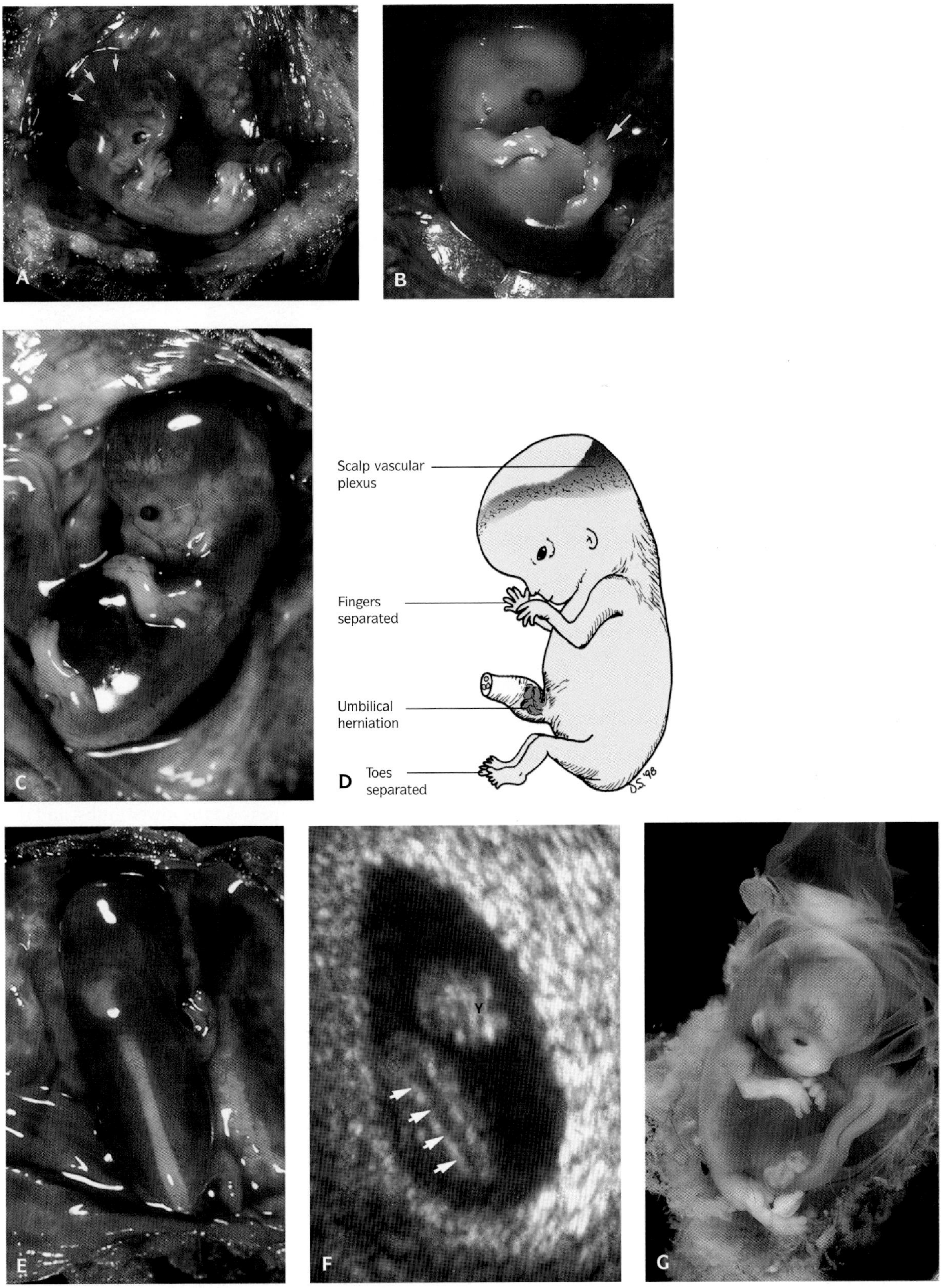

1.9. (*cont.*) such as a rounder head and completed development of the face, hands and feet. **(D)** Drawing of a human embryo at stage 23. **(E)** Posterior view of the embryo shown in **(C)** with an intact neural tube. **(F)** Ultrasound showing a posterior view of an embryo with the characteristic appearance of an intact neural tube (arrows) (Y, yolk sac). **(G)** Fetus at beginning of the fetal period (9 developmental weeks).

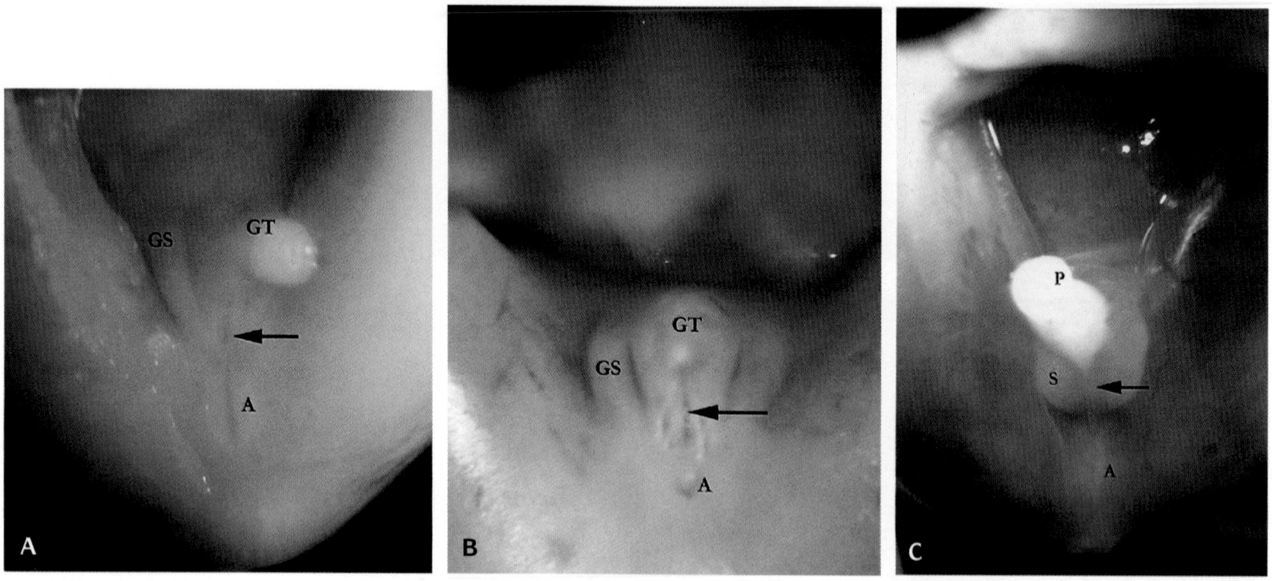

1.10. **(A)** Sexual differentiation of male and female cannot be determined until the 12th week of fertilization age. At 9 weeks the genitalia are ambiguous (GT, genital tubercle; urogenital groove, arrow; GS, genital swelling; A, anus). **(B)** Female at 12 weeks fertilization age (GT, genital tubercle; urogenital groove, arrow; GS, genital swelling; A, anus). **(C)** Male at 12 weeks fertilization age (P, penis; S, scrotum; A, anus; arrow, scrotal raphe).

Seventh Week of Development (Stages 18 and 19)

At the end of the 7th week, the embryo attains a CR length of 20 mm. The head continues to enlarge rapidly and the trunk straightens. **Elbow regions** can be recognized on upper limbs, toe rays appear on the lower limbs, and the nipples become visible. **Physiological herniation of the intestinal tract into the umbilical cord** occurs (Figures 1.8 to 1.10). The intestinal loops normally return to the abdomen by the end of the 10th week.

Eighth Week of Development (Stages 20–23)

At this stage, the **fingers are distinct but are still webbed**. There are **notches between the toe rays**, and a **scalp vascular plexus** appears. Toward the end of week 8, the fingers become free and longer and the development of hands and feet approach each other. The head becomes more rounded and shows typical human characteristics. The embryo has a CR length of 20 mm at the beginning of the 8th week and is 30 mm in CR length at the end of the 8th week. All major organ systems are formed by the end of the 8th week – the completion of blastogenesis, organogenesis, and embryonic development. Then the fetal period begins.

Prenatal Evaluation of Growth by Ultrasound

Prenatal evaluation is usually possible 3 weeks after fertilization.

Embryonic development and growth start with fertilization and progress through 4 weeks, blastogenesis (postconception days 0–28), and organogenesis (days 29–56). In humans, fusion of the eyelids (days 56–60) is regarded as an arbitrary end of the embryonic period.

Evaluation by ultrasound is dated from the first day of the last menstrual period, which is termed "gestational age" (2 weeks longer than embryonic age).

A gestational sac can usually be identified at 5 weeks and is an early indication of an intrauterine pregnancy. Ultrasound evaluation of the embryo reveals the following:

1. At 6 weeks, gestational age, embryonic structures and heart activity are almost always visible.
2. At 7 weeks, the embryo is 10 mm at a minimum and fetal heart activity should be visible in 100% of viable pregnancies.
3. At 8 weeks, fetal structures are visible and the yolk sac is identified as a circular structure measuring 5 mm in diameter. The detection of a yolk sac excludes the diagnosis of a blighted ovum because a viable embryo is necessary for yolk sac development.
4. An empty gestational sac with a mean diameter greater than 30 mm with no visible embryonic structures means that a nonviable pregnancy (blighted ovum) exists.
5. At 9–11 weeks, progressive ossification occurs with major centers in the calvaria and ilium.

The CR length is measured from the outer edge of the cephalic pole to the outer edge of the fetal rump. This measurement predicts the gestational age with an error of ±3 days (90% confidence limits) after 7–10 weeks. The error increases to ±5 days between 10 and 14 weeks of gestation. Fetal flexion may decrease maximal CR length by 5%.

The cephalic index is the ratio of the biparietal diameter (BPD) divided by the occipital frontal diameter. A normal ratio is 0.75 to 0.85. After 20 weeks of gestation, the BPD is less reliable for gestational dating because of changes in shape, growth disturbances, and individual variation.

The femur can be measured as early as 10 weeks gestational age.

Fetal BPD and femur length for gestational age dating have a confidence interval of ±1 week from 12 to 22 weeks, ±2 weeks from 22 to 32 weeks, and ±3 weeks from 32 to 41 weeks.

Small for gestational age (SGA) is defined as a birth weight less than the 10th centile. Therefore, the SGA group includes most normal but small infants. Large for gestational age (LGA) is defined as birth weight greater than the 90th centile. This LGA group also includes normal but large infants.

Examination of Products of Conception

Fetal weight can be estimated by ultrasound with established charts comparing

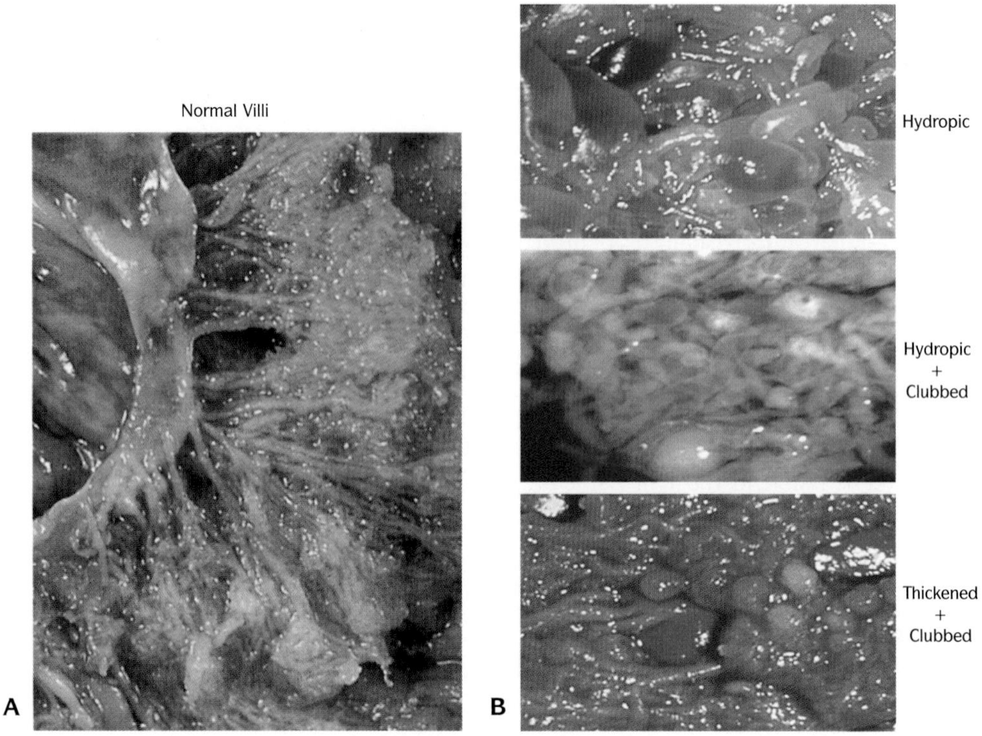

1.11. Illustration of **(A)** normal and **(B)** abnormal villi.

the BPD and abdominal circumference (AC). The BPD exceeds the AC until 38 weeks of gestation, when they become equal. The AC then exceeds the BPD.

Adequate examination and evaluation of products of conception can yield important information that may benefit future pregnancies. The fate of the fertilized ova can be quite grim within the embryonic period; about 16% of those exposed to sperm fail to divide either because they are not penetrated by sperm or because the meiotic mechanism is not functioning. Another 15% fail to implant. Grossly abnormal embryos (27%) are spontaneously aborted at previllous stages with another 20% estimated to die after the first missed period for a total loss rate of 70–80%. Abortion is defined as the premature expulsion or removal of the conceptus from the uterus before it is able to sustain life on its own. Clinically, the term takes on many definitions, such as threatened abortion, incomplete abortion, missed abortion, recurrent abortion, and induced/therapeutic abortion. Early spontaneous abortion occurs in the embryonic period up to the end of the 8th developmental week.The embryonic period is from conception to the end of the 8th week, the fetal period from the 9th week to birth. Late spontaneous abortion occurs between the 9th week to the 20th week of development.

Initial examination of the products of conception should begin with assessing the villous component of the gestational sac (Figures 1.11 to 1.13). Normal

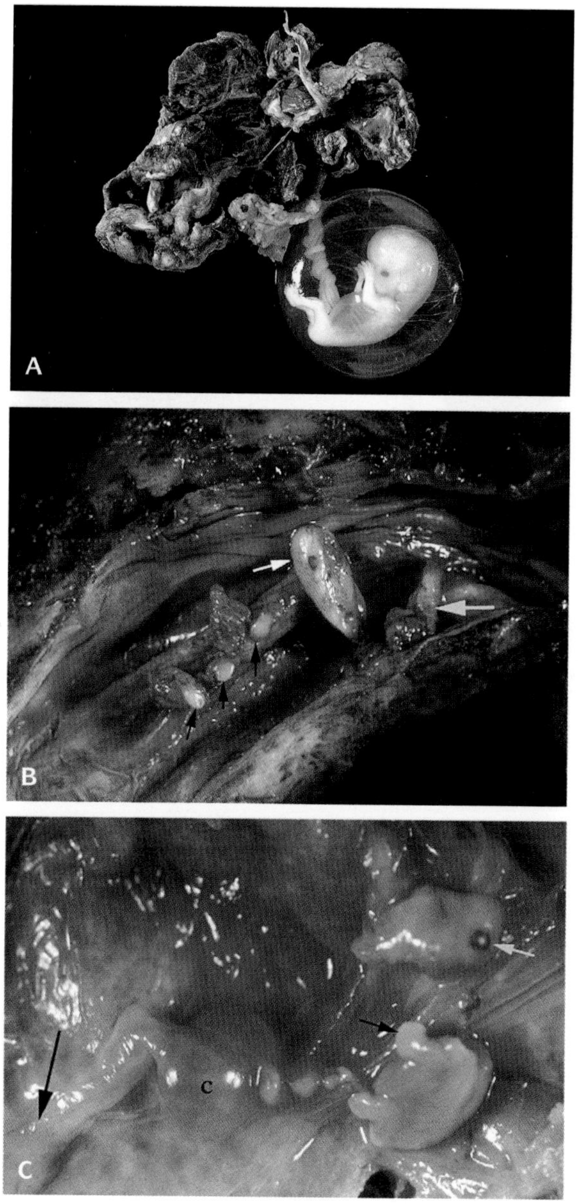

1.12. **(A)** Example of a complete specimen. The chorionic sac has been ruptured but the amniotic sac and embryo are still intact. **(B)** Cross-section of a complete specimen showing artifactual separation of the embryo from the umbilical cord (yellow arrow) secondary to maceration. The embryo is also fragmented (black arrows = limbs, white arrow = malformed head with retinal pigment). This embryo is a GD IV. **(C)** A complete specimen showing a macerated embryo (yellow arrow = head with retinal pigment, small black arrows = upper limb). Note the constricted, twisted, cystic (C) umbilical cord. (Large arrow at cord insertion.)

villi are very lush, fine and hairlike, covering the entire surface of the sac. Abnormal villi can appear hydropic, clubbed, and/or thickened and are usually sparse. A complete specimen consists of an intact chorionic sac that may be empty or contain various embryonic or extraembryonic tissues. The diagnosis

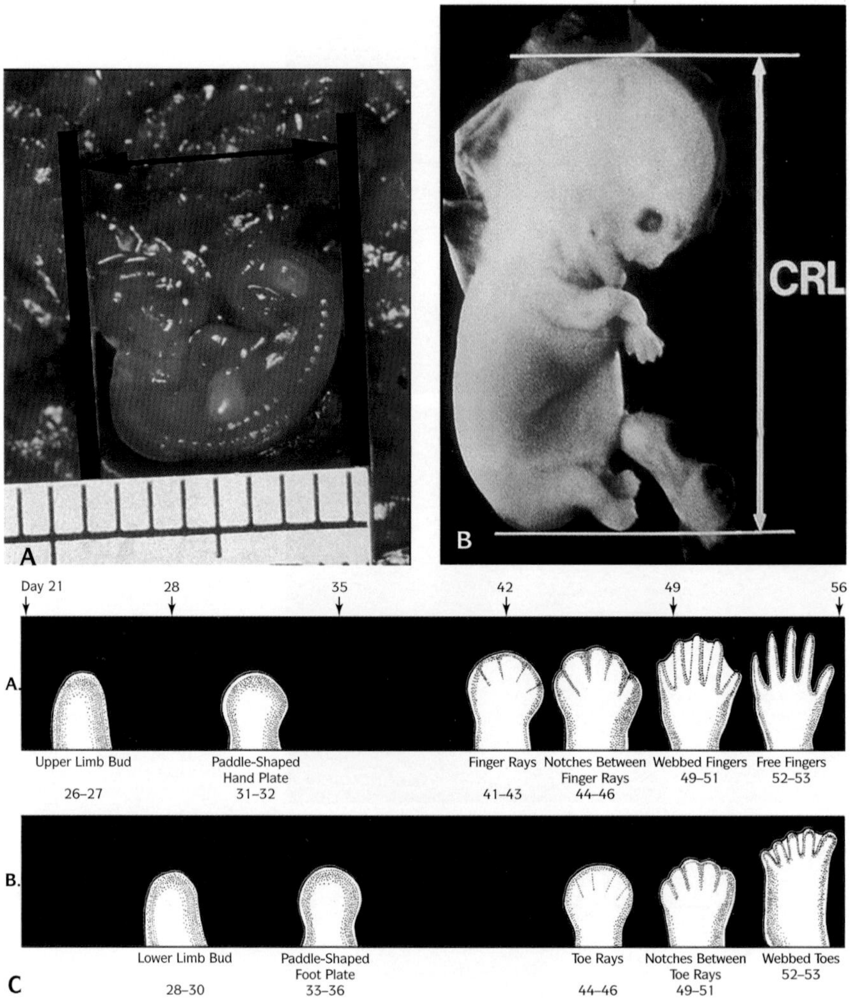

1.13. CR measurement of embryos. **(A)** Early embryo (32 days developmental age). **(B)** Embryo at about 7 weeks developmental age. **(C)** Illustrations demonstrating development of the hand and foot.

of a blighted ovum is an intact but empty sac without a trace of an embryo. Incomplete specimens consist of an opened or ruptured chorionic sac without an identifiable embryo. Curetted specimens are most often incomplete. When an embryo is identified, it should be measured and assessed for all developmental features, such as limb development, eyes, branchial arches, etc. (Tables 1.6 to 1.8). The embryo is measured in its natural position, from the curvature of the head to the curvature of the rump in younger embryos and from the crown to the rump in older embryos as they begin to straighten. Examination of the hand and foot also determines embryonic age. Under normal circumstances developmental age can be based primarily on length of hands and foot length.

Growth Disorganization (GD)

Four types of growth disorganization (GD) have been established by Poland

Table 1.6 Criteria for estimating developmental stages in human embryos

Age (days)	Carnegie stage	No. of somites	Length (mm)	Main characteristics
20–21	9	1–3	1.5–3.0	Deep neural groove and first somites present. Head fold evident.
22–23	10	4–12	2.0–3.5	Embryo straight or slightly curved. Neural tube forming or formed opposite somites but widely open at rostral and caudal neuropores. First and second pairs of branchial arches visible.
24–25	11	13–20	2.5–4.5	Embryo curved owing to head and tail folds. Rostral neuropore closing. Otic placodes present. Optic vesicles formed.
26–27	12	21–29	3.0–5.0	Upper limb buds appear. Rostral neuropore closed. Caudal neuropore closing. Three pairs of branchial arches visible. Heart prominence distinct. Otic pits present.
28–30	13	30–35	4.0–6.0	Embryo has C-shaped curve. Caudal neuropore closed. Upper limb buds are flipper-like. Four pairs of branchial arches visible. Lower limb buds appear. Otic vesicles present. Lens placodes distinct. Attentuated tail present.
31–32	14	*	5.0–7.0	Upper limbs are paddle-shaped. Lens pits and nasal pits visible. Optic cups present.
33–36	15		7.0–9.0	Hand plates formed. Lens vesicles present. Nasal pits prominent. Lower limbs are paddle shaped. Cervical sinuses visible.
37–40	16		8.0–11.0	Foot plates formed. Pigment visible in retina. Auricular hillocks developing.
41–43	17		11.0–14.0	Digital rays appear in hand plates. Auricular hillocks outline future auricle of external ear. Trunk beginning to straighten. Cerebral vesicles prominent.
44–46	18		13.0–17.0	Digital rays appear in foot plates. Elbow region visible. Eyelids forming. Notches between digital rays in the hands. Nipples visible.
47–48	19		16.0–18.0	Limbs extend ventrally. Trunk elongating and straightening. Midgut herniation prominent.
49–51	20		18.0–22.0	Upper limbs longer and bent at elbows. Fingers and thumb distinct but webbed. Notches between digital rays in the feet. Scalp vascular plexus appears.
52–53	21		22.0–24.0	Hands and feet approach each other. Fingers are free and longer. Toes distinct but webbed. Stubby tail present.
54–55	22		23.0–28.0	Toes free and longer. Eyelids and auricles of external ears are more developed.
56	23		27.0–31.0	Head more rounded and shows human characteristics. External genitalia still have sexless appearance. Distinct bulge still present in umbilical cord: caused by herniation of intestines. Tail has disappeared.

* At this and subsequent stages, the number of somites is difficult to determine and so is not a useful criterion.

Source: Moore KL. *Before We Are Born; Basic Embryology and Birth Defects*, WB Saunders Co., p. 60, 1989.

Table 1.7 Criteria for estimating fertilization age during the fetal period

Age (weeks)	CR length (mm)*	Foot length (mm)*	Fetal weight (g)†	Main external characteristics
Previable Fetuses				
9	50	7	8	Eyes closing or closed. Head more rounded. External genitalia still not distinguishable as male or female. Intestines in umbilical cord.
10	61	9	14	Intestine in abdomen. Early fingernail development.
12	87	14	45	Sex distinguishable externally. Well-defined neck.
14	120	20	110	Head erect. Lower limbs well developed. Early toenail development.
16	140	27	200	Ears stand out from head.
18	160	33	320	Vernix caseosa present.
20	190	39	460	Head and body hair (lanugo) visible.
Viable Fetuses‡				
22	210	45	630	Skin wrinkled and red.
24	230	50	820	Fingernails present. Lean body.
26	250	55	1,000	Eyes partially open. Eyelashes present.
28	270	59	1,300	Eyes open. Good head of hair. Skin slightly wrinkled.
30	280	63	1,700	Toenails present. Body filling out. Testes descending.
32	300	68	2,100	Fingernails reach finger tips. Skin pink and smooth.
36	340	79	2,900	Body usually plump. Lanugo hairs almost absent. Toenails reach toe tips. Flexed limbs; firm grasp.
38	360	83	3,400	Prominent chest; breasts protrude. Testes in scrotum or palpable in inguinal canals. Fingernails extend beyond finger tips.

* These measurements are averages and so may not apply to specific cases; dimensional variations increase with age.

† These weights refer to fetuses that have been fixed for about 2 weeks in 10% formalin. Fresh specimens usually weigh about 5% less.

‡ There is no sharp limit of development, age, or weight at which a fetus automatically becomes viable or beyond which survival is ensured, but experience has shown that it is uncommon for a baby to survive whose weight is less than 500 g or whose fertilization age is less than 22 weeks. Even fetuses born during the 26- to 28-week period have difficulty surviving, mainly because the respiratory and central nervous systems are not completely differentiated. The term abortion refers to all pregnancies that terminate before the period of viability.

Source: Moore KL. Before We Are Born; Basic Embryology and Birth Defects, WB Saunders Co., p. 74, 1989.

et al. (Tables 1.9 to 1.10). Most spontaneous abortions are found to have some type of growth disorganization, the frequency of which is listed in Table 1.8. To adequately evaluate the inconsistent morphologic development in aborted embryos, the specimen must be complete. This consists of an intact chorionic sac or a ruptured sac with an embryo. All growth disorganized embryos have a high percentage of chromosome anomalies – up to 80%.

Table 1.8 Causes of early abortion

- Abnormal uterine anatomy
- Hormonal dysfunction
- Autoimmune and alloimmune abnormalities
- Excessive genomic sharing
- Chromosome abnormalities
- Mutations (lethal)
- Infections
- Dysmorphic and other disruptive events
- Teratogens

Table 1.9 Growth disorganization

Classification (Poland and Kalousek)

GD I: intact chorionic or amniotic sac with no evidence of embryo

GD II: piece of embryonic tissue 1–4 mm with no recognizable external structures and no caudal or cephalic poles

GD III: grossly disorganized embryo up to 10 mm long, morphology not distinguishable but caudal and cephalic poles present

GD IV: major distortion of body shape always involving head 3–17 mm, not consistent with any one stage of development

Table 1.10 Correlation between embryonic morphology and cytogenetic findings

Embryonic morphology	Abnormal cytogenetics %	Specimen morphology	Frequency (%)
GD I	60	Complete specimens	50
GD II	73	Embryos with growth disorganization	37–73
GD III	52	Normal embryos	20
GD IV	37	Embryos with localized defects	92
Apparently normal embryo	20	Degenerated embryos	8
Focal defects	92	Incomplete specimens	50
		Ruptured/fragmented sacs	38
		Decidua only	12

Source: Embryonic morphology and abnormal cytogenetic data from Gilbert-Barness E. (Editor) *Potter's Pathology of Fetus and Infant*, Mosby-Year Book, Inc. 1997.

GD type I (GD I) consists of an intact chorionic or amniotic sac with no evidence of an embryo or body stalk (Figure 1.14). The yolk sac is absent. The amnion and chorion are abnormal structurally and usually are fused or closely apposed. Fusion of the amnion and chorion before 10 weeks gestation is abnormal. The chorionic villi are abnormal and are often sparse. Grossly they are clubbed or cystic; microscopically they are avascular and hydropic.

GD type II (GD II) consists of a chorionic sac containing a piece of embryonic tissue 1–4 mm long (Figure 1.15). This embryo has no recognizable external features and is without an identifiable cephalic or caudal pole. It is usually

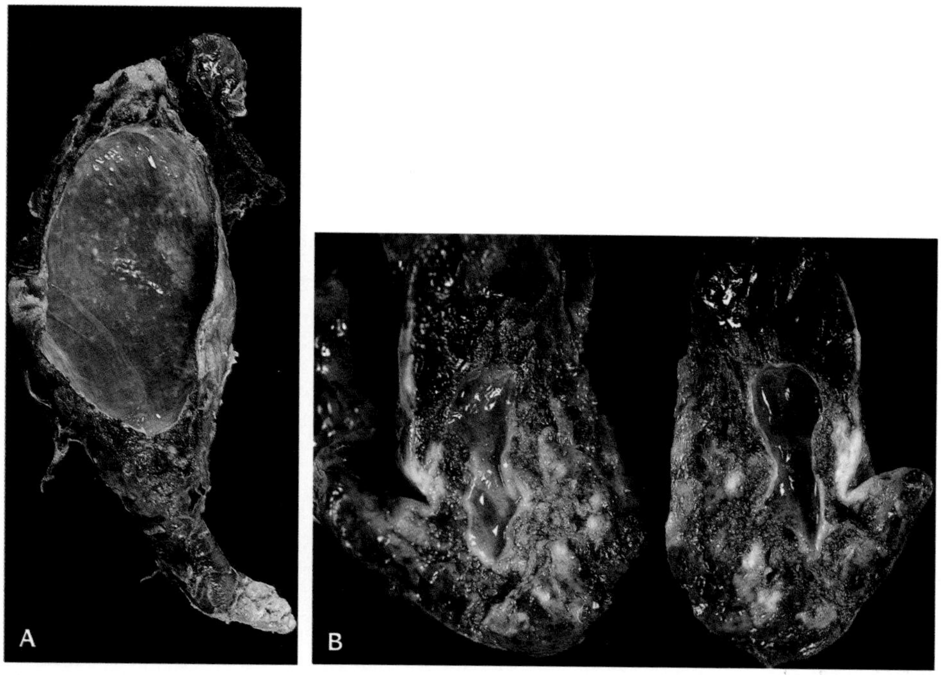

1.14. (A) Empty gestational sac with scant villus tissue. **(B)** Empty gestational sac with fibrotic villi and hemorrhage.

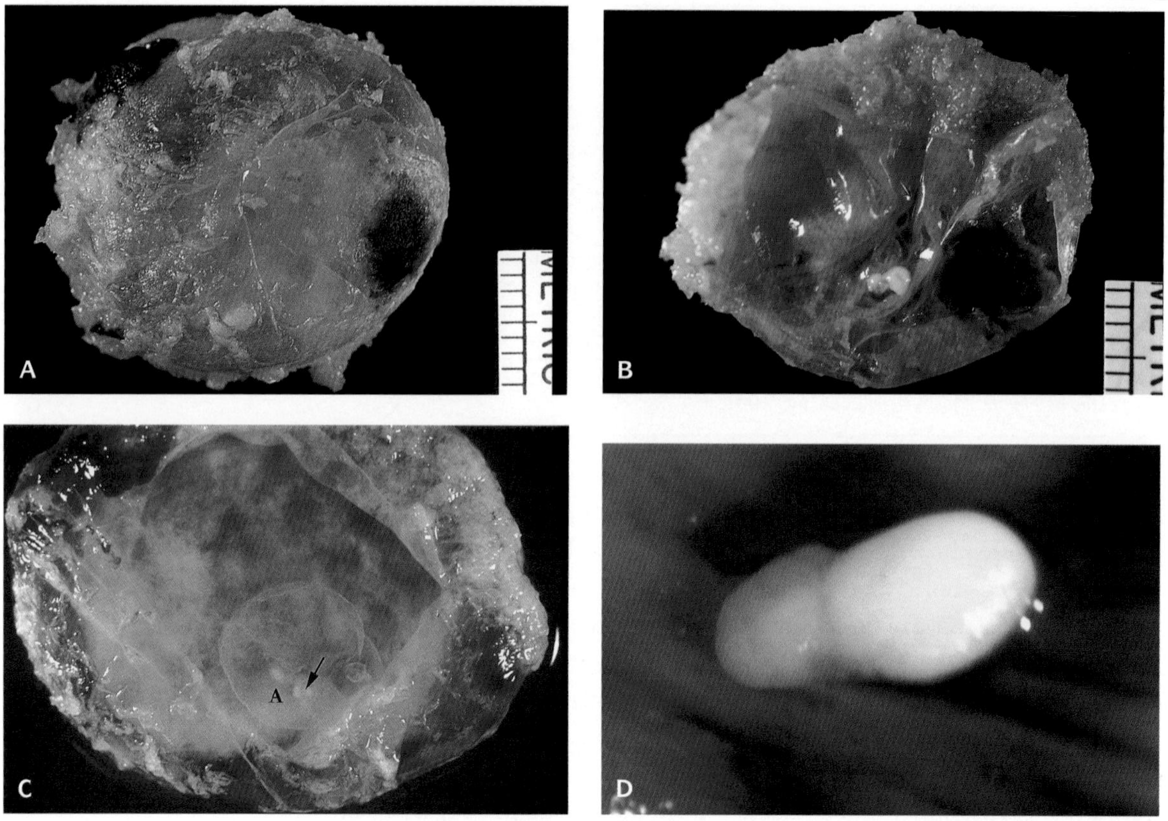

1.15. **(A)** Intact chorionic sac with sparse villi. **(B)** Opened sac containing a piece of embryonic tissue with no recognizable external features. **(C)** Opened sac showing an amniotic sac (A) that is considerably smaller than the surrounding chorionic sac. The amniotic sac contains a portion of embryonic tissue (arrow) consistent with a GD II. **(D)** Close up of a GD II embryo. There are no recognizable external features.

directly attached to the amnion, or it may have a short body stalk. A yolk sac can be identified and is distinguished from the embryo by its position between the amnion and chorion.

GD type III (GD III) consists of a chorionic sac containing a disorganized embryo up to 10 mm long. This embryonic tissue has recognizable cephalic and caudal poles (Figure 1.16). Retinal pigment may be present. A short body stalk is present and limb buds are absent.

GD type IV (GD IV) consists of an embryo that has a CR length from 3 to 17 mm. There is major distortion of the body shape always involving the head (Figure 1.17). These embryos have a recognizable head, trunk, and limb buds and the morphologic characteristics are not consistent with any one stage of development. The head is usually small and cervical flexion is absent or abnormal.

Growth disorganization without chromosome abnormalities: Submicroscopic lethal genetic defects preventing normal embryogenesis or teratogenic effects interfering with normal embryogenesis.

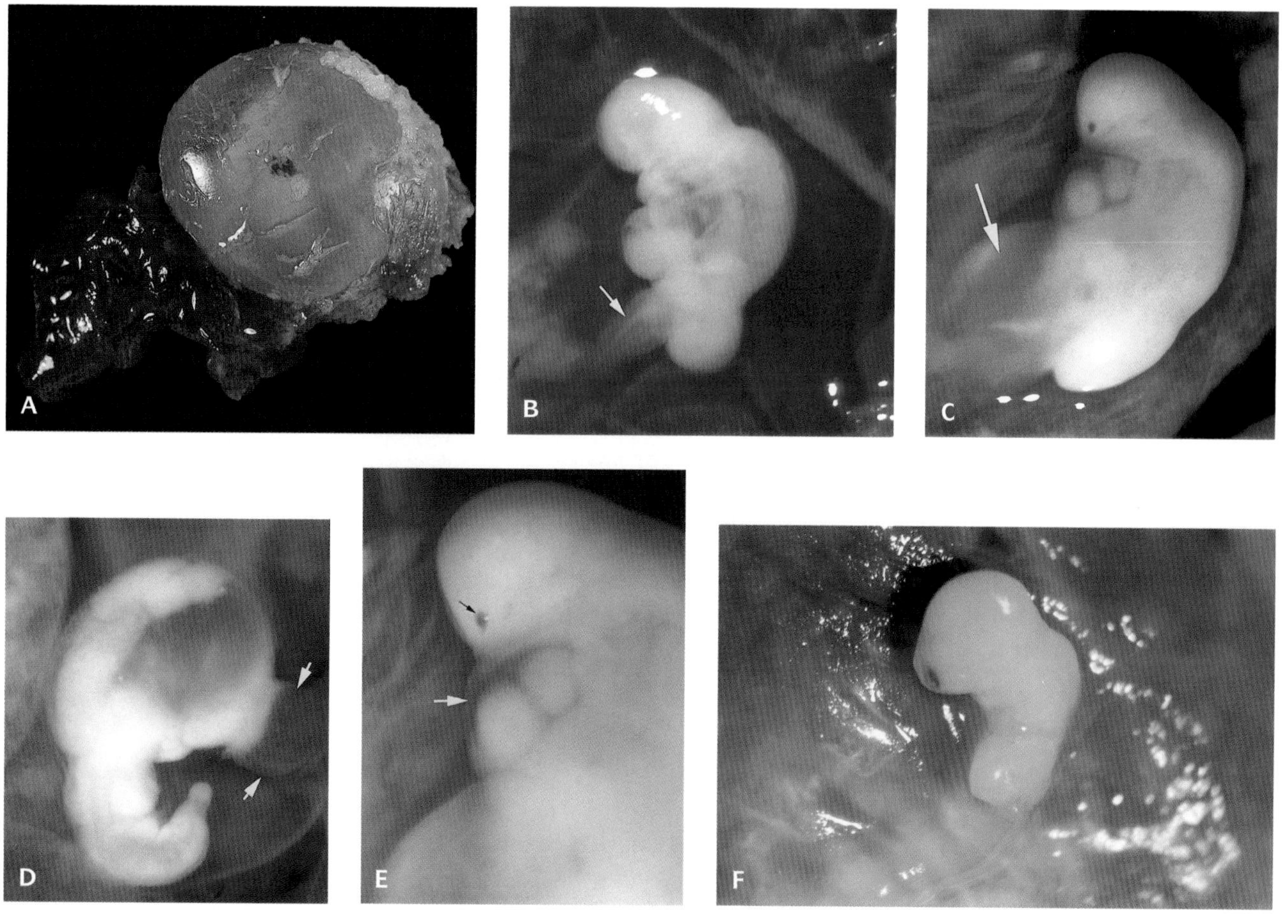

1.16. **(A)** Intact chorionic sac with sparse villi. (**B**, **C**, and **D**) Embryos with recognizable cephalic and caudal poles. A short body stalk (arrow) is identified in **(B)** and **(C)**. Note the frontal cyst (arrows) at the cephalic pole in **(D)**. **(E)** Closeup of **(C)** showing a small cephalic pole and cardiac prominence with a translucent chest wall (yellow arrow). A small hemorrhage is at the cephalic bud (black arrow), this is not retinal pigment. Microscopically this was a collection of red blood cells. **(F)** Growth disorganization III (GD III) with retinal pigment.

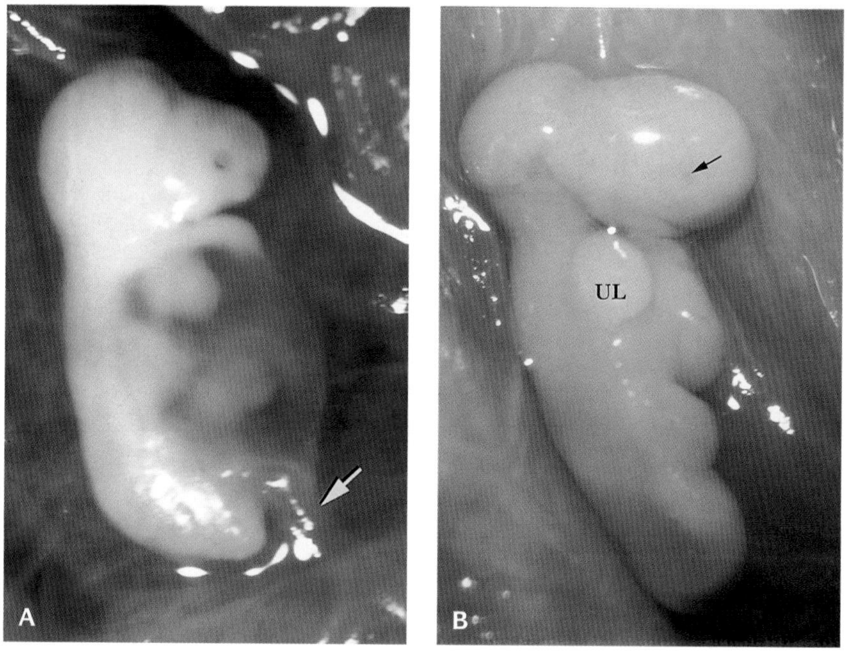

1.17. **(A)** Embryo with small, distorted head, absent cervical flexion, absent limb buds, short body stalk (arrow), translucent thoracoabdominal wall, and faint retinal pigment. The presence of retinal pigment and absence of limbs is dyssynchronous. **(B)** Elongated embryo with a small head and abnormal cervical flexion. An upper limb bud (UL) is identified along with a lens vesicle (arrow) showing inconsistent development.

REFERENCES

England MA: *Color Atlas of Life Before Birth Normal Fetal Development.* Chicago, Year Book, 1983.

Glass RH, Giolbus MS: Habitual abortion. *Fertil Steril* 29:257, 1987.

Hertig AT, Rock J: A series of potentially abortive ova recovered from fertile women prior to the first missed menstrual period. *Am J Obstet Gynecol* 58:968–93, 1949.

Ho MN, Gill TJ III, Hseih RP, et al.: Sharing of human leukocyte antigens (HLA) in primary and secondary recurrent spontaneous abortions. *Am J Obstet Gynecol* 163:178, 1990.

Kalousek DK: The pathology of abortion: the embryo and previable fetus. In Gilbert-Barness E (ed): *Potter's Pathology of the Fetus and Infant*, Philadelphia, Mosby-Year Book, 1997, pp. 106–127.

Kalousek DK, Fitch N, Paradice BA: *Pathology of the Human Embryo and Previable Fetus – An Atlas.* Springer-Verlag, 1990.

Kalousek DK, Neave C: Pathology of abortion, the embryo and the previable fetus. In Wigglesworth JS, Singer DB (eds): *Textbook of Fetal and Perinatal Pathology*, Boston, Blackwell Scientific Publications, 1991, pp. 123–160.

Larsen WJ: *Essentials of Human Embryology*, 3rd ed, Australia, Harcourt, 2001.

Larsen WJ: *Human Embryology*, 3rd ed, New York, Churchill Livingstone, 2001.

Moore KL: *Before We Are Born-Basic Embryology and Birth Defects.* WB Saunders Co., 1989.

Moore KL, Persaud TVN, Schmitt W: *Before We Are Born: Essentials of Embryology and Birth Defects*, 5th ed, Philadelphia, WB Saunders, 1998.

Moore KL, Persaud TVN, Schmitt W: *The Developing Human Clinically Oriented Embryology*, 6th ed, Philadelphia, WB Saunders, 1998.

Moore KL, Persaud TVN: *The Developing Human: Clinically Oriented Embryology*, 5th ed, Philadelphia, WB Saunders, 1993.

Nishimura M, Takano K, Tanimura T, Yasuda M: Normal and abnormal development of human embryos. *Teratology* 1:281–90, 1968.

On-Line Mendelian Inheritance in Man. OMIM (http://www3.ncbi.nlm.nih.gov/omim/).

O'Rahilly R, Muller F: *Developmental Stages in Human Embryos*, Publication 637, Washington, DC, Carnegie Institute of Embryology, 1987.

Orahilly R, Müller F: *Human Embryology and Teratology*, 3rd ed, NY, Wiley-Liss, 2001.

Paul NW, Opitz JM (ed): *Blastogenesis: Normal and Abnormal. Proceedings of the Second International Workshop on Fetal Genetic Pathology*, Big Sky, Montana, October 12–16, 1991, 29(1), 1993.

Poland BJ, Miller JR, Harris M, Livingston J: Spontaneous abortion: a study of 1961 women and their conceptuses. *Acta Obset Gynecol Scand* 102:5–32, 1981.

Rushton DI: Examination of products of conception from previable human pregnancies. *J Clin Pathol* 34:819–35, 1981.

Sadler TW: *Langman's Medical Embryology*, 8th ed, Lippincott, Williams & Wilkins, 2000.

Simpson JL: Aetiology of pregnancy failure. In Chapman M, Grudzinskas S, Chand T (eds): *The Embryo Normal and Abnormal Development and Growth*, Berlin, Springer-Verlag, 1991, pp 11–39.

Thomas ML, Harger JH, Wagener DK, et al.: HLA sharing and spontaneous abortion in humans. *Am J Obstet Gynecol* 151:1053, 1985.

Wilson RD: Prenatal evaluation of growth by ultrasound. *Growth Genetics and Hormones*, Volume 9, 1993.

TWO

Late Fetal Death, Stillbirth, and Neonatal Death

Stillbirth or fetal death is the delivery of an infant with no signs of life between 20 weeks gestational age and term. The infant does not breathe or show any evidence of life: heart beat, pulsation of the umbilical cord, or definite movement of voluntary muscles.

Perinatal death includes stillbirths and early neonatal deaths (less than 7 completed days from birth) (Tables 2.1 and 2.2). World Health Organization national statistics include fetal deaths with a fetus weighing 500 g or more, or gestation > 22 weeks, or crown-heel length > 25 cm. International statistics include fetal deaths with a fetus weighing > 1,000 g, gestation > 28 weeks, or crown-heel length > 35 cm.

Late intrauterine fetal death with stillbirth accounts for 1% of pregnancies.

PLACENTAL ABNORMALITIES ASSOCIATED WITH LATE FETAL DEATH

Umbilical Cord

- Cord accidents comprise 15–18% of fetal demise.
- Long cord – entanglement around a fetal part, cord prolapse, cord compression, true knots, and excessive spiraling (sometimes may be a postmortem artifact) (Figure 2.1).
- Short cord may indicate a central nervous system abnormality; it is more frequent with congenital anomalies. Delay in completion of the second stage

Table 2.1

	Weight	Gestational age
Immature	<1,000 g	20–28 weeks
Premature	1,000–2,499 g	29–36 weeks
Mature	>2,500 g	36–42 weeks
Post-mature		>42 weeks

Abortion is pregnancy loss between conception and the end of the 19th week.
Fetal death occurs *in utero* between the 20th and 36th week or later.
Neonatal death occurs anytime between complete delivery of the infant and the end of 28th day of extrauterine life.
Perinatal deaths include fetal deaths and neonatal deaths.

of labor, abruption, inversion of the uterus, or cord rupture at delivery may be complications (Figures 2.2 to 2.4).

- Nuchal cord may cause fetal strangulation – functionally significant if two or more loops are around the neck, with associated plethora of the face and scalp.
- True knots – 1% of pregnancies. Significant if there is differential congestion on either side of the knot or an associated mural thrombus and evidence of hemorrhage.
- Cord prolapse and compression cannot be confirmed pathologically.
- Umbilical cord insertion: velamentous insertion – 1.6% of placentas; increased risk of tearing of the vessels with exsanguination; frequency is increased in multiple pregnancies with a single umbilical artery (Figures 2.5 to 2.6).

Table 2.2 Causes of fetal death

Cause of death	Percentage of deaths
Hypertensive disease (pre-eclampsia and pregnancy-induced hypertension)	25
Maternal medical complications	10
Maternal diabetes	
Connective tissue disorders	
Erythroblastosis fetalis	5
Umbilical vessel thrombosis and cord and placental complications	30
Abruptio placental	
Placenta infarction	
Maternal smoking with placental fibrin deposition	
Maternal floor infarction	
Congenital malformation	10
Intrauterine infection	15
Unexplained	5

Source: Pitkin RM: Fetal death: Diagnosis and management. *Am J Obstet Gynecol* 157:583, 1987.

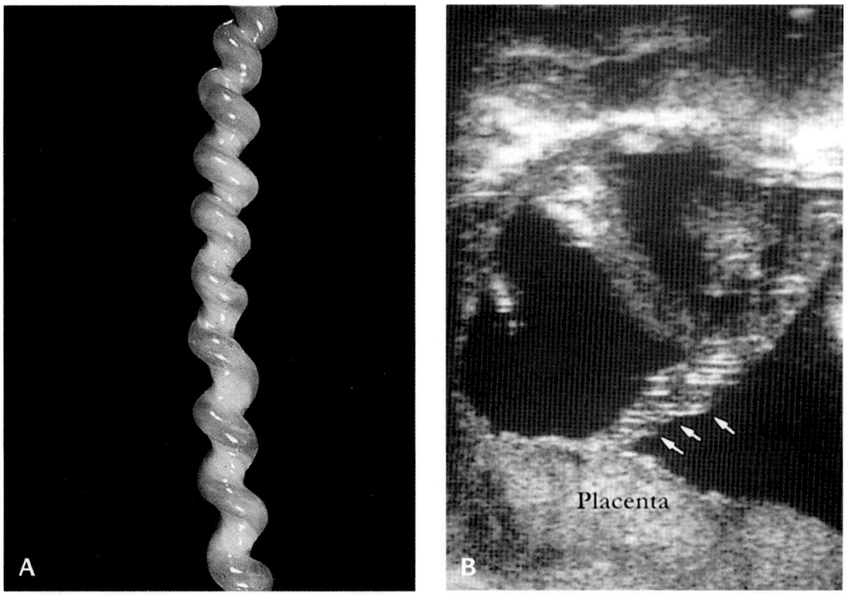

2.1. **(A)** Hypercoiled umbilical cord (corkscrew). **(B)** Ultrasound of hypercoiled umbilical cord (arrows).

Membranes

- Chorioamnionitis – increased preterm labor, fetal hypoxia (placental villus edema)
- Placenta extrachorialis
- Amniotic bands ensnare fetal parts of the umbilical cord and may result in umbilical cord compression, amputations, or numerous congenital malformations.

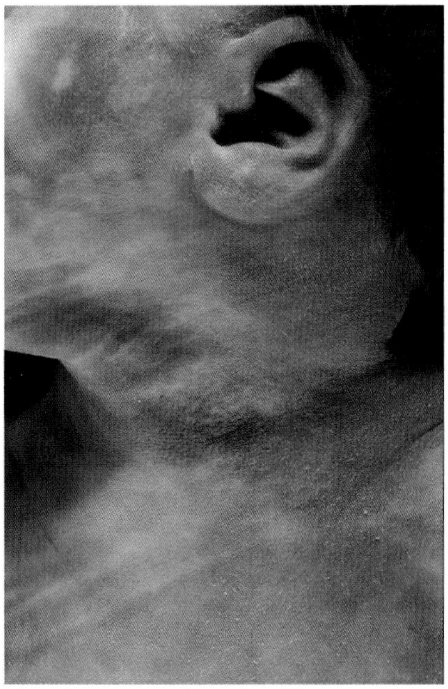

2.2. Nuchal cord. Note constriction around neck that had caused fetal death.

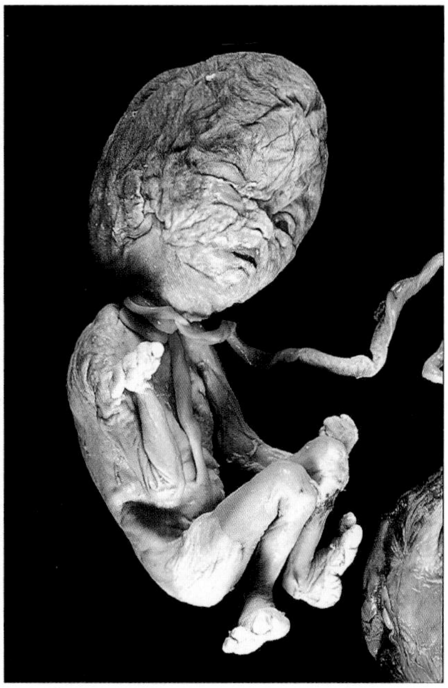

2.3. Nuchal cord with intrauterine death and maceration.

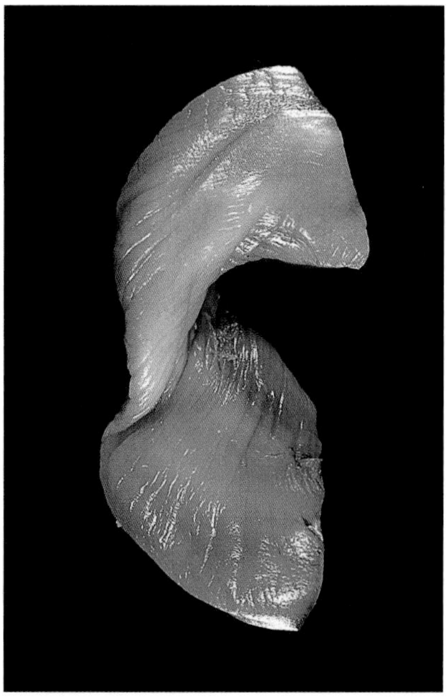

2.4. Twist of umbilical cord resulting in vascular constriction.

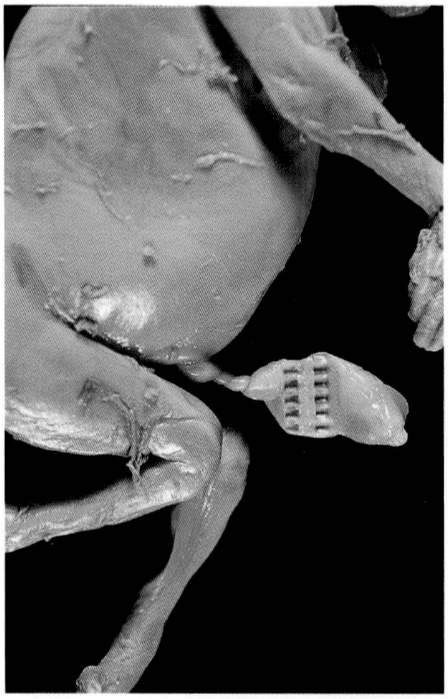

2.5. Constriction and twisting of umbilical cord at abdominal insertion of cord.

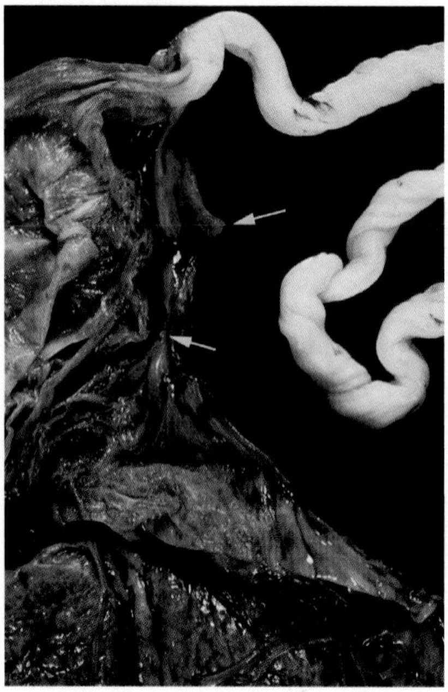

2.6. Vasa previa. The umbilical cord has a velamentous insertion with site of hemorrhage due to vascular rupture (arrows).

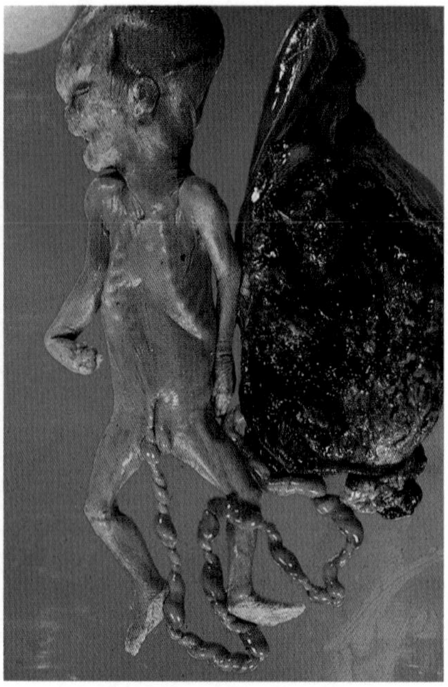

2.7. Retroplacental hemorrhage due to abruption with attached twisted umbilical cord (postmortem event) and macerated fetus.

Placental Disc Abnormalities

- Abruptio placentae is related to 15% of fetal deaths. It may be due to abdominal trauma; uterine tumors; hydramnios, short umbilical cord, sudden decompression of the uterus; occlusion or compression of the inferior vena cava, lupus erythematosus; and the use of anticoagulants (Figure 2.7). Other causes include acute chorioamnionitis, coitus, increased maternal age (more frequent arterial and arteriolar damage), maternal cigarette smoking, and maternal hypertension.
- Placental infarction > 20%; indication of compromised uteroplacental blood flow. Causes and associations include pregnancy-induced hypertension, lupus anticoagulant, and antiphospholipid antibodies.
- Maternal floor infarct has an incidence of 1/200. Heavy deposition of fibrin in the decidua basalis occurs and encases villi; 17% of fetuses are stillborn; chorioamnionitis and intrauterine growth retardation are strongly associated.

Fetal Abnormalities in Stillbirths

Maceration occurs if there is intrauterine fetal retention after fetal death. Maceration (Latin macerate – to soften by soaking) is characterized by softening and peeling of the skin, discoloration and softening of the viscera, and fluid accumulation in body cavities. The changes of maceration are nonputrefactive

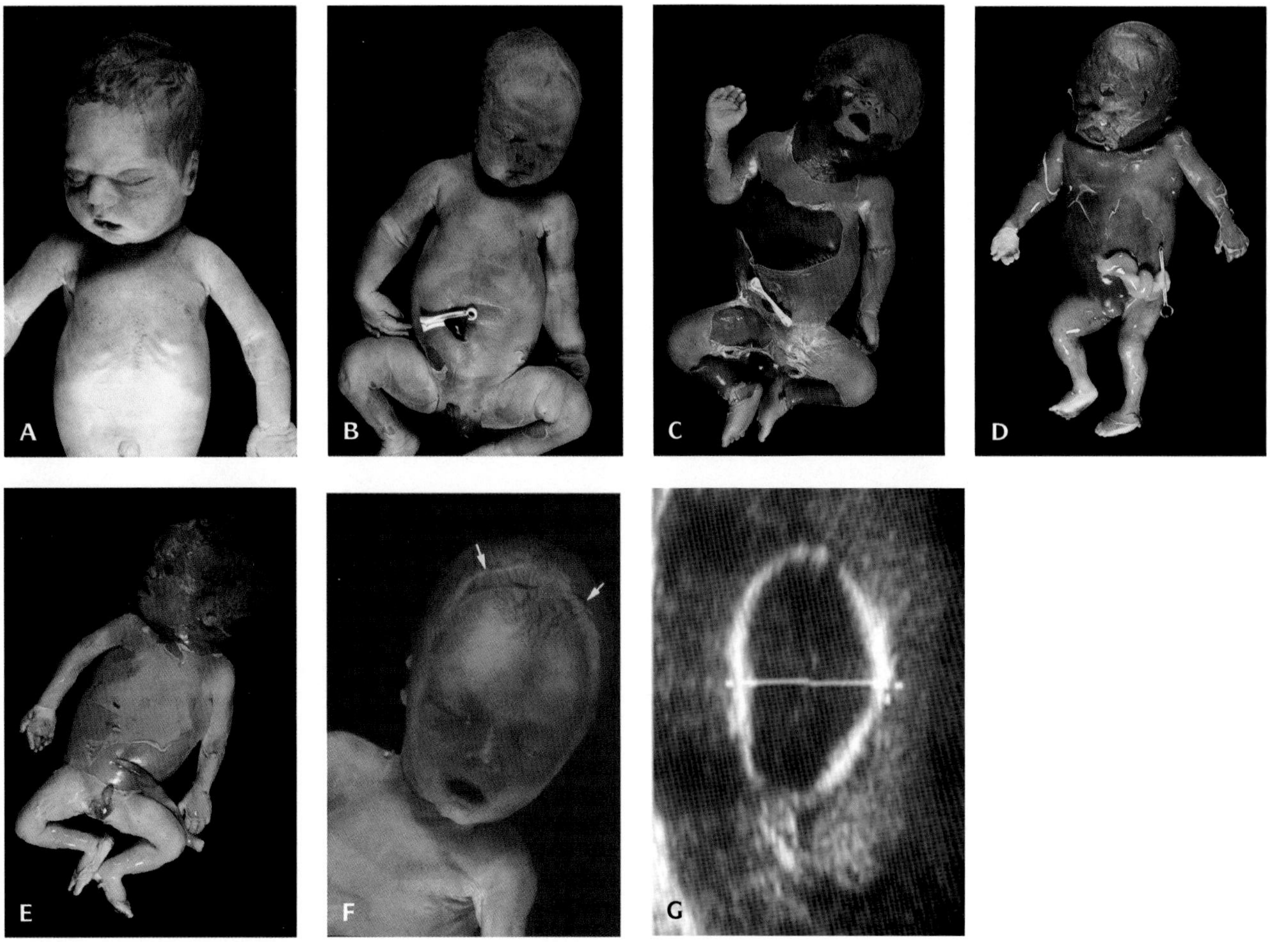

2.8. Degrees of maceration in stillbirths. **(A)** Early death less than 6 hours. Hyperemia of skin of face and petechial hemorrhages on chest. **(B)** Desquamation of skin patches about 1 cm in diameter with blebs. Fetal death approximately 8 hours. **(C)** Fetus with skin slippage and cranial compression death approximately 36 hours. **(D)** Extensive desquamation of skin, fetal death 3–4 days. **(E)** Desquamation of skin, overlapping sutures and gaping mouth. Fetal death approximately 1 week. **(F)** Overlapping sutures (arrows) of fetus. **(G)** Ultrasound demonstrating spalding sign.

and result from fetal immersion in amniotic fluid and digestion of fetal tissues by autolytic enzymes. The extent of maceration in stillborn fetuses may be a rough indicator of the time interval from fetal death to delivery; however, its rate may be influenced by maternal fever, fetal or placental infection, fetal hydration at the time of death, amniotic fluid volume, and delay from delivery to postmortem examination. Maceration may hinder, but does not negate, the pathological investigation of the stillbirth. Placental changes after fetal death appear to be more constant; if cytotrophoblasts are increased without stromal changes, fetal death has occurred in <7 days. Stromal fibrosis, calcifications, syncytial knotting, and thickening of the basement membrane occur >7 days after the death of the fetus (Figure 2.8, Table 2.3).

Table 2.3 Timetable of changes caused by maceration after intrauterine fetal death

Intrauterine duration of retention	Gross fetal examination	Histology of fetal organs	Histology of placenta
4 hours		Kidney: loss of tubular nuclear basophilia	
6 hours	Desquamation of patches 1 cm; brown or red discoloration of umbilical stump		Intravascular karyorrhexis
8 hours		Loss of basophilia in gastrointestinal tract	
12 hours	Desquamation on face, back, or abdomen		
18 hours	Desquamation of 5% body, or two, or more body regions	Desquamation of bronchial epithelium	
24 hours	Brown or tan skin discoloration on abdomen Moderate desquamation	Liver: loss of hepatocyte nuclear basophilia. Inner one-half of myocardium: loss of nuclear basophilia	
36 hours	Cranial compression		
48 hours	Desquamation of >50% of body	Outer one-half of myocardium: loss of nuclear basophilia	Multifocal stem vessel luminal abnormalities
72 hours	Desquamation of >75% of body		
96 hours	Overlapping cranial sutures (4–5 days)	Loss of nuclear basophilia in bronchial epithelial cells and in all liver cells	
1 week	Widely open mouth Collapse of calvarium Laxity and dislocation of joints	Gastrointestinal tract: maximal loss of nuclear basophilia Adrenal glands: maximal loss of nuclear basophilia. Trachea: chondrocyte loss of nuclear basophilia	
2 weeks	Mummification (dehydration, compression, tan color)		Extensive vascular luminal change (see 48-hour findings). Extensive fibrosis of terminal villi
28 days		Kidney: maximal loss of nuclear basophilia	

Modified from data of Genest DR, William Ma, Greene MF: Estimating the time of death in stillborn fetuses: I. Histologic evaluation of fetal organs: An autopsy study of 150 stillborns, *Obstet Gynecol* 80:575, 1992; Genest DR: Estimating the time of death in stillborn fetuses: II. Histologic evaluation of the placenta: A study of 71 stillborns, *Obstet Gynecol* 80:585, 1992; Genest DR: Estimating the time of death in stillborn fetuses: III. External fetal examination: A study of 86 stillborns, *Obstet Gynecol* 80:593, 1992.

Major malformations – 4–26% of stillbirths:

- Central nervous system (failure of closure of the neural tube)
- Abdominal wall and gastrointestinal tract defects
- Premature closure of the foramen ovale or ductus arteriosus
- Hypoplastic left heart

- Single umbilical artery occurs in 1% of stillborn twins
- Mendelian disorders that occur in stillborns are usually recessive or X-linked. Dominant mutations are rarely lethal except those due to a new mutation.

Chromosomal defects – 5–10% of stillbirths:

- Confined placental mosaicism – two or more karyotypically different cell lines within the placenta. Increased risk of poor perinatal outcome.

Multiple pregnancies:

- Twins – 11 times greater risk of fetal death.
- Second trimester loss due to incompetent cervix and premature dilatation, ascending infection, or premature placental separation.
- Third trimester – growth retardation, fetal anomalies. Mortality rate two to three times higher for monozygous than dizygous twins.
- Intrauterine growth retardation (IUGR)
  - 7–15% of stillborns
  - Relatively large head compared to body size
  - Normal brain/liver ratio is 3 : 1; may increase to 6 : 1
  - Common cause of asymmetric IUGR is uteroplacental insufficiency
  - Symmetric growth restriction seen in chromosomal abnormalities
- Fetomaternal hemorrhage
  - 75% of all pregnancies but usually a small volume. If large may cause:
    - fetal death
    - fetal distress
    - hypovolemic shock
    - anemia with cardiac failure
    - hydrops (Figure 2.9)

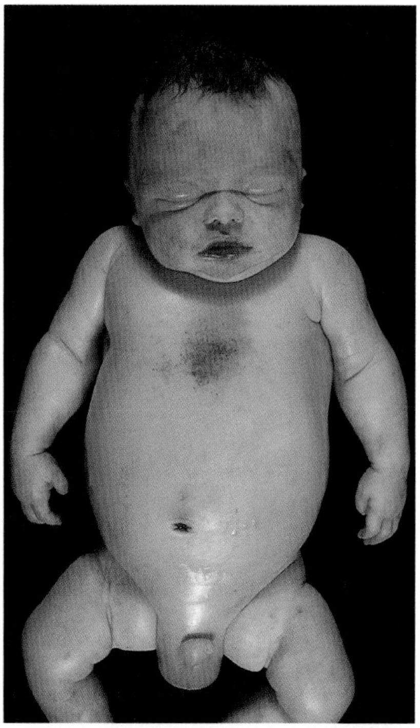

2.9. Feto-maternal hemorrhage. The fetus is anemic, pale, and hydropic.

The standard method of testing for fetal erythrocytes in maternal circulation is **Kleihauer-Betke** staining of a peripheral blood smear. This test is based on different acid elution characteristics of fetal and adult hemoglobin. The test should be done routinely in all cases of unexplained stillbirth, fetal distress, and neonatal anemia. Immediate transfusion may be lifesaving, and testing of the mother during the puerperium is still important.

The size of the hemorrhage can be calculated on the basis of the percentage of fetal red cells present (number of fetal cells in 2,000 total red cells divided by 20), an estimated average maternal blood volume of 5,800 mL, an average maternal hematocrit of 0.35, and an average normal fetal hematocrit of 0.45. For example, if 5% of the red cells in the maternal circulation are fetal in origin, the size of the hemorrhage is calculated as $5{,}800 \times 0.05 \times 35/45 = 225$ mL of fetal blood; 80 mL (approximately one-third of the infant's blood volume) or greater is considered significant for fetomaternal transplacental hemorrhage. (The average blood volume of a term infant is 250 mL).

Kleihauer-Betke Test

Estimation of the volume of fetal hemorrhage percent of fetal cells in maternal circulation × 50 – e.g., 5% × 50 = 250 mL.

The estimation of the total blood volume of a full-term infant (approximately 3 kg) is 3.0 kg × 100 mL = 300 mL.

MATERNAL FACTORS IN STILLBIRTH

- Maternal age < 20 years or > 35 years
- Hypertensive disease may cause
  - uteroplacental insufficiency
  - placental abruption
- Diabetes mellitus
  - Up to 17% of fetal deaths
  - Causes intrauterine hypoxia
  - Congenital malformation
- Systemic lupus erythematosus
  - Fetal loss
  - Preterm birth
  - Increased maternal lupus activity
  - Hemolysis, elevated liver enzymes, low platelets (HELLP)
  - Placental thromboses
  - Infarcts
  - Maternal antibodies may result in heart block, fetal hydrops, and stillbirth.
- Maternal drug abuse
  - Tobacco, drugs, and alcohol are implicated in fetal deaths.
  - Fetal deaths increased by as much as 50% if mothers smoke three or more cigarettes per day.
  - Cocaine – acute and massive placental separation due to vasoconstriction.
- Intrauterine asphyxia (Table 2.4)
  - Acute asphyxia (Figure 2.10) is associated with
    retroplacental hemorrhage (abruption)
    transfusion syndrome
    umbilical cord complication (prolapse, compression)
    birth trauma
  - Subacute asphyxia is associated with
    infections
    fetal heart failure
    blood group incompatibility
    tumors of the placenta or umbilical cord
    diabetes
  - Chronic asphyxia is associated with
    placental pathology due to long-standing circulatory insufficiency
  - Postmaturity

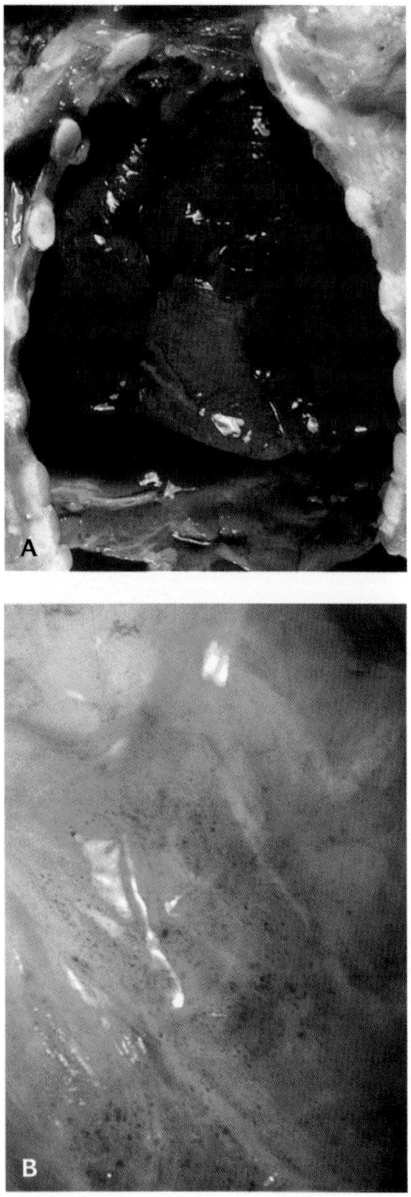

2.10. Acute intrauterine asphyxia. **(A)** Opened thoracic cavity showing dark purple lungs with petechial hemorrhages. **(B)** Petechial hemorrhages over the epicardial surface.

Table 2.4 Correlation of pathological changes in fetal death with time of intrauterine asphyxia

Mode	Acute	Subacute	Chronic
Time	<24 hours	Few days to 3 weeks	>3 weeks
External features	Normally developed	Excessive edema	Too small for age with wrinkled skin
Petechiae	Skin		
Meconium	Present on skin and fetal surface of placenta		
Internal features			
Subcutaneous fat	Normal		
Body cavities	Excessive fluid		
Organs	Congested		
Stomach	Dilated with mucus, meconium may be present		
Distal colon	Devoid of meconium		
Asphyctic hemorrhages	Thymus, epicardium, pericardium, pleural surfaces		
Adrenal glands	Fatty transformation of fetal zone adjacent to central vein	Distinct fatty change of cells of fetal cortex, fat-free zone between definitive cortex and abnormal fat containing central zone of fetal cortex	Complete fatty transformation of fetal zone
Lungs	Irregular acinar air space expansion, squames and meconium present Congestion of vessels and subpleural hemorrhages	Aspiration of amniotic fluid and meconium	
Thymus	Starry-sky appearance	Small involuted ranging from starry sky appearance to distinct cortical depletion of lymphocytes	Decreased weight, calcified Hassal corpuscles
Kidneys	Proximal tubular degeneration		
Spleen	Sporadic iron deposits	Increased hematopoiesis, iron in trabeculae and splenic capsule	
Liver	Congestion	Degeneration – color difference between left and right lobes Diffuse glycogen depletion. Occasionally there is diffuse accumulation of iron especially in the right lobe. Depletion of glycogen especially in the left lobe and fatty change. May see increased hematopoiesis	Decreased weight. Absence of glycogen Decreased iron. May see diffuse fatty transformation of hepatocytes
Costochondral junction			Small chondral proliferative zone

Modified from: Becker MJ, Becker AE: *Pathology of Late Fetal Stillbirth*. New York, Churchill Livingstone, Inc., 1989.

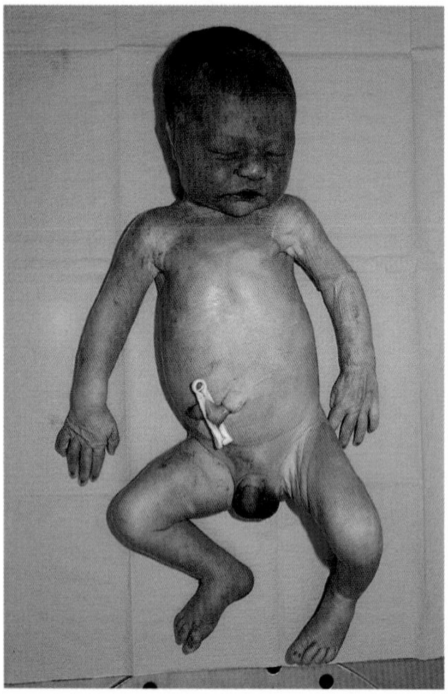

2.11. Postmature infant. The skin is wrinkled and meconium stained.

Postmaturity is a gestation > 42 weeks. The infant is at risk for placental insufficiency and perinatal hypoxia, intrauterine distress, respiratory distress syndrome, and stillbirth. Features of postmaturity are meconium staining, scaly wrinkled skin, and long fingernails. Placental signs of this condition include chronic meconium staining, numerous nucleated red blood cells (NRBCs) in fetal vessels, degenerate amnionic epithelium with squamous balls, and wrinkled or finely ulcerated umbilical cords whose Wharton jelly by light microscopy has increased eosinophilia. Placental insufficiency implies low uteroplacental blood flow. Some postdate newborns have no biochemical, physiologic, or other signs of placental dysfunction.

NEONATAL DEATHS

Neonatal deaths are defined as deaths of live-born infants that occur in the first 4 weeks after birth. A live birth is defined by the World Health Assembly as "the complete expulsion or extraction from its mother of a product of conception which, after separation breathes or shows any other evidence of life, such as beating of the heart, pulsation of the umbilical cord, or definite movement of the voluntary muscles."

Prematurity and Complications of Preterm Birth

The most common cause of neonatal mortality is prematurity. In the United States, 20% occur in the African-American population and 9% in the white population. The major complications of prematurity are hyaline membrane disease that may progress to bronchopulmonary dysplasia, necrotizing enterocolitis, and germinal matrix and intraventricular hemorrhage.

Prematurity is defined as a weight of 2,500 g or less or a gestational age of <37 weeks (Figures 2.13 and 2.14, Tables 2.5 to 2.11). It accounts for 7% of

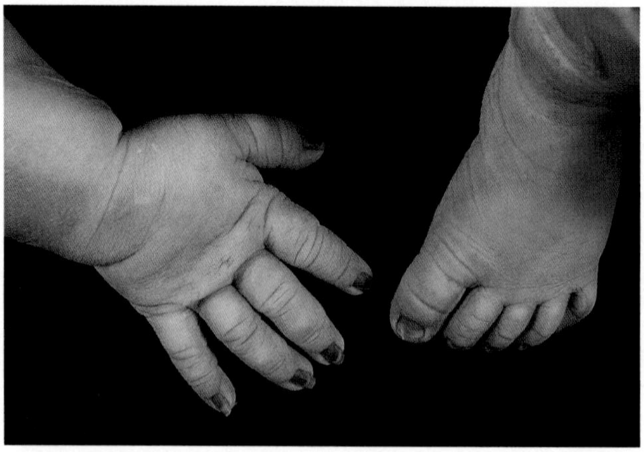

2.12. Postmature infant. The hand and foot show nails extending beyond the tips of the digits and meconium staining of skin and nails.

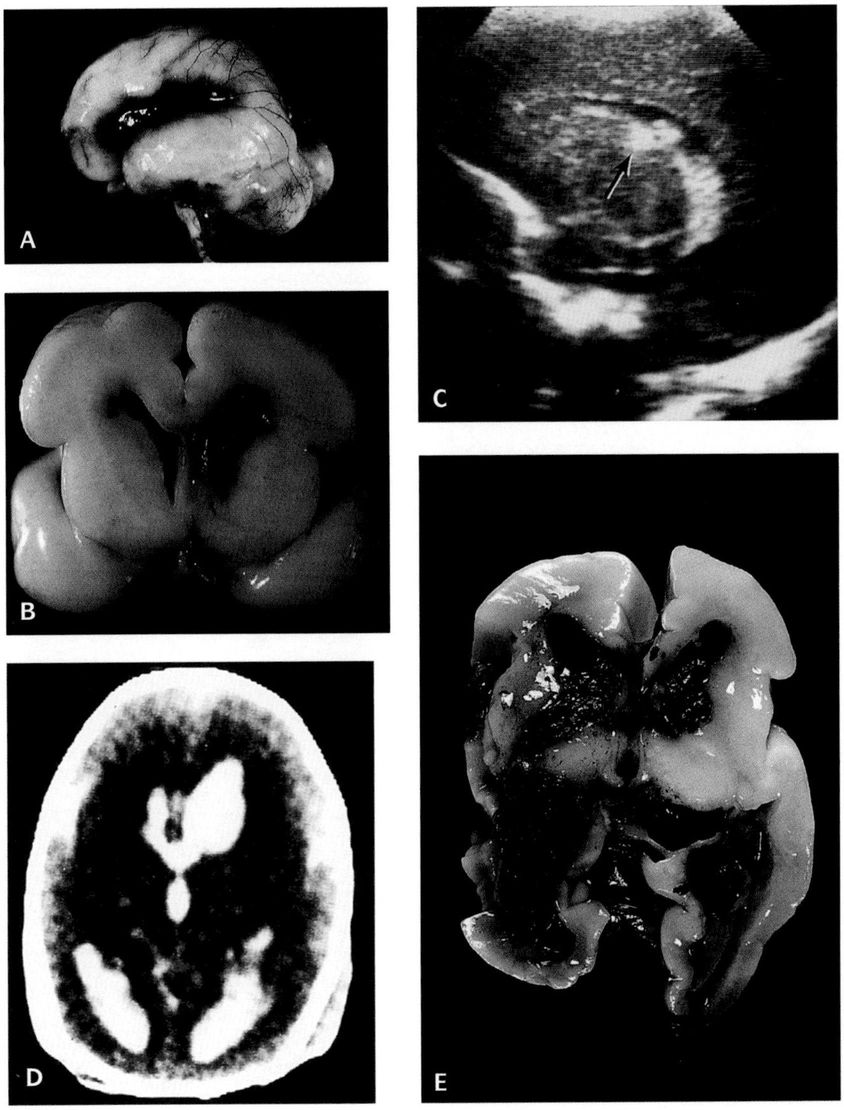

2.13. Infant brain 22 weeks' gestation. **(A)** External surface showing hemorrhage within the operculum. **(B)** Cut surface showing germinal matrix and intraventricular hemorrhage. **(C)** Ultrasound showing an intraventricular hemorrhage (arrow) in the sagittal plane. **(D)** CT scan showing hemorrhage into the lateral ventricles and a suggestion of hemorrhage spreading into the brain parenchyma. **(E)** Extensive intracerebral hemorrhage in an infant 25 weeks' gestation.

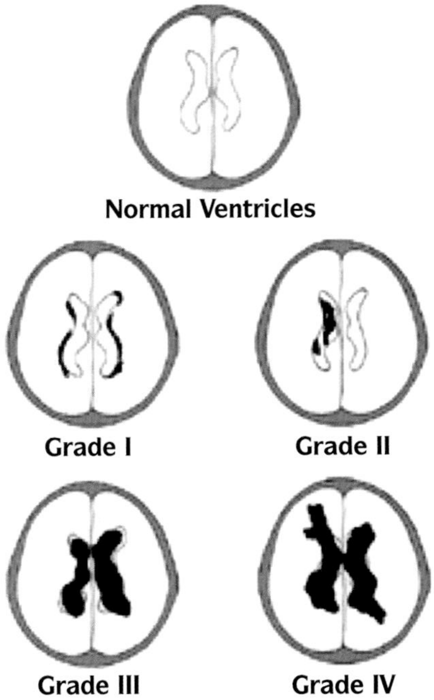

2.14. Intraventricular hemorrhage (IVH), classification. Grade I, hemorrhage in germinal matrix only. Grade II, IVH without ventricular dilatation. Grade III, IVH with ventricular dilatation: 35–45% incidence of motor/intellectual impairment. Grade IV–IVH with parenchymal extension: 65–80% incidence of motor/intellectual impairment.

all live births in the United States. Very-low-birth weight infants weigh 1,500 g or less and constitute 1% to 2% of all live births. There is about 2% survival at 501 to 600 g and 85% to 95% at 1,200 to 1,500 g. Only 2% of those born at 23 weeks, 21% at 24 weeks, and 69% at 25 weeks survive without intracranial hemorrhage.

The major risk factors for prematurity are premature rupture of membranes (PROM), chorioamnionitis, low uteroplacental blood flow, and multiple gestation.

Table 2.5 Effects of postmaturity

Fetus ceases growing and loss of soft tissue and low birth weight result
Absence of lanugo hair
Long nails
Abundance of scalp hair
Pale skin with desquamated epithelium
Decreased vernix caseosa
Increased alertness
High hematocrit
Dehydration
Hypoglycemia

Table 2.6 Leading causes of neonatal death in order of frequency

1. Prematurity and complications of preterm birth
   - Hyaline membrane disease and bronchopulmonary dysplasia
   - Intracranial hemorrhage
   - Necrotizing enterocolitis
   - Diffuse pulmonary hemorrhage
2. Congenital anomalies
3. Dysplasia
4. Infections: frequently a complication of chorioamnionitis
5. Perinatal hypoxia/asphyxia
6. Maternal complications of pregnancy
   - Age
   - Parity
   - Complications of placenta/cord/membrane
   - Smoking
   - Hypertension and preeclampsia
   - Postmaturity
   - Diabetes mellitus
   - Thyrotoxicosis
   - Collagen vascular diseases
7. Sudden infant death, excluding SIDS
   - Accidental suffocation
   - Infections
   - Congenital cardiac defects
   - Cardiac conduction defects
8. Amniotic fluid and meconium aspiration
9. Neonatal hemorrhage – coagulation defects
10. Birth trauma
11. Intrauterine growth retardation
12. Blood dyscrasias of newborn
13. Metabolic disorders

Table 2.7 Ten leading causes of infant mortality, birth to 1 year old, United States, 1995

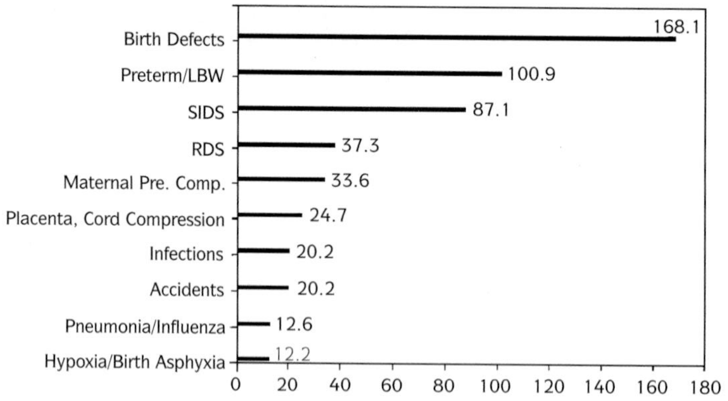

Source: Data from U.S. Office of Vital Statistics

Table 2.8 Risk factors for neonatal mortality

- Majority related to low birth weight and its risk factors
  - Prematurity
  - Intrauterine growth retardation
- In developing countries, infant mortality rates range from 18 to 200 per 1,000 live births
- Causes of death in developing countries are diarrhea, vaccine preventable illness, and acute respiratory infections

Table 2.9 Maternal risk factors for poor fetal outcome

Absent or inadequate prenatal care
Smoking
Poor nutritional status
Heavy alcohol consumption
Illicit drug use
Other toxin exposure (DES, occupational hazards)
High altitude

Table 2.10 Premature birth risk factors during pregnancy

Multiple pregnancy	Fetal anomalies
Placental problems (abruptio, previa)	Isoimmunization
Short interpregnancy interval	Premature rupture of membranes (PROM)
Hypertension/preeclampsia	Hyperemesis
Selected infections (urinary tract infection), rubella, cytomegalovirus	Oligo/Polyhydramnios
Bleeding first/second trimester	Anemia
	Cervical Incompetence
	Poor Weight Gain

Table 2.11 Leading causes of infant deaths due to congenital anomalies/ birth defects, 1998

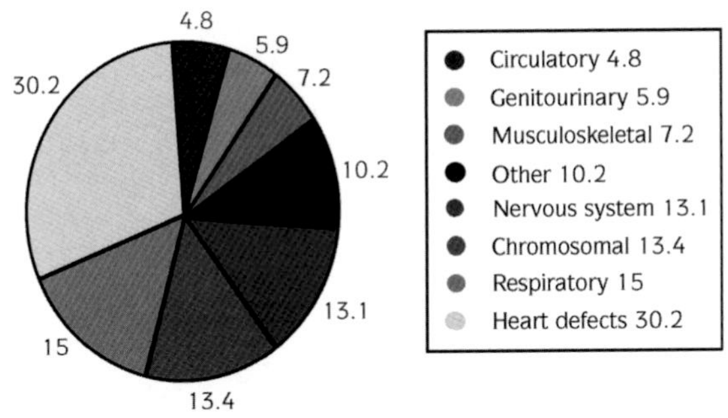

Source: National Center for Health Statistics as prepared by March of Dimes, 1998.

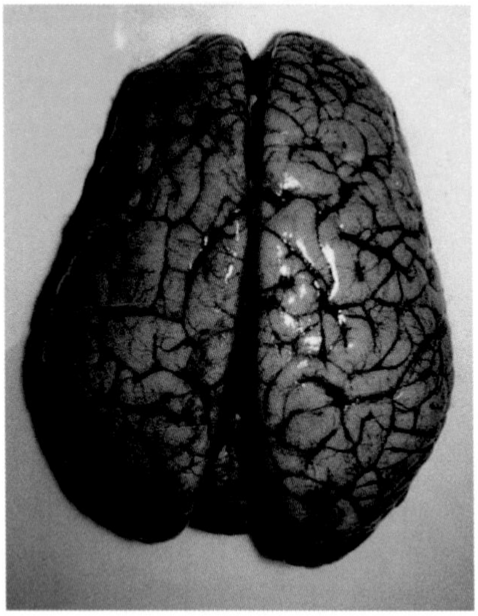

2.15. Severe cerebral edema of brain in a newborn who sustained severe birth anoxia.

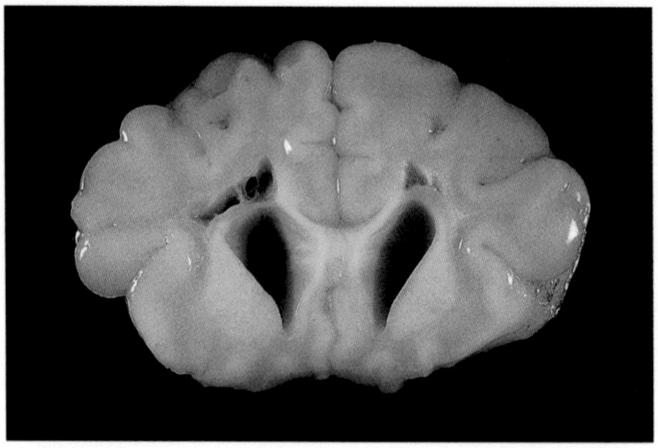

2.16. Periventricular leukomalacia. Coronal section of brain in a 6-week infant who had hypoxia at birth.

Chorioamnionitis is a major risk factor for PROM, as well as maternal cigarette smoking during pregnancy, vigorous motor activity by the fetus, a long umbilical cord, and diffuse fibrin beneath the chorionic plate.

With prolonged preterm PROM, there is an increased risk for abruption of the placenta. PROM leads to leakage of amniotic fluid and oligohydramnios. Oligohydramnios for only 1 week can lead to pulmonary hypoplasia.

Antibiotics administered prophylactically after PROM delay the onset of labor and reduce the incidence of infections in neonates.

Hypoxic Ischemic Encephalopathy

Hypoxic ischemic encephalopathy is the result of perinatal asphyxia usually occurring at or shortly before birth. It is preceded by cerebral edema and followed by neuronal necrosis. The cortex, basal ganglia hippocampus, brain stem, and cerebellar Purkinje cells are primarily affected. The neurons are shrunken with pyknotic nuclei and karyorrhexis.

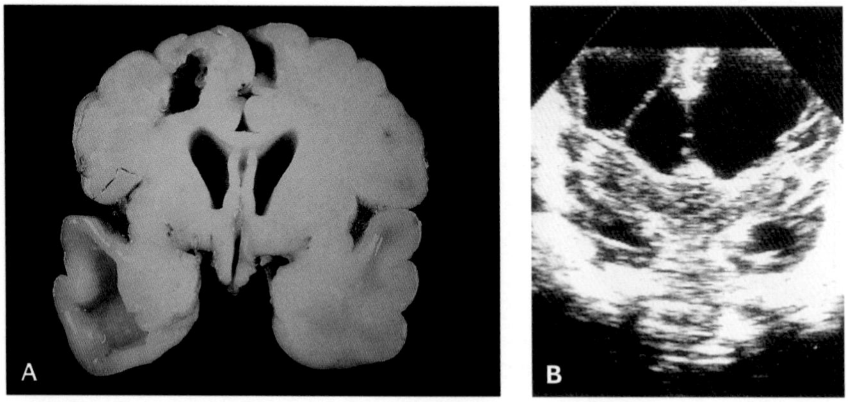

2.17. **(A)** Coronal section of brain with porencephalic cysts in an infant with hypoxic ischemic encephalopathy at 3 months of age. Note the septum cavum pellucidum. **(B)** Ultrasound showing porencephalic cysts following hypoxic ischemic encephalopathy. Initially the cysts were separate from the ventricles, but communication subsequently developed.

Table 2.12 Pathogenesis of necrotizing enterocolitis

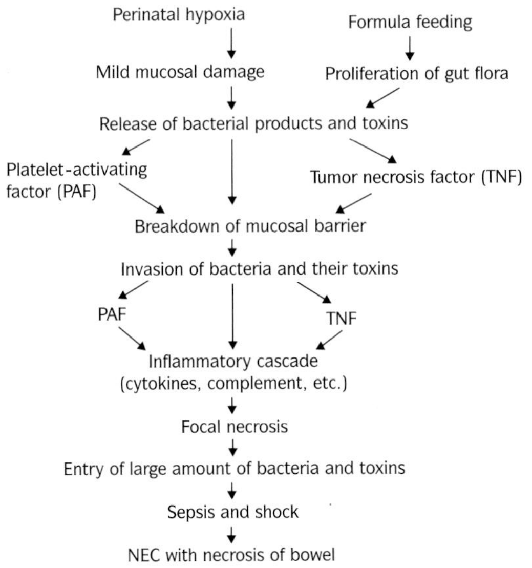

Perivascular Leukomalacia

Perivascular leukomalacia is a form of hypoxic encephalopathy. It usually is a complication of hypoxia in a premature infant but may occur in full-term infants. It is characterized by chalky white, small cystic lesions circummarginating the lateral ventricles.

Porencephaly

Perivascular leukomalacia may progress to porencephaly with coalescence of small cysts to form large cystic spaces that may communicate with the ventricles.

Necrotizing Enterocolitis (NEC)

NEC affects neonates with severe, necrotizing injury to the intestine (Table 2.12 and Figure 2.18). NEC is a leading cause of morbidity and mortality with a reported incidence of 10% among very-low-birthweight infants (<1,500 g) and a mortality of 26%. NEC may cause multisystem organ failure. Twenty-five hundred cases occur annually in the United States and 20% to 60% require surgical treatment. Eighty percent of patients are preterm or have low, or very low, birthweight. Those infants 28 weeks or less of gestational age are at greatest risk. In preterm infants, NEC begins 10–15 days after birth. Symptoms are staged. In stage I, the infant manifests abdominal distension, vomiting, increased gastric residual, lethargy, apnea, bradycardia, or guaiac-positive stools. In stage II, pneumatosis intestinalis or free air is present in the portal vein. Stage III is manifested by shock, disseminated intravascular coagulation, acidosis, thrombocytopenia, and sometimes intestinal perforation.

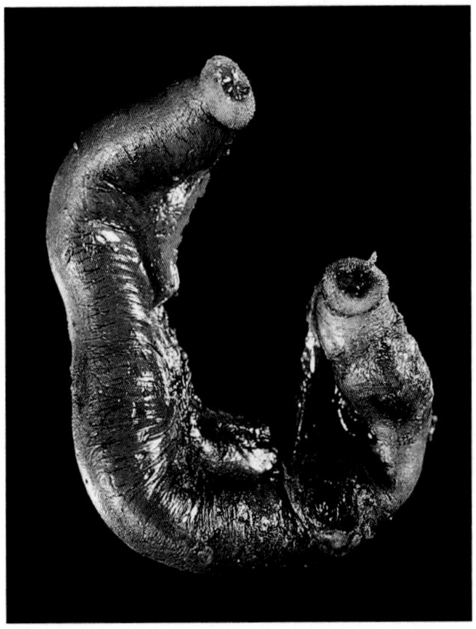

2.18. Necrotizing enterocolitis. Surgically resected segment of bowel with hemorrhage necrosis and perforation.

The pathologic lesion of NEC is coagulative or ischemic necrosis, usually at the ileocolic region; in about half the cases necrosis involves both the small and large intestine; it may be a continuous or a discontinuous involvement. The bowel is grossly distended, dark purple or black in areas containing extensive hemorrhage; the soft, friable wall may perforate when the involvement is severe and transmural. Perforation occurs at a junction between normal and necrotic bowel or in a devitalized region.

In neonates with severe anoxic episodes, blood is diverted to the heart and the brain and the bowel are exposed to severe ischemia. Necrosis of the bowel in some cases may be secondary to mesenteric thromboembolism.

Bacteria are important in causing NEC, because it does not occur before colonization of the intestine by bacteria. Microorganisms isolated from the stools include *Escherichia coli*, *Klebsiella*, *Enterobacter*, *Pseudomonas*, *Salmonella*, *Clostridium perfringens*, *Clostridium difficile*, *Clostridium butyricum*, coaglulase-negative staphylococci, coronavirus, rotavirus, and enteroviruses.

Regenerative changes in NEC are replacement of the mucosa by a cuboidal or tall columnar epithelium with hyperchromatic nuclei, absent mucin production, and mitotic activity overlying a layer of granulation tissue.

Congenital Malformations

Congenital malformations are a leading cause of death in neonates. Causes of neonatal deaths from major organ system anomalies include cardiovascular, pulmonary, renal, central nervous system, musculoskeletal, and gastrointestinal malformations as well as chromosomal defects and multiple congenital anomaly syndromes.

Infections in the Newborn

Infections in the newborn are either complications of an ascending infection from chorioamnionitis, including aspiration of infected amniotic fluid, or maternal placental transmission, including TORCH (toxoplasmosis, rubella, cytomegalovirus, herpes virus), coxsackie virus, human immunodeficiency virus, and syphilis. Bacterial infections may result in neonatal pneumonia, meningitis, or encephalitis. The most likely bacterial infections in the newborn are group B streptococcus (GBS), *Haemophilus influenzae, E. coli, Bacteroides fragilis*, and *Streptococcus faecalis.*

Risk factors include PROM more than 18–24 hours before labor, chorioamnionitis, prematurity, maternal colonization with *Mycoplasma* (*Ureaplasma urealyticum*), and male gender.

Neonatal mortality due to GBS infection is relatively high, 15–30%.

Infant of Diabetic Mother

The infant of a diabetic mother is at particular risk for severe hypoglycemia, hyperinsulinemia with pancreatic islet cell hyperplasia, malformations, and

Table 2.13 Abnormalities in the infant of a diabetic mother

Placenta	Prematurity
Heavy, bulky, edematous	Intrapartum asphyxia, acidosis, apneic spells
Amnion nodosum (oligohydramnios)	Asphyxia, acidosis, apneic spells
Fetal vascular thrombosis	Respiratory distress → hyaline membrane disease
Single umbilical artery	Hyperinsulinemia → hypoglycemia
Immature villi	Hypocalcemia
Dysmaturity of villi	Hypomagnesemia
Cytotrophoblastic hyperplasia	Neuromuscular excitability
Increased syncytial knots	Polycythemia
Thick trophoblastic basement membranes	Hyperbilirubinemia → jaundice
Fibrinoid necrosis beneath trophoblast membrane	Infections: septicemia, peritonitis, meningitis, cellulitis, adenitis Urinary tract, skin, and conjunctival infections Hemorrhage, intracranial
Organs and tissues Brain – Weight below average Heart – Cardiomegaly, hypertrophy and hyperplasia Cardiomyopathy –Obstructive hypertrophic –Dilated, congestive	Congenital Malformations First and second branchial arch anomalies Cleft palate Microtia Diaphragmatic hernia Anal atresia
Liver – Increased weight Increased hematopoiesis Increased fat and glycogen	Contractures Costovertebral defects Anencephaly
Pancreas – Increased size and number of islets of Langerhans Eosinophilic infiltrate and Charcot–Leyden crystals Peri-insular connective tissue Increase in number of beta cells	Hydrocephalus Meningomyelocele Holoprosencephaly Caudal regression syndrome–sirenomelia
Spleen – Splenomegaly Hematopoiesis	Congenital cardiac defects Small left colon syndrome
Adrenals – Increased weight Cytomegaly Hematopoiesis	Urinary tract abnormalities Limb reduction defects Hypoplasia of bones
Thyroid – Increased size Delayed maturation Increased colloid content	 Genital tract Female – Follicular cysts of ovaries
Pituitary – Increased number of acidophils	Decidual stromal change of endometrium Endometrial hyperplasia
Kidneys – Increased weight Immature glomeruli Renal vein thrombosis	Male – Increase in Leydig cells Vacuolization of prostatic epithelium
General Appearance Abundant vernix caseosa Nasal milia Hirsutism	Disorders of Fetal Growth Intrauterine growth retardation (rare) Large for gestational age Macrosomia (increase in adipose tissue and organomegaly)
Thymus Increase in size Hematopoiesis Lymphoid depletion	Bones and Teeth Bone osteosclerotic Reduced osteoclastic activity Hypoplasia of teeth enamel
Eyes Cataracts Microphthalmia Opaque cornea Anterior chamber dysgenesis	Lungs Immature Thrombosis Renal vein

particularly caudal dysgenesis, sirenomelia, holoprosencephaly, Vater association, and anencephaly.

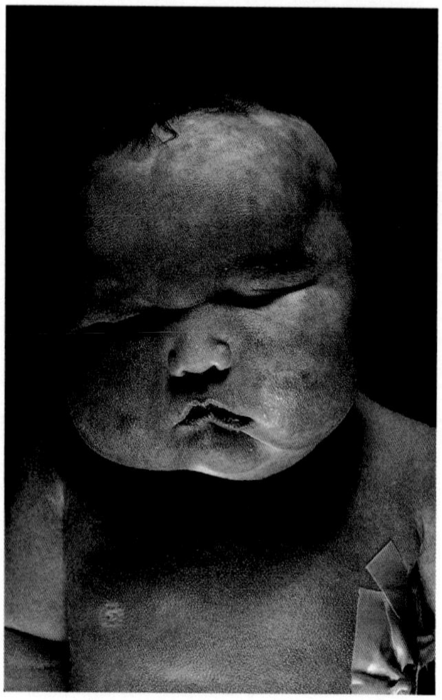

2.19. Infant of a diabetic mother. This infant weighed 6.2 kg, was hypoglycemic, and died 2 hours after birth.

Complications of Amniocentesis (see Chapter 10)

Amniotic Fluid and Meconium Aspiration

Amniotic fluid aspiration is most likely to occur in a hypoxic infant. Meconium aspiration occurs in 5–15% of births and is most common in term or postterm infants. It usually improves within 48 hours of birth, but if severe it carries high mortality. Meconium aspiration syndrome occurs in 9 per 1,000 births; 59% have been attributed to severe acute chorioamnionitis and less frequently to low uteroplacental blood flow and abruptio placentae.

Birth Trauma

Birth trauma, including skull fractures (Figure 2.20A and B); extracranial, extradural, and intraparenchymal hemorrhages; and occipital diastasis may result in neonatal death. Face and breech presentation carry a high risk of trauma to the infant.

Occipital Osteodiastasis

Occipital diastasis (separation of the squamous and lateral parts of the occipital bone) (Figure 2.20C and D) is the most important form of disruption of the cranial bones but is missed at autopsy unless specifically sought. At autopsy, reflection of the scalp downward as far as the foramen magnum is necessary to explore fully the occipital bone. The squamous and lateral parts of the occipital bone are widely separated by cartilage until about 36 weeks' gestation and do not fuse until the second year of life. Excessive pressure on the suboccipital region during birth causes traumatic separation of the cartilaginous joint between the squamous and lateral parts of the bone on one or both sides. The lower edge of the squamous occipital bone is then displaced and rotated forward. The dura and occipital sinuses are torn, resulting in subdural hemorrhage in the posterior fossa and laceration of the cerebellum.

Table 2.14 Complications of amniocentesis

Stimulation of uterine contractions with the induction of premature labor
Maternal sensitization of fetal blood
Fetal skin puncture with healing to form small scars or dimples
Peritoneal adhesions
Ileal atresia
Fetal intracranial hemorrhage resulting in porencephalic cysts

Table 2.15 Immune hemolytic anemia

Rh isoimmunization
Fetal-maternal ABO blood group incompatibility
Kell antigen isoimmunization

Blood Dyscrasia

1. Hemolytic disease of the newborn due to blood group incompatibility (Figures 2.21 and 2.22, Table 2.15) with high bilirubin levels may result in kernicterus (Figure 2.23).
2. Vitamin K deficiency (hemorrhagic disease of the newborn)
3. Anemia due to fetomaternal hemorrhage
4. Twin-to-twin transfusion
5. Maternal transfer of antiplatelet antibodies
6. Maternal lupus with anticardiolipin and/or RO antibodies transferred to the fetus
7. Protein S, protein C, and antithrombin deficiencies

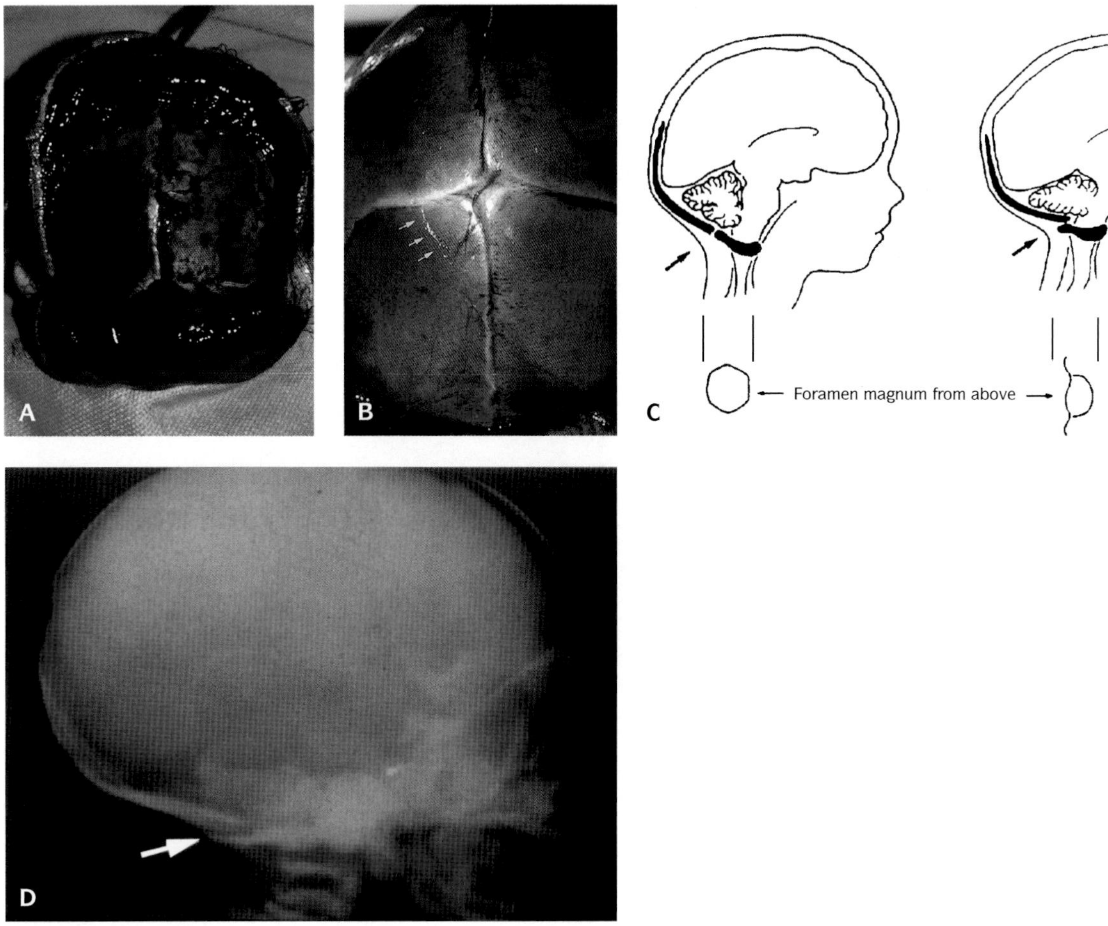

2.20. **(A)** Birth trauma. Extensive subgaleal hemorrhage that was due to suction extraction. **(B)** Skull fracture (arrows) due to a difficult forceps delivery. **(C)** Occipital diastasis. Mechanism of injury. **(D)** Occipital diastasis (arrow) demonstrated on a lateral skull radiograph.

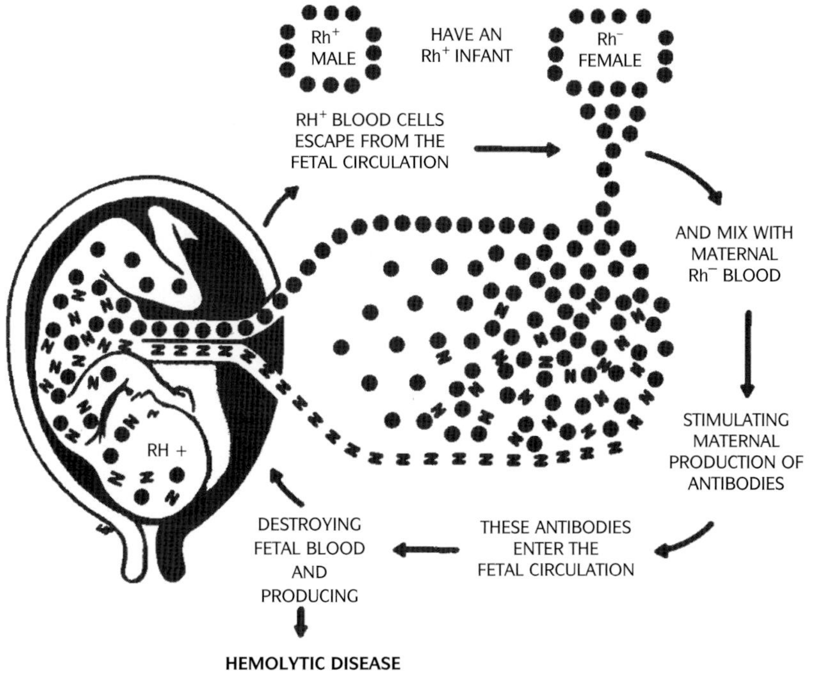

2.21. Mechanisms of erythroblastosis fetalis.

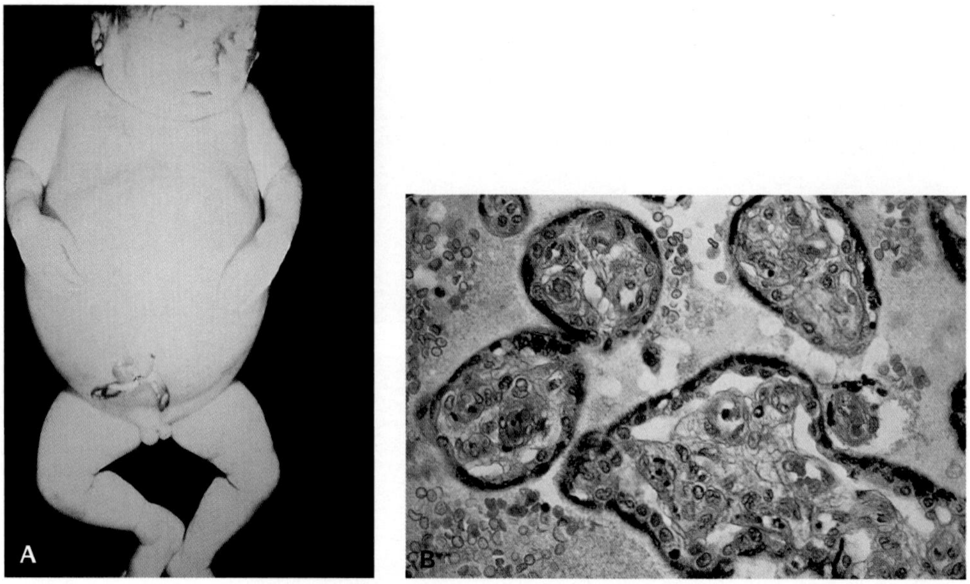

2.22. Erythroblastosis fetalis. **(A)** Hydropic infant with anemia due to Rh blood group incompatibility. The mother was Rh negative and had not received Rhogam at a previous delivery. **(B)** Microscopic section of the placenta showing persistence of the cytotrophoblasts and nucleated red blood cells in the villus capillaries.

Metabolic Disorders (see Chapter 24)

Metabolic disorders have been related to unexpected death in newborns. In these disorders, there is usually a normal period immediately after birth followed by hypoglycemia, respiratory difficulty, vomiting, and acidosis.

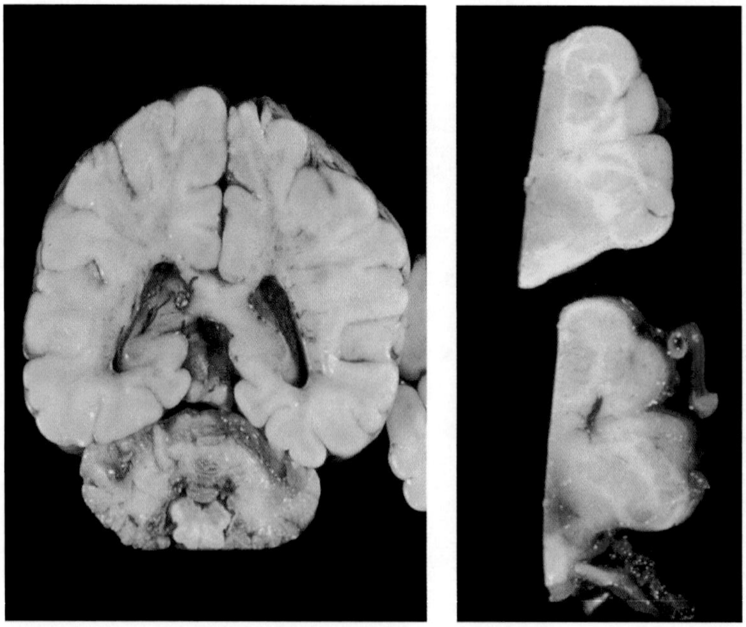

2.23. Kernicterus. Bilirubin staining of basal ganglia (left) and the olivary nuclei (right) in an infant with erythroblastosis fetalis.

NEONATAL REFERENCES

Allen MC, Donohue PK, Duisnau AE: The limit of viability: neonatal outcome of infants born at 22 to 25 weeks' gestation. *N Engl J Med* 329:1597, 1993.

Gerdes JS: Clinicopathologic approach to the diagnosis of neonatal sepsis. *Clin Perinatol* 18:361, 1991.

Hsueh W, Caplan MS, Tan X, et al.: Necrotizing enterocolitis of the newborn: pathogenetic concepts in perspective. *Perspectives Pediatr Pathol* 21:9, 1999.

Liggins D, Thurlbeck WM: Conditions altering normal lung growth and development. In Thibeault DW, Gregory GA (eds): *Neonatal Pulmonary Care*, 2nd ed, Norwalk, CT, Appleton-Century-Crofts, 1986, p. 3.

Miller HC, Jekel JF: Epidemiology of spontaneous premature rupture of membranes: factors in pre-term births. *Yale J Biol Med* 62:241, 1989.

Naeye RL: Functionally important disorders of the placenta, umbilical cord and fetal membranes. *Hum Pathol* 7:680, 1987.

Naeye RL: *Disorders of the Placenta, Fetus, and Neonate: Diagnosis and Clinical Significance*, St. Louis, Mosby-Year Book, 1992.

Nelson DM, Stempel LE, Zuspan FP: Association of prolonged, preterm premature rupture of the membranes and abruptio placentae. *J Reprod Med* 31:249, 1986.

Phelps DL, Brown DR, Tung B, et al.: 28-day survival rates of 6676 neonates with birth weights of 1250 grams or less. *Pediatrics* 87:7, 1991.

Rotschild A, Ling EW, Puterman ML, et al.: Neonatal outcome after prolonged preterm rupture of the membranes. *Am J Obstet Gynecol* 162:46, 1990.

Verber IG, Pearce JM, New LC, et al.: Prolonged rupture of the fetal membranes and neonatal outcome. *J Perinat Med* 17:469, 1989.

FETAL, STILLBORN, AND NEONATAL DEATH REFERENCES

Allen MC, Donohue PK, Dusinau AE: The limit of viability; neonatal outcome of infants born at 22 to 25 weeks' gestation. *N Engl J Med* 329:1597, 1993.

Becker MJ, Becker AE: *Pathology of Late Fetal Stillbirth*, New York, Churchill Livingstone, Inc., 1989.

Bergsjo P: Introducing two international studies on perinatal and infant growth, morbidity and mortality. *Acta Obstet Gynecol Scand* 68:3, 1989.

Dimmick JE, Kalousek DK (eds): *Developmental Pathology of the Embryo*, Philadelphia, JB Lippincott, 1992.

Fretts RC, Boyd ME, Usher RH, Usher HA: The changing pattern of fetal death, 1961–1988. *Obstet Gynecol* 79:35, 1992.

Gerdes JS: Clinicopathologic approach to the diagnosis of neonatal sepsis. *Clin Perinatol* 18:361, 1991.

Gilbert ER, Zugibe FT: Torsion and constriction of the umbilical cord. A cause of fetal death. *Arch Pathol* 97:58, 1974.

Golding J: Epidemiology of fetal and neonatal death. In Keeling JW (ed): *Fetal and Neonatal Pathology*. London, Springer Verlag, 1993.

Hsueh W, Caplan MS, Tan X, et al.: Necrotizing Enterocolitis of the newborn: pathogenetic concepts in perspective. *Perspectives Pediatr Pathol* 21:9, 1999.

Johnson A, Townsend PA, Yudkin P, et al.: Functional abilities at 4 years of children born before 24 weeks of gestation, *Br Med J* 306:1715, 1993.

Kalousek DK, Gilbert-Barness E. Causes of stillbirth and neonatal death. In Gilbert-Barness E (ed): *Potter's Pathology of the Fetus and Infant*, 2nd ed, St. Louis, Mosby, 1997.

Layde PM, Erickson JD, Falek A, McCarthy BJ: Congenital malformations in twins. *Am J Hum Genet* 32:69, 1980.

Liggins D, Thurlbeck WM: Conditions altering normal lung growth and development. In Thibeault DW, Gregory GA (eds): *Neonatal Pulmonary Care*, 2nd ed, Norwalk, CT, Appleton-Century-Crofts, 1986, p. 3.

Machin GA, Ackerman J, Gilbert-Barners E: Abnormal umbilical cord coiling is associated with adverse perinatal outcomes. *Ped Devel Pathol* 3: 2000.

Miller HC, Jekel JF: Epidemiology of spontaneous premature rupture of membranes: factors in pre-term births. *Yale J Biol Med* 62:241, 1989.

Naeye RL: Functionally important disorders of the placenta, umbilical cord and fetal membranes. *Hum Pathol* 7:680, 1987.

Naeye RL: *Disorders of the Placenta, Fetus, and Neonate: Diagnosis and Clinical Significance*, St. Louis, Mosby-Year Book, 1992.

Nelson DM, Stempel LE, Zuspan FP: Association of prolonged, preterm premature rupture of the membranes and abruptio placentae. *J Reprod Med* 31:249, 1986.

Phelps DL, Brown DR, Tung B, et al.: 28-day survival rates of 6676 neonates with birth weights of 1250 grams or less. *Pediatrics* 87:7, 1991.

Rotschild A, Ling EW, Puterman ML, et al.: Neonatal outcome after prolonged preterm rupture of the membranes. *Am J Obstet Gynecol* 162:46, 1990.

Singer DB, Macpherson T: Fetal death and the macerated stillborn fetus. In Wigglesworth JS, Singer DB (eds): *Textbook of Fetal and Perinatal Pathology*. Boston, Blackwell Scientific Publications, 1991.

Verber IG, Pearce JM, New LC, et al.: Prolonged rupture of the fetal membranes and neonatal outcome. *J Perinat Med* 17:469, 1989.

Whitfield CR, Smith NC, Cockburn F, Gibson AAM: Perinatally related wastage-a proposed classification of primary obstetric factors. *Br J Obstet Gynecol* 93:694, 1986.

THREE

Fetal Autopsy

The normal anatomy of the adult and child are similar; however, the perinatal autopsy is significantly different. The variety and complexity of the congenital anomalies found in perinatal and fetal autopsies is endless and the prosector must be prepared to spend the necessary time demonstrating these anomalies. This detailed procedure can be altered to preserve any anomaly encountered without deforming the body itself. Most of the anomalies found in this population never survive to adulthood. Together with the clinical information this meticulous examination provides the necessary information to educate the families about future pregnancies.

PLACENTAL CHANGES AFTER FETAL DEATH

After the intrauterine death of the fetus, the placenta remains vital until it is expelled. However, changes occur that resemble vascular insufficiency but are diffuse, affecting fetal structure and all villi (Figure 3.1). Focal lesions suggest a preexisting abnormality (Tables 3.1).

Fetal death results in complete interruption of the fetal circulation. Vascular spaces within the villi are empty and collapsed. Within weeks, ingrowth of fibroblasts ultimately completely obliterate the vessels. Thrombosis does not occur and if present indicates preexistent pathology.

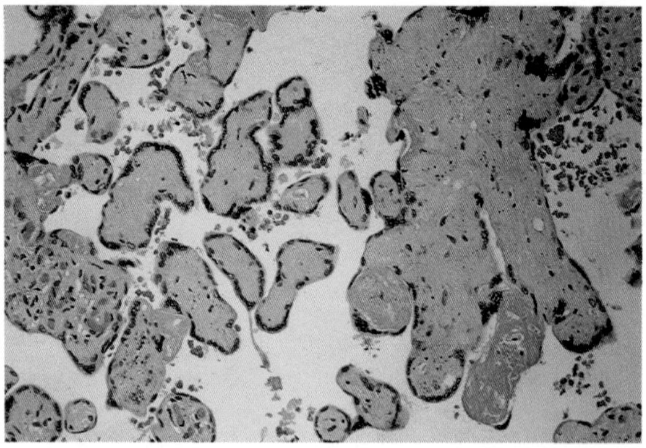

3.1. Microscopic appearance of placenta after fetal death. The chorionic villi are shrunken and fibrotic. Loss of fetal perfusion leads to stromal fibrosis, loss of capillaries with retention of trophoblasts from maternal perfusion.

Calcification may be observed in addition to fibrosis as a postmortem change within villi. It presents as fine granules deposited along the basal membrane of the trophoblast, sometimes almost in linear fashion. The fine granules contrast with the coarse deposits that sometimes occur in villi during physiological maturation. After fetal death, there are excessive syncytial knots that are diffuse. Primary vascular insufficiency is usually focal.

The villi are eventually clustered more closely together and the intervillous spaces become almost completely obliterated.

EXAMINATION OF THE PLACENTA

The immature placenta should be examined in a similar fashion to the mature placenta (see Chapter 4). When the fetus is severely macerated, amniotic membranes can be used for karyotypic analysis.

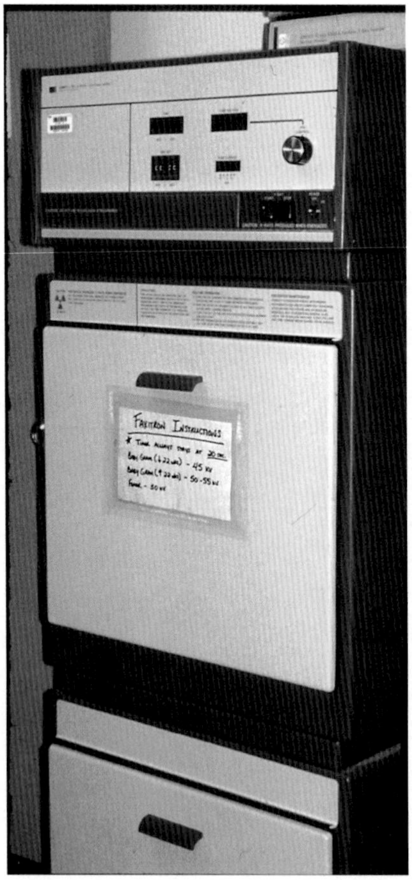

3.2. Faxitron.

Table 3.1 Placental changes

Stillbirth	Prematurity
Maternal vascular disease	Chorioamnionitis
Retroplacental hemorrhage	Retroplacental hemorrhage
Cord occlusion/hemorrhage	Circumvallation
Hematogenous infection	Marginal hemorrhage
Ascending infection, severe	Shape abnormalities
Extensive fibrinosis	Hydrops
Maternal floor infarction	Decidual vascular disease
Fetal vascular thrombosis	Villous ischemic change
VUE (villitis of unknown etiology)	Chronic villitis
Hydrops	
Dysmaturity	

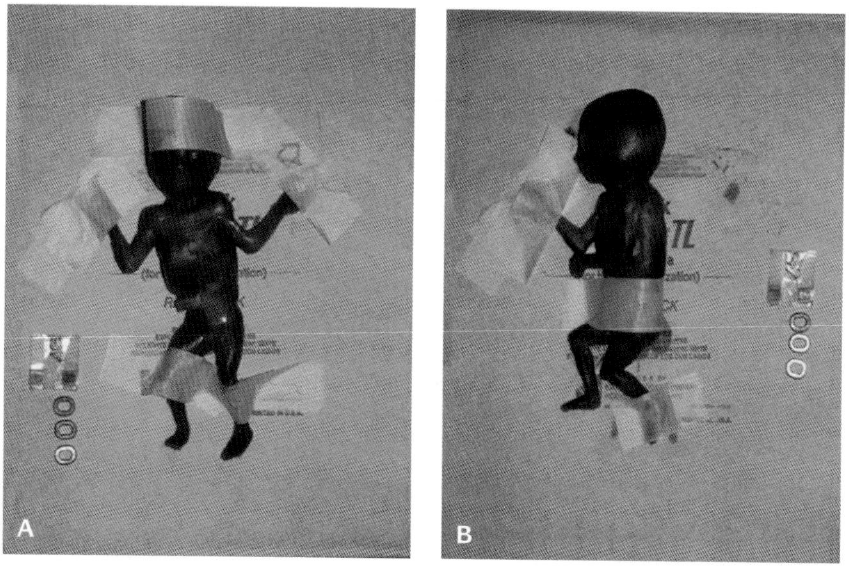

3.3. Mammogram films used in the faxitron with a fetus of 18 weeks gestation positioned to obtain anteroposterior **(A)** and lateral **(B)** views.

ROENTGENOGRAPHIC EXAM

Roentgenographic examination including anteroposterior and lateral views of the entire body is necessary with a faxitron (Figures 3.2 to 3.4 and Table 3.2). If a faxitron is not available, conventional x-ray studies can be performed. The faxitron is not limited to bony surveys and can be used to demonstrate visceral anomalies through injection studies. By injecting a radiopaque liquid, such as barium or an ionotropic contrast, fistulas can be demonstrated, particularly for bronchial morphology and extrahepatic and intrahepatic biliary ducts without disrupting the anatomy. This is most beneficial in small fetuses (<20 weeks gestation) where the structures are extremely small. Malformations are thus demonstrated before dissection commences. Several sizes of small catheter tubing should be available. X-rays are taken with mammogram film.

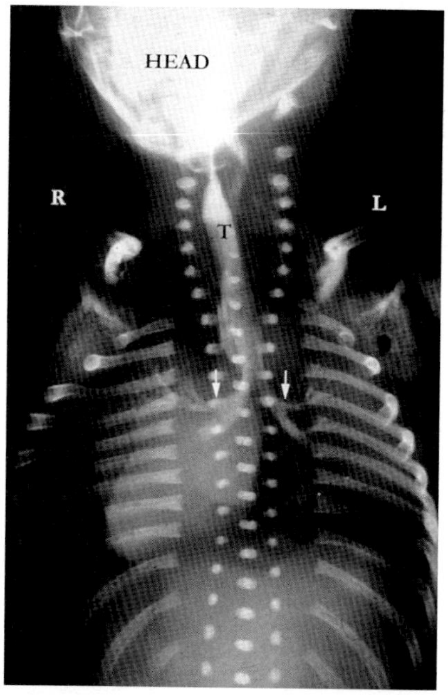

3.4. Injection study to determine bronchial morphology in a fetus at 14 weeks gestation, with asplenia. There are bilateral morphologic right bronchi (arrows). (R = right, L = left).

PHOTOGRAPHS

Photographs are of the utmost importance when performing a fetal or infant autopsy. The external features may provide the only information necessary to make the diagnosis of a malformation syndrome. The photographs must be close enough to depict the abnormal features with adequate points of reference remaining in the field. In situ photographs can be very beneficial, preserving anatomic relationships and depicting the initial presentation of visceral lesions before fixation. In the autopsy a good photograph is often more valuable than any number of microscopic sections (Table 3.3).

Table 3.2 Faxitron settings and exposure times for embryos and fetuses*

Gestational age: 10–12 weeks	
Head	28 kV/20 seconds
Chest and Long Bones	24 kV/18 seconds
Hands and Feet	23 kV/17 seconds
Gestational age: 13 weeks	
Chest and Long Bones	20 kV/17 seconds
Gestational age: 14 weeks	
Head	29 kV/21 seconds
Chest and Long Bones	20 kV/17 seconds
Gestational age: 15 weeks	
Head	34 kV/22 seconds
Chest and Long Bones	30 kV/22 seconds
Hands and Feet	25 kV/22 seconds
Gestational age: 16 weeks	
Head	31 kV/23 seconds
Chest and Long Bones	31 kV/23 seconds
Hands and Feet	27 kV/22 seconds
Gestational age: 17 weeks	
Chest and Long Bones	30 kV/26 seconds
Gestational age: 18 weeks	
Head	30 kV/35 seconds
Chest and Long Bones	27 kV/35 seconds
Hands and Feet	24 kV/30 seconds
Gestational age: 19–20 weeks	
Head	34 kV/31 seconds
Chest and Long Bones	34 kV/31 seconds
Hands and Feet	26 kV/30 seconds
Gestational age: 21 weeks	
Head	35 kV/30 seconds
Chest and Long Bones	35 kV/30 seconds
Hands and Feet	26 kV/30 seconds
Gestational age: 22 weeks	
Head	35 kV/30 seconds
Chest and Long Bones	30 kV/30 seconds
Hands and Feet	26 kV/28 seconds
Gestational age: 23 weeks	
Head	37 kV/40 seconds
Chest and Long Bones	30 kV/28 seconds
Gestational age: 24 weeks	
Head	35 kV/40 seconds
Chest and Long Bones	32 kV/30 seconds
Hands and Feet	26 kV/28 seconds
Gestational age: 25–28 weeks	
Head	40 kV/40 seconds
Chest and Long Bones	37 kV/40 seconds
Hands and Feet	29 kV/28 seconds
Gestational age: 29 weeks	
Head	30 kV/45 seconds
Chest and Long Bones	28 kV/25 seconds
Hands and Feet	20 kV/18 seconds
Gestational age: 30 weeks	
Head	48 kV/38 seconds
Chest and Long Bones	40 kV/35 seconds
Hands and Feet	27 kV/24 seconds
Gestational age: 31–32 weeks	
Head	47 kV/31 seconds
Chest and Long Bones	36 kV/28 seconds
Hands and Feet	28 kV/26 seconds
Gestational age: 33–39 weeks	
Head	47 kV/55 seconds
Chest and Long Bones	34 kV/30 seconds
Gestational age: 40–41 weeks	
Head	53 kV/60 seconds
Chest and Long Bones	45 kV/60 seconds
Hands and Feet	28 kV/32 seconds

* Data from Department of Pathology, Magee Hospital for Women, University of Pittsburgh, Pittsburgh, PA Courtesy of Dr. Trevor McPherson.

Table 3.3 Equipment for perinatal autopsy

Charts providing normal weights and measurements for newborns and stillborns
Sterile and nonsterile syringes and needles (multiple sizes)
Sterile packs including scissors and forceps for cultures and karyotype
Magnifying glass
Dissecting microscope, preferably with a camera attached
Dissecting board (cork or plastic)
Pins or tacks
Sponge (8 × 4 × 2.5). This will serve as a movable work area for dissecting the organ block
Gauze or absorbent paper towels
String
A large scale for weighing the fetus
A small scale, preferably digital, with a small balance scale as an alternative
Tape measure (flexible) and at least one 15-cm plastic ruler
Scalpel handles (two) and blades
Large knife (brain cutting knife)
Small forceps with teeth (one) and without teeth (one)
Medium forceps with teeth (one) and without teeth (one)
Stout scissors for cutting bone
Metzenbaum scissors (one)
Small scissors with at least one sharp point (one)
Small scissors with both points sharp (one)
Fine probe with rounded ends (one)
Hemostats (several of various sizes)

Table 3.4 Clinical information and autopsy checklist

Autopsy/Surgical #:			
Autopsy consent authorized by:		Restrictions:	
Date:			
Infant			
Last name:		Gestational age:	
Sex:		Postnatal age at time of death:	
Race:		Birthweight:	
Liveborn/Stillborn:		Birth date:	Time:
Mother			
Age:		Para:	Gravida:
Prenatal care:			
Folic acid supplementation (periconceptual):			
Medications during pregnancy:			
Complications of pregnancy:			
Labor:		Spontaneous:	
		Induced:	
Duration of labor:			
Rupture of membranes (date and time):			
Complications of labor:		Fetal monitoring:	
Presentation:		Delivery (date and time):	
Complications of delivery:			
Neonatal			
Apgar scores:	1 min,	5 min,	10 min,
Clinical problems:			
Diagnosis:			
Treatment:			
Autopsy Measurements			
Weight:			
CR:	CH:	FL:	
HC:	CC:	AC:	
IP:	IC:	OO:	
Notes:			

EQUIPMENT

Special instruments must be used when performing a perinatal autopsy, because of the small size of the fetus. These small instruments are too small for general autopsy purposes and can be destroyed by using them for even one adult autopsy. Ophthalmic instruments are excellent for these small dissections.

CLINICAL INFORMATION

A complete examination cannot be performed without the necessary clinical information (Table 3.4). The necessary permits should be in order and properly signed before beginning the autopsy. A good family history is very important, especially any information about other perinatal or neonatal deaths.

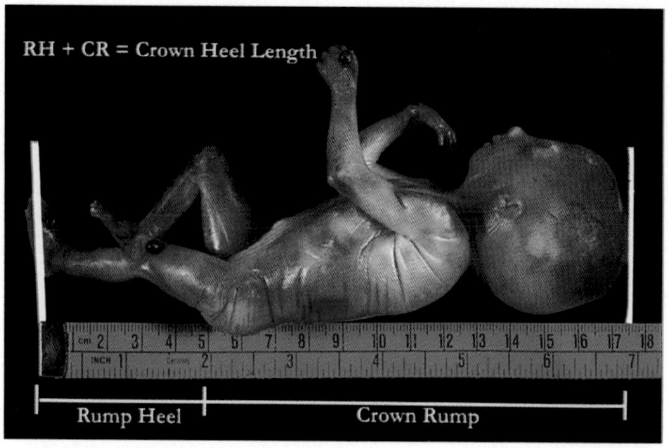

3.5. Measurement of crown rump, rump heel, and crown heel lengths.

EXTERNAL EXAM

The external examination includes weighing and measuring the fetus, the measurements consist of: head circumference (HC), chest circumference (CC), abdominal circumference (AC), crown–rump (CR) length, crown–heel (CH) length, foot length, inner and outer canthal distance, interpupillary distance and mesurements of the cranial fontanels (Figures 3.5 to 3.8). The CR length is usually two-thirds that of the CH length. The CR length and HC usually do not differ by more than 1.0 cm; major differences indicate megencephaly or microencephaly. A large abdomen may indicate autosomal recessive polycystic kidney disease. Foot length is particularly useful in fetuses of early gestational age, in severely macerated fetuses, in infants with major abnormalities (anencephaly), and in dilatation and evacuation (DE) specimens, where an intact foot may be the only measurement available. Facial measurements are helpful in determining hypo- or hypertelorism. The size, shape, and orientation of the eyes are assessed. The length of the philtrum should be measured.

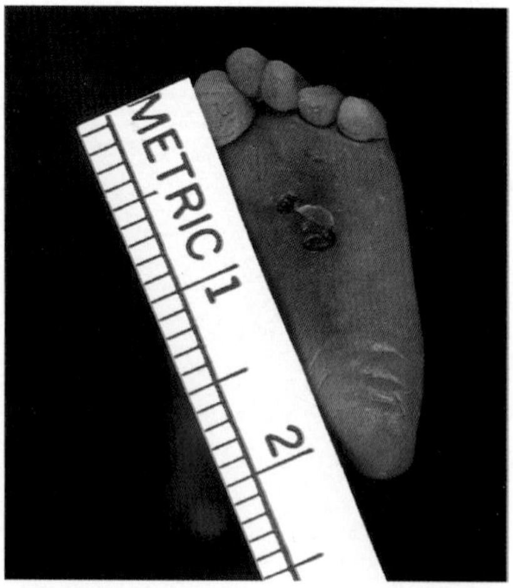

3.6. Measurement of foot length.

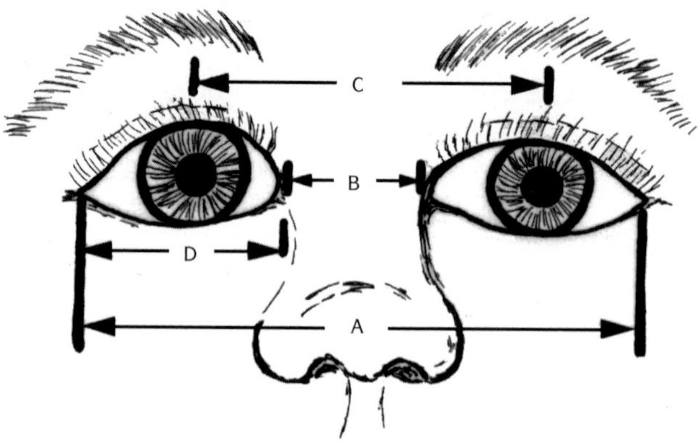

3.7. Illustration demonstrating outer (A) and inner (B) canthal and interpupillary distances (C); (D = length of the fissures).

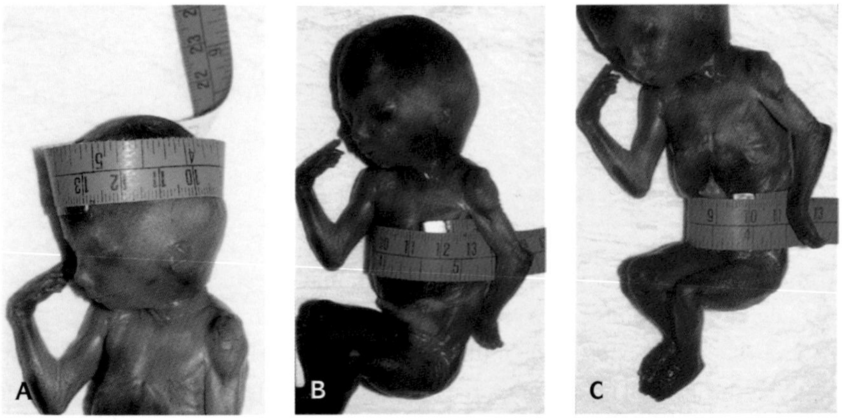

3.8. **(A)** Method for obtaining head circumference. **(B)** Method for obtaining chest circumference. **(C)** Method for obtaining abdominal circumference.

The external exam is systematically performed on all fetuses regardless of gestational age (Figures 3.9 and 3.10). Timing of fetal death is determined by the degree of maceration (see Chapter 2). Vernix caseosa can be detected from approximately 30 weeks gestation. In early fetal stillbirth, there is no, or only a small amount of vernix caseosa. In macerated fetuses, it is present for a considerable length of time in skin creases, such as the axillae, groins, and behind the ears. The usual color of the vernix caseosa is yellow-white. Green color is due to meconium impregnation. When meconium is suspected, a cotton swab can be placed in the external auditory canal and/or the nostrils.

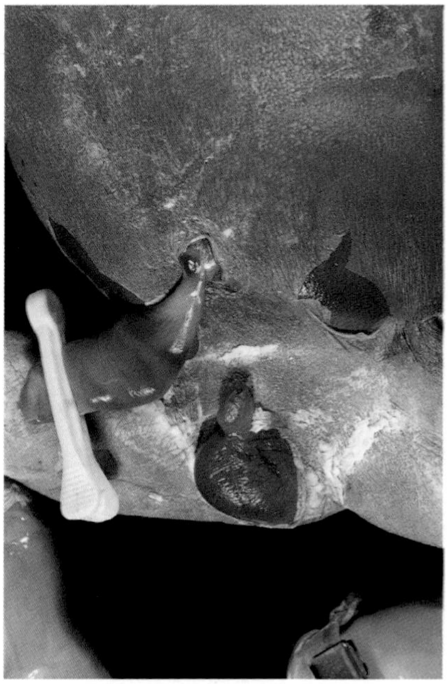

3.9. Typical yellow-white appearance of vernix caseosa in the groin areas of a macerated, stillborn fetus at 37 weeks gestation.

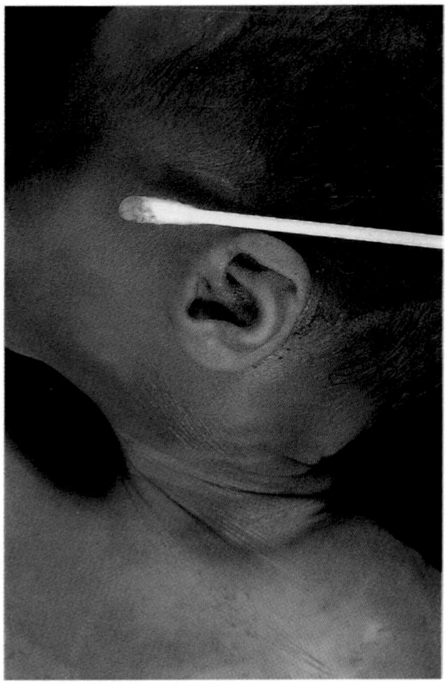

3.10. Cotton swab demonstrating meconium from the external auditory canal in a stillborn fetus at 39 weeks gestation.

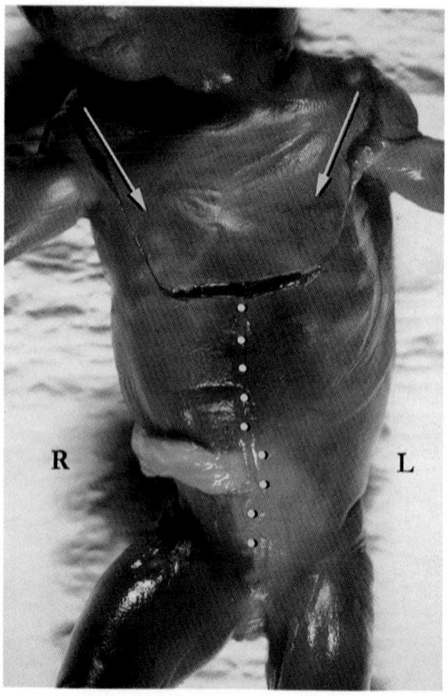

3.11. Illustration of the initial (Y-shaped) incision. Arms of the Y (arrows) extend from the tops of the shoulders. In the midline, a vertical incision (yellow dots) extends from the xiphoid process to the symphysis pubis.

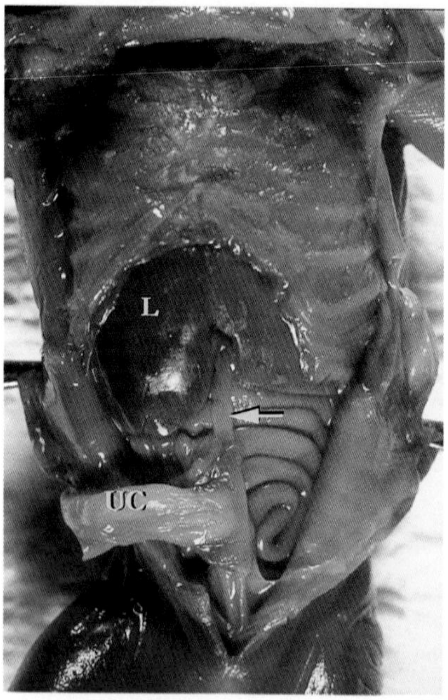

3.12. Reflection of the abdominal skin flaps with an intact umbilical arteries and vein (arrow). The umbilical cord (UC) is left intact by making an elliptical incision along its right side. (L = liver).

Table 3.5 Indications for cytogenetic studies

Congenital malformations, including ambiguous genitalia or dysgenetic gonads
Any suspicious embryo, tiny or macerated fetus
Nuchal cystic hygroma
Congenital neoplasm, e.g., leukemia or teratoma
Suspect fetus on which no autopsy has been performed

If meconium is present, the swab will be stained green. The fingernails and toenails can be examined for the presence of meconium.

The systematic external examination should be performed with an autopsy protocol in hand. This ensures that no component is omitted. Jaundice can best be assessed in the sclera and cyanosis in the fingernail beds and vermilion border. All catheters and tubes should be left in place until the distal end can be observed or palpated during the internal examination. These can be removed and weighed and then subtracted from the initial weight of the infant to equal the true weight.

CYTOGENETICS

Indications for chromosome analysis include clinical evidence suggestive of, or a number of anomalies suspicious for, a chromosome abnormality (Table 3.5). The tissue should be taken by a sterile technique, cleaning the skin with sterile saline and not alcohol. The best sources of tissue for culture are skin, fascia, lung, chorionic villi from the placenta, and cartilage. Fibroblast cultures for metabolic and enzymatic studies as well as electron microscopy can be obtained by the same method.

INITIAL INCISION

A Y-shaped incision is used, extending the arms of the Y to the tops of the shoulders to free up the skin over the anterior aspect of the neck (Figure 3.11). The arms of the Y meet inferiorly in the midline, at the xiphoid process. The skin flap over the chest is pulled upward while incising its attachments to the chest wall. The muscle and fibrous tissues should be entirely stripped to reveal the ribs and the clavicles. A vertical incision is made in the midline, from the xiphoid process to the symphysis pubis. The incision should extend around the left side of the umbilicus. A small nick is made near the umbilical vein and scissors are used to open the abdominal cavity. Lifting upward on the abdominal wall will eliminate cutting into the abdominal organs. One finger is inserted inferior to the umbilicus and along the inner abdominal wall to palpate the umbilical arteries, which extend on either side of the urinary bladder. An ellipse is made around the right side of the umbilicus to preserve the umbilical arteries and/or vein (Figure 3.12). Some prefer to cut the umbilical vein and leave the arteries with the bladder and others cut the umbilical arteries leaving the vein attached to the liver. This decision can also depend on the known or suspected anomalies, to best preserve them. The skin and subcutaneous tissues are dissected away from the anterior lateral aspects of the lower ribs exposing the abdominal organs.

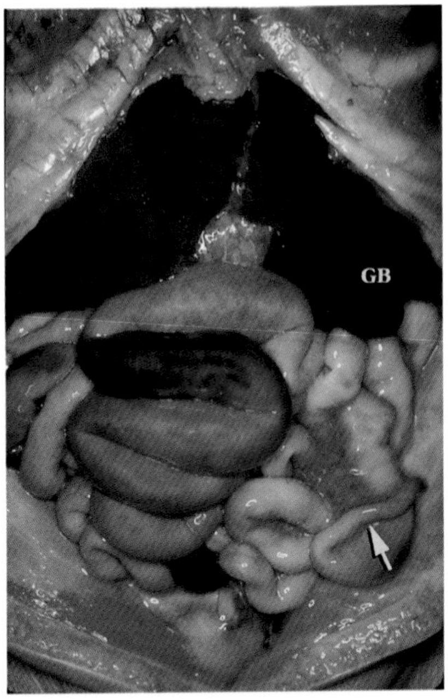

3.13. In situ examination of abdominal organs with situs inversus. Note the symmetrical liver, left-sided gallbladder (GB) and malrotated intestine with the appendix (arrow) in the left lower quadrant of the abdomen.

IN SITU EXAMINATION OF THE ABDOMEN

If a pneumothorax is suspected the leaf of the diaphragm on the affected side is usually displaced inferiorly and is flat or bulging into the abdominal cavity.

The abdominal organs are first inspected for situs (Figure 3.13). Abnormalities in the abdominal situs very often predict the thoracic situs and the presence of congenital heart disease. The color, size, and relationships of the organs are noted. The mesenteric attachments are examined and the position of the appendix is noted.

IN SITU EXAMINATION OF THE THORAX

Before incising the chest plate, test for a pneumothorax by 1) inserting a sterile syringe with a 22-gauge needle containing a small amount of sterile saline into an intercostal space on the anterolateral aspect of the side in question, or 2) filling the gutter next to the rib and reflected skin with water and incising an intercostal space below the water line. In both cases, bubbles will be produced in the presence of a pneumothorax.

The chest plate is removed by separating the sternoclavicular joint on each side (Figures 3.14 and 3.15). This is best done with a scalpel blade. The chondral portions of the ribs are incised in an upside-down V-like pattern, approximately 4 mm from the costochondral junction. This flared cut allows for maximum exposure of the thoracic organs. The ribs are lifted off the thoracic organs by grasping the xiphoid process with toothed forceps and cutting away the fibrous attachments as close to the bone as possible.

In some cases lung cultures may be necessary. This should be performed as soon as the chest plate is removed, keeping the field as sterile as possible. One or both lungs may be cultured as follows: The edge of the lung can be clamped with a hemostat and the lung pulled from the pleural cavity. With a sterile blade and forceps, a wedge of lung is removed and placed in the appropriate medium for bacterial, fungal, or viral culture.

Exposing the great vessels and the heart is achieved by removing the pericardium and thymus together. The pericardium is nicked and a cut is made parallel to the diaphragm, extending to the base of the inferior vena cava (IVC) on the right and the pulmonary veins (PV) on the left. The pericardium is cut away on the right as close

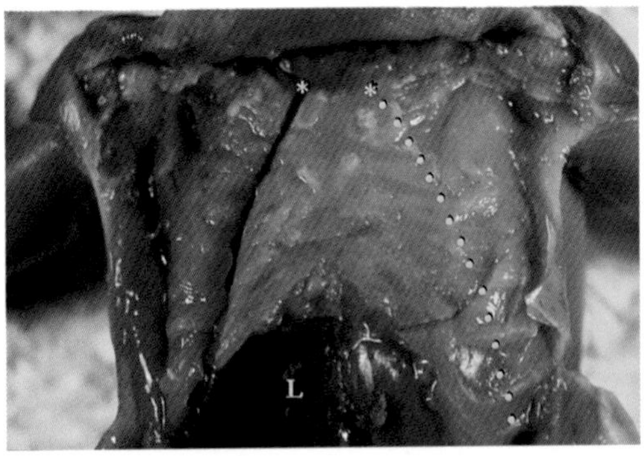

3.14. The chest plate is removed with an upside down V-shaped incision that begins at the sternoclavicular joint (*) and flares laterally on each side. The incision is made on the right, leaving at least 4 mm of cartilage at the tip of each rib. The left portion of the incision is indicated with yellow dots. (L = liver).

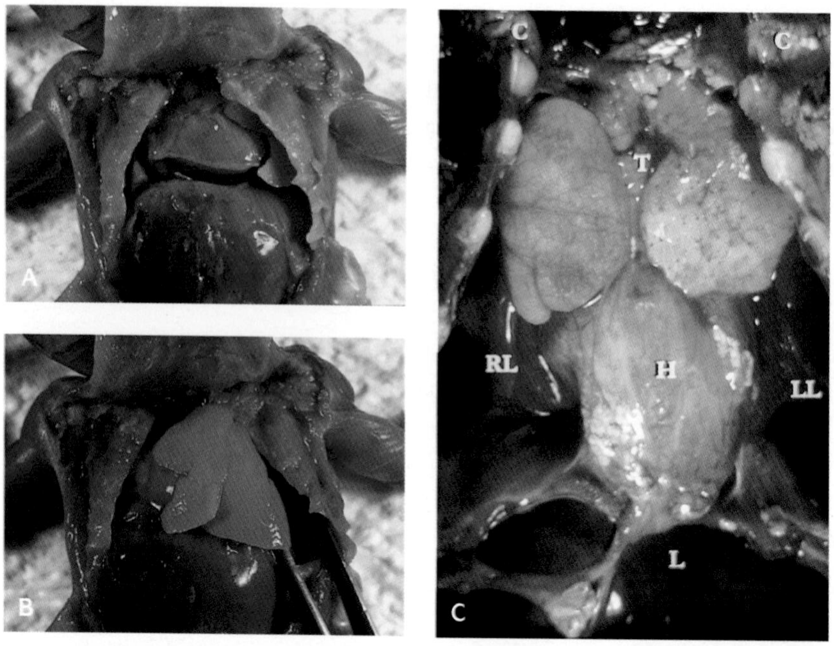

3.15. **(A)** View of the thoracic organs in a premature fetus after removal of the chest plate. Note the apex of the heart pointing to the left. **(B)** Examination of the lungs in situ. Each lung can be easily lifted from the pleural cavity. **(C)** View of the thoracic organs in a full-term fetus. Note the large thymus gland (T) lying over the superior anterior portion of the heart (H) and great vessels. (L = liver, RL = right lung, LL = left lung, C = clavicle).

as possible to the IVC, along the lateral aspect of the right atrium (RA) and superior vena cava (SVC) to the level of the left innominate vein. On the left the scissors are placed perpendicular to the diaphragm and flat against the PVs as they exit the left atrium (LA). A continuous cut is made to the level of the left pulmonary artery with no loose pericardial flaps left to obstruct the view. At this point, a blood culture can be taken, if necessary. A sterile needle and syringe can be inserted into the lateral wall of the RA. Pressing up on the liver may make it easier to obtain blood. Raising the head may also allow some blood to drain toward heart. The pericardium, with the thymus attached, is carefully dissected off the left innominate vein. The dissection continues into the neck; the superiormost portions of the thymus often extend to the inferior aspect of the thyroid. The thymus is then dissected away from the pericardium and weighed. If a left innominate vein is not identified, a persistent left superior vena cava (PLSVC) should be suspected.

The thoracic situs is determined, noting the lobation of the lungs, position of the cardiac apex, and atrial morphology. Before evisceration the heart should be opened in situ.

IN SITU EXAMINATION OF THE HEART

A thorough examination of the external appearance of the heart and vascular connections can predict the presence of congenital abnormalities. The location

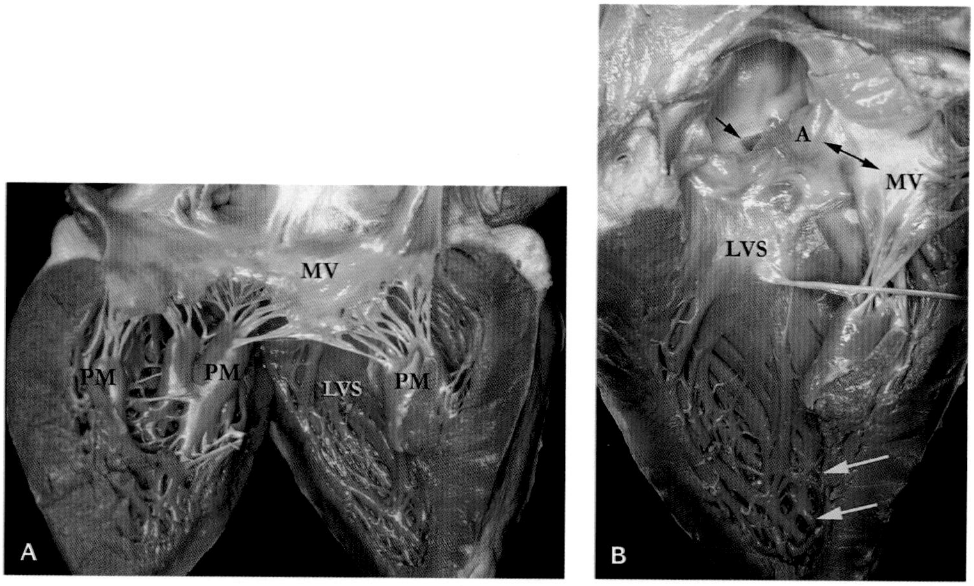

3.21. Morphological left ventricle. **(A)** The mitral valve is in its inlet portion (MV) and has only papillary muscle (PM) attachments. (LVS = left ventricular septal surface). **(B)** The atrioventricular (MV) and arterial (A) valves are in fibrous continuity and the septal surface (LVS) is smooth with a fine apical trabecular component (arrows).

SPECIAL PROCEDURES

Removal of the Tongue

The trachea and esophagus can be lifted from the vertebral column with blunt dissection. Lift the trachea and esophagus with your index finger, and use scissors to cut along the vertebral column, freeing all soft tissues posterior and lateral to the esophagus, up into the neck. Separate the tongue from the inner edge of the mandible with the tip of a scalpel blade, guided by the tip of the index finger. The soft tissues are cut from the inner rim of the bone (mandible) anteriorly and the tongue can then be pulled into the chest with toothed forceps. Posteriorly a curved cut is made to include the tonsils, uvula, pharynx, and larynx with the block.

REMOVAL OF THE EXTERNAL GENITALIA

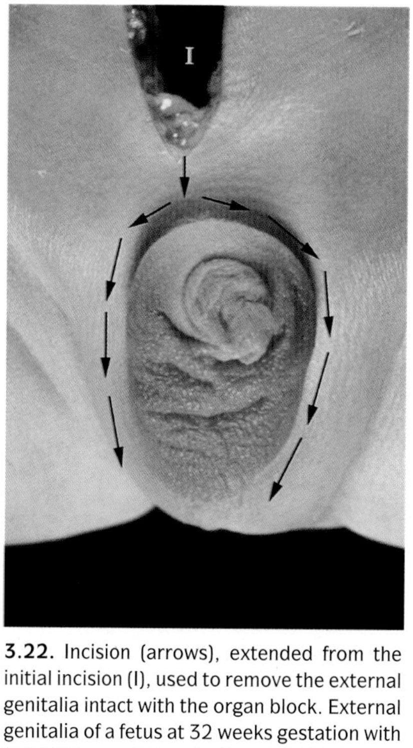

3.22. Incision (arrows), extended from the initial incision (I), used to remove the external genitalia intact with the organ block. External genitalia of a fetus at 32 weeks gestation with CHARGE association (polytopic field defect). There is a shawl scrotum and an imperforate anus that is not in view.

This procedure is warranted in cases with genitourinary anomalies, ambiguous genitalia, anal atresia and suspected fistulas (Figure 3.22). Begin with a curved cut on each side of the external genitalia to include the anus or probable site of the anal opening in cases with anal agenesis. The symphysis pubis is incised in the midline with a scalpel blade, and the hips are gently pushed posteriorly to spread the pelvis. The entire length of the urethra and colon can be freed from the surrounding tissues with blunt dissection with scissors. This blunt dissection will lead to the margin of the curved cuts initially made in the skin and subcutaneous tissues, allowing the genitourinary/anorectal block to be removed, attached to the organ block.

In males with posterior urethral valves, the entire urethra can be removed without disrupting the external genitalia. The symphysis pubis is split as described above and the urethra is dissected from the pelvis. As the urethra becomes externalized, blunt dissection is used to circumferentialy free it from the penile skin. The penile skin is left intact.

The gonads should always have a gross and microscopic examination. In females they are easily removed with the block at evisceration. In males, a cut across the inguinal triangle and gentle pressure, pushing upward on the scrotal sac, will produce the testicles at the margin of the inguinal triangle. The soft tissues surrounding the testes can be grasped with toothed forceps; they are pulled from the inguinal canal and cut free.

EXAMINATION OF THE CARDIAC CONDUCTION SYSTEM

The examination of the cardiac conduction system is best performed using the technique of Davies and colleagues (Figure 3.23). The pacemaker or sinoatrial node, lies immediately beneath the epicardium of the sulcus terminalis at the base of the SVC at its junction with the RA. It is supplied by the first branch of the right coronary artery in 55% of cases and usually can be located by dissecting this artery to its termination. The sinoatrial node can be sectioned as a single block or as multiple sequential blocks in a plane perpendicular or parallel to the long axis of the SVC.

The AV node lies beneath the right atrial septal endocardium above the insertion of the medial leaflet of the TV. In infant hearts the conduction tissues can be examined with a single block of tissue, that contains all the components of the conduction system except for the distal ventricular bundle branches. Elastic-van Gieson or Masson trichrome stains may be helpful in identifying the conduction tissues. Routinely, every tenth section is examined with hematoxylin and eosin.

In larger hearts the conduction tissues can be split up into three blocks for easier sectioning. This procedure can be used in smaller hearts to selectively section portions of the conduction system.

OTHER PROCEDURES

Several standard procedures should be performed after evisceration:

1. The ribs on each side are counted and recorded.
2. Two ribs are removed including the costochondral junction. Each sample should be at least 1 cm.
3. Sample the abdominal skin in the area adjacent to the initial incision.
4. Sample the psoas muscle.

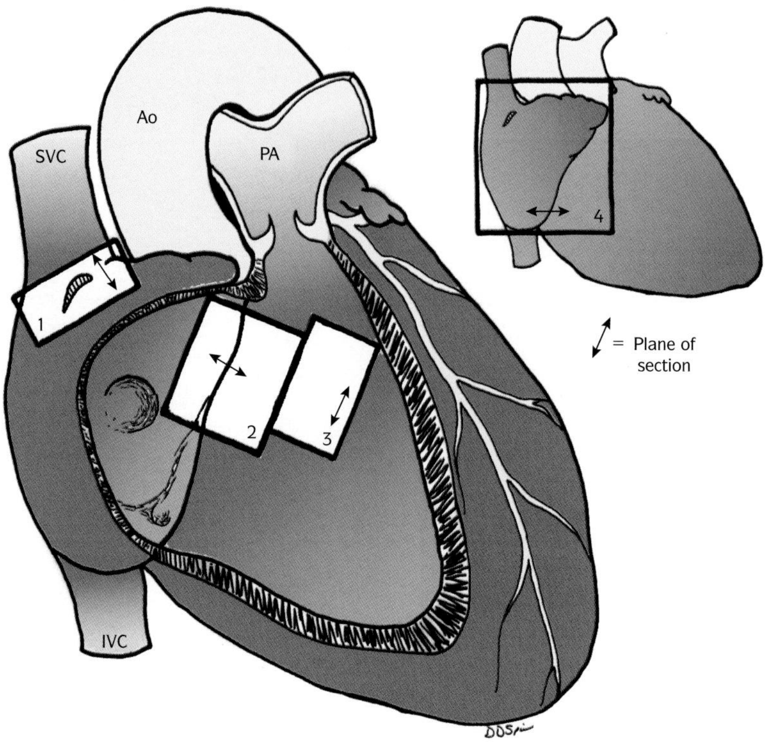

3.23. Tissue blocks removed for examination of the conduction tissues: 1, sinus node; 2, atrioventricular node, penetrating and branching atrioventricular bundle; 3, proximal ventricular bundle branches. In larger hearts, blocks 1–3 allow for easier examination of the conduction tissues. A single block (Block 4 = insert) can be used in infant hearts. This block contains all the conduction tissues except the distal ventricular bundle branches.

5. Remove a submandibular gland. (This can be done while removing the tongue.)
6. Breast tissue can be removed by taking an ellipse of skin, including the nipple, adjacent to the initial incision on the chest.

REMOVING THE BRAIN

The incision in the skin should extend from behind one ear, upward, over the top of the cranium and then down behind the other ear (Figure 3.24). The skin of the scalp is reflected anteriorly over the eyes and posteriorly in a caudal direction. Inspection of the fontanels can be critical in some cases. The degree of tension (sunken or tense and bulging), particularly of the anterior fontanel, should be noted in each case. The length and breadth of the fontanels are measured. To open the skull, begin with two small nicks, one in each lateral corner of the anterior fontanel. Scissors with slightly rounded points are inserted into the nick on each side and a nearly complete oval is cut, leaving a portion intact on the lateral aspects (Figure 3.25). This intact portion will act as a hinge allowing the bony flap to be folded away from the brain. The cuts are made through the bone just lateral to the sagittal sinus, leaving it intact.

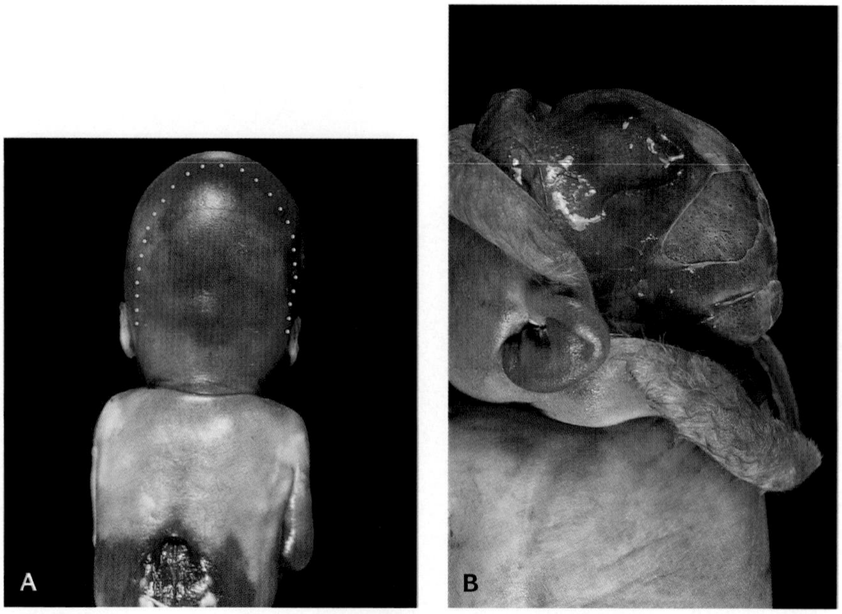

3.24. **(A)** Most common incision path (dots) used to reflect the scalp when removing the brain. **(B)** Reflected skin of the scalp, anteriorly over the eyes and posteriorly in a caudal direction.

The brain should be inspected in situ by tilting the head forward, backward, and to each side. The falx and the tentorium are cut away from their bony attachments with a scalpel and/or scissors. To remove the brain, position your left hand over the occiput, cradling the skull and brain in the palm of your hand, so that the skull bone does not cut into the brain. Gently tilt the head back and the brain will fall away from the calvarium. The first cranial nerves are inspected and removed with the brain. The cerebral hemispheres can be gently retracted with the index and middle finger of your right hand and the remaining cranial nerves can be transected, working from anterior to posterior. The optic nerves are cut close to the skull and the pituitary stalk, close to the brain. As the brain falls free from the calvarium, your hand should support it so that no stretching artifact of the midbrain occurs. The undersurface of the brainstem and the anterior spinal cord should be in view. The cervical spinal cord can be transected (with a sharp scalpel blade) as far down as possible. The brain should easily fall into your hand. It is inspected, weighed, and placed into formalin. The brain can be fixed by placing it into a bed of cotton or by placing a string beneath the basilar artery to suspend the brain in the container. The brain should fix for up to 10 days.

Markedly macerated or hydrocephalic brains can be removed under water by the method described above. The brain will float in the water, eliminating tearing of the parenchyma that is caused by gravity and the weight of the brain itself.

An alternative method for removing the brain is to make a circular cut in the calvarium and then remove the brain along with the skull cap. The brain can then be floated out of the calvarium under water or formalin. This preserves

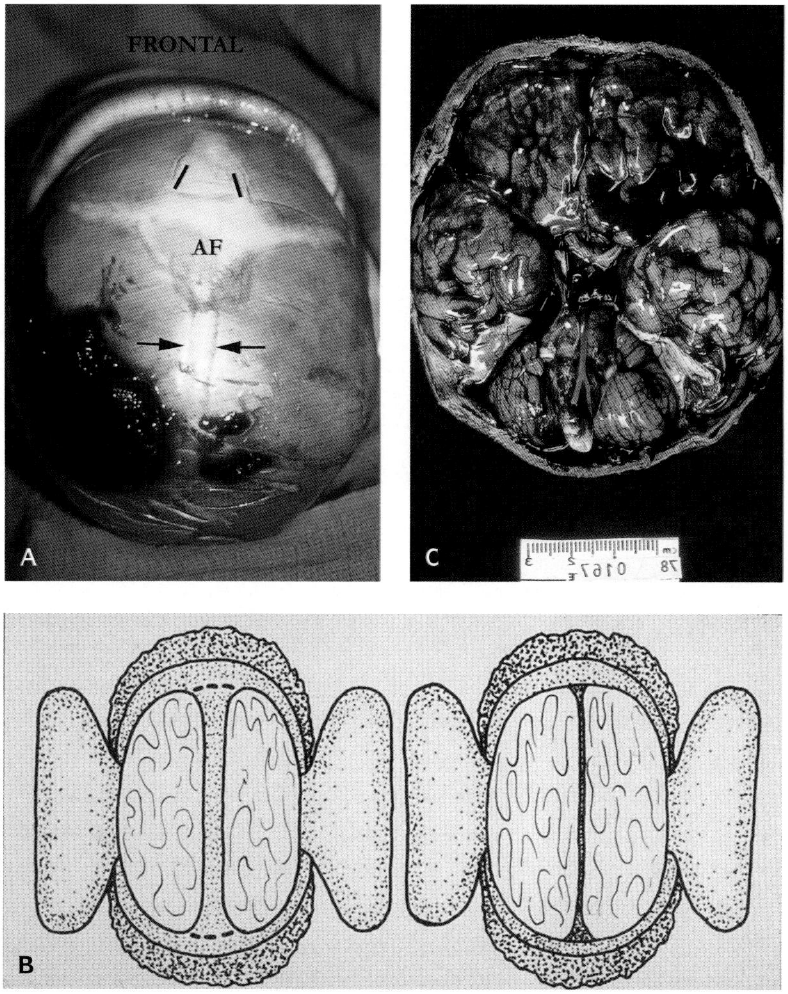

3.25. **(A)** Top of the skull with the skin reflected. The anterior fontanel (AF) is easily visualized as is the sagittal sinus (arrows). On either side of the frontal bone (black lines) the dura is nicked, allowing for insertion of the scissors to cut the calvarium open. **(B)** Oval cuts made on each side to expose and remove the brain. **(C)** Brain removed along with the calvaria. This method protects the brain during removal and is achieved with a single, circumferential cut around the calvarium.

the brain intact without it ever being handled. The brain can be weighed with the skull, and after flotation of the brain the weight of the skull cap can be subtracted.

After removal of the brain the base of the skull is inspected and the dural sinuses opened.

REMOVING THE SPINAL CORD – ANTERIOR APPROACH

After evisceration the thoracic and lumbar portions of the spinal column are in full view. Using a scalpel blade, transect one of the lowermost lumbar intervertebral disks. Insert one end of a rounded pair of scissors into this opening and make a continuous cut cephalad. The dura is left intact; the cut is made

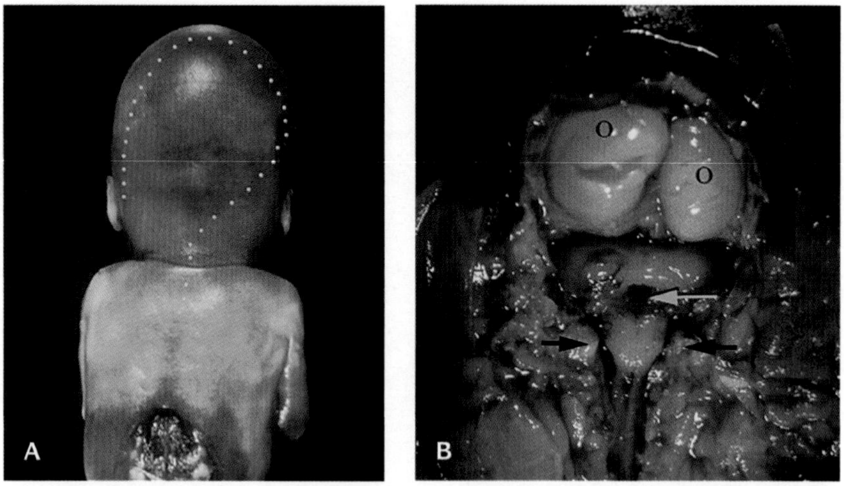

3.26. **(A)** Question mark incision (dots). **(B)** Posterior view of a Dandy-Walker cyst (yellow arrow) with herniation of the cerebellum (black arrows are at the margin of the foramen magnum). Using this technique in fetuses below 20 weeks gestation allows the prosector to preserve the anatomy, leaving the brain mostly contained in the calvarium. (O = occipital lobes).

between the dura and the bone. Once all the spinal pedicles have been cut (up to the base of the skull), the same procedure is performed on the other side. Lift the freed vertebral bodies, exposing the spinal cord, and cut it off as far into the neck as possible. With a sharp scalpel blade, transect the cord at the lumbar end and gently lift the dura surrounding it with toothed forceps. Dissect the dura and the cord from the spinal canal from the lumbar to cervical portion, without exerting any tension on the cord. Once in the cervical region, the dissection becomes blind; damage to the cord can be prevented by keeping the scissors close to the bone. The cervical region can also be approached from the base of the skull, through the foramen magnum.

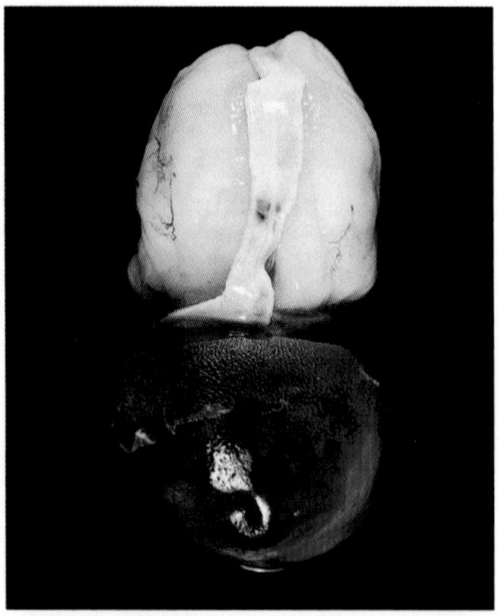

3.27. Brain with an occipital encephalocele. The brain and encephalocele after removal intact following the question mark incision and continuing the cut in the skin at the base of the encephalocele.

REMOVING THE BRAIN AND SPINAL CORD INTACT – POSTERIOR APPROACH

This approach is used when there are anomalies of the skull or spinal column that need to be preserved, such as occipital encehalocele, Dandy-Walker malformation, Arnold-Chiari malformation, and myelomeningoceles anywhere along the length of the spine (Figures 3.26 to 3.28). The incision in the skin is in the form of a question mark; this procedure was described by Emery. The portion extending over the neck can be extended caudally as far as needed to preserve the defect. The skin over the skull is reflected, as previously described. The muscle over the occiput is carefully removed and the soft tissues over the rami of the upper cervical vertebrae are dissected away. The atlas is cut away along with the second and third cervical vertebrae if necessary. The exposed dura is carefully incised without cutting the arachnoid. This prevents the

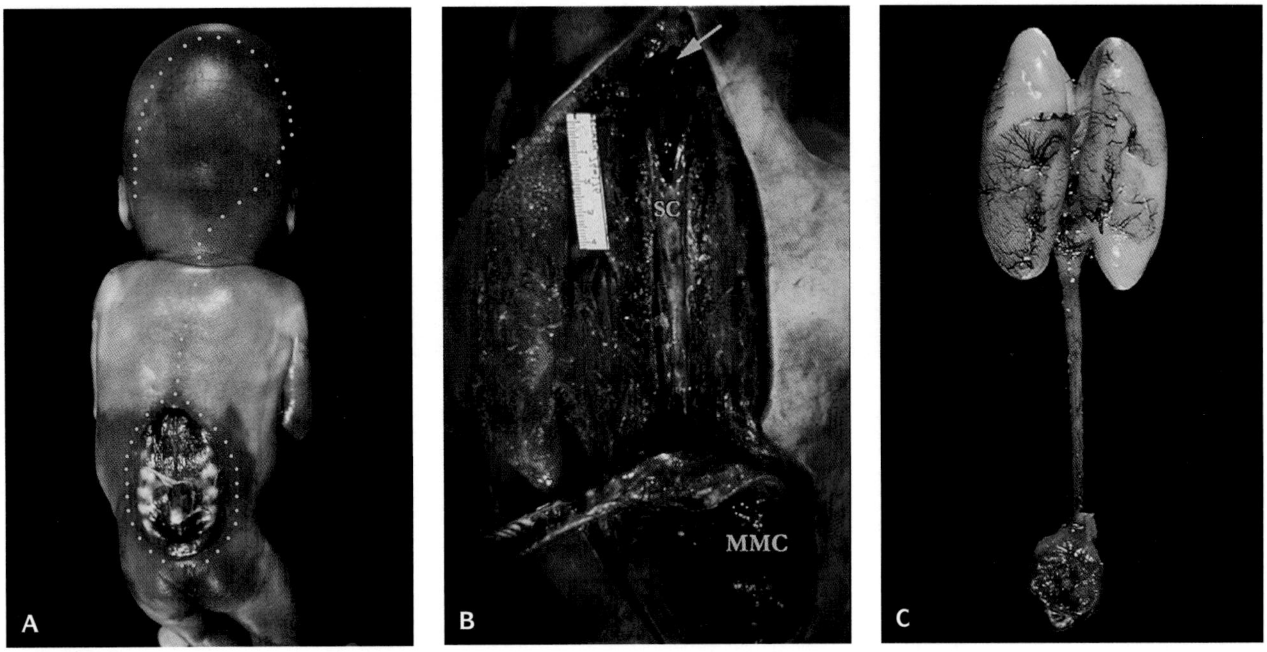

3.28. **(A)** Question mark incision extended down the middle of the back to surround a myelomeningocele (yellow dots). **(B)** Removal of the spinal cord and brain intact, along with the myelomeningocele (MMC) via the posterior approach. **(C)** Brain, spinal cord, and MMC intact.

cerebrospinal fluid from escaping and a culture can be draw at this time with a sterile needle and syringe. The dural incision is enlarged to expose the cervical cord and foramen magnum. In a normal setting, the cavity of the fourth ventricle is obvious and the cerebellar tonsils can be just visualized. The cerebellar tonsils will be approximated with mild to moderate edema and will be herniated through the foramem magnum when there is severe edema.

To continue removing the cord, with or without a spinal defect, blunt scissors are placed between the bone and dura and the bone is cut on each side. The bone surrounding the defect is also cut. The spinal cord is carefully dissected from the spinal canal, leaving it attached to the skin and bone surrounding the defect, if present. Do not cut the cervical cord. The cord can be placed back into the spinal canal and the skin folded over it, held together with several hemostats (Figure 3.29). The brain is removed as previously described, with an additional cut in the midline of the occipital plate allowing the brain and cord to be removed as one. Once the brain is free the hemostats holding the protective flaps of skin are removed, allowing for easier removal of the cord.

THE PITUITARY

The pituitary is a very delicate organ and should be removed along with a portion of the adjacent sella turcica. This avoids direct handling of the gland itself.

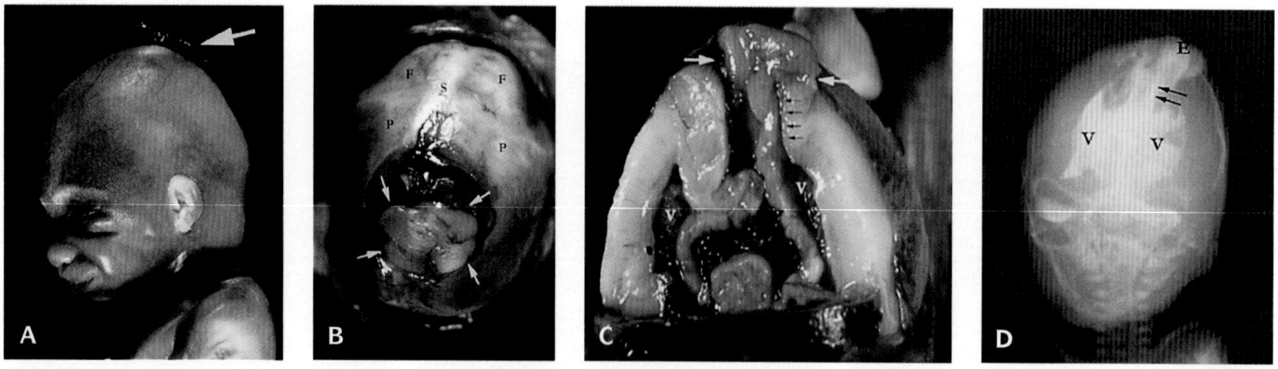

3.29. Injection study and special dissection to confirm ultrasound suspicion of the right ventricle communicating with the parietal encephalocele. **(A)** Side view of the fetus at 19 weeks gestation with a parietal encephalocele (arrow). **(B)** The scalp skin is reflected revealing the encephalocele (arrows). (F = frontal bones, P = parietal bones, S = sagittal sinus). **(C)** A cross section of the brain while still in the skull, following reflection of the cranial bones. The cut is through the mid portion of the encephalocele (yellow arrows) and shows the ventricular communication (black arrows) with the encephalocele. **(D)** Before examining the brain, a syringe was filled with radiopaque liquid and a needle was inserted through the occipital bone, into the right ventricle (v). The radiopaque liquid was injected and an x-ray was taken, demonstrating the ventricular communication (arrows) with the encephalocele before opening the skull. (E = encephalocele).

REMOVING THE EYES

Removing the eyes is not a routine procedure and can be performed via an anterior or posterior approach (Figure 3.30). The posterior approach is performed after removal of the brain. The thin bony plate overlying the orbit is cut away with scissors with at least one sharp tip. In older fetuses, a saw may be required. Once the orbit has been unroofed, the globe can be pushed backward and upward by exerting pressure on it through the closed eyelids. The eye can be retracted by grasping some of the attached fibroadipose tissue surrounding it with toothed forceps. The fat and extraocular muscles surrounding the globe are dissected away, taking care not to cut the eyelids.

Anteriorly, the eyes are removed with the aid of an ophthalmic surgical tray. The eyelids are separated with retractors and the globe is detached from the extraocular muscles and fibroadipose tissue. The sclera is incised circumferentialy and the optic nerve is cut, allowing the eye to be lifted from the orbit. This procedure can be done without ophthalmic instruments.

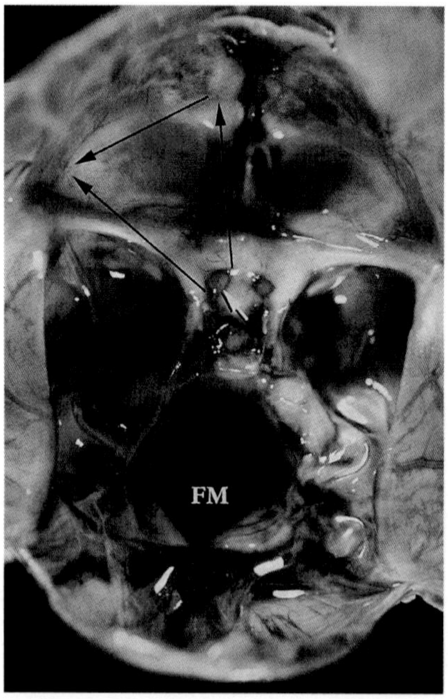

3.30. Base of the skull illustrating the necessary cuts (black arrows) for removing the eyes via the posterior approach. (FM = foramen magnum, yellow arrow = optic nerve).

REMOVING THE TEMPORAL BONE

Removing the petrous portion of the temporal bone allows for the examination of the middle ear (Figure 3.31). With stout scissors, or a saw in older infants, the first cut is made along the lateral aspect (squamous portion) of the temporal bone, perpendicular to the petrous ridge and parallel with the skull. The next cut is made at the medial aspect of the petrous ridge, just medial to the carotid canal and including the internal acoustic meatus. Placing the scissors into the superior and inferior aspects of the two previous cuts and cutting parallel with the petrous ridge will produce the temporal bone. The specimen is roughly rectangular and when lifted out the middle ear will be in view. Culture any pus that is visualized. The temporal bone can be decalcified and sectioned.

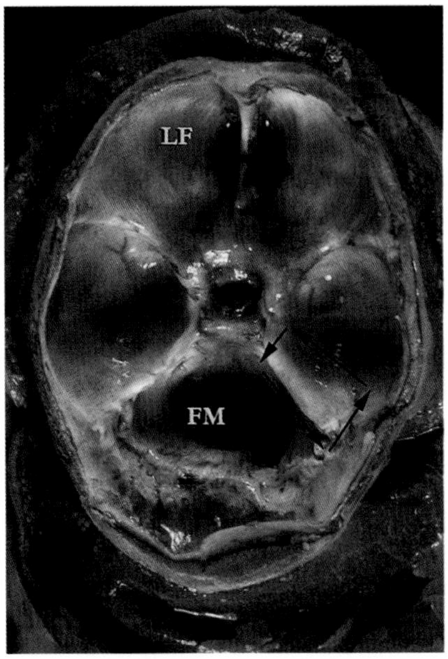

3.31. Base of the skull illustrating the necessary cuts (arrows) for removing the temporal bone. (FM = foramen magnum, LF = left frontal bone).

DISSECTING THE ORGAN BLOCK

The organ block is placed on its ventral surface. The aorta is opened posteriorly to the aortic arch. The renal arteries are opened and can be left attached to the kidneys and a segment of aorta or cut, separating the kidneys. Reflect the aorta off the block and cut it just distal to the left subclavian artery. Open the IVC to the porta hepatis and open the renal veins. The renal veins can be left attached or separated. Reflect the leaves of the diaphragm away from the adrenals and remove each adrenal. Removing the adrenals at this point allows for easy identification, while the kidneys are still in their anatomic position. Weigh the adrenals together. The kidneys can be dissected away from the block, taking care to preserve the ureters. The urinary bladder and internal genitalia in the case of a female can be dissected free from the rectum, unless there is an anomaly (i.e., rectovesical fistula). The urinary bladder, vagina, and uterus are opened along with the ureters. The kidneys are weighed. The porta hepatis is examined by first opening the bile ducts, extending the cut throughout the common duct to the ampulla of Vater. Squeezing gently on the gallbladder should express some bile through the cystic duct, confirming its patency. The hepatic artery and portal vein are opened. The umbilical vein and the sinus venosus (if patent) should be opened. The splenic vein is opened as it extends from the portal vein and the spleen is removed. Examine the perisplenic fat for accessory spleens and weigh the spleen. The intestine can be removed from its mesentery and cut at the duodenum. It is opened and the contents and mucosa examined. The esophagus is always opened before it is reflected from the trachea. This eliminates transecting a fistula. Once the esophagus is dissected away from the trachea, the diaphragm can be cut away and the esophagus, stomach, duodenum, and pancreas can be removed as one block. The stomach and duodenum are opened – the stomach along the greater curvature – and the pancreas is sectioned. The liver and diaphragm are removed from the thoracic organs, and the diaphragm is dissected free from the liver. The liver is weighed and the gallbladder opened.

The heart and lungs are left in one block and can be weighed together. The trachea is opened posteriorly to the carina and into each large bronchus. The bronchial morphology is assessed. The lungs are sectioned and the heart is examined again, following the flow of blood. At this point, demonstration of congenital anomalies of the heart can be performed by removing portions of the myocardium or vascular connections (windowing) to better show the anatomy for teaching or photographic purposes.

Table 3.6 Routine microscopic sections

Thymus	Pancreas (head and tail)
Thyroid	Liver (right and left lobes)
Tongue	Spleen
Salivary gland	Kidney (right and left)
Trachea	Urinary bladder
Lung (at least one section from each lobe)	Prostate
Heart (two sections):	Testis or ovary
Right atrium, tricuspid valve, and right ventricle	Uterus, cervix and vagina
Left atrium, mitral valve, and left ventricle	Breast
(These are taken along the incisions made when opening the heart)	Diaphragm
	Psoas muscle
Gastroesophageal junction	Skin
Pylorus	Umbilicus
Small intestine	Vertebra
Large intestine	Rib with costochondral junction
Mesenteric lymph nodes	

PERFUSION FIXATION AND WINDOWING OF THE HEART

If you decide to perfuse the heart, do not open it in situ.

To prepare the specimen for perfusion, all the great vessels arising from the aortic arch are tied along with the IVC. The IVC can be secured with a pursestring suture and pulling the ends of the suture to tightly seal it. The distal end of the aorta is left open. The free end of the tubing that is attached to the perfusion bottle is inserted into the SVC and well into the RA. A double suture tie just above the RA secures it. The perfusion bottle is lifted above the specimen (15 cm) and the clamp is opened on the tubing. The heart will immediately begin to enlarge and fluid will soon be flowing from the opened end of the aorta. The perfusion bottle is first filled with saline and will test the system and flush all the blood. Two bottles of saline are used to flush the system and the perfusion bottle is then filled with formalin. The distal aorta is tied and the specimen is placed in a plastic container, at least 12 cm deep and 17 cm in diameter. The container should be placed in a sink for adequate drainage and the perfusion bottle is placed about 60 cm above the specimen. When the perfusion bottle is nearly empty, fill it with formalin again and allow it to perfuse the heart. It is fixed for 12–24 hours.

After fixation, windowing can be performed. Assess the external appearance of the heart or use prenatal ultrasound findings to make calculated cuts to adequately demonstrate the anatomy. Initially, a window should be cut in the convexity of each atrium so the heart can be rinsed. The windows should be cut as large as possible without damaging any important internal structures or vascular connections. The atrial structures and the AV valves are inspected. Using a scalpel blade, create a window in the convexity of the ventricles. This cut is initially made about halfway between the apex and the base and as far as possible from the septum. The window can then be enlarged as

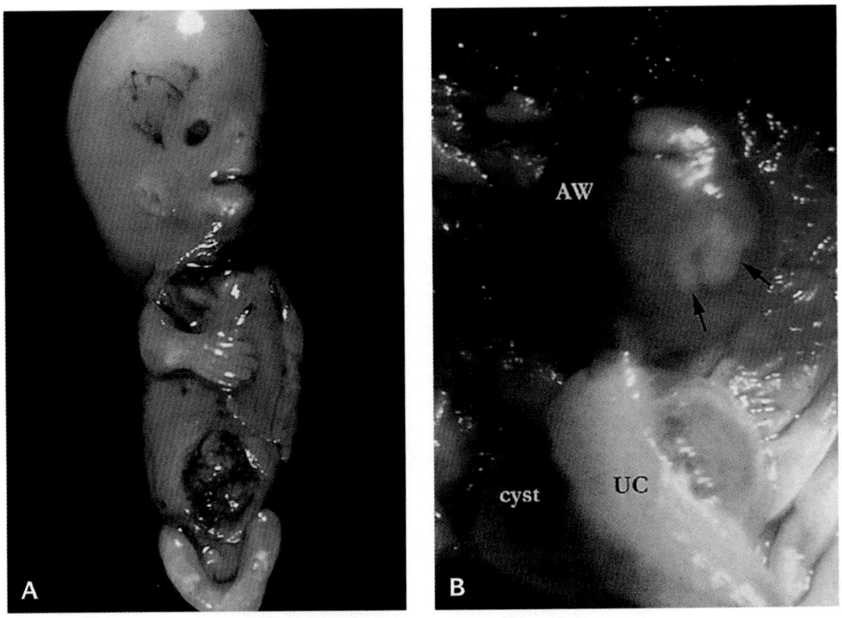

3.32. **(A)** Fetus with an artifactual abdominal wall defect. **(B)** Umbilical cord (UC) from the same fetus with attached abdominal wall (AW) and the normal, physiologic herniation of the intestine (arrows). The umbilical cord has a cyst.

needed to examine and demonstrate any anomalies. Care must be taken so that no important structures are damaged. A window is created in the wall of each great vessel, just above the valve ring. The only portion of the heart not accessible when windowing is the inferior aspect of the aortic valve.

This preparation produces an excellent specimen for teaching.

MICROSCOPIC EXAMINATION

Routine microscopic exam is an important part of the autopsy, particularly in liveborn and well-preserved fetuses (Table 3.6). In severely macerated fetuses, microscopic sections may be helpful in estimating the time of fetal death. The morphology is poorly preserved, precluding accurate histologic exam and for this reason sectioning does not need to be extensive. Bone is usually well preserved in macerated fetuses.

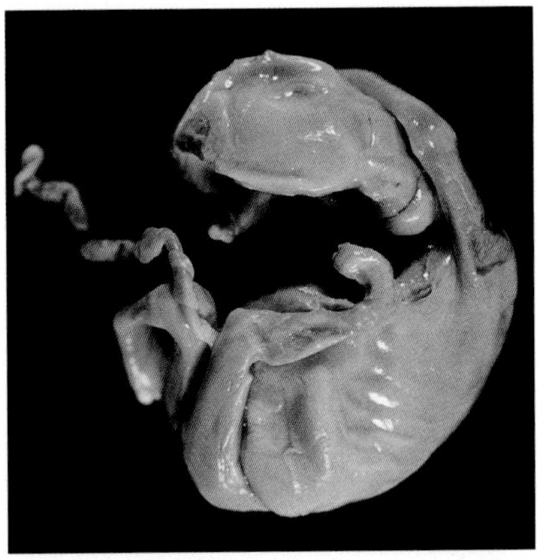

3.33. Macerated fetus at 16 weeks gestation with prolonged uterine retention showing squash artifact secondary to absent amniotic fluid and marked distortion of the limbs.

ARTIFACTS

Differentiating between an artifact and a true defect can be a problem, particularly when dealing with embryos and early fetal death (Figures 3.32 to 3.34). A common artifact in embryo/fetuses occurs between 7 and 10 weeks of gestation. The embryo/fetus at this stage has the physiologic herniation of the intestine into the base of the umbilical cord. In some cases, the cord is torn from the

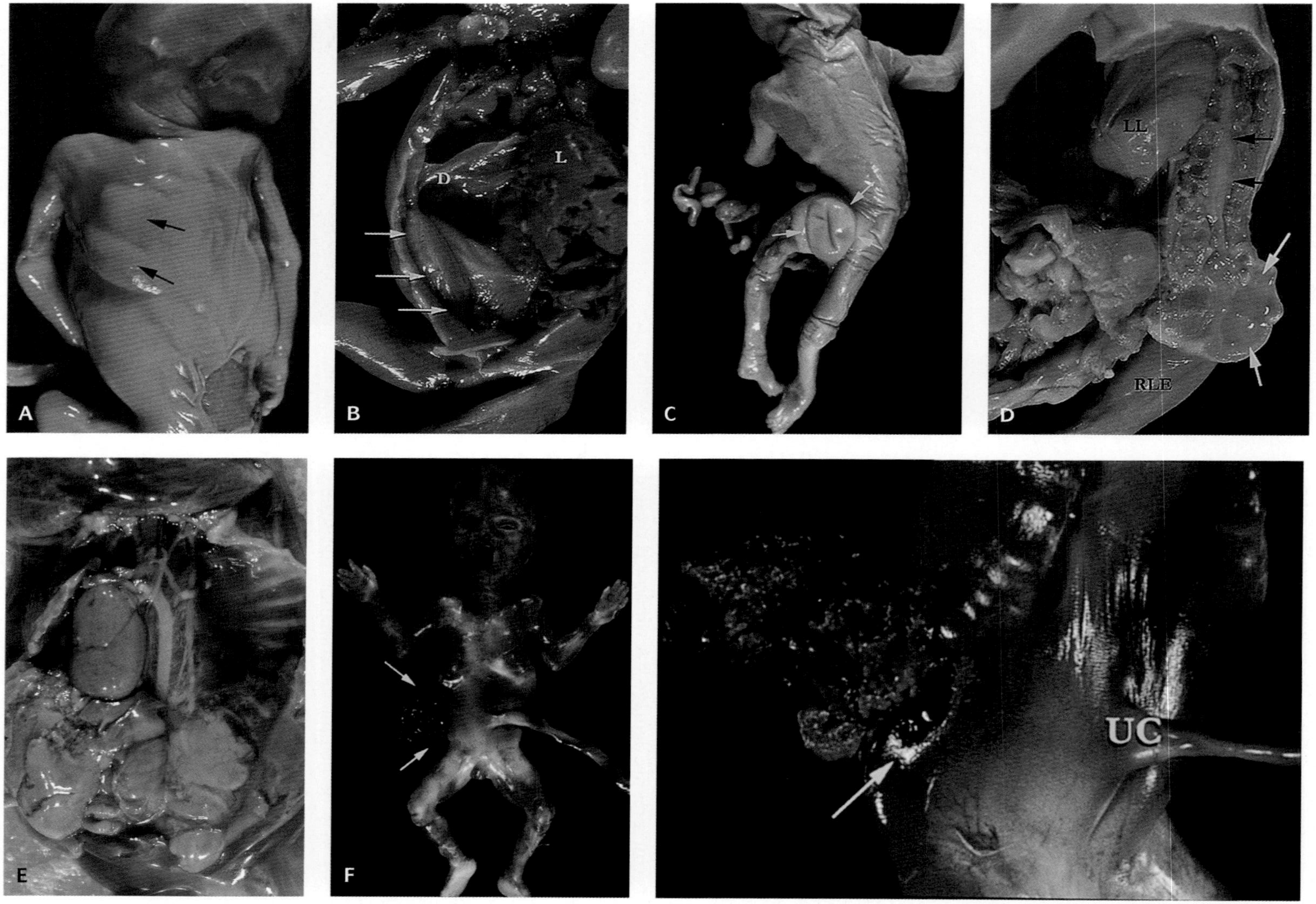

3.34. Mass-like lesions filled with macerated brain. **(A)** Bulges (arrows) in the skin of the upper back. **(B)** A right retroperitoneal mass (arrows). (D = diaphragm, L = liver). **(C)** A sacrococygeal mass (arrows). **(D)** A midline cross-section of the mass in **(C)** revealing a multiloculated structure (yellow arrow) filled with cloudy material. Black arrows indicate budging dura surrounding the spinal cord; this area filled with the same material. (LL = left lung, RLE = right lower extremity). **(F)** A markedly macerated fetus at 17 weeks gestation with a tear (arrows) in the right abdomen, lateral to the umbilical cord (left). A close up of the artifactual abdominal wall defect (arrows) (right) (uc = umbilical cord). **(E)** Lateral view of the aorta and thoracic lymphatics filled with macerated brain tissue in a markedly macerated fetus at 21 weeks gestation.

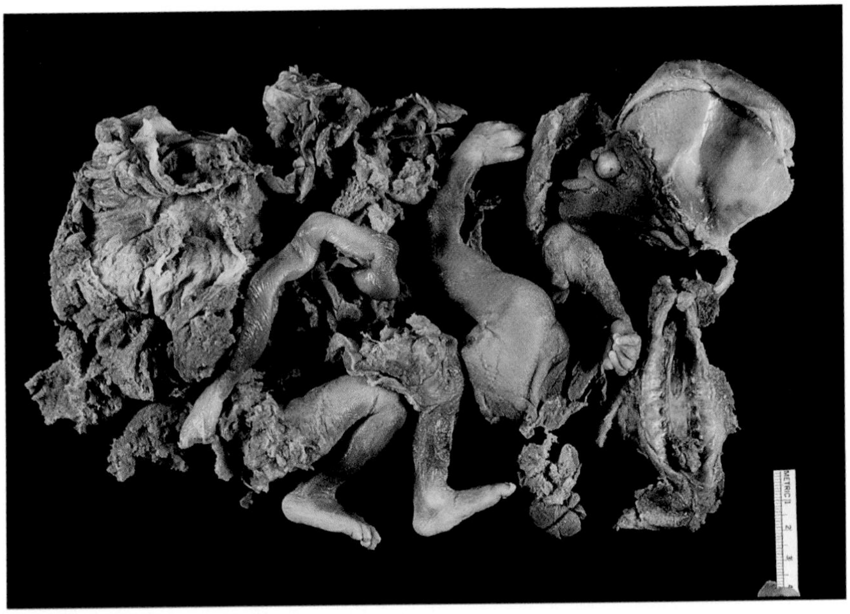

3.35. Typical appearance of the tissues received with a dilatation and evacuation (DE) specimen. This case has complete spinal rachischisis (lower right) and the face (upper right) exhibited a large tongue and prognathism of the lower jaw.

abdominal wall leaving a defect in the skin with intestinal loops protruding. The edges of the defect are often ragged, whereas those of a true defect are usually smooth. If a placenta or gestational sac is received, the attached portion of the umbilical cord should be examined. Very often, loops of bowel will be attached to it.

Early fetal death (<20 weeks) can exhibit a number of artifacts; the most common are secondary to a prolonged interval between intrauterine fetal death

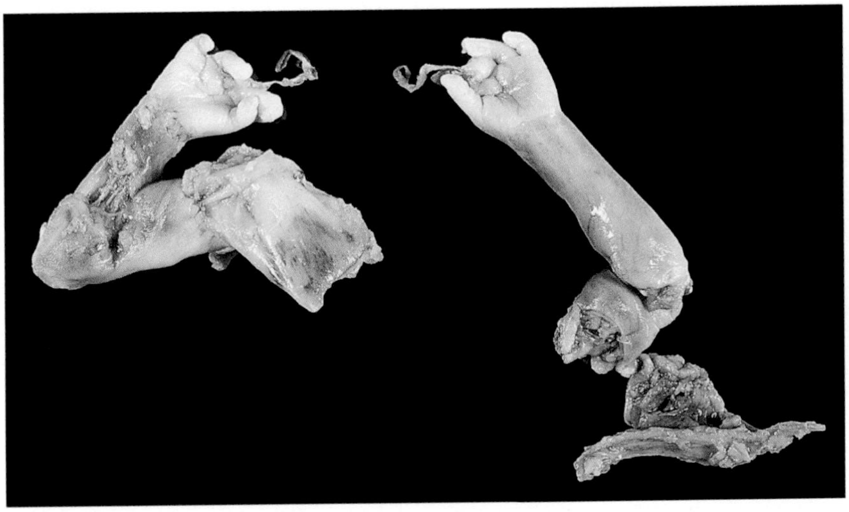

3.36. Upper limbs from a dilatation and evacuation (DE) specimen showing partial amputation of the third digit on the right hand and the second digit on the left hand with an abnormal palmar crease on the left caused by amniotic bands.

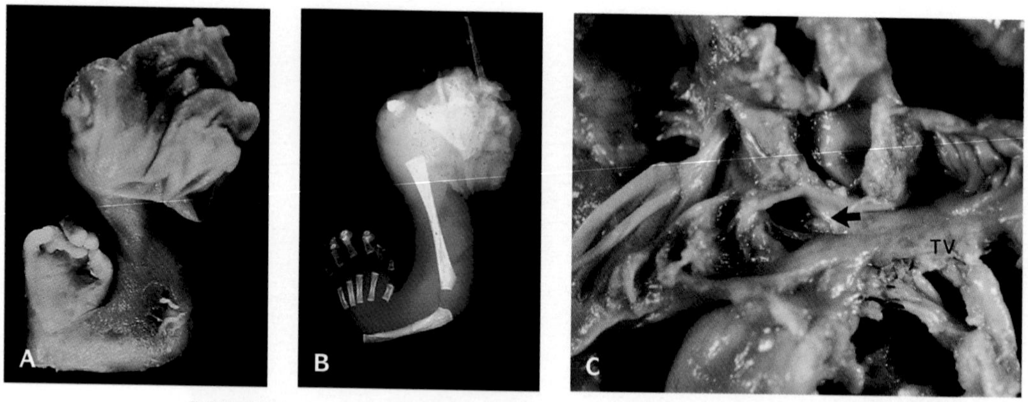

3.37. Dilatation and evacuation (DE) specimen with the diagnosis of Holt-Oram syndrome. **(A)** Right arm with radial aplasia. **(B)** X-ray of **(A)**. **(C)** Septum secundum ASD (arrow). (TV = tricuspid valve).

and expulsion. That time frame can be predicted by using the clinical information (estimated gestational age) and the foot length taken at autopsy. These fetuses can exhibit a wide range of deformations from being compressed in the uterine cavity with no amniotic fluid. The limbs often appear twisted and the head and chest flattened. There may be mass-like lesions in the retroperitoneum and protruding from the abdomen or back. These are often mistaken for a tumor. When these are incised they are filled with cloudy gray-white material that represents macerated brain that has seeped through the soft tissues and aggregates in one or more sites. This gray-white material can be seen in the chambers of the heart or along the posterior pleural cavities, exhibiting a beaded appearance.

Irregular tears in the abdominal wall are a frequent occurrence. These occur secondary to maceration or manual delivery. The edges of the tear are usually irregular and if near the umbilicus should not be confused as a gastroschisis or omphalocele. Large dilated urinary bladders, secondary to posterior urethral valves, have been known to rupture as well. A good delivery history from the obstetrician will usually clear up any questions.

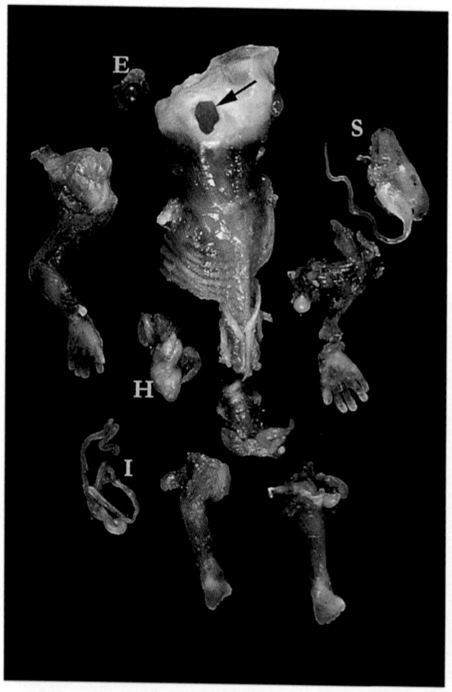

3.38. DE specimen submitted to rule out Meckel syndrome. Note the skull defect (arrow) where there was an occipital encephalocele. There was no polydactyly and a fragment of kidney was microscopically normal. (E = eye, H = heart, S = stomach, I = intestinal loops).

DILATATION AND EVACUATION

Dilatation and evacuation (DE) can be a valuable pathologic specimen (Figures 3.35 to 3.39). This procedure yields a fragmented specimen consisting of placenta and fetal parts. A meticulous examination should be performed, separating the placental and fetal tissues into groups. The placental fragments can be described and any unusual findings submitted for microscopic exam. The fetal tissues may require a closer examination and usually will consist of intact limbs and organs. Important diagnostic information can be obtained including number of umbilical vessels, foot length

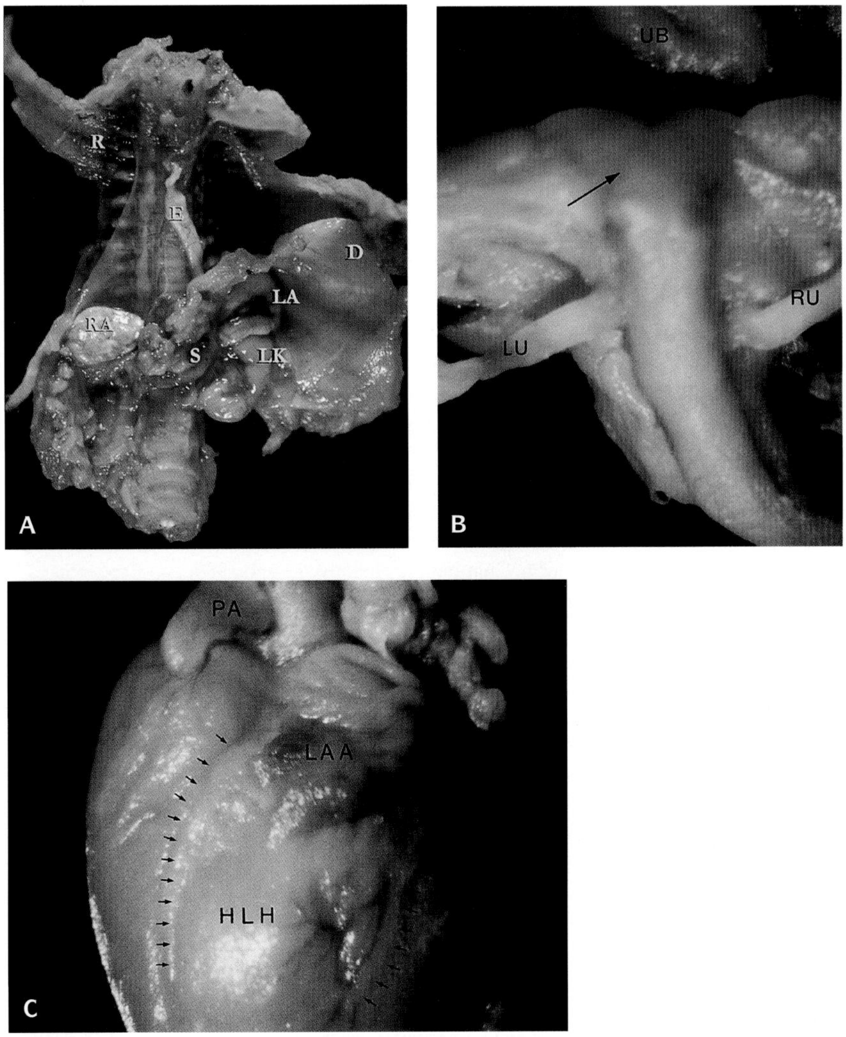

3.39. DE specimen submitted to rule out absent right kidney and with suspected hypoplastic left heart (HLH). **(A)** A portion of thoracolumbar spine with attached ribs (R), diaphragm (D), esophagus (E), and stomach (S). Normal appearing and intact left adrenal (LA) and kidney (LK) were identified. A normally shaped, and positioned right adrenal (RA) was identified. **(B)** The internal genitalia and the urinary bladder (UB) with a right (RU) and left (LU) ureter were identified. Both ureters were the same size, suggesting the presence of a right kidney. Note the bicornate uterus (arrow), an incidental finding. **(C)** Confirmation of a HLH ventricle with the coronary arteries (arrows) outlining a small left ventricle. The pulmonary artery (PA) is very large, which is also an expected finding in HLH syndrome. (LAA = left atrial appendage).

to determine gestational age, limb abnormalities, congenital heart disease, and so on. X-rays are important in ruling out skeletal or limb abnormalities and may confirm a diagnosis. A dissecting microscope is helpful. Receiving the tissues fresh allows for cytogenetic analysis, although examination of the tissue for fetal parts is optimal after fixation.

The meticulous pathologic exam along with utilization of the clinical history, ultrasound studies, and cytogenetics can provide genetic counselors with important information that may have an impact on future child-bearing decisions.

REFERENCES

Berry CL: The examination of embryonic and fetal material in diagnostic histopathology laboratories. *J Clin Pathol* 33:317, 1980.

Chi JG, Dooling EHG, Gilles FH: Gyral development of the human brain. *Ann Neurol* 1:86, 1977.

Clayton-Smith J, Farndon PA, McKeown C, et al.: Examination of fetuses after induced abortion for fetal abnormality. *Br Med J* 300:295, 1990.

Davies MJ, Anderson RH, Becker AE: *Appendix: The Conduction System of the Heart.* London, Butterworth, 1983.

Davies MJ, Anderson RH, Becker AE: *The Conduction System of the Heart*, Boston, Butterworth, 1983.

Devine WA, Debich DE, Anderson RH: Dissection of congenitally malformed hearts – with comments on the value of sequential segmental analysis. *Ped Pathol* 11:235, 1991.

Emery JL: The postmortem examination of a baby. In Mason JK (ed): *Pediatric Forensic Medicine and Pathology.* London, Chapman & Hall, pp. 72–84, 1989.

Hudson REB: The human conducting system and its examination. *J Clin Pathol* 16:492, 1963.

Jacot FRM, Poulin C, Bilodeau AP, et al.: A 5-year experience with second trimester inducted abortions: no increase in compliation rate as compared to the first trimester. *Am J Obstet Gynecol* 168:633, 1993.

Jones KL, Harrison JW, Smith DW: Palpebral fissure size in newborn infants. *J Pediatr* 92:787, 1978.

Kalousek DK, Fitch N, Paradice BA: *Pathology of the Human Embryo and Previable Fetus. An Atlas*, New York, Springer-Verlag, 1990.

Klatt EC: Pathologic examination of fetal specimens from dilatation and evacuation procedures. *Am J Clin Pathol* 103:415, 1995.

Klatt EC: Pathologic examination of fetal specimens from dilatation and evacuation procedures. *Am J Clin Pathol* 103(4):415, 1995.

Knowles SAS: Examination of products of conception terminated after prenatal investigation. *J Clin Pathol* 39:1049, 1986.

MacPherson TA, Valdes-Dapena M: The perinatal autopsy. In Wigglesworth JS, Singer D (eds): *Perinatal Pathology*, Philadelphia, WB Saunders, pp. 93–122, 1998.

O'Rahilly R, Muller F: *Developmental Stages of Human Embryos*, Publication 637, Washington, DC, Carniegie Institution, 1987.

Ornoy A, Borochowitz Z, Lachman R, Rimoin LD: *Atlas of Fetal Skeletal Radiology*, Chicago, Year Book, 1988.

Rushton DI: Examination of products of conception from previable human pregnancies. *J Clin Pathol* 34:819, 1981.

Scammon RE, Calkins LA: *The Development and Growth of the External Dimensions of the Human Body in the Fetal Period*, Minneapolis, University of Minnesota Press, 1929.

Shulman LP, Ling FE, Meyers CM, et al.: Dilatation and evacuation for second trimester genetic pregnancy termination. *Obstet Gynecol* 75:1037, 1990.

Szulman AE: Examination of the early conceptus. *Arch Pathol Lab Med* 115:696, 1992.

Valdes-Dapena M, Huff D: *Perinatal Autopsy Manual*, Washington, DC, Armed Forces Institute of Pathology, 1983.

Wigglesworth JS: *Perinatal Pathology*, Philadelphia, WB Saunders, 1984.

FOUR

Part I. Ultrasound of Embryo and Fetus: General Principles

Mark Williams and Kathy B. Porter

ABSTRACT

The area of obstetric ultrasonography has undergone rapid and dramatic evolution over the past three decades. Initial imaging studies were limited to rudimentary evaluations of fetal position and identification of amniotic fluid pockets to the current state of the art, which offers the potential for three-dimensional image reconstructions and targeted Doppler sonographic interrogation of the heart and cerebral vascular structures. Because of the rapid pace of change within the field, several professional organizations offer guidance about routine performance of obstetric ultrasound. In the United States, the American College of Obstetrics and Gynecology (ACOG), the American College of Radiology (ACR), and the American Institute of Ultrasound in Medicine (AIUM) have offered guidelines for obstetric sonography, while in the British Commonwealth, the Royal College of Obstetrics and Gynecology (RCOG) of England, and the Society of Obstetrics and Gynecology of Canada (SOGC) offer recommendations and guidance. Potential resources include the following publications: ACOG, *Practice Bulletin 27*; ACOG, *Technical Bulletin 187, Ultrasonography In Pregnancy* (12/93) (*http://www.acog.org*); ACR, *Standard for the Performance of Antepartum Obstetrical Ultrasound* (*http://www.acr.org*); AIUM, *Standards for Performance of the Antepartum Obstetrical Ultrasound Examination* (*http://www.aium.org*); RCOG, *Ultrasound Screening for Fetal Anomalies and the Value of Ultrasound in Pregnancy* (*http://www.rcog.org.uk*); SCOG, *Guidelines of Ultrasound as*

Part of Routine Prenatal Care (8/99), *Obstetrics/Gynecologic Ultrasound* (7/97) (*http://www.sogc.medical.org*).

PHYSICS AND SAFETY CONSIDERATIONS

Ultrasound is a form of physical energy, and exposure to ultrasonic fields results in increased amounts of regional energy, usually resulting in locally increased temperatures. Initial experience with high-frequency sound waves caused some concern about their use as an imaging modality, and the destructive potential of ultrasound has since been harnessed with ultrasonic lithotripsy. Theoretical concerns over the safety of ultrasound centered on the potential biological effects of local thermal effects and of cavitation. Cavitation involves the sudden expansion of gas microbubbles, which can have locally destructive effects. Such effects have been created in vitro by moving solid specimens in acoustic fields but have not been documented in biological systems at normal diagnostic acoustic power levels.

Before widespread adoption of intensive ultrasound diagnostic modalities, the potential biologic effects were reviewed by the National Institutes of Health (NIH), and a consensus report was created (*NIH Consensus Report on Safety of Ultrasound 1984*). In this report, potential effects of ultrasound exposure on biological included alterations in immune response, alterations in sister chromatid exchange frequencies, altered cell membrane function and cell death, degradation of macromolecules, increased free radical formation, and reduced cell reproductive potential. At that time, the consensus panel questioned the applicability of in vitro laboratory studies to in vivo human imaging because some of the findings cited could not be reproduced, and laboratory experiments often used higher power levels than were found in clinical imaging modalities.

In the past, the U.S. Food and Drug Administration (FDA) limited acoustic output for the fetal application to 94 mW/cm^2 spatial peak temporal average for fetal imaging. Over time the need for improved color and Doppler imaging required higher power densities, and machines are now only limited to a higher 720 mW/cm^2 spatial peak temporal average. To allow safe use of potentially higher power densities, two indices were developed to characterize the acoustic energy, the thermal index and the mechanical index, and safe levels of acoustic energy were defined by various entities, including the FDA, ACOG, AIUM, and the National Electrical Manufacturers Association (ACOG Committee on Obstetric Practice, Opinion Number 180, November 1996). One of the two measurements should be displayed at all times if machines are capable of generating potentially dangerous levels of sonic energy. If only one is displayed, the thermal index should be displayed during normal imaging and the mechanical index during Doppler studies.

The thermal index (TI) is a calculated estimate of local temperature rise due to ultrasound energy. TI values < 1.0 are not generally of concern, while greater values may result in local thermal effects even after only several minutes of exposure. The sensitivity of a particular region to thermal effects is related to its composition (soft tissue versus bone) and its relative vascularity. Increased vascularity and perfusion will conduct heat away and mitigate the effects of the acoustic energy. Currently available sonographic equipment must provide a graphic warning if TI exceeds 1.0. Subsets of TI include TS (soft tissue, appropriate for first-trimester fetal examinations), TIB (TI, bone; used in second- and third-trimester fetal examinations), and TIC (TI, cranial; for use with transcranial Doppler).

The mechanical index, calculated as the peak rarefactional pressure of the acoustic pulse divided by the square root of the transducer center frequency, is a relative measure of the mechanical effects of compression and decompression related to the ultrasound field. Values < 1.0 are considered generally safe, while insonnation intensities of 1.0 should be used with caution for appropriate clinical purposes.

In operation, the ultrasound unit generates a sound pulse, awaits a return signal for a fixed interval, and then generates another pulse. In standard real-time imaging, the ultrasound transducer is in a transmitting or "sending" mode for $<0.1\%$ of the time, limiting the total energy exposure to the region being insonnated. When color or pulsed Doppler is used a much greater portion of the duty cycle (a cycle of one transmission and reception) is spent applying acoustic energy to the region being assessed and has much greater potential for causing local bioeffects. Recently, new forms of sonographic imaging have been developed. One involves harmonic imaging, in which the insonnation pulse causes harmonic oscillations in the targeted tissues, which are then imaged directly from the oscillations that have been generated. This technology offers great promise for improved imaging of various organ systems (Lencioni et al. 2002).

Insonnation frequencies range from 2 or 3 mHz to 8–9 mHz or higher, and scanning depths typically range from 2 or 3 cm to 10–15 cm from the transducer. Lower frequencies yield lower resolution but offer greater tissue penetration, while higher frequencies carry greater energy and yield better resolution, but do not penetrate as deeply as lower frequencies. The impact of maternal obesity on image resolution can often be minimized by imaging via the vagina (especially for first trimester imaging), the maternal suprapubic area, or umbilicus. Image resolution is also subject to interference by high sonodensity objects such as fetal spine, ribs, or limbs in the foreground between the transducer and target area. Such structures absorb acoustic energy and yield areas of sonic shadowing and diminished imaging resolution for structures behind them. In the second trimester, such shadowing is usually intermittent because of frequent fetal position changes, but in the late third trimester, such imaging obstructions may persist for much longer time intervals.

At all times, sonographic imaging should be obtained with adherence to the ALARA standard, using power densities, as low as reasonably achievable, to yield useable images and information. Prudent use of equipment is the responsibility of the operator, and scan modes and power outputs that result in the lowest possible energy exposures compatible with completion of the diagnostic study should be used.

In spite of the theoretical potential for bioeffects and fetal injury, no significant effects on birthweight or length, childhood growth, cognitive function, acoustic or visual abilities, or incidence of neurologic impairments have been found associated with clinical applications of ultrasound imaging in pregnancy.

Various types of sonographic image generation have been used. They include A mode (only of historical interest), real-time B mode, color flow, pulsed Doppler, and three-dimensional sonography. The ability to provide and interpret sonograms other than real-time B mode differs widely by clinical setting. Both relatively recent, high-quality equipment and an experienced technician and interpreting physician are required to perform the other sonographic procedures.

A mode (amplitude modulation) sonography was the first sonographic application used in obstetric sonography. It offered visualization of points and relative distances as determined by time delay from transmission to reception, but only objects returning strong signals were represented and were usually displayed as spikes on an oscilloscope. This modality was rapidly supplanted by B mode (brightness modulation), in which the proportional strength of the returning signal is displayed in a gray scale of tones ranging from black (minimal signal return indicating no evident tissue densities) to white (indicating high sonographic tissue density). These gray tones are displayed as a linear, curvilinear, or radial array with distance from the transducer indicating insonnation depth and provide the traditional cross-sectional images associated with sonographic imaging, usually in real time. Linear images are generated by imaging directly below a transducer, while a radial or sector transducer probe depicts a variable angular range (typically 10°–80° of arc) of information in regions that extend radially away from the transducer. This allows visualization of structures that cannot be viewed in a direct linear fashion, often because of interposed structures, such as the pubic bone, but some experience is required to adapt to the radial spatial orientation of images. Curvilinear images combine characteristics of linear imaging in central regions and sector (radial) images on lateral margins of the scanned region.

M mode (motion mode) displays sonographic information from a narrow region (several millimeters wide) over time information from a fixed area over time, allowing evaluation of valve function or structural dimensions (such as aortic diameter, ventricular wall thickness, or ventricular diameter) during a cardiac cycle.

Color flow ultrasonography uses Doppler shift information to assess average velocities relative to the ultrasound transducer within an area of insonnation. These velocity estimates are usually coded on a scale ranging from one color to another, often deep blue to deep red, and the color images generated are superimposed on a real-time B mode or M mode image of the same area.

Color-coded flow characteristics allow evaluation of flow characteristics such as direction, velocity, and turbulence within the heart, placenta, or various organs. Flow characteristics may be used to characterize risk for malignancy near cystic lesions.

Doppler information can also be used to assess flow velocity relative to the probe in a small area several millimeters wide and deep. The velocity characteristics can then displayed as velocity over time. If the direction of flow is within several degrees of parallel to the angle of insonnation (i.e., $0^\circ \pm 3^\circ$–5°), relatively precise estimates of flow velocity can be obtained. As the angle of insonnation increases from parallel, accuracy of velocity estimation diminishes rapidly because smaller proportions of the flow vector (those parallel to the insonnation beam) are being used to project the overall flow velocity. When flow is perpendicular to insonnation, no component of flow velocity relative to the transducer and flow velocity cannot be assessed with Doppler sonography.

In addition to velocity estimation at narrow angles of insonnation, useful information can also be obtained at relatively great angles of insonnation by comparing systolic and diastolic velocities from the same site. These characteristics are reported as ratios of systolic to diastolic flow velocity (the S/D ratio), or by computing indices such as the ratio of systolic velocity to the mean flow velocity (the pulsatility index), or the ratio of the difference between systolic and diastolic velocity and the systolic velocity (the resistance index). The S/D ratio is often preferred because it is conceptually easier to visualize and compute, but it is statistically a poor characteristic because it ranges from 1 to an unreal number ($n/0$). As a result, the other two indices are more commonly used in most publications. Flow characteristics of the umbilical artery are easily obtained by the most basic Doppler equipment and help in identifying fetuses with increased placental resistance. Increased placental resistance results in high umbilical S/D ratios and increased pulsatility. Conversely, redistribution of cerebral flow in fetal growth restriction is often associated with lower cerebral artery S/D ratios and less pulsatility then is found in normal infants. Evaluations of flow in the cerebral circulation require relatively high-quality Doppler equipment, but such equipment is becoming increasingly more readily available as sonographic equipment becomes more advanced and prices decrease.

Three-dimensional sonography has only recently become available. It requires an ultrasound transducer capable of rapidly generating a sequence of images that are then processed and analyzed by a computer in a fashion similar to the methods used for generating computed tomographic (CT) images. The reconstructed images can then be rotated and viewed from many different aspects. The ability to manipulate the images in this fashion allows certain structural anomalies such as neural tube anomalies and facial clefts to be viewed much more easily and from more favorable angles. They also offer the advantage of generating an image that is much more easily understood and interpreted by the lay public and that facilitates understanding of the high degree of anatomic disarrangement often present in severe anomalies. At this time, sonographic units capable of generating rapidly sequenced three-dimensional renderings of the fetus allow the equivalent of a three-dimensional cinematographic image, further enhancing the diagnostic capabilities of such sonographic studies.

Routine Antepartum Sonography

It is estimated that basic ultrasonography is performed in 60–70% of pregnancies, but in the United States, sonography of low-risk patients has never been established as a requisite of routine care (Dooley 1999). This may relate to the relatively low incidence of anomalies, the rather poor sensitivity of ultrasound screening for identifying structural anomalies as described below, and the limited options available for correction of the problems identified. Additionally, many clinical situations, such as multiple gestations, excessive fetal growth, fetal growth restriction, oligohydramnios, and polyhydramnios will present clinical findings that initiate a process of evaluation resulting in their diagnosis by ultrasound evaluation.

Although antepartum sonographic screening has been found associated with lower perinatal mortality at term, most of that reduction has been ascribed to voluntary terminations of infants with severe anomalies that otherwise would be included in perinatal mortality statistics. After assessing the benefits and risks of antenatal screening, ACOG recently reported that antepartum sonographic evaluations are an optional aspect of prenatal care rather than a requisite evaluation (ACOG Practice Pattern 5, August 1997, *Routine Ultrasound in Low-Risk Pregnancy*, Washington, DC).

Patterns of sonographic utilization vary internationally. In England, patients often undergo an initial sonographic evaluation at the time of their first prenatal visit to confirm menstrual dating, followed by an anatomic survey in the early second trimester, and a sonogram to confirm normal fetal growth and development in the early third trimester. Although, such utilization patterns may not yield statistically improved morbidity and mortality statistics, they afford unquestionable opportunities for parents to bond with their children, identify fetal growth restriction before it is clinically evident, and in cases of major anomalies, may offer the advantages of more prompt prenatal diagnosis.

Indications for Antenatal Sonography

As with other tests, sonography is usually performed to answer a clinical question such as excluding the possibility of ectopic gestation, surveying for structural anomalies or abnormalities of placentation, assessing size/gestational age disparities (as might occur if the gestational age has been incorrectly assessed, in cases of multiple gestation, with aberrant fetal growth, or if the amniotic fluid volume is abnormal), or to evaluate fetal well-being. Although fetal size can be estimated clinically to a reasonable degree of accuracy in low-risk pregnancies, this is sometimes impossible (in multiple gestation) or impractical (in cases of morbid maternal obesity). Additionally, sonographic serial fetal growth assessment is often recommended if conditions strongly predisposing to fetal growth abnormalities such as hypertension, collagen vascular disease, and advanced stage diabetes are present. Serial sonographic estimates in these circumstances are more sensitive early markers of aberrant fetal growth than clinical size assessment. Also, newer Doppler sonographic techniques can be used to document circulatory changes associated with ongoing fetal nutritional stress such as the shift of fetal circulation to the cerebral vasculature in growth restriction and the increased flow velocity in the middle cerebral artery associated with fetal anemias due to rhesus and other atypical forms of isoimmunization.

Indications for sonography include the following:

- Estimation of gestation age in patients with uncertain clinical dates, who plan to deliver by indicated induction of labor or scheduled repeat elective cesarean, or who plan to electively terminate their pregnancies.
- Evaluation of fetal growth in pregnancy in cases of maternal disease that predisposes to anomalous fetal growth, in multiple gestation, and to aid estimation of fetal weight and presentation in premature rupture of membranes or premature labor
- Evaluation of cases of vaginal bleeding in pregnancy of undetermined etiology such as suspected abruptio placentae, placenta previa, or ectopic pregnancy
- Evaluation of the fetal condition in late registrants for prenatal care
- Assessment of the fetal presentation if malpresentation is suspected
- Evaluation of significant uterine size/clinical dates discrepancies possibly due to multiple gestation, amniotic fluid volume disturbance, or abnormal fetal growth
- Evaluation of suspected uterine anomalies, pelvic masses, suspected hydatidiform moles, or to locate intrauterine contraceptive devices
- As an adjunct to cervical cerclage placement, amniocentesis, percutaneous umbilical blood sampling, chorionic villus sampling, fetal urinary stent placement, external cephalic (breech) version, or placement of cervical cerclage
- Evaluation of fetal well-being by biophysical profile, of intrapartum events, and suspected fetal death
- For evaluation of patients at risk for congenital structural fetal anomalies, investigation of suspected fetal anomalies, evaluation of cases in which abnormal maternal serum screening results suggest increased risk of aneuploidy or neural tube abnormalities, and evaluation of fetuses with cardiac rhythm disturbances
- Evaluation of placental location in prior cases of identified placenta previa

Assessment of Fetal Well-being

In addition to assessments of fetal structures or Doppler and color sonographic evaluations of blood flow patterns and velocities, sonography is widely used for antenatal assessment of fetal well-being. Initially, well-being assessment centered on sonographic evaluations of amniotic fluid volume after increased rates of morbidity and mortality were noted in post-term fetuses with abnormally low amniotic fluid volume. Criteria such as absence of a fluid pocket greater than 1 cm^2 or 2 cm^2 eventually gave way to assessments of the amniotic fluid index, computed as the sum of the deepest amniotic fluid pocket from the four quadrants of the amniotic cavity. Amniotic fluid indices were then evaluated as falling above or below certain critical values (values < 5 or 6 often characterized as oligohydramnios, values >25 considered polyhydramnios) or assessed with gestationally specific norms (Moore and Cayle 1990).

Sonography also allows the possibility of dynamic, real-time assessment of the fetus. A system of sonographic assessment pioneered by Manning et al. (1980), the biophysical profile, used four sonographic criteria scored as either present or absent, with 2 or 0 points awarded, respectively, and a fifth criterion derived from electronic fetal heart rate pattern assessment termed "non-stress testing". The sonographic criteria to be evaluated over a 30-min interval included presence of fetal breathing movements of 30 seconds or greater, fetal tone, gross body movements, and presence of a normal amniotic fluid volume (various criteria have been used over time). The fifth heart rate pattern criterion required a normal amount of fetal heart rate variability, termed reactivity, to be present to allow an award of 2 points to the overall score. After evaluation in over 15,000 pregnancies, it is well established that biophysical profile scores of 8 or 10 are associated with very low rates of fetal demise in utero, perinatal morbidity, or perinatal morality. Scores of 6 are considered to be equivocal and require further assessment within 12–24 hours, while scores of 4 or less are strongly associated with impending demise of the fetus (Manning 1999, 2002; Manning et al. 1980, 1985).

Because non-stress tests cannot be performed without special electronic fetal monitoring equipment and infants with scores of 8 and 10 fared equally well, variations of the biophysical score have been investigated. Some clinicians use a strictly sonographic profile, with only the four sonographic criteria and maintaining the original 8-point criterion for a normal study; others use an abbreviated sonogram with assessment only of the amniotic fluid volume in combination with an electronic fetal non-stress test. In the latter test, presence of a normal amniotic fluid volume and a reactive fetal heart rate tracing are considered to be a normal well-being assessment.

The most intriguing uses of sonography for fetal assessment now utilize Doppler sonography to document changes in flow of the umbilical arteries (Divon and Ferber 2001; Westergaard et al. 2001; Harrington et al. 1999), the ductus venosus (Baschat et al. 2001; Sterne et al. 2001; Baschat et al. 2002; Muller et al. 2002; Hofstaetter et al. 2002), and the middle cerebral arteries (Stefos et al. 2002; Mari et al. 2002; Detti et al. 2002; Cosmi et al. 2002; Madazli et al. 2001). These studies allow advanced clinicians to more fully assess fetuses suspected of fetal growth restriction or anemia (postinfectious or due to isoimmunization) and in some cases allow the clinician to delay invasive procedures such as fetal blood sampling in cases of suspected fetal anemia. The information afforded by these sonographic techniques often presages more common markers of impending fetal compromise by days or weeks (Baschat et al. 2001), and thus allow the ability to stratify patients and treatment protocols by risk, to investigate potential treatment regimens for conditions assessed, and to monitor fetal response to treatments such as in utero fetal transfusions (Stefos et al. 2002) and anti-arrhythmic therapy.

Sonographic Study Profiles

There are several categorizations of obstetric sonographic evaluations. Traditionally, obstetric sonographers using guidance from ACOG have recognized at least two levels of sonography – basic and advanced or targeted – while other organizations such as ACR and AIUM recognize only one standard of sonographic imagery (Seeds 1996). Other organizations such as RCOG of England, and SOGC also offer guidance as to potential sonographic examination strategies.

Limited studies are focused examinations of limited scope and constitute a subset of basic evaluations. Limited studies may involve evaluations to establish an intrauterine pregnancy or fetal presentation, to look for evidence of placental abruption, or to confirm amniotic fluid volume or cardiac activity. Such studies are often performed on an urgent basis, perhaps by sonographers with limited expertise, and may or not have been preceded by a more extensive evaluation. The limitations inherent in such studies should be recognized, and a more thorough study should be ordered at a later date if clinically indicated.

Basic studies are intended to provide a general survey of fetal biometry and anatomy. Parameters such as the biparietal diameter, head circumference, abdominal circumference, and femur length are usually measured, and an assessment of amniotic fluid volume by measurement or visual inspection is performed. The number of fetuses and their presentation are recorded, and an attempt is made to inspect anatomic features of the fetal head, face, chest, and abdomen, placenta, and umbilical cord. Factors that may limit the performance of basic studies include oligohydramnios, maternal obesity, and fetal positioning. Follow-up of commonly obtained basic images with a later study is often performed but may depend on individual clinical circumstances.

An advanced or comprehensive study will include most or all of the details noted previously for a basic study (if not previously performed) but also will include a more extensive evaluation of some aspect of the fetal-placental unit. This study is usually prompted by information from family histories, past medical histories, or prior diagnostic evaluations that suggest fetal abnormalities amenable to further sonographic evaluation. These may include

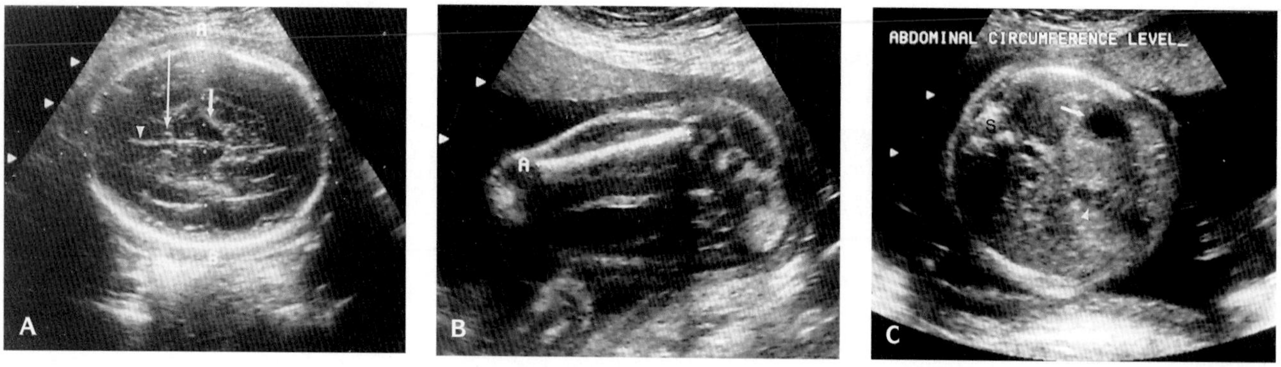

4.1. **(A)** Axial image at 31 weeks: measurement of the BPD and head circumference at the level of the thalami (arrow), cavum septum pellucidum (long arrow) and falx cerebri (arrowhead). (A – B = biparietal diameter). **(B)** Axial image at 24 weeks: measurement of the femur length (+ → +). **(C)** Axial image at 24 weeks: abdominal circumference taken at the level of the stomach (arrow) and the umbilical vein (arrowhead) (S = spine).

suspected neural tube abnormalities, aneuploidy, chondrodystrophies, or congenital abnormalities of the gastrointestinal, genitourinary, central nervous system (CNS), or cardiac systems. Additionally, newer sonographic techniques may be used to characterize blood flow within the heart or CNS structures and give guidance as to the severity and progression of problems as diverse as fetal anemia and fetal growth restriction.

Components of Sonographic Studies

In the first trimester, the crown–rump length (CRL) is measured from the top of the head to the rump. Average values of the CRL range from 3.7 mm at 6 weeks gestation to 21.9 mm at 9 weeks gestation and 51.7 mm at 12 weeks gestation. It provides the most accurate estimator of gestational age, with ±3 days accuracy at 7–10 weeks gestation and ±5 days at 10–14 weeks gestation. Nuchal fold thickness offers a highly useful screening tool for both aneuploidy and congenital heart disease, but measurement of this characteristic must be performed in a standardized fashion to allow good correlation with adverse outcomes. The Fetal Medicine Foundation of England (London, England; www.fetalmedicine.com) is administering this process in the United States by providing didactic lectures and ongoing quality assurance of images obtained. Finally, sonography in the first trimester is also of paramount importance for guidance during chorionic villus sampling to perform fetal karyotypic evaluation at 10–12 weeks gestation. Chorionic villus samples allow karyotypic determinations in 3 or 4 days, and they provide this information up to 6 weeks before similar information can be obtained by traditional amniocentesis at 15 weeks or beyond.

A variety of characteristics and structures may be evaluated in the second and third trimesters of pregnancy depending on indications for the study. These include fetal number, lie, and presentation, an assessment of amniotic fluid volume, site of placentation, gestational age assessment by measurement of biparietal diameter (BPD), head circumference (HC), femur length (FL), and abdominal circumference (AC) (Figure 4.1).

The head normally has an elliptical appearance in cross section. Head shape may be altered in cases of open neural tube disorder (frontal-temporal narrowing causes the head to look lemon-like in cross section, the lemon sign). The cerebral ventricles should be evaluated for abnormal size, symmetry, and the presence of choroid plexus cysts. In open neural tube disorders, the lateral ventricles are often dilated, and the cerebellum often appears fused (the banana sign) rather than showing two characteristic spheres.

The spine is optimally evaluated in longitudinal and transverse planes (Figures 4.2 and 4.3). The fetal chest should be visualized with particular attention to the diaphragmatic contour, situs and intrathoracic angle of the cardiac axis, the size of the heart relative to the chest, and the presence of a four-chamber cardiac silhouette. The stomach bubble should be located caudad to the heart just below the diaphragm and with situs concordant with the heart (Figure 4.4). The urinary bladder, and kidneys (Figure 4.5) should be evaluated, and special attention should be given to evaluation of these structures if the amniotic fluid volume is decreased. The umbilical cord should have three vessels, and the umbilical cord should insert directly to the abdominal wall. A normal appearing umbilical cord (Figure 4.6) insertion site effectively excludes the possibility of ventral wall abnormalities such as gastroschisis and omphalocele, and its location relative to a ventral wall defect may help distinguish between these two entities. The length of the cervix and the appearance of the cervical canal can be evaluated either transabdominally or endovaginally (Colombo and Iams 2000; Iams et al. 1996). Cervical lengths average 3.4 cm in nulliparous women and 3.6 cm in parous women at 24 weeks gestation, and 3.3 cm and 3.5 cm, respectively, at 28 weeks gestation (Iams et al. 1996). At 24 weeks gestation, cervical lengths of 2.8–3.2 cm are associated with an approximately 4-fold increased risk of delivery before 35 weeks gestation and an 8-fold risk or more for cervical lengths <2.4 cm (Colombo and Iams 2000). Dilation of the internal junction of the lower uterine segment and the proximal cervix (funneling) indicates increased risk for incompetent cervix or preterm labor (Figure 4.7). Although the association between these cervical findings and preterm delivery appears robust, it is not clear whether cervical cerclage for abnormal cervical length in suspected incompetent cervix is justified (Harger 2002).

When possible, the umbilical cord should be evaluated in cross section. It normally has three vessels, one large vein conducting blood from the placenta to the fetus, and two smaller arteries that arise from the fetal iliac arteries (Figure 4.10). If a two vessel cord (single umbilical artery) is present, the risk of structural fetal anomalies and aneuploidy is increased. Single umbilical artery in combination with any other anomaly indicates a high risk of other structural abnormalities and aneuploidy.

Umbilical artery Doppler velocimetry is not normally performed during routine sonographic evaluations but is recommended if fetal growth restriction

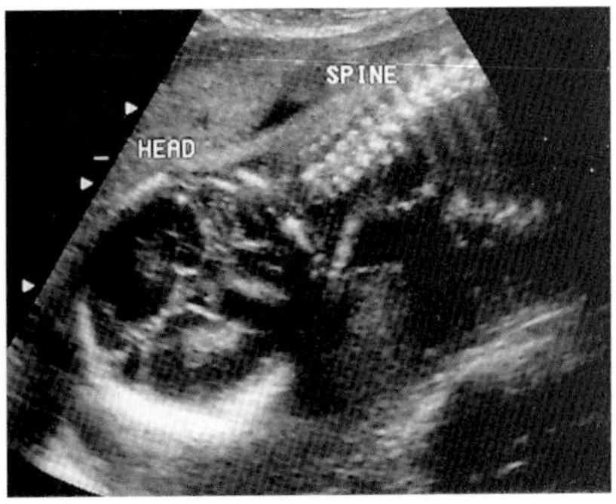

4.2. Coronal image of the fetal head and spine at 24 weeks.

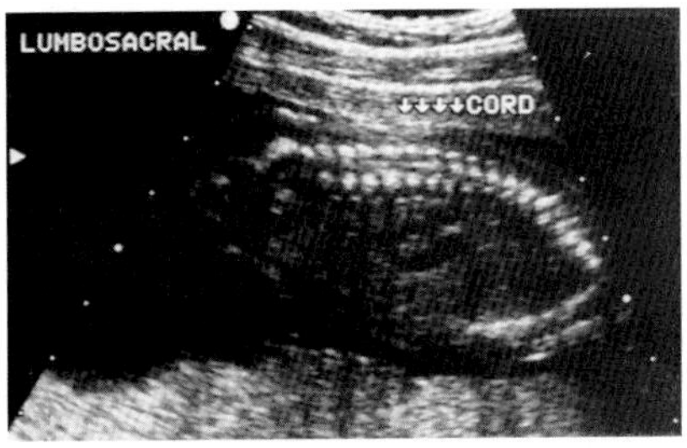

4.3. Sagittal image at 19 weeks of the lumbosacral spine; the linear spinal cord can be seen between the bony processes.

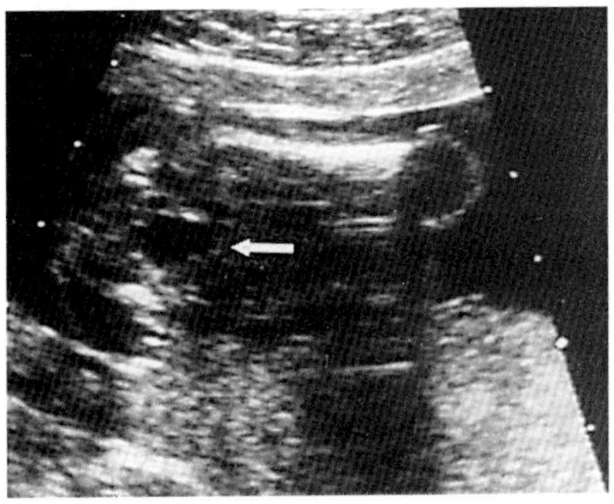

4.4. Axial image at 19 weeks: fetal urinary bladder (arrow).

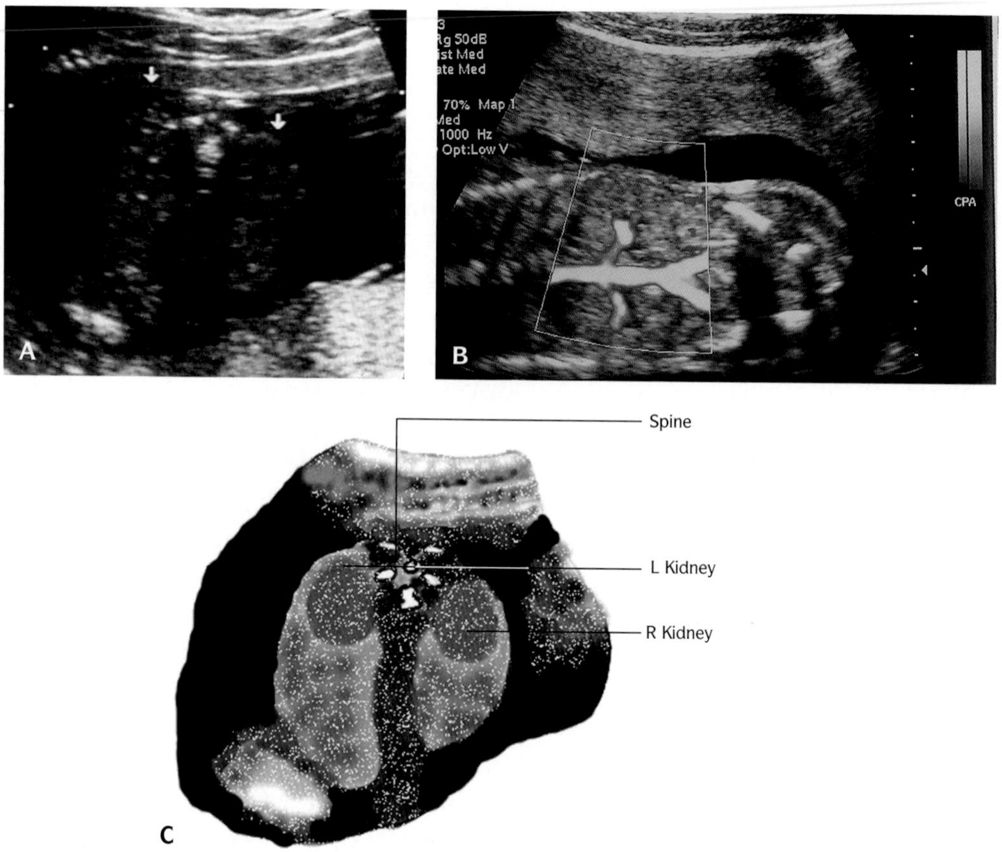

4.5. **(A)** Axial image of the fetal kidneys at 19 weeks (arrows). **(B)** Normal renal arteries branching from aorta (color). **(C)** Schematic.

is suspected. Increased S/D ratios are believed to be caused by increased placental vascular resistance, while absent or reversed end-diastolic flow are strongly correlated with imminent fetal death (Divon and Ferber 2001; Westergaard et al. 2001; Harrington et al. 1999). Conversely, because the process

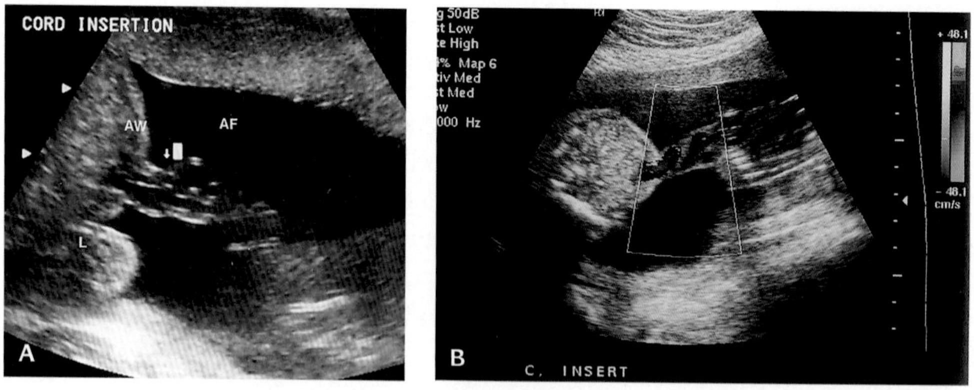

4.6. **(A)** Axial image at 24 weeks: cord insertion into the fetal abdomen (arrow) (AW = abdominal wall, AF = amniotic fluid, L = limb). **(B)** Doppler ultrasound of a normal umbilical cord insertion showing normal blood flow.

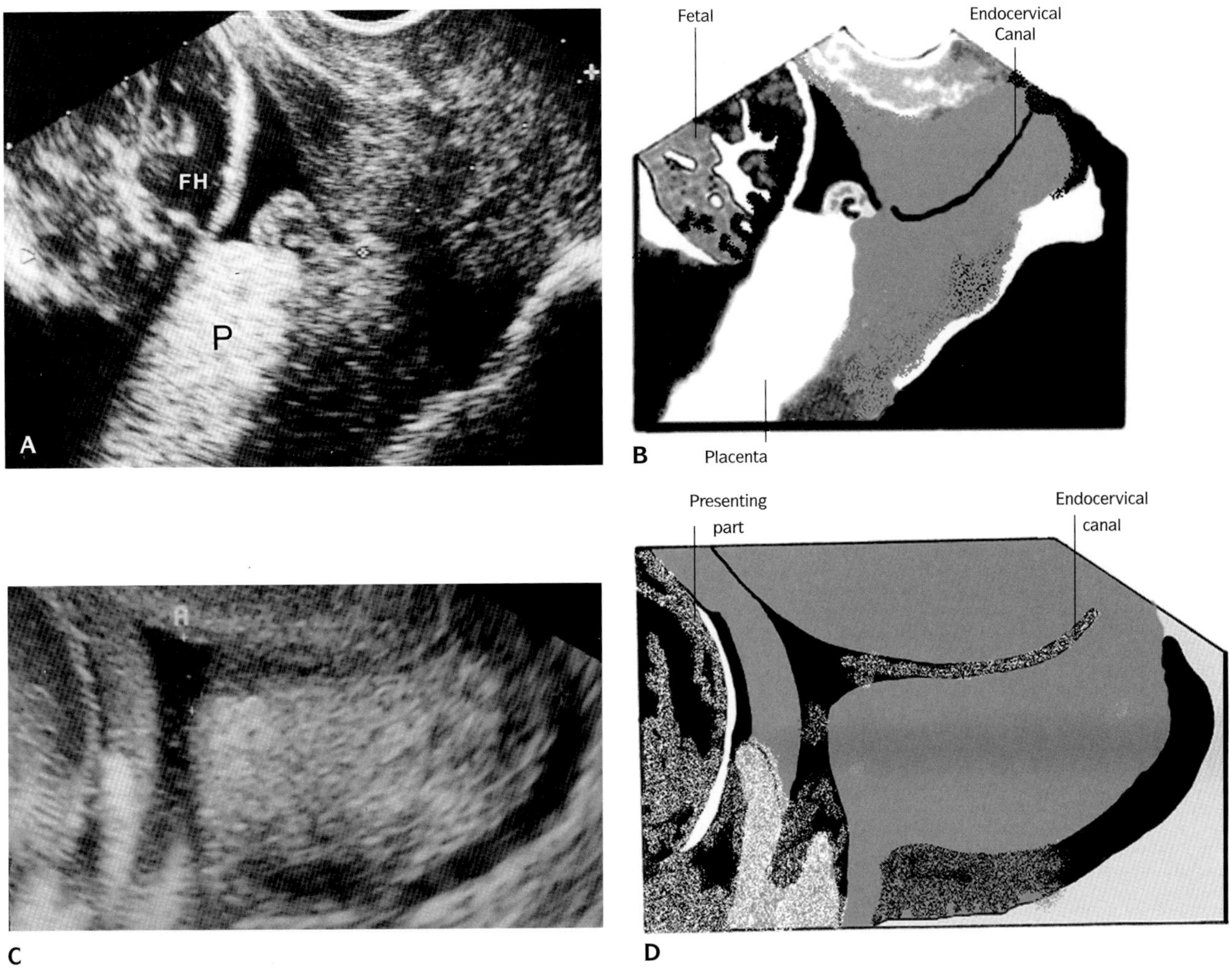

4.7. **(A)** Sagittal image of the cervical length marked by calipers measuring 4.22 cm at 19 weeks (FH = fetal head, P = placenta). **(B)** Schematic. **(C)** Sagittal image of the cervix demonstrates funneling at 20 weeks gestation. Small calipers measure funneling of the cervix at 0.69 cm in the anterior/posterior dimension; large calipers measure the cervical length at 3.50 cm in length. **(D)** Schematic.

of cerebral sparing, flow velocity waveforms in the middle cerebral artery show decreased pulsatility and lower S/D ratios when growth restriction or other fetal stressors are present (Bahado-Singh et al. 1999). If growth retardation is present and umbilical artery Doppler velocimetry is normal, there may be an increased risk of aneuploidy.

In multiple gestations, membranes dividing the fetuses should be assessed (Figure 4.9), because cord entanglement is very unlikely if each fetus is contained in a separate amniotic sac. Some information may be derived from looking at the placental insertion of dividing membranes. If they join in a perpendicular fashion with no interposed tissue near the placenta, they are likely monochorionic. Conversely, if some tissue is present at the base of the membranes, the site of union with the placenta has the appearance of the Greek

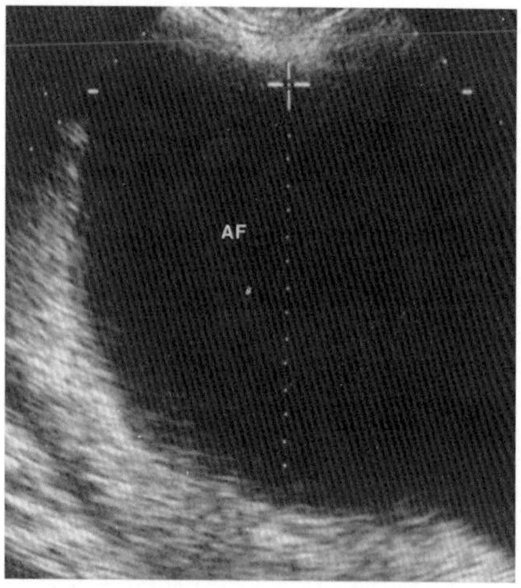

4.8. Sagittal image: polyhydramnios (AF = amniotic fluid).

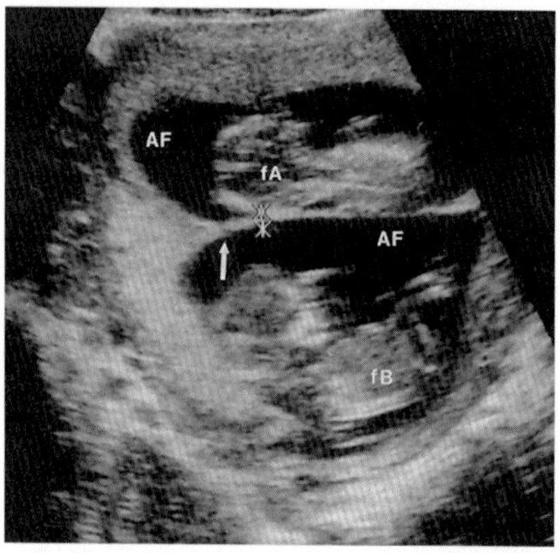

4.9. "Twin-peak" sign of a multiple gestation (arrow). Calipers measure membrane thickness (AF = amniotic fluid, fA = fetus A, fB = fetus B).

letter λ, the lambda sign. This finding indicates that the placentas are likely separate and unlikely to have shared fetal circulatory systems within the placenta.

After fetal biometry has been obtained, an estimate of gestational age should be undertaken. Accuracy of the menstrual history should be verified. If the patient has irregularly timed menses, if she has received contraceptive hormonal therapy in the preceding several months, if the last menses was abnormal in duration or began unexpectedly, or if there is more than a 10% difference between the menstrual and sonographic dating, it may be best to use a sonographically determined gestational age. Sonographic dating is best accomplished by using information from the first reliable sonographic evaluation of the fetus for the balance of the pregnancy. Dates should not be reassigned based on subsequent sonographic biometric measures. Highly accurate dating can be achieved by crown-rump lengths before the second trimester, and measures of biparietal diameter, head circumference, and femur length give excellent assessment of gestational age in the second and third trimesters. If a biometric parameter is likely affected by underlying pathology, such as the biparietal diameter or head circumference with evidence of hydrocephaly present, that parameter should not be used for gestational age assessment. Additionally, aberrant fetal growth (either excessive or restricted growth) is more common after 20–22 weeks gestation and abdominal circumference measures are more affected by such processes than either head or long bone measures. For this reason, in the second half of pregnancy, the abdominal circumference is not ideally suited for gestational age estimations.

Sonographic estimations of gestational age are accurate to ±10% of the gestational age in weeks determined, but patients with significant size/dates discrepancy occurring after 22 or 23 weeks gestation should be carefully evaluated. Growth disturbances before 22 weeks gestation are quite rare, but later in pregnancy growth disturbances of the fetus may be present, which will both complicate the assignment of gestational age and may cause growth restriction

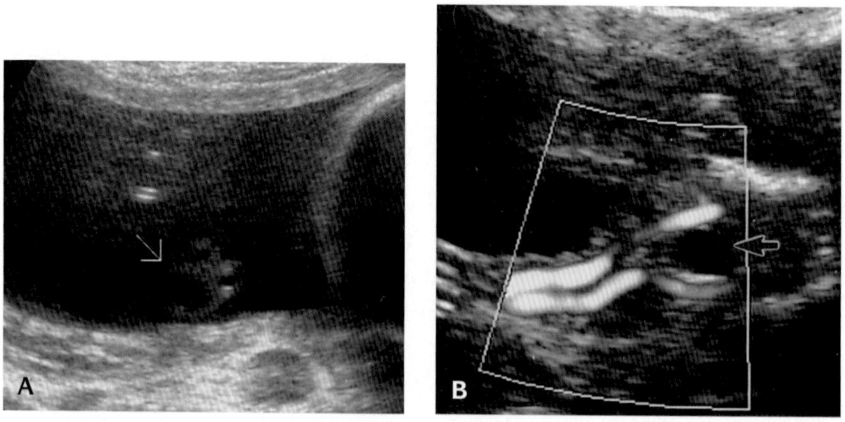

4.10. **(A)** Sagittal image of the three-vessel umbilical cord (arrow). (Mickey mouse sign). **(B)** Blood flow in umbilical vessels with normal cord insertion (arrow = urinary bladder).

or macrosomia to remain undiagnosed. For example, a fetus at 28 weeks gestation by a purportedly accurate menstrual history and with symmetric sonographic measurements of 24 weeks gestation will most often truly be 24 weeks gestation but on occasion may represent a symmetrically growth-restricted fetus. Further evaluation of such pregnancies, looking for other evidence of normal or abnormal fetal growth and development, will often help establish which of these two diagnoses is more appropriate.

The placenta is first visible at 8–9 weeks gestation as a thickened portion of gestational ring. Its appearance gradually changes over the course of pregnancy. These changes usually are assigned to one of four grades, 0–3: homogeneous echo pattern bounded by the smooth chorionic plate (Grade 0) are usually present until 31–33 weeks; nonhomogenous echo patterns are then observed (Grade 1); increased amounts of basilar and intraplacental calcifications (Grade 2); and development of diffuse calcifications and indentations of the chorionic and basilar plates into the intraplacental perivillous septa (Grade 3).

Placental depth normally ranges from 1.5 to 5 cm. Abnormally thin placentas (<1.5 cm) are found more often in pregnancies complicated by intrauterine growth restriction, placental insufficiency, polyhydramnios, and preeclampsia while placental depth of more than 5 cm occur in association with pregnancy complications such as maternal diabetes, rhesus isoimmunization, cytomegalovirus infection, abruption, aneuploidy (triploidy), chorioangioma, and multiple gestations.

Because of the relatively small volume of the uterine cavity before 12 weeks, placental location is difficult to assess in the first trimester. In the early second trimester, placentas are often identified in close proximity to the cervix but usually appear more normally situated later in pregnancy. Placentas with margins in close proximity to the cervix are termed low lying, while those that abut the cervical canal are termed marginal placenta previas. Increasing degrees of association with the cervical canal are termed partial or complete placenta previa. Abnormal situs may be associated with fetal growth abnormalities and abruption, and the placenta may grow into a prior cesarean scar. Lesser degrees of abnormal situs often resolve as the lower uterine segment lengthens and the placenta appears to migrate, particularly if such findings were noted in the first 12 weeks of pregnancy. Suspected cases of abnormal situs should be reevaluated at 30–32 weeks gestation, or sooner if vaginal bleeding is noted. Abnormal situs persisting after 30–32 weeks gestation places the patient at significant risk for abnormal placental situs at delivery and merits special management considerations during the last weeks of pregnancy and at delivery.

Amniotic fluid originates as a transudate from placental membranes, the pulmonary tree, and across the fetal skin in the first weeks of pregnancy. It has an electrolyte concentration and osmolarity similar to sea water. After 15–17 weeks of gestation, the urinary system becomes the primary source of amniotic fluid, and amniotic fluid volume will drop precipitously if an abnormal genitourinary tract is present. The amniotic fluid volume is most commonly estimated by inspection. If more accurate characterization of the fluid volume is required, an amniotic fluid index (the sum of the deepest vertical pocket depth in the four uterine quadrants) can be calculated. The amniotic fluid index normally rises predictably over the course of pregnancy (Moore and Cayle 1990). Subjective estimates of fluid volume by experienced technicians correlate well with numerical quantitations of the amniotic fluid index. Commonly used criteria for oligohydramnios include the absence of any 2 cm × 2 cm fluid pocket or four-quadrant amniotic fluid indices of <5 or 6, while amniotic fluid indices of >25 are considered polyhydramnios.

Although oligohydramnios is sometimes a sporadic event, it commonly occurs in association with another pregnancy complication, such as uteroplacental insufficiency, ruptured amniotic membranes, a fetal genitourinary abnormality such as renal agenesis or obstructive uropathy, or chronic abruption sequence (if found in association with persistent, irregular vaginal bleeding). If oligohydramnios occurs before approximately 24 weeks gestation, the fetus may exhibit features of the Potter's sequence (facial malformations, joint mobility limitation, and pulmonary hypoplasia), which are reminiscent of the findings in renal agenesis (Potter's syndrome). In post-term pregnancy, oligohydramnios is strongly associated with perinatal morbidity and is considered an indication for delivery, but recent reports indicate that this association is not nearly as strong before 40 weeks of gestation and may not hold beyond 40 weeks of gestation in carefully selected, normal pregnancies (Sherer 2002; Conway et al. 1998; Kreiser et al. 2001).

Polyhydramnios (Figure 4.8) is more common in diabetic pregnancies and also may develop as a result of abnormal fetal amniotic fluid homeostasis. Fetal conditions that can produce polyhydramnios include conditions causing excessive urine production such as diabetes insipidus and disorders associated with decreased swallowing such as CNS abnormalities, tracheo-esophageal abnormalities, and bowel atresia.

Prenatal Diagnostic Screening

The value of ultrasound imaging for prenatal screening is quite controversial, because it has not been found to significantly improve obstetric outcomes, and it is not considered an intrinsic component of normal obstetric care in low-risk patients (Dooley 1999).

Although a high percentage of abnormalities can be successfully detected under ideal circumstances, the ability of routine imaging under ordinary circumstances to reliably detect major fetal structural malformations is much more suspect (see below for discussion of the RADIUS study). Factors that affect the potential sensitivity of a given sonographic study include machine characteristics (resolution, availability of ancillary modalities such as harmonic imaging, color flow Doppler, pulsed Doppler velocimetry, three-dimensional imaging) and patient characteristics such as maternal body habitus, presence of an anterior placenta, fetal positioning and mobility, and an adequate amount of amniotic fluid surrounding the fetus. The skill and experience of the sonographic technician performing the study and the interpreting physician (sometimes the same person) are also critical to optimal screening accuracy. Finally, patient historical factors that serve to increase the index of suspicion may be very helpful by focusing attention to details that ordinarily would not be aggressively pursued. Familial predisposition to congenital cardiac disease, suspicion of aneuploidy or a neural tube disorder after prior maternal serum screening, and suspected aberrant fetal growth are examples of clinical circumstances that often would result in a much more thorough fetal evaluation than might occur absent such a prior history.

Certain epidemiologic factors also appear to influence the utility of sonographic screening. Detection rates are higher in referral centers and in infants with multiple anomalies. The predictive value of anomalous findings is influenced by population prevalence rates for those findings. For example, echogenic intracardiac focus is weakly associated with aneuploidy in many populations, but it is a relatively common finding in Asian populations. In addition to benefitting from often more experienced personnel and better equipment, studies performed in referral populations tend to be more focused and extensive because of concern for the historical factors and prior findings that prompted the initial referral.

Major structural congenital anomalies occur in 12–18 per 1,000 live births, with published rate estimates that range from 6 to 26 per 1,000. Prenatal rates of anomalies are higher than live birth statistics because of increased rates of pregnancy loss among anomalous infants. In addition to the institutional factors that affect the sensitivity of sonographic evaluation, detection rates vary by the organ system involved. Anderson et al. report that up to 90% of CNS anomalies were detected, while 30–40% of cardiac and genitourinary anomalies were diagnosed, and only 20% of craniofacial anomalies were identified (Anderson et al. 1995).

A large national survey of value and benefits of routine diagnostic ultrasound in pregnancy was recently described. The RADIUS Study (routine antenatal diagnostic imaging with ultrasound) prospectively evaluated the sensitivity of screening ultrasound evaluations to detect structural fetal malformations at an amalgam of tertiary referral centers and community diagnostic centers, which voluntarily participated in the study. The study provides a reasonably accurate depiction of current sonographic capabilities as practiced on a day-to-day basis in this country, but the results were disappointing to many proponents of broadly based sonographic screening of pregnancies. Anomaly detection rates were higher in screened pregnancies, but only 35% of all anomalous fetuses were detected by screening compared with detection rates of 11% of anomalies in unscreened pregnancies. In screened infants, 71 of 232 (31%) major structural anomalies were found in screened infants, with only 35 of 232 (15%) identified before 24 weeks gestation. In unscreened pregnancies, 24 of 198 (12%) major anomalies were detected in unscreened fetuses, and only 10 of 198 (5%) were detected before 24 weeks. Diagnostic sensitivity varied substantially by organ system, ranging from high sensitivity for CNS anomalies such as anencephaly (3 of 3, 100%) and spina bifida (3 of 4, 75%) to rather low sensitivity for cardiac lesions (0 of 19 isolated atrial or ventricular septal defects and only 5 of 19 infants with complex heart disease). Tertiary diagnostic sonographic sites involved had better detection rates than lower acuity sonography sites (6.8 versus 1.7 anomalies detected per 1,000 screened infants, $P < 0.00001$) (Crane et al. 1994; Ewigman et al. 1993; LeFevre et al. 1993; DeVore 1994).

Clinical Significance of Anomalous Findings

Over the course of an ultrasonographic evaluation, numerous fetal characteristics are evaluated, both qualitatively and quantitatively. In addition to major malformations such as omphalocele and central facial or CNS anomalies, numerous minor abnormalities have been identified that occur more frequently in infants with aneuploidy than in euploid infants. These include nuchal thickness, fetal renal pyelectasis, shortened long bones, choroid plexus cysts, cranial ventriculomegaly, malposition of fingers or toes, cardiac malformations, echogenic foci within the cardiac ventricles, and increased echogenicity of the bowel. After screening for these characteristics, risk adjustment can be performed by using either the absence or presence of these characteristics. Although the negative predictive value associated with their absence has been widely used (Nyberg et al. 1995, 2001; Nyberg and Souter 2001; Vintzileos et al. 2001, 2002; Bromley et al. 2002; Benacerraf 1998), the ideal method of utilizing positive findings to adjust risk has been controversial for clinicians and confusing for some patients (Shipp et al. 2002).

It is most instructive to consider the addition of sonographic anomaly screening information to patients of two types, use of the negative predictive value of a negative study in patients with borderline or marginally increased a priori anomaly risk, and the positive predictive value of abnormal findings in patients otherwise at low risk of aneuploidy after other considerations have been accounted for.

A Priori Risk

The a priori (prescreening) risk of aneuploidy in a given patient requires individualized assessment. In patients with no familial predisposition toward aneuploidy evident after a family history is obtained, it usually consists of the age-based risk for a given chromosomal anomaly or anomalies. In cases of balanced translocations or in circumstances such as a history of prior children with trisomies occurring in younger women (recurrence risk often 1% or more), higher risks are present and are best evaluated by a clinical geneticist. With this underlying baseline risk established, serum screening for aneuploidy risk is performed (usually between 14 and 22 weeks of gestation, although earlier screening paradigms are now being implemented). A new modified risk for given anomalies is established, and patients are classified as being in increased or decreased risk groups for the clinical circumstance in question. Similar considerations must be undertaken for risk screening for open neural tube anomalies.

Although screening tests by nature may assign a bimodal result (positive or negative), determination of whether a given result and its assigned risk are high are often accepted as fact, but should more accurately be considered somewhat arbitrary. The criterion for assigning a positive or increased post-screening risk assessment for most screening tests related to aneuploidy is often related to the approximated risk of severe complications from further diagnostic procedures that might then be performed. Commonly, risks in excess of 1/200 to 1/280 are considered positive. This range of risk approximates the risk of pregnancy loss after a mid-second trimester amniocentesis (which is variously estimated to be between 1/100 and 1/300 or higher) and is similar to the likelihood of trisomy 21 or other aneuploidy during the mid-second trimester in a 35-year-old woman (approximately 1/200). Using this knowledge, clinicians may allow patients to participate in deciding whether to proceed with more invasive diagnostic procedures. Some patients may opt for more sensitive criteria (i.e., invasive testing with risks otherwise considered low or negative), while other patients may forgo investigation of risks considered elevated by usual criteria.

If a higher-morbidity invasive diagnostic evaluation such as chorionic villus sampling or percutaneous blood sampling (approximated pregnancy loss rates of 0.5–1% per procedure) is contemplated, the higher risks should be compared relative to the likelihood of detecting the anomaly in question. An extra benefit provided by invasive karyotypic diagnosis is a much more comprehensive evaluation of the fetus than a mere confirmation of a given diagnosis. Such testing occasionally may uncover other conditions that were unanticipated in the initial phases of the evaluation.

In patients with a borderline to marginally increased risk for aneuploidy, screening for multiple markers of aneuploidy has been widely advocated (Nyberg et al. 1995, 2001; Nyberg and Souter 2001; Vintzileos 2002, Bromley et al. 2002; Benacerraf 1998). Factors potentially evaluated include posterior nuchal thickening, short humerus, short femur, echogenic bowel, pyelectasis, echogenic intracardiac focus, choroid plexus cysts, hypoplastic middle phalanx of the 5th digit, wide space between great and 2nd toe, and two vessel umbilical cord. Some of these markers are bimodal (i.e., present or absent), while others such as shortened long bones require adjustment for gestational age and possibly race. It is also possible to change an analog characteristic into a bimodal marker by using a cut point defined in a way that gives diagnostic value. Examples of this include the use of discrete criteria such as nuchal fold >5 mm or femur length <91% of average for gestation (Snijders et al. 2000), or comparisons with other criteria such as BPD/FL ratio >95% (Snijders et al. 2000). It is also possible to create a marker of proportional risk by using markers such as multiples of the median, as is done with maternal serum markers for aneuploidy screening.

The various criteria must be well studied and used with a degree of caution. Factors specific to given criteria may reduce the predictive value of some screening markers, and these limitations are not necessarily obvious. In the case of shortened femur length as a marker for aneuploidy, for instance, Snijders (2000) found that a fixed cutoff of 91% of expected femur length yielded 12% false positives at 15–17 weeks and 6% at 18–20 weeks for trisomy 21 screening, with detection rates of 29% and 38%, respectively, at those two gestational age. Similarly, shortened femur length was also found to have substantial variation by maternal ethnicity [Asians on average had shorter femur lengths, and average femur lengths in whites differed significantly from those of blacks and Asians (Kovac et al. 2002)], maternal stature (short maternal stature predisposed to abnormally low BPD/FL ratios at 18–19 weeks gestation but not before that (Pierce et al. 2001)), and femur lengths measured at 15–17 weeks were predisposed to appear shortened more so than at later gestational ages (Pierce et al. 2001; Snijders 2001).

Sonographic markers of aneuploidy are believed to be relatively independent of variations in the serum markers used to screen for trisomy 21 (Souter et al. 2002), allowing these adjusted risks combined in a risk assessments with minimal concern for interaction between the two screening modalities. If all screened sonographic markers are negative, it has been estimated that the prescreening risk is decreased by half or more (Nyberg et al. 1995; Bromley et al. 2002), while the presence of any positive marker is considered to invalidate any associated risk reduction of the other negative screening parameters and may actually increase the risk of aneuploidy somewhat.

Nyberg evaluated six minor markers of aneuploidy (nuchal thickening, hyperechoic bowel, shortened femur, shortened humerus, echogenic intracardiac focus, and renal pyelectasis) and found that single isolated minor markers for aneuploidy were more likely in infants with trisomy 21(42 of 186 infants, 22.6%) than in euploid control infants (987 of 8,728, 11.3%). Although use of such information in isolation would yield unacceptably high rates of amniocentesis (11.3% screen positive rates in euploid infants) and its attendant complications, such a characteristic can be used to adjust a priori risks that have already accounted for other factors such as maternal age and adjustment for serum screening results (Nyberg 2001).

In patients with a low a priori risk of aneuploidy before sonographic screening, the best method of using sonographic information to provide more accurate risks for aneuploidy is poorly established (Winter et al. 2000). The magnitude of increased risk associated with these findings varies by the population studied, the way information was obtained, and the number of criteria evaluated. Posterior nuchal thickening has been estimated to increase the risk of trisomy 21 by 11- to 17-fold, while shortened femur increased risks by 5- to 7.5-fold and pyelectasis increased risks by 1.5- to 1.9-fold. The best way to use these findings has not been fully validated, and a substantial degree of intercorrlelation among the factors may be present. In such circumstances, direct combination of the risks will give falsely high estimates of aneuploidy risk.

Over the past 10–15 years, various scoring systems have been proposed that assign point scores to sonographic markers of aneuploidy (Winter et al. 2000). Patients with single major markers or more than one minor findings were judged at increased risk of aneuploidy and considered for invasive diagnosis. These systems were useful but did not integrate well with the method of using sequentially adjusted risks (i.e., age risk × multiplier for genetic risks × multiplier for serum screening × multiplier for sonographic risk). As a result of such problems, some patients with single abnormal findings may have been considered for invasive diagnosis because of concerns for aneuploidy. This could occur if maternal age, medical history, and serum screening gave a low risk categorization, while single isolated sonographic findings raised concerns about aneuploidy. The significance of isolated sonographic findings as predictors of aneuploidy is unclear (ACOG 2001). Recently, Smith-Bindman et al. (2001) evaluated published studies of minor aneuploidy markers and found that only nuchal thickening was found to have a positive predictive value sufficient to merit consideration of further evaluation (Nyberg 2001).

In cases of two or more risk factors, karyotypic screening is often offered in a manner consistent with the original scoring systems proposed by Benacerraf and others (Benacerraf et al. 1992, 1994; Bromley et al. 1999). The proper manner of adjusting risk for an isolated single abnormal finding and multiple normal findings is not yet well established, because the overall effect on risk of disparate markers (most negative with one positive) is unclear (ACOG 2001).

Care must also be taken to avoid falsely negative sono screening in cases with one identified anomaly. If one or more anomalies are present but not detected, falsely low risk assessments will result. For example, if choroid plexus cysts are seen in a mid-trimester sonogram in a 20-year-old woman, the risk for trisomy 18 is about 1/4,015 if no other anomalies are present, 1/341 if one other anomaly is present, and 1/6 if two or more anomalies are present. The relevant risks of trisomy 18 in a 26-year-old woman with 0, 1, and 2 or more other anomalies are 1/3,267, 1/277, and 1/5, respectively (Snijders and Nicolaides 1996). The rapid rise in estimated risks associated with multiple anomalies highlights the validity of offering invasive diagnosis in such circumstances and underscores the need to identify all potential anomalies when such patients are scanned.

Special Considerations on Early Pregnancy Sonography

Sonography in the first trimester is very helpful in identifying intrauterine pregnancies and in assessing patients at risk for ectopic pregnancy. Recent advances in prenatal diagnosis also offer the possibility of sonographic screening for nuchal thickness as a marker of aneuploidy and congenital heart abnormalities and for combined screening for aneuploidy by serum marker and nuchal thickness, as previously noted.

Critical landmarks in early pregnancy include implantation at 20 or 21 menstrual days (6 or 7 days postconception) and evidence of Beta human Chorionic Gonadotropin (BhCG) at 8–10 days after conception, and usually sooner. The first sonographic evidence of pregnancy is the presence of a 2- to 5-mm-diameter gestational sac at 4 or 5 menstrual weeks, followed by the presence of a visible fetal pole at 5 or 6 menstrual weeks, and a fetal heart beat evident at 6 weeks of gestation.

Bree et al. (1989) evaluated 53 patients with 75 transvaginal sonographic examinations. Using BhCG determinations standardized with the first international reference preparation, they observed gestational sacs in all patients with BhCG levels of 1,000 milli-international units (mIU)/mL, uniformly visualized yolk sacs at BhCG levels of 7,200 mIU/mL, and formed visible embryos with heart beats in all patients with BhCG levels of 10,800 mIU/mL or more. Similarly, Nyberg et al. (1988) reported finding evidence of an intrauterine gestational sac in 17 of 17 patients eventually found to have ongoing intrauterine gestations when BhCG levels of 1,000 mIU/mL (using the Second International Standard) were present. Recently, Barnhart et al. (2002) recommended using a threshold of 2,000 mIU/mL with no evidence of an intrauterine pregnancy by sonogram as diagnostic of the minimal likelihood for subsequent normal pregnancy. Such a recommendation, largely depends on the skill of the diagnostic sonographer and likely varies among institutions and practitioners. Instead of relying on published norms, it is preferable for institutions to evaluate their own experience and establish institution-specific BhCG cut points at which the absence of sonographic evidence of an intrauterine pregnancy will reliably exclude the subsequent presence of a gestational sac or more advanced fetal structures (Peisner and Timor-Tritsch 1990).

Such an organized plan for the evaluation of early pregnancy has become increasingly more important as sonography has taken a primary role in the management of complications of early pregnancy, and as nonsurgical therapies have become available for ectopic pregnancy. Apart from the traditional role of identifying ectopic gestations in high-risk patients (prior ectopic pregnancy or tubal surgery, vaginal bleeding, and uterine cramping combined with a positive pregnancy test) to identify candidates for surgical management, sonography is also now used to identify early ectopic gestations that may be managed nonsurgically with methotrexate. It is very important to exclude the presence of a normal intrauterine pregnancy before using methotrexate because of the devastating effects of methotrexate on the developing fetus.

The diagnostic accuracy of endovaginal sonography varies by the evaluation attempted. Enk et al. (1990) found that endovaginal sonography was 81% sensitive and 97% specific for identifying viable intrauterine pregnancies but 96% sensitive and 71% specific when determining ectopic pregnancy. If judged medically stable, patients in such circumstances often undergo serial BhCG testing and serial sonography. A doubling BhCG value over 48 hours is most consistent with a normally developing pregnancy and lesser increases or decreases indicate increased risk for either miscarriage or ectopic pregnancy (Letterie and Hibbert 2000), but neither of these tendencies is absolute and normally rising titers are not a substitute for sound clinical judgment. Some early ectopic pregnancies show normal doubling, and some normal pregnancies do not demonstrate a normal doubling pattern. The issue is further confused by various estimates of the minimum BhCG titers [usually 1,000–2,000 mIU, depending on imaging modality (Nyberg et al. 1988; Lehner et al. 2000)] at which intrauterine gestational sacs potentially can be identified. As previously noted, these estimates may not fully characterize the minimum BhCG level at which an intrauterine gestational sac will not ultimately be visualized, and institution-specific criteria may provide the best means of minimizing false diagnoses. A final element is added by the various standardizations that have been used in the literature to standardize BhCG titers, including the two methodologies previously referenced.

Unfortunately, some clinicians overestimate the ability of sonography to reliably exclude intrauterine pregnancy after BhCG has been quantitated. This may be due to confusion about what BhCG level allows such a determination to be derived from a negative sonogram. Because of poor characterization of BhCG in the literature and among practitioners, absence of a sonographic intrauterine gestational sac has been taken to represent strong evidence of an early ectopic pregnancy, without further evaluations to exclude an ongoing intrauterine pregnancy, and methotrexate therapy has been initiated. (Methotrexate is much more effective in early gestations with small gestational tissue masses and is much less effective as the tissue mass increases in size.) In this manner, some intrauterine pregnancies have been inadvertently exposed to methotrexate. To avoid such a sequence of events, care must be taken to consider emergency surgical interventions if appropriate, measure serial BhCG quantitations to evaluate for a normal increase in time, and use endovaginal sonography to assess for evidence of both an ectopic gestation and an intrauterine pregnancy. If the gestational mass appears to be increasing in size, if the serum BhCG titer is higher than about 2,500 mIU/mL, or if the tube appears to have ruptured surgery is usually required (Lehner et al. 2000).

Rarely, ectopic pregnancies may coexist with a normal intrauterine pregnancy. Heterotopic gestations occur in about 1/50,000 pregnancies. They are potentially highly morbid, because evidence of an intrauterine pregnancy will cause delay in diagnosis of the component ectopic gestation. Such a diagnosis often will be achieved only by constant vigilance on the part of the clinician.

Sonography can provide useful information about the health of early pregnancies. Healthy gestational sacs usually have a smooth contoured, round, or oval shape and often are located in the fundal or central portion of the endometrial cavity. The sac wall is echogenic and may measure 3 mm or more thick. By the time the sac diameter is greater than 10 mm in diameter, a yolk sac usually is present, while a fetal pole should be evident for sacs of >18 mm by transvaginal sonography and >30 mm in diameter by abdominal sonography

(Cacciatore 1990). Characteristics of an abnormal sac that suggest increased risk for early pregnancy failure include an irregularly shaped gestational sac, sac growth of <0.6 mm per day, no evident yolk sac for sac diameters of >8 mm, and no evident embryo with sac diameters of >18 mm. Additionally, the fetal crown-rump length is >5 mm and no heart beat is observed, fetal demise is strongly suggested.

SUMMARY OF ULTRASOUND EVALUATION IN PREGNANCY

In summary, sonography offers important diagnostic information throughout the course of pregnancy. Initial sonographic screening is not necessarily mandated in all pregnancies, but it offers potential benefit when properly performed. In certain circumstances, epidemiologic considerations, familial risk factors, results of other screening procedures, exposure to various teratogens, and threatened pregnancy complications may necessitate sonographic evaluation of the fetus and pregnancy.

Detailed sonography often is best performed at referral centers, which frequently benefit from better equipment and often are staffed with more experienced technicians and diagnosticians.

Abnormalities evaluated and treated often are best managed by a multidisciplinary group, which may include specialists from a wide range of specialties, including obstetricians/gynecologists, maternal–fetal medicine specialists, sonographers, neonatologists, pediatric cardiologists, pediatric surgeons, social workers, and pathologists.

REFERENCES

Allan L, Hornberger L, Sharland G (eds): *Textbook of Fetal Cardiology*, London, Greenwich Medical Media Unlimited, 2000.

American College of Obstetrics and Gynecology: *Practice Bulletin: Clinical Management Guidelines for Obstetrician-Gynecologists*, 27:2001.

Anderson N, Boswell O, Duff G: Prenatal sonography for the detection of fetal anomalies: results of a prospective study and comparison with previous studies. *Am J Roentgenol* 65:943, 1995.

Bahado-Singh RO, Kovanci E, Jeffres A, Oz U, Deren O, Copel J, Mari G: The Doppler cerebro placental ratio and perinatal outcome in intrauterine growth restriction. *Am J Obstet Gynecol* 180:750, 1999.

Barnhart KT, Katz I, Hummel A, Gracia CR: Presumed diagnosis of ectopic pregnancy. *Obstet Gynecol* 100(3):505, 2002.

Baschat AA, Gembruch U, Harman CR: The sequence of changes in Doppler and biophysical parameters as severe fetal growth restriction worsens. *Ultrasound Obstet Gynecol* 18:571, 2001.

Baschat AA, Gembruch U, Viscardi RM, Gortner L, Harman CR: Antenatal prediction of intraventricular hemorrhage in fetal growth restriction: what is the role of Doppler? *Ultrasound Obstet Gynecol* 19:334, 2002.

Benacerraf BR: *Ultrasound of Fetal Syndromes*, New York, Churchill Livingstone, 1998.

Benacerraf BR, Nadel A, Bromley B: Identification of second-trimester fetuses with autosomal trisomy by use of a sonographic scoring index. *Radiology* 193:135, 1994.

Benacerraf BR, Neuberg D, Bromley B, Frigoletto FD, Jr: Sonographic scoring index for prenatal detection of chromosomal abnormalities. *J Ultrasound Med* 11:449, 1992.

Berman MC, Cohen HL: *Diagnostic Medical Sonography: A Guide to Clinical Practice, Obstetrics and Gynecology*, 2nd ed, Philadelphia, Lippincott-Rowen, 1997.

Bree RL, Edwards M, Bohm-Velez M, Beyler S, Roberts J, Mendelson EB: Transvaginal sonography in the evaluation of normal early pregnancy: correlation with HCG level. AJR 153:75, 1989.

Bromley B, Lieberman E, Shipp TD, Benacerraf BR: The genetic sonogram: a method of risk assessment for Down syndrome in the second trimester. *Ultrasound Med* 21:1087, 2002.

Bromley B, Shipp T, Benacerraf BR: Genetic sonogram scoring index: accuracy and clinical utility. *J Ultrasound Med* 18:523, 1999.

Cacciatore B, Tiitnen A, Steinman UH, Ylostalo P: Normal early pregnancy serum hCG levels and vaginal ultrasongraphy findings. *Br J Obstet Gynecol* 97:899, 1990.

Callen PW: *Ultrasonography in Obstetrics and Gynecology*, 3rd ed, Philadelphia, WB Saunders, 1994.

Chervenak FA, Kurjak A, Comstock CH (eds): *Ultrasound and the Fetal Brain. Progress in Obstetrics and Gynecological Sonography Series.* New York, Parthenon Publishing Group, 1995.

Colombo DF, Iams JD: Cervical length and preterm labor. *Clin Obstet Gynecol* 43:735, 2000.

Conway DL, Adkins WB. Schroeder B, Langer O: Isolated oligohydramnios in the term pregnancy: is it a clinical entity? *J Maternal-Fetal Med* 7(4):197, 1998.

Cosmi E, Mari G, Delle Chiaie L, Detti L, Akiyama M, Murphy J, Stefos T, Ferguson JE 2nd, Hunter D, Hsu CD, Abuhamad A, Bahado-Singh R: Noninvasive diagnosis by Doppler ultrasonography of fetal anemia resulting from parvovirus infection. *Am J Obstet Gynecol* 187:1290, 2002.

Crane JP, LeFevre ML, Winborn RC, Evans JK, Ewigman BG, Bain RP, Frigoletto FD, McNellis D: A randomized trial of prenatal ultrasonographic screening: impact on the detection, management, and outcome of anomalous fetuses. The RADIUS Study Group. *Am J Obstet Gynecol* 171:392, 1994.

Detti L, Mari G, Akiyama M, Cosmi E, Moise KJ Jr, Stefor T, Conaway M, Deter R: Longitudinal assessment of the middle cerebral artery peak systolic velocity in healthy fetuses and in fetuses at risk for anemia. *Am J Obstet Gynecol* 187:937, 2002.

DeVore GR. The routine antenatal diagnostic imaging with ultrasound study: another perspective. *Obstet Gynecol* 84(4):622, 1994.

Divon MY, Ferber A: Umbilical artery Doppler velocimetry – an update. *Semina Perinatol* 25:44, 2001.

Dooley SL. Routine ultrasound in pregnancy. *Clin Obstet Gynecol* 42:737, 1999.

Enk L, Wieland M, Hammarberg K, Lindblom B: The value of endovaginal sonography and urinary human chorionic gonadotropin tests for differentiation between intrauterine and ectopic pregnancy. *Clin Ultrasound* 18:73, 1990.

Ewigman BG, Crane JP, Frigoletto FD, LeFevre ML, Bain RP, McNellis D: Effect of prenatal ultrasound screening on perinatal outcome. The RADIUS Study Group. *N Engl J Med* 329(12):821, 1993.

Fleischer AC, Romero R, Manning FA, et al.: *The Principles and Practice of Ultrasonography in Obstetrics and Gynecology*, 4th ed, Norwalk, CT, Appleton & Lange, 1991.

Hedrick WR, Hykes DL, Starchman DE: *Ultrasound Physics and Instrumentation*, 3rd ed, St. Louis, Mosby-Year Book, 1995.

Hickey J, Goldberg F: *Ultrasound Review of Obstetrics and Gynecology*, Philadelphia, Lippincott-Raven, 1996.

Harger JH: Cerclage and cervical insufficiency: an evidence-based analysis. *Obstet Gynecol* 100:1313, 2002.

Harrington K, Thompson MO, Carpenter RG, Nguyen M, Campbell S: Doppler fetal circulation in pregnancies complicated by pre-eclampsia or delivery of a small for gestational age baby: 2. Longitudinal analysis. *Br J Obstet Gynecol* 106:453, 1999.

Hofstaetter C, Gudmundsson S, Hansmann M: Venous Doppler velocimetry in the surveillance of severely compromised fetuses. *Ultrasound Obstet Gynecol* 20:233, 2002.

Iams JD, Goldenberg RL, Meis PJ, et al.: The length of the cervix and the risk of spontaneous premature delivery. *N Engl J Med* 334:567, 1996.

Kovac CM, Brown JA, Apodaca CC, Napolitano PG, Pierce B, Patience T, Hume RF Jr, Calhoun BC: Maternal ethnicity and variation of fetal femur length calculations when screening for Down syndrome. *J Ultrasound Med* 21:719, 2002.

Krebs CA, Giyanani VL, Eisenberg RL: *Ultrasound Atlas of Disease Processes*, Norwalk, CT: Appleton & Lange, 1993.

Kreiser D, el-Sayed YY, Sorem KA, Chitkara U, Holbrook RH Jr, Druzin ML: Decreased amniotic fluid index in low-risk pregnancy. *J Reprod Med* 46:743, 2001.

LeFevre ML, Bain RP, Ewigman BG, Frigoletto FD, Crane JP and McNellis D: A randomized trial of prenatal ultrasonographic screening: impact on maternal management and outcome. The RADIUS (Routine Antenatal Diagnostic Imaging with Ultrasound) Study Group. *Am J Obstet Gynecol* 169(3):483, 1993.

Lehner R, Kucera E, Jirecek S, Egarter C, Husslein P: Ectopic pregnancy. *Arch of Gynecol Obstet* 263:87, 2000.

Lencioni R, Cioni D, Bartolozzi C: Tissue harmonic and contrast-specific imaging: back to gray scale in ultrasound. *Euro Radiol* 12:151, 2002.

Letterie GS, Hibbert M: Serial serum human chorionic gonadotropin (hCG) levels in ectopic pregnancy and first trimester miscarriage. *Arch Gynecol Obstet* 263:168, 2000.

Madazli R, Uluda S, Ocak V: Doppler assessment of umbilical artery, thoracic aorta and middle cerebral artery in the management of pregnancies with growth restriction. *Acta Obstet Gynecol Scand* 80:702, 2001.

Manning FA, Platt LD, Sipos L: Antepartum fetal evaluation: development of a fetal biophysical profile. *Am J Obstet Gynecol* 136:787, 1980.

Manning FA: Fetal biophysical profile: a critical appraisal. *Clin Obstet Gynecol* 45:975, 2002.

Manning FA: Fetal biophysical profile. *Obstet Gynecol Clin North Am* 26:557, 1999.

Manning FA, Morrison I, Lange IR, Harman CR, Chamberlain PF: Fetal assessment based on fetal biophysical profile scoring: experience in 12,620 referred high-risk pregnancies. I. Perinatal mortality by frequency and etiology. *Am J Obstet Gynecol* 151:343, 1985.

Mari G, Detti L, Oz U, Zimmerman R, Duerig P, Stefos T: Accurate prediction of fetal hemoglobin by Doppler ultrasonography. *Obstet Gynecol* 99:589, 2002.

McGahan JP, Porto M: *Diagnostic Obstetrical Ultrasound*, Philadelphia, Lippincott, 1994.

Moore TR, Cayle JE: The amniotic fluid index in normal human pregnancy. *Am J Obstet Gynecol* 162:1168, 1990.

Muller T, Nanan R, Rehn M, Kristen P, Dietl J: Arterial and ductus venosus Doppler in fetuses with absent or reverse end-diastolic flow in the umbilical artery: correlation with short-term perinatal outcome. *Acta Obstet Gynecol Scand* 81:860, 2002.

Nyberg DA, Mack LA, Laing FC, Jeffrey RB: Early pregnancy complications: endovaginal sonographic findings correlated with human chorionic gonadotropin levels. *Radiology* 167:619, 1988.

Nyberg DA, Luthy DA, Cheng EY, Sheley RC, Resta RG, Williams MA: Role of prenatal ultrasonography in women with positive screen for Down syndrome on the basis of maternal serum markers. *Am J Obstet Gynecol* 173:1030, 1995.

Nyberg DA: Ultrasound markers of fetal Down syndrome. *JAMA* 285:2856, 2001.

Nyberg DA, Souter VL, El-Bastawissi A, Young S, Luthhardt F, and Luthy DA: Isolated sonographic markers for detection of fetal Down syndrome in the second trimester of pregnancy. *J Ultrasound Med* 20:1053, 2001.

Nyberg DA, Souter VL: Sonographic markers of fetal trisomies: second trimester. *J Ultrasound Med* 20:655, 2001.

Peisner DB, Timor-Tritsch IE: The discriminatory zone of beta-hCG for vaginal probes. *J Clin Ultrasound* 18:280, 1990.

Pierce BT, Hancock EG, Kovac CM, Napolitano PG, Hume RF Jr, Calhoun BC: Influence of gestational age and maternal height on fetal femur length calculations. *Obstet Gynecol* 97:742, 2001.

Seeds JW: The routine or screening obstetrical ultrasound examination. *Clin Obstet Gynecol* 39:814, 1996.

Sherer DM: A review of amniotic fluid dynamics and the enigma of isolated oligohydramnios. *Am J Perinatol* 19:254, 2002.

Shipp TD, Benacerraf BR: Second trimester ultrasound screening for chromosomal abnormalities. *Prenatal Diagnosis* 22:296, 2002.

Smith-Bindman R, Hosmer W, Feldstein VA, Deeks JJ, Goldberg JD: Second-trimester ultrasound to detect fetuses with Down syndrome: a meta-analysis. *JAMA* 285:1044, 2001.

Snijders RJM, Nicolaides KH: *Ultrasound Markers for Fetal Chromosomal Defects. Frontiers in Fetal Medicine*, New York, Parthenon Press, 1996.

Snijders RJ, Platt LD, Greene N, Carlson D, Krakow D, Gregory K, Bradley K: Femur length and trisomy 21: impact of gestational age on screening efficiency. *Ultrasound Obstet Gynecol* 16:142, 2000.

Souter V, Nyberg DA, El-Bastawissi A, Zebelman A, Luthhardt F, Luthy DA: Correlation of ultrasound findings and biochemical markers in the second trimester of pregnancy in fetuses with trisomy 21. *Prenatal Diagnosis* 22:175, 2002.

Stefos T, Cosmi E, Detti L, Mari G: Correction of fetal anemia on the middle cerebral artery peak systolic velocity. *Obstet Gynecol* 99:211, 2002.

Sterne G, Shields LE, Dubinsky TJ: Abnormal fetal cerebral and umbilical Doppler measurements in fetuses with intrauterine growth restriction predicts the severity of perinatal morbidity. *J Clin Ultrasound* 29:146, 2001.

Timor-Tritsch IE, Monteagudo A, Cohen HL (eds): *Ultrasonography of the Prenatal and Neonatal Brain*, Stamford, Appleton and Lange, 1996.

Vintzileos AM, Guzman ER, Smulian JC, Yeo L, Scorza WE, Knuppel RA: Down syndrome risk estimation after normal genetic sonography. *Am J Obstet Gynecol* 187:1226, 2002.

Vintzileos AM, Guzman ER, Smulian JC, Yeo L, Scorza WE, Knuppel RA: Second-trimester genetic sonography in patients with advanced maternal age and normal triple screen. *Obstet Gynecol* 99:993, 2002.

Westergaard HB, Langhoff-Roos J, Lingman G, Marsal K, Kreiner S: A critical appraisal of the use of umbilical artery Doppler ultrasound in high-risk pregnancies: use of meta-analyses in evidence-based obstetrics. *Ultrasound Obstet Gynecol* 17:466, 2001.

Winter TC, Uhrich SB, Souter VL, Nyberg DA: The "genetic sonogram": comparison of the index scoring system with the age-adjusted US risk assessment. *Radiology* 215:775, 2000.

Part II. Major Organ System Malformations

Mark Williams and Kathy B. Porter

Obstetric ultrasonography is widely used for both general screening for underlying anomalies in low-risk infants and for detailed screening of suspected abnormalities. One principle goal is to identify conditions that present opportunities to improve the fetal outcome, such as in fetal growth restriction or obstructive uropathy, or that present high risk for adverse fetal outcomes. To achieve these goals, it is necessary to understand how various combinations of sonographic findings may suggest syndromic fetal abnormalities.

To identify the forms of aneuploidy least compatible with life, it is important to be aware of findings that are characteristic of these syndromes. Infants with trisomy 13 often have structural, such as cardiac, anomalies, midline facial anomalies, microcephaly, holoprosencephaly, polydactyly, rocker-bottom feet, and single umbilical artery. In cases of trisomy 18, structural cardiac anomalies, growth retardation, cleft lip, single umbilical artery, cystic hygroma, hydrocephaly, overlapping fingers, and rocker-bottom feet are often observed. Infants with polyploidy often experience severe early-onset asymmetric growth retardation, molar degeneration of the placenta, cardiac anomalies, central nervous system defects, and oligohydramnios; they may present with early onset severe preeclampsia. These syndromes are associated with high prevalence rates (often 20–30%) for the major structural anomalies listed, and they often have multiple structural anomalies. As a result, such infants often are identified by abnormal sonographic findings, and, in common with low baseline prevalence rates, a normal screening sonogram makes such syndromes very unlikely in a given fetus.

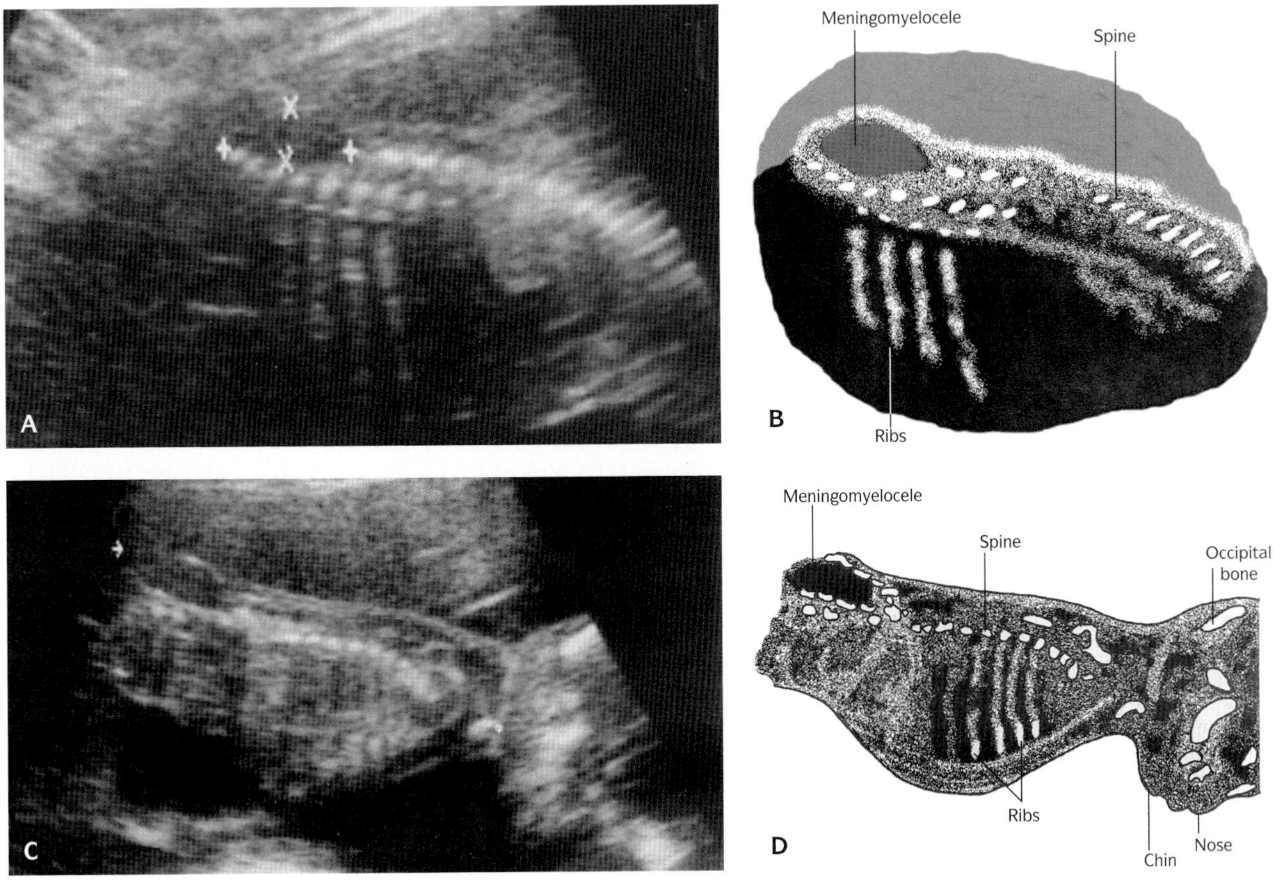

4.11. **(A)** Sagittal image: calipers delineate a myelomeningocele. **(B)** Schematic. (open neural tube defect) at the lumbosacral area of the spine. **(C)** Sagittal image: a myelomeningocele at the lumbosacral area of the spine (arrow). **(D)** Schematic.

Certain major structural malformations and findings place the fetus at very high risk for aneuploidy. These include CNS anomalies such as cystic hygroma (60–75%), hydrops (30–80%), and holoprosencephaly (40–60%); cardiac structural anomalies (5–30%); abdominal abnormalities such as diaphragmatic hernia (20–25%), omphalocele (30–40%); duodenal atresia (20–30%); and bladder outlet obstruction (20–25%) (ACOG 2001). Early diagnosis of such conditions allows assessment of the fetal karyotype and offers important help in managing the ongoing pregnancy, especially if a highly morbid karyotype is identified. When a condition with an extremely poor prognosis is identified, such as trisomy 13 or 18, pregnancy termination may be considered, or cesarean section at term for fetal distress may be avoided (as it will offer little benefit to the fetus and significant potential morbidity to the mother).

If screening for fetal structural anomalies is elected, it is generally most efficient to do an initial, broad assessment of fetal anatomy, and then pursue any further anomalous findings that may have been uncovered. The following sections describe differential diagnostic considerations for various fetal anomalies that may be encountered.

ULTRASONOGRAPHY OF THE HEAD AND NECK

Standard images of the head and spine include a cross-sectional image of the head and posterior fossa, and images of the spine in longitudinal and (multiple) transverse planes. The standard cross-sectional view of the head is obtained in a generally axial orientation and provides measures of the head circumference (HC) and biparietal diameter (BPD). The image is obtained in a plane showing the medial walls of the cerebral lateral ventricles, the cavum septum pellucida, and the thalamic nuclei. Sometimes the middle cerebral artery can be seen to pulsate. This image should be evaluated for discontinuities as might be seen with encephaloceles, bi-fronto-temporal narrowing (an abnormality termed a "lemon sign" because it gives the calvaria a cross-sectional appearance reminiscent of a lemon), which is often associated with open neural tube abnormalities (ONTDs), or other abnormal shape characteristics suggestive of other disorders (see below).

Basic evaluation of the head usually includes a brief evaluation of head shape and of the symmetry of intracranial structures, ensuring that no shift of midline structures is present. The lateral ventricles, thalami, and other midline structures should be observed. Views of the face, with attention to the mouth and palate (if possible), may be obtained and the posterior fossa evaluated. The cervical spinal area may then be observed. If other abnormalities are noted on the sonogram, care should be taken to evaluate organ systems that might result in the abnormal findings noted. Polyhydramnios, for example, might prompt further evaluation of the tracheo-esophageal disorders or bowel atresias.

As previously noted, cerebral structures should be assessed for symmetry and shift of midline CNS structures. If the ventricles and CNS structures are not symmetric within the calvaria, verify that a proper scanning plane has been obtained (Figure 4.12A). Assuming proper imaging orientation, shifts of midline structures suggest a local mass effect, perhaps from isolated ventriculomegaly.

Lateral ventricular diameters greater than 8 mm at 15–24 weeks and greater than 10 mm at 25 weeks or more are uncommon (Farrell et al. 1994). The cerebral ventricles normally do not exceed 10 or 11 mm in diameter, and values in excess of 11 mm usually indicate ventriculomegaly (Pretorius et al. 1985). The proportionality between the lateral ventricles and the hemispheric diameter can also be used to help identify abnormal ventricular dilation. Ventricle/hemisphere ratios vary by gestational age, ranging (± 2 standard deviations) from 0.45 to 0.69 at 16 weeks to from 0.22 to 0.37 at 22 weeks of gestation or thereafter (Johnson et al. 1983).

It is possible for normal brain tissue to give the appearance of ventriculomegaly (pseudoventriculomegaly) if there is sonographic dropoff (poor acoustic return) posterior to the distal ventricular wall margin. This acoustic loss may give the false impression of excessive ventricular diameter and an abnormally large ventricle. A means of confirming ventriculomegaly involves

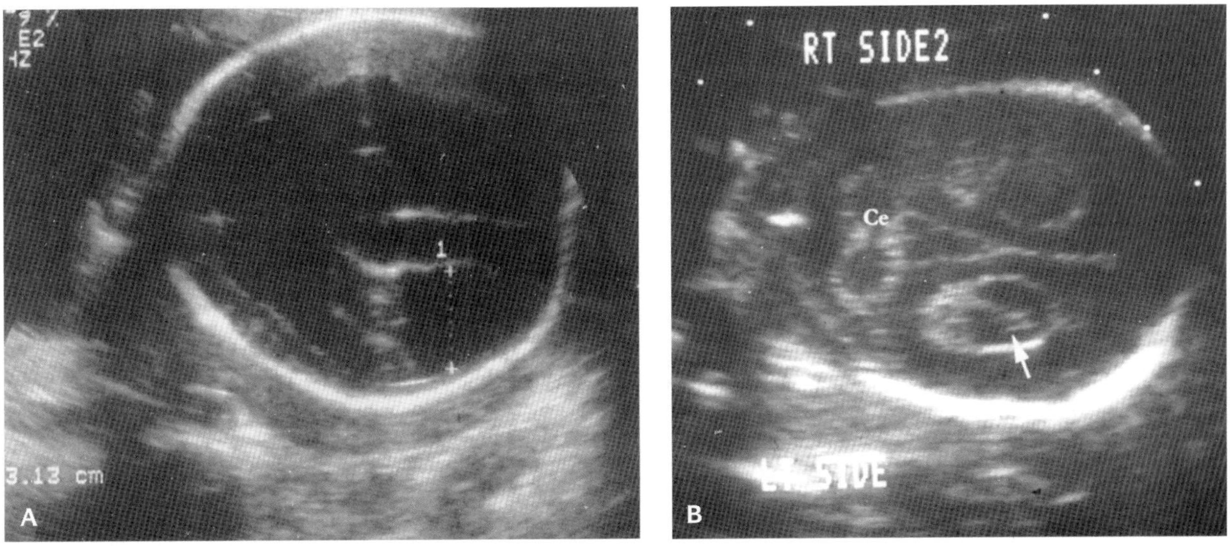

4.12. **(A)** Axial image of ventriculomegaly. Note the atrium, which measures 3.13 cm and is above normal limits. **(B)** Sagittal image of mild hydrocephalus showing dangling choroid plexus (arrow) (Ce = cerebellum).

observation of the choroid plexus, a vascular structure found within the lateral cerebral ventricles. The choroids fill the ventricles until 16–18 weeks gestation, gradually occupy a smaller proportion as pregnancy proceeds, and usually are oriented relatively parallel to the long dimension of the ventricle. They are never normally oriented at acute angles or perpendicular to the ventricle, and a dangling choroid crossing most of the width of the ventricle strongly suggests ventriculomegaly (Figure 4.12B).

If ventriculomegaly is identified, the fetus should be evaluated for other structural abnormalities, which are found in 70–85% of fetuses with ventriculomegaly. These include CNS abnormalities in 50–60%, and extra-CNS anomalies involving the heart, thorax, kidneys, face, ventral abdominal wall, and extremities. Aneuploidy is found in 2% of infants with isolated ventriculomegaly and in 17% if one or more other structural abnormalities are present.

Ventriculomegaly occurs in 9–18% of infants with trisomy 21, 18, 13, fragile X, and triploid infants. It is associated with a variety of syndromes, including neural tube defects (spina bifida and Arnold-Chiari II malformation); CNS anomalies such as Dandy-Walker malformation, agenesis of the corpus callosum, and lissencephaly; aqueductal stenosis (X linked recessive, autosomal, sporadic, postinflammatory); inherited syndromes including Meckel-Gruber, Apert syndrome, nasal-facial-digital syndrome, Robert syndrome, and Walker-Warburg syndrome); various chondrodystrophies (achondroplasia, osteogenesis imperfecta, thanatophoric dysplasia); and conditions that result in obstructed flow within the cerebral ventricles after infection, hemorrhage, or other inflammatory states. It is important to note that, although most causes of ventricular dilation in pregnancy cannot be treated until after delivery, toxoplasmosis is an exception. Toxoplasmosis may present with ventriculomegaly and is sometimes treatable in utero with potential salvage of fetal neurologic development. Evaluation usually consists of a search for infectious etiologies such as TORCH infections and consideration of karyotypic evaluation. If patients are unwilling to risk pregnancy loss by amniocentesis before 24 weeks gestation, later amniocentesis at about 34 weeks gestation should be considered. Amniocentesis at this time risks only preterm emergency delivery, will usually allow chromosomal determination in time to optimize delivery management, and may facilitate management of the neonate after birth.

The choroid plexuses normally have a rather homogenous appearance. Choroid plexus cysts are found in 0.7–1% of patients in the late second trimester. Choroid cysts appear as single or multiple 2- to 5-mm cysts and may be unilateral or bilateral. They are a normal variant but also occur much more often in aneuploid fetuses. As a result, they constitute a potential marker for increased aneuploidy risk. This is especially true if any other sonographic abnormalities are noted. Choroid cysts resolve in 90% of patients by 26–28 weeks gestation regardless of karyotype, and their resolution does not indicate any decreased association with aneuploidy. Aneuploid karyotypes have been reported in 8% of infants with choroid cysts (1% aneuploidy in cases of isolated cysts but 46% aneuploidy if other anomalies are present). Choroid cysts occur in 47% of infants with trisomy 18, and with lesser frequency in trisomy 21 (8%) and trisomy 13 (2%).

As isolated abnormalities, the risk of trisomy 18 for choroid cysts does not exceed 1/280 until the maternal age is 40 or greater (the risk at age 40 is 1/238). If any other single abnormality is identified, the risk for trisomy 18 is 1/277 in women 26 years of age, but the risk of trisomy 18 is 1/6 in women 20 years old if two or more abnormalities are present (Snijders 1996). Counseling for patients with fetal choroid cysts varies by maternal age and the ability to accurately detect other sonographic findings.

As previously noted, the risk of aneuploidy rises precipitously if other anomalies are present. The potential for falsely low risk assessments due to false-negative sonographic screening should be discussed with patients during the process of their evaluation. Because of problems with ascertainment of structural anomalies in many community sonographic sites documented by the RADIUS study (see the discussion of the RADIUS findings in Part I of this chapter, page 91), follow-up targeted evaluation in circumstances such as these should be performed by sonographers and physicians experienced in such evaluations.

The most common additional findings in trisomy 18 are ventricular septal defects and abnormalities of the extremities, which may be subtle and difficult to detect. Proper risk assessment for the risk of aneuploidy in the presence of choroid cysts is highly dependent on the degree of skill of the sonographer and, to a certain degree, on advantageous fetal positioning and imaging

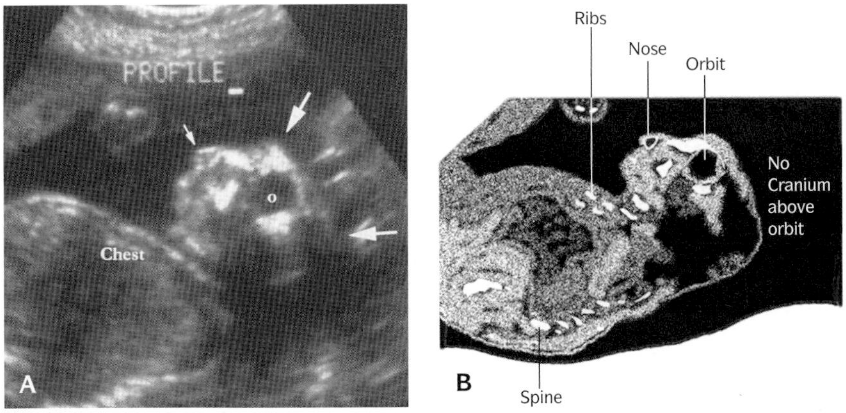

4.13. **(A)** Sagittal image of an anencephalic fetus with no cranium or ossification beyond the orbit (large arrows) (O = orbit, small arrow-nose). **(B)** Schematic.

opportunities. In cases of isolated choroid plexus cysts, amniocentesis has variously been recommended as a consideration for women 32 years and older (Gupta et al. 1997), or in women 35 years or older at the time of delivery (Brown et al. 1999; Sullivan et al. 1999).

Numerous other abnormalities may be uncovered by sonographic evaluation of the head and CNS structures. Anencephaly (Figure 4.13) results from a defect in the closure of the neural groove, which is usually complete by 28 days of gestation and may not be evident on sonograms performed before 9 or 10 weeks gestation. Anencephaly should be suspected if images of the fetus show it to be closely approximated to the uterine wall and clear views of the head above the level of the lower and central face and orbits cannot be obtained. It should also be considered if maternal α-fetoprotein levels are very elevated when screened at 14–22 weeks gestation.

Cephaloceles (encephaloceles, meningoceles) (Figure 4.14) represent a protrusion of cerebral structures outside the cranium and occur in 1/2,000 live births. Isolated protrusion of only meningeal structures is termed meningocele, while involvement or the encephalon as well is termed encephalocele. Anterior

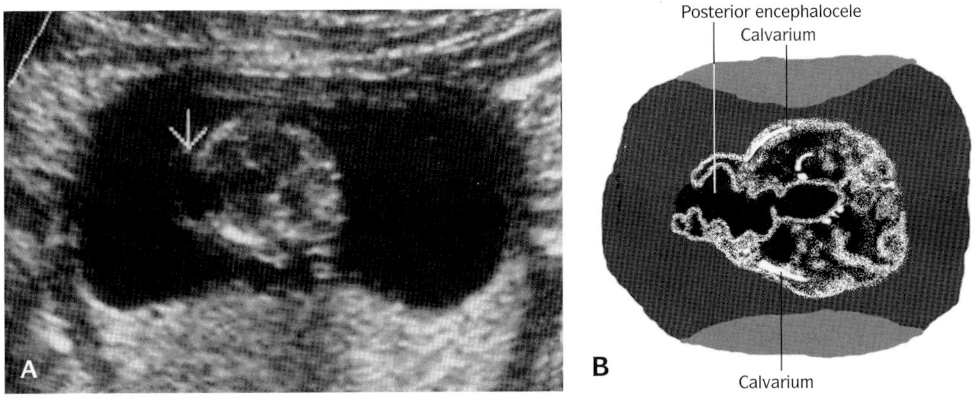

4.14. **(A)** Axial image of a posterior encephalocele (arrow). **(B)** Schematic.

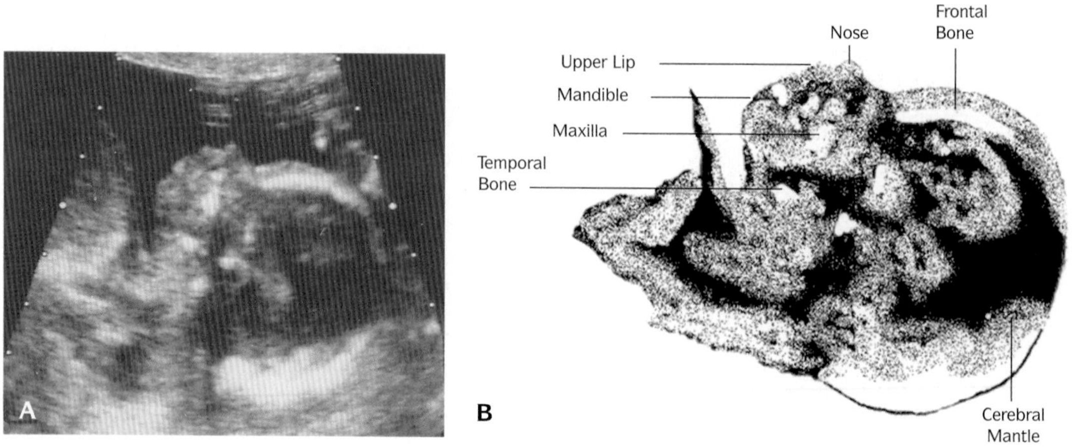

4.15. **(A)** Sagittal image of the fetal profile at 19 weeks. **(B)** Schematic.

cephaloceles occur more often in Asian patients (75%), while occipital lesions predominate in the Western world.

Cephaloceles usually result from failure of closure of the rostral end of the neural tube during the fourth week of gestation but may also result from disruption by amniotic bands, or as a component of autosomal recessive conditions such as Meckel-Gruber, Robert, Chemke-Knoblock, cryptophthalmus syndromes, and in dyssegmental dwarfism. They are usually located in the midline anteriorly or posteriorly, although those associated with amniotic bands may be asymmetric and occur in atypical locations. Posterior encephaloceles sometimes present as masses in the posterior neck and should be distinguished from cystic hygroma and meningocele in the neck.

Evaluation of the face in coronal and sagittal planes aids in evaluation of encephaloceles and oral clefts (Figures 4.15 and 4.16) On occasion, frontal cephaloceles may not be evident in the normally obtained images. Occipital cephaloceles often are not easily seen on views of the cerebral cross section but may be detected when the posterior fossa is evaluated. Temporal bulging of cranial structures found in the cloverleaf skull of thanatophoric dysplasia has been falsely diagnosed as an encephalocele.

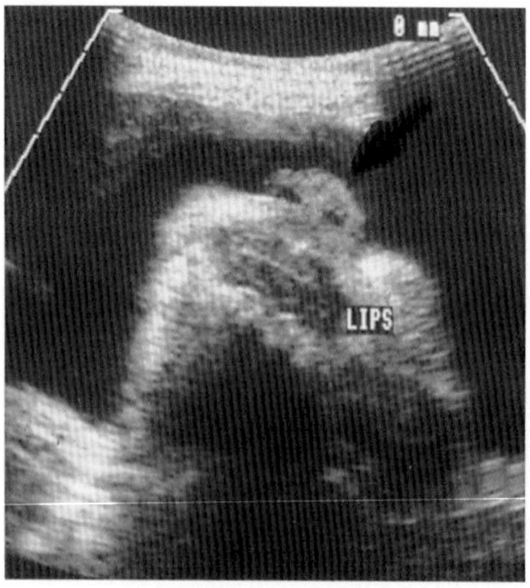

4.16. Coronal image of fetal lips and nose (arrow). Nostrils can be visualized just above the lips.

Cephaloceles are often accompanied by hydrocephaly (seen in 60–80% of posterior lesions and 20% of anterior lesions) or spina bifida (present in 15% of cases). The prognosis depends on the presence and quantity of brain outside the cranium. Almost 50% of infants with isolated meningoceles have normal development after surgical repair of their defects, while fetuses with large amounts of brain protruding out of the skull have a very poor prognosis. Delivery by cesarean section should be considered for anomalies sufficiently large and solid enough to cause dystocia, when indications relating to maternal health or another (twin) fetus are present, or if an isolated cephalocele is present and it is believed that minimization of birth trauma may improve neonatal outcome.

Holoprosencephaly encompasses a group of disorders that result from abnormal differentiation of the prosencephalon (forebrain) into the cerebral hemispheres and lateral ventricles. It is present in 1/5,000 to 1/16,000 liveborn infants and in up to 1/250 conceptuses. The three most common forms are alobar, semilobar, and lobar. Holoprosencephaly often is found in association with hydrocephaly or in combination with severe distortions of the overall cerebral sonographic architecture or with structural facial abnormalities. Holoprosencephaly is common (present in up to 50%) in fetuses with karyotypic abnormalities such as trisomy 13, trisomy 18, triploidy, 13q-, and 18p-. Aneuploidy is found in 4% of cases of isolated holoprosencephaly but in 39% of cases if other abnormalities are present. Holoprosencephaly is present in 39% of infants with trisomy 13 and in 3% of infants with trisomy 18. It occurs more often in cases of maternal diabetes (a 200-fold increased risk) and is also a commonly observed feature of numerous syndromes, including Pallister-Hall syndrome, Kallman syndrome, Meckel-Gruber syndrome, Vasadi syndrome, and camptomelic dysplasia. The prognosis for alobar and semilobar holoprosencephaly is very poor, as most infants die at birth or within 1 year of life. If a prior infant had holoprosencephaly unrelated to karyotypic abnormalities, the estimated recurrence rate is 6%, although some families appear to exhibit either autosomal recessive (25% recurrence) or dominant (50%) inheritance.

The shape of the skull may offer important clues about underlying fetal disorders. Some fetuses display a cross-sectional skull shape reminiscent of a lemon (the lemon sign), which results from bilateral frontoparietal narrowing of the skull. This finding is closely associated with open neural tube disorders. When present, such findings suggest a thorough evaluation for open neural tube defects.

Fetuses with excessively round skull morphology, brachycephaly, are at increased risk of trisomy 21. Twenty percent of trisomy 21 infants have fronto thalamic/BPD ratios less than the 5th percentile due to the decreased growth of the frontal lobes. Fetuses with skulls having a clover-leaf shape (kleeblattschädel) should have careful assessment of long bone structure because of the strong association of this finding with thanatophoric dysplasia.

Hypoplasia of the facial bones may result in proportionately narrowed anterior skull dimensions, giving the skull a strawberry shaped appearance (strawberry skull). Strawberry skull deformity is strongly associated with aneuploidy. Nicolaides et al. (1992) found 81% of infants with strawberry skull had karyotypic abnormalities, most often trisomy 18.

Although fetuses with head circumferences less than the 10th centile usually have excellent outcomes, those with more severe restriction of head size, microcephaly, do not. Microcepahaly is strongly associated with adverse neonatal outcomes and is a clinically useful marker for underlying aneuploidy, hereditary conditions, in utero infection, teratogen exposure, and radiation injury. Various criteria have been offered to characterize microcephaly, including head circumference $<$ 5th centile, biparietal diameter $<$ the 1st centile, and head

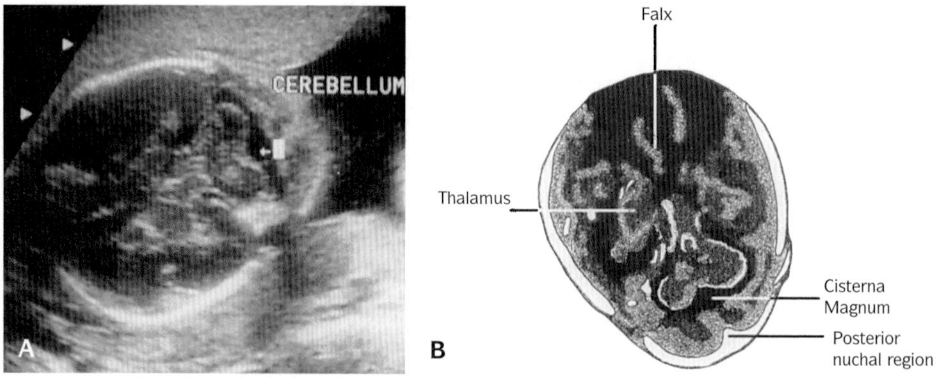

4.17. (A) Axial image of the cerebellum (arrow). **(B)** Schematic.

circumference/femur length ratios < 2.5th centile for gestation in infants with otherwise normal growth of the abdomen and femur. It may not be evident until the third trimester. Twenty percent of microcephalic fetuses have karyotypic abnormalities and trisomy 13 is the most common chromosomal abnormality found.

The posterior fossa view offers a cross-sectional assessment of the cisterna magna, cerebellum, and the posterior nuchal fold, which can be measured from this plane (Figure 4.17). It is obtained at a 30°–45° angle from the plane used for the BPD view. Characteristic findings include a cisterna magna, with an average depth of 5 mm (Figure 4.18). The plane of imaging is highly angle dependent, and improper tangential images may yield falsely elevated cisterna depths of 13 mm or more. The cerebellum can be nicely visualized and the nuchal thickness measured in this same plane.

The cisterna magna ranges from 1 to 10 mm in depth over gestational age from 15 to 36 weeks and from 4 to 10 mm at term. Decreased cisterna magna depths may result from herniation of the brainstem down the spinal canal, which may occur in association with neural tube abnormalities. Cisterna magna depths of less than 3 or 4 mm suggest the possibility of open neural tube defects

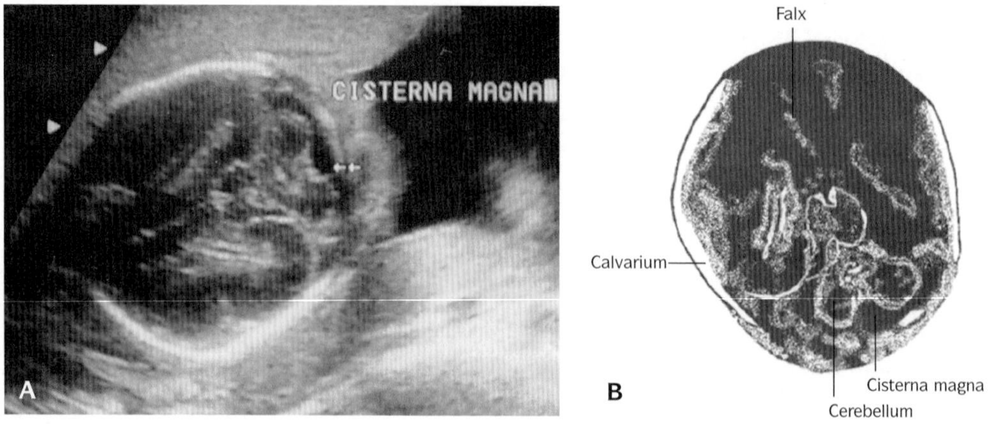

4.18. (A) Axial image of the cisterna magna (double arrows). **(B)** Schematic.

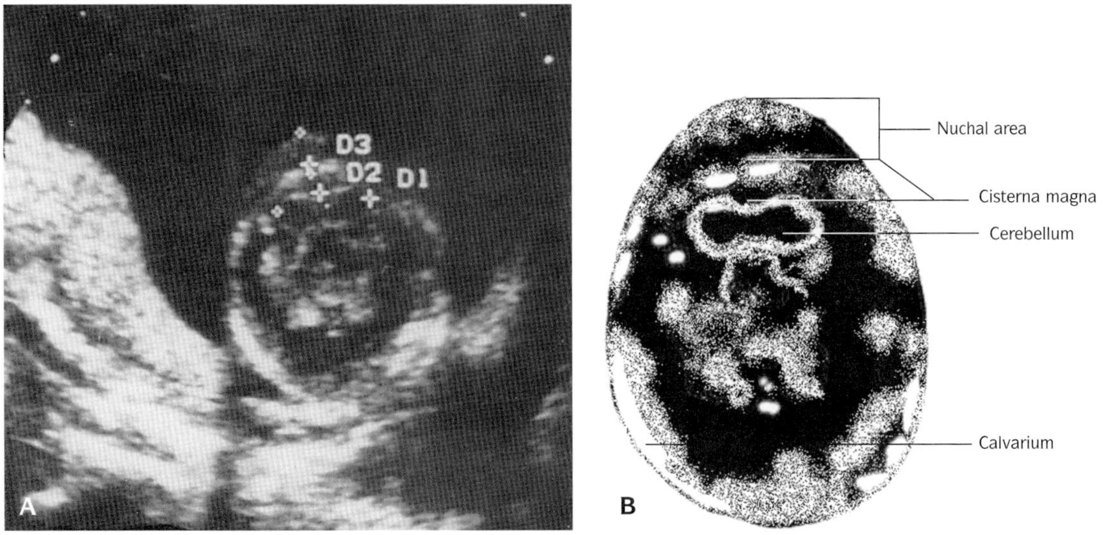

4.19. **(A)** Axial image at 19 weeks indicates measurements of the cerebellum (D1), cisterna magna (D2), nuchal area (D3). **(B)** Schematic.

(ONTD), especially if the cerebellum (see below) appears fused with a shape similar to a banana (the banana sign) (Figure 4.20). Cerebellar abnormalities are found in 95% of cases of ONTD. Banana sign cerebellar deformities are present in 70% of infants before 24 weeks gestation with ONTD but in only 17% of infants at later gestational ages. Unfortunately, although cerebellar abnormalities are highly predictive of ONTD, the cerebellum can not be visualized in 27% of infants before 24 weeks and often is not adequately available for imaging at later gestational ages.

Cisterna magna depths > 11 mm in rare cases may be a normal variant and sometimes result from inappropriate imaging with excessive angulation of the ultrasound imaging plane. When observed, the CNS structures also should be

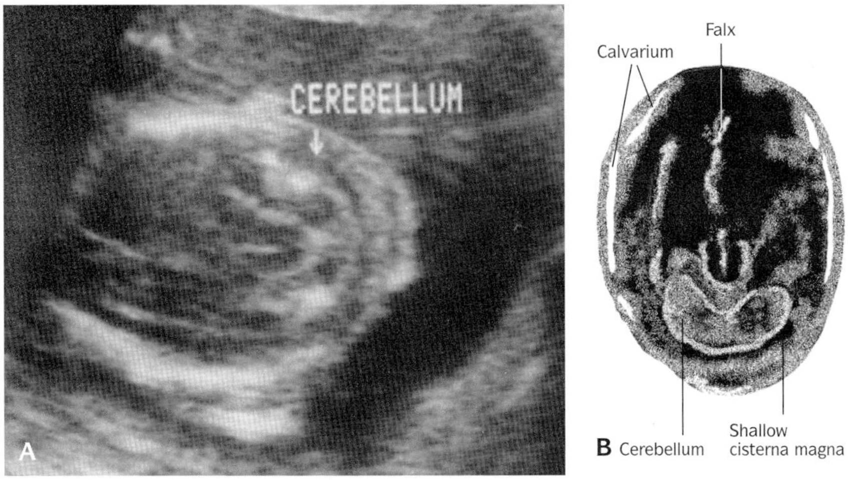

4.20. **(A and B)**. Axial image: banana sign – cerebellum (arrow).

evaluated for evidence of other posterior fossa abnormalities such as Arnold Chiari malformations, Dandy-Walker malformations, and aneuploidy. Forty percent of fetuses with excessively deep cisterna magna have been found to be aneuploid (most with trisomy 18). Posterior fossa cysts are present in 10% of infants with trisomy 18, 15% of those with trisomy 13, 1% of those with trisomy 21, and in 6% of infants with triploidy.

The cerebellum normally has a bilobed or dumb-bell shaped appearance, but in cases of neural tube abnormalities, it may assume a fused appearance similar in shape to a banana (the banana sign). Cerebellar transverse diameter varies with gestational age and can be affected by fetal growth retardation. The cerebellar vermis can also be viewed in a similar imaging plane but may not be easily imaged in many patients.

Dandy-Walker malformations are characterized by partial or complete absence of the cerebellar vermis and a characteristic cystic dilation of the fourth ventricle often accompanied by hydrocephaly. The Dandy-Walker anomaly is associated with a variety of underlying conditions, including autosomal recessive conditions such as Aicardi syndrome, Meckel-Gruber syndrome, Walker-Warburg syndrome; aneuploidy (trisomy 18); infections such as toxoplasmosis, cytomegalovirus, and rubella; maternal diabetes, exposure to compounds such as coumadin and ethanol, agenesis of the corpus callosum, porencephaly, and schizencephaly.

Increased nuchal thickness is an important marker of aneuploidy and is perhaps the only commonly observed minor sonographic finding with a positive predictive value high enough to independently indicate consideration of fetal karyotypic evaluation (Smith-Bindman 2001), although this is analysis has been widely debated (Nyberg 2001). In the second and third trimesters, the nuchal fold is best measured in the same plane used to evaluate the posterior fossa. Care must be taken to obtain an optimal imaging plane, because estimates of the nuchal fold width and cisterna magna depth vary widely if inaccurate images are created. Inadequate angulation relative to the axial plane will result in falsely low estimates of these characteristics, while excessive angulation will result in falsely large estimations. In practice, the best estimates of these parameters will be obtained from images that optimally image the cerebellum.

Nuchal thickness greater than 6 mm at 15–23 weeks gestation are associated with trisomy 21 and other aneuploidies and are also associated with increased risk for cardiovascular malformations (Bahado-Singh et al. 2002). Upper normal range values (5.0–5.9 mm) may also be at increased risk of aneuploidy, especially if other risk factors such as advanced maternal age or borderline abnormal antenatal serum screening risk for trisomy 21 are present. Unfortunately (for purposes of aneuploidy screening), nuchal thickness gradually increases over this range of gestational ages in normal pregnancies. (A nuchal thickness of 6 mm is more closely associated with aneuploidy at 15 weeks than at 23 weeks gestation.) To improve the predictive value of nuchal thickness, various investigators have attempted to normalize this characteristic for

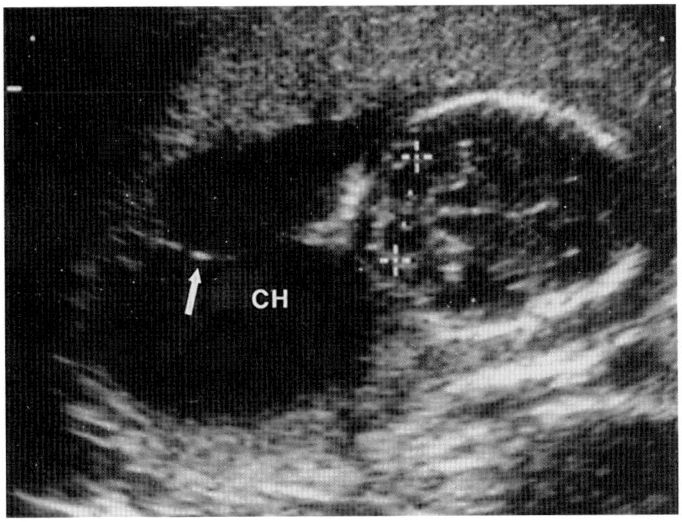

4.21. Axial image: cystic hygroma (CH) with septation (arrow). Calipers mark the cerebellum.

gestational age by establishing gestational age specific tables for multiples of median nuchal thickness for gestational age (Bahado-Singh et al. 1999), or by identifying biological correlates to compare with, such as the ratio of nuchal fold width to humerus length (Bahado-Singh et al. 2001).

In the first trimester, increased nuchal thickness is also correlated with both aneuploidy and congenital heart disease. It is optimally imaged in a sagittal plane with the fetal head in a neutral position (not flexed or overly extended). Unfortunately, measurements of this characteristic are very prone to operator variation, and this technical issue has limited the general applicability of early pregnancy nuchal thickness screening. To remedy this shortcoming, the Fetal Medicine Foundation (London, UK; www.fetalmedicine.com) has assumed worldwide responsibility for standardization of this screening test. They offer a certification process at numerous sites worldwide that provide didactic teaching and ongoing quality control of nuchal thickness images generated. With properly obtained images, Pandya et al. (1995) found that the odds of trisomy 21 and 18 in the late first trimester increased rapidly with increasing nuchal thickness (3.2 and 3.1 if >3 mm, 19.8 and 14.0 if >4 mm, 28.6 and 27.8 if >5 mm, 21.7 and 69.2 if >6 mm, respectively). The association between increased nuchal translucency and aneuploidy is also valid in multiple gestations. As a result, nuchal lucency screening offers a means of antenatal aneuploidy screening in multiple gestation not offered by standard serologic methods such as maternal serum triple or quadruple marker screening, which, for the most part, are confounded by problems engendered by assessing the risk of aneuploidy in two fetuses from the same pooled maternal serum sample. In chromosomally normal infants, other potential infectious causes such as toxoplasmosis, parvovirus, and coxsackievirus B should be considered.

Cystic hygroma (Figure 4.21) is the most common neck mass. It results from failure of the lymphatic system in the neck to connect with the venous system, either due to abnormal embryonic sequestration of lymphatic tissue or due to abnormal budding of the lymphatic epithelium between 6 and 9 weeks of gestation. It occurs in about 1/6,000 pregnancies and usually presents as bilateral, asymmetric, thin-walled, often multiseptate cystic masses located posterior and lateral to the high cervical vertebrae. Generalized fetal hydrops is also often present. In severe hydrops, skin thickening may be in excess of 3–5 mm. The skull and spine should appear normal and without defect.

Cystic hygromas may represent normal developmental events but usually result from aberrant development due to aneuploidy or early infections. They are most commonly found in association with aneuploidy (monosomy X, trisomy 21, trisomy 18). Septations within the hygroma are associated with increased risk for cephalocele. Cystic hygromas due to aneuploidy or infection have a high propensity for fetal demise in utero. All fetuses with cystic hygroma should be considered for karyotypic evaluation.

A variety of other tumors of the neck are occasionally encountered, including thyroid goiter, hemangiomas, teratomas, branchial cleft cysts, lipomas, fibromas, neuroblastomas, and posterior mediastinal thyroglossal duct cyst. Perhaps the most important of these from an obstetric perspective is fetal thyromegaly or goiter. Fetal goiter may present as a massive enlargement of the thyroid as a result of therapy with maternal thyroid blocking medications, ingestion of iodides, due to transplacental passage of long-acting thyroid stimulant (LATS), or in association with congenital hypothyroidism (1/3,700 births). The enlarged thyroid usually presents as a solid, bilobed, homogenous mass in the anterior neck, and hydramnios (present in 30%) may occur due to impaired fetal swallowing. The carotids may be displaced posteriorly, or the neck may be hyperextended. Delivery at a high-risk neonatal facility is recommended because of the high risk of airway obstruction at birth (Stocks et al. 1997; Ramirez et al. 1992).

Hemangiomas also represent rare but clinically important fetal neck masses. They result from a localized proliferation of vascular tissue that rarely presents as a discrete fetal neck mass. They usually have a complex sonographic appearance with many small vascular channels and an almost solid appearance. Color flow and pulsed Doppler show heavy vascular flow patterns and offer the potential for a highly specific diagnosis. Over time, high blood flow through this lesion may cause high output cardiac failure. Close surveillance for hydrops, skin edema, ascites, and pleural effusion should be maintained, and newer methods of fetal cardiac assessment may be considered. Falkensammer and Huhta recently described the use of the Tei-index (isovolumetric time/ejection time) and a cardiac function score, which assessed 5 factors related to cardiac function (presence of hydrops, venous Doppler flow profile, heart function, arterial Doppler flow characteristics, and heart size) to characterize changes in cardiac function. Using these indices and serial evaluations, it may be possible to identify early fetal cardiac dysfunction, and institute therapy before overt failure is present. (Falkensammer et al. 2001) Cesarean section for cervical hemangioma has been reported as a means of facilitating prompt airway management, sometimes before interruption of the placental-fetal circulation (Schwartz and Silver 1993). Such measures should be considered if large lesions are present.

Cervical teratomas are rarely identified before birth. They are usually unilateral and situated in the anterolateral portion of the neck, often presenting as cystic lesions that enlarge and increase in complexity over the course of pregnancy, sometimes achieving 8–10 cm in diameter. Calcifications are present in 45%. Most teratomas (90%) are benign but present difficult clinical problems. Untreated cervical teratomas have high mortality rates (80–100%), but operative mortality of 9–15% is not negligible. The presence of large neck masses may limit mobility of the neck, which in turn may contradict breech delivery. Large masses may also necessitate consideration of cesarean delivery for vertex-presenting infants, as has been described for goiter and hemangiomas (Stocks et al. 1997; Ramirez et al. 1992; Schwartz and Siver 1993).

CRANIOFACIAL ANOMALIES

Views of the face are often obtained in a complete basic sonogram but should definitely be attempted if a history suggestive of increased risk for craniofacial abnormalities is present. Clefting of the upper lip is relatively easy to assess, while abnormalities of the palate are more difficult to evaluate. If major chromosomal abnormalities are suspected, care should be taken to exclude the possibility of central facial abnormalities. Measurement of inter- and intraorbital diameters and careful evaluation of the nose and mouth are recommended. Facial clefts not due to underlying syndromic causes occur in about 1/800 births. They occur more often in males (60–80% male predominance) and are associated with advanced maternal age. They occur more commonly in Asians and Native Americans and are uncommon in blacks. If one first-degree relative is affected, a 4% recurrence risk is observed. The association between facial clefts and aneuploidy varies by the timing of the evaluation. Aneuploidy is found in up to 40% of antepartum evaluations for facial clefting (usually either trisomy 13 or 18) but in only 1% of newborns with facial clefts. Clefting is found in 40% of infants with trisomy 13, 10% of infants with trisomy 18, and in 1–2% of infants with either trisomy 21 or triploidy. These differences occur because of higher pregnancy wastage rates in aneuploid fetuses.

SPINAL COLUMN

Evaluation of the spinal column usually includes longitudinal views of the various spinal segments, and a brief evaluation of the axial (transverse) anatomy of the various vertebral bodies (Figure 4.11A and B). Posterior elements of vertebral processes should be located in the midline and should not appear excessively separated from each other. The images should be evaluated to identify any bulging, sac-like protrusions, or if abnormal thickening of the skin posterior to the spine is present, which might suggest a neural tube abnormality. If an elevated maternal serum α-fetoprotein screen has been identified, or if sonographic markers of neural tube abnormalities such as bitemporal narrowing (the lemon sign), cerebellar fusion (the banana sign), or ventriculomegaly are present, special care should be taken to evaluate for abnormalities of the neural tube.

Abdominal Sonography

Evaluation of the abdomen should include documentation of the stomach bubble in its proper situs (and concordant with the heart in the thoracic cavity). Inspection of the abdominal contents such as bowel lumen size, ascites, proper appearance of the umbilical cord insertion site, overall contours of the diaphragm and anterior abdominal wall, and appearance of the kidneys is recommended. The primary cross-sectional abdominal image should be obtained in a plane almost perpendicular to the major axis of the spine. The optimal image should include the stomach bubble and hepatic vein in an area close to (but not at) the umbilical cord insertion site and should not include cross sections of the heart, kidneys, bladder, or the actual umbilical cord insertion into the abdomen. This view is best localized by aligning the transducer with the spinal column, rotating the transducer 90° and sliding the transducer cephalad or caudad to obtain a scanning plane inferior to the heart and superior to the renal poles.

The stomach bubble is normally found situated on the left of the abdomen, caudad to the heart but with concordant situs. Absent stomach bubble suggests tracheo-esophageal abnormalities, thyromegaly, or an abnormal swallowing mechanism (which in turn may suggest CNS abnormalities). Esophageal atresia and other small bowel atresias are associated with aneuploidy (usually trisomy 21 and 18). Esophageal atresia is also associated with cardiac, gastrointestinal, and genito-urinary abnormalities. A right-sided stomach bubble suggests possible situs inversus or complete transposition of the great vessels (depending on cardiac situs).

The size of the stomach increases with fetal swallowing activity and by gestational age. Average dimensions at 16–18 weeks gestation are 13 × 6 × 8 mm and increase to 28 × 14 × 16 mm at 34–36 weeks of gestation (Goldstein et al. 1987). When two stomach-like bubbles (Figure 4.22) are seen adjacent to each other (the double-bubble sign), duodenal atresia may be present (see below). This finding strongly suggests aneuploidy, usually trisomy 21, and necessitates consideration of amniocentesis. Swallowed particulate material within the stomach suggests possible meconium passage in utero.

On abdominal imaging, the fetal stomach bubble at times may not be seen. If the stomach is not seen on several follow-up attempts, various clinical

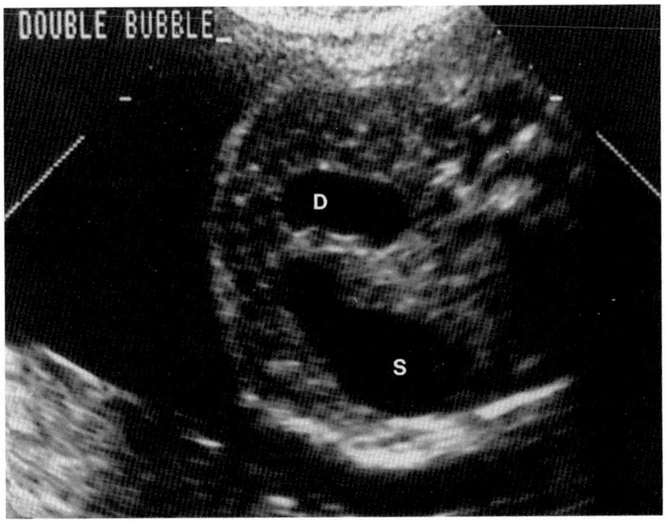

4.22. Axial image: "Double-bubble sign" of duodenal atresia (S = stomach, D = duodenum).

syndromes are suggested, including esophageal atresia, congenital diaphragmatic hernia, situs inversus, and neurologic or musculoskeletal conditions, which might affect swallowing. Attempts should be made to investigate these potential abnormalities.

Esophageal atresia occurs in 1/800 to 1/5,000 deliveries. It results from abnormal division of the primitive foregut into the trachea and esophagus during weeks 3–8 of embryonic life.

Esophageal atresia should be suspected if polyhydramnios develops and the stomach bubble cannot be identified. In 10% of cases, an associated tracheoesophageal fistula may allow filling of the stomach, or gastric secretions may be present in sufficient quantity to distend the stomach and allow its visualization. Other structural congenital anomalies are present in 50–70% of cases, including tracheal abnormalities in 90% of cases, cardiac abnormalities in about 30%, gastrointestinal abnormalities in 28%, musculoskeletal abnormalities in 11%, central nervous system abnormalities in 7%, and facial abnormalities in 6%. Aneuploidy is present in 3–4% of infants with esophageal atresia at birth, principally trisomy 21 and 18. Higher rates would be expected if such infants were assessed earlier in pregnancy.

Bowel Echogenicity

During abdominal sonography, increased echogenicity of bowel or abdominal structures may be noted. This is a subjective finding that occasionally is associated with karyotypic abnormalities but at times may be overdiagnosed because of technical considerations. The combination of high ultrasound gain and low dynamic range should be avoided when evaluating possibly echogenic bowel to limit falsely positive diagnoses. If the echo density of the structures in question approximates the brightness of local pelvic bone and sonographic gain and dynamic range are appropriately selected, hyperechogenicity is judged present

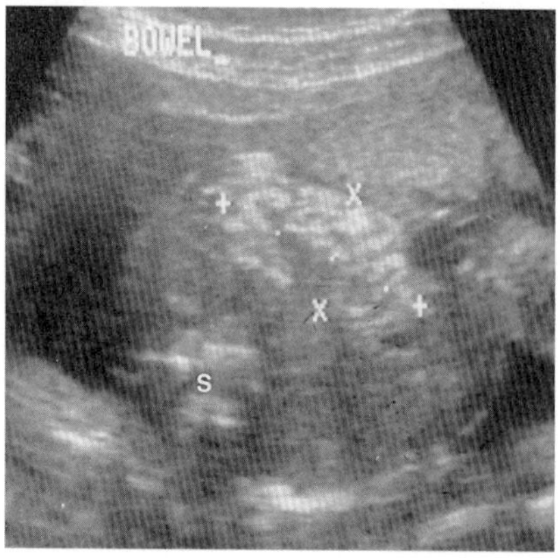

4.23. Axial image: Calipers delineate the area of echogenic bowel (S = spine).

(Figure 4.23). Potential causes of this sonographic appearance include normal variation, aneuploidy (present in 20% of cases), infections such as toxoplasmosis, meconium ileus due to cystic fibrosis, prior intra-amniotic hemorrhage with ingestion of red blood cells, and uteroplacental insufficiency. If echogenic bowel is found as an isolated anomaly, aneuploidy is expected in 2–7% of fetuses, while if any other structural abnormality is present, 36–42% of fetuses may have karyotypic abnormalities. Echogenic bowel in association with growth retardation usually is not associated with chromosomal abnormalities.

Abdominal calcifications are bright specular intra-abdominal echos with evidence of posterior shadowing. A wide variety of conditions are associated with such calcifications, including infections such as toxoplasmosis and cytomegalovirus, neoplasms (neuroblastoma, teratoma, hemangioma, and hepatoblastoma), fetal cholelithiasis, and complications from meconium peritonitis and meconium plugging. Meconium peritonitis may be focal or diffuse, and meconium pseudo-cysts may develop. Meconium plugs commonly are found with cystic fibrosis and also sometimes occur in association with small bowel atresias and anorectal atresia (very distal lesions may not show dilated loops of bowel).

Excessive bowel dilation suggests distal obstruction, and dilated bowel loops are sometimes confused with hydroureters. At 5 weeks of embryonic life, proliferating bowel epithelium obliterates the duodenal lumen, with subsequent restoration of patency within 6 weeks. Failures of vacuolation, vascular accidents, and interruption of the bowel lumen by a diaphragm or membrane may interrupt the recannulation of the duodenum. Historically, duodenal atresia occurred after exposure to thalidomide at 30–40 days of gestation. Duodenal atresia occurs in 1/500 to 1/10,000 live births. In the presence of atresia, amniotic fluid swallowed by the fetus does not transit further than the stomach or proximal duodenum, and these structures fill with amniotic fluid. As the pylorus is relatively nondistensible, the dilated stomach and proximal duodenum connected by the pylorus give a characteristic double-bubble appearance. Atresia is often noted near the ampulla of Vater, and common bile duct obstruction may also be present. Duodenal atresia often develops after 24 weeks gestation and may not be noted on sonograms performed at 16–20 weeks of gestation, as is traditionally done. Rarely, a central web within the stomach may obstruct flow out of the stomach, leaving a single bubble.

Duodenal atresia is strongly associated with aneuploidy, which is present in 57% of cases diagnosed antenatally (trisomy 21 is present in 8–30% of liveborn infants with duodenal atresia, while trisomy 13 is present in 2% of affected infants). Aneuploidy is found in 38% of cases of isolated duodenal atresia, and in 64% of infants with aneuploidy and any other anomalies. Duodenal atresia is often accompanied by a variety of other abnormalities. These include skeletal anomalies (present in 50%), skeletal defects involving vertebral and rib abnormalities, sacral agenesis, radial abnormalities, and talipes equinovarus; gastrointestinal anomalies such as esophageal atresia, tracheo-esophageal fistula,

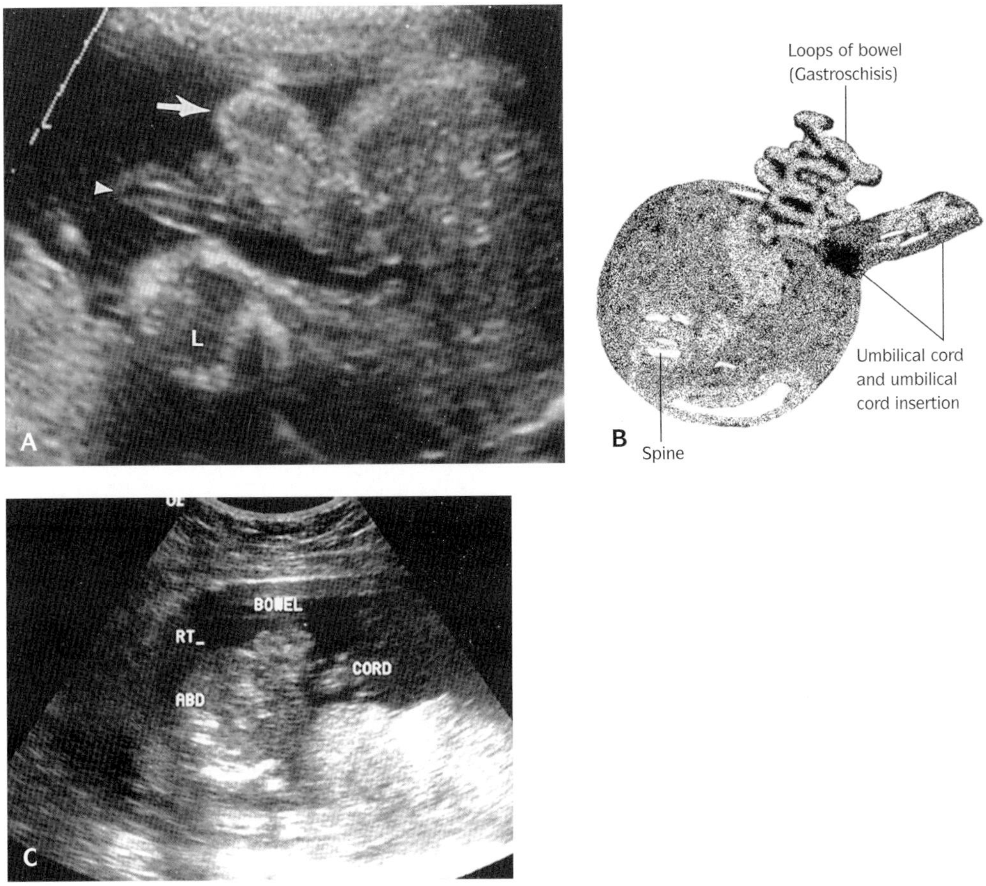

4.24. **(A** and **B)**. Axial image of gastroschisis (arrow). Note the cord insertion into the fetal abdomen (arrowhead) lateral to the gastroschisis (L = limb).

intestinal malrotation, Meckel diverticulum, and anal-rectal atresia; and renal abnormalities. Mortality from duodenal atresia is approximately 36%, primarily in infants with multiple anomalies.

The colon can be visualized by 28 weeks in most fetuses, and it increases in diameter with gestational age, averaging 5 mm at 26 weeks gestation and 17 mm at term gestation (Goldstein et al. 1987). Colonic diameters in the range of 3–5 cm are considered abnormally dilated. This may result from imperforate anus, volvulus, bowel perforation and meconium ileus, and Hirschsprung disease. Dilated bowel does not necessarily constitute an indication for emergency delivery (Sipes et al. 1990; Alysulyman et al. 1996; Albert et al. 2001).

Most ventral wall abnormalities are located near the umbilical cord insertion into the abdomen. Gastroschisis (Figure 4.24) is a ventral wall defect that is usually situated to the right of the umbilicus and does not involve the region of the umbilical cord insertion. It occurs in 1/10,000 to 1/15,000 live births and often is found in association with elevation of maternal serum α-fetoprotein. Gastroschisis may result from vascular compromise of either the umbilical vein or the omphalomesenteric artery. Premature involution of the right umbilical

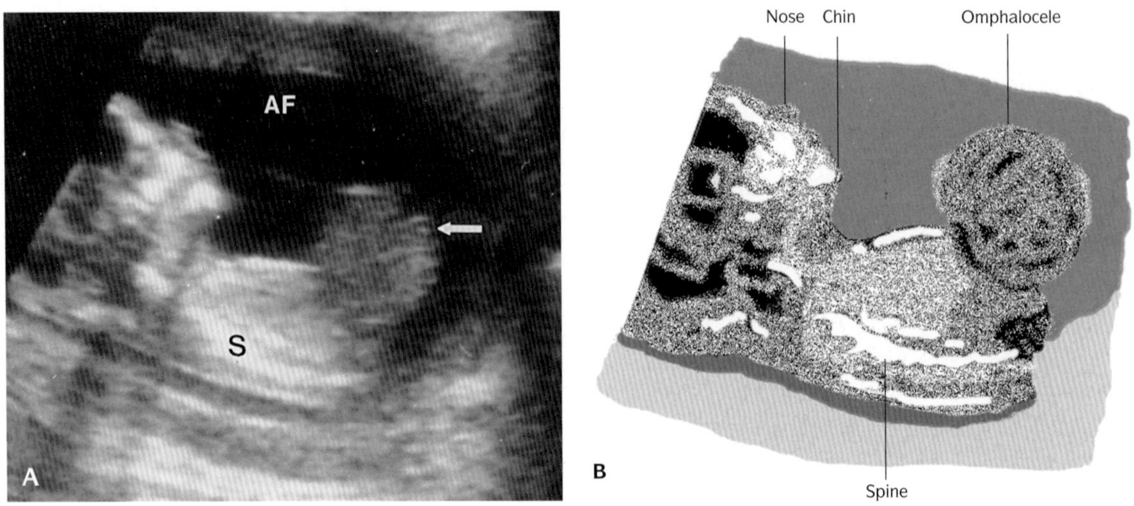

4.25. **(A** and **B)**. Sagittal image: well-circumscribed omphalocele. Arrow points to the bowel extruding outside the abdomen (AF = amniotic fluid, S = spine).

vein, before 28–32 conceptual days, may lead to ischemia and resultant mesodermal and ectodermal defects. Ischemic injury to the region of the superior mesenteric artery may explain high rates of jejunal atresia found in association with gastroschisis.

Defects in gastroschisis are generally small, <4 cm in diameter, and bowel loops are often covered by an inflammatory exudate. The defects are usually situated in the right paraumbilical area and free-floating bowel often is noted in the peritoneal cavity. The fetal liver is rarely involved, bowel obstruction is common, and associated syndromes and anomalies are generally rare. Be careful in evaluating masses of bowel floating freely in the amniotic cavity. Although this usually indicates gastroschisis, an omphalocele sac may have ruptured and no longer be evident, obscuring the diagnosis of omphalocele. One key to this differentiation is the normal close association between omphaloceles and the umbilical cord, while abdominal wall defects to the right of the umbilicus may indicate gastroschisis. The risk for aneuploidy is 1%, or less, and many believe gastroschisis has no significant association with chromosomal abnormalities. If amniocentesis is not elected, care should be taken to ensure that the observed defect conforms closely to the above description. If defects are situated to the left of the midline, are moderate or large in size, involve the liver or other abdominal structures, or if other sonographic findings are present, the possibility of a ruptured omphalocele should be considered and appropriate evaluation considered (the association between omphalocele and aneuploidy is much greater than the association between gastroschisis and aneuploidy).

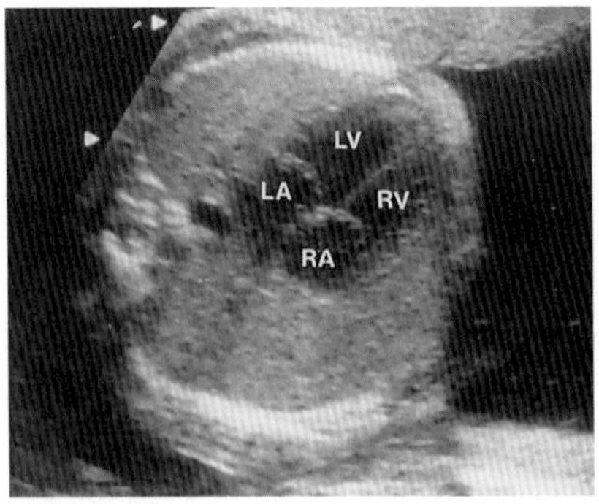

4.26. Axial image of the four-chamber heart at 24 weeks (LV = left ventricule, RV = right ventricule, LA = left atrium, RA = right atrium).

Omphalocele (Figure 4.25) occurs in 1/300 livebirths and is characterized by a midline defect with intra-abdominal contents that herniate within a peritoneal sac into the amniotic cavity thorough the base of the umbilical cord, often in association with other structural abnormalities. Bowel loops, stomach, and liver are commonly involved, and the size of the defect ranges from small to sacs containing most of the abdominal contents. The sac consists of peritoneum and amnion. The anterior abdominal wall normally is formed by fusion of the cephalic folds. Isolated omphaloceles develop from defective fusion of the lateral folds (between the 2nd and 4th conceptual weeks), while fusion of the cephalic folds with the lateral folds yields omphalocele with ectopia cordis, diaphragmatic, and sternal defects. Failed fusion of the caudal and lateral folds results in bladder exstrophy and cloacal exstrophy. Nyberg et al. (1989) believe omphaloceles should be categorized as either herniation, which is limited to bowel (possibly associated with persistence of the primitive body stalk), or herniation of the bowel, liver, and other organs (possibly due to failure of body wall closure).

Aneuploidy is common in omphalocele, often as trisomy 13, trisomy 18, or trisomy 21. If isolated omphalocele is present, aneuploidy occurs in 13% of cases, while aneuploidy rates of 46% have been reported if omphalocele is complicated by other structural abnormalities. Up to 95% survival should be expected if the omphalocele is the sole structural abnormality present.

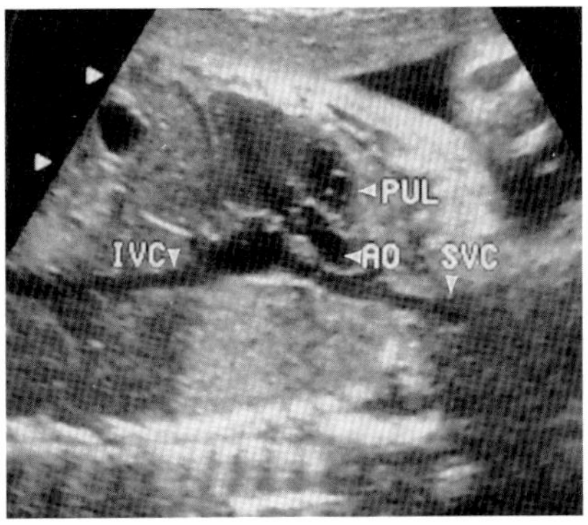

4.27. Sagittal image of the great vessels of the heart: pulmonary artery (PUL), aorta (AO), superior vena cava (SVC), and inferior vena cava (IVC).

Bowel

The small bowel and colon increase in average diameter over the course of pregnancy. The average diameter is 3–4 mm at 20 weeks gestation and increases to about 1.5 cm at 40 weeks gestation. (Nyberg et al. 1997). Normal small bowel rarely exceeds 6 mm in diameter, and colonic diameter normally is <2.3 cm (Nyberg 1987; Parulekar 1991). Abnormally dilated bowel loops on occasion should be distinguished from severely dilated ureters. Age-appropriate tables can often be used to evaluate bowel dilation and other characteristics (Goldstein et al. 1987). Strong associations with aneuploidy for major abdominal malformations such as omphalocele and duodenal atresia should be given consideration when such findings are present.

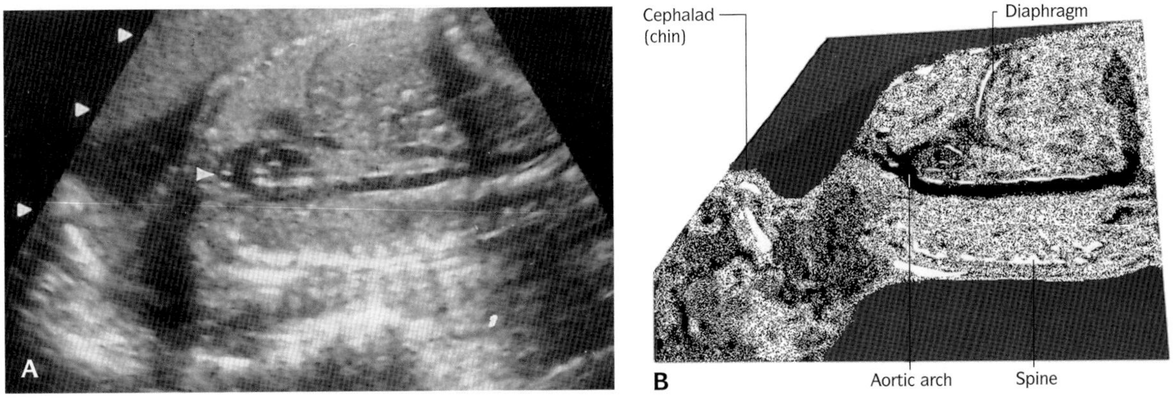

4.28. (A and B). Sagittal image of the aortic arch. Strap vessels can be seen superior to the arch (arrowhead).

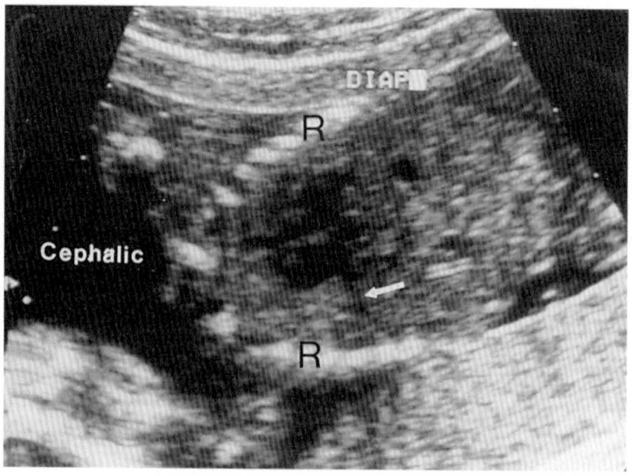

4.29. Sagittal image of the fetal diaphragm (arrow) (ribs).

Hepatomegaly

Abnormally enlarged fetal liver and splenic structures are uncommonly encountered and merit careful evaluation. Potential causes include immune hydrops, nonimmune hydrops, congenital hemolytic anemias, congenital TORCH infections (toxoplasma, rubella, cytomegalovirus, syphilis), maternal metabolic disorders such as hypothyroidism, hereditary disorders (glycogen storage disorders, Beckwith-Wiedemann syndrome, Zellweger (cerebral-hepatorenal) syndrome, hepatic hemangioma, and tumors such as hepatoblastoma (the most common malignancy in the neonatal period), hemangioendothelioma, mesenchymal hamartoma, and metastatic neuroblastoma.

Syndromic Associations of Gastrointestinal Anomalies

Various hereditary conditions may be suggested by combinations of gastrointestinal anomalies with other sonographic features. Fetal macrosomia in combination with increased renal and liver size suggest Beckwith-Wiedemann syndrome, an autosomal recessive condition (with possibly other inheritance patterns as well) that usually also presents with macroglossia. Presence of a Dandy-Walker malformation in combination with features such as encephalocele, enlarged echogenic kidney, polydactyly, cleft lip, suggests Meckel-Gruber, an autosomal recessive condition. Cloacal exstrophy may present with absent urinary bladder, a lumbosacral neural tube defect, and a single umbilical artery. Pentalogy of Cantrell, often associated with underlying trisomy 13, trisomy 18, or monosomy X (Turner) syndrome presents with omphalocele, ectopia cordis, diaphragmatic hernia, pericardiac defect, and structural cardiac anomalies.

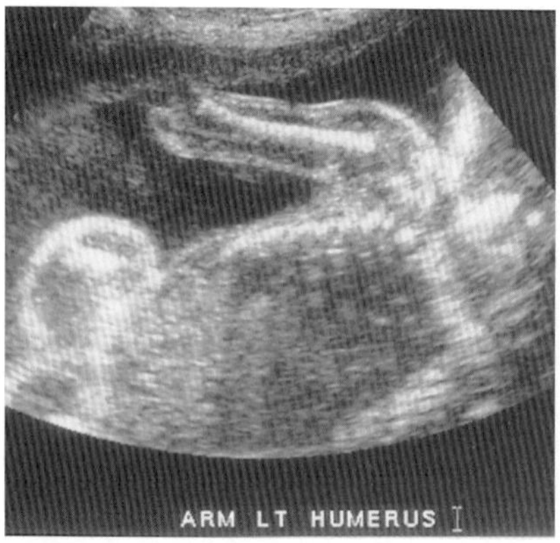

4.30. Axial image at 19 weeks: measurement of the humerus.

THE GENITOURINARY SYSTEM

Images of the kidneys are usually available during basic sonograms performed after 15–16 weeks gestation (Figure 4.31). Abnormal dilation may highlight an

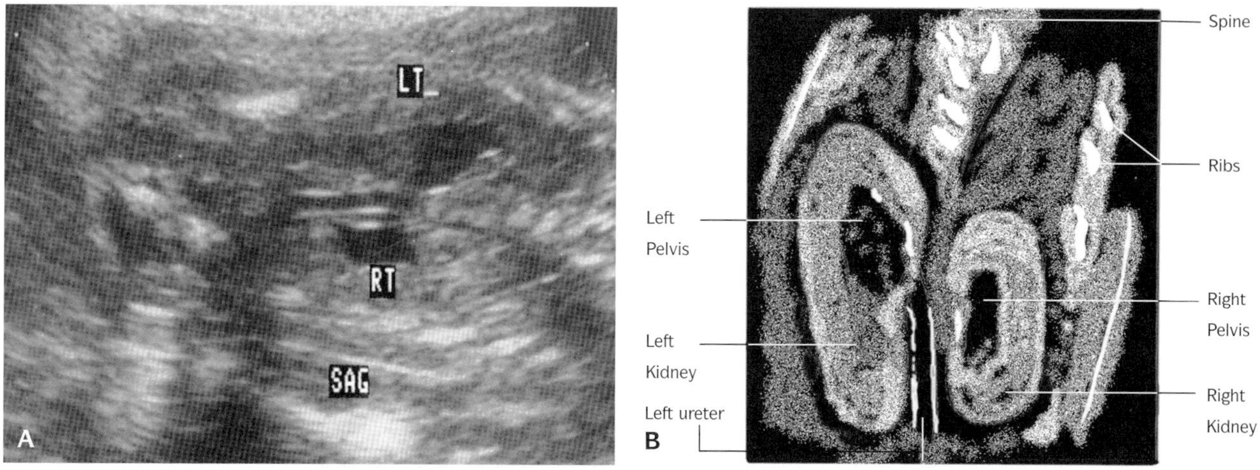

4.31. (A and B). Sagittal image: hydronephrosis demonstrated in both the right and left kidneys.

increased risk for aneuploidy or may indicate obstruction of the renal system distal to the observed finding. Decreased amniotic fluid production after 15 or 16 weeks is often associated with abnormal renal function but may also be due to premature rupture of membranes (Figure 4.32). The particularly high morbidity associated with anhydramnios before 20 weeks gestation is partly due to pulmonary hypoplasia, which is a component of Potter's sequence. Potter's sequence is a group of physical findings and fetal deformities characteristic of renal agenesis that may also develop if severe oligohydramnios of any origin is present. Elements of Potter's sequence include pulmonary hypoplasia, abnormal facies (low-set ears, flattened nose, recessed chin), and positional abnormalities of the limbs, including clubfeet, joint contractures, and hip dislocation.

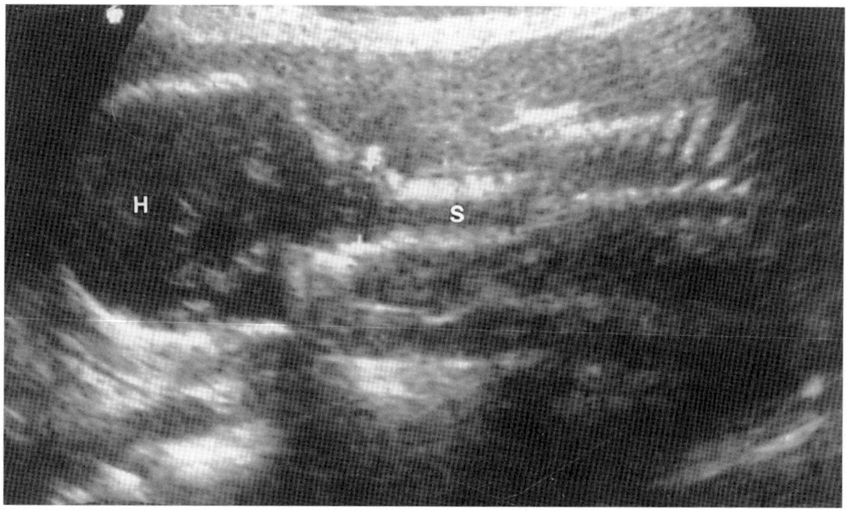

4.32. Sagittal image of the cervical spine and posterior head demonstrating anhydramnios – absence of amniotic fluid (H = head, S = spine).

Renal abnormalities are present in 2–3% of pregnancies. Renal dimensions gradually increase over the course of pregnancy. In the last several weeks of the second trimester (21–25 weeks gestation), the average anterior-posterior diameter and transverse diameter are about 1.5 cm, the average circumference 5.4 cm, and the kidney circumference/abdominal circumference ratio is 0.30. At 36 weeks gestation and beyond, the average anterior-posterior diameter is 2.4 cm, the average transverse diameter is 2.6 cm, and average circumference is 8.4 cm, and the kidney/abdominal circumference ratio is 0.27(Grannum et al. 1980).

On sonographic evaluation, fetal kidneys normally have the appearance of doughnuts, with a circumferential ring of cortical tissue surrounding a small circular fluid filled renal pelvis. The renal pelvis or calyx averages 2 or 3 mm in diameter or less in the mid-second trimester, and is several millimeters wider at term. The bladder should also be observed. Amniotic fluid before 16–18 weeks gestation is usually present as a result of transfer of fluid across the placental membranes and does not give helpful information about renal function. The presence of an identifiable bladder and amniotic fluid after 16–18 weeks gestation imply a functioning renal system has been present in the fetus at some time. If the bladder is not easily imaged, it will usually become apparent after 30 minutes to 1 hour, as urine is produced by the fetus.

If the renal calyx or calyces appear severely widened, pyelectasis or caliectasis is considered present, and a variety of conditions should be considered. These include distal urinary tract obstruction or malformations such as a uretero-pelvic junction abnormalities, ureteral atresia, duplication of the ureters, and posterior urethral valves (usually associated with megacystis and hydroureter). On the whole, dilation of the renal pelvis is associated with aneuploidy in 11% of cases (usually trisomy 21, 18, or 13). Isolated renal anomalies have comparatively low rates of associated aneuploidy (3%), but much higher rates (24%) are seen if other abnormalities are present. When used to estimate relative risk for aneuploidy, isolated mild pyelectasis is associated with a 3-fold increased risk for aneuploidy, while mild pyelectasis in combination with other renal or structural anomalies increases the aneuploidy risk 30-fold.

Abnormal dilation of the renal pelvis may also progress over the course of pregnancy. Ongoing sonographic surveillance of the kidneys has been suggested if renal pelvic diameters are >4 mm at 15–20 weeks gestation, >8 mm at 20–30 weeks gestation, and >10 mm at 30–40 weeks gestation (Mandell, et al. 1991). In cases of severe obstructive uropathy, such as that associated with posterior urethral valves, placement of in-dwelling catheters to effect drainage of enlarged urinary bladders may be considered to attempt to retain renal function before delivery and postnatal surgical correction. In utero interventions are preferred for recently, relatively acute uropathy rather than long-standing disease because the potential maternal complications of such therapy may outweigh the minimal anticipated fetal benefit if more chronic lesions are treated.

Renal function can be assessed by sampling urine directly from the urinary bladder with amniocentesis and then analyzing urinary electrolytes. Characteristics suggestive of a favorable long-term prognosis and that are most suitable for in utero intervention include moderate or mild oligohydramnios, the renal parenchyma having a normal to echogenic appearance, a filling rate greater than 2 mL/min in the urinary bladder, and urinary electrolytes consistent with normal glomerular function (Na < 100 mg/dl, Cl < 90 mg/dl, and osmolarity < 210 mmole/liter). Conversely, findings suggestive of an adverse outcome and possibly nonreversible renal injury include moderate to severe oligohydramnios, an echogenic or cystic appearance of the renal parenchyma, urinary output less than 2 mL/hour, and abnormal urinary electrolyte studies (Na > 100 mg/dl, Cl > 90 mg/dl, and osmolarity > 210 mmole/liter) (Glick et al. 1985). If severe, bilateral pyelectasis is seen in combination with acutely worsening severe oligohydramnios near term, delivery may be considered after discussion with the pediatric urologist who will treat the child.

Pyelectasis due to distal obstruction of the urinary tract is frequently associated with the eventual postnatal diagnosis of congenital hydronephrosis. The likelihood of postnatal renal compromise is suggested by the degree of renal pyelectasis. Pyelectasis of more than 6 mm at 14–23 weeks gestation is associated with renal function compromise or the need for corrective surgery in 40–73% of infants. High risks of renal function deficit or the need for surgery are also associated with pyelectasis of >10 mm at 24–32 weeks gestation (72% adverse outcomes or need for surgery) and in 50% or more of infants when pyelectasis of >6 mm is noted after 32 weeks of gestation (Corteville et al. 1991).

Apart from postobstructive renal disease, a variety of hereditary disorders may affect the kidneys. These include adult polycystic disease, infantile polycystic kidney disease, and multicystic kidney disease. Numerous other syndromes often present with cystic renal abnormalities as well, including Meckel syndrome, Ivemark syndrome, retinal-renal dysplasia, asphyxiating thoracic dysplasia, Zellweger syndrome, Ehlers-Danlos syndrome, Laurence-Moon-Bardet-Biedl syndrome, Kaufman-McKusick syndrome, Von Hippel-Lindau syndrome, Fryns syndrome, branchio-oto-renal syndrome, trisomy 13, and trisomy 18 (Zerres 1984, 1985). When counseling patients with cystic renal abnormalities detected, care should be taken to exclude acquired renal disease from inherited conditions (Zerres 1984).

Adult polycystic disease is one of the most common genetic disorders. It usually presents in adulthood but on occasion is noted in neonates as well. Prenatal diagnosis is possible but often not until the third trimester. It usually manifests as multiple cysts of various sizes that replace the renal parenchyma. It usually is a bilateral process, although it may first appear to involve only one kidney.

Infantile polycystic kidney disease creates renal parenchymal cystic changes similar to adult polycystic disease but is inherited as an autosomal recessive disorder. The cystic changes are always bilateral and consist of multiple cysts

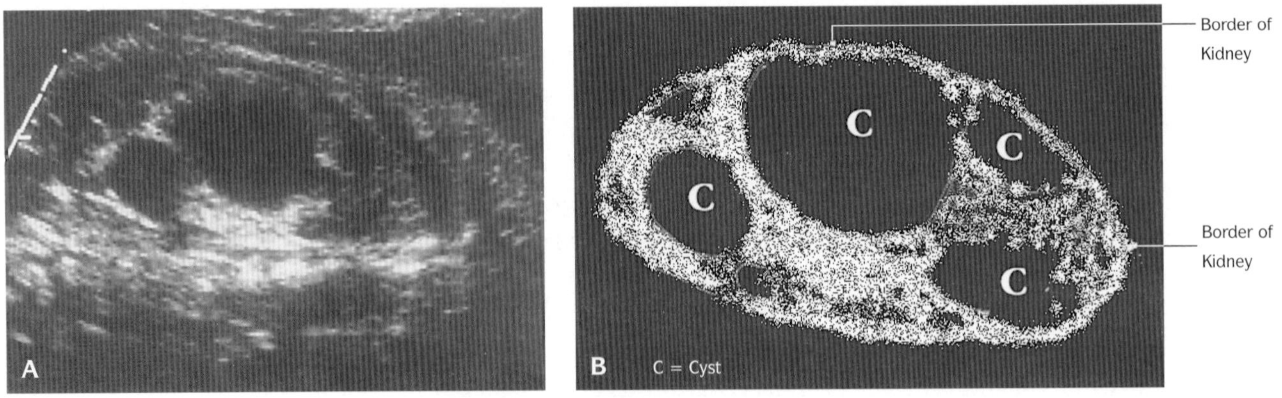

4.33. (A and B). Sagittal image of the kidney demonstrating multicystic dysplastic kidney (MCDK).

of various sizes. It is not related to obstruction of the urinary system. There are three common presentations: perinatal, neonatal, and infantile. Perinatal infantile polycystic disease presents with massively dilated fetal kidneys, cystic changes in 90% of the renal parenchyma, in utero renal failure, and associated with high neonatal mortality rates. Neonatal infantile polycystic disease usually presents more than 1 month after birth and has cystic changes in about 60% of the renal parenchyma. Renal enlargement is less pronounced than with perinatal onset disease, mild hepatic fibrosis is often present, and death often occurs within one year of life. Infantile polycystic kidney disease presents at 3–6 months of age, shows less cystic involvement of the renal parenchyma, but has a disease course similar to the infantile form of the disorder.

Multicystic kidney disease (Figure 4.33) is characterized by renal dysplasia ranging from segmental to bilateral involvement with dilation of the collecting tubules. The dilated tubules present as multiple, round, variably sized cysts arranged peripherally around the renal parenchyma in a grape-like fashion, do not communicate with each other, and obliterate the renal parenchyma. The kidneys are usually enlarged. If bilateral disease is present, the fetal bladder does not fill over time or with maternal administration of furosemide. Oligohydramnios is usually present. Bilateral disease is a fatal condition, while those with unilateral disease are at increased risk for hypertension.

Multicystic kidney disease may result from either early obstructive uropathy or from developmental failure of the mesonephric blastema. It occurs sporadically or within families and occasionally is reported with maternal diabetes; often it is found in association with hereditary conditions such as Meckel-Gruber, Dandy-Walker, Zellweger, Roberts, Fryns, Smith-Lemli-Opitz, and Apert syndromes, and with some trisomies. The differential diagnosis for multicystic kidney disease includes infantile polycystic kidney disease and ureteropelvic junction obstruction.

In cases of severe oligohydramnios, renal agenesis should be considered. In such cases, imaging quality is often severely limited and care should be taken to evaluate structures in the renal fossa. Renal agenesis may occasionally be falsely excluded because, in the absence of kidneys, the adrenals assume a more spheroid shape and may be falsely identified as kidneys. The use of fluid instilled transabdominally into the amniotic cavity to assist with visualization of fetal structures has been reported (Lameier and Katz 1993).

THORAX

The cross-sectional anatomy of the chest is evaluated in planes perpendicular to the long axis of the torso. A thoracic sonographic evaluation usually includes an appraisal of the general shape of the chest (characteristically abnormal in some chondrodystrophies), the appearance of the lungs, presence of any pleural or pericardiac effusions, an evaluation of the cardiac size, axis and position within the thorax, and a comparison of the thorax with the overall fetal body size. The continuity of the diaphragm on the left and right should be verified, and the chest should be surveyed for abnormal structures such as bowel loops, cystic anomalies, or the stomach bubble. The heart usually occupies approximately the central one-third of the cross-sectional area of the thoracic cavity and its main axis is angled at 45° to the midline. Deviation of the heart or alteration of the cardiac axis due to a mass defect of anomalous organs in the thorax may suggest the presence of other structures such as bowel or stomach within the thorax, and diaphragmatic hernia. Only very minimal amounts of pleural or pericardiac fluid should be present on inspection.

The chest circumference is measured in the transverse plane at the level of the four-chambered cardiac view but is of limited value in clinical practice because of the difficulty estimating gestational age in some cases and because of the poor correlation between it and pulmonary hypoplasia. Chest circumference ranges from an average of 12.8 cm (2 SD; range 9.5–16 cm) at 20 weeks gestation to 30 cm (2 SD; range 27.7–34.2 cm) at 40 weeks gestation. Ratios of thoracic diameter to other body dimensions may be helpful in evaluating the size of the chest with relation to gestational age, especially when considering certain chondrodystrophies, such as asphyxiating thoracic dysplasia. The thoracic/abdominal circumference ratio varies minimally over pregnancy (mean 0.89, 2 SD; range 0.77–1.01), and after 20 weeks gestation is >0.80 in nearly all normal pregnancies. Similarly, the thoracic/head circumference varies minimally over pregnancy (mean 0.80, 2 SD; range 0.56–1.04). Abnormal thoracic shape may be due to skeletal dysplasia and spinal abnormalities such as kyphoscoliosis, and oligohydramnios. The fetal lungs usually appear as hypoechogenic regions.

The fetal cardiac evaluation performed for most basic sonograms usually includes at least one view of the heart, the four-chamber view, documentation of a normal cardiac rate and rhythm, and an assessment of the cardiac axis. Other standardized images of the heart may also be obtained, including views of the great vessel arches and a five-chamber view. It is not clear what the minimum evaluation of the heart should consist of, but even a single normal four-chamber image will exclude up to 90% of cardiac structural anomalies. The number of cardiac images performed may vary by the circumstances of the study (i.e., less intensive imaging if no history suggestive of increased risk for cardiovascular anomalies) and also may depend on factors such as the quality of the sonographic equipment utilized, fetal positioning, and maternal body habitus. In the best circumstances, significant cardiac structural abnormalities are missed on occasion (Anderson et al. 1995). To a certain degree, the sensitivity of cardiac anomaly screening depends on the severity of the cardiac disease present. In the RADIUS study, 43% of fetuses with complex congenital heart diseases were identified, but none of the 21 fetuses with isolated ventricular or atrial septal defects was recognized (Crane et al. 1994). Additionally some cardiac lesions may actually develop after fetal cardiac imaging has been performed (Allan et al. 1989).

The most commonly obtained image of the heart is the four-chamber view. Characteristics of a normal four-chamber cardiac view include symmetric atria and ventricles, intact intraatrial and intraventricular septa, a foramen ovale with its flap oriented into the left atrium, and a cardiac axis oriented to the left at about a 45° angle to the sagittal plane. The left atrium is usually closest to the spine, the tricuspid valve inserts slightly lower on the interventricular septum than the mitral valve, and the heart occupies about one-third of the chest. The four-chamber view is helpful for documenting disorders such as right or left ventricular hypoplasia, ventricular septal defects, tetralogy of Fallot, coarctation of the aorta, Ebstein's anomaly, pericardial effusion, dextrocardia, cardiac hypertrophy, situs inversus, ectopia cordis, and single ventricle. The four-chamber view of the heart is obtained from an imaging plane that is at an approximate 45° angle from the view used to obtain the abdominal circumference view. The heart and stomach bubble should have concordant situs. A more thorough description of fetal cardiac images and structures assessed is provided on pages 133–137.

A wide range of conditions cause an increased risk for congenital heart disease (CHD). Increased rates of CHD are found if siblings or parents have a history of CHD. If one sibling is affected, 2% of other siblings are affected, while rates of 10% affected are found if there are two siblings or relatives affected, and 9% affected infants if one parent is affected. Disorders such as Ehlers-Danlos syndrome (increased risk of aortic and carotid aneurysms due to decreased strength of collagen tissues), Ellis-vanCreveld syndrome (associated with single atrium), Holt-Oram (predisposes to atrial and ventricular septal defects), Kartagener syndrome (associated with dextrocardia), and Leopard syndrome (increased risk of pulmonary stenosis) are also associated with increased risk for CHD.

Maternal illnesses also play a role in CHD. CHD is seen in 2% of infants of diabetic mothers, with a predominance of ventricular septal defects, coarctation, cardiomegaly, cardiomyopathy, transposition of the great vessels, and patent ductus arteriosus as neonates. Increased rates of tetralogy of Fallot are seen in patients with maternal phenylketomuria, while systemic lupus is associated with congenital heart block. Infection with rubella (wild type, not accidental vaccination during pregnancy) is associated with increased rates of ventricular septal defect, transposition of the great vessels, and patent ductus arteriosus.

Medication and substance exposures can also predispose to CHD. Trimethadione is associated with a 20% risk of CHD, including transposition, tetralogy of Fallot, and hypoplastic left heart. Patients receiving diphenylhydantoin are at increased risk for fetal pulmonic stenosis, aortic stenosis, coarctation, and neonatal patent ductus arteriosus. Amphetamine use is associated with increased risk for ventricular septal defect, transposition of the ductus arteriosus, and patent ductus arteriosus as a neonate. Lithium use has been reported associated with with Ebstein anomaly (although this association recently has been called into question), tricuspid atresia, and atrial septal defect. Use of retinoic acid, sex steroids, and excessive amounts of alcohol have all been reported associated with CHD. Tachyarrhythmias usually are not associated with CHD. Bradycardia due to congenital heart block is associated with a 50% risk for CHD with somewhat less predisposition to CHD if a maternal connective tissue disorder is present. Finally, before being removed from the market, thalidomide exposure was found associated with tetralogy of Fallot, ventricular and atrial septal defects, and truncus arteriosus.

In addition to maternal disease states, genetic syndromes, and familial hereditary risk factors, aneuploidy also may cause CHD. Aneuploidy may be present in up to 30% of fetuses with CHD, with somewhat lower rates (16%) if isolated cardiac abnormalities are present and higher rates (66%) if two or more abnormalities are present. Infants with structural cardiac anomalies should be considered for karyotypic evaluation.

Chest Masses

Masses within the fetal chest may be characterized by their appearance as either primarily solid, cystic, or combined solid/cystic. Chest tumors presenting as primarily solid tumors include bronchial atresias, bronchogenic cysts with obstruction, and congenital cystic adenomatoid malformations (CCAM). Primarily cystic chest abnormalities include bronchogenic or neuroenteric cysts, diaphragmatic hernias, and mediastinal meningoceles. Tumors with a mixed solid/cystic appearance include congenital cystic adenomatoid malformations, neuroenteric cysts, pulmonary sequestrations, and pericardiac teratomas.

Bronchial atresia is rare and is usually not diagnosed before birth. It presents with focal obliteration of a portion of the segmental, lobar, or main-stem bronchus lumen and probably results from a vascular accident in the 15th week of gestation. It may be detected after 24 weeks gestation as a dilated, fluid-filled cyst (bronchus) located in the left upper lobe or right upper and middle lobes. Lesions in the lower lobes are more likely extralobar pulmonary sequestration or due to underlying diaphragmatic herniation.

Bronchogenic cysts and neuroenteric cysts are uncommon anomalies that result from abnormal development in the branching of the tracheobronchial tree at the 26th to 40th day of gestation, probably as a result of abnormal budding of the diverticulum of the foregut. Bronchogenic cysts result from abnormal development of the anterior diverticulum of the foregut. They commonly are located in the anterior mediastinum or (rarely) in the pulmonary parenchyma and usually are not associated with other structural abnormalities. Bronchogenic cysts characteristically present as a single unilocular cyst, with mediastinal shift, and evidence of bronchial obstruction. In one case report of antenatal diagnosis, an enlarged, obstructed lung was identified that ultimately led to the discovery of a bronchogenic cyst. Posterior mediastinal neuroenteric cysts occur due to anomalous development of the dorsal foregut and notochord, probably in the 4th week of gestation. They often are associated with spinal abnormalities and may compress the trachea or communicate with the bowel through a diaphragmatic defect.

CCAM are large, bulky lesions that are typically unilobar and involve segments or lobes of the lung. They rarely fill the entire lung or involve both lungs. The ultrasound appearance of CCAM's ranges from multiple large 2- to 10-cm macrocysts (Type 1) to confluent, 3- to 5-mm microcysts resembling bronchioles (Type 3). Spontaneous regression in utero has been reported. Microcystic forms (Type 3) and CCAM in combination with hydrops appear to have a worse prognosis. Infants with isolated CCAM who survive after delivery are often asymptomatic in the neonatal period and can then undergo surgical correction at a later date.

Diaphragmatic hernias (Figure 4.29) occur in 1/200 to 1/5,000 live births. These hernias may occur in several characteristic locations. The most common is posterolateral (Bochdaleck) herniation through the pleuroperitoneal canal or foramen of Bochdaleck. Bochdalek hernias are usually located on the left and comprise up to 92% of diaphragmatic hernia cases. Other potential hernia sites include parasternal (Morgagni) herniation through the costal and sternal origins of the diaphragm; septum transversum hernias, which herniate through the central tendon; and esophageal hiatal hernias. Diaphragmatic hernias are often associated with other structural abnormalities, including CNS anomalies in 28% of cases and abnormalities of the gastrointestinal tract, skeleton, genitourinary system, or the heart in 9–23% of cases. Aneuploidy, usually trisomy 21 or 18, occurs in 4% of cases. Diaphragmatic hernias are often fatal (75%), depending on the presence of other associated abnormalities, often as a result of pulmonary hypoplasia or inadequate diaphragmatic musculature for pulmonary function. Infants diagnosed with diaphragmatic hernias should be delivered at a facility that provides intensive care for neonates. Extracorporeal membranous oxygenation is often useful in maintaining the most severely affected of these infants in the peripartum interval.

Pulmonary sequestration consists of a mass of pulmonary tissue supplied by systemic circulation and isolated from normal bronchial and pulmonary vascular connections. It results from abnormal differentiation of the primitive foregut. On sonographic evaluation, it appears as a homogenous, echogenic lung mass. If a feeding vessel from the aorta can be demonstrated, pulmonary sequestration is considered more likely. Two forms of pulmonary sequestration have been described: extralobar and intralobar. Extralobar sequestration is more common in prenatal diagnosis than the intralobar variety and is associated with increased rates of diaphragmatic hernia, cardiac abnormalities, and gastric duplication. Ninety percent are left sided, located in the posterobasal region in the costophrenic sulcus. Extralobar sequestration results in complete anatomic and physiologic separation or the sequestered structures from other pulmonary structures. The sequestered tissue is surrounded by a separate pleural structure, and drainage occurs via the systemic vasculature, usually the hemiazygous or portal veins. Intralobar sequestration is rare in fetuses but accounts for 75% of sequestrations in children and adults. In intralobar sequestrations, a portion of the lung is separated from the bronchial tree but it shares a common pleura with the other ipsilateral lung tissue, and venous drainage is usually to pulmonary veins.

Teratomas are tumors derived from all three embryonic cellular layers. They have a highly disorganized appearance, often with both solid and cystic components, and are capable of elaborating most body components, including hair, bone, cartilage, muscle, nervous tissue, and other less-differentiated structures. If bone or cartilage are elaborated, they appear highly echogenic when evaluated with ultrasound.

Tracheal or laryngeal atresia in the fetus may result in high degrees of laryngeal or tracheal obstruction, resulting in trapping of pulmonary secretions within the lungs. The bronchi become distended and filled with trapped secretions, giving the lungs a hyperechoic appearance bilaterally. Ascites is common, and morality in reported cases is 100%.

SKELETON AND LIMBS

Imaging of selected fetal limbs is commonly performed. Although the femur length is almost always obtained, full measurements of all limbs are rarely performed if there is no concern for underlying skeletal abnormalities or syndromes affecting long-bone development. If abnormally shaped bones or shortened long-bones are observed during the course of a routine sonogram, careful assessment of the long bones is indicated. A firmly established gestational age is essential to properly interpret long-bone measurements.

Skeletal Anomalies

Evaluation of the fetal limbs and digits can yield important information relative to fetal structural abnormalities and the possible presence of syndromic abnormalities or aneuploidy. Limb shortening, usually defined as limb dimensions less than the 1st centile for gestational age (Figure 4.30), is associated with a wide variety of chondrodystrophic syndromes. Chondrodystrophies potentially detected include the following:

Syndrome	Rate/livebirths	Syndrome	Rate/livebirths
Achondrogenesis (all types)	1/75,000	Hypophosphatasia (severe)	1/110,000
Camptomelic dysplasia	1/150,000	Osteogenesis imperfecta	1/55,000
Chondrodysplasia punctata	1/85,000	Thanatophoric dysplasia	1/30,000

When diminished fetal long-bone measurements are noted, it is important to distinguish them from symmetric growth retardation. Skeletal dysplasias generally are autosomally mediated inherited conditions, while severe symmetric growth retardation also may result from early fetal infections, chromosomal abnormalities, and severe uteroplacental insufficiency. Morphologically, most skeletal dysplasias do not affect head circumference, abdominal circumstance, or fetal foot length. Tables that describe average long-bone length for head circumference or abdominal circumference or biparietal diameter and gestational age assess symmetry and are useful. They assist in determining whether long bones are small relative to other body characteristics – as in skeletal dysplasia, or whether body proportions are generally symmetric, indicating symmetric growth retardation. The femur/foot ratio is a helpful and easily understood biometric characteristic. It discriminates rather well between chondrodystrophy and symmetric growth retardation because foot length generally is not reduced in chondrodystrophy. The ratio of the fetal femur/foot length approximates 1.0 over the course of gestation. Femur/foot ratios are <0.84 in only $<10\%$ of normal infants, and femur/foot ratios <0.84 are associated with increased likelihood of skeletal dysplasia.

If gestational age is known with some accuracy, the relative long-bone length can be evaluated. Long bones less than the 1% or less than 3–4 SD for gestational age are highly suggestive of skeletal dysplasia. These are clinically efficacious criteria, because the degree of long-bone shortening usually is profound in the most skeletal dysplasias. Lesser degrees of shortening of the humerus has also been proposed as a means of screening for chromosomal aberrations. Mild shortening of the humerus may be present in up to 60% of trisomy 21 fetuses. Ratios of long bones such as the femur with the BPD or HC have also been evaluated. Values of the BPD/femur ratio falling above the 1.5 SD range from 1.9 at 16 weeks to 1.58 at 20 weeks gestation and 1.47 at 22 weeks of gestation. The Harris birthright center also has evaluated the utility of HC/femur length ratios greater than the 95th centile and found this to be a useful marker of skeletal dysplasia. This characteristic is approximately 6.5 at 16 weeks, 5.9 at 20 weeks, 5.5 at 24 weeks, and 5.4 at 28 weeks of gestation.

There appears to be an association between short femur length and chromosomal abnormalities. Trisomy 21 fetuses often have HC/femur length ratios >97.5% for gestation. Increased rates of relative shortening of the femur are seen in fetuses with triploidy (60%), Turner syndrome (59%), trisomy 18 (25%), and trisomy 13 (9%). Potential pitfalls in the use of long bones to screen for aneuploidy are discussed in Part I, page 94.

Single Umbilical Artery

A single umbilical artery occurs in 1–3% of normal pregnancies. It may result from primary agenesis or secondary atrophy of one of the umbilical arteries or from persistence of the original single allantoic artery of the body stalk. A single umbilical artery is more common in white fetuses, in autopsy series, in placentas with marginal or velamentous insertions, and in fetuses with aneuploidy or other structural abnormalities. Although it occurs more often in twins, monozygotic twin fetuses are usually discordant for single umbilical artery.

Umbilical artery evaluation should be performed near the abdominal cord insertion in the fetal abdomen. Isolated single artery findings at the placental insertion site do not appear to have the same negative associations as this same finding more proximally in the cord. Additional structural abnormalities are found in 20–50% of cases, and multiple anomalies are noted in 20% of fetuses. Associated anomalies in single umbilical artery include musculoskeletal abnormalities in 23%, genitourinary abnormalities in 20%, cardiovascular abnormalities in 19%, gastrointestinal abnormalities in 10%, and central nervous system anomalies in 8%. As previously noted, single umbilical artery is also associated with aneuploidy, most often trisomy 18, but also with trisomy 13, monosomy X (Turner's syndrome), and triploidy. The risk of aneuploidy is proportional to the presence of other anomalies. If other anomalies are present, rates of aneuploidy range from 33% to 43%. The combination of CNS abnormalities and single umbilical artery is associated with aneuploidy in 50% of cases.

Targeted Fetal Echocardiography

Certain patients will benefit from a targeted or more comprehensive evaluation of the fetal cardiac system. Fetal echocardiograms are usually beyond the capabilities of a general obstetric sonographer and are most often performed by a clinician skilled in evaluation of fetal cardiac structures, such as a pediatric cardiologist, maternal–fetal medicine specialist, or radiologist with a special interest in fetal cardiac disease. The more common risk factors for CHD were previously described in this chapter on pages 128 and 129.

The targeted fetal cardiac sonogram usually includes views such as the four-chamber view (Figure 4.26), images of the great vessels (the left and right ventricular outflow tracts or pulmonary artery and aorta, respectively) (Figure 4.27), the aortic arch (Figure 4.28), the arch of the ductus arteriosus (which has a hockey stick appearance), and a view of the short axis of the heart. In certain circumstances, further Doppler evaluation of valve function or synchronicity of the atria and ventricles may be undertaken. Simultaneous M-mode evaluation of the atria and ventricle may be performed to characterize chamber wall thickness, a pericardial effusion, or to determine whether synchronous cardiac contractions are occurring. Doppler sampling also may be placed near valve structures to document regurgitation or to assess synchrony between atrial and ventricular contractions.

The four-chamber view is obtained at about a 45° angle (more caudad anteriorly and more cephalad posteriorly) to the plane of scanning used for the standard abdominal circumference view. This image will capture the four-chambers of the heart with the left atrium closest to the fetal spine and the cardiac axis at about 45° to the midsagittal plane. Relative sizes of atria and ventricles, position of AV valve relative to atria and ventricles (abnormal in Ebstein's anomaly), interatrial and interventricular septa can be evaluated. The cardiac rate and rhythm can be monitored and dyssynchrony of atrial and ventricular contractions further evaluated with M mode and pulsed Doppler.

The five-chamber view is found adjacent to the four-chamber view, and combines elements of the four cardiac chambers with a view of the origin of the aortic root to allow better evaluation of the continuity between the intraventricular septum, the aortic valve, and the aortic root. It is also helpful, if possible, to image the orientation between the aorta and pulmonary artery. If these structures are oriented in a parallel fashion, transposition of the great vessels should be suspected, while if they are arrayed in a transverse or crossing fashion, transposition of the great vessels is unlikely.

The cardiac axis (the axis of the intraventricular septum) should be at a 30° to 59° angle from the midsagittal plane. Cardiac axis angles outside this range indicate possible cardiac abnormalities, possibly due to a mass effect from intrathoracic masses or diaphragmatic hernia, or other abnormalities. Crane found cardiac axis outside of the normal range as 79% sensitive and 97% specific for congenital cardiac abnormalities, and 5 of 23 infants with structural cardiac anomalies and an abnormal axis were initially thought to have a normal four-chamber view of the heart (Crane et al. 1997). Cardiac axis to the right is rare but strongly associated with underlying cardiac abnormalities. Comstock found 22 such infants among 16,562 fetuses evaluated over a 6-year period. Twelve infants had isolated rotation of the heart axis, six fetuses had mirror-image hearts with situs inversus, and four had inversion of the ventricles. Fourteen of the 22 infants had structural cardiac defects, most of which were atrioventricular septal defects, double outlet right ventricles, or common atria. The chromosomes and/or phenotypes of all 22 were normal. Neonatal outcomes were good in 16 of the infants, while 4 infants with polysplenia or asplenia, and 2 infants with other severe extracardiac malformations died (Comstock et al. 1998).

The intraventricular septum should be intact from the cardiac apex to the crux. The membranous septal portion of the intraventricular septum, located immediately adjacent to the cardiac crux, is anatomically very thin. If imaged in anything other than an ideal imaging plane, the membranous septum may appear discontinuous, having a tendency to simulate a membranous ventricular septal defect. Further imaging from slightly different angles and evaluation with color Doppler color flow or pulsed Doppler will usually exclude such false positive diagnoses. Small ventriculoseptal defects may also go undetected, but this is often of minimal clinical significance, as small defects often resolve spontaneously during the first months and years of life.

Several other views are useful to fully evaluate the heart. These include the left ventricular outflow view and short axis great vessel views, which are usually obtained by rotating the longitudinal axis of the transducer from the four-chamber view by 30°–45° to the right or left, resulting in imaging planes that transect the scapula and torso at 30°–45° angles from the midsagittal plane.

In addition, the five-chamber view is a modification of the four-chamber imaging plane in which the aortic root origin in the left ventricle is imaged (one chamber), as well as accompanying views of the other four standard chambers giving a five-chamber appearance. The ventricular septum should make a smooth transition into the aorta.

The left ventricular outflow tract view shows left atrium, left ventricle, the mitral valve, and the aorta. Some septal defects can be detected in this view. The right ventricular outflow tract view shows the right ventricle, the pulmonic valve, the pulmonary artery, and a portion of the ductus arteriosus. A crossing view of the pulmonary artery and aorta in which the pulmonary artery and right outflow tract can often be shown to cross the aorta and left ventricular outflow tract in a transverse fashion at an angle of about 30° generally excludes the transposition of the great vessels.

The short axis great vessel view demonstrates the right cardiac structures (right atrium, tricuspid view, right ventricle, and pulmonic valve) arrayed circumferentially around the aortic root, with the bifurcation of the pulmonary artery into the ductus and the right pulmonary artery clearly seen. The aortic root can be viewed as the eye of the hurricane. The triple leaf pattern of the aortic valve (resembling the letter Y) is often seen. This view is helpful to show the discrete origin of the major great vessels and assists with evaluation of complex cardiac abnormalities.

The aortic arch begins centrally within the heart, initially crosses from left to right, then curves from right to left, travels somewhat anteriorly to form the transverse arch, and then continues curving inferiorly and posteriorly to form the descending aorta. Its shape has been compared with that of a candy cane. The three strap vessels (the left subclavian artery, the left common carotid artery, and the brachiocephalic trunk) arising from the aortic arch help distinguish the aortic from the ductal arch. Discontinuities in the arch lead to coarctation, and asymmetry in right and left ventricular volumes suggest possible alterations in the relative flow through the pulmonary and systemic circulatory systems, which will become more significant later in pregnancy or after birth. In cases of disordered flow, abnormalities of the heart may become more obvious as time progresses (Allan et al. 1989).

The ductal arch arises as the principle extension of the pulmonary artery. It forms a broad, gently curved arch, which is similar to a hockey stick in appearance. The ductal arch is much more prominent in fetuses than infants after birth, because it conducts blood from the pulmonary artery to the aorta and then (under normal circumstances) closes soon after delivery. In utero, the ductus arteriosus allows right heart structures to process blood volumes approximating postpartum levels and at levels far in excess of volumes passing through the fetal lungs before delivery. The fetal lungs then expand after delivery and blood flow through the lungs increases dramatically. Subsequently, prostaglandin production by lung tissues decreases after increased local oxygen tension has been achieved, and the ductus arteriosus normally then closes. In this manner, the right heart and pulmonary vessels are prepared for the eventual transition to normal adult circulatory patterns.

Fetal Cardiac Dysrhythmias

Both bradyarrhythmias and tachyarrhythmias are occasionally noted on auscultation or direct observation of the fetal heart. Bradycardia may result from transient positional maternal hypotension, as a sporadic fetal event of minimal clinical significance, in a prolonged acute fashion potentially related to fetal compromise, or as a chronic finding related to maternal diseases or structural cardiac abnormalities. Transient bradycardias often occur as a result of supine maternal positioning during sonographic evaluations. They normally resolve after repositioning in a more lateral when initial maternal symptoms of warmth and faintness are noted. Transient bradycardias are also noted during prolonged intervals of fetal cardiac monitoring and are not related to maternal hypotension. They usually last 60–90 seconds, occur sporadically, and do not occur more often than every several hours. Bradycardic events occurring with greater frequency or as new onset bradycardia without resolution should be evaluated from the perspective of possible impending fetal compromise.

Bradycardia may also occur as a result of disordered or disrupted conduction within the heart. Dysfunction of the cardiac conduction system may result from disruption by structural abnormalities of cardiac valves or septa, or may be caused by autoimmune damage to these structures. Antiphospholipid antibodies such as anti-Sjogren's Syndrome A (or anti-Rho) are often found, although antibodies against SS-B (anti-La) are also sometimes identified. When bradycardia occurs in this way, it usually persists chronically, although medical therapy with steroids has been reported to be beneficial in isolated cases. Bradycardia with hydrops has a high associated mortality. In the absence of structural abnormality, chronic heart rates of 70–80 may be well tolerated over the course of pregnancy if signs of cardiac failure do not develop. Structural cardiac abnormalities occur in 50% of infants with heart block, but maternal collagen vascular disease is present in up to 70% of such infants if the heart appears structurally normal.

Fetal cardiac dysrhythmias such as premature ventricular and premature atrial contractions are sometimes auscultated. These are usually sporadic events but generally are referred for fetal echocardiography to exclude the possibility of underlying congenital heart disease. Pulse Doppler is helpful in evaluating PVCs (premature ventricular contractions) and PACs (premature atrial contractions). The Doppler sampling area is placed near the site of the origin of the aorta or pulmonary artery and an associated atrial-ventricular valve. The timing of blood flow from atrium to ventricle and out of the ventricular outflow tract can then be assessed from the same image and the origin of the dysrhythmia established.

Fetal tachycardia is usually defined as a fetal heart rate > 170 beats per minute. It is a relatively rare complication of pregnancy and accounts for about 15% of fetal cardiac rhythm disturbances. The most common tachyarrhythmia is supraventricular tachycardia. Other potential etiologies include atrial flutter and atrial fibrillation. Tachycardia may also result from problems such as maternal fever, infection, or as a consequence of early uteroplacental insufficiency. During the initial evaluation of fetal tachycardia, it is important to determine whether the rhythm disturbance is possibly related to one of the later causes, as these may require acute management, or even delivery.

The cases associated with very high ventricular rates commonly develop cardiac failure and hydrops, sometimes progressing on to death. The hydrops results from progressively shortened diastolic filling intervals as the atrial rate increases. This forces the fetal heart to be less efficient, and hydrops may then develop. Two complementary methods of monitoring fetal cardiac function have recently been evaluated by Falkensammer. They allow noninvasive serial fetal assessment and offer the potential to treat fetuses if they appear to be developing heart failure (Falkensammer et al. 2001).

Treatment of tachyarrhythmias centers around assessment of fetal status, correction of the rhythm disturbance by pharmacologic measures (using digoxin, propranolol, verapamil, or other medications), and ongoing assessment of the fetal status as measures to control the disturbance are undertaken.

Evaluation for IUGR

Fetal growth restriction is an important obstetric complication that may result from a wide variety of causes. When incorrect dates have been excluded from consideration, growth restricted fetuses are at increased risk of aneuploidy, increased rates of fetal demise in utero and neonatal mortality, numerous forms of perinatal morbidity, and cerebral palsy. Conversely, if suspected growth restriction is in fact due to incorrect pregnancy dating, patients will be subjected to needless worry, undergo unnecessary testing, and may even undergo unnecessary expense and risks related to procedures such as umbilical blood sampling, amniocentesis, premature delivery, or cesarean section. It is clearly in the patient's and fetus's best interest to accurately assess the fetal growth status.

Fetal growth and development consist of overlapping phases of cellular activity. Fetal growth in the early stages of pregnancy consists primarily of cellular hyperplasia. In mid-second trimester, growth consists of both cellular hyperplasia and hypertrophy, while in the latter portion of the third trimester fetal cellular activity consists, for the most part, of cellular hypertrophy (Winnick 1971). Diseases that affect fetal growth and development early in pregnancy will tend to result in symmetric growth anomalies (most or all parameters are smaller than expected for gestation) because cellular hyperplasia will be affected, while abnormalities occurring later in pregnancy will tend to result in asymmetric growth because of effects that influence the fetus while cellular hypertrophy is supposed to be occurring. As fetal growth restriction begins in later pregnancy, the fetus often attempts to adapt by increasing perfusion to the head and decreasing perfusion to abdominal circulation. The head circumference remains relatively unaffected by initial growth restriction and appear appropriate for gestational age, while the abdominal circumference is smaller than would normally be expected. This circulatory pattern leaves the fetus with asymmetric body proportions.

Fetal growth restriction is most often diagnosed by identifying fetal biometric characteristics that are abnormally small for gestational age. To make such determinations, it is of paramount importance to establish the gestational age to the highest degree of certainty possible. Without accurate pregnancy dating, the process of identifying aberrant fetal growth is made much more difficult, is often delayed significantly, and may require serial electronic fetal well-being assessments and evaluation with relatively complex sonographic techniques, such as pulsed Doppler evaluation of the middle cerebral artery velocity waveforms. Such advanced ultrasonographic techniques may not be available at many community sonographic sites.

Estimated fetal weights are calculated by using one of numerous equations available for the purpose. The abdominal circumference in combination with the BPD, the head circumference, the femur length, or some combination of the three factors is used to estimate fetal weight. If the gestational age is known from other criteria, the derived weight can be compared with standardized tables and a birth weight centile for that gestational age can be assigned. When possible, tables appropriate for the local population and specific for the relevant locale should be used. Tables developed at sea level are not appropriate for fetuses delivered at high altitude, and ascertainment of fetal growth abnormalities in certain ethnic groups will be more accurate as well. Black infants average lower birth weights than white infants, and infants born at altitudes above 5,000 feet, such as in Denver, have been found to weigh approximately 10% less than other infants.

If the estimated weight and estimated gestational age are derived from the same sonographic information, there will be a tendency to find the fetus at some weight centile approximating the 50th centile, because the same normed numbers have been used for both determinations. In many cases, no other option is available. If such circumstances do exist, care should be taken to look for evidence of fetal growth aberrations, especially if the estimated fetal gestational age places the fetus in the third trimester.

Estimated fetal weights are usually within 15–20% of their actual value, with the majority (58%) actually falling within 10% of the predicted value. In term or postterm infants, clinical estimations of fetal weight are for the most part as accurate as sonographic methods, while sonographic methods appear to be superior in fetuses that are preterm, or that weigh <2,500 g (Chauhan et al. 1998). Estimated fetal weights also tend to be less accurate in rather small (<1,500 g) or heavy (>4,000 or 4,500 g) infants. Some authors believe estimated fetal weight with coexistent oligohydramnios may tend to underestimate the actual fetal weight; also, recent research calls this into question (Chauhan et al. 1999). It is technically very difficult to estimate fetal weights in fetuses with conditions such as gastroschisis or omphalocele, because the mathematic formulae used for weight prediction require accurate abdominal circumference estimations. Nevertheless, care should be taken to look for evidence of other pathological processes that may have caused abnormal (restricted) fetal growth rather than ascribing differences to problems with estimation of the abdominal circumference (Rode et al. 2002).

Gestational age should be assigned with data from an accurate menstrual history and the earliest accurate fetal evaluation available. In practice, if the menstrual history is considered accurate, and the menstrual gestational age falls within 10% of the sonographic estimate of gestational age, the menstrual gestational age is accepted for pregnancy dating. If any uncertainty about the accuracy of the menstrual dating is noted, or if the menstrual age estimate falls outside the 10% margin of error, the earliest accurate sonographic age estimate should be used to establish the estimated gestational age.

Gestational age estimations from crown–rump lengths (CRL) obtained at 6–10 weeks gestation are accurate to <1 week gestation, while gestational age determinations later in pregnancy are proportionately less accurate. The mean CRL ranges from approximately 1.9 mm at 5.5 weeks to 3.1 cm at 10 weeks gestation and 6.4 cm at 13 weeks of gestation. The CRL is accurate to +3 days at 7–10 weeks gestation and +5 days at 10–14 weeks gestation. As previously noted, gestational age estimations before 22 weeks gestation are accurate to approximately 10% of the age determined. Slightly greater errors in gestational age estimation may occur after 22 weeks gestation. Fetal growth disturbances such as insufficient or excessive fetal growth, when present, will cause erroneous estimations of gestational age.

If gestational age dating information is poorly established, the overall pattern of sonographic findings should be taken into account. Reduced amniotic fluid,

Grade 3 placental morphology, and elevated FL/AC all suggest the possibility of ongoing pathology and possible fetal growth restriction, while a normal appearing amniotic fluid volume, Grade 1 placental morphology, symmetric body measurements, and a normal range FL/AC are as a group more consistent with a normal fetal nutritional status.

Although not as specific or sensitive as direct biometric measures, ratios of several fetal parameters are also useful in identifying aberrant fetal growth. The femur/abdomen ratio normally falls between 0.20 and 0.24 throughout the third trimester. Values of >0.24 indicate an abnormally small abdominal circumference, a hallmark of asymmetric fetal growth restriction. The ratio of head circumference to abdominal circumference varies by gestational age, ranging from 1.05 to 1.20 (± 2 SD range) at 28 weeks gestation to 0.9–1.15 at 36 weeks gestation and 0.8–1.05 at 40 weeks gestation. If the gestational age is uncertain, the FL/AC ratio is more useful for fetal evaluation.

Doppler sonography now offers the ability to assess for uteroplacental insufficiency and redistribution of flow. These methods have been described in the section on general sonographic techniques.

REFERENCES

Albert A, Sancho MA, Julia V, Diaz F, Bombi JA, Morales L: Intestinal damage in gastroschisis is independent of the size of the abdominal defect. *Pediatr Surg Int* 17:116, 2001.

Allan LD, Sharland G, Tynan MJ: The natural history of the hypoplastic left heart syndrome. *Int J Cardiol* 25:341, 1989.

Alsulyman OM, Monteiro H, Ouzounian JG, Barton L, Songster GS, Kovacs BW: Clinical significance of prenatal ultrasonographic intestinal dilatation in fetuses with gastroschisis. *Am J Obstet Gynecol* 175:982, 1996.

American College of Obstetrics and Gynecology: *Practice Bulletin, Clinical Management Guidelines, Number 27: Prenatal Diagnosis of Fetal Chromosomal Abnormalities*, Washington, DC, May 2001.

Anderson N, Boswell O, Duff G: Prenatal sonography for the detection of fetal anomalies: results of a prospective study and comparison with prior series. *Am J Roentgen* 165:943, 1995.

Bahado-Singh RO, Oz UA, Kovanci E, Deren O, Feather M, Hsu CD, Copel JA, Mahoney MJ: Gestational age standardized nuchal thickness values for estimating midtrimester Down's syndrome risk. *J Maternal-Fetal Med* 8:37, 1999.

Bahado-Singh RO, Oz U, Hsu CD, Deren O, Copel JA, Mahoney MJ: Ratio of nuchal thickness to humerus length for Down syndrome detection. *Am J Obstet Gynecol* 184:1284, 2001.

Bahado-Singh RO, Rowther M, Bailey J, Mendilcioglu I, Choi SJ, Oz U, Copel J: Midtrimester nuchal thickness and the prediction of postnatal congenital heart defect. *Am J Obstet Gynecol* 187:1250, 2002.

Brown T, Kliewer MA, Hertzberg BS, Ruiz C, Stamper TH, Rosnes J, et al.: A role for maternal serum screening in detecting chromosomal abnormalities in fetuses with isolated choroid plexus cysts: a prospective multicentre study. *Prenat Diagn* 19:405, 1999.

Chauhan SP, Hendrix NW, Magann EF, Morrison JC, Kenney SP, Devoe LD: Limitations of clinical and sonographic estimates of birth weight: experience with 1034 parturients. *Obstet Gynecol* 91:72, 1998.

Chauhan SP, Scardo JA, Hendrix NW, Magann EF, Morrison JC: Accuracy of sonographically estimated fetal weight with and without oligohydramnios. A case-control study. *J Reprod Med* 44:969, 1999.

Comstock CH, Smith R, Lee W, Kirk JS: Right fetal cardiac axis: clinical significance and associated findings. *Obstet Gynecol* 91:495, 1998.

Corteville JE, Gray DL, Crane JP: Congenital hydronephrosis: correlation of fetal ultrasonographic findings with infant outcome. *Am J Obstet Gynecol* 165:384, 1991.

Crane JM, Ash K, Fink N, Desjardins C: Abnormal fetal cardiac axis in the detection of intrathoracic anomalies and congenital heart disease. *Ultrasound Obstet Gynecol* 10:90, 1997.

Crane JP, LeFevre ML, Winborn RC, Evans JK, Ewigman BG, Bain RP, Frigoletto FD, McNellis D: A randomized trial of prenatal ultrasonographic screening: impact on the detection, management, and outcome of anomalous fetuses. The RADIUS Study Group. *Am J Obstet Gynecol* 171:392, 1994.

Drugan A, Johnson MP, Isada NB, Holzgreve W, Zador IE, Dombrowski MP, Sokol RJ, Hallak M, Evans MI: The smaller than expected first-trimester fetus is at increased risk for chromosome anomalies. *Am J Obstet Gynecol* 167:1525, 1992.

Falkensammer CB, Paul J, Huhta JC: Fetal congestive heart failure: correlation of Tei-index and Cardiovascular-score. *J Perinat Med* 29:390, 2001.

Farrell TA, Hertzberg BS, Kliewer MA, Harris L, Paine SS: Fetal lateral ventricles: reassessment of normal values for atrial diameter at US. *Radiology* 193:409, 1994.

Geirsson RT, Busby ERM: Certain dates may not provide a reliable estimate of gestational age. *Br J Obstet Gynaecol* 98:108, 1991.

Glick PL, Harrison MR, Golbus MS, Adzick NS, Filly RA, Callen PW, Mahoney BS, Anderson RL, deLorimer AA: Management of the fetus with congenital hydro nephrosis II: Prognostic criteria and selection for treatment. *J Pediatric Surgery* 20:376, 1985.

Grannum P, Bracken M, Silverman R, Hobbins JC: Assessment of fetal kidney size in normal gestation by comparison of ratio of kidney circumference to abdominal circumference. *Am J Obstet Gynecol* 136:249, 1980.

Goldstein I, Lockwood C, Hobbins JC: Ultrasound assessment of fetal intestinal development in the evaluation of gestational age. *Obstet Gynecol* 70:682, 1987.

Goldstein I, Reece EA, Yarkoni S, Wan M, Green JL, Hobbins JC: Growth of the fetal stomach in normal pregnancies. *Obstet Gynecol* 70:641, 1987.

Gupta JK, Khan KS, Thornton JG, Lilford RJ: Management of fetal choroid plexus cysts. *Br J Obstet Gynaecol* 104:881, 1997.

Johnson ML, Pretorius D, Clewell WH, Meier PR, Manchester D: Fetal hydrocephalus: diagnosis and management. *Semin Perinatol* 7:83, 1983.

Kuhn P, Brizot ML, Pandya PP, Snijders RJ, Nicolaides KH: Crown-rump length in chromosomally abnormal fetuses at 10 to 13 weeks' gestation. *Am J Obstet Gynecol* 172:32, 1995.

Lameier LN, Katz VL: Amnioinfusion: a review. *Obstet Gynecol Surv* 48:829, 1993.

Lynch L, Berkowitz GS, Chitkara U, Wilkins IA, Mehalek KE, Berkowitz RL: Ultrasound detection of Down syndrome: is it really possible? *Obstet Gynecol* 73:267, 1989.

Mandell J, Blyth BR, Peters CA, Retik AB, Estroff JA, Benacerraf BR: Structural genitourinary defects detected in utero. *Radiology* 178:193, 1991.

Nicolaides KH, Azar G, Snijders RJ, and Gosden CM: Fetal nuchal oedema: associated malformations and chromosomal defects. *Fetal Diagn Ther* 7:123, 1992.

Nicolaides KH, Salvesen DR, Snijders RJ, Gosden CM: Strawberry- shaped skull in fetal trisomy 18. *Fetal Diagn Ther* 7:132, 1992.

Nyberg DA, Fitzsimmons J, Mack LA, Hughes M, Pretorius DH, Hickok D, Shepard TH: Chromosomal abnormalities in fetuses with omphalocele. Significance of omphalocele contents. *J Ultrasound Med* 8:299, 1989.

Nyberg DA, Mack LA, Laing FC, Jeffrey RB: Early pregnancy complications: endovaginal sonographic findings correlated with human chorionic gonadotropin levels. *Radiology* 167:619, 1988.

Nyberg DA, Mack LA, Patten RM, Cyr DR: Fetal bowel: normal sonographic findings. *J Ultrasound Med* 6:3, 1987.

Nyberg DA, Resta RG, Hickok DE, Hollenbach KA, Luthy DA, Mahony BS: Femur length shortening in the detection of Down syndrome: is prenatal screening feasible? *Am J Obstet Gynecol* 162:1247, 1990.

Nyberg DA: Ultrasound markers of fetal Down syndrome. *JAMA* 285:2856, 2001.

Pandya PP, Kondylios A, Hilbert L, Snijders RJ, Nicolaides KH: Chromosomal defects and outcome in 1015 fetuses with increased nuchal translucency. *Ultrasound Obstet Gynecol* 5:15, 1995.

Parulekar SG: Sonography of normal fetal bowel. *J Ultrasound Med* 10:211, 1991.

Pretorius DH, Davis K, Manco Johnson ML, Manchester D, Meier PR, Clewell WH: Clinical course of fetal hydrocephalus: 40 cases. *Am J Roentgenol* 144:827, 1985.

Ramirez A, Espinosa de los Monteros A, Parra A, De Leon B: Esophageal atresia and tracheo-esophageal fistula in two infants born to hyperthyroid women receiving methimazole (Tapazol) during pregnancy. *Am J Med Genet* 44:200, 1992.

Rode ME, Jackson GM, Jenkins TM, Macones GA: Ultrasonographic measurement of the abdominal circumference in fetuses with congenital diaphragmatic hernia. *Am J Obstet Gynecol* 186:321, 2002.

Schwartz MZ, Silver H, Schulman S: Maintenance of the placental circulation to evaluate and treat an infant with massive head and neck hemangioma. *J Pediatr Surg* 28:520, 1993.

Sipes SL, Weiner CP, Williamson RA, Pringle KC, Kimura K: Fetal gastroschisis complicated by bowel dilation: an indication for imminent delivery? *Fetal Diagn Ther* 5:100, 1990.

Smith-Bindman R, Hosmer W, Feldstein VA, Deeks JJ, Goldberg JD: Second-trimester ultrasound to detect fetuses with Down syndrome: a meta-analysis. *JAMA* 285:1044, 2001.

Snijders RJ, Sherrod C, Gosden CM, Nicolaides KH: Fetal growth retardation: associated malformations and chromosomal abnormalities. *Am J Obstet Gynecol* 168:547, 1993.

Snijders RJM and Nicolaides KH: *Ultrasound Markers for Fetal Chromosomal Defects*, New York, Parthenon Publishing Group, 1996.

Stocks RM, Egerman RS, Woodson GE, Bower CM, Thompson JW, Wiet GJ: Airway management of neonates with antenatally detected head and neck anomalies. *Arch Otolaryngol Head Neck Surg* 123:641, 1997.

Sullivan A, Giudice T, Vavelidis F, Thiagarajah S: Choroid plexus cysts: is biochemical testing a valuable adjunct to targeted ultrasonography? *Am J Obstet Gynecol* 181:260, 1999.

Wald NJ, Smith D, Kennard A, Palomaki GE, Salonen R, Holzgreve W, Pejtsik B, Coombes EJ, Mancini G, MacRae AR, et al.: Biparietal diameter and crown-rump length in fetuses with Down's syndrome: implications for antenatal serum screening for Down's syndrome. *Br J Obstet Gynaecol* 100:430, 1993.

Winnick M: Cellular changes during placental and fetal growth. *Am J Obstet Gynecol* 109:166, 1971.

Zerres K, Albrecht R, Waldherr R: Acquired cystic kidney disease – a possible pitfall in genetic counseling. *Hum Genet* 71:267, 1985.

Zerres K, Volpel MC, Weiss H: Cystic kidneys. Genetics, pathologic anatomy, clinical picture, and prenatal diagnosis. *Hum Genet* 68:104, 1984.

Part III. Advances in First Trimester Ultrasound

Susan Guidi

Throughout the last 25 years, revolutionary advances in obstetrical ultrasound imaging have continued to surpass our expectations of what was possible in imaging the embryo and fetus. In the late 1970s, linear real-time technology was our first leap forward, allowing us to appreciate movement for the first time. The introduction of endovaginal technology in the late 1980s, once again revolutionized our imaging capabilities. This technology not only gave outstanding clarity to the image, it gave birth to the phrase sonoembryology.

Three-dimensional endovaginal ultrasound renders images that rival those in morphologic embryology texts. The focus in ultrasound moves to the embryonic period, because most major anatomic structures and organ systems are formed during this period. Three-dimensional endovaginal ultrasound provides a view of the embryo in sculpture-like reconstruction mode. Three-dimensional ultrasound is a valuable, noninvasive imaging tool for the first trimester of pregnancy.

MORPHOLOGICAL DEVELOPMENT OF THE EMBRYO

Note: Periods are given as gestational age, which is 2 weeks greater than the developmental age.

Five Weeks

Gestational sac can be seen as a small spherical cystic structure inside the

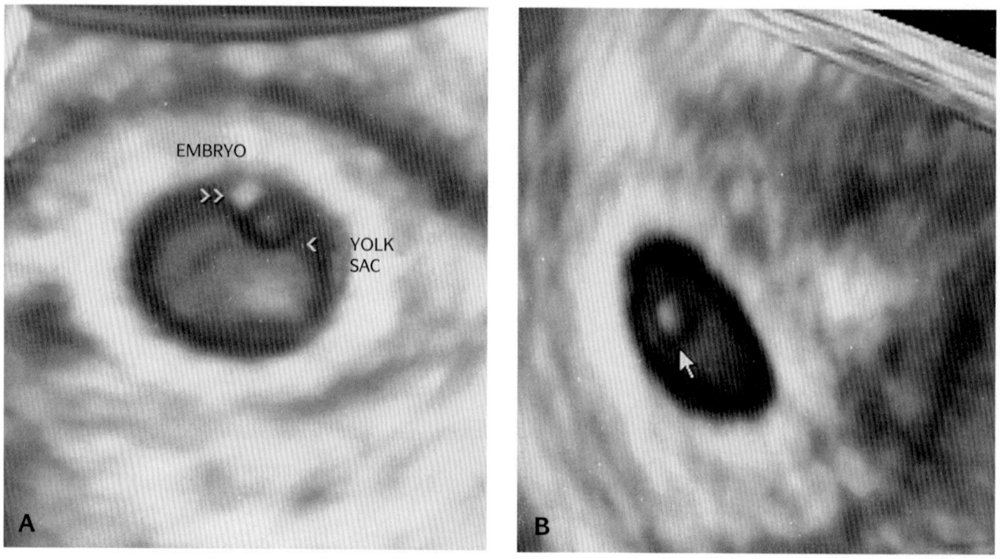

4.34. **(A)** Three-dimensional transvaginal imaging of a gestational sac at 6 weeks. Note the yolk sac (arrow). **(B)** Three-dimensional transvaginal imaging at 6 weeks gestation by surface mode. The embryo and yolk sac are depicted in various grayscale images.

endometrial cavity from the 5th week of gestation (the last menstrual period, 3 weeks developmental age).

Multiplanar images can distinguish between the early gestational sac and free fluid between the endometrial leaves (pseudogestational sac).

Three-dimensional ultrasound can be used to calculate the volume of the gestational sac in the multiplanar mode.

Three-dimensional ultrasound can also be used to calculate **yolk sac** volume and will further enhance the capability of the diagnosis of normal versus abnormal yolk sac.

The **embryo** can be seen 24–48 hours after visualization of the yolk sac. The embryo can be seen as a straight line, adjacent to the yolk sac at 2–3 mm in CRL.

The planar mode will allow better detection of the embryonic pole within the gestational sac.

Six Weeks

Typical characteristics of the 6-week embryo include a rounded bulky head and a thinner body (Figure 4.34). The head is bulky due to the developing forebrain

- The limb buds are rarely visible.
- The umbilical cord and vitelline duct are clearly visible.
- The amnion is visible.
- At this stage of pregnancy the planar mode will allow for more accurate assessment of multiple pregnancies.

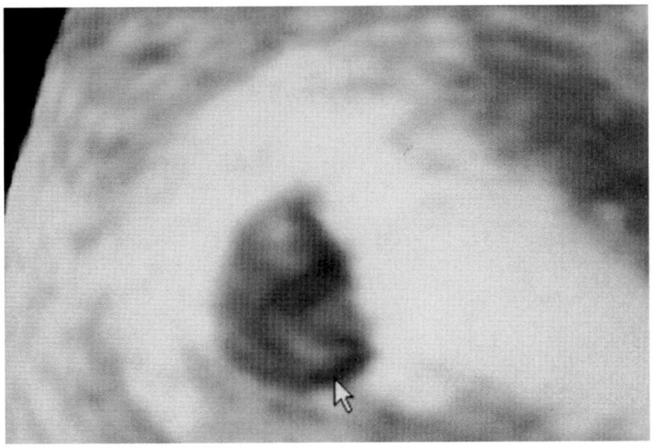

4.35. Three-dimensional surface view of a normal embryo (arrow) at 7 weeks gestation.

Seven Weeks

The embryonic head is still prominent because the rapid development of the rhombencephalon (Figure 4.35). The developing primary vesicles of the brain can be well delineated by the planar mode and are depicted as cystic structures. The head is strongly flexed anteriorly. The hypoechoic brain cavities are visible, particularly the lateral ventricles. Planar mode will allow for more accurate assessment of gestational age by crown–rump determination.

Eight Weeks

The most dramatic change at this gestational age is the complete delineation of limb buds (Figures 4.36 to 4.38). The shape of the face is becoming apparent but the flexion of the cranial pole still makes it very difficult to view the face entirely.

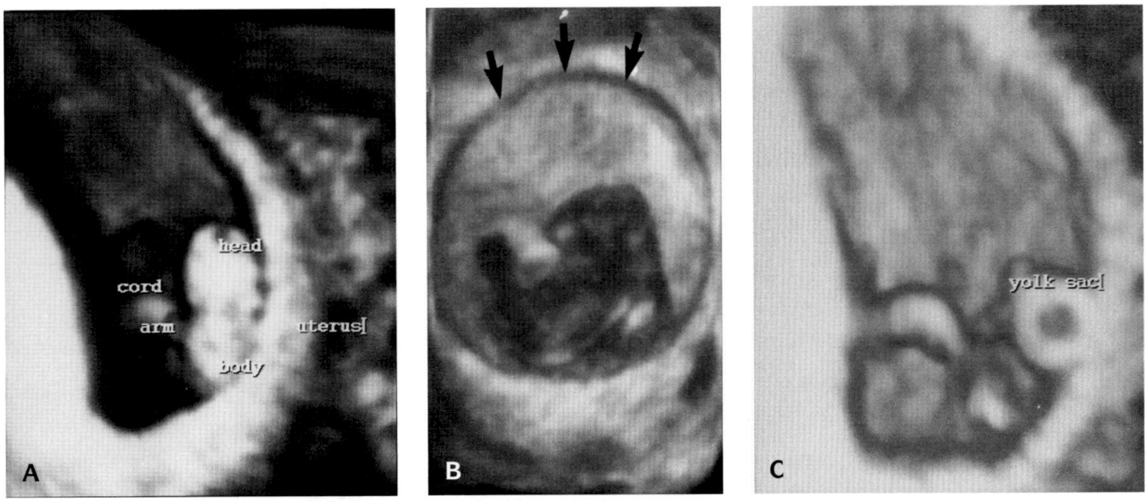

4.36. **(A)** Three-dimensional surface view of a normal embryo at 8 weeks gestation. Note the limb buds, and the detail of the yolk sac. **(B)** Three-dimensional view of the amnion (arrows). **(C)** Three-dimensional view of the yolk sac.

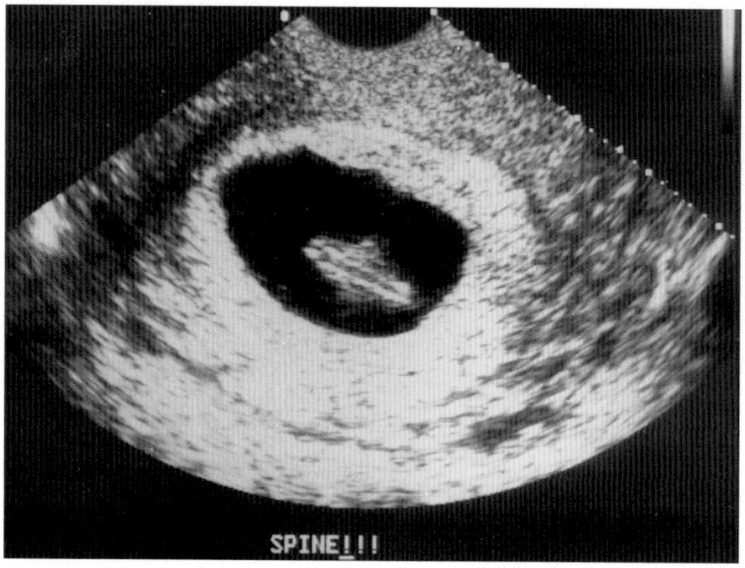

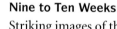

4.37. Two-dimensional images of a coronal scan of an 8 week 0 day embryo. Coronal scans of the neural tube.

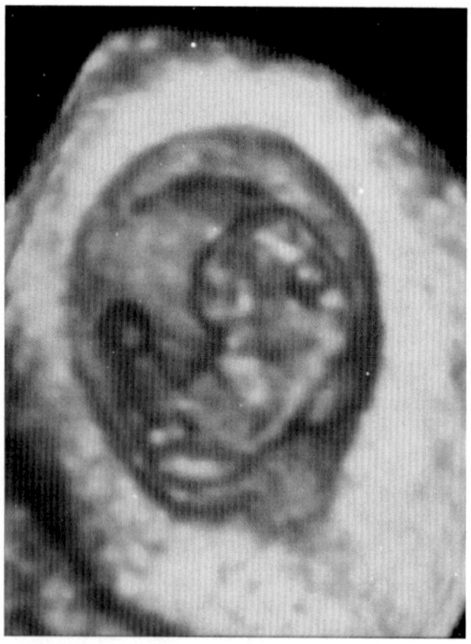

4.38. Three-dimensional surface view of an 8 week 3 day embryo. Note the anterior flexion of the head and excellent delineation of the amniotic sac.

Various authors have now described detailed imaging of the brain, and the anterior and posterior contours of the embryo can be well delineated to enhance early detection of anomalies such as anencephaly.

The amnion can be clearly seen and the extraembryonic coelom is still larger in volume than the amniotic sac. The extraembryonic space will appear more echogenic than the amniotic sac. The yolk sac is a very prominent structure. The ventricular cavities are characteristically cystic, particularly the rhombencephalon. This should not be confused with an early diagnosis of Dandy Walker cyst.

Nine to Ten Weeks

Striking images of the fetal face can now be obtained by the surface-rendering mode and the external ear can often be demonstrated (Figure 4.39).

Mid-gut herniation is quite apparent and should not be mistaken for omphalocele.

The dorsal column and spine can be examined in its whole length.

The arms and legs with the knees are clearly visible and the feet can be seen.

From the 8th to the 9th week dramatic changes in the fetus can be observed in the surface-rendering mode. The external ear can often be demonstrated. The fetal face can now be visualized. Mid-gut herniation is normally present as a physiologic phenomenon.

Eleven to Twelve Weeks

During the last phases of the end of the first trimester striking changes in the development of the head and neck continue (Figures 4.40 and 4.41).

Details in the face such as the nose, orbits, maxilla, and mandible are visible.

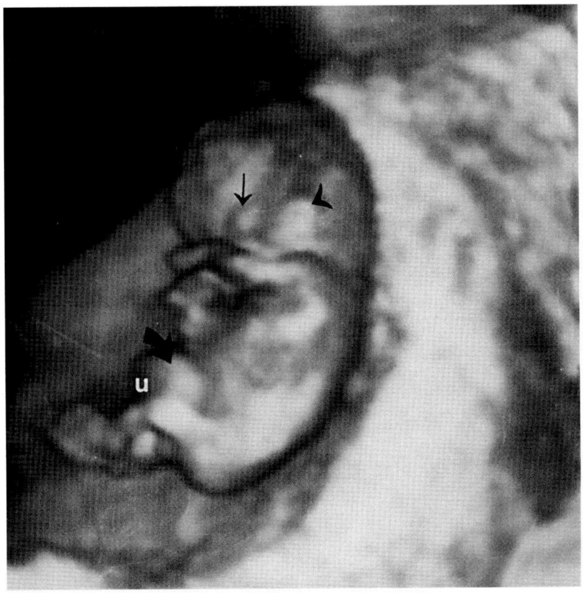

4.39. Three-dimensional surface image of a fetus at 9 weeks, 6 days. The eye (thin arrow) and external ear (arrow head) are depicted. Note the definition in the fetal profile. Herniation of the mid-gut is present (thick arrow) (U = umbilical cord). Note the regular morphology of the fetal head, body and extremities.

The herniation of the gut is no longer visible and its persistence should be presumptive of omphalocele.

The planar mode allows for visualization of the embryonic body and the stomach, kidneys, and bladder are often visible.

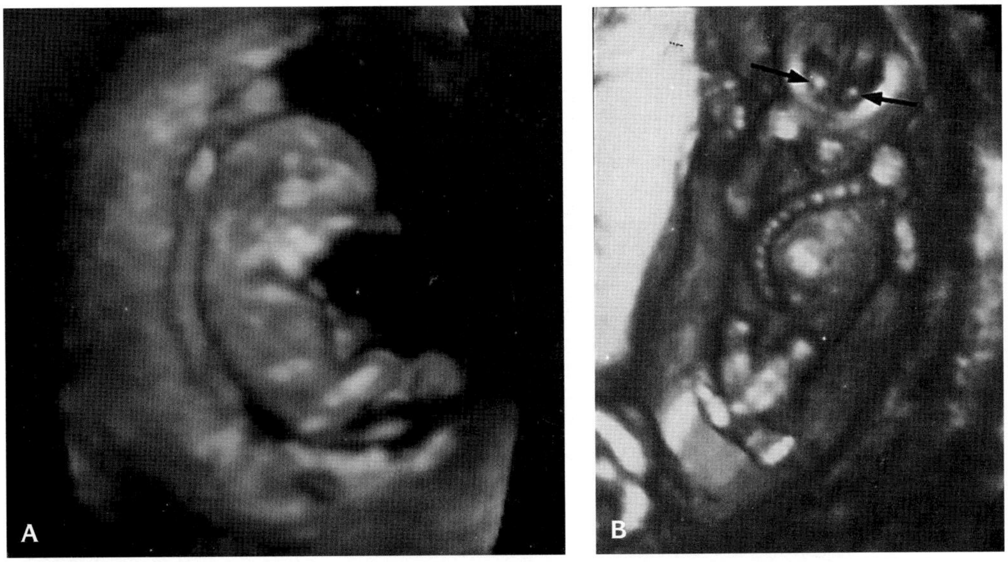

4.40. **(A)** Three-dimensional surface view of the fetus at 12 weeks gestation. Note the regularity of the anterior abdominal wall, since the mid-gut has returned into the abdomen. **(B)** Three-dimensional surface view of a fetus at 12 weeks gestation. Note the choroid plexus (arrows) within the brain and the well demarcated umbilical cord and its insertion into the abdominal wall.

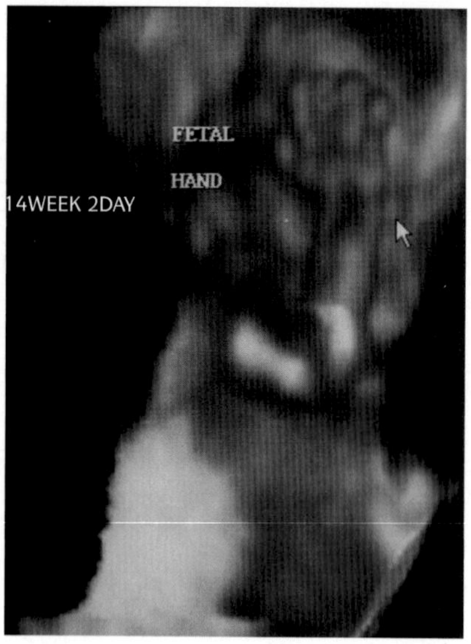

4.41. Three-dimensional surface view of the fetal hand (arrow) at 14 weeks of gestation.

The fetal limbs can be seen with great detail and the ability to distinguish fingers and toes is better with three-dimensional than with two-dimensional ultrasound.

The long bones can be visualized inside the upper and lower extremities and detailed analysis of the fetal spine, chest, and limbs is possible with the transparent/x-ray system.

The lateral ventricles dominate the brain structures seen at this gestational age and the choroid plexus is very prominent. The rhombencephalic cavity filled with the growing cerebellum is clearly visible. Multiplanar reconstruction is more complex, even though this measurement begins to be performed.

FETAL NUCHAL TRANSLUCENCY AND THE USE OF THREE-DIMENSIONAL ULTRASOUND

The technique of measuring nuchal translucency between the 11th and 14th weeks of pregnancy has allowed an amazingly high rate of detection of chromosomal abnormalities (Figure 4.42). The technique is often difficult and the ability of three-dimensional ultrasound to reorient the fetal position using the multiplanar mode will only improve our ability to obtain the measurement consistently. The amniotic membrane is often a problem area. The ability of three-dimensional ultrasound to distinguish between the nuchal region and the amnion will aid greatly in this very important screening exam. Transabdominal scanning is often a more reliable method for obtaining measurement of nuchal thickness because of the lack of flexibility of movement of the endovaginal

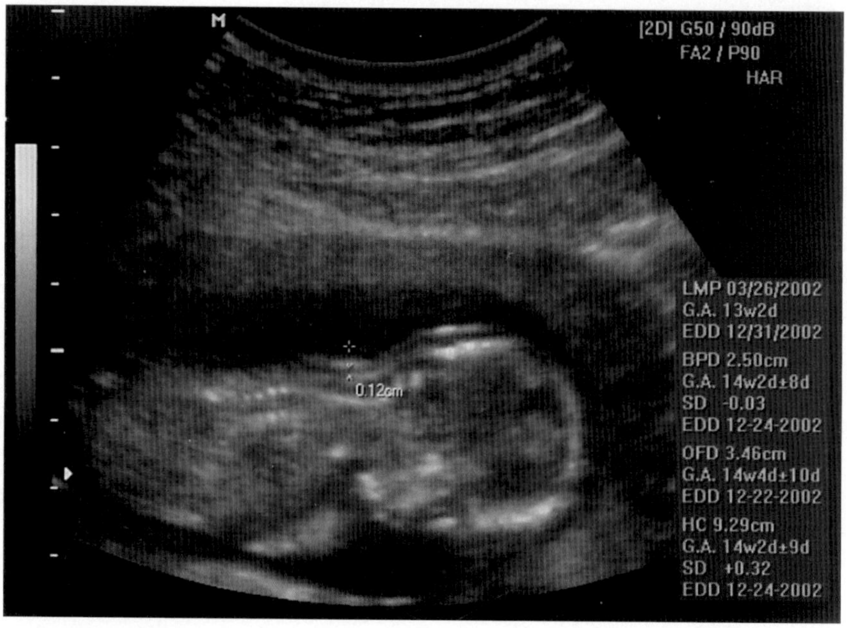

4.42. Measurement of nuchal thickness.

probe in the vaginal vault. Even though endovaginal ultrasound is superior for assessing anatomic detail, the capacity to move around the fetus with the transabdominal probe is distinctly an advantage. The added component of the surface view with three-dimensional scanning allows the anterior and the posterior contours of the fetus to be detailed with outstanding clarity.

REFERENCES

Blaas HG, Eik-Nes SH, Kiserud T, Hellevik LR: Early development of the forebrain and midbrain: a longitudinal study from 7 to 12 weeks of gestation. *Ultrasound Obstet Gynecol* 5:151, 1995.

Bonilla-Musoles F, Raga F, Osborne N, Blanes J: The use of three-dimensional (3D) ultrasound for the study of normal and pathological morphology, of the human embryo and fetus: preliminary report. *J Ultrasound Med* 14:757, 1995.

Braithwaite JM, Economides DL: The measurement of nuchal translucency with transabdominal and transvaginal sonography – success rates, repeatability and level of agreement. *Br J Obstet Gynaecol* 68:720, 1995.

Bree RL, Marn CS: Transvaginal sonography in the first trimester: embryology, anatomy, and hCG correlation. *Semin Ultrasound CT MR* 12:11, 1990.

Fujiwaki R, Hata T, Hata K, Kitao M: Intrauterine sonographic assessments of embryonic development. *Am J Obstet Gynecol* 173:1770, 1995.

Kurchak A, Kupesic S: *Clinical Application of Three-Dimensional Sonography*, Carnforth, UK, Parthenon Publishing, 2000, pp. 109–126.

Merz E: Three-dimensional ultrasound in the evaluation of fetal anatomy fetal malformations. In Chervenak FA, Kurjak A, (eds): *Current Perspectives on The Fetus as a Patient.* Carnforth, UK, Parthenon Publishing, 1996, pp. 75–87.

Nelson TR, Pretorius DH: Three-dimensional ultrasound of fetal surface features. *Ultrasound Obstet Gynecol* 2:166, 1992.

Pretorius DH, House M, Nelson TR: Fetal face visualization using three-dimensional ultrasonography. *J Ultrasound Med* 14:349, 1995.

Pretorius DH, Nelson TR: Three-dimensional use in obstetrics. In Fleischer AC, Manning FA, Jeanty P, Romero R, (eds): *Principles and Practice of Ultrasonography in Obstetrics and Gynecology*, 5th ed, Norwalk, CT, Appleton Lange, 1995, pp. 119–26.

Roberts LJ, Bewley S, Mackinson AM, Rodeck CH: First trimester nuchal translucency: problems with screening the general population I. *Br J Obstet Gynaecol* 102:381, 1995.

Steiner H, Staudach A, Spitzer D, Schaffer H: Three-dimensional ultrasound in obstetrics and gynecology: technique, possibilities and limitations. *Hum Reprod* 1773, 1994.

FIVE

Abnormalities of Placenta

EXAMINATION OF PLACENTA

The placenta should be examined fresh and weighed after the removal of the cord and membranes. Cord length is measured in toto. The cord's insertion site is noted. The placental membranes are examined for both completeness and color. The chorionic vasculature is studied, and notes on aberrancies should be recorded. The cord and membranes are trimmed from the placenta before its weight is determined. The parenchyma of the placenta is examined in "bread loaf" sections to identify irregularities.

A membrane roll is made, which is derived from spiral rotation of the membranes with the point of rupture at the center. This is sectioned (Figure 5.1 and Tables 5.1 to 5.3).

Sections to be microscopically examined include a cross section of the cord, the membrane roll, and three sections from the parenchyma including central and peripheral areas of the placental disc. Any grossly abnormal lesions should also be sectioned.

PLACENTA

The placental parenchyma consists of the villous tissue beneath the chorionic plate and the intervillous space.

Table 5.1 Indications for placental evaluation

Maternal	Prematurity
Diabetes mellitus	Intrauterine growth retardation
Pregnancy-induced hypertension	Congenital anomalies
Premature rupture of membranes	Erythroblastosis fetalis
Preterm delivery before 36 weeks	Transfer to a neonatal intensive care unit
Post term delivery greater than or equal to 42 weeks	Ominous fetal heart rate tracing
Unexplained fever	Presence of meconium
Poor previous obstetric history	Apgar scores below 5 at 1 minute or below 7 at 5 minutes
Oligohydramnios	**Placenta and umbilical cord**
History of drug abuse	Infarcts
Fetus/newborn	Abruptio
Stillborn	Vasa previa
Neonatal death	Placenta previa
Multiple gestation	Abnormal appearance of placenta or cord

Table 5.2 Placenta: gross examination

General features	Umbilical cord
Abnormally large or small placenta	Abnormally short (<32 cm at term)
Abnormal shape	Abnormally long (>100 cm at term)
Visible or palpable abnormalities (infarcts, retroplacental hematoma/abruption, fibrin, calcification, hematomas)	Thrombosis, torsion, absent Wharton jelly
Meconium, heavy staining with thick membrane	True knots, SUA, velamentous insertion

Table 5.3 Placenta: microscopic examination

General features	Membranes	Villi	Inflammation
Intervillous fibrin	Squamous metaplasia	Maturation	Chorioamnionitis
Infarctions	Amnion nodosum	Vessels – chorangiosis	Funisitis
Calcifications	Meconium staining	N.B.C. – fetal distress	Villitis
Fetal stem vessels	Twin gestation	anemia	Deciduitis
Decidual and spiral arteries		hypoxia	
		Edema	

NBC, nucleated red blood cells.

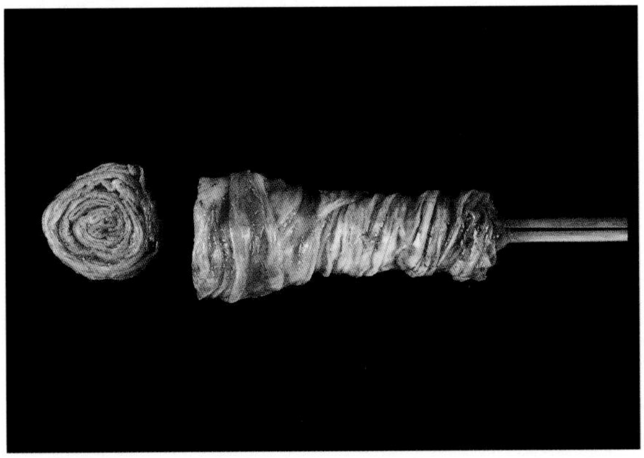

5.1. Membrane roll prepared for microscopic examination with cross section at left.

Table 5.4 Ratio of placental: fetal weight according to gestational age

Age in lunar months	Weight placenta: fetal
6	1:3
7	1:4
8	1:5
9	1:6
10	1:7

Table 5.5 Mean placental weights for normal fetuses, developmental ages 8–18 weeks

Fetal age (wk)	Placental weight (gm)	Fetal age (wk)	Placental weight (gm)
8	1.5	14	83
9	15	15	97
10	29	16	110.5
11	42	17	124
12	56	18	138
13	70		

Data from the Embryofetopathology Laboratory, B.C. Children's Hospital.

ABNORMAL PLACENTAL WEIGHT

Fetal placental weight ratios have been established for various gestational ages (Tables 5.4 to 5.10). At 24 weeks, this ratio is equal to four and increases to seven at term. Small placentas are seen in preeclampsia, low birth weight, and accelerated villous maturation.

Large placentas are seen with villous edema, severe maternal anemia, fetal anemia, syphilis, large intervillous thrombi, maternal diabetes, subchorionic thrombosis, toxoplasmosis, congenital fetal nephrosis, idiopathic fetal hydrops, and multiple placental chorangiomas (Table 5.11).

ABNORMAL COLOR

Pallor is seen in fetal anemia, and, with fetal plethora, deeper hues of bright red are noted.

Severe anemia of the fetus is seen with large amounts of fetal–maternal hemorrhage. Anemia of the fetus may be secondary to hemorrhage from

Table 5.6 Mean weights for singleton placentas

Fetal age (wk)	Placental weight (gm)	Fetal age (wk)	Placental weight (gm)
19	143	30	364
20	157	31	387
21	172	32	411
22	189	33	434
23	208	34	457
24	227	35	478
25	248	36	499
26	270	37	519
27	293	38	537
28	316	39	553
29	340		

Table 5.7 Mean weights for twin placentas

Fetal age (wk)	Placental weight (gm)	Fetal age (wk)	Placental weight (gm)
19	212	31	600
20	218	32	644
21	231	33	687
22	251	34	727
23	276	35	764
24	307	36	798
25	341	37	827
26	380	38	850
27	421	39	868
28	464	40	879
29	509	41	882
30	554		

Table 5.8 Placental ultrasound

Location	Sonographic features	Pathology
Fetal plate	Multiple sonolucent areas to placental periphery	Circumvallate placenta;
	Single sonolucent or hypoechoic area surrounded by thin membrane	Subamniotic cyst; old subamniotic hematoma
	Single hyperechoic area surrounded by thin membrane	Recent subamniotic hematoma
	Heterogenous mass protruding into amniotic cavity	Chorangioma; teratoma
Placental tissue	Small sonolucent area in center of cotyledon	Centrocotyledonary cavity
	Hypoechoic round mass, well circumscribed	Chorioangioma; old infarct
	Large sonolucent area	Cavern; recent thrombosis; septal cyst
	Large hyperechoic area	Old thrombosis; recent infarct
	Multiple sonolucent areas of various sizes and shapes	Hydatidiform-like transformations
Maternal plate	Large hyperechoic area	Recent retroplacental hematoma
	Large hypoechoic area	Old retroplacental hematoma

Table 5.9 Cord lengths for normal fetuses, developmental ages 8–18 weeks

Fetal age (wk)	Cord length (cm)	Fetal age (wk)	Cord length (cm)
8	6.5	14	16
9	8.0	15	18
10	10	16	19
11	11	17	21
12	13	18	23
13	14.5		

Data from the Embryofetopathology Laboratory, B.C. Children's Hospital.

Table 5.10 Umbilical cord length through second half of gestation

Gestational age (wk)	Mean umbilical cord length (cm)
20–21	32
22–23	36
24–25	40
26–27	42.5
28–29	45
30–31	48
32–33	50
34–35	52.5
36–37	56
38–39	57
40–41	60
42–43	61

(Naeye RL: Umbilical cord length: clinical significance. *J Pediatr* 107:278, 1985)

Table 5.11 Causes of placentomegaly

Maternal
Maternal diabetes mellitus
Maternal malnutrition
Anemia

Fetal
Chronic intrauterine infection
Immunohemolytic anemia
- Rh isoimmunization
- Fetal-maternal ABO blood group incompatibility
- Kell antigen isoimmunization

Fetomaternal hemorrhage
α-Thalassemia
Twin-to-twin transfusion syndrome
Renal vein thrombosis
Other causes for nonimmunologic hydrops
Fetal cardiac failure
- premature closure of foramen ovale
- premature closure of ductus arteriosus
- endocardial fibroelastosis
- myocarditis
- hypoplastic left heart syndrome
- large atrioventricular malformation
- intrauterine heart block (due to maternal systemic lupus erythematosus)

Fetal hypoproteinemia
- congenital nephrosis (Finnish type)
- chromosomal errors/partial molar change
- open neural tube defects
- metabolic storage diseases
- osteochondrodystrophies
- Wiedemann-Beckwith syndrome

Placental
Placental tumors (chorangioma)

unprotected velamentous vessels or to an abruption and placenta previa. Congenital infections, such as parvovirus B19, will produce anemia and is seen as pallor in the placenta.

ABNORMAL PLACENTAL SHAPE

Placentas are usually discoid. They may be bilobed or have multiple accessory lobes (succenturiate) (Figures 5.2 to 5.4).

In placenta membranacea, the entire chorion laeve persists and covers the membranes. Little or no free membranes are evident. These abnormal placentas are often associated with placenta accreta, second-trimester bleeding, and fetal and neonatal complications. Incidence is approximately 1/40,000 gestations.

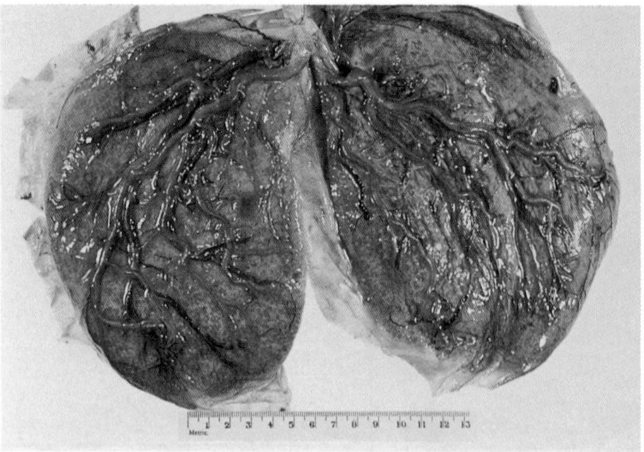

5.2. Bilobate placenta (placenta duplex).

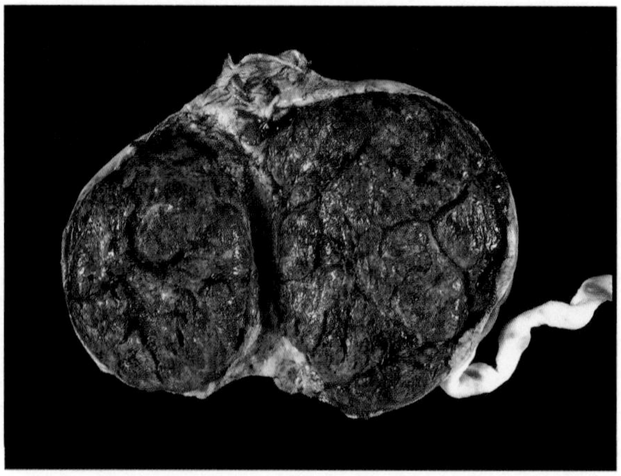

5.3. Succenturiate lobe of placenta.

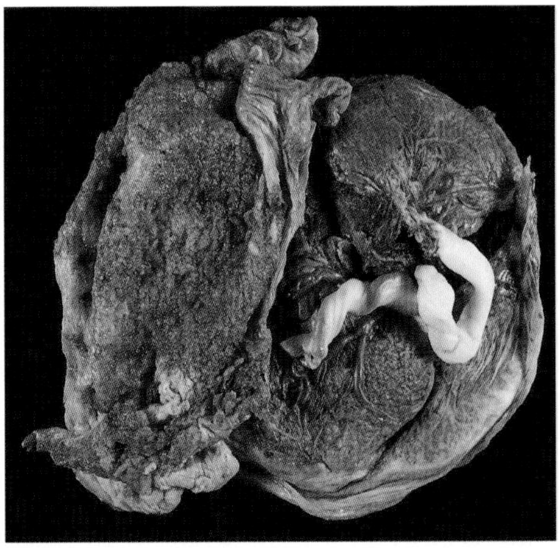

5.4. Placenta membranacea. The chorion laeve has persisted and covers the membranes on left.

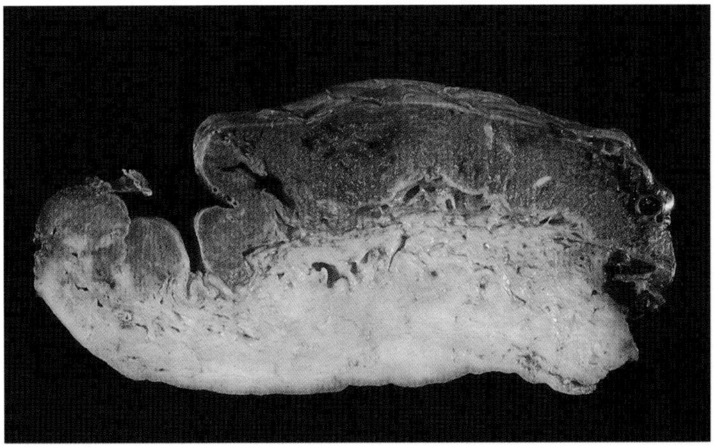

5.5. Placenta increta. The placenta has penetrated into the muscularis of the uterus.

PLACENTA ACCRETA, INCRETA, PERCRETA

The hallmark of placenta accreta is the failure of normal decidua to be juxtaposed between implanting villi on the uterine myometrium (Figures 5.5 and 5.6). The absence of decidual tissue focally creates an implantation in the myometrium that cannot be cleaved postpartum and thus results in a retained placenta. If the villous tissue implants within the myometrium, placenta increta

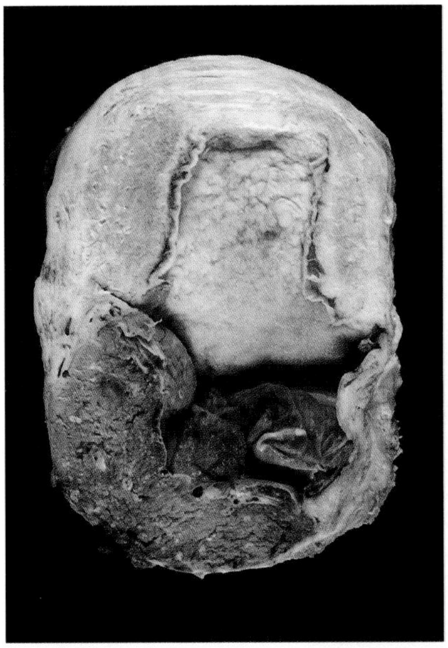

5.6. Placenta percreta. The placenta has penetrated through the full thickness of the uterus.

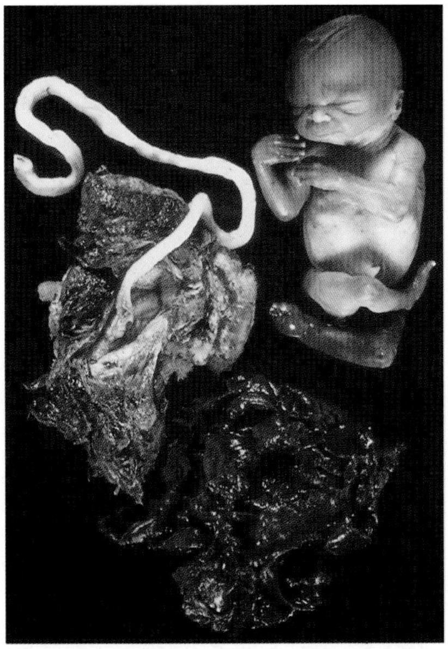

5.7. Retroplacental hemorrhage on maternal surface resulting in abruption. The fetus is macerated.

Table 5.12 **Placental changes: bleeding**

Retroplacental hemorrhage
Marginal hemorrhage
Circumvallation
Ascending infection
Retromembranous hemorrhage
Marginal previa
Ruptured velamentous vessel

occurs; where the parenchymal tissue actually erodes through the serosa of the uterus is a placenta percreta.

PLACENTA PREVIA

Low implantations of the placenta may cover the entire cervical os and be a complete placenta previa or border the internal cervical os and be a marginal placenta previa (Table 5.12). Placental findings include atrophy or infarction of villi near the cervical os because many such pregnancies are marked by second- and third-trimester bleeding, retroplacental hemorrhage, or hemosiderin deposition in the membranes. Preterm birth, as well as chronic bleeding and associated maternal and fetal anemia, increase the risk of hypoxia. There is also a positive correlation between cigarette smoking and the finding of placenta previa.

PLACENTAL ABRUPTION

Abruptio placentae results in retroplacental hematoma or hemorrhage. Findings in the placenta include characteristic intervillous hemorrhage and associated early changes of infarction (Figures 5.7 to 5.9). Thrombotic material is often found adherent to the base of the placenta that will depress its surface. Causes of placental abruption include chorioamnionitis, hypertensive disease, inflammation of the decidual vasculature, and trauma. A long umbilical cord, congenital malformations, preeclampsia, and smoking during pregnancy result in an increased risk of placental abruption. There is increased association of preterm birth, stillbirth, and neonatal death. Other causes for placental bleeding should be considered.

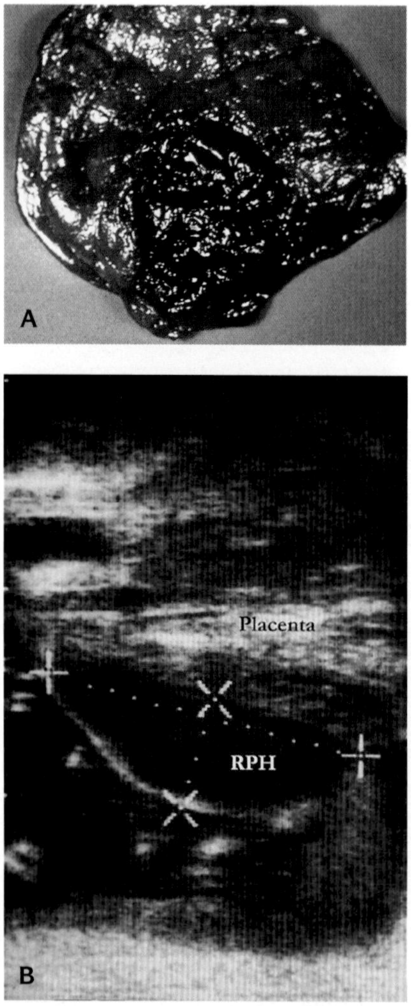

5.8. **(A)** A large retroplacental hematoma on the maternal surface. **(B)** Ultrasound of a large retroplacental hematoma (RPH) outlined by calipers.

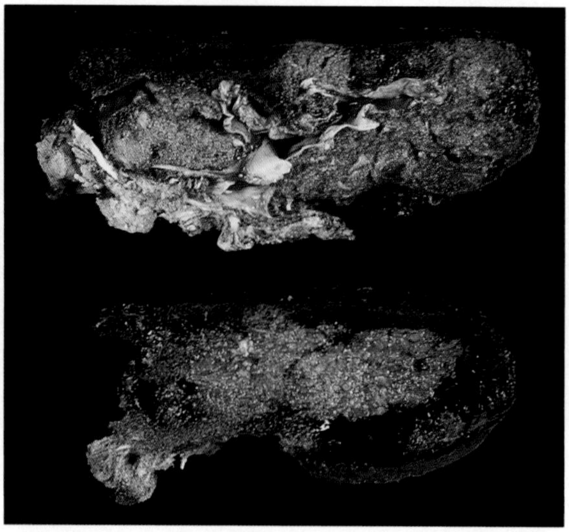

5.9. Retroplacental hemorrhage penetrated into the substance of the placenta.

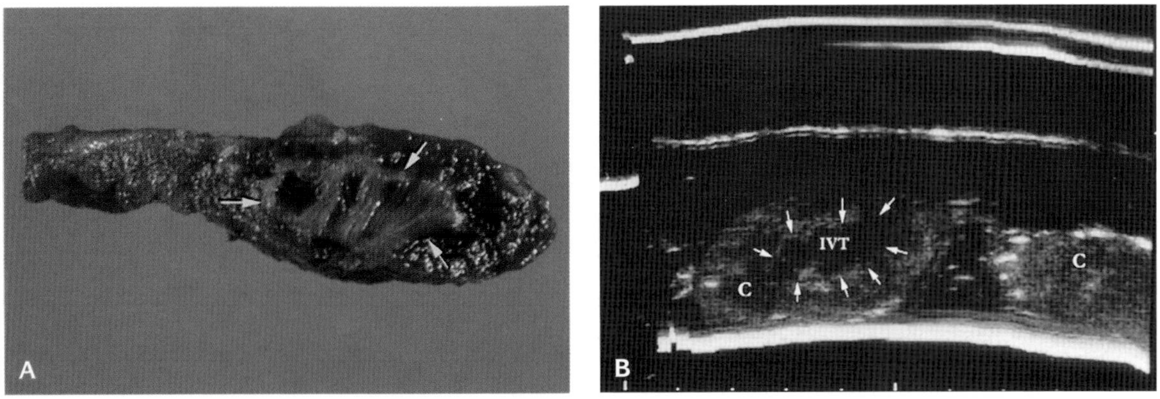

5.10. **(A)** Intervillous thrombus (arrows). **(B)** Ultrasound of intervillous thrombus (IVT, arrows) at mid cotyledon (c).

INTERVILLOUS THROMBUS

A thrombus in the intervillous space is composed of both maternal and fetal blood. Intervillous thrombi are responsible for fetal–maternal hemorrhage and associated fetal anemia (Figure 5.10). The Kleihauer-Betke test is used for detection of fetal red blood cells. Maternal systemic lupus erythematosus has circulating antiphospholipid and anticardiolipin antibodies and is associated with second trimester abortions. The placenta shows much intervillous fibrin and immunoglobulin deposits of principally IgG and IgM.

INFARCTION

Infarction of the placenta is very common. Acute or early infarction involves villus crowding and congestion and is followed by necrotic changes and the deposition of intervillous polymorphonuclear leukocytes (PMNs) (Figures 5.11 to 5.15 and Table 5.13). Older infarctions are characterized by "ghost" villi

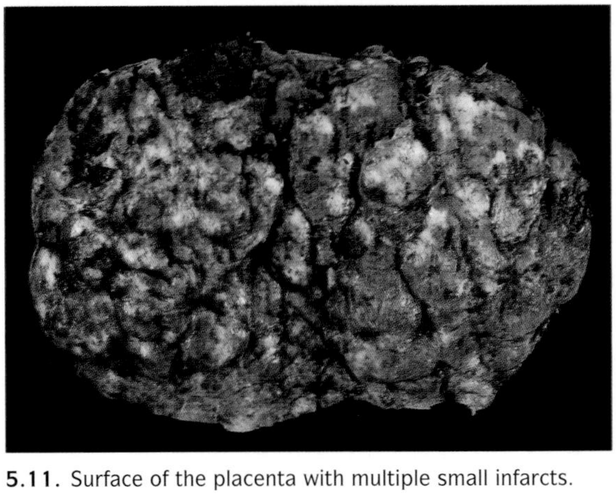

5.11. Surface of the placenta with multiple small infarcts.

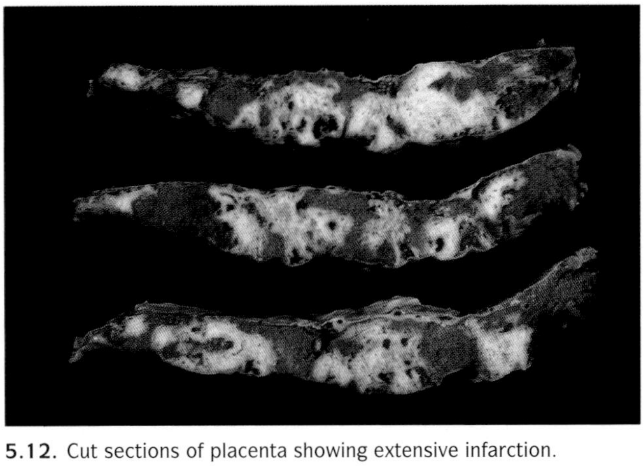

5.12. Cut sections of placenta showing extensive infarction.

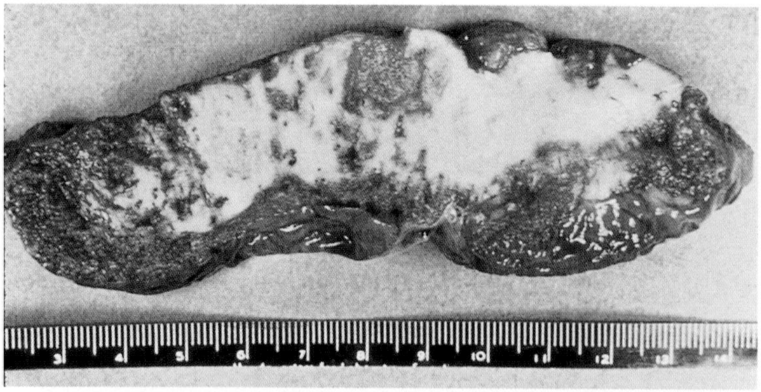

5.13. Cut section of placenta with infarction of approximately 70% of the placenta. The mother had pre-eclampsia and the infant was stillborn.

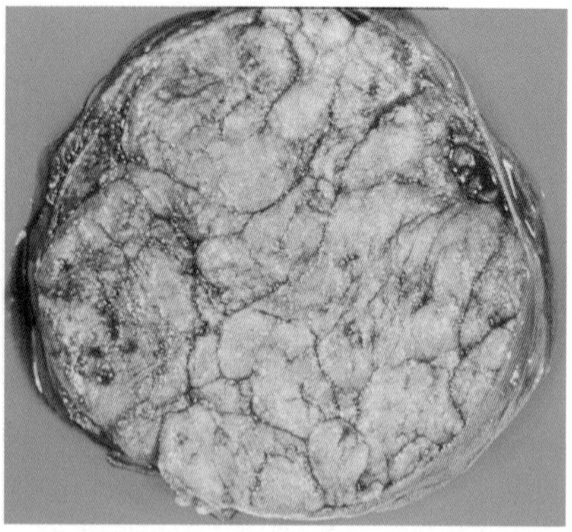

5.14. Extensive ischemia of the placenta with infarction. There was a history of heavy maternal smoking during pregnancy.

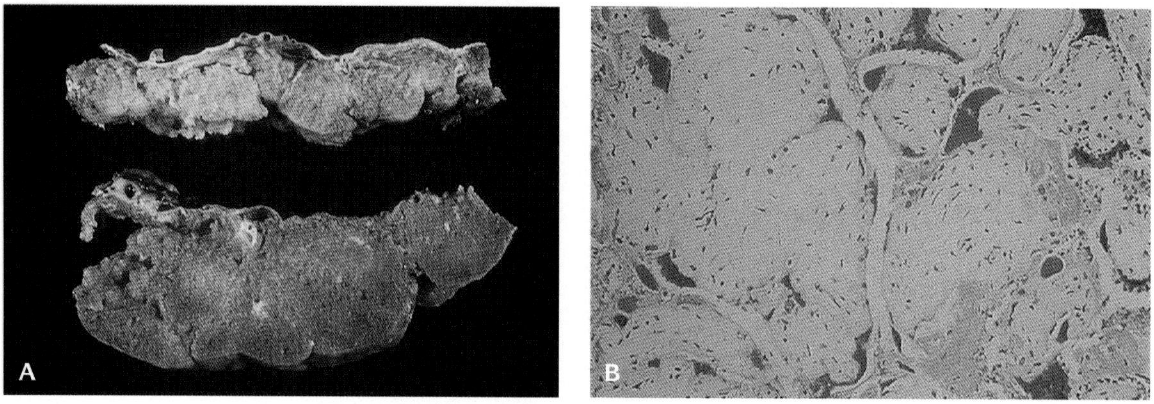

5.15. **(A)** Cut section (above) of placenta with history of heavy maternal smoking with extensive infarction compared to normal placenta (below). **(B)** Microscopic section of infarcted placenta.

without villous stromal fibrosis. Early infarction is red, granular, and firm. Old infarcts appear yellow to white and are also granular. In hypertensive pregnancies, characteristic decidual vascular disorders diminish blood flow to the villous parenchyma and result in infarction. Abruption, infection, immunologic disorders, smoking, and possibly cocaine all correlate with villous ischemia and infarction. Infarction, which tends to be minimal and peripheral in the disk, generally has no ill effects on the fetus. If infarction is more centrally located and involves more than 20% of the placental disk, there is an increased association of intrauterine fetal growth restriction, increased incidence of intrauterine fetal demise, and hypoxic ischemic complications.

MATERNAL FLOOR INFARCTION

Maternal floor fibrin deposition results in fetal growth restriction and intrauterine fetal demise (Figure 5.16). The term maternal floor infarction is a

Table 5.13 Timing of the presence of meconium and Fetal distress: Meconium

Duration of Exposure

Immediate – color – green-yellow

– 1 hour – amniotic epithelial disorganization/necrosis
– amniotic macrophages

– 3 hours – chorionic macrophages
– gross staining

– 6 hours – meconium staining of fetal skin

– 16 hours – meconium induced vascular necrosis and ulceration

Types of meconium – first passage – viscid
later – thin

misnomer. Excessive fibrin deposition occurs along the maternal floor. This deposition chokes the villi. The condition is associated with major basic protein, a substance identified in these massive fibrin deposits derived from intermediate trophoblasts (X cells). There is a high propensity for recurrence in subsequent gestations.

NONHYDROPIC VILLOUS EDEMA

Focal villous edema and individual swollen, edematous villi are seen microscopically. Hydrops of the placenta is a uniform diffuse hydropic swelling of villous tissues. Villous edema is especially associated with preterm delivery. There is an extremely high incidence of stillbirth, neonatal death, and neurologic abnormalities as well as motor abnormalities and severe mental retardation at 7 years of age.

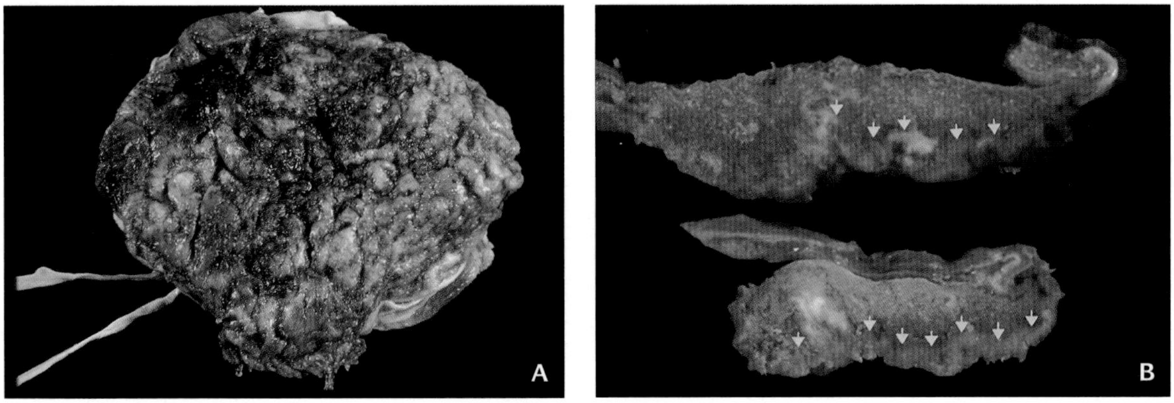

5.16. Maternal floor infarction. This is a misnomer. **(A)** The maternal surface of the placenta is covered by an uneven layer of fibrin. **(B)** The cut surface shows fibrin deposition (arrows).

NUCLEATED RED BLOOD CELLS AND FETAL VESSELS

After 30 weeks of gestation, nucleated red blood cells (NRBC) within the vasculature is abnormal. Causes include erythroblastosis, fetal anemia, infection, intrauterine growth retardation, and hypoxic ischemic events in utero. The presence of cord blood erythrocytic precursors, normoblasts, and lymphocytes is a response to hypoxic and ischemic events in utero. Two thousand NRBC/cu mm occurs within 2 hours of the hypoxic events and returns to normal by 24–36 hours.

A level of 10,000 lymphocytes/CMM occurs within 2 hours of the hypoxic event and returns to normal by 24 hours.

Increase in syncytial knots is also a manifestation of hypoxia.

CHORANGIOSIS

Chorangiosis is defined histologically as 10 vessels per 10 villi per × 10 fields in 10 microscopic fields. It is associated with chronic hypoxia, maternal diabetes, and placental villitis with increased association of perinatal morbidity and mortality and fetal malformations.

VILLITIS

Villitis is inflammation/infection of the placental villi. It is either acute villitis, chronic villitis, villitis of unknown etiology or noninflammatory villitis (Figures 5.17 to 5.19).

In acute villitis, the most common antigen is *Listeria monocytogenes.* Prominent microabscesses occur within the villous parenchyma.

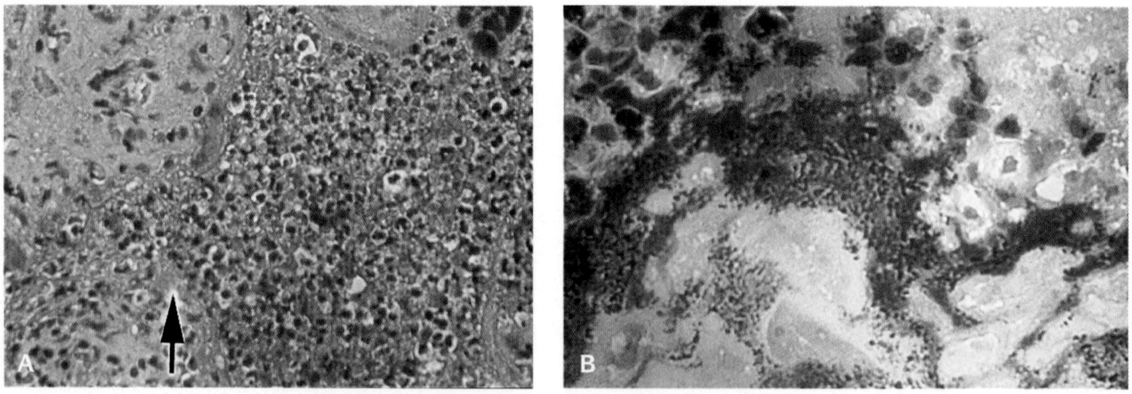

5.17. (A) Microscopic section of placenta in listeria infection showing microabscesses (arrow). **(B)** Gram stain showing gram and coccobacilli of *Listeria*.

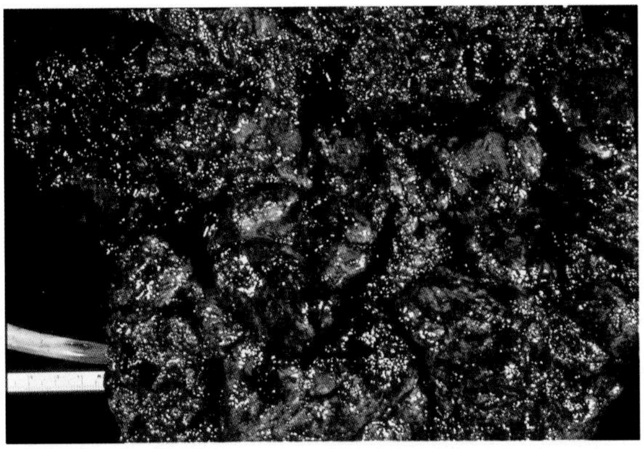

5.18. Syphilis of the placenta. The placenta is large and bulky.

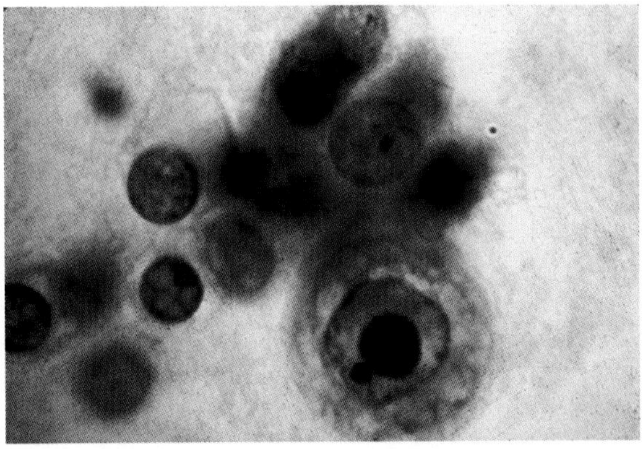

5.19. Microscopic appearance of smear of amniotic membranes showing intranuclear inclusion of cytomegalovirus.

Chronic villitis is generally associated with nonbacterial infectious agents; syphilis, cytomegalovirus (CMV), and rubella are the most common. In syphilis, villi appear club shaped with a mononuclear chronic inflammatory infiltrate including plasma cells. Spirochettes may be readily found by the Warthin-Starry stain. In CMV, the inflammatory infiltrate may have noncharacteristic CMV inclusions. Silver stains may identify spirochetes in syphilis. Immunohistochemical stains are valuable in CMV and herpes virus.

Villitis of unknown etiology is the presence of mononuclear inflammatory cells, generally in the absence of plasma cells. The infectious agent may be nondeterminable; however, a fetal–maternal immunologic phenomenon may also be present.

Noninflammatory villitis occurs with an inflammatory infiltrate. The most common cause is HIV infection; however, in situ hybridization or immunohistochemistry will identify the nucleic acids or antigens of the organism.

ABNORMAL MATURATION

Accelerated maturation occurs in hypertensive conditions and is presumed to be a physiologic response to hypoxemia. Increased syncytial knotting is an abortive attempt to increase the villous surface. Growth restriction, placental infarction, and decidual vasculopathy are commonly associated. Retarded maturation of villous development may be present in maternal diabetes, fetal anemia, fetal heart failure, and hydrops. A third-trimester pregnancy may have the histologic appearance of the second trimester.

Irregular maturation is a combination of varying immature and advanced maturational forms. These are commonly associated with genetic abnormalities, including trisomy 18 and chronic villitis.

Extensive villous fibrosis is commonly seen in cases of intrauterine fetal demise.

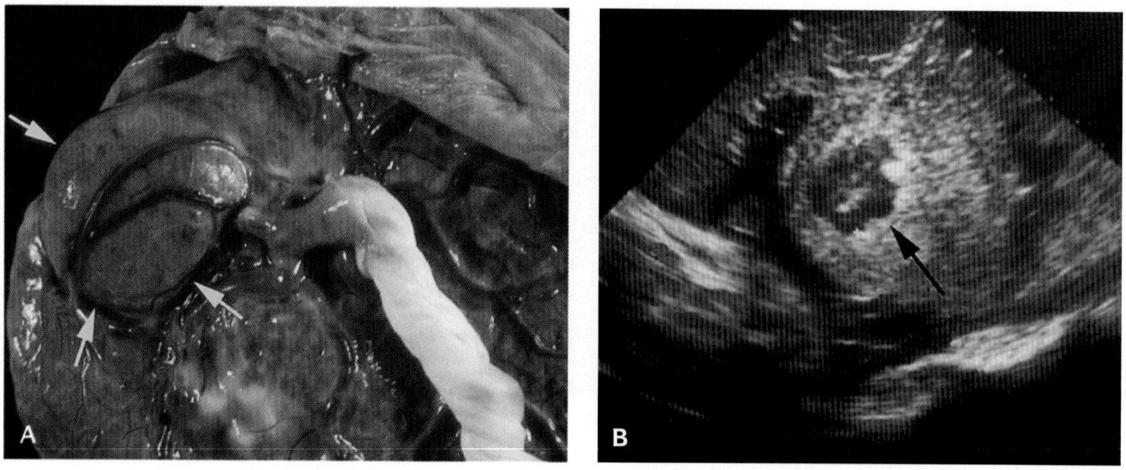

5.20. **(A)** Placenta showing chorioangioma (arrows). **(B)** Ultrasound of chorangioma (arrow).

CHORANGIOMAS

Chorangiomas are vascular tumors of the placenta and are analogous to hemangiomas (Figures 5.20 and 5.21). Larger lesions have associated fetal morbidity and even mortality. High-output congestive heart failure may develop with large lesions. The small-caliber vasculature may result in microangiopathic hemolytic anemia and even disseminated intravascular coagulation.

INTERVILLOUS FIBRIN DEPOSITION

In its minor forms, intervillous fibrin deposition is without pathologic significance (Figure 5.22). Large amounts of intervillous fibrin may be associated with intrauterine demise and growth restriction. The intervillous fibrin deposition

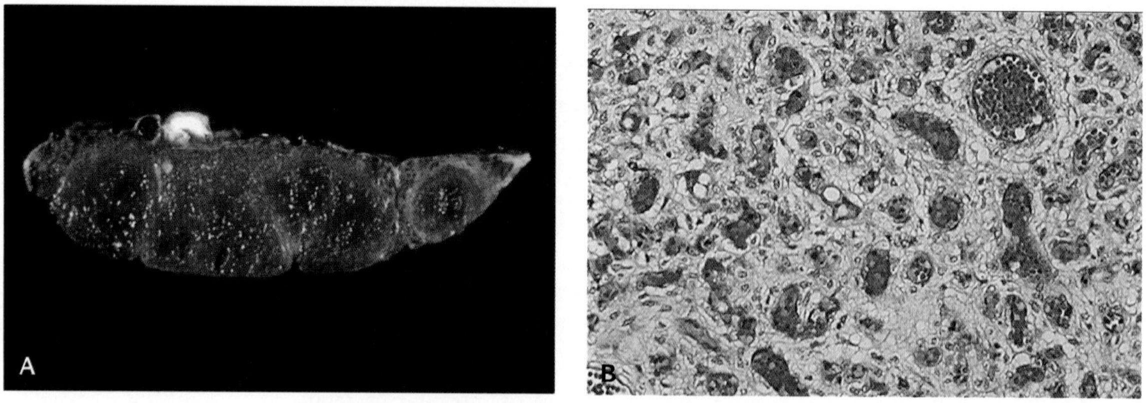

5.21. **(A)** Multiple chorangiomas of placenta. **(B)** Microscopic appearance of chorangioma showing small capillary vascular spaces.

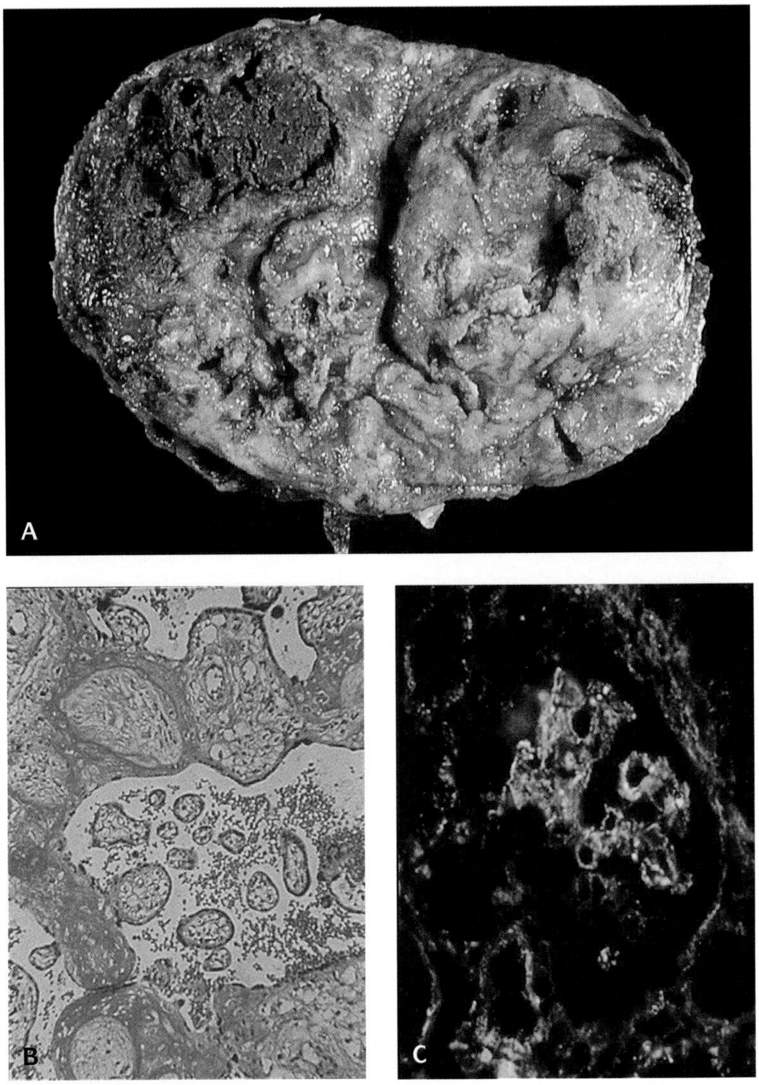

5.22. Placenta of maternal lupus. **(A)** Extensive fibrin deposition. **(B)** Microscopic section showing intervillous fibrin deposition (immunostain for fibrin). **(C)** Immunofluorescent stain for immunoglobulin in intervillous spaces.

may account for more than 30% of the placental substance. It has been termed "gitterinfarkt." Maternal floor infarction is a subcategory of this condition.

ABNORMAL CELLS IN THE INTERVILLOUS SPACE

In sickle cell anemia and in sickle cell trait, sickled erythrocytes may be noted in the intervillous space (Figure 5.23). At this site, there is decreased oxygen tension that induces sickling not only in sickle cell anemia but also in sickle cell trait. Infectious disease agents such as *Plasmodium faciparum*-infected erythrocytes may also be noted.

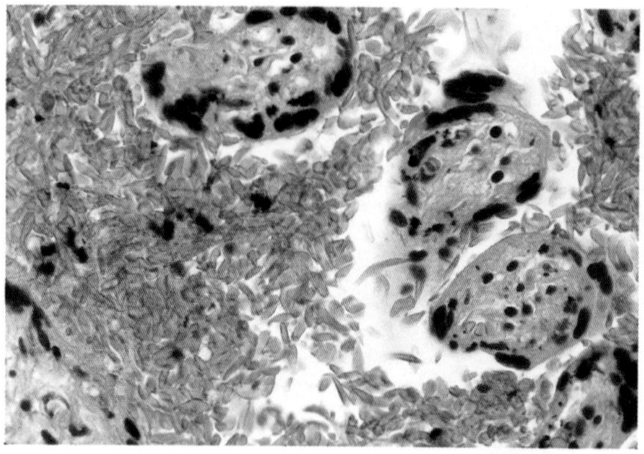

5.23. Sickled red blood cells in the intervillous spaces.

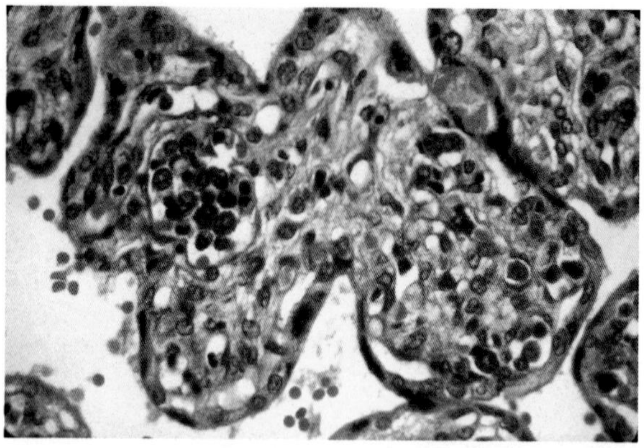

5.24. Microscopic appearance of neuroblastoma in placental capillaries.

Metastatic maternal lesions such as breast carcinoma and melanoma may metastasize to the intervillous spaces (Figure 5.24).

Fetal neoplasia may be identified within villi. The most common are neuroblastoma and fetal leukemia.

DECIDUAL VASCULOPATHY

Maternal medical conditions affecting the decidual vasculature include hypertension and systemic lupus erythematosus (Figure 5.25). Hypertension characteristically affects the decidual vessels by atherosis with lipid-laden atheromatous change (foam cells) in the normal endothelium of the spiral arterioles. Similar changes may be noted in lupus. In lupus, a perivascular inflammatory infiltrate is associated with intervillous fibrin and immunoglobulin deposition resulting in placental insufficiency and hypoxic change within the placenta. Small placentas, increased syncytial knotting, and infarction may occur. Decidual vasculopathy carries a higher than expected rate of spontaneous

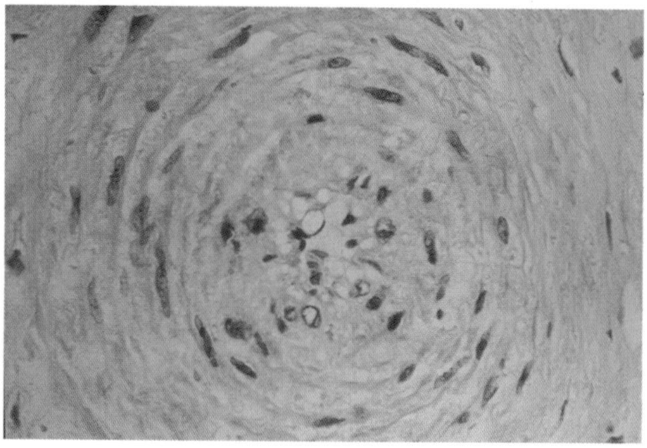

5.25. Arteriole from stem cell villous showing atherosis with vacuolization of the endothelial cells and obliteration of lumen in pre-eclampsia.

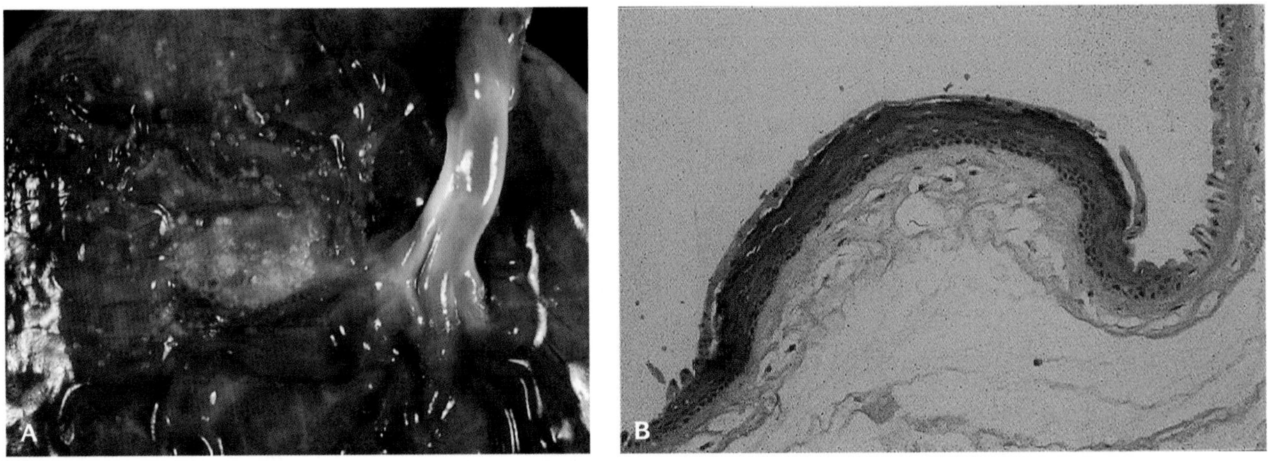

5.26. **(A)** Squamous metaplasia of amniotic membranes. **(B)** Microscopic appearance.

abortion, stillbirth, placental abruption, preterm birth, and growth-retarded infants.

DECIDUAL INFLAMMATION

Decidual inflammation is part of the ascending infection seen in chorioamnionitis.

VILLOUS HYDROPS

Placentas that are large because of diffuse villous hydrops are most commonly associated with infections (including syphilis, toxoplasmosis, and CMV), anemia, heart failure, and hypoxia.

MEMBRANES

The membranes are composed of the inner amnion and outer chorion. The amnion develops from ectodermal layers and the chorion from trophoblastic derivatives.

SQUAMOUS METAPLASIA

Squamous metaplasia of the amnion is very common. It should be distinguished grossly from amnion nodosum (Figure 5.26). It may be associated with traumatization of the amnion by fetal malformations such as a large encephalocele. When immersed in water, squamous metaplasia beads water and does not hydrate. It is very difficult to excoriate squamous metaplasia from the surface of the placenta.

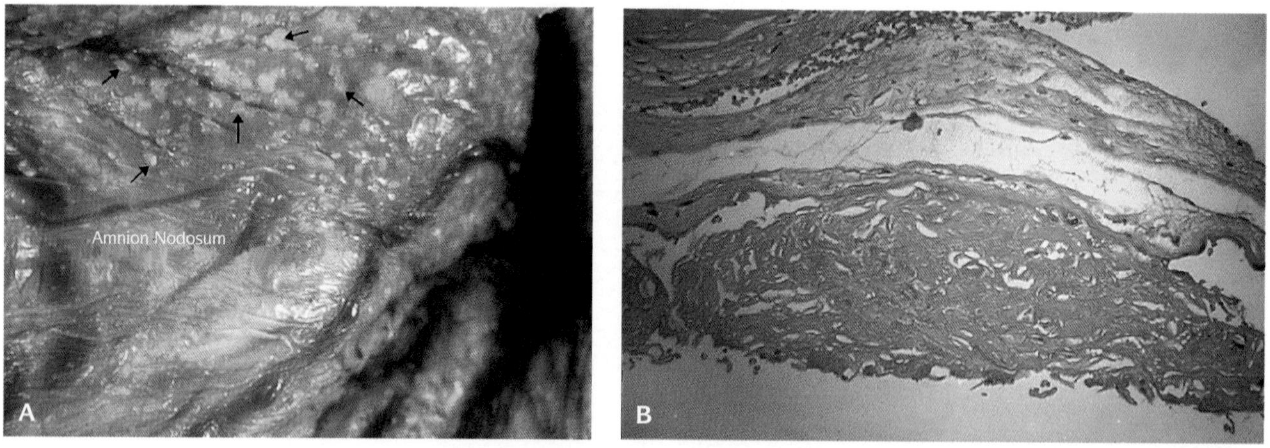

5.27. Amnion nodosum. **(A)** Surface of amniotic membranes. **(B)** Microscopic appearance of vernix caseosa of amnion nodosum.

AMNION NODOSUM

Amnion nodosum occurs in conditions of long-standing oligohydramnios. Chronic leakage of amniotic fluid, as well as its failure of production, as in renal agenesis is a well-known antecedent of this phenomenon (Figure 5.27). Fetal epidermal cells, hair, and amnion coalesce on the surface of the amnion to form innumerable papules pathognomonic of amnion nodosum.

MECONIUM STAINING

Meconium is generally not present until 32–34 weeks gestation. Meconium should be histologically distinguished from heme pigment by a special staining

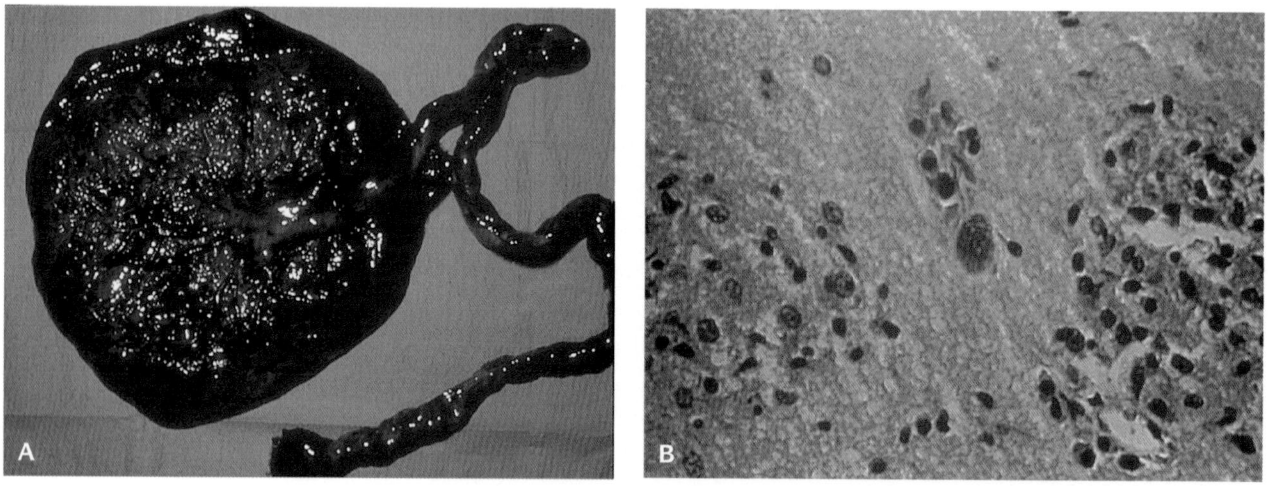

5.28. **(A)** Meconium staining of the amniotic membranes. **(B)** Microscopic appearance showing pigment in macrophages.

of placental sections for iron (Figure 5.28). Meconium is periodic acid–schiff positive.

After 34 weeks, motilin is present in the fetal gut, and stimulation of peristalsis through normal physiologic events may result in *in utero* evacuation of meconium; meconium evacuation may be the result of intrauterine distress.

Amnion macrophages will pick up meconium within 1 hour of exposure and may be seen in the chorion within 3 hours and even extend into the decidua as the time of exposure increases. The temporal relationship of meconium may explain the timing of adverse fetal or hypoxic events (Table 5.13).

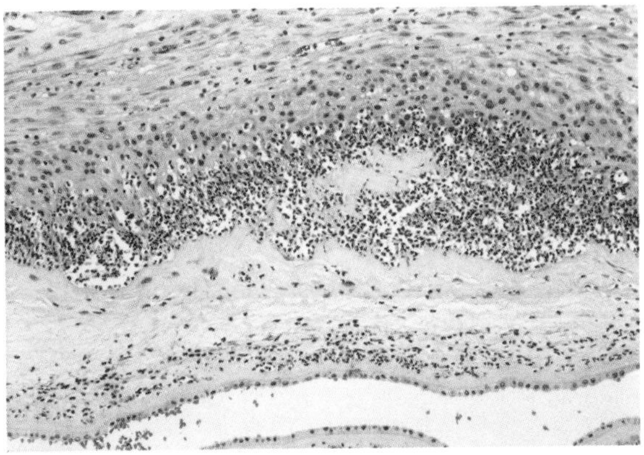

5.29. Acute stage three chorioamnionitis.

CHORIOAMNIONITIS

With ascending intra-amniotic infection, decidual margination of PMNs results in chemotactic migration toward the amniotic cavity (Figures 5.29

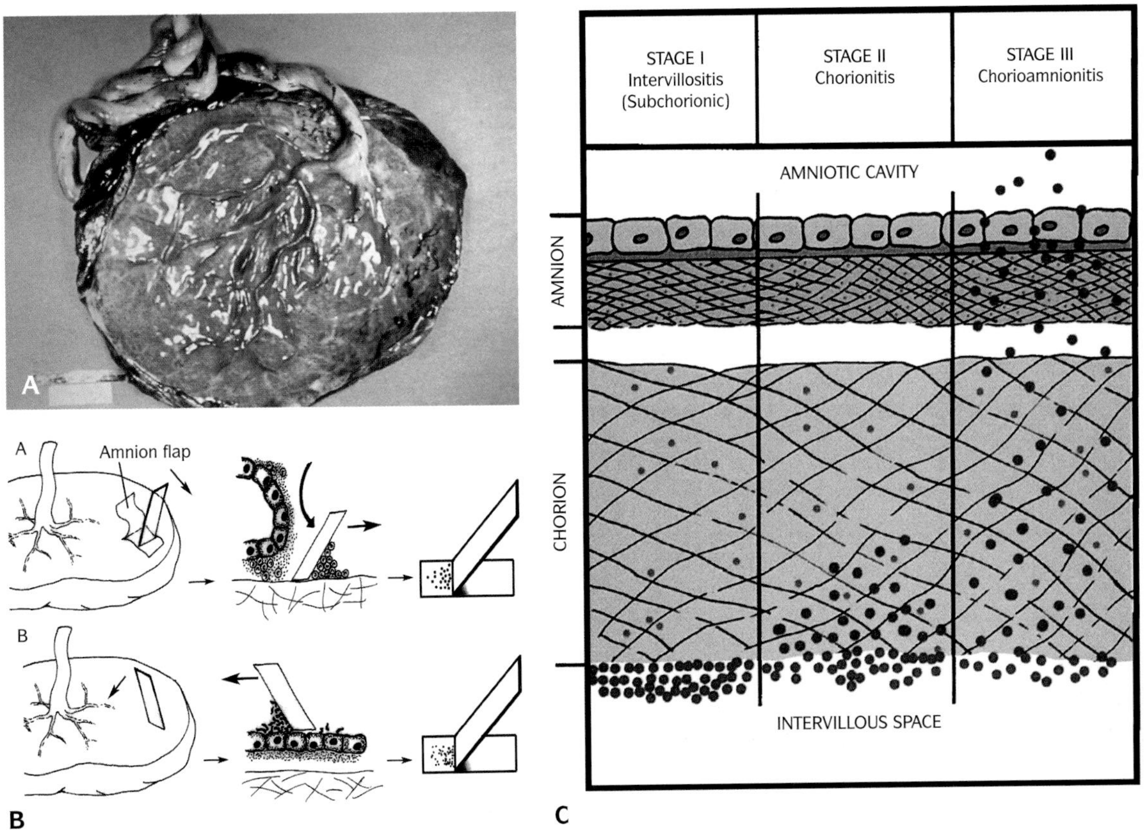

5.30. **(A)** Gross appearance of thick opaque membranes in acute chorioamnionitis. **(B)** Preparation of amniotic and chorionic smears for quick diagnosis of inflammation and bacteriologic screening. **(C)** Stages of inflammation of the placental surface.

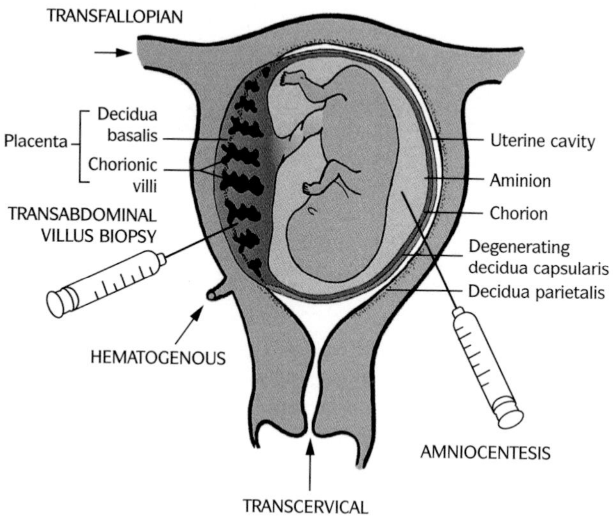

5.31. Routes of fetal infection.

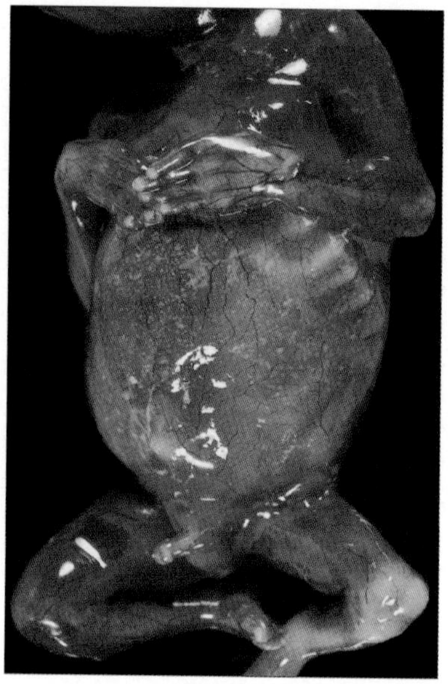

5.32. *Candida* infection of the infant.

to 5.33 and Tables 5.14 and 5.15). The decidua, then the chorion, and finally the amnion will show an inflammatory response. PMNs may migrate into the intra-amniotic cavity and produce an intra-amniotic infection syndrome in which aspiration of bacteria and inflammatory cells by the fetus may result in severe pneumonitis and sepsis. Group B streptococcal sepsis is generally associated with a severe outcome in neonates.

There is a strong association between chorioamnionitis with premature rupture of membranes, preterm delivery, and chorionic and umbilical thrombosis.

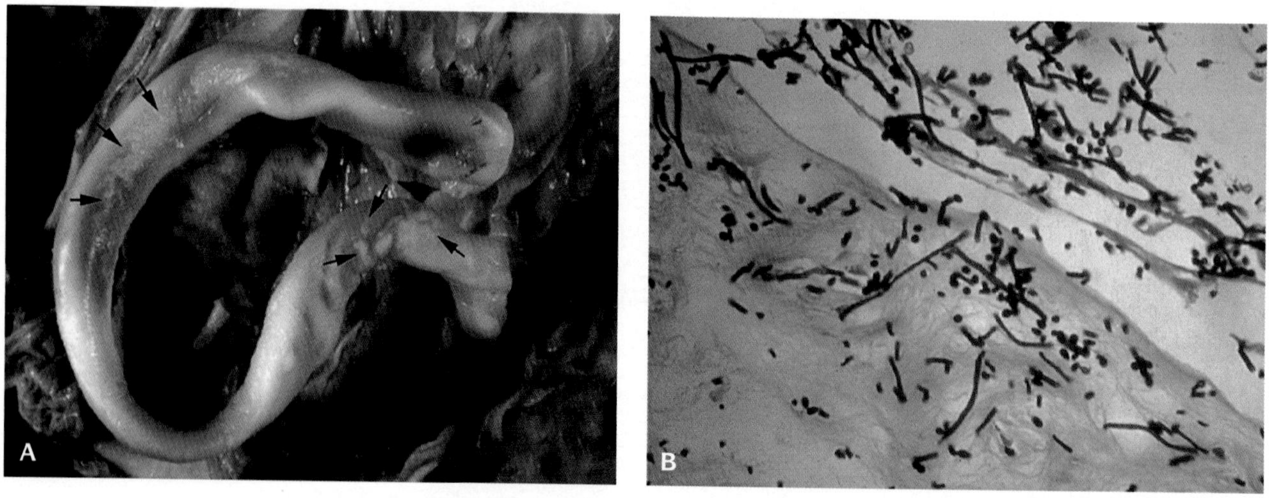

5.33. **(A)** *Candida* infection of the umbilical cord (arrows-white plaques). **(B)** Microscopic sections of the umbilical cord showing mycelial and yeast forms of candida albicans (Gomori silver stain).

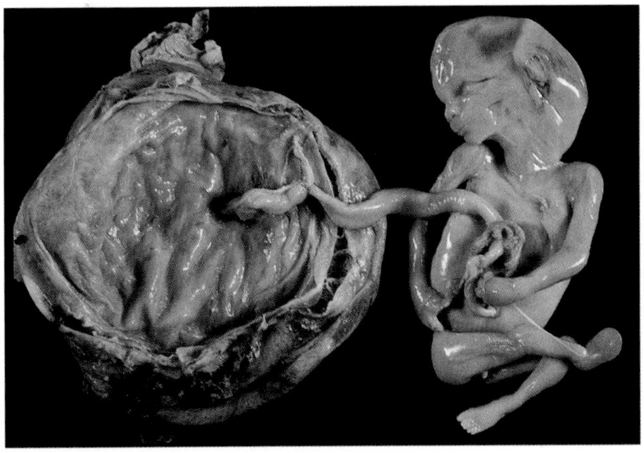

5.34. Amniotic bands constricting the umbilical cord between both hands and extending to right ankle.

Table 5.14 Most common causes for chorioamnionitis

Group B Strep
Chlamydia
Trachomatis
Mycoplasma
Urea Urealyticum
Fusobacterium
Candida (most commonly involves umbilical cord with funisitis)

Table 5.15 Staging of chorioamnionitis

Stage 1:	Polymorphs confined to the deep connective tissue above the chorionic plate
Stage 2:	Polymorphs through the placental chorionic surface
Stage 3:	Polymorphs all the way through the chorion and the amnion
Stage 4:	Necrotizing chorioamnionitis

AMNIOTIC BANDS

Chronic rupture of the amnion results in the formation of amniotic bands. The amnion is most densely adherent to the umbilical cord at its insertion in the placental disk (Figure 5.34). With early amniotic rupture, bands that remain under tension because of continued adherence to the surface of the cord insertion are prone to characteristic malformations and amputations.

EXTRACHORIAL PRESENTATION

Circummarginate and circumvallate placentas are examples of extrachorial placentas (Figures 5.35 and 5.36). In circumvallate placenta, the amnion enfolds upon itself and is encased in fibrin. Circummarginate and circumvallate placentas are associated with major fetal malformations. Circumvallate placentas occur in approximately 6% of pregnancies and are associated with growth retardation, preeclampsia, and acute or chronic bleeding in the first and second trimesters. Circumvallation also carries an increased risk of premature rupture of membranes, preterm delivery, and oligohydramnios.

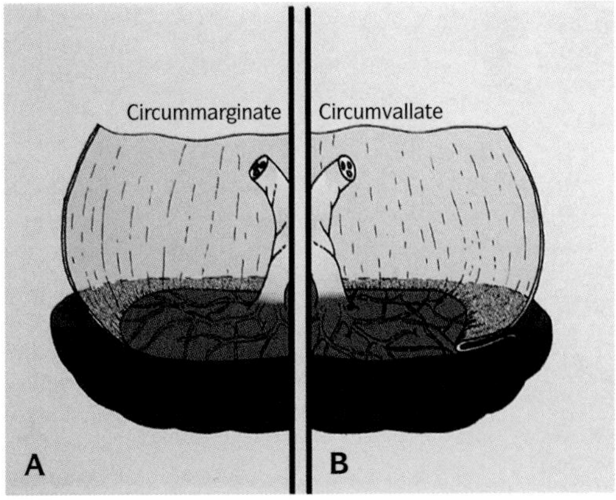

5.35. **(A)** Circummarginate placenta. The membranes do not extend to the edge of the placenta. **(B)** Circumvallate placenta. The membranes form a plica beneath which is a thick rim of fibrin.

CHORIONIC VASCULAR THROMBOSIS

Faint linear white streaks along the margins of chorionic vessels or more prominent thromboses occlude the vasculature with consequent proximal vascular dilatation *in utero*, causing hypoxia or ischemia to the fetus.

MULTIPLE GESTATIONS

Increased malformations noted in twins and maternal complications include pregnancy-induced hypertension, hydramnios,

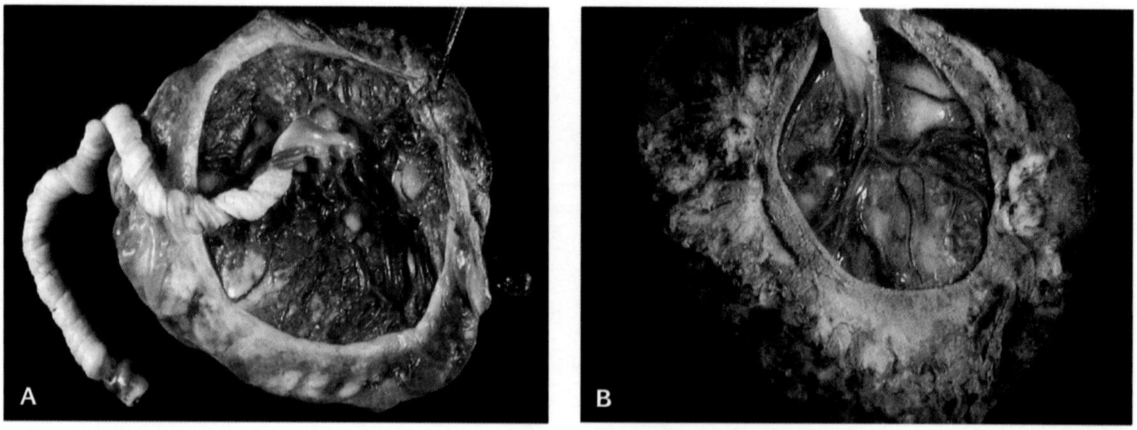

5.36. **(A)** Gross appearance of circummarginate placenta. **(B)** Gross appearance of circumvallate placenta.

retroplacental bleeding (abruptio placentae), placenta previa, and prolapsed umbilical cord. Placental findings include infarction, increased syncytial knots, decidual vasculopathy, cord prolapse, and increased frequency of velamentous vessels.

In monozygotic twins there is a monochorionic placenta. The greatest risk to the fetus is twin-to-twin transfusion and cord entanglement, which carries 50% mortality. Monochorionic monoamniotic twin gestation is more rare accounting for approximately 3% of twin gestations.

In twin-to-twin transfusion syndrome, the most common vascular anastomoses are vein to vein. In twin-to-twin transfusion, the placenta from the donor twin appears pale because of anemia, and the parenchyma is edematous secondary to high-output cardiac failure. The recipient placenta is dark and congested. Villous tissue from the anemic twin has abundant macrophages and vascular spaces containing nucleated hematologic precursors. Villi from the placenta of the recipient twin often appear dramatically congested. Injection studies delineate the anastomotic patterns in the chorionic vasculature of the placenta.

Examination of the dividing membrane determines the chorionicity of twin gestations. In monochorionic placenta, the membrane will be thin and translucent. When the membranes are diamniotic, dichorionic, they are thick and nontranslucent. In approximately one-third of diamniotic dichorionic placentas, the gestations will be monozygotic. This occurs with very early splitting of the zygote (before 3 days of development).

Fetus Papyraceous

Fetus papyraceus results from intrauterine twin death usually in the second trimester. The dead fetus shrinks, becomes flattened and necrotic (Figure 5.37). It may occur in both monochorionic and dichorionic twin gestations.

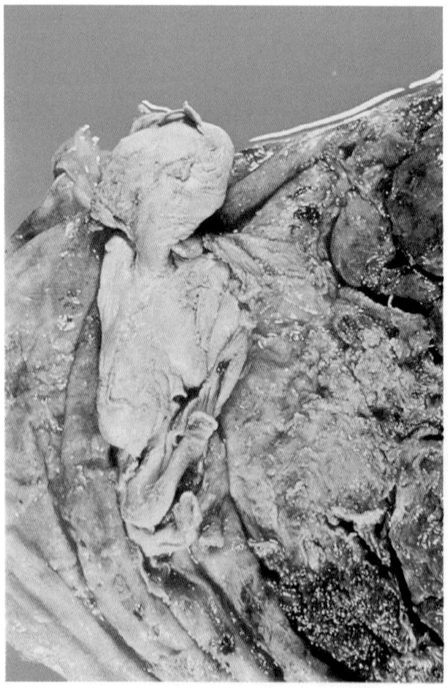

5.37. Fetus papyraceous.

UMBILICAL CORD

Remnants of the allantoic duct, omphalomesenteric duct, and embryonic vessels may persist; however, there is no pathologic significance except that

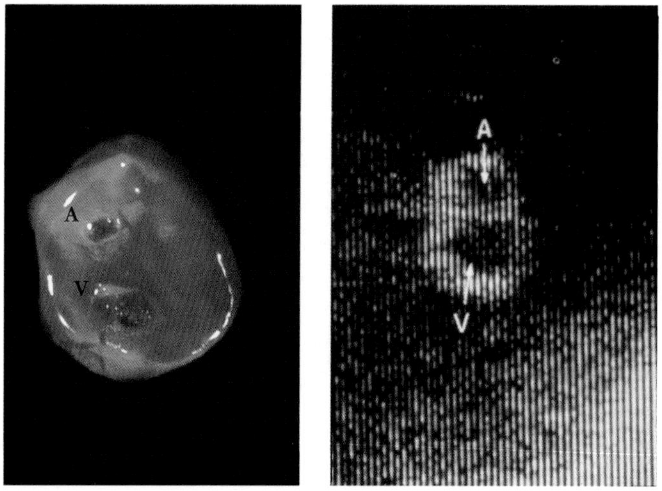

5.38. Cross section of an umbilical cord with a single umbilical artery (A) (V = vein), right. Ultrasound of a single umbilical artery (A), (V = vein), left.

occasionally a prominent omphalomesenteric duct may be seen in association with an omphalocele and trapped enteric contents may be traumatized. Vitelline vascular remnants may at times rupture and cause hemorrhage within the cord substance; this results in occlusion of vascular flow with resultant vascular insufficiency or demise.

SINGLE UMBILICAL ARTERY

The incidence of single umbilical artery (SUA) is 1 percent in neonates (Figure 5.38). This anomaly is caused by either developmental agenesis or marked hypoplasia.

Female infants are more commonly affected than males. There is an increased tendency for male fetuses with SUA to be malformed. The incidence of SUA in twins is three times that of singletons. Urologic malformations are considered the most common abnormalities. Sirenomelia may be associated with SUA.

Determination of SUA should be made at a point on the umbilical cord close to its insertion at the umbilicus. It is not unusual for two arteries to fuse near the insertion of the umbilical cord into the placental disk.

Velamentous Insertion of the Cord

One to 2% of umbilical cords are velamentous. The vessels of the cord insert with the chorion of the reflected fetal membranes (Figures 5.39 and 5.40). The umbilical vasculature remains unprotected by Wharton jelly. These vessels are prone to inadvertent rupture through amniotomy as well as fetal compression, with resultant umbilical or chorionic vascular thrombosis. Furcate cord insertion occurs in 1/40,000 pregnancies. The umbilical vessels branch before their insertion in the placental disk (and are also devoid of Wharton jelly) and are subject to compression and thrombosis. Velamentous cords are

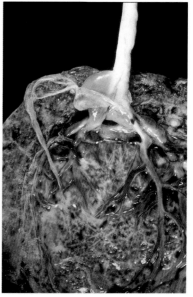

5.39. Furcate insertion of the umbilical cord into the placenta.

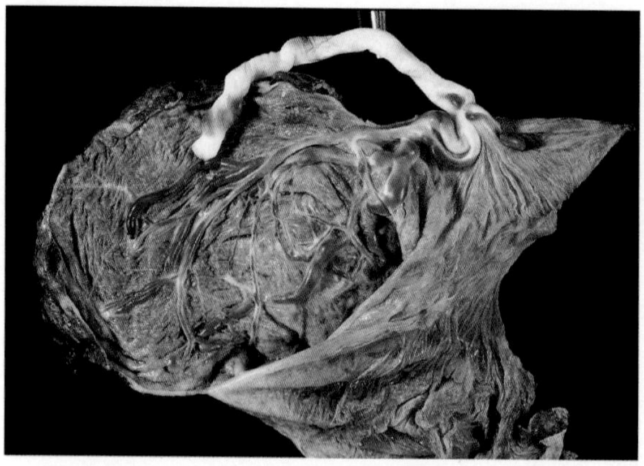

5.40. Velamentous insertion of the umbilical cord into the membranes. This may result in rupture of the umbilical vessels with hemorrhage and fetal death in utero.

associated with multiple gestations and a variety of congenital syndromes. Diabetes, smoking, and advanced maternal age are correlated. Adverse pregnancy outcomes and preterm delivery with velamentous insertions are found in 3/1,000 live births. Neurologic abnormalities at 7 years of age as well as hyperactivity syndromes occur with twice the incidence as in the normal population.

KNOTS

Loose knots occurring from increased fetal movement *in utero* are seen more frequently in conjunction with long umbilical cords (Figures 5.41 and 5.42). Knots occur in approximately 1% of gestations. When a knot is "tight," fetal demise may result from complete obstruction of the vasculature with proximal vascular dilation, as well as notching within the grooves of the knot itself.

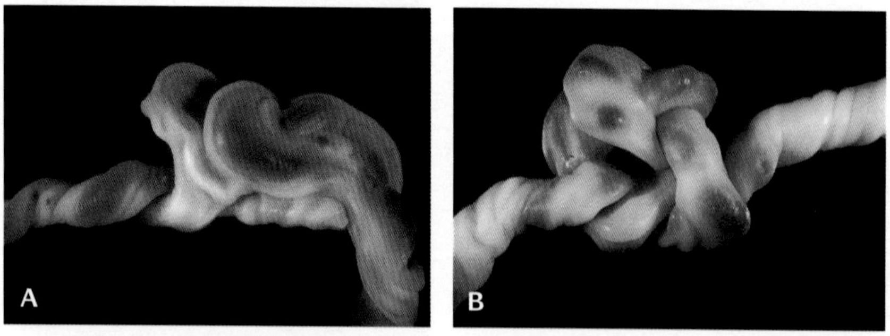

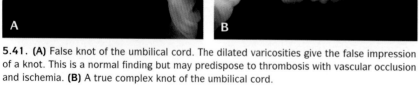

5.41. **(A)** False knot of the umbilical cord. The dilated varicosities give the false impression of a knot. This is a normal finding but may predispose to thrombosis with vascular occlusion and ischemia. **(B)** A true complex knot of the umbilical cord.

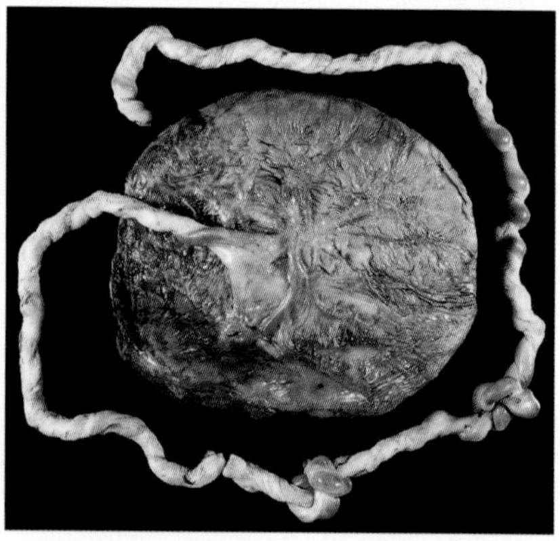

5.42. True knots on the umbilical cord.

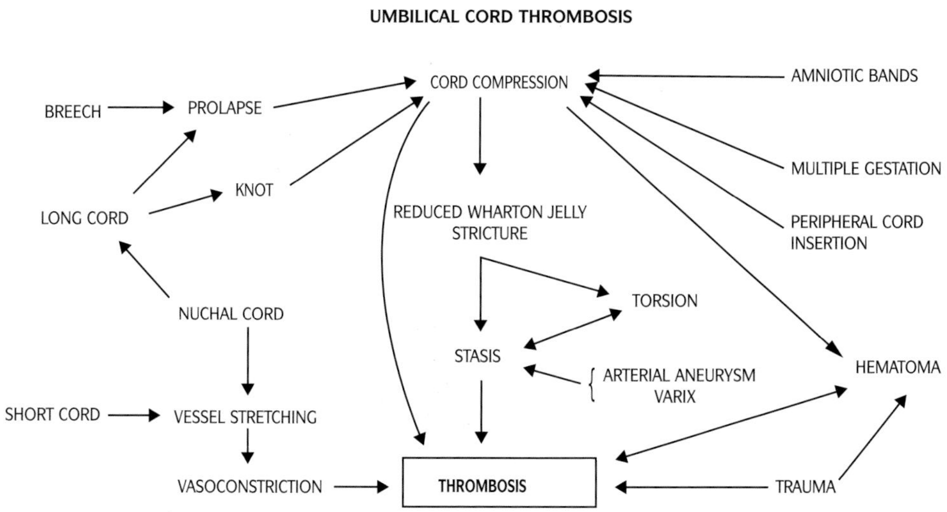

5.43. Umbilical cord thrombosis algorithm.

UMBILICAL VASCULAR THROMBOSIS

The causes of umbilical vascular thrombosis include velamentous cord insertions, which may be affected by vascular thrombosis, marked cord inflammation (funisitis), tangled cords in twin pregnancies, intravascular exchange transfusions *in utero*, protein C and protein S deficiency, antithrombin III, lupus anticoagulant, and anticardiolipin antibodies (Figures 5.43 and 5.44). Adverse pregnancy outcomes include stillbirth, preterm delivery, and neonatal death. The occurrence of umbilical vascular thrombosis occurs in 7/1,000 deliveries.

UMBILICAL CORD HEMATOMA

At term, long umbilical cords are considered to be those >70 cm, and short cords are <32 cm (Figure 5.45).

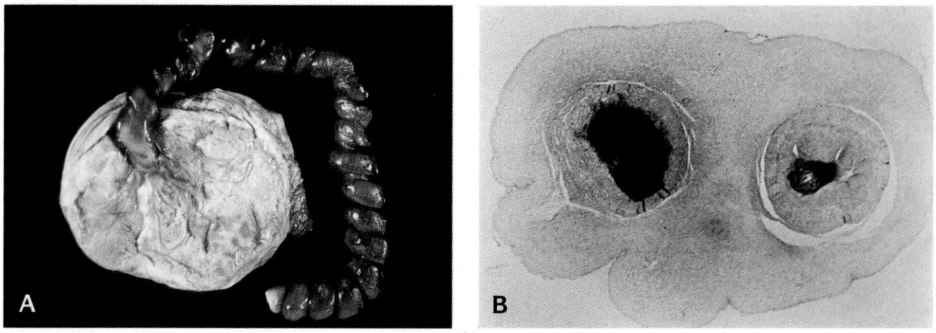

5.44. **(A)** Corkscrew coiling of the umbilical cord. This may result in fetal death *in utero* but may also occur after death of the fetus. **(B)** Microscopic section of the umbilical cord showing thrombosis of the umbilical vein.

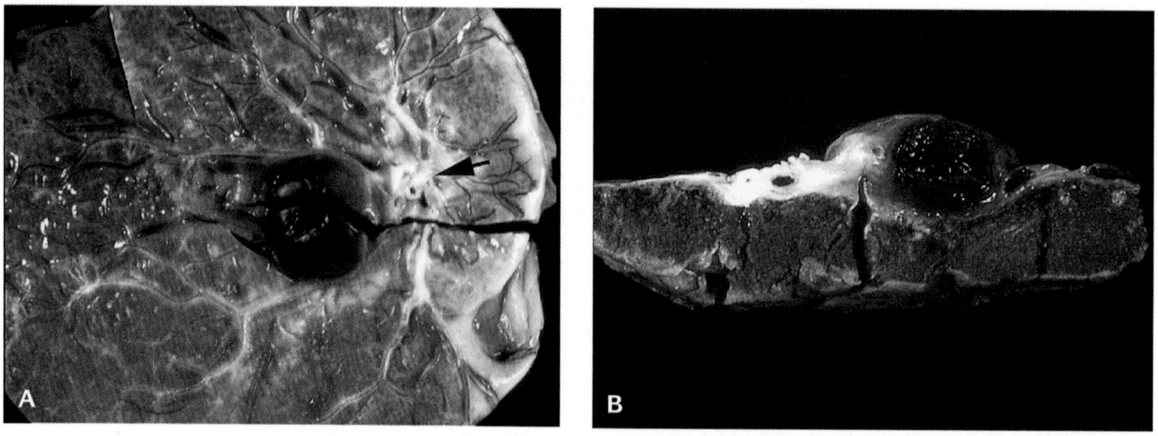

5.45. **(A)** Hematoma of the umbilical cord. (Arrow = umbilical cord insertion.) **(B)** Cross section of the hematoma.

Cord Length

Cord length appears to be directly related to fetal activity in utero. Short cords are seen in fetuses with hypokinesia, and long cords are seen in fetuses with increased activity (Figures 5.46 to 5.50).

Long umbilical cords carry an increased risk of thrombosis, entanglement, knots, and increased propensity for prolapse.

UMBILICAL CORD STRICTURE

Specific narrowing in the umbilical cord is associated with loss of Wharton jelly in that region and commonly occurs near the cord insertion at the umbilicus. Most frequently, this is secondary to excessive torsion and results in intrauterine fetal demise. There is associated fetal growth restriction. Diffusely narrow umbilical cords are also associated with maternal smoking. The placentas of fetuses with unusually narrow cords are also small and their villous development is abnormal.

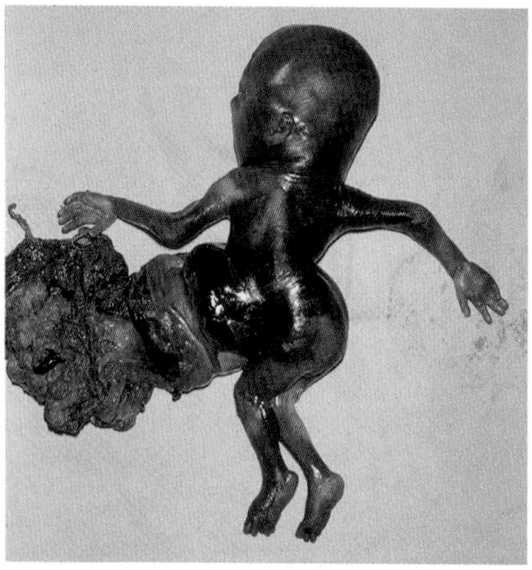

5.46. A short umbilical cord with an omphalocele.

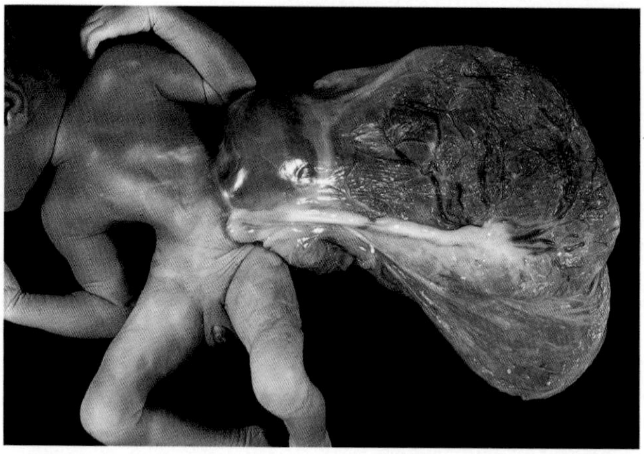

5.47. A short umbilical cord attached to the fetus with omphalocele and cord tethered to the placenta.

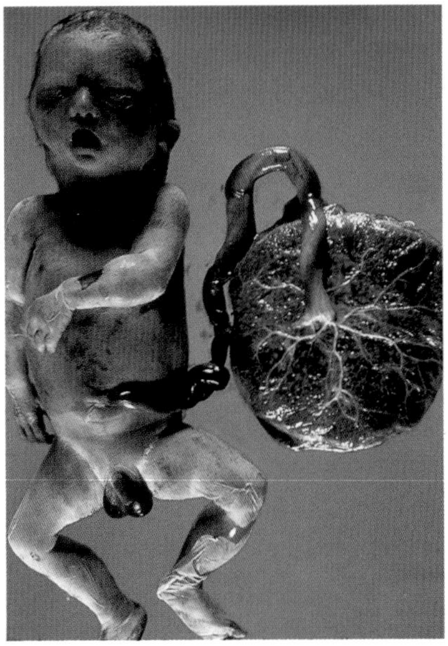

5.48. A short umbilical cord 20 cm long.

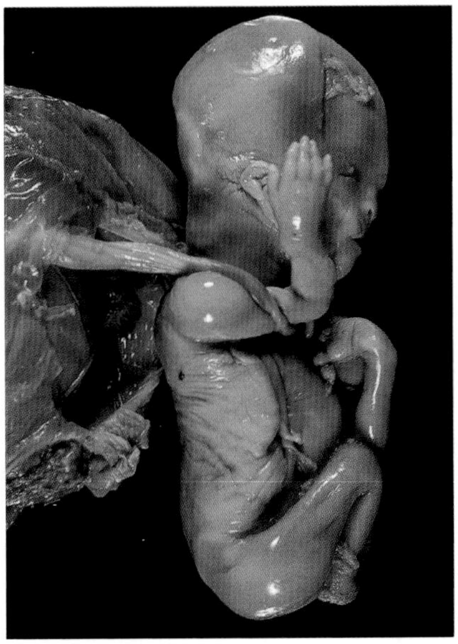

5.49. A tight nuchal cord that caused intrauterine fetal death.

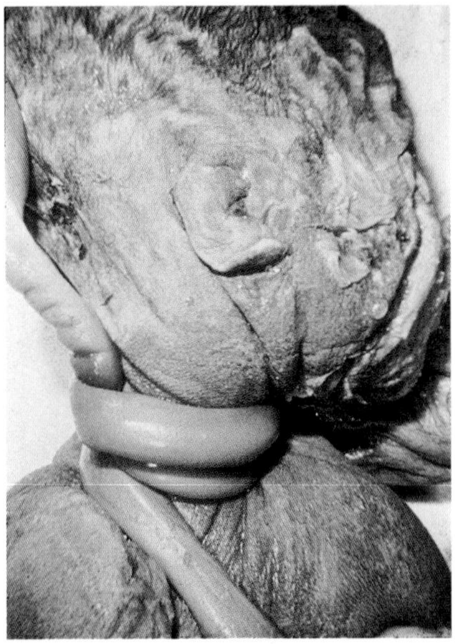

5.50. A tight umbilical cord that caused fetal death and maceration.

UMBILICAL CORD TORSION

The umbilical cord normally twists in a left-to-right fashion, a so-called left-handed twist. The left-sided twist probably occurs because the right umbilical artery is slightly larger than the left. Increased spiraling is associated with increased fetal activity and torsion, and, when excessive torsion occurs, fetal death may result. Cords without spiraling and no twists are seen in infants with an increased risk of fetal distress in utero, as well as growth restriction.

Edema of the umbilical cord occurs in about 3% of all deliveries (Figure 5.51). It is seen in conjunction with hypertensive and preeclamptic pregnancies, uteroplacental insufficiency, and chorioamnionitis.

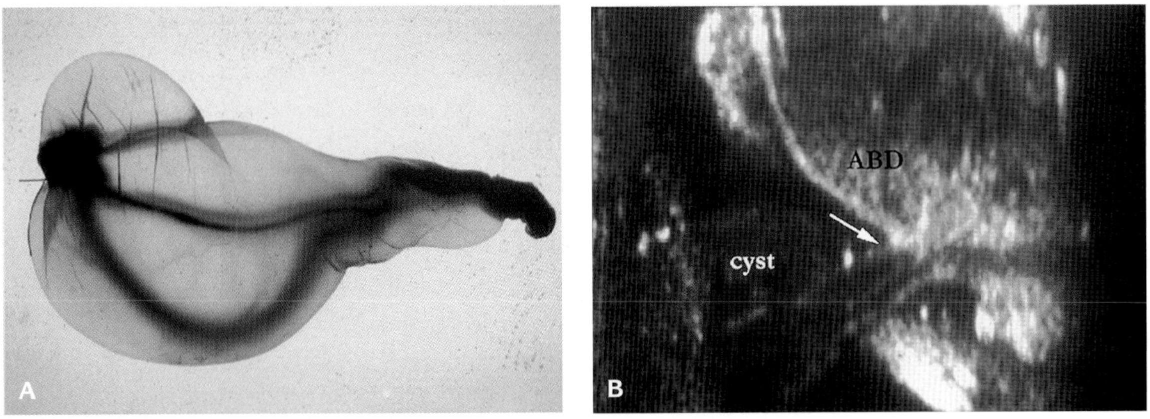

5.51. **(A)** Severe edema of the umbilical cord. **(B)** Ultrasound of an edematous umbilical cord with a cystic appearance. (ABD = abdominal wall, arrow = umbilical cord insertion.)

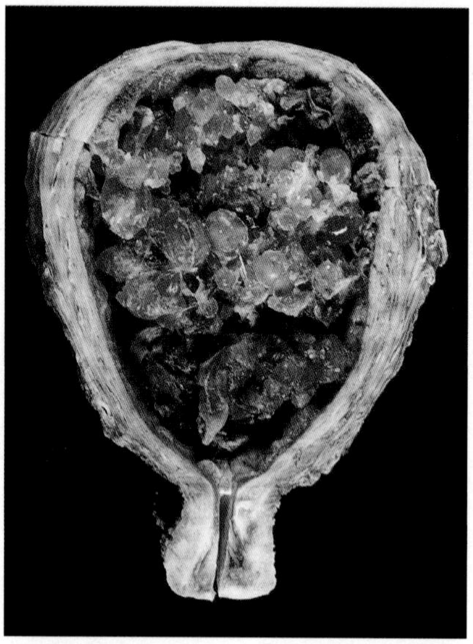

5.52. Complete hydatidiform mole. Uterine cavity is filled with grape-like vesicular chorionic villi.

Cord Inflammation

Funisitis is inflammation of the umbilical cord. Fetal circulating PMNs permeate Wharton jelly; PMNs usually emanate first from the umbilical vein and then from the umbilical arteries. When in excess, thrombosis of the umbilical vessels may occur. It predisposes to spasm of the umbilical vascular media, thereby resulting in ischemic and anoxic changes. With necrotizing funisitis, calcium deposition may occur peripheral to the umbilical cord vessels.

MECONIUM

Meconium in the umbilical cord causes umbilical vascular spasm and subsequent fetal ischemia. Meconium may induce myonecrosis of umbilical vascular media and result in spasm. Intense meconium staining of the umbilical cord may be associated with intrauterine fetal hypoxia.

MOLAR PREGNANCY

Complete Hydatidiform Mole (CMM)

The incidence of CMM is approximately 1/2,000 pregnancies and presents between the 11th and 25th weeks of pregnancy (Figures 5.52 and 5.53 and Table 5.16). The human chorionic gonadotropin level is markedly elevated. Ultrasonography discloses a classic "snowstorm" appearance. It is often voluminous with 300 to 500 mL or more of tissue and is characterized by gross generalized villous edema forming grapelike transparent vesicles measuring up to 2 cm. Only rarely is an embryo or fetus associated with CMM and in all instances, this finding represents a twin gestation. Ten to 30% of the cases of CMM result in persistent gestational trophoblastic disease that may result in invasive mole or choriocarcinoma.

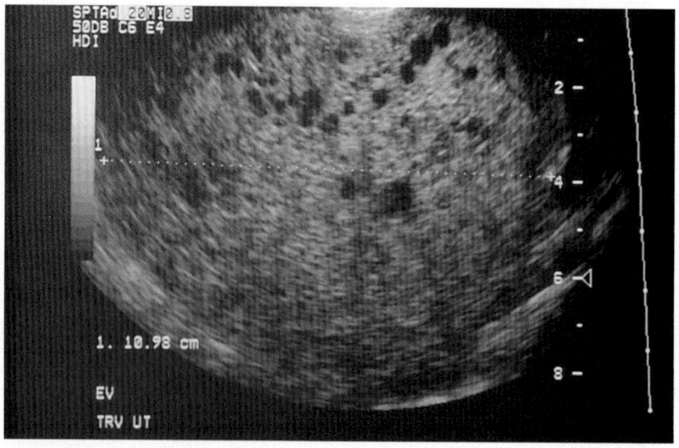

5.53. Ultrasound of a complete hydatidiform mole showing the typical "snowstorm" appearance.

Table 5.16 Complete and partial moles: differential features

Feature	Partial	Complete
Clinical presentation	Missed or spontaneous abortion	Spontaneous abortion
Gestational age	18–20 weeks	16–18 weeks
Uterine size	Often small for dates	Often large for dates
Serum BhCG	+	++++
Cytogenetics	Triploid XXY (58%), XXX (4%), XXY (2%) 2/1 paternal/maternal	XX (over 90%) or XY (<10%) All paternal
Persistent gestational trophoblastic disease	4–11%	10–30%
Trophoblastic proliferation	Focal, minimal	Circumferential
Trophoblastic atypia	Absent	Often present
Hydropic swelling	Less pronounced	Marked
Villous outline	Scalloped	Round
Immunochemistry		
β-hCG	+	++++
α-hCG	++++	+
PLAP	++++	+
PL	++++	++

hCG – human chorionic gondotropin; PLAP – placental alkaline phosphatase; PL – placental lactogen

Trophoblastic proliferation is variable; it may be exuberant or focal and minimal. It is usually circumferential around the villi. Most complete moles have a 46, XX karyotype, resulting either from dispermy or from duplication of haploid sperm in an anuclear ovum (diploid androgenesis). XY moles, which represent only some 4% of cases of CMM, originate from the fertilization of an anuclear ovum by two spermatozoa. Molar gestations are associated with an empty gestational sac.

Partial Hydatidiform Mole (PHM)

In PHM an embryo or fetus is usually present, the microcystic pattern may be diffuse or focal and is not as prominent as in CMM, and trophoblastic hyperplasia is less prominent and sometimes strikingly focal (Figure 5.54). PHMs are usually triploid with two paternal and one maternal haploid complements. The malignant transformation rate in PHM is the same as in any nonmolar pregnancy.

Hydropic villi like those seen in CMM mixed with nonmolar placental tissue are grossly visible.

Microscopically, a mixture of large, edematous villi and small, normal-sized villi without edema are seen with central acellular cisterns and small villi that are often fibrotic. Trophoblastic hyperplasia is focal and often confined to the syncytiotrophoblasts. The villi have irregular, scalloped outlines with infoldings of trophoblastic cells into the villous stroma. Stromal vasculature and vessels may

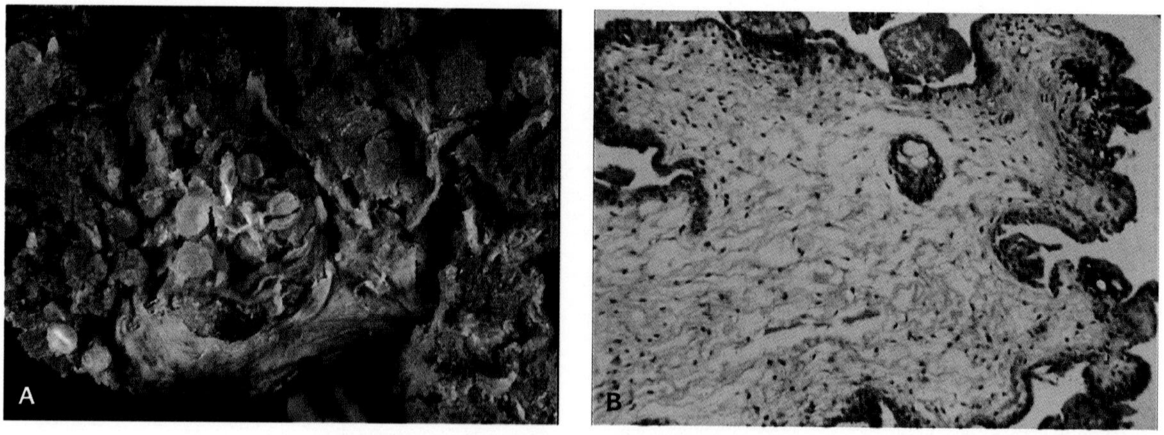

5.54. (A) Partial hydatidiform mole. Scattered vesicular chorionic villi can be seen. **(B)** Microscopic appearance of partial hydatidiform mole. The chorionic villus is distended with scalloping of the border and trophoblastic inclusion.

contain nucleated erythrocytes. There are two fetal phenotypes: type I fetuses with paternal chromosome dominance are associated with a large cystic placenta and have relatively normal fetal growth and microcephaly; type II fetuses with maternal chromosome dominance are associated with small noncystic placentas, are markedly growth retarded, and have a disproportionately large head.

REFERENCES

Ackerman J, Gilbert-Barness E: Immunological studies of the placenta in maternal connective tissue disease. *Pediatr Pathol Lab Med* 17:513, 1997.

Baldwin VJ: *Pathology of the Embryonic Fetus*, Philadelphia, JB Lippincott, 1992.

Baldwin VJ: *Pathology of Multiple Gestation*, New York, Springer-Verlag, 1993.

Benirschke K, Fox H: Thrombosis of fetal arteries in the human placenta. *Brjobeste Gynecol* 73:961, 1966.

Benirschke K, Kaufmann P: *The Pathology of the Human Placenta*, 3rd ed, New York, Springer-Verlag, 1995.

College of American Pathologists: The examination of the placenta: patient care and risk management. College of American Pathologists' Conference XIX. *Arch Pathol Lab Med* 115:7, 1991.

Fox H: Placenta accreta, 1945–1969. *Obstet Gynecol Surg* 27:475, 1992.

Gilbert-Barness E, ed: *Potter's Pathology of the Fetus and Newborn*, St. Louis, Mosby, 1997.

Gilbert-Barness E. The significance of the placenta in assessment of the newborn. *Crit Res Clin Lab Sci*, 2002.

Heifetz SA: Single umbilical artery: A statistical analysis of 237 autopsy cases and review of the literature. *Perspect Pediatr Pathol* 8:345, 1984.

Heifetz SA: The pathology of the umbilical cord in the placenta. In Lewis SH, Perrine E (eds), *Contemporary Issues in Surgical Pathology*, 2nd ed, New York, Churchill Livingstone, 1998.

Hyde S, Altschuler G: Infectious disorders of the placenta. In Lewis SH (ed), *The Placenta*, New York, Churchill Livingstone, 1998.

Lewis SH, Richard RM: Chorioangioma of the placenta. *Contemp Obstet Gynecol* 36:95, 1991.

Lewis SH, Gilbert-Barness E: Placenta and its significance for neonatal outcome. In Barness LA (ed), *Advances in Pediatrics, 45:223*, Philadelphia, Mosby, 1998.

Lewis SH, Gilbert-Barness (eds): *The Membranes and Pathology of the Placenta*, New York, Churchill Livingston, 1999.

Lewis SH, Perrin E: *Pathology of the Placenta*, 2nd ed, New York, Churchill Livingstone, 1999.

Molteni RA, Styes SJ, Battaglia FC: Relationship of fetus and placental weight in human beings: fetal/placental weight ratios at various gestational ages and birth weight distributions. *J Reprod Med* 21:327, 1978.

Naeye RL: Umbilical cord length: clinical significance. *J Pediatr* 107:278, 1985.

Naeye RL: *Disorders of the Placenta, Fetus, and Neonate: Diagnosis and Clinical Significance*, St. Louis, Mosby, 1992.

Naeye RL, Localio AR: Determining the time before birth when ischemia and hypoxemia initiated cerebral palsy. *Obstet Gynecol* 86:713, 1996.

Naeye RL, Shen-Scwartz S, Ruchelli E, et al.: Villous edema of the placenta: a clinical pathologic study. *Placenta* 10:297, 1989.

Smith CR, Chan HSL, deSa DJ: Placental involvement in congenital neuroblastoma. *J Clin Pathol* 34:785, 1981.

SIX

Chromosomal Abnormalities in the Embryo and Fetus

Structural chromosomal abnormalities include translocations, inversions, deletions, ring chromosomes, isochromosomes, intrachromosomal duplications, insertions, and dicentric chromosomes (Figures 6.1 and 6.2).

Inversions involve two breaks within a single chromosome with the intervening segment inverted.

Deletions are the result of a distal break or two internal breaks on the chromosome, allowing portions of chromosomal material to be lost. When two breaks occur, a ring chromosome can be formed.

Isochromosomes are usually mirror image chromosomes that result from single breaks close to the centromere, thus eliminating the whole of a long or short arm.

Chromosome abnormalities represent the largest category of causes of deaths in humans (Table 6.1). Abortuses that have reached a 2-week stage of development are estimated to have a 38% rate of chromosome abnormalities. In liveborn infants, the rate of chromosome defects is 1:200.

In stillbirths ($\geq$20 gestational weeks), the rate of chromosome abnormalities is between 6.6% and 11.7%. In fetuses between 9 and 20 weeks, the rate of chromosome abnormalities is around 7%. The average rate of chromosome defects of spontaneously aborted embryos earlier than 9 weeks is about 60% (59.1%) and above 60% in abortuses of a developmental age less than 7 weeks. It is conceivable to the rate of chromosome abnormalities before 2 weeks

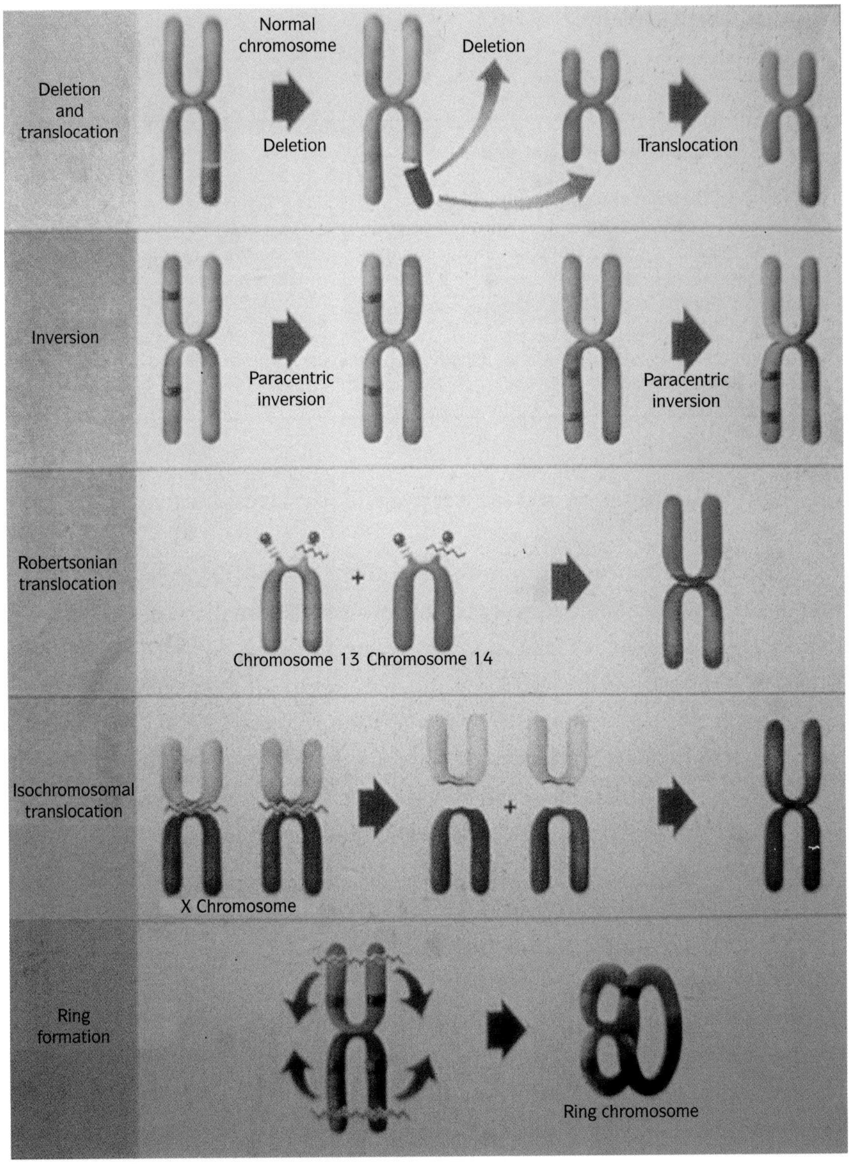

6.1. Structural abnormalities of chromosomes. (From Rubin E and Farber JL: *Pathology*. Philadelphia, Lippincott-Raven, 1997.)

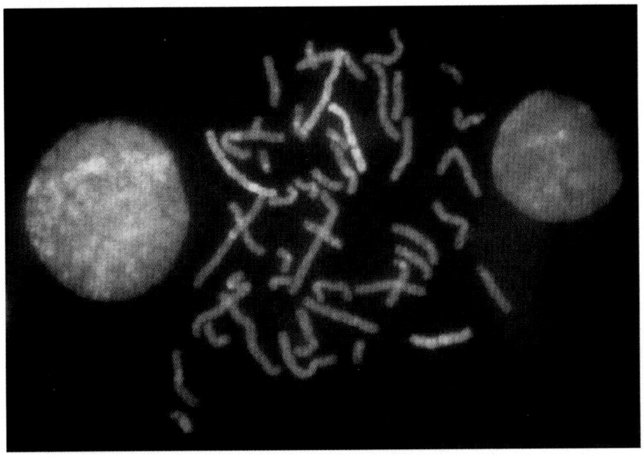

6.2. Fluorescent in situ hybridization (FISH) technology. Chromosome painting probes for chromosome 3 (spectrum orange) and chromosome 7 (spectrum green) confirm an insertional translocation of chromosome 7 material into the chromosome 3 long arm.

Table 6.1 Chromosomal defects

At birth 1:200 have chromosomal defects
38% of all 2 week embryos have chromosomal defects
50% of all embryos from the time of conception are estimated to have chromosomal defects
High % of chromosomal defects represent trisomies
Trisomy 16 – lethal
Most aborted 7–8 weeks, although usually stop their development at approximately 4 weeks

(i.e., between fertilization and the early previllous stages shortly after implantation) is 82%.

Fetuses with abnormal chromosomes are encountered after termination of pregnancy for prenatal detection of a chromosome anomaly; after termination of pregnancy when major fetal anomaly or intrauterine fetal death has been diagnosed by ultrasound examination; and, less commonly, in a second trimester spontaneous abortus. In most of the rare trisomies (mostly 2, 6, 11, 19, and 20), an embryo does not form. These are blighted ova with a developmental arrest around 3 weeks. The commonest autosomal trisomy is chromosome 16; it allows formation of a chorionic vesicle of 2–3 cm, a small amnion of 5 mm, and a tiny embryonic rudiment arrested at the embryonic disk stage. In trisomies 4, 5, 7, 8, 9, 10, and 22, disorganized embryos of a developmental age of 25–35 days are generally seen. Aborted trisomy 13, 14, and 15 embryos generally reach a 40- to 45-day stage of development. Alobar holoprosencephaly field defect is seen not only in trisomy 13 but also in trisomy 14 embryos. First trimester death of trisomy 21 fetuses usually occurs at a developmental age of 6–7 weeks. Gross abnormalities are rarely observed. Triploidy occurs in about 1% of all recognized human conceptions but is observed in only 1 of 10,000 live births – i.e., has a mortality rate of 99%. Most triploids are either 69,XXY (the most common) or 69,XXX; 69,XYY is very rare. About three-fourths of triploids represent dispermy or diandry (i.e., a paternal defect in meiosis I or II). About one-fourth represent digyny I or II. Most (86%) triploids are associated with formation of a partial mole with large amniotic sac containing an embryo with cord and membranes and with placenta showing hydatidiform changes, focal trophoblastic scalloping of villi, and formation of trophoblastic inclusions or microcysts. Most particularly, partial moles are paternally derived triploids; digyny II maternally derived triploids are nonmolar. Even if retained for a long time in utero, partial moles do not seem to be responsible for malignant sequelae but may be associated with high human chorionic gonadotropin levels and preeclampsia. On the other hand, complete moles have, in 90% of cases, a 46,XX chromosome constitution, with both haploid spermatozoa, or, more likely, a duplication of a haploid sperm entering an anucleate egg (which, however, retains all its maternal mitochondrial DNA). Tetraploidy seems to represent a postzygotic event resulting from failure of karyokinesis at first cell division. The commonest chromosome anomaly encountered during the second trimester is 45X (Turner syndrome). Fetuses with this anomaly are often identified on routine scans because of postnuchal fluid accumulation or generalized fetal hydrops. Women of 37 years and over, particularly those women of more than 40 years of age, are at increased risk of bearing a fetus with a chromosome abnormality. The autosomal trisomies, particularly trisomy 21, are commonly encountered, as are fetuses with sex chromosome anomalies. The observation that a trisomic pregnancy is associated with a low level of α-fetoprotein in maternal serum offers another method of prenatal identification, useful because it is independent of maternal age. Investigation of pregnancies in which a potentially treatable malformation, such as exomphalos, has been identified, and those pregnancies complicated by growth retardation will also lead to the identification of some chromosomally abnormal fetuses. Fetal growth retardation is more likely to be identified beyond 21 weeks gestation, although fetuses with a triploid karyotype may be severely growth retarded in the second trimester.

A wide range of anomalies are encountered in the offspring of individuals with balanced translocations, particularly when more than two chromosomes are involved.

About 99% of all conceptuses with chromosomal abnormalities die prenatally, including almost all cases of monosomy X, polyploidy, and autosomal trisomy; one-half of fetuses with trisomy 21 die prenatally. Forty percent of liveborn Down syndrome children die by the end of the first year of life. Nondisjunction appears to be nonrandom because women who have had a chromosomally unbalanced fetus are more likely to have another aneuploid fetus if they miscarry again than women whose first miscarried fetus was chromosomally normal.

The risk of recurrence after one affected child with a standard trisomy is about 1% for a baby with some form of trisomy (trisomy 21 would be the most common).

Approximately 25% of liveborn infants with chromosomal abnormalities have autosomal trisomy, and approximately 40% have a structural chromosomal defect. Those with balanced structural chromosomal defects are phenotypically normal but have some 15% fewer liveborn offspring than their chromosomally normal siblings.

The phenotypic expression of chromosome abnormalities can be readily observed in the fetus. Dermatoglyphics are also discernible by 13 weeks of gestation. The pathologic changes can be recognized and some pathologic markers for specific chromosome abnormalities may be apparent in early fetal life such as cystic and calcified Hassal corpuscles in trisomy 21, gelatinous multivalvular disease in trisomy 18, partial hydatidiform mole of the placenta in triploidy, and cystic hygromas in Turner (45,X) syndrome. Although chromosome

Table 6.2 Fates of fertilized ova

- Approximately 16% of ova exposed to sperm fail to thrive
- Another 15% fail to implant
- Approximately 27% are aborted spontaneously at previllous stages, presumably because they are grossly abnormal
- Of the 42% of fertilized human ova that survive the first missed menstrual period, approximately one fourth are aborted spontaneously
- 68.5% total reproductive loss. 31.5% of ova exposed to sperm in women of proven fertility survive to be born alive

Table 6.3 Incidence of types of chromosomal abnormalities in 1500 spontaneous abortions

Abnormalities	Rate of occurrence (%)
Autosomal trisomies	52.00
Triploidy	19.86
45X	15.30
Tetraploidy	6.18
Double trisomy	1.73
Translocations	3.80
Mosaicism	1.08

Adapted from Boue J, Boue A, Lazar P: Retrospective and prospective epidemiological studies of 1500 karyotyped spontaneous human abortions, *Teratology* 12:11, 1975.

Table 6.4 Incidence of major chromosomal abnormalities in liveborn infants

Trisomy 13:1 in 5000
Trisomy 21:1 in 300 at age 35 (1:1000 at age 20; 1:95 at age 40)
del(5p) (cri-du-chat syndrome): 1 in 50,000
Klinefelter syndrome: 1 in 850 male births
Monosomy X: 1 in 2500 female births
Fragile X syndrome: 1 in 1000 male births

Table 6.5 Mild malformations in chromosome defects

Bipartite uvula
Abnormal lobation of lungs
Intrahepatic gallbladder
Stenosis and abnormal branching of bile ducts
Annular pancreas
Malrotation of gut
Meckel diverticulum
Kinky ureters
Megaureters and megapelvis
Renal microcysts
Single umbilical artery
Mingling of different organ tissues
Abnormal lobulation of spleen
Accessory spleens
Abnormal lobation of liver
Costal defect (x-ray)

Table 6.6 Chromosomal syndromes: pathologic examination

Careful observation for minor anomalies on external examination
Facial dysmorphism
Ear morphology
Good photographs*
X-rays
Dermatoglyphics
Careful anatomic dissection for minor and major anomalies

studies confirm the diagnosis, if the specimen has been placed in fixative or is autolyzed (precluding chromosome analysis) pathologic studies are helpful in the recognition of chromosome abnormalities.

The fate of fertilized human ova is shown in Table 6.2. The total reproductive loss due to aneuploidy or polyploidy is greater than 50%. The incidence and types of chromosome abnormalities in spontaneous abortions are listed in Table 6.3. The incidence of chromosome defects in liveborn infants is seen in Table 6.4 and the developmental effects of aneuploidy are shown in Table 6.4. These include multiple mild and major malformations with the most severe effects being on the central nervous system (CNS) with frequent gross malformation prenatally and mental retardation postnatally. Disturbance of growth results in intrauterine growth retardation or a small-for-gestational-age infant. Aneuploidy has more or less severely deleterious developmental effects on gonads. Turner syndrome is associated with gonadal dysgenesis of late fetal ovarian degeneration, and Klinefelter syndrome is associated with congenital microorchidism. The increased incidence of dysplasia in aneuploidy results in a greater risk for the development of neoplasia; for example, there is an association of (del)13q with retinoblastoma; del(11p) with Wilms tumor; trisomy 21 with leukemia, retinoblastoma and CNS and testicular tumors; Klinefelter syndrome with breast cancer; trisomy 13 with retinal dysplasia, retinoblastoma, and leukemia; and trisomy 18 with Wilms tumor.

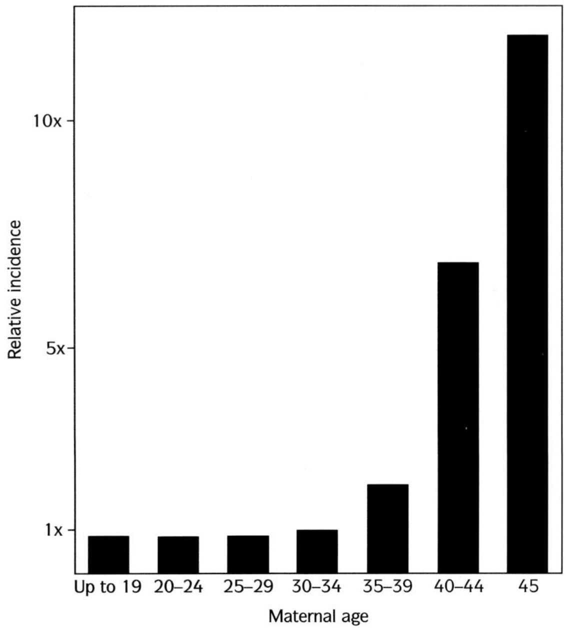

6.3. Trisomy 21 and maternal age.

Mild malformations are also common in aneuploidy syndromes. A mild malformation is an anomaly of morphogensis and should be viewed as a reduced expression of a major anomaly. They are all-or-none traits. A list of the more common mild malformations seen in chromosomal defects is shown in Table 6.5. The pathologic examination in chromosomal defects includes procedures mentioned in Table 6.6.

Some pathologic markers can be identified in some of the aneuploidy syndromes. The characteristic appearance of trisomy 21 is evident in the fetus and can be identified by 14 weeks' gestation. Cystic and calcified Hassal corpuscles recognized as well as gelatinous valvular tissue in the heart. This involves all valves (multivalvular) and represents persistence of early fetal valvular development. In triploidy, partial hydatidiform mole is constantly present.

TRISOMY 21

Trisomy 21 is the most common autosomal trisomy encountered in pregnancies that extend beyond the first trimester. Lower than normal α-fetoprotein levels

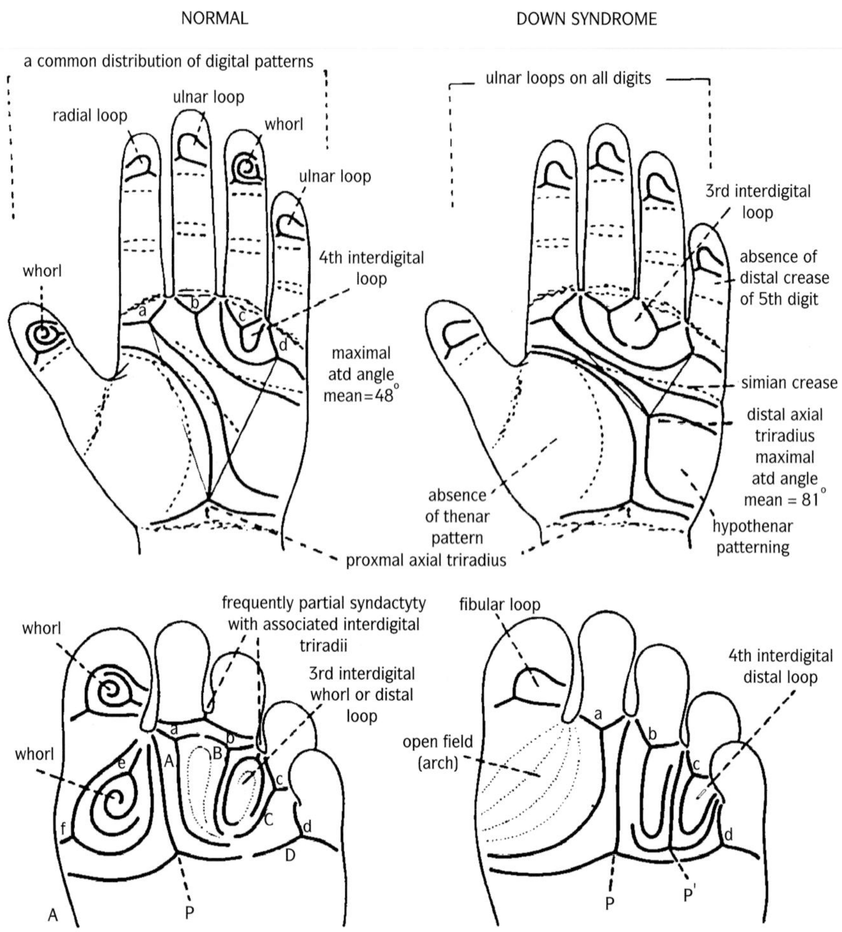

6.4. Dermatoglyphics of Down syndrome (trisomy 21) (right) compared with the normal (left). (From Jones KL: *Smith's Recognizable Patterns of Malformation Syndromes*. Philadelphia, WB Saunders, 1988, p 673, with permission.)

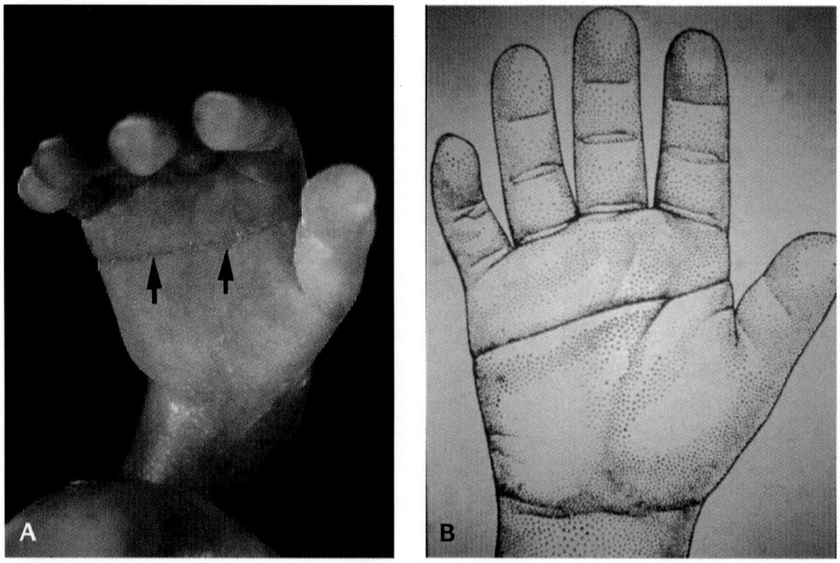

6.5. **(A)** Stillborn fetus at 24 weeks gestation with trisomy 21 with a simian crease (arrow). **(B)** Illustration of a simian crease.

Table 6.7 Trisomy 21 (Down syndrome)

Trisomy 21	94%
Translocations D/G and G/G	4%
Trisomy 21/normal mosaicism	2%

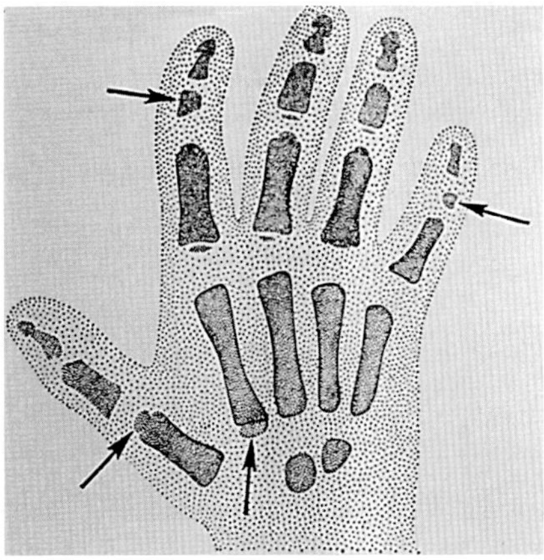

6.6. Down syndrome – bones of hand in x-ray. Middle phalanx of fifth finger is hypoplastic; a proximal epiphysis is present on the second and distal epiphysis on the first finger (arrows).

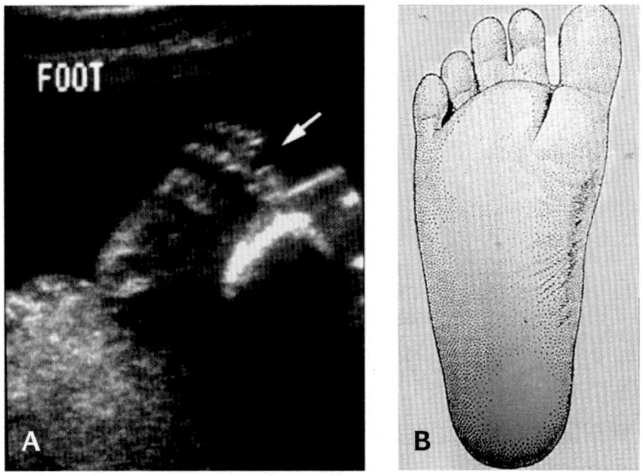

6.7. **(A)** Down syndrome – an ultrasound of a foot with space (arrow) between 1st and 2nd toes. **(B)** Illustration of a foot characteristic for trisomy 21.

in maternal serum in the second trimester of pregnancy may occur in the presence of a 21 trisomic fetus.

Genetic Aspects

Ninety-five percent of cases have regular trisomy 21, about 3% of cases have mosaicism, and 2% have translocations (Figures 6.3 to 6.12 and Tables 6.7 to 6.8). General features of abnormalities observed in trisomy 21 include intrauterine growth retardation; diminished sucking and swallowing reflexes;

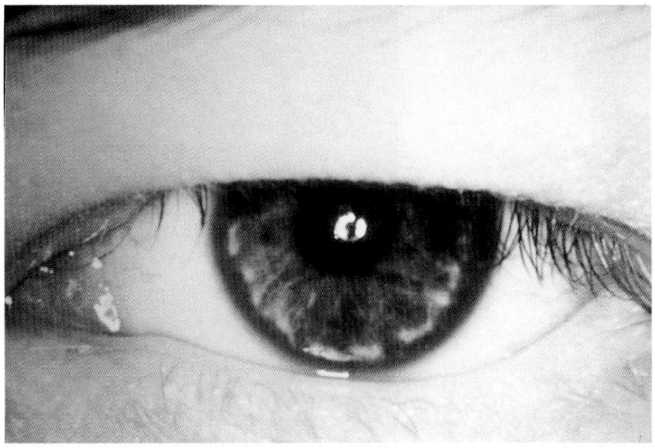

6.8. Down syndrome – brushfield spots of iris.

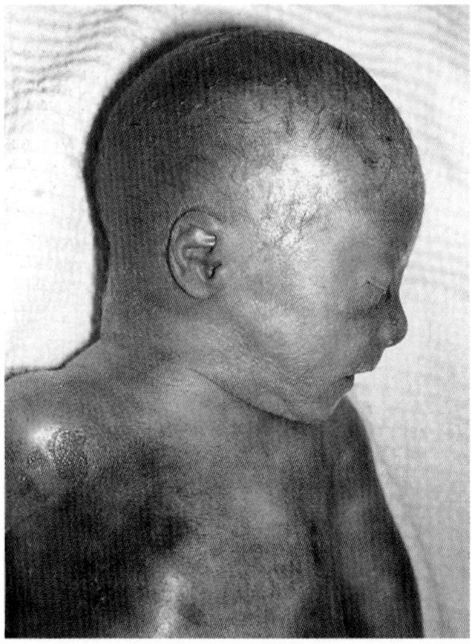

6.9. Down syndrome profile. Fetus of trisomy 21 at 22 weeks gestation with typical facial features.

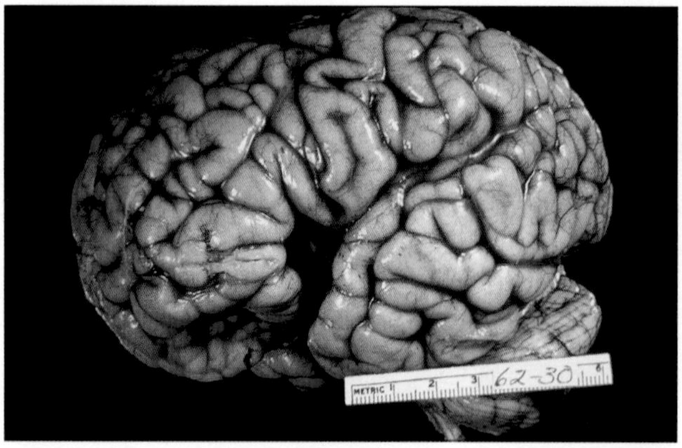

6.10. Brain in Down syndrome. There is a short anteroposterior diameter, an open operculum, and a hypoplastic superior temporal gyrus.

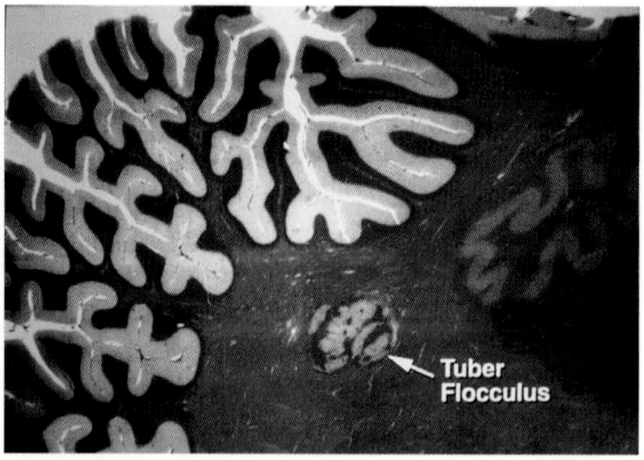

6.11. Brain in Down syndrome showing a tuber flocculus within the cerebellum.

mental retardation; and a specific dermatoglyphic pattern. A 14:21 Robertsonian translocation is the most common. A small percentage of translocation cases have an isochromosome for the long arm of chromosome 21 t(21q:21q).

Maternal nondisjunction is responsible for 95% of trisomic cases. The risk of a liveborn infant with Down syndrome increases with the age of the mother.

If the mother carries a 14:21 translocation, recurrence risks are 10% and if the father carries such a translocation, the risks are 2%. In the rare t(21q:21q)

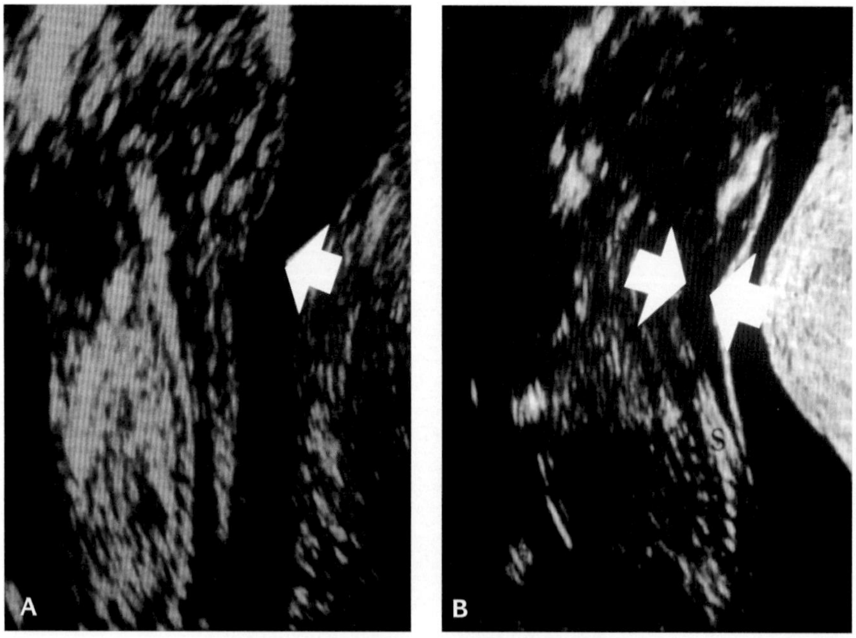

6.12. Sagittal transvaginal ultrasonographic image. **(A)** Normal fetus at 13 weeks gestation with no translucency of the neck. **(B)** Zone of nuchal translucency of 6 mm (arrows) in a 14-week fetus with trisomy 21. (Courtesy *N Eng J Med* 337:1655, 1997.)

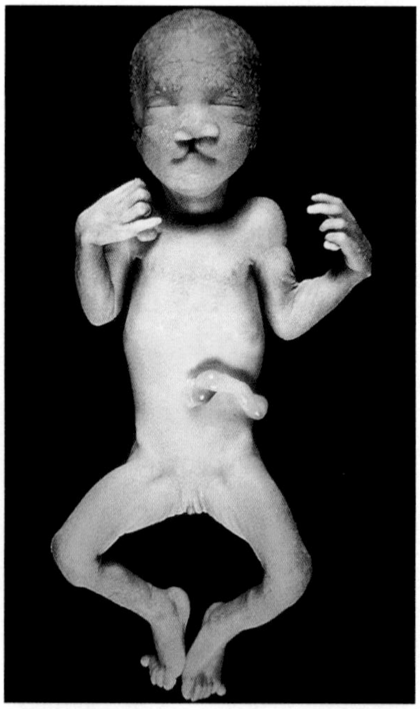

6.13. Trisomy 13: midline facial defect, hypertelorism and polydactyly.

Table 6.8 Abnormalities observed in trisomy 21

Cardiac	Visceral	Renal
Endocardial cushion defects	Large liver	Stricture at ureteropelvic junction
Tetralogy of Fallot	Moderate to severe fatty change	Hydronephrosis
Ventricular septal defect	Esophageal atresia 1%	Focal cystic malformation of collecting tubules
Double-outlet right ventricle	Duodenal atresia 30%	Immature glomeruli
Pulmonary hypertension	Annular pancreas	Renal dysplasia
Pulmonary vascular stenosis	Congenital intestinal aganglionosis (Hirschsprung disease) 2%	Nephrogenic rests
	Diastasis recti	Kidneys small
	Umbilical hernia	Hemangiomas of kidney

Endocrinologic	Hematologic	Immune system	Central nervous system – brain
Hypothyroidsm	Polycythemia	T-cell immunodeficiency	Weight usually less than normal
Precocious puberty	Leukemia (1%): congenital acute myelobastic, acute lymphoblastic in childhood, and acute megakaryocytic	Thymus usually small: large Hassall corpuscles, with calcification and cystic changes	Delayed maturity
Diabetes mellitus	Transient myeloproliferative syndrome	Spleen: lymphocyte depletion	Convolutions small
Hyperthyroidism		Lymph nodes: depleted T-dependent zones	Myelination retarded
Hypogenitalism		Hepatitis B surface antigenemia	Cerebral convolutions: flat
Penis and testes small			Frontal and temporal poles compressed
Crytorchidism			Gyri: frontal poles flattened
Macrogenitosomia precox			Hypoplastic brachycephalic brain
Adrenal hyperplasia			Hypoplasia of superior temporal gyrus
Testes: interstitial fibrosis, hypoplasia of seminiferous tubules			Open operculum
Ovaries usually small			Short corpus callosum
Hypoplasia with persistence of atretic corpora lutea			Hypoplasia of brainstem and medulla
Development of axillary and pubic hair, and breasts deficient			Hypoplasia of cerebellar hemispheres

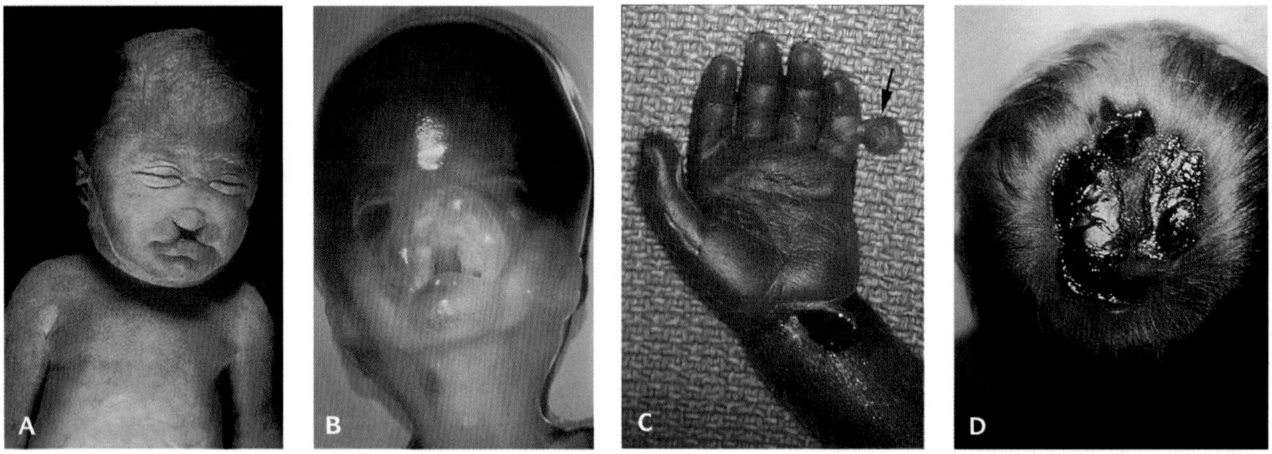

6.14. Fetus at **(A)** 34 weeks with bilateral cleft lip and other abnormalities. **(B)** 16 weeks with bilateral midline cleft and protrusion of premaxilla. **(C)** post-axial polydactyly. **(D)** Midline scalp defect.

translocation cases in which one parent carries the translocation chromosome, recurrence risks are 100%.

TRISOMY 13

Forty-five percent of cases die within the first month, 70% die within 6 months, and 86% die within 12 months (Figures 6.13 to 6.19 and Tables 6.9 to 6.13). Few survive beyond 5 years.

Genetic Aspects

Seventy-five to 80% of cases are simple trisomies. Twenty percent of cases have translocations. A few cases are mosaic.

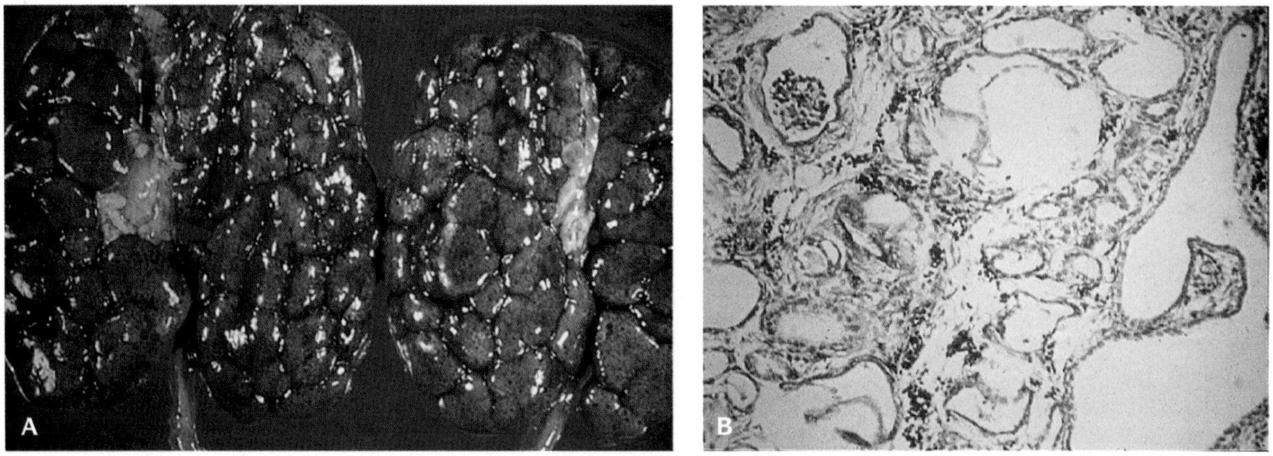

6.15. Trisomy 13. **(A)** Kidney with excessive fetal lobulation and multiple cortical cysts. **(B)** Micromulticystic kidney.

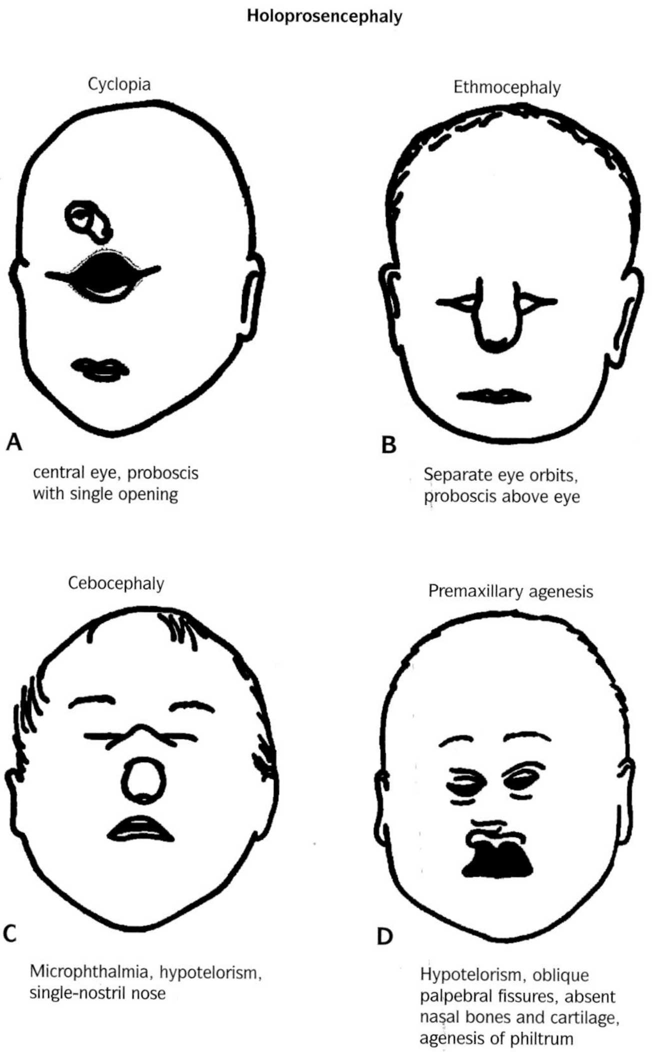

6.16. Cartoon – spectrum of holoprosencephaly. **(A)** Cyclopia with two eyes in single orbit (proboscis above). **(B)** Ethmocephaly with proboscis. **(C)** Cebocephaly with single nostril. **(D)** Bilateral cleft lip, premaxillary aplasia, and hypotelorism.

Table 6.9 Trisomy 13

Incidence 1:6,000 births
Females slightly higher
50% die by one month of age
20% survive to one year

Table 6.10 Trisomy 13: dermatoglyphics

Distal axial triradius
Single palmar crease
Fibular arch pattern – toes

Table 6.11 Holoprosencephaly: genetics

Sporadic pattern
Recessive trait
Dominant trait
Association with chromosomal abnormality; trisomy 13, del(13q), del(18p), trisomy 21, triploidy

Table 6.12 Holoprosencephaly

Median cleft lip	Hypotelorism with separate orbits Hypoplastic nose Absence of median portion of upper lip Lobar or semilobar holoprosencephaly
Cebocephaly	Hypotelorism with separate orbits Proboscis-like nose, single nostril Holoprosencephaly
Ethmocephaly	Severe hypotelorism with two separate orbits Absence of nose or proboscis Holoprosencephaly
Cyclopia	Single or partially divided eye in single orbit Absence of nose or proboscis Holoprosencephaly

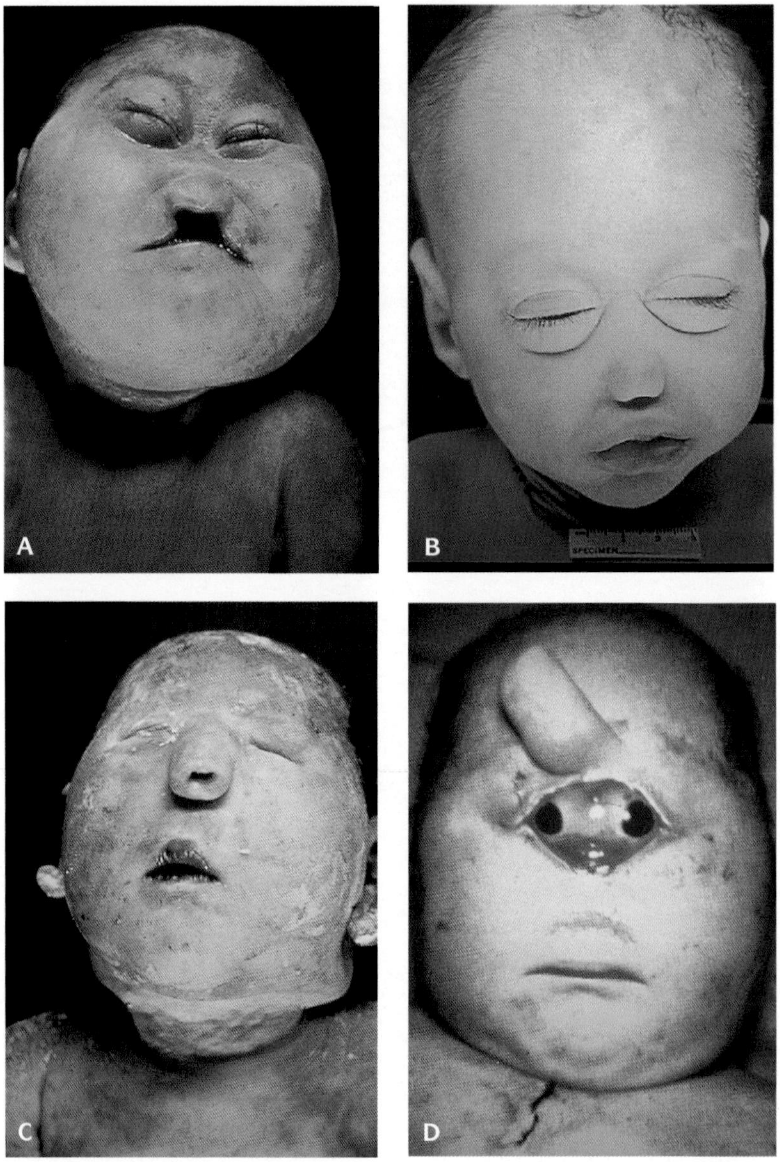

6.17. Holoprosencephaly with **(A)** midline facial defects in trisomy 13. **(B)** Cebocephaly. **(C)** Ethmocephaly. **(D)** Cyclopia.

TRISOMY 18

There is a low birthweight, a prominent occiput, narrow palpebral fissures, and a small chin (Figure 6.20). The finger nails are small, the index finger overlaps the middle finger, and the fifth finger overlaps the fourth (Figure 6.21). The feet are rocker bottom and the heel prominent. Other common malformations include cleft lip, omphalocele, exomphalos, radial aplasia, congenital heart defects, horseshoe kidney (Figure 6.22), multivalvular thickened, and rolled valve leaflets (Figure 6.23 and Table 6.14).

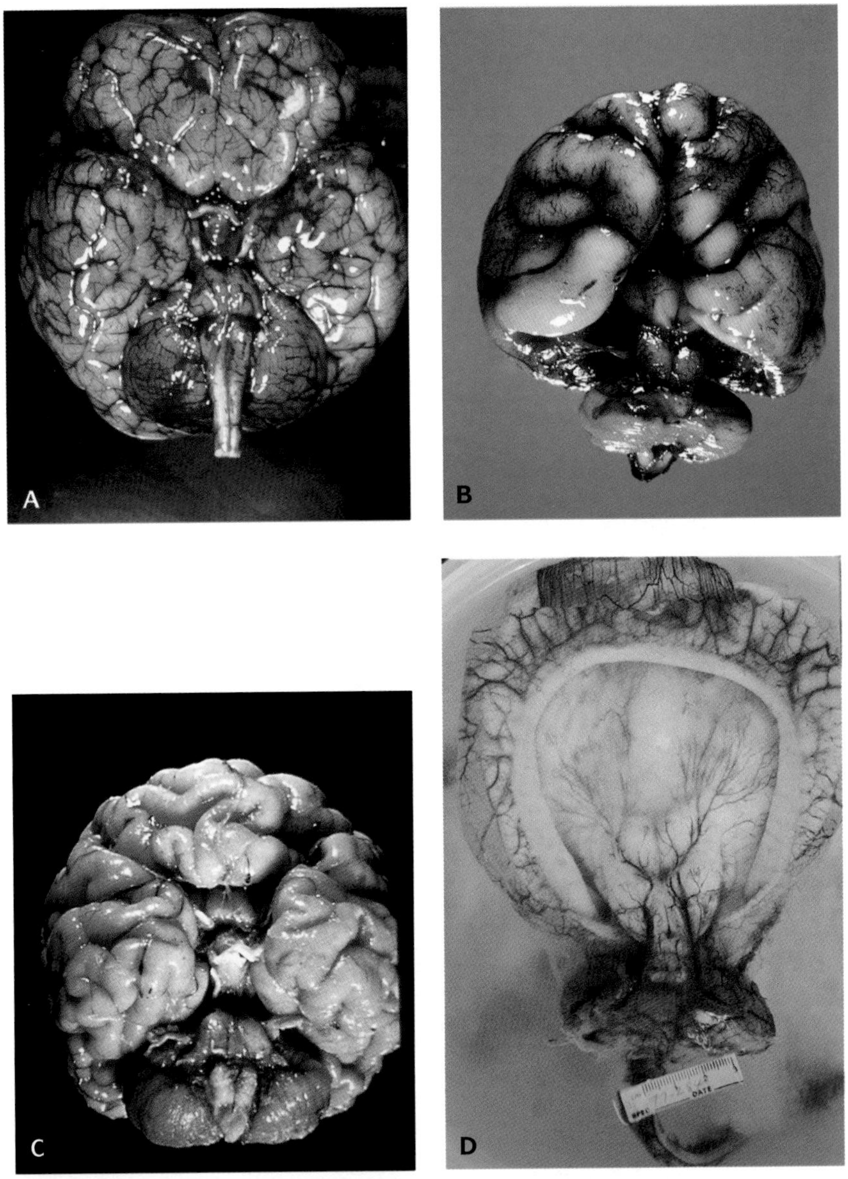

6.18. Trisomy 13. Brain spectrum of holoprosencephaly. **(A)** Arrhinencephaly (absence of olfactory bulbs and tracts). **(B)** Lobar holoprosencephaly. **(C)** Alobar holoprosencephaly. **(D)** Alobar holoprosencephaly (basket brain).

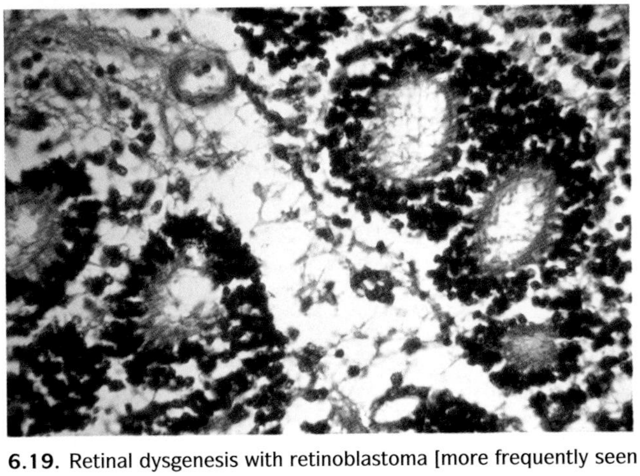

6.19. Retinal dysgenesis with retinoblastoma [more frequently seen with 13q del (25%)].

Table 6.13 Abnormalities observed in trisomy 13

External	Visceral	Cardiovascular
Inrauterine growth retardation	Abnormal lobation of lungs	Ventricular septal defects
Microcephaly	Pulmonary hypoplasia	Patent ductus arteriosus
Receding forehead	Abnormal lobation of liver	Atrial septal defect
Epicanthal folds	Malrotation of intestines	Dextrocardia/dextroposition
Deep-set eyes	Elongated, hypoplastic, malrotated or hydropic gallbladder	Patent foramen ovale
Absent philtrum	Cholestasis	Pulmonic valvular stenosis
Midline facial defect, cleft lip/palate	Focal hepatic calcification	Pulmonic valvular atresia
Hypotelorism	Ectopic pancreas in spleen	Bicuspid aortic valve
Rocker-bottom feet	Omphalocele	Transposition of the great vessels
	Gastroschisis	Truncus arteriosus
	Meckel diverticulum	Double outlet right ventricle
	Absent mesentery	Aortic coarctation
	Inguinal and/or umbilical hernia	Polyvalvular dysplasia
	Adrenal hypoplasia	
	Ectopic adrenal tissue	

Genitourinary	Ocular	Central nervous system
Micromulticystic kidneys	Microphthalmia/anophthalmia	Arrhinencephaly-holoprosencephaly
Double kidney	Cataracts	Cerebellar anomalies
Double ureter	Corneal opacities	Corpus callosum defects
Hydronephrosis and hydroureter	Retinoschisis	Heterotopias
Renal dysplasia	Hypoplasia of optic nerve	Arnold-Chiari malformation
Horseshoe kidney	Premature vitreous body	Vascular malformations
Renal hypoplasia	Coloboma of iris or retina	Anencephaly
Renal dysplasia	Aniridia	Migration defects
Male	Retinal dysplasia	Dandy-Walker malformation
Cryptorchidism	Retinoblastoma	
Agenesis of testes		
Hypospadias		
Female		
Bicornuate uterus		
Double separate vagina		
Uterus didelphis		

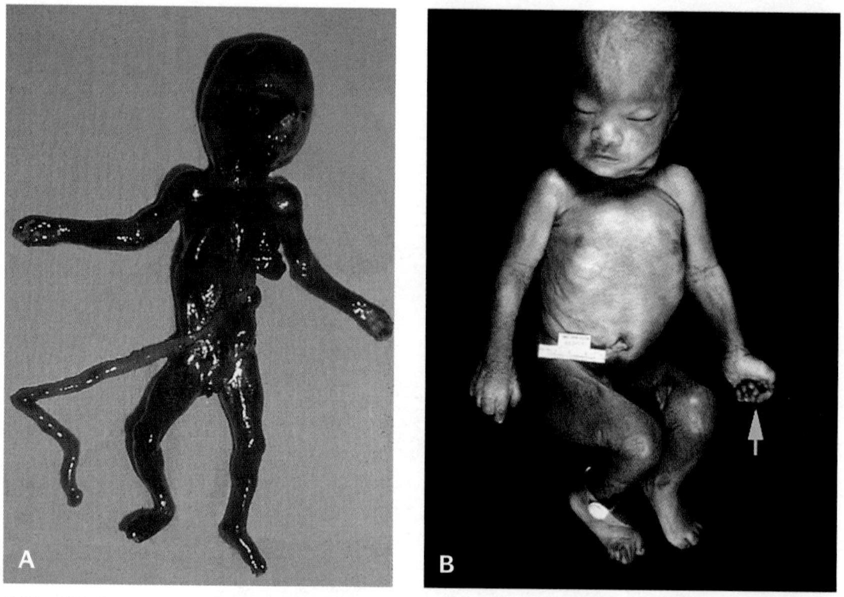

6.20. (A) Fetus at 14 weeks – note overlapping index over 3rd fingers and typical phenotype. **(B)** Fetus at 32 weeks. This male infant shows the typical phenotype of trisomy 18 including micrognathia, low-set ears, slender bridge of the nose, short sternum, narrow pelvis, clenched fists with the index finger overlapping the 3rd finger, and rocker-bottom feet.

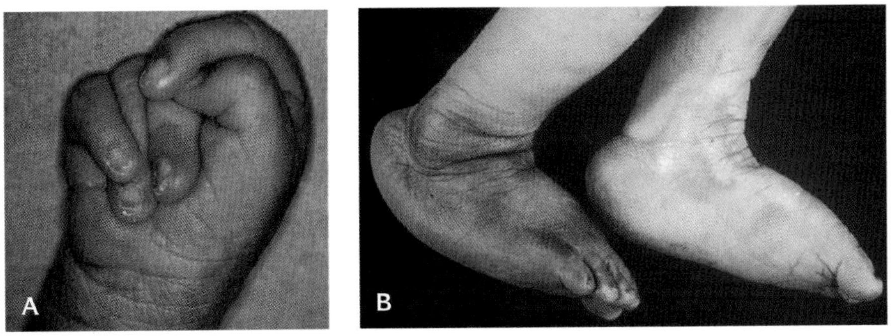

6.21. **(A)** Trisomy 18. Overlapping of the index finger over the middle finger. **(B)** Trisomy 18. Rocker-bottom feet.

TRISOMY 22

The clinical features are a coloboma of the iris, pre-auricular pits and tags, anal abnormalities (a covered anus, anal atresia, or an anteriorly placed anus), congenital heart defects, kidney abnormalities, and variable mental retardation, although intelligence can be normal.

TRISOMY 8

The main clinical clues to the diagnosis (Figures 6.26 and 6.27 and Table 6.15) are:

1. Expressionless face with hypertelorism and deep-set eyes.
2. Deep skin creases in palms and soles.
3. A long narrow trunk.
4. Small or absent patellae.

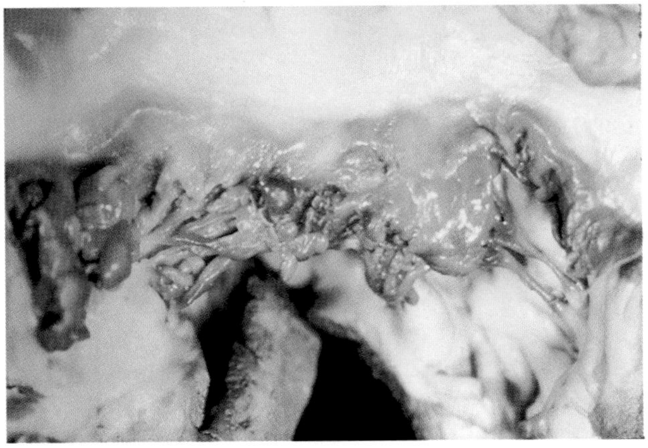

6.22. Multivalvular heart abnormality in trisomy 18. The tricuspid valve leaflets are thickened, rolled, and distorted.

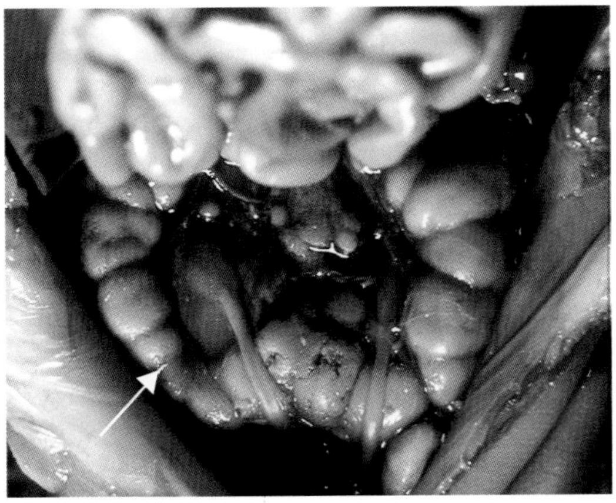

6.23. Horseshoe kidney.

Table 6.14 Abnormalities observed in trisomy 18

Visceral	Cardiovascular	Central nervous system	Gastrointestinal
Pulmonary hypoplasia	Ventricular septal defect with or without overriding aorta	Meningomyelocele	Meckel diverticulum
Abnormal lobation of lung	Patent ductus arteriosus	Cerebellar anomalies	Malrotation
Pyloric stenosis	Pulmonic stenois/bicuspid valve	Abnormal gyri	Pyloric stenosis
Omphalocele	Bicuspid aortic valve	Hydrocephalus	Hypoplasia of intestine
Common mesentery	Atrial septal defect	Arnold-Chiari malformation	Accessory spleen
Hypoplasia of intestine	Dysplastic valves	Corpus callosum defects	Abnormal lobation of liver
Exstrophy of cloaca	Coarctation of aorta	Holoprosencephaly	Ectopic pancreas
Adrenal hypoplasia	Double outlet right ventricle	Frontal lobe defect	Hypoplastic gallbladder
Thymic hypoplasia	Hypoplastic left heart	Migration defect	T-E fistula with or without esophageal atresia
Thyroid hypoplasia	Abnormal coronary artery	Anencephaly	Biliary atresia
Diaphragmatic eventration			Imperforate anus
Umbilical and inguinal hernia			Bile duct stenosis
Prominent extramedullary hematopoiesis			
Adrenal hypoplasia			

Urogenital	Skeletal	Ocular
Horseshoe kidney	Flexion contractures	Abnormal retinal pigmentation
Double ureter	Short or abnormal sternum	Cataract
Cystic kidney	Limited hip adduction	Coloboma
Double kidney	Rocker-bottom feet	Clouding of cornea
Hypoplastic ovaries	Syndactyly	Microphthalmia
Unilateral absent or hypoplastic kidney	Hammer toes	
Ectopic kidney	Hypoplastic toes	
Uterus bicornis	Small pelvis	
Uterus bicollis	Talipes equinovarus	
Cryptorchidism	Abnormal nails	
	Ulnar deviation	
	Hyperextensible joints	
	Hypoplastic thumbs	
	Hypoplastic clavicles	
	Phocomelia	

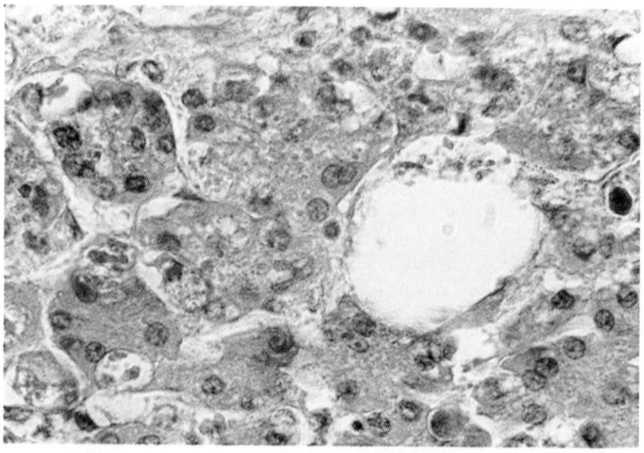

6.24. Microscopic section of liver showing giant cell transformation of hepatocytes and cholestasis not infrequently seen in trisomy 18.

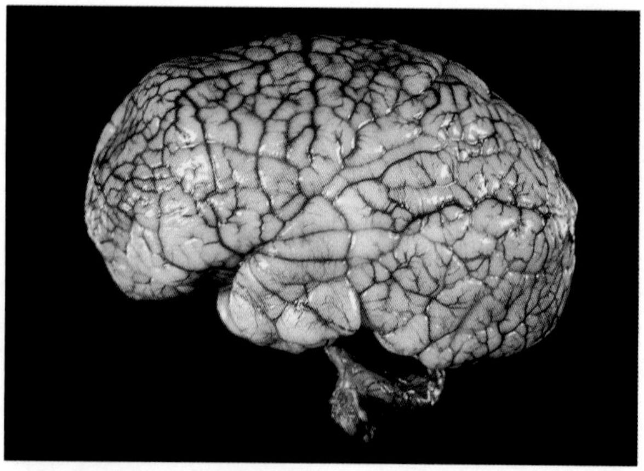

6.25. Brain with polymicrogyria.

Table 6.15 Abnormalities observed in trisomy 8 mosaicism

Craniofacial	Limb and trunk	Skeletal	Visceral
Scaphocephaly	Clinodactyly	Hemivertebrae	Interrupted aortic arch
Dysmorphic ears	Deep skin furrows on soles and/or palms	Extra vertebrae	Diaphragmatic hernia
Hypertelorism	Camptodactyly	Butterfly vertebrae	Esophageal atresia
Strabismus	Syndactyly of toes	Spina bifida occulta	Malrotation or absence of gallbladder
Broad-bridged, upturned nose	Narrow pelvis	Broad dorsal ribs	
Thick, everted lower lip	Long slender trunk	Narrow and hypoplastic iliac wings	
Micrognathia		Absent patellae	
High-arched palate		Kyphoscoliosis	
Coarse, pear-shaped nose		Pectus carinatum	
Down-slanting palpebral fissures		Radioulnar synostosis	
		Normal or advanced growth	

Genitourinary	Central nervous system	Ocular
Hydronephrosis	Hydrocephalus	Micropthalmia
Ureteral obstruction	Agenesis of corpus callosum	Iridal coloboma
Horseshoe kidney	Large sella turcica	Glaucoma
Unilateral agenesis of kidney		Corneal or lenticular opacities
Cryptorchidism		
Testicular hypoplasia		
Hypospadias		

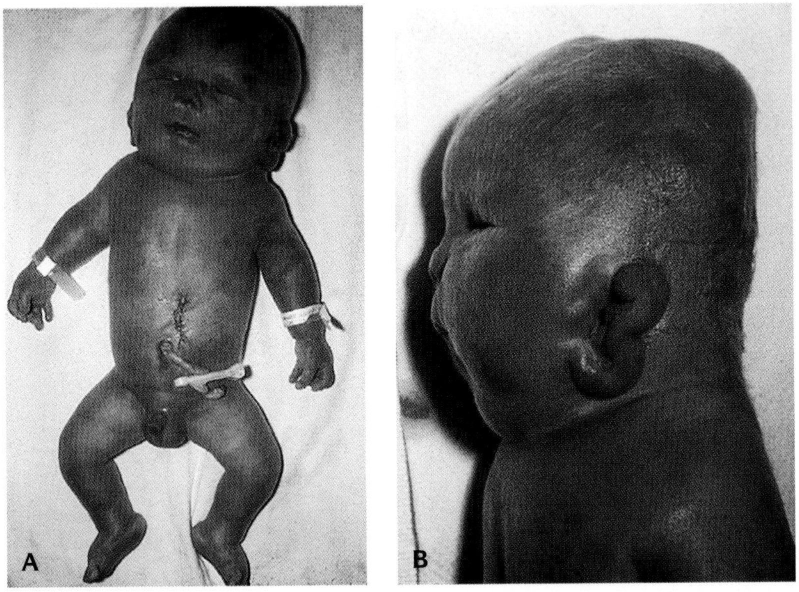

6.26. **(A)** Complete trisomy 8 in an infant who died shortly after birth with lymphedema and multiple anomalies. **(B)** Trisomy 8. The ears are malformed and edematous.

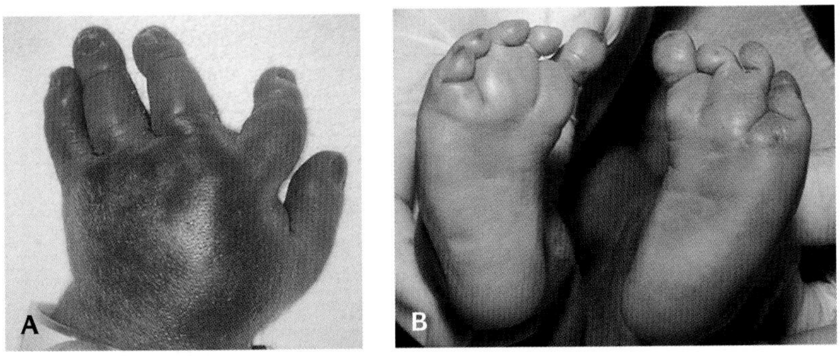

6.27. **(A)** Trisomy 8. The hands are broad and the fingers short and malformed. (**B**) Trisomy 8. Deep plantar furrows and malpositioned toes (four on the left foot).

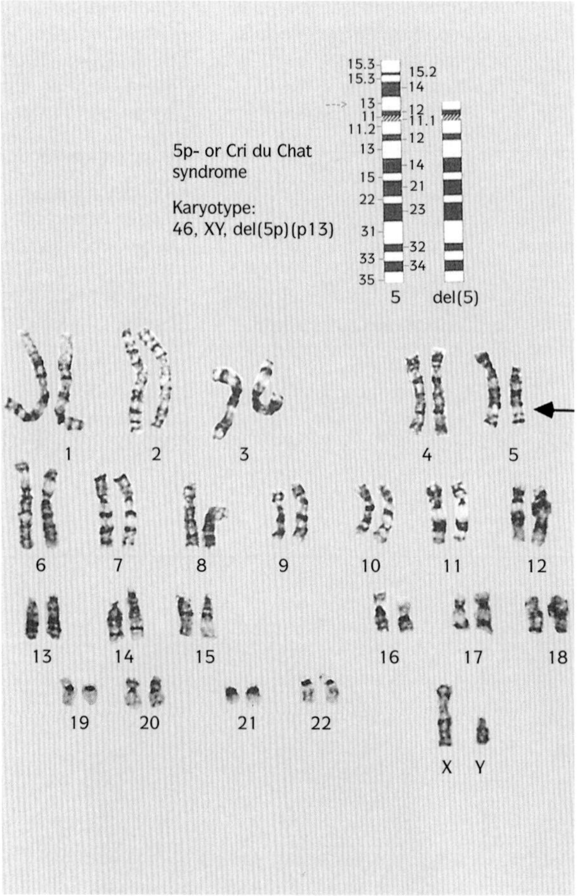

6.28. Karyotype of cri du chat (5p del) syndrome.

Genetic Aspects

Two-thirds of cases have a low-frequency mosaicism.

5P- [CRI DU CHAT]

This condition has a frequency of about 1 in 50,000 live births (Figures 6.28 and 6.29 and Tables 6.16 and 6.17). There is a cat-like cry, which can disappear

Table 6.16 Cri-du-chat syndrome (partial deletion of the short arm of chromosome 5)

General	Performance	Craniofacial
Low birthweight	Mental deficiency	Microcephaly
Slow growth	Hypotonia	Round face
Cat-like cry		Hypertelorism
		Downward slanting of palpebral fissures
		Strabismus
		Poorly formed ears

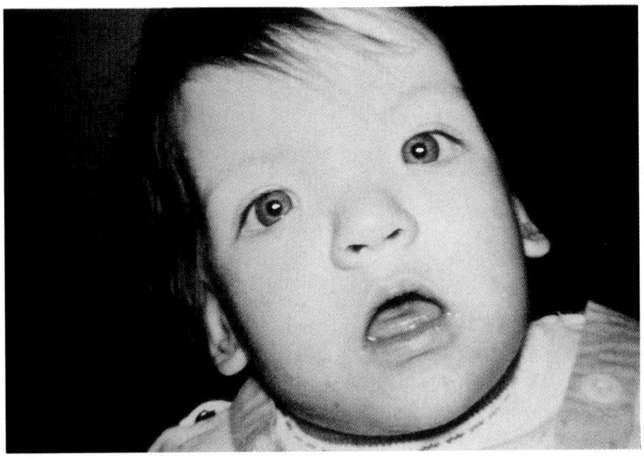

6.29. Cri du chat syndrome: hypertelorism, oval face, antimongoloid slant of the eyes and large ears.

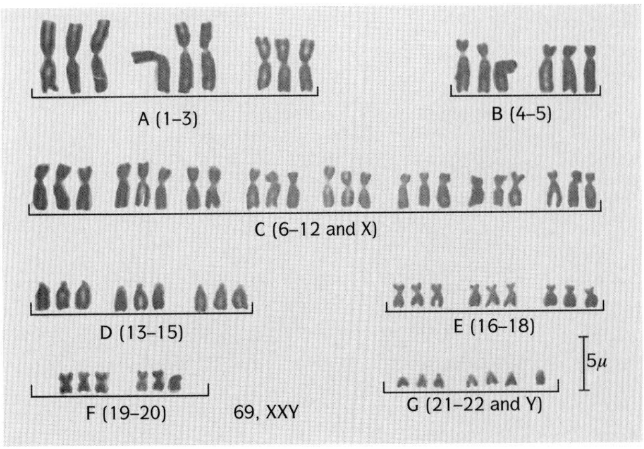

6.30. Karyotype 69 XYY.

later in life, microcephaly and a moon face, hypertelorism, epicanthal folds, flat nasal bridge, and severe mental retardation.

Genetic Aspects

Deletion of band 5p15. If parental chromosomes are normal, recurrence risks are about 1%.

TRIPLOIDY

The extra haploid set of chromosomes in triploidy is the result of double fertilization of the ovum (diandry) or failure of the ovum to extrude a polar body (digyny); 66% of triploidies are the result of dispermy; 24% are the result of fertilization of a haploid ovum by a diploid sperm (Figures 6.30 to 6.34 and Tables 6.18 to 6.21). There are two types of triploidy.

Table 6.17 Abnormalities observed in cri du chat (cat-cry) syndrome

At birth	Childhood
Growth retardation	Small, narrow, often asymmetric face
Microcephaly	Malocclusion
Mewing cry (cat cry)	Scoliosis
Full cheeks, round face	Muscle tone normal or increased
Depressed nasal bridge	Shortening of metacarpals three through five
Downward slant of palpebral fissures	Premature graying of hair
Cleft palate	
Preauricular fistulas	
Hypospadias	
Cryptorchidism	
Syndactyly of second and third toes and fingers	

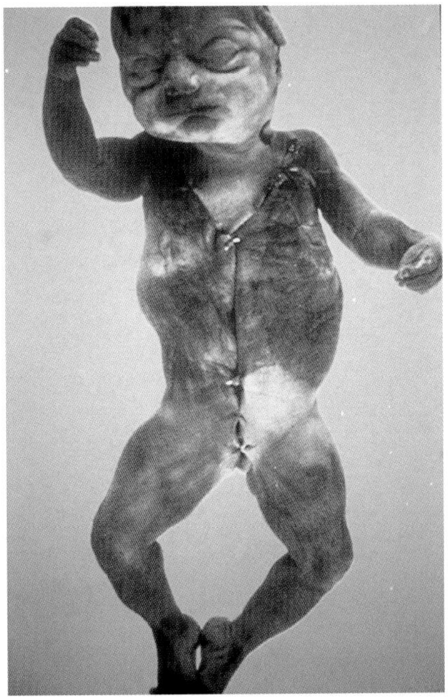

6.31. Triploid fetus: hypertelorism, bulbous nose, sloping forehead, and small mouth.

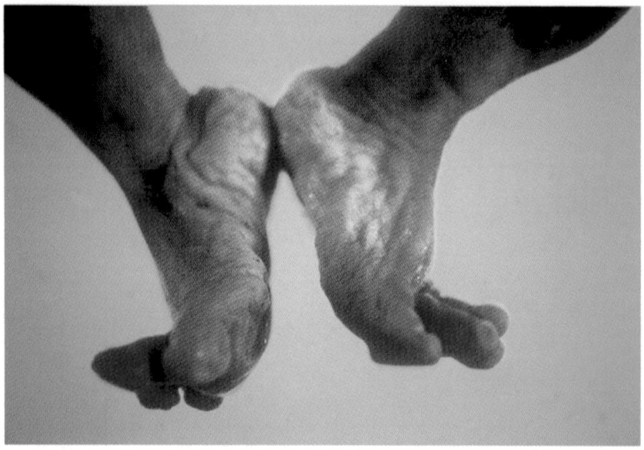

6.32. Triploidy. Bizarre appearance of toes.

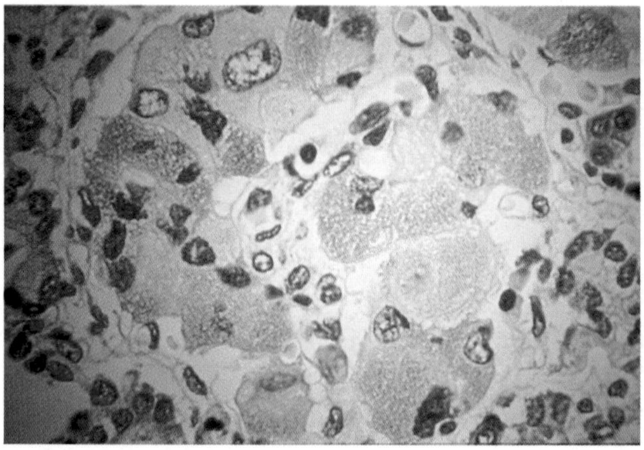

6.33. Microscopic appearance of a pancreatic islet; cytomegaly of the cells that are somatostatin positive by immunoperoxidase staining.

Type 1: 85%, extra haploid set of chromosomes of paternal origin, normal fetal growth, microcephaly, and a partial hydatidiform mole.

Type 2: 15%, extra haploid set of maternal origin, severe intrauterine growth retardation, relative macrocephaly, and a small noncystic placenta.

MONOSOMY X (TURNER SYNDROME)

At birth there is short stature, cystic hygromas, webbing of the neck (develops later), wide-spaced nipples, pedal edema, and a congenital heart defect (coarctation) (Figures 6.35 and 6.36 and Tables 6.22 to 6.26). There is an increased carrying angle at the elbows and shield-shaped chest, gonadal dysgenesis with absent or delayed and scanty menstruation and infertility develop later.

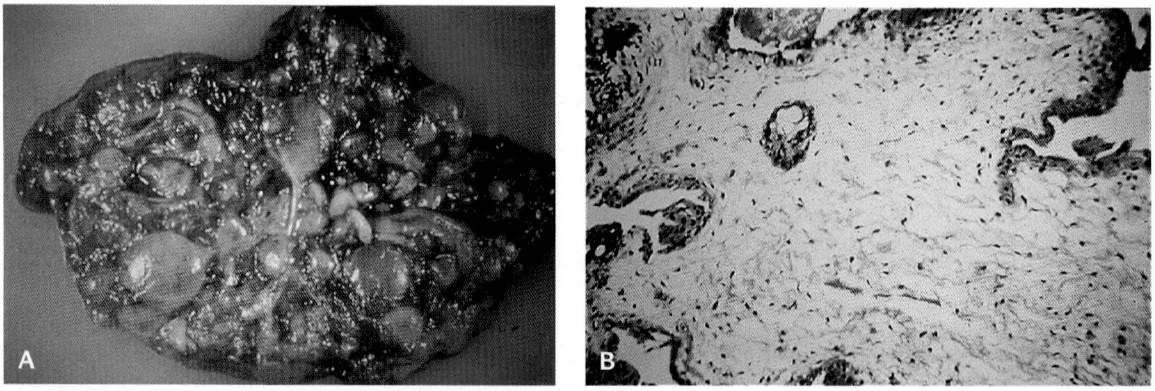

6.34. **(A)** Placenta in triploidy with partial hydatidiform mole. **(B)** Triploidy. Microscopic section of the placenta. The chorionic villi are large, with scalloping at the margins, trophoblastic inclusion, and an edematous stroma.

Table 6.18 Triploidy: two percent of all pregnancies

Diandry – paternal origin of extra haploid set	
dispermy (2 sperm fertilize single ovum)	65%
fertilization by a diploid sperm	25%
Digyny – maternal origin of extra haploid set	
fertilization of diploid ovum	10%

Table 6.19 Triploidy

Usually spontaneous abortion
Some stillborn – rarely liveborn
Meningomyelocele
Congenital heart defects
Cleft lip/palate
Syndactyly of hands and/or feet
Growth retardation
Hydatidiform degeneration of placenta

There are 50,000 to 75,000 girls and women with Turner syndrome in the United States. It is the most common sex-chromosome abnormality in females and affects an estimated 3% of all females conceived. In live-born female infants, the incidence is only 1/1,500 to 1/2,500. Fifteen percent of spontaneous miscarriages have a 45,X karyotype. It is estimated than only 1/100 embryos with a 45,X karyotype survive to term. Maternal X is retained in two-thirds of patients with Turner syndrome. More than half of all patients with Turner syndrome have a mosaic chromosomal complement (e.g., 45,X/46,XX). The identification of mosaicism depends directly on the method of ascertainment. The use of fluorescence in situ hybridization increases the detected prevalence from 34% with conventional cytogenetic techniques to 60%, and the use of reverse transcription–polymerase chain reaction assays as well, further increases the detected prevalence to 74%. Mosaicism with a normal cell line in the fetal membranes may be necessary for adequate placental function and fetal survival.

Table 6.20 Abnormalities observed in triploidy

Maternal and placental	External craniofacial	Extremities and skeletal	Cardiopulmonary
Midtrimester preeclampsia	Malformed ears	Transverse palmar crease	Ventricular septal defect
Polyhydramnios	Large, bulbous nose	Large posterior fontanelle	Retroesophageal right subclavian artery
Proteinuria, hypertension	Cleft lip and palate	Incomplete ossification of calvarium	Tetralogy of Fallot
Partial hydatidiform mole	Fetal growth retardation	Syndactyly between third and fourth fingers	Atrial septal defect, secundum type
Mild trophoblastic proliferation		Talipes equinovarus	Persistent left superior vena cava
Hydropic villi with scalloping		Proximal displacement of thumbs	
Large cisternae within villi		Lumbosacral myelomeningocele	
Trophoblastic inclusions			

Gastrointestinal	Genitourinary	Central nervous system and ocular
Malrotation of colon	Renal hypoplasia and cysts	Hydrocephalus
Aplasia of gallbladder	Hypospadias	Arnold-Chiari malformation
	Cryptorchidism	Meningomyelocele
	Leydig cell hyperplasia of testes	Holoprosencephaly
	Hydronephrosis	Hypoplasia of basal ganglia, cerebellum, and occipital lobe
	Micropenis	Aplasia of corpus callosum
	Bifid scrotum	Iris coloboma
	Hypoplasia of ovaries	Microphthalmia

Table 6.21 Typical features of partial hydatidiform mole

Gross findings	Microscopic findings	Genetics
Both placenta and embryo or fetus present	Focal trophoblastic hyperplasia	69 chromosomes with XXX, XXY, or rarely XYY complements
	Scalloping of villous outline	Dominance of two paternal sets (diandric triploidy)
	Focal villous swelling with cistern formation	
	Trophoblastic inclusions present	
	Embryonic or fetal vasculature with red blood cells present	

Table 6.22 45 X – Turner syndrome

50,000 – 75,000 with Turner syndrome in U.S.
Most common chromosome abnormality in females – 3% of all females conceived
–liveborn 1 in 1,500–2,500
15% spontaneous abortions have 45X
–1 in 100 embryos with 45X survive to term
Maternal X retained in 2/3
–50% are mosaic (45X/46XX) by fluorescent in situ hybridization and polymerase chain reaction
Mosaicism with a normal cell line. Fetal membranes necessary for placental function and fetal survival

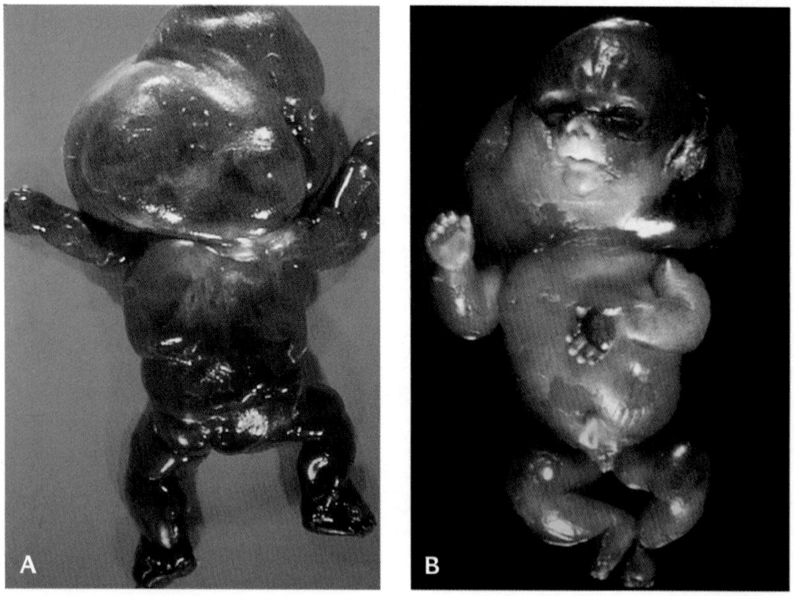

6.35. **(A)** 45,X fetus with huge cystic hygroma and fetal hydrops. **(B)** 45,X fetus showing bilateral cystic hygromas of the neck.

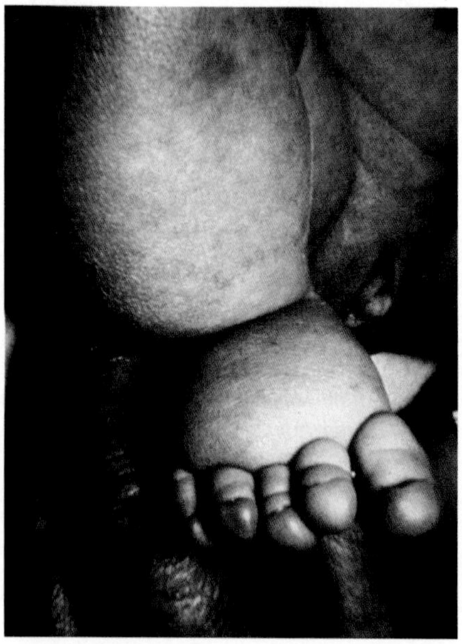

6.36. Characteristic edema seen on both hands and feet in monosomy X.

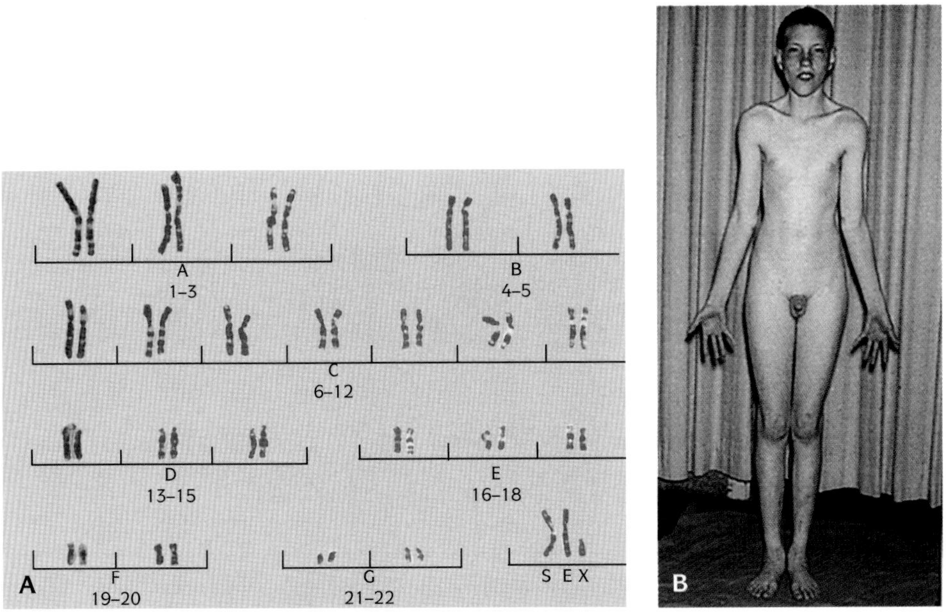

6.37. **(A)** Karyotype 47,XXY, the most common karyotype in Klinefelter syndrome. **(B)** Phenotype: tallness with arachnodactyly and small testes.

Prenatal diagnosis can be made with ultrasonography. Typical findings include thickening of the nuchal fold, cystic hygroma, renal (horseshoe kidney), and left-sided cardiac abnormalities (coarctation of the aorta). There is a very high likelihood of short stature and ovarian failure.

Genetic Aspects

Mosaic patterns are 45,X/46,XX and 45,X/47,XXX. The presence of a cell line with a Y chromosome causes a 30% risk of dysgerminoma or a gonadoblastoma in a streak gonad. Removal of the gonads is important.

KLINEFELTER SYNDROME

Klinefelter syndrome includes 47,XXY, 48,XXYY, and 49,XY/XXY mosaicism and other rarer forms such as 48,XXXY, 49,XXXYY (Figures 6.37 and 6.38).

Table 6.23 45 X – Turner syndrome: ultrasonography

Thickening of nuchal fold
Cystic hygroma
Horseshoe kidney
Left-sided cardiac abnormalities

Table 6.24 Monosomy X

Serum estrogens ↓
Serum pregnanediol ↓
Follicle-stimulating hormone ↑
Urinary 17 ketosteroids ↓

Table 6.25 Turner syndrome

Infant	Childhood and adolescence
Small for gestational age	Small stature
Lymphedema of dorsum of hands and feet	Short, webbed neck
Deep-set nails	Low posterior hair line
Excess skin on nape of neck (becomes pterygium coli later in life)	Cubitus valgus
	Multiple nevi
Cystic hygroma	

Table 6.26 Turner syndrome

Genitourinary	Cardiovascular	Endocrinologic	Central nervous system	Ocular
Infantile female external genitalia Pubic hair scanty or absent Streak gonads Hypoplastic, sometimes bifid uterus Failure of development of secondary sex characteristics Horseshoe kidney Micromulticystic kidneys Membranoproliferative glomerulonephritis Gonadal malignancy if Y chromsomosomal component present	Coarctation of the aorta Cystic medial necrosis of aorta Dissecting aneurysm Floppy mitral or aortic valves (myxoid degeneration) Aortic valvular stenosis	Low serum levels of estrogens and pregnanediol; increased follicle-stimulating hormone Low urine levels of 17-ketosteroids Hashimoto thyroiditis (autoimmune)	Slight cortical dysplasia Gray matter heterotopia Hydrocephalus	Severe myopia Congenital cataracts Congenital deafness

There is hypogonadism, azoospermia, mild mental deficiency, tall stature, atrophic testes with hyalinization of tubules and clusters of Leydig cells, gynecomastia, elevated urinary gonadotropins, low concentrations of urinary 17-ketosteroids, kidney cysts, and hydronephrosis.

CONFINED PLACENTAL MOSAICISM

This results from mutations occurring in the trophoblast or extraembryonic progenitor cells of the inner cell mass (Figure 6.39). It is found in 1–2% of pregnancies. Some progress to term uneventfully but it may be associated with intrauterine fetal death, intrauterine growth retardation, and prenatal mortality. Three types have been identified:

Table 6.27 Confined placental mosaicism

Mutations in Trophoblast or Extraembryonic Progenitor Cells of the Inner Cell Mass – 3 types:
- Type 1: Abnormal cell line in placenta and fetus
- Type 2: Abnormal cell line in placenta, fetus normal
- Type 3: Placenta normal (abnormal cells lost), fetus, abnormal cell line

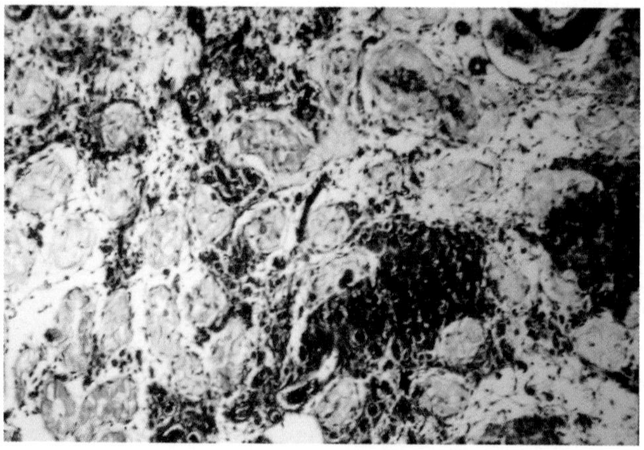

6.38. Testes in Klinefelter syndrome. Tubular atrophy with increased Leydig cells.

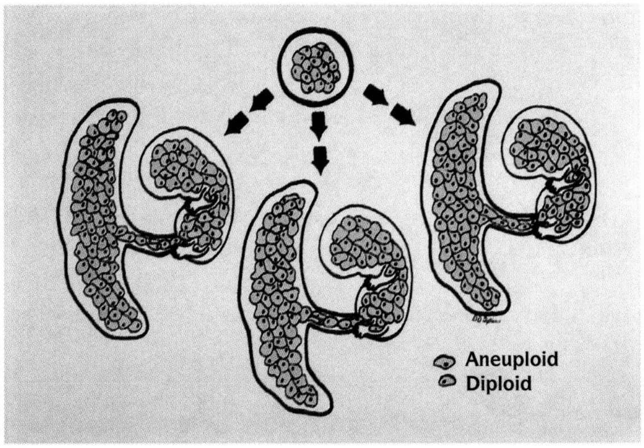

6.39. The three patterns of confined placental mosaicism. Type 1: Abnormal cell line in cytotrophoblast associated with chromosomally normal placental stroma; the most common type. Type 2: Abnormal cell line in placental stroma associated with diploidy in cytotrophoblast and embryo and fetus. Type 3: Diploidy in fetus associated with mosaic or nonmosaic cell line in placental stroma and cytotrophoblast.

Type 1: Abnormal cell line in cytotrophoblast associated with chromosomally normal placental stroma; the most common type.

Type 2: Abnormal cell line in placental stroma associated with diploidy in cytotrophoblast and embryo and fetus.

Type 3: Diploidy in fetus associated with mosaic or nonmosaic cell line in placental stroma and cytotrophoblast.

REFERENCES

Baldwin VJ, Kalousek DK, Dimmick JE, et al.: Diagnostic pathologic investigation of malformed conceptus. *Perspect Pediatr Pathol* 7:65, 1982.

Bauld R, Sutherland GR, Bain AD: Chromosome constitution of 500 infants dying during the perinatal period. *Humangenetik* 23:183, 1974.

Boué J, Boué A: Anomalies chromosomiques dans les avortements spontanés. In Boué A, Thibault CD (eds): *Les Accidents Chromosomiques de la Reproduction*, Paris, Inserm, 1973, p 29.

Boué J, Philippe E, Giroud A, et al.: Phenotypic expression of lethal chromosomal anomalies in human abortuses. *Teratology* 14:3, 1976.

Dimmick JE, Kalousek DK: *Developmental Pathology of the Embryo and Fetus*, Philadelphia, JB Lippincott, 1992.

Gilbert EF: *Potter's Pathology of the Fetus and Infant*, Philadelphia, Mosby-Year Book, 1997.

Gilbert EF, Opitz JM: Developmental and other pathologic changes in syndromes caused by chromosome abnormalities. *Persp Pediatr Pathol* 7:1, 1982.

Gilbert EF, Opitz JM: Chromosomal abnormalities. In Wigglesworth J, Singer D (eds): *Textbook of Fetal and Perinatal Pathology*, 2nd ed, Boston, Blackwell Science Publications, 1998, p 291.

Hubbard JD: Down's syndrome – Dilated Hassall's corpuscles as a histopathologic marker. Pediatric Pathology Club Interim Meeting, Providence, Rhode Island, October 11–13, 1979.

Jacobs PA: Epidemiology of chromosome abnormalities in man. *Am J Epidemiol* 105:180, 1977.

Jacobs PA, Hunt PA, Matsuura JS, Wilson CC: Complete and partial hydatidiform moles in Hawaii: cytogenetics, morphology and epidemiology. *Br J Obstet Gynaecol* 89:258, 1982.

Jacobs PA, Szulman AE, Funkhouser J, et al.: Human triploidy: relationship between parental origin of the additional haploid complement and development of partial hydatidiform mole. *Ann Hum Genet* 46:223, 1982.

Kalousek DK, Dill FJ: Chromosomal mosaicism confined to the placenta in human conceptions. *Science* 221:665, 1983.

Kalousek DK, Fitch N, Paradice BA: *Pathology of the Human Embryo and Previable Fetus – An Atlas*, New York, Springer-Verlag, 1990.

Karayalcin G, Shanske A, Honigman R: Wilms' tumor in a 13-year-old girl with trisomy 18. *Am J Dis Child* 135:665, 1981.

Keeling JW: Chromosome anomalies. In *Fetal and Neonatal Pathology*, 2nd ed, NY, Springer-Verlag, 1993, p 139.

Kuleschov NP, Alekhin VI, Egoliana NA, et al.: Frequency of chromosomal anomalies in children dying in the perinatal period [Plenum translation]. *Genetika* 11:107, 1975.

Machin GA, Crolla JA: Chromosome constitution of 500 infants dying during the perinatal period. *Humangenetik* 23:138, 1974.

Matsuoka R, Matsuyama S, Yamamoto Y, et al.: Trisomy 18q: A case report and review on karyotype-phenotype correlations. *Hum Genet* 57:78, 1981.

Moerman P, Fryns JP, Goddeeris P, Lauweryns JM: Spectrum of clinical and autopsy findings in trisomy 18 syndrome. *J Genet Hum* 30:17, 1982.

Rodrigues MM, Punnet HH, Valdes-Dapena M, et al.: Retinal pigment epithelium in a case of trisomy 18. *Am J Ophthalmol* 76:265, 1973.

Rushton DI, Faed M, Richards S, et al.: The fetal manifestations of the 45,XO karyotype. *J Obstet Gynaecol* 89:258, 1982.

Szulman AE, Philippe E, Boué JG, Boué A: Human triploidy: association with partial hydatidiform moles and nonmolar conceptuses. *Human Pathol* 12:1016, 1981.

Vander Putte SCJ: Lymphatic malformations in human fetuses. A study of fetuses with Turner's syndrome or status Bonnevie-Ullrich. *Virch Arch Path Anat* 376:233, 1977.

SEVEN

Terminology of Errors of Morphogenesis

MALFORMATION

A malformation is a qualitative, structural end result of a disturbance of embryogenesis leading to a (congenital) defect of an organ, body part, or body region. Such defects can be mild or severe, common or rare. They arise either during blastogenesis (first 4 weeks of development) or during organogenesis (2nd half of embryogenesis, weeks 5–8). Defects of blastogenesis tend to be severe, to be frequently lethal, and to involve several parts of the developing organism sharing a common inductive molecular pathway (polytopic anomalies; i.e., DiGeorge anomaly) (Figure 7.1 and Tables 7.1 to 7.5). Defects of organogenesis tend to involve single structures (monotopic anomalies) – i.e., isolated polydactly, cleft palate, distal hypospadias, etc. Regardless of how mild or common in the population, malformations are never normal. Mild malformations (cleft uvula or xiphisternum, agenesis of palmaris longus muscle or of upper lateral incisors, spina bifida occulta of L5) are common in the population and tend to be dominantly inherited.

Developmental Fields

Developmental (or embryogenic or morphogenetic) fields are the parts of the embryo that react as a unit in response to normal inductive, teratogenic, or mutational causes (Tables 7.6 and 7.7). During early blastogenesis the entire pluripotent embryo is the primary field. A midline, axis formation and the

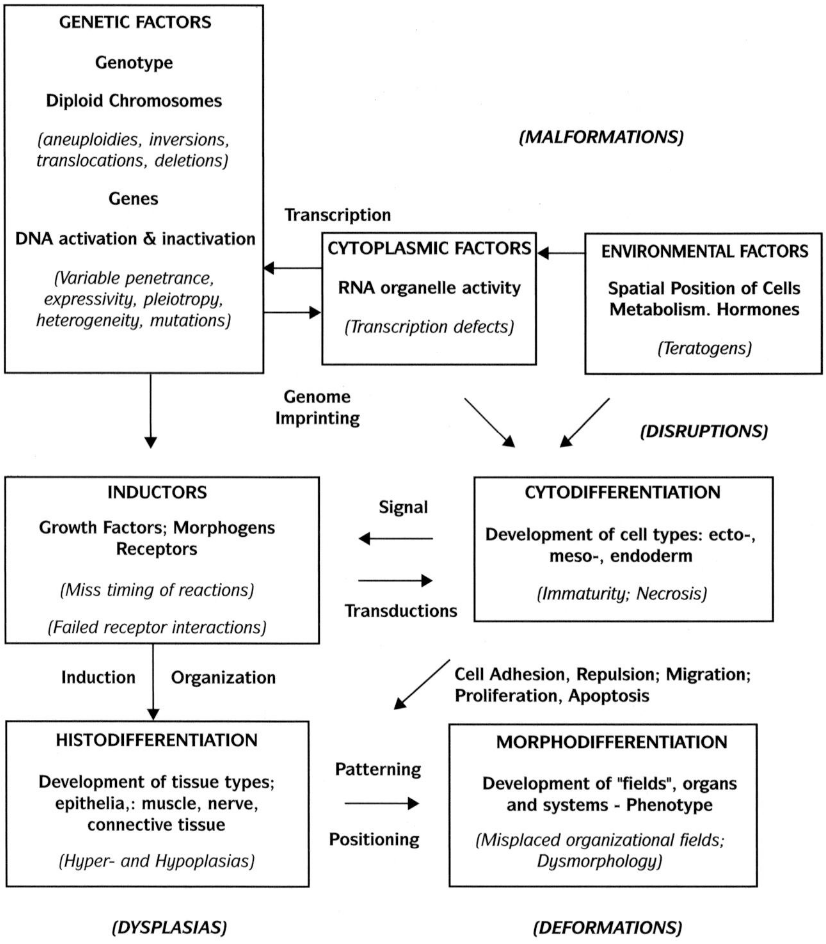

7.1. Schema of embryogenesis and possible sources of anomalies.

initial events of gastrulation are its most important morphogenetic characteristics. Progenitor fields (Davidson) arise in the primary field and represent upstream expression domains of combinations of molecular inductive systems including transcription factors (e.g., *HOX*, *SOX*, *TBX* genes), growth factors (FGF, BMPs), and secreted morphogens (i.e., SHH). These combinations are specific for the anlage induced whether this is neural tube, heart, or gonadal ridge. The secondary or epimorphic fields are those subdivisions of the progenitor fields giving irreversible rise to the final structure. They remain fields so long as they are still capable of reactivity to causes of normal or abnormal development.

Events in developmental fields are epimorphically hierarchical, temporally syndromized, spatially coordinated, and morphogenetically constrained. They are dynamic reaction units and phylogenetically highly co-adapted with all other fields in the body.

Table 7.1 Defects of blastogenesis

Monozygotic (MZ) twinning correlates with aneuploidy as in the Ullrich-Turner and Down syndromes and acephaly/acardia, parasitic twinning, conjoined twins, facial/body axis duplications.

Polytopic field defects

- Acrorenal
- Laterality defects
- Cardiomelic
- Gastromelic
- Lumbosacral agenesis
- Ulnar-mammary, etc.
- Pulmonary agenesis [Cunningham and Mann, 1997]

Associations: Multiple polytopic field defects. Delimitation of individual entities such as VATER, MURCS etc. is an arbitrary exercise since all overlap. Common in infants of diabetic mothers.

Malformations: appearing to be monotopic, but probably arising during blastogenesis:

- Sirenomelia and all forms of caudal dysgenesis including sacral agenesis
- Otocephaly
- Anencephaly, rachischisis, and other gross neural tube defects
- Holoprosencephaly (with or without otocephaly)
- Renal agenesis
- Anal, colonic atresia
- Tracheo-esophageal fistula, tracheal agenesis, esophageal atresia
- Pentalogy of Cantrell (involving upper abdominal wall, lower sternum, diaphragm, pericardium, heart, and ectopia cordis).
- Conotruncal septation defects
- Vertebral segmentation defects
- DiGeorge anomaly
- Ectopia cordis
- Limb-body wall complexes
- OEIS complex: omphalocele, exstrophy, imperforate anus, spinal defects
- Diaphragmatic defects
- Exstrophy of bladder/cloaca
- Goldenhar complex (or anomaly)
- Gross limb defects (amelias, phocomelias, etc.)
- Severe facial clefts
- Currarino "triad": imperforate anus, sacral defects, and presacral teratoma
- Sacrococcygeal teratomas, epignathus

Anomalies of body stalk/wall, umbilical cord formation, and placentation

Time and place of action of many midline mutations:

- HPE3: holoprosencephaly (AD)
- XLOS (X-linked Opitz or G/BBB syndrome) due to M1D1 mutations
- Many other XLB (X-linked blastogenesis) mutations [Opitz 1993, 1997]

Source: Opitz JM, Zanni G, Reynolds JF, Gilbert-Barness E: *Defects of Blastogenesis, Seminars in Medical Genetics-Development and Malformations*, *Am J Med Genet*, 115:269, 2002.

The Midline

The midline is the phylogenetically oldest part of the metazoan body; it is not a field per se but rather the most important morphogenetic landmark of the primary field. It is a real biologic entity and not just the (mid) sagittal plane of the body. An enormous number of extremely important inductive events occur at the midline including gastrulation with formation of notochord, laterality formation, neurulation, cardiogenesis, etc. In humans the early midline is highly unstable as witnessed by the common occurrence of monozygotic

Table 7.2A Timing of malformations

Tissues	Malformations	Defect in	Before developmental age	Comment
Craniofacial	Cleft lip	Closure of lip	36 days	42% associated with cleft palate
	Cleft maxillary palate	Fusion of maxillary palatal shelves	10 weeks	
	Branchial sinus and/or cyst	Resolution of branchial arch	8 weeks	Preauricular and cyst cleft along the line anterior to sternocleidomastoid
Heart	Transposition of great vessels	Directional development of bulbus cordis septum	34 days	
	Ventricular septal defect	Closure of ventricular septum	6 weeks	
	Patent ductus arteriosus	Closure of ductus arteriosus	9–10 months	
Gastrointestinal	Esophageal atresia plus tracheoesophageal fistula	Lateral septation of foregut into trachea and foregut	30 days	
	Rectal atresia with fistula	Lateral septation of cloaca into rectum and urogenital sinus	6 weeks	
	Duodenal atresia	Recanalization of duodenum	7–8 weeks	
	Malrotation of gut	Rotation of intestinal loop so that cecum lies to right	10 weeks	Associated incomplete or aberrant mesenteric attachments
	Omphalocele	Return of midgut into abdomen	10 weeks	
	Meckel diverticulum	Obliteration of vitelline duct	10 weeks	May contain gastric and/or pancreatic tissue
Genitourinary	Diaphragmatic hernia	Closure of pleuroperitoneal canal	6 weeks	
	Exstrophy of bladder	Migration of infraumbilical mesenchyme	30 days	Associated Müllerian and Wolffian duct defects
	Bicornuate uterus	Fusion of lower portion of Müllerian ducts	10 weeks	
	Hypospadias	Fusion of urethral folds (labia minora)	12 weeks	
	Cryptorchidism	Descent of testicle into scrotum	7–9 months	
Limb	Aplasia of radius	Agenesis of radial bone	38 days	Often accompanied by other defects of radial side of distal limb and also defects of kidney
	Syndactyly, severe	Separation of digital rays	6 weeks	

Table 7.2B Definitions in abnormal morphogenesis

1. DEVELOPMENTAL FIELD DEFECT: One or more defects developmentally interrelated in a organ or region – develop at the same and relate to the same cause, e.g., Pierre Robin complex
   Monotopic Field Defect occurs within a single developmental field.
   Polytopic Field Defect incorporates more than one developmental field but occurs within the same time during development.
2. MALFORMATION: Primary structural defect resulting from a localized error in morphogenesis, e.g., cleft palate.
3. MALFORMATION SYNDROME: A recognized pattern of malformation presumably having the same etiology, e.g., Down syndrome.
4. DEFORMITY: Alteration in shape and/or structure of a previously normal formed part, e.g., torticollis, arthrogryposis.
5. DYSPLASIA: Abnormality of tissue organization (dyshistogenesis) and occurs in connective tissue, bone, skin, or blood vessels.
6. ASSOCIATION: Non-random association of defects currently not considered to be a malformation syndrome. Most associations are now classified as Polytopic Field Defects.

Table 7.3 Causes of birth defects

Category	Types	Usual characteristics	Example
Chromosome abnormalities	Polyploidy	Multiple defects, mental retardation	Triploidy (e.g., partial moles)
	Aneuploidy		Down syndrome
	Mixoploidy		Ullrich-Turner mosaicism
	UPD		Silver-Russell syndrome (UPD 17)
	Contiguous gene deletions		DiGeorge complex
Mendelian abnormalities	Autosomal dominant traits	Vertical patterns	Achondroplasia mostly sporadic
	Autosomal recessive traits	Horizontal patterns	Stickler syndrome
	X-linked dominant traits	Oblique pattern, male lethality	Smith-Lemli-Opitz syndrome
	X-linked recessive traits	Oblique pattern, males affected	Incontinentia pigment
	Y-linked traits	Vertical pattern, males affected	Coffin-Lowry syndrome
			Swyer (del or mutation SRY) syndrome
Abnormalities exhibited atypical inheritance	Mitochondrial diseases	Maternal inheritance	MELAS syndrome
	Disorders of imprinting	Parent-of-origin effects	Angelman syndrome
	Triplet repeat expansion	Anticipation of defect	Myotonic dystrophy
Multifactorial abnormalities	Common birth defects	Environmental modification Empiric recurrence risks Sex predilection Moderate twin concordance (monozygotic greater than dizygotic)	Cleft palate, spina bifida, etc.
Environmental abnormalities	Chemicals (teratogens)	Sporadic occurrence	Fetal alcohol syndrome
	Physical agents	High twin concordance (monozygotic equals dizygotic)	Hyperthermia sequence
	Infectious agents		Congenital rubella syndrome
	Maternal metabolism		Maternal PKU, diabetes mellitus

UPD, uniparental disomy; MELAS, mitochondrial, encephalopathy, lactic acidosis, and stroke-like episodes; PKU, phenylketonuria

Table 7.4 **Polygenic (multifactorial) interaction of environmental factors with genetic predisposition**

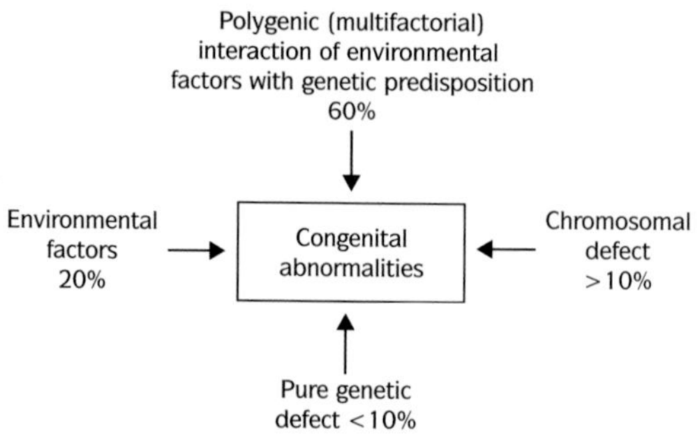

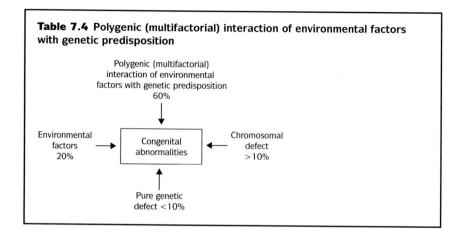

Table 7.5 **Etiology of congenital abnormalities**

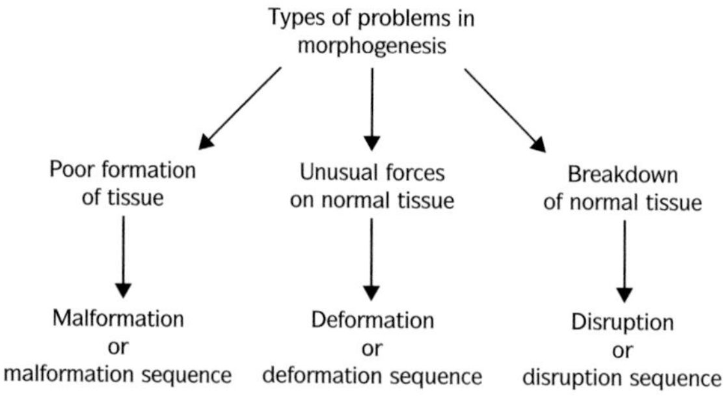

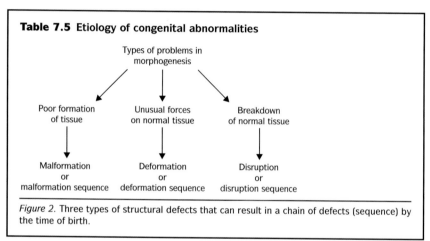

Figure 2. Three types of structural defects that can result in a chain of defects (sequence) by the time of birth.

Table 7.6 **Midline as a developmental field**

Midline – Generalized developmental midline weakness morphogenesis poorly buffered site of division and fusion

- Division of lung bud
- Development of neuraxial commissures
- Fusion of palatal shelves
- Mullerian ducts
- Urethral folds
- Closure of umbilical ring

Midline defects include:

- Schisis defects
- Caudal regression complex
- Clefting defects

Table 7.7 **Developmental field defects**

Monotopic – Contiguous anomalies in the same developmental field – e.g., cyclopia with holoprosencephaly, cleft lip and cleft palate.

Polytopic – Disturbed mutual induction during morphogenesis results in more distantly located defects – e.g., acro-renal field defect results from inductive effect of mesonephros on limb-bud development.

Table 7.8 Minor anomalies

Minor anomalies are normal developmental variants and variations of final structure.
Minor anomalies are defects of phenogenesis.
They are the traits that constitute our morphologic uniqueness, which are also the heritage of ethnic groups and of family inheritance.
May occur in the normal population as developmental variants.
They can be regarded as the failure of end-stage fine tuning.
Common in chromosomal defects.

twinning and conjoined twinning of mild to severe midline malformations ranging from total neurorachischisis to minimal hypospadias.

The morphogenetic lability of the midline increases the probability of multiple midline anomalies in the same individual (as in the trisomy 13 syndromes).

Midline morphogenetic events include segmentations (rhombomeres), branchings (lung buds), decussations (corpus callosum), programmed cell death with morphogenetic resorptions (buccopharyngeal and anal membranes, tail), morphogenetic movements (d-looping of cardiac tube), cell migrations (neural crest, primodial cells), etc.

Mild Malformations Versus Minor Anomalies

Minor anomalies are quantitative changes occurring during phenogenesis (i.e., fetal life, last 20 days of intrauterine life) affect growth, ethnic characteristic, and family resemblance (Table 7.8). Subjective minor anomalies include abnormal ties of facial structure and appearance; objective minor anomalies include any trait that can be measured or counted – i.e., cephalic index, intraorbital distance, and dermatoglyphic total ridge count. Mild malformations are evident as such per se; apparent minor anomalies must always be evaluated on the basis of the family. Minor anomalies shade into normality; mild malformations are never normal. Multiple minor anomalies and apparent absence of family resemblance are a highly sensitive indicator of aneuploidy; indeed, many Down syndrome individuals have only growth and minor anomalies. Minor anomalies become more evident the later the age of gestation. In embryos no minor anomalies can be seen.

Holoprosencephaly

The range of arrhinencephaly/holoprosencephaly brain defects is reflected by the midline facial defects (Figure 7.2). In the third week of development, the mesoderm migrates anterior to the notochord and is responsible for the induction and differentiation of the forebrain and the midline facial structures. Failure of this migration produces a developmental field defect, including arrhinencephaly/holoprosencephaly with midline facial defects.

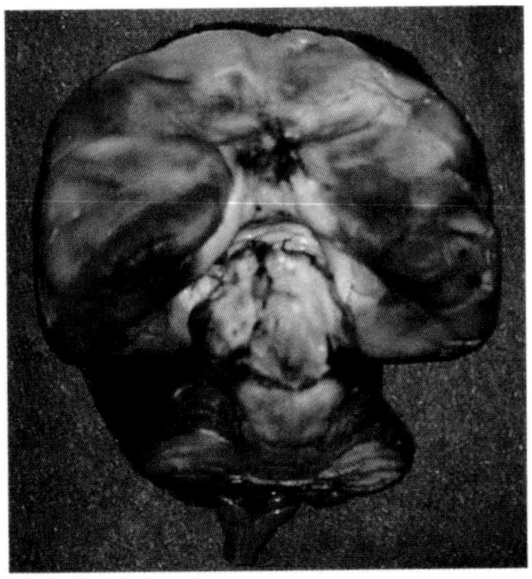
7.2. Brain in alobar holoprosencephaly.

Otocephaly

Otocephaly is a first branchial arch developmental field defect that affects structures in the face and upper neck and comprises absence of the mandible and

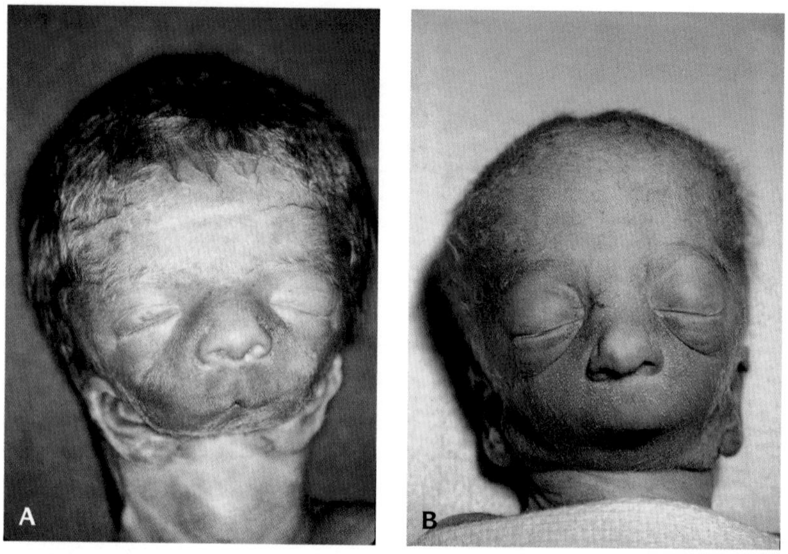

7.3. **(A)** and **(B)** Otocephaly. Extreme mandibular hypoplasia, microstomia and contiguous ears (A) beneath the mandible.

approximation of the ears in the midline region normally occupied by the mandible (Figure 7.3 and Table 7.4). It has been related to defects of the neural crest cells of cranial origin or to defects in the underlying mesodermal support elements of these cells. Patients with otocephaly may have associated cardiac defects, renal anomalies, bilateral pulmonary agenesis, and esophageal atresia. Most cases have occurred sporadically, although its rare presence in sibs suggests autosomal recessive inheritance in a few cases.

Robinson Defect

In Robinson defect, agenesis of the cloacal membrane creates a persistent cloaca without external genitalia and urinary, genital, and anal orifices (Figure 7.4). The bladder may be massively distended or ruptured, and hydroureters, hydronephrosis, and cystic renal dysplasia may occur.

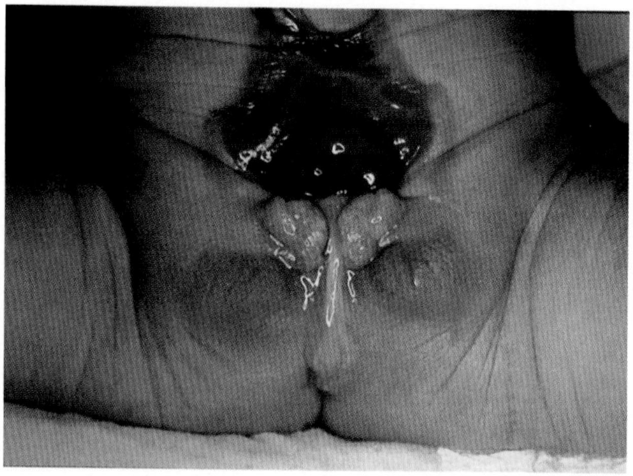

7.4. Robinson defect showing exstrophy of the cloaca.

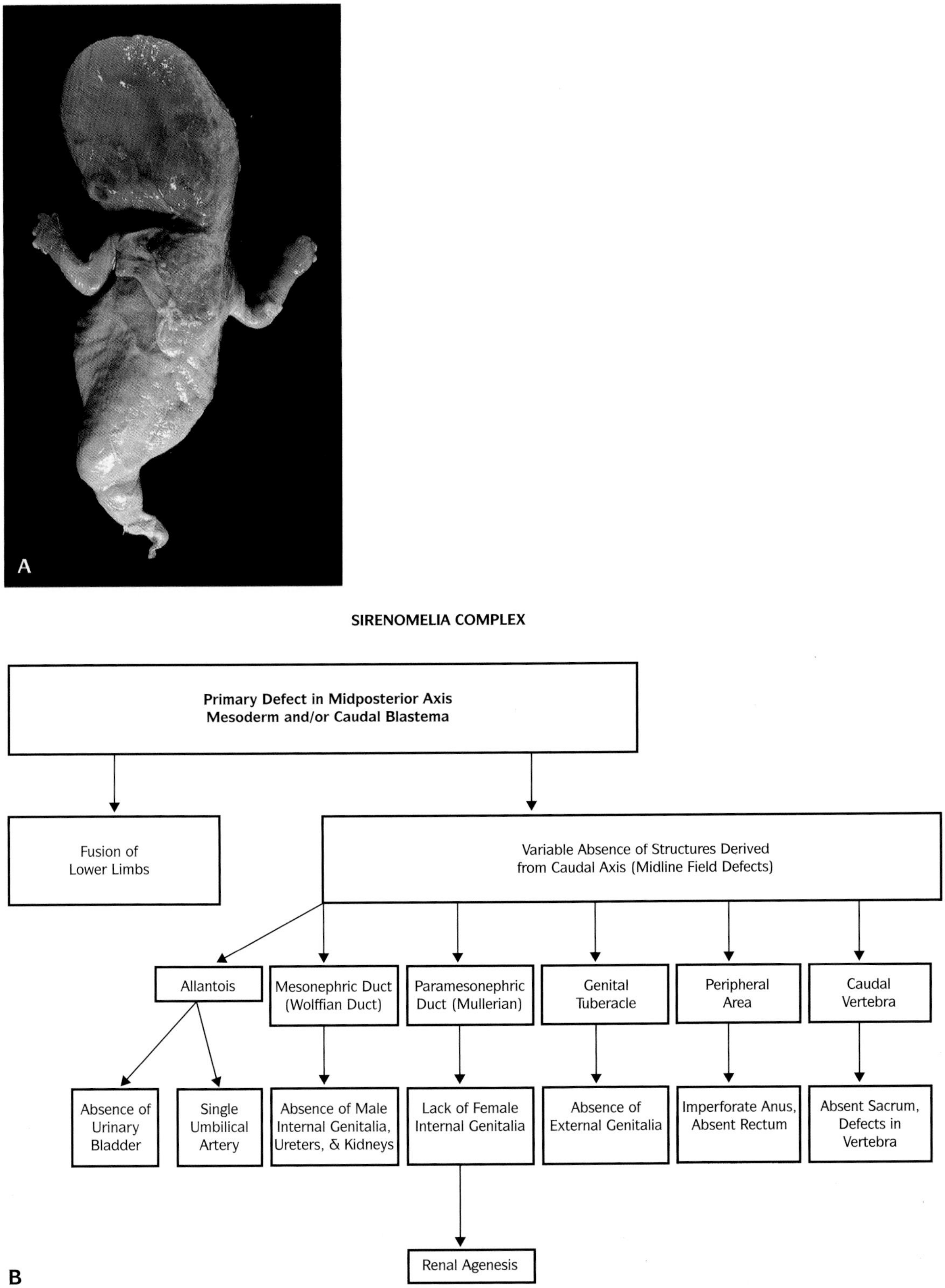

7.5. **(A)** Sirenomelia. 10-week gestation fetus. **(B)** Sirenomelia complex.

Table 7.9 Pathogenesis of otocephaly

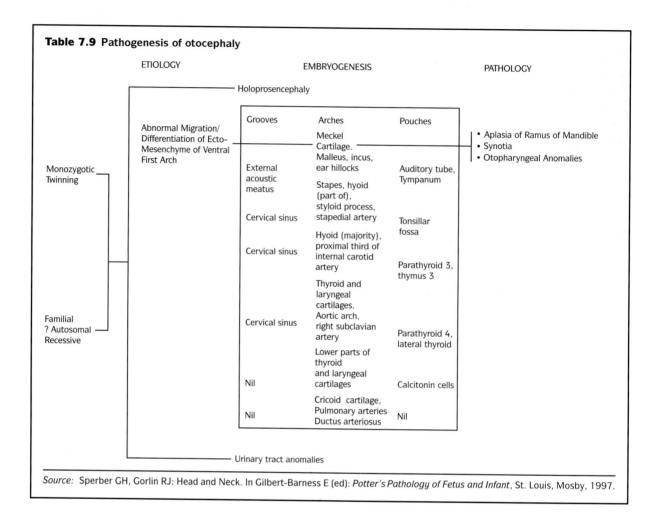

ETIOLOGY: Monozygotic Twinning; Familial ? Autosomal Recessive

EMBRYOGENESIS: Holoprosencephaly; Abnormal Migration/ Differentiation of Ecto-Mesenchyme of Ventral First Arch; Urinary tract anomalies

Grooves	Arches	Pouches
External acoustic meatus	Meckel Cartilage. Malleus, incus, ear hillocks	Auditory tube, Tympanum
Cervical sinus	Stapes, hyoid (part of), styloid process, stapedial artery	Tonsillar fossa
Cervical sinus	Hyoid (majority), proximal third of internal carotid artery	Parathyroid 3, thymus 3
Cervical sinus	Thyroid and laryngeal cartilages. Aortic arch, right subclavian artery	Parathyroid 4, lateral thyroid
Nil	Lower parts of thyroid and laryngeal cartilages	Calcitonin cells
Nil	Cricoid cartilage, Pulmonary arteries Ductus arteriosus	Nil

PATHOLOGY:
- Aplasia of Ramus of Mandible
- Synotia
- Otopharyngeal Anomalies

Source: Sperber GH, Gorlin RJ: Head and Neck. In Gilbert-Barness E (ed): *Potter's Pathology of Fetus and Infant*, St. Louis, Mosby, 1997.

Sirenomelia

This midline defect of blastogenesis occurs in about 1 of 60,000 newborn infants; it occurs more often in males and is more common in one of identical twins (Figure 7.5). It is a severe developmental field defect of the posterior axis caudal blastema, resulting in apparent fusion of the lower limb buds. It occurs in the primitive streak stage during week 3 of gestation, before development of the allantois, and the allantoic vessels are usually absent. There may be a single umbilical artery that arises directly from the aorta but two symmetrical umbilical arteries have been observed severally. Other defects of the caudal axis include imperforate anus, lower vertebral defects, and genitourinary anomalies. Cardiovascular, respiratory, and upper gastrointestinal tract malformations occur in 20–35% of these cases. The radial aplasia, esophageal atresia, and tracheoesophageal fistula in some cases suggest that the VATER polytopic field defect (PFD) (Tables 7.10 and 7.11) may represent a lesser degree of the caudal dysgenesis sequence. Caudal dysgenesis is a defect that is most commonly seen in infants of diabetic mothers. Renal agenesis or cystic renal dysplasia occurs in virtually every case and is accompanied by pulmonary hypoplasia.

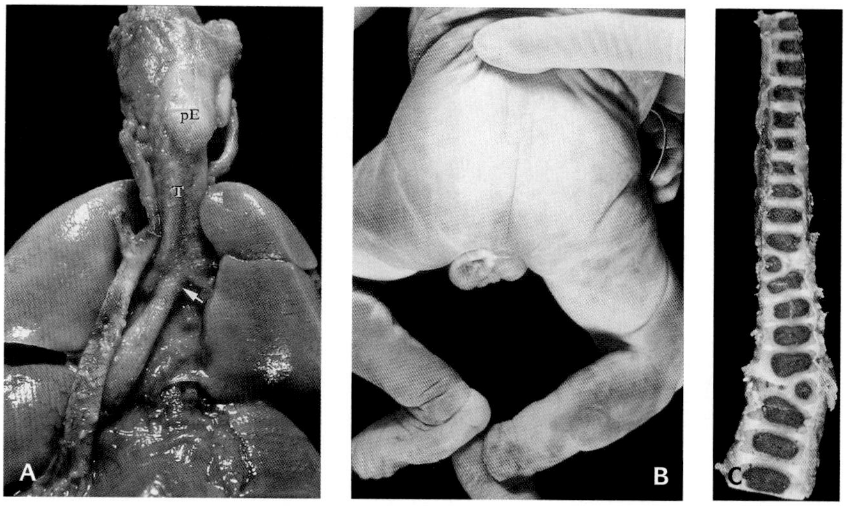

7.6. **(A)** Dissected organs in VATER polytopic field defect showing esophageal atresia (PE = proximal esophagus, T = trachea) with T-E fistula (arrow), renal agenesis. **(B)** Anal atresia. **(C)** Longitudinal section of "butterfly" vertebrae.

Polytopic Developmental Field Defect (PFD)

An arbitrarily defined combination of defects of blastogenesis that has been shown to be causally heterogeneous (Figure 7.6). Most associations are now considered multiple polytopic field defects.

Associations

The concept of association is defined as a nonrandom occurrence in two or more individuals of multiple congenital anomalies not known to a sequence or syndrome; however, it has been suggested that so-called associations are usually PFDs. The term association should be restricted to the idiopathic occurrence of multiple congenital anomalies apparently not of blastogenetic origin.

MURCS Association (Polytopic Field Defect)

MURCS is an acronym for Müllerian duct aplasia, renal aplasia, and cervicothoracic somite malformation with cervicothoracic vertebral defects, especially from C5 to T1. It is a sporadic disorder. Absence of the vagina, absence or hypoplasia of the uterus, and renal abnormalities, including agenesis and ectopy, also occur.

CHARGE Association (Polytopic Field Defect)

CHARGE (coloboma, heart disease, atresia choanae, and retarded growth and ear anomalies) may also include genital anomalies, tracheoesophageal fistula, facial palsy, micrognathia, cleft lip, cleft palate, omphalocele, congenital cardiac defects, and holoprosencephaly (Figure 7.7). It has been suggested that CHARGE is not an association or PFD but a syndrome.

Schisis Association (Polytopic Field Defect)

The schisis PFD (Table 7.12) includes midline defects such as neural tube

Table 7.10 Schisis association and sirenomelia

Neural tube defects
Cleft lip and palate
Abdominal wall defects
Diaphragmatic hernia
Oies complex
Midline abdominal and pelvic defects of omphalocele
Extrophy of bladder
Spine abnormalities
Sirenomelia
Short umbilical cord

Table 7.11 VATER association (polytopic field defect)

V – Vertebral defects
A – Anal atresia
T – Tracheoesophageal fistula
E – Esophageal atresia
R – Radial dysplasia renal defects
Probability of chance concurrence of 3 or 4 of these defects: Exceedingly small – suggests nonrandom selection.

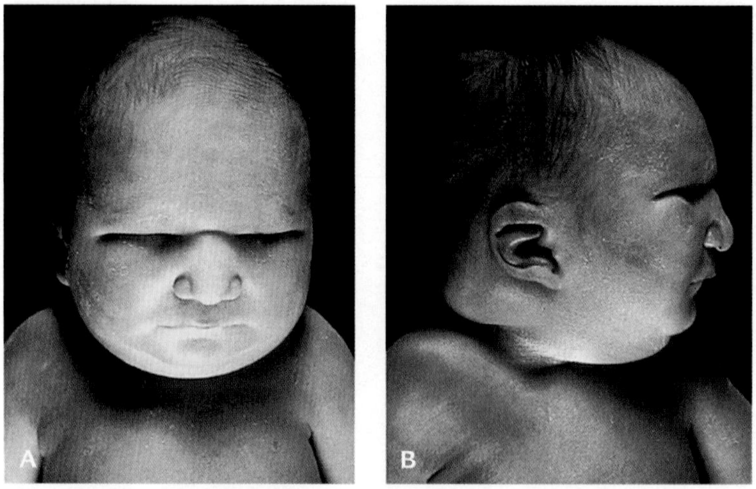

7.7. CHARGE polytopic field defect. This newborn infant had colobomas, atresia choanae, retarded growth and ear anomalies. **(A)** Anterior view. **(B)** Profile.

defects (i.e., anencephaly, encephalocele, meningomyelocele), oral clefts, omphalocele, and diaphragmatic hernia. It occurs more often in girls, in twins (4.6%), and in breech presentations. Schisis PFD may include congenital cardiac defects, limb deficiencies, and defects of the urinary tract, mainly renal agenesis. Schisis-type abnormalities appear to occur nonrandomly.

Disruption (See Chapter on Disruptions)

A disruption, or secondary malformation, is a morphologic defect of an organ, part of an organ, or larger region of the body resulting from an extrinsic breakdown of, or interference with, an originally normal developmental process (Table 7.13).

Sequence

A sequence is a pattern of multiple anomalies derived from a single known or presumed prior anomaly. A sequence has a cause, pathogenesis, and phenotype. Cause is heterogeneous, pathogenesis uniform, and phenotype variable.

Potter Sequence

The cause may be a gene mutation (e.g., HRA) leading to a malformation such as renal agenesis or infantile polycystic kidneys (an autosomal recessive disorder)

Table 7.12 VATER association (polytopic field defect)

Nonrandom association – due to common developmental pathogenesis
Defect in mesoderm in early development before 35 days
All the following occur prior to 35 days:

- Rectum and anus formed by mesodermal shelf, which divides cloaca into urogenital sinus and rectum and anus
- Mesodermal sinus separates trachea from esophagus
- Radius formed by condensation of mesodermal tissue in limb bud
- Vertebrae formed by migration and organization of somite mesoderm

Table 7.13 Disruption

A disruption is a morphologic defect of an organ, part of an organ, or larger region of the body resulting from the extrinsic breakdown of, or an interference with, an originally normal developmental process.

Disruptions tend to be sporadic occurrences.

Examples:

- Ischemic disruptions – porencephalic cysts or ileal atresia
- Radiation disruption
- Infectious disruptions – caused by viruses and toxoplasmosis
- Amniotic adhesion – the ADAM syndrome (amniotic-deformities-adhesions-mutilation)
- Caused by teratogenic drugs – thalidomide syndrome
- Mechanical disruptions – caused by bicornuate uterus or intrauterine myomata

resulting in oligohydramnios (pathogenesis) (Table 7.14). The lack of amniotic fluid restricts fetal movement and causes fetal compression, producing the typical phenotype of the Potter sequence.

Pierre Robin Sequence

Robin sequence can be malformational when based on intrinsic mandibular hypoplasia, or deformational when based on constraint. There is micrognathia, glossoptosis, and cleft soft palate. The lack of intrauterine movement causes micrognathia that results in glossoptosis and cleft palate (Figure 7.8 and Table 7.15).

Prune-Belly Sequence and Related Defects

Prune-belly sequence occurs sporadically as a triad of apparent absence of abdominal muscles, urinary tract defects, and cryptorchidism (Figure 7.9). The urinary tract is greatly dilated, usually with urethral or bladder neck obstruction. Megalourethra, megacystis, megaureters, renal hypoplasia, and hydronephrosis may occur.

Table 7.14 Potter sequence

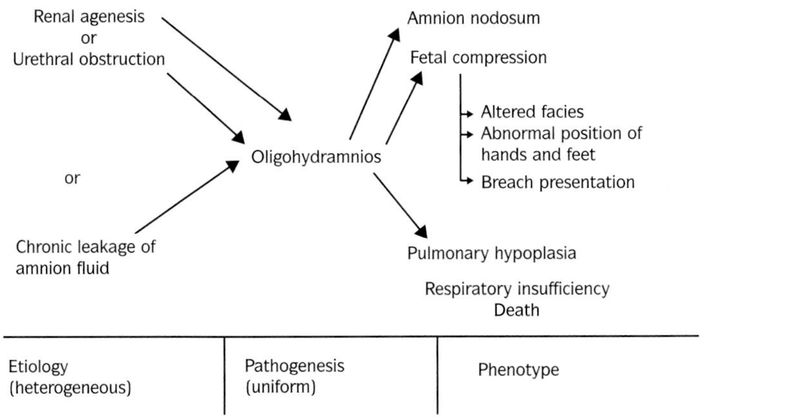

Source: Gilbert-Barness E (ed): *Pathology of the Fetus and Infant*, St. Louis, Mosby Co., 1997.

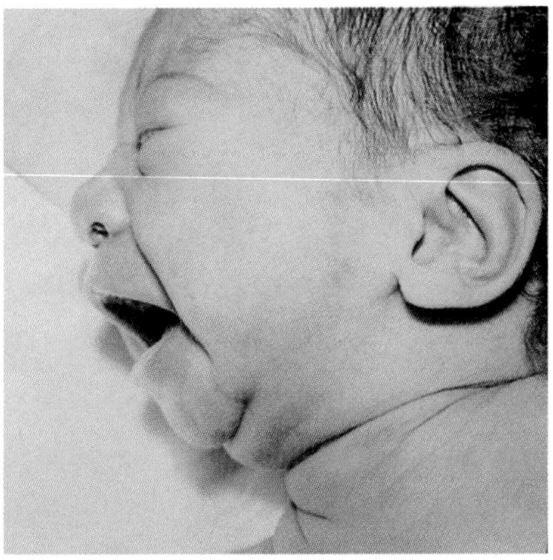

7.8. Pierre Robin sequence. Infant with retrognathia due to small mandible. Glossoptosis and cleft palate were also present.

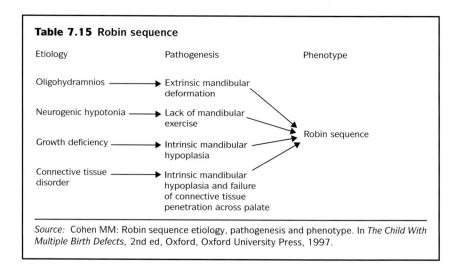

Table 7.15 Robin sequence

Etiology	Pathogenesis	Phenotype
Oligohydramnios →	Extrinsic mandibular deformation →	Robin sequence
Neurogenic hypotonia →	Lack of mandibular exercise →	Robin sequence
Growth deficiency →	Intrinsic mandibular hypoplasia →	Robin sequence
Connective tissue disorder →	Intrinsic mandibular hypoplasia and failure of connective tissue penetration across palate →	Robin sequence

Source: Cohen MM: Robin sequence etiology, pathogenesis and phenotype. In *The Child With Multiple Birth Defects,* 2nd ed, Oxford, Oxford University Press, 1997.

DiGeorge Sequence

The primary defect in DiGeorge sequence involves the fourth branchial arch and derivatives of the third and fourth pharyngeal pouches with defects of the thymus, parathyroids, conotruncal defect of the heart, occasionally the thyroid (Table 7.16). This complex is associated with congenital absence of the thymus, absence of the parathyroid glands, and immunodeficiency. Because of the role played by the cephalic neural crest in the morphogenesis of the heart, conotruncal heart defects are commonly seen in the DiGeorge sequence. The neural crest has a midline pathogenetic origin and DiGeorge sequence is frequently associated with other midline sequences, schisis anomalies, and arrhinencephaly. Causally, it also may be related to fetal alcohol and fetal-Accutane-induced disruptions as well as to the effects of maternal diabetes. A common (1/4,000 liveborn infants) microdeletion of chromosome 22 has been identified as is also seen in the velocardiofacial and conotruncal face syndromes.

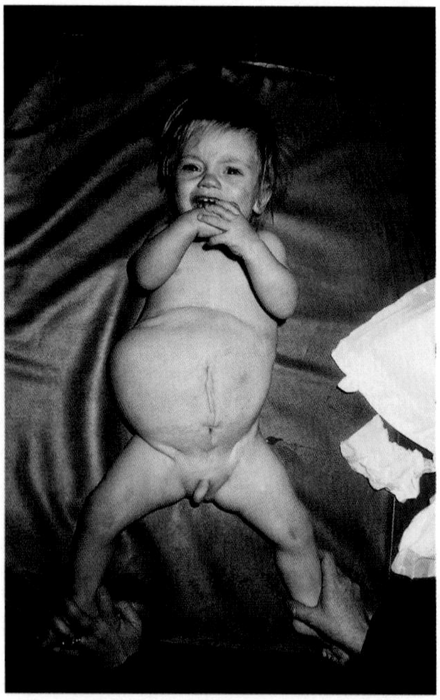

7.9. Prune belly syndrome. Infant with markedly distended abdomen.

Dysplasia (See Chapter 9)

Dysplasia is the process and the consequences of dyshistogenesis. It is an abnormal differentiation of tissue (Table 7.17). A dysplasia demonstrates a sporadic pattern. Dysplasias can be induced environmentally, and many are dominantly inherited.

PERIODS OF HUMAN DEVELOPMENT

Blastogenesis

Blastogenesis refers to all stages of development from the time of karyogamy and the first cell division to the end of gastrulation [(stage 13), day 28]. This is the time of closure of the caudal neuropore and the end of the formation of the intraembryonic mesoderm from the primitive streak. The events of gastrulation during the first 4 weeks of development are:

Table 7.16 Pathogenesis of DiGeorge sequence

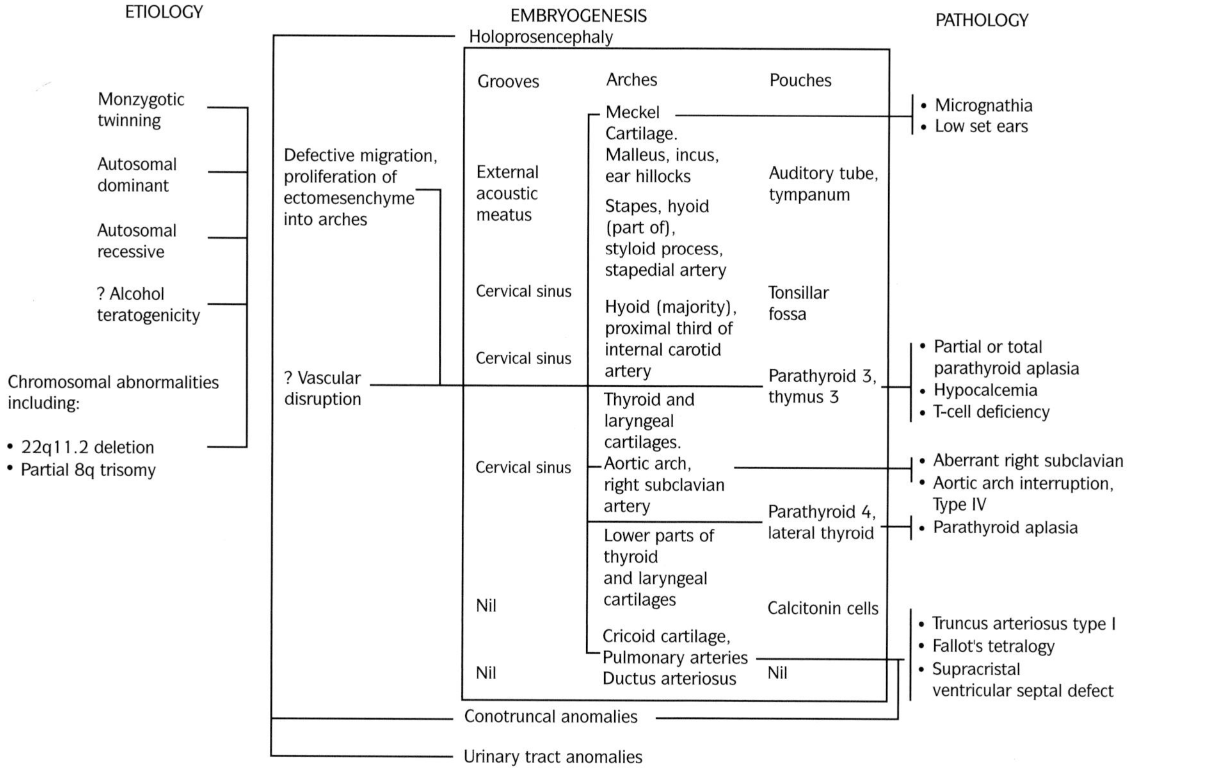

Source: Sperber GH, Gorlin RJ: Head and Neck. In Gilbert-Barness E (ed): *Potter's Pathology of Fetus and Infant*, St. Louis, Mosby, 1997.

Week 1. Formation of a unilaminar embryo – i.e., of the inner cell mass within the blastocyst and the beginning of implantation – Carnegie stages 1–4 and beginning stage 5.

Week 2. Formation of the bilaminar embryo (epiblast/hypoblast) with the amniotic cavity and secondary yolk sac; appearance of primary villi and primitive streak – stages 5 and 6.

Week 3. Formation of the trilaminar embryo (ectoderm, mesoderm, and endoderm). This stage extends from stage 7 to stage 9. Present at this stage is

Table 7.17 Dysplasias: abnormal growth of tissues

Frequently caused by autosomal dominant mutations, rarely by the homozygous state of recessive mutations
Occasionally caused by teratogens
Not biochemically defined
Primarily expressed as extensive multiple or generalized abnormalities of one type of tissue
Principally involves:

- Connective tissue
- Blood vessels
- Bone
- Skin

a primitive streak with notochordal process and notochord; the first somites in the paraxial mesoderm; neural plate, neural folds, and neuromeres in presumptive brain vesicles; primitive heart tube and intraembryonic coelom, and primitive blood vessels and villi.

Week 4. At the cephalic end, development is more advanced than at the caudal end (stages 10–13).

Development during the fourth week of gastrulation includes:

- Fusion of neural folds
- Ultimate closure of rostral (first) and caudal neuropores
- Formation of the branchial arches
- Formation of the myocardium with beginning heartbeat (days 19) and later formation of the cardiac septa
- Beginning formation of the gastrointestinal tract with rupture of the buccopharyngeal membrane
- Appearance of hepatic plate and of dorsal pancreatic bud and spleen
- Formation of the urorectal septum and appearance of ureteric buds
- Appearance of lung buds and optic vesicles with later lens placode
- Closure of the otic vesicle with beginning detachment from the overlying ectoderm
- Formation of limb buds and extension of somites 28–30

Blastogenesis includes the first 4 weeks of development. It encompasses the following:

- **Gastrulation**, which occurs with the formation of mesoderm and the appearance of the midline, cranial/caudal, right/left, and dorsal/ventral body axes; segmentation; neurulation; and initiation of all developmental processes including neurogenesis, angiogenesis, and (meso)nephrogenesis.
- **Initiation of laterality**.
- **Initiation of placentation**.

Comparison of anomalies of blastogenesis and of organogenesis*:

1. Anomalies of blastogenesis tend to be severe, those of organogenesis less severe.
2. Anomalies of blastogenesis tend to be complex, those of organogenesis less complex.
3. Anomalies of blastogenesis tend to be multisystem anomalies or complex polytopic field defects such as the acrorenal field defect; those of organogenesis are more likely to be localized, monotopic field defects.
4. Anomalies of blastogenesis are frequently lethal; anomalies of organogenesis are less commonly lethal.
5. Anomalies of blastogenesis frequently involve defects of placentation or cord formation; except for the presence of a single umbilical artery, the umbilical cord, placenta, and body wall are usually normal in defects of organogenesis.

6. Defects of blastogenesis are frequently associated with monozygotic twinning, which is, by definition, an abnormality of blastogenesis; twinning is less common or not a factor in organogenetic malformations.
7. Sex differences in occurrence appear to be less conspicuous in blastogenetic malformations. In organogenetic malformations there are frequently striking sex differences, an apparent indicator of multifactorial determination.
8. Anomalies of blastogenesis are defects of the embryonic midline; defects of organogenesis are not confined to the midline.
9. Abnormalities of blastogenesis may constitute a cancer risk such as teratomas anywhere along the midline from the skull to the tip of the coccyx; organogenetic malformations are rarely associated with a cancer risk.
10. Multiple congenital anomalies of blastogenesis are usually polygenic field defects or associations; multiple congenital anomalies of organogenesis are more likely to be syndromes representing pleiotropy due to Mendelian mutations and/or chromosome abnormalities.
11. A mild abnormality in blastogenesis may not produce grave defects but may extend into organogenesis, as in mildly affected infants of diabetic mothers or those with the fetal alcohol or retinoic acid (Accutane) syndromes; thus, some apparent organogenetic anomalies may in fact represent mild defects of blastogenesis.
12. Primitive, initially poorly hemoglobinized, short-lived, permanently nucleated red blood cells of yolk sac origin do not appear in the villous capillaries until 4.5 weeks after fertilization; even though the embryonic heart starts beating at 19–21 days after fertilization, vascular abnormalities are probably less likely a pathogenetic abnormality of blastogenesis than of organogenesis.
13. *From: Opitz JM: Blastogenesis and the "primary field" in human development. In Opitz JM (ed): *Blastogenesis – Normal and Abnormal*, New York, 1993, Wiley-Liss for The March of Dimes Birth Defects Foundation, BD, OAS XXIX (1):3–37.

DEFORMITIES

Deformations of extrinsic cause are more frequently isolated defects and have a better prognosis, while deformations of intrinsic origin are more frequently associated with other congenital anomalies and, generally, have a poor prognosis (Table 7.18).

Deformities result from a bending out of shape of usually normally developed structures due to excessive extrinsic pressure, or weakness (intrinsic inability to resist the deforming tendencies of normal extrinsic pressure) or lack of movement. **Oligohydramnios** is an important and common cause of deformity exemplified in the **Potter sequence**. Intrinsic weakness or hypotonia as in the

Table 7.18 Deformities

Predominant clinical manifestations are secondary to functional and mechanical disturbances

Congenital hypotonia: Micrognathia, microglossia, highly arched palate, deformities of feet

Arthrogryoposis: Due to disorders of intrauterine movements – defects in central or peripheral innervation

Potter sequence: Oligohydramnios, Potter facies, abnormal positioning of limbs, bowing of limbs

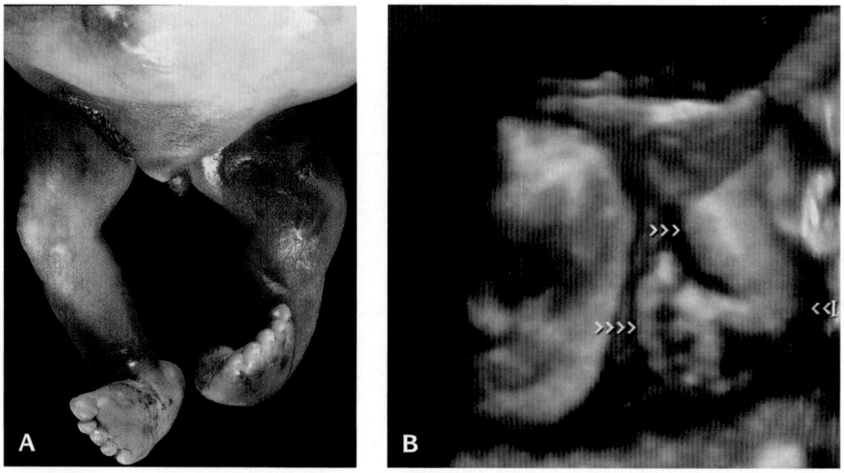

7.10. **(A)** A 32-week gestation fetus with arthrogryposis. **(B)** Three-dimensional ultrasound of a fetus at 31 weeks gestation with a club foot (four arrows) (two arrows = knee, three arrows = rump).

arthrogryposis or hypotonia (hypokinesia) sequence results in immobility and at times in webbing across the joints.

Pena and Shokeir first described early lethal neurogenic arthrogryposis and pulmonary hypoplasia as the Pena-Shokeir phenotype (Pena-Shokeir I syndrome, or fetal akinesia sequence deformation). Facial abnormalities include prominent eyes, hypertelorism, telecanthus, epicanthal folds, malformed ears, depressed tip of the nose, small mouth, high arched palate, and micrognathia. Polyhydramnios, small placenta, and a relatively short umbilical cord are frequent findings.

Pena-Shokeir type II syndrome (cerebro-oculo-facio-skeletal) is an autosomal recessive disorder with degenerative brain and spinal cord defects.

A common deformity is talipes equinovarus deformity (club foot). Many deformities improve with age, differential growth, and normal use.

Fetal Akinesia/Hypokinesia. Any situation which limits the intrauterine space or movement of the embryo or fetus may result in fetal akinesia deformation

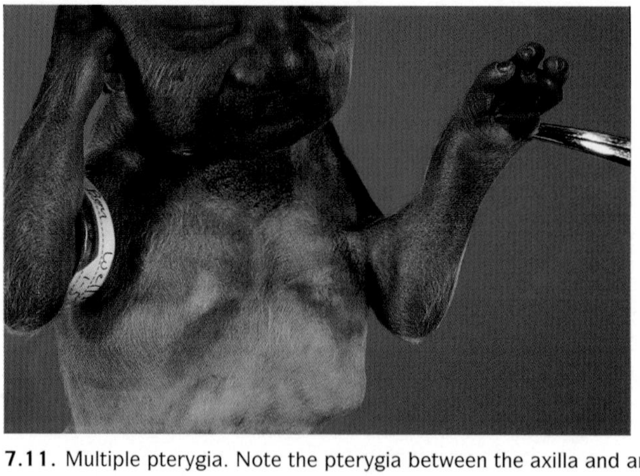

7.11. Multiple pterygia. Note the pterygia between the axilla and antecubital fossa.

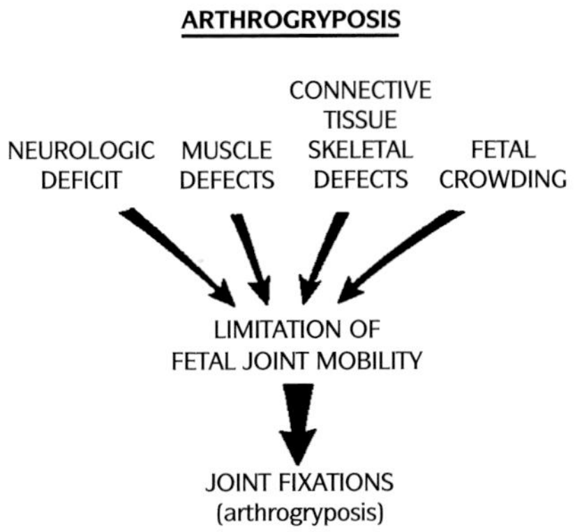

7.12. Causes of arthrogryposis. (From Jones KJ: *Smith's Recognizable Patterns of Human Malformation*, 5th ed, Philadelphia, Saunders, 1997.)

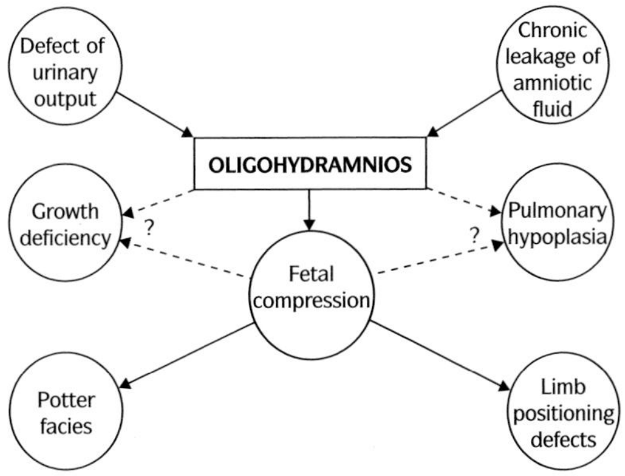

7.13. Oligohydramnios. (From Jones KJ: *Smith's Recognizable Patterns of Human Malformation*, 5th ed, Philadelphia, Saunders, 1997.)

sequence (FADS) (Figures 7.10 to 7.12). Akinesia may be produced extrinsically by mechanical factors such as oligohydramnios, oligohydramnios sequence (OS) – which produce fetal compression and retardation of movement of the fetus – or may be secondary to intrinsic lesions of the nervous or muscular systems.

Arthrogryposis may result from extrinsic or intrinsic immobilization of the joints during embryonic or fetal development (Figure 7.13). Increased mechanical pressure in oligohydramnios can restrain the movements of the limbs in utero. The limbs so confined become rigidly fixed in the position imposed by external forces.

Lack of movement beginning early in gestation is associated with pterygium or webbing of the skin surrounding the affected joint. The earlier the insult, the more severe the consequences with severe webbing and lethality; the skin lacks the normal wrinkles and creases that are a function of movement. Absence of normal skin creases has been noticed in most patients with FADS; however, it does not occur in OS because immobilization comes later during gestation. In OS there is an overgrowth of skin due to constraint.

Restriction of fetal movements by oligohydramnios leads to a short umbilical cord and short gut.

Infants with muscular weakness and intrauterine akinesia have a reduced bone mass. Fetuses with akinesia due to oligohydramnios, but preserved muscle function, have normal bone mass.

Impairment of lung movement secondary to compression of the thoracic cage in OS or to muscular weakness in FADS reduces the expansion of the pulmonary cavity and the lungs will remain hypoplastic and immature.

REFERENCES

Buyse MI, ed: *Birth Defects Encyclopedia.* Cambridge, Blackwell Scientific, 1990.

Cohen MM Jr: *The Child with Multiple Birth Defects.* Oxford, Oxford Press, 1997.

Cohen MM Jr: Editorial comment: Robin sequences and complexes: causal heterogeneity and pathogenetic/phenotypic variability. *Am J Med Genet* 84:311, 1999.

Cunningham ML, Mann N: Pulmonary agenesis: a predictor of ipsilateral malformations. *Am J Med Genet* 70:391, 1997.

Davis JE, Kalousek DK: Fetal akinesia deformation sequence in previable fetuses. *Am J Med Genet* 29:77, 1988.

Gilbert-Barness E, ed: *Potter's Pathology of the Fetus and Infant.* St. Louis, Mosby, 1997.

Gilbert-Barness E, ed: *Potter's Atlas of Fetal and Infant Pathology*. St. Louis, Mosby, 1998.

Gilbert-Barness E, Opitz J: *Congenital Anomalies and Malformation Syndromes in Pediatric Pathology*, Lippincott, Philadelphia, 1999.

Hall JG, Reed SD, Rosenbaum KN, et al.: Limb pterygium syndromes: a review and report of eleven patients. *Am J Med Genet* 12:377, 1982.

Hall JF: Invited editorial comment: Analysis of Pena-Shokeir phenotype. *Am J Med Genet* 25:99, 1986.

Larsen WJ: *Essentials of Human Embryology*, 3rd ed, NY, Churchill Livingstone, 2001.

Martinez-Frias ML, Bermejo E, Frias JL: Analysis of deformations in 26,810 consecutive infants with congenital defects. *Am J Med Genet* 84:365, 1999.

Martinez-Frias ML, Frias JL, Opitz JM: Errors of morphogenesis and developmental field theory. *Am J Med Genet* 76:291, 1998.

McKusick VA: *Mendelian Inheritance in Man: A Catalog of Human Genes and Genetic Disorders*, 12th ed, Baltimore, John Hopkins University Press, 1998.

Moore KL, Persaud TVN: *The Developing Human: Clinically Oriented Embryology*, 5th ed, Philadelphia, WB Saunders, 1993.

Moore KL, Persaud TVN, Shiota K: *Color Atlas of Clinical Embryology*, Philadelphia, WB Saunders, 1994.

Opitz JM: The Farber lecture: Prenatal and perinatal death: the future of developmental pathology. *Pediatr Pathol* 7:363, 1987.

Opitz JM: Blastogenesis and the "primary field" in human development. In *Blastogenesis – Normal and Abnormal*, Opitz JM (ed): New York, Wiley-Liss for The March of Dimes Birth Defects Foundation, 1993, vol. 1, Birth Defects, original article series vol. XXIX, pp. 3–37.

Opitz JM, Gilbert-Barness E: Editorial comment: CNS anomalies and the midline as a "developmental field." *Am J Med Genet* 12:443, 1982.

Opitz JM, Gilbert EF: The developmental field concept. *Am J Med Genet* 21:1, 1985.

Opitz JM, Wilson GN, Gilbert-Barness E: Abnormalities of blastogenesis, organogenesis, and phenogenesis. In Gilbert-Barness E (ed): *Potter's Pathology of the Fetus and Infant*, St. Louis, Mosby-Year Book, 1997, p. 65.

Opitz JM, Zanni G, Reynolds JF, Gilbert-Barness E: Defects of Blastogenesis, Seminars in Medical Genetics-Development and Malformations. *Am J Med Genet* 115:269, 2002.

Palacios J, Rodriguez JI: Extrinsic fetal akinesia and skeletal development. A study in oligohydramnios sequence. *Teratology* 42:1, 1990.

Rodriguez JI, Palacios J, Garcia-Alix A, et al.: Effects of immobilization on fetal bone development. A morphometric study in newborns with congenital neuromuscular diseases with intrauterine onset. *Calcif Tissue Int* 43:335, 1988.

Spranger J, Benirschke K, Hall JG, et al.: Errors of morphogenesis: concepts and terms. *J Pediatr* 100:160, 1982.

Stern CD, Ingham PW: *Gastrulation.* Cambridge, The Company of Biologists, Ltd, 1992.

Thomas IT, Smith DW: Oligohydramnios, cause of the non-renal features of Potter's syndrome, including hypoplasia. *J Pediatr* 84:811, 1974.

Wilson GN: Genomics of human dysmorphogenesis. *Am J Med Genet* 42:187, 1992.

Wilson GN: Atypical inheritance. *Neurol Clin North Am* 12:663, 1994.

Wilson GN: Mechanisms of development and growth: molecular genetics. In Gilbert-Barness E (ed): *Potter's Pathology of the Fetus and Infant*, St. Louis, Mosby-Year Book, 1997, p. 3.

EIGHT

Malformation Syndromes

Syndromes are causally identified entities. The multiple manifestation of those with a syndrome reflect pleiotropy (Table 8.1 and Figure 8.1). In (genetic) syndromes this phenomenon most likely reflects the several primary and secondary effects of a disturbance of a specific molecular system required for normal development. Thus, in Smith-Lemli-Opitz (SLO) syndrome microencephaly, cleft palate, cataracts, total anomalous pulmonary venous return, polysyndactyly, intersex genitalia, and Hirschsprung anomaly all seem to represent the primary and secondary effects of disturbed sonic hedgehog (SHH) signaling during ontogeny. No structural component anomaly of any malformation syndrome is obligatory and no one component is pathognomonic of any syndrome. Malformation syndromes consist or two or more developmental field defects or a single major field defect and several minor anomalies.

Hanhart and Poland-Möbius Complexes

Hanhart anomaly usually includes severe limb defects of at least one hand or foot and frequently is associated with severe oral abnormalities (Figure 8.2). The form of the condition associated with cranial nerve palsy is called the Hanhart-Möbius complex. It appears to be sporadic.

Beckwith-Wiedemann Syndrome (BWS) (OMIM #130650)

BWS is a multigenic disorder caused by dysregulation of imprinted growth regulatory genes within the 11p15 region. The clinical features include

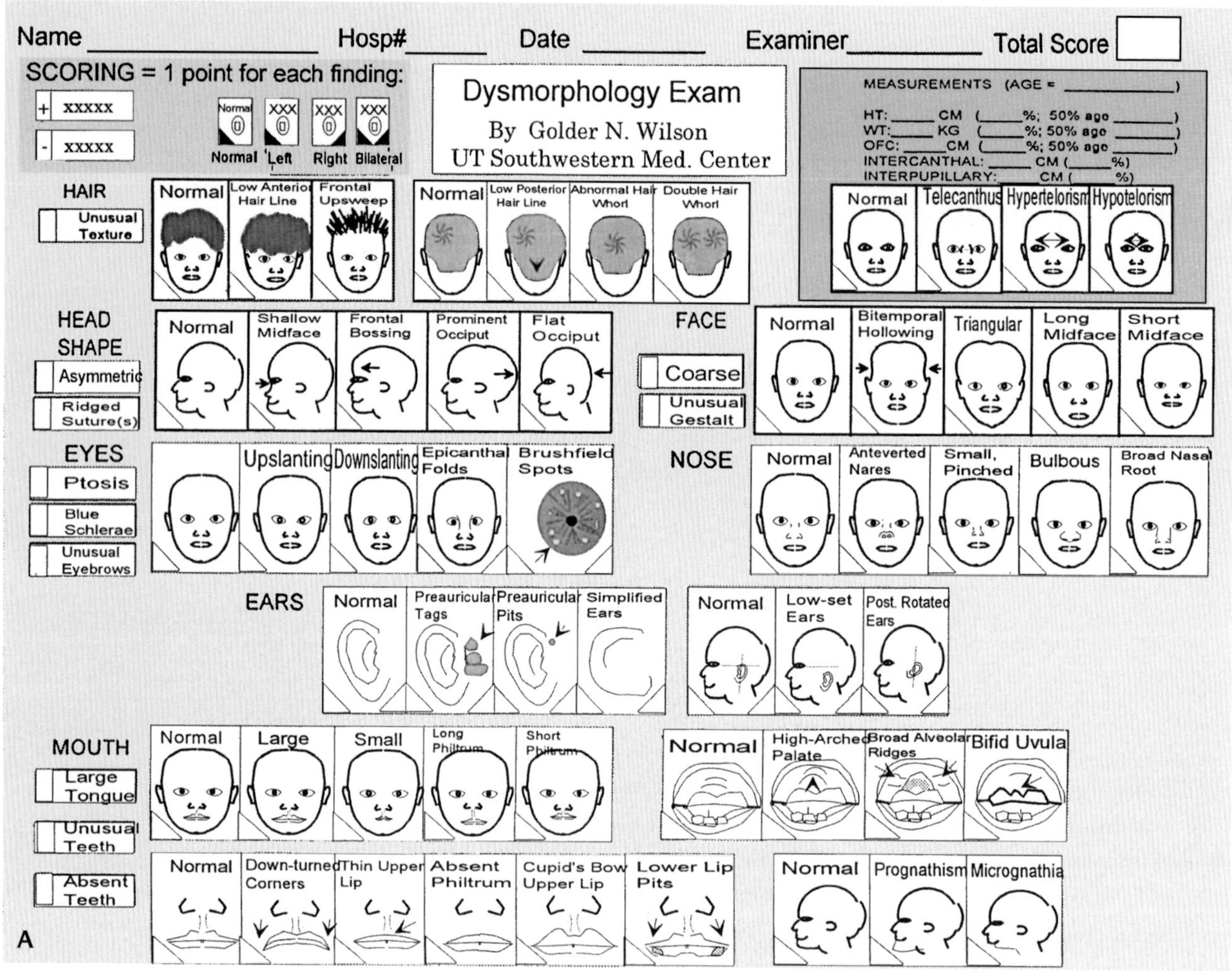

8.1. **(A)** and **(B)** Dysmorphology examination (Courtesy of Dr. Golden N. Wilson).

macroglossia, omphalocele, postnatal somatic gigantism, and neonatal hypoglycemia (Figures 8.3 to 8.5 and Table 8.2). Mean birth weight is about 3,900 g, although prematurity occurs in about 25%. Eventually height and weight are above the 90th centile and most exhibit advanced bone age. Hemihypertrophy has been noted in about 15%. Mild to moderate mental retardation is frequent and mild microcephaly occurs in about 50%. The tongue, which may also protrude from the mouth, eventually is included within the dental arch.

Table 8.1 Malformation syndrome

A **syndrome** is a pattern of multiple anomalies thought to be pathogenetically related.
Malformation syndromes tend to have definite cause – include chromosomal abnormality disorders and gene-determined errors of morphogenesis.
Recognition of malformation syndromes is pattern recognition.
There is no one obligatory malformation in a malformation syndrome.

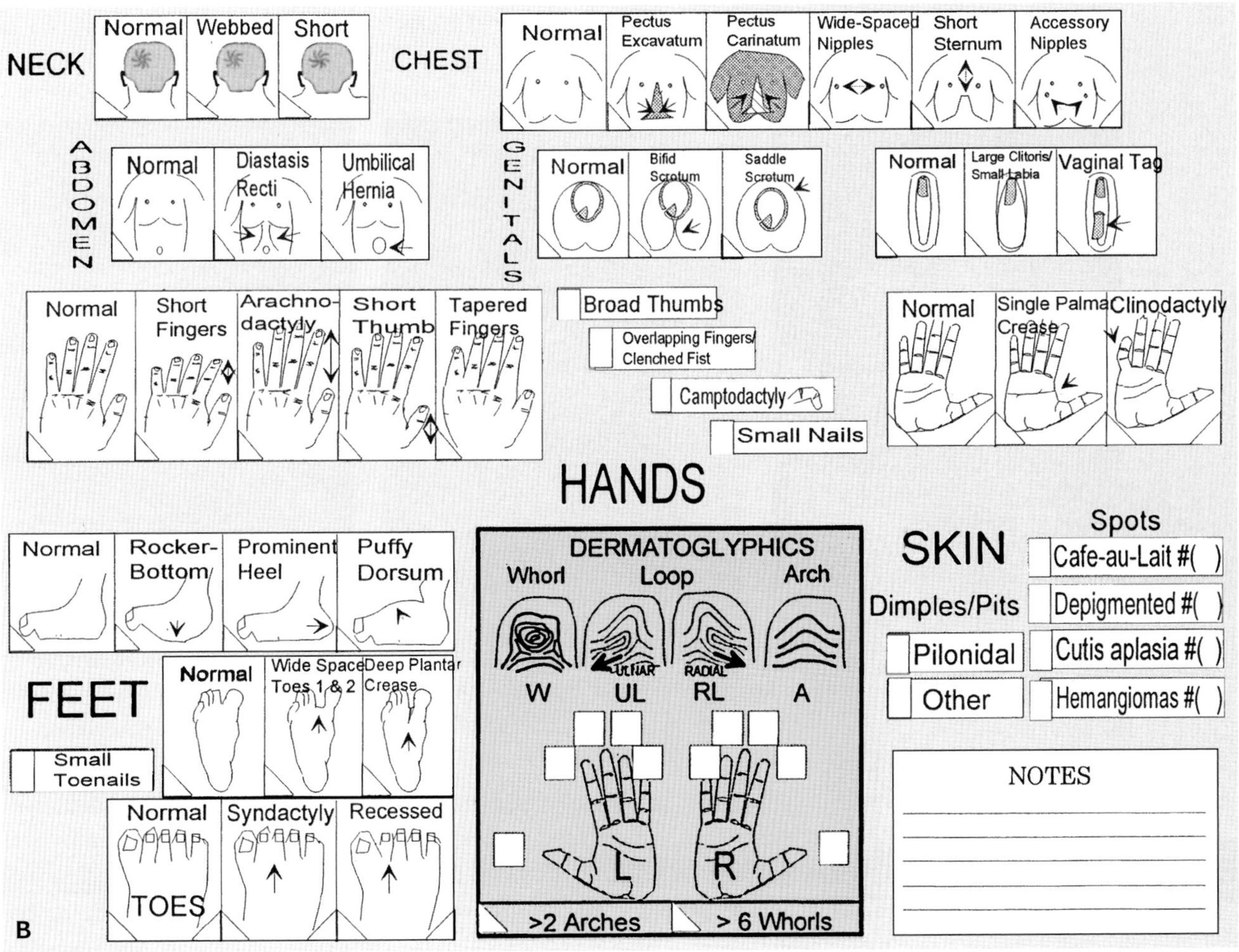
NECK
Normal
Webbed
Short
CHEST
Normal
Pectus Excavatum
Pectus Carinatum
Wide-Spaced Nipples
Short Sternum
Accessory Nipples
ABDOMEN
Normal
Diastasis Recti
Umbilical Hernia
GENITALS
Normal
Bifid Scrotum
Saddle Scrotum
Normal
Large Clitoris/ Small Labia
Vaginal Tag
Normal
Short Fingers
Arachnodactyly
Short Thumb
Tapered Fingers
Broad Thumbs
Overlapping Fingers/ Clenched Fist
Camptodactyly
Small Nails
Normal
Single Palmar Crease
Clinodactyly
HANDS
Normal
Rocker-Bottom
Prominent Heel
Puffy Dorsum
DERMATOGLYPHICS
Whorl
Loop
Arch
ULNAR
RADIAL
W
UL
RL
A
L
R
>2 Arches
> 6 Whorls
SKIN
Spots
Cafe-au-Lait #( )
Dimples/Pits
Depigmented #( )
Pilonidal
Cutis aplasia #( )
Other
Hemangiomas #( )
NOTES
FEET
Normal
Wide Space Toes 1 & 2
Deep Plantar Crease
Small Toenails
Normal
Syndactyly
Recessed
TOES
B

8.1. (*continued*)

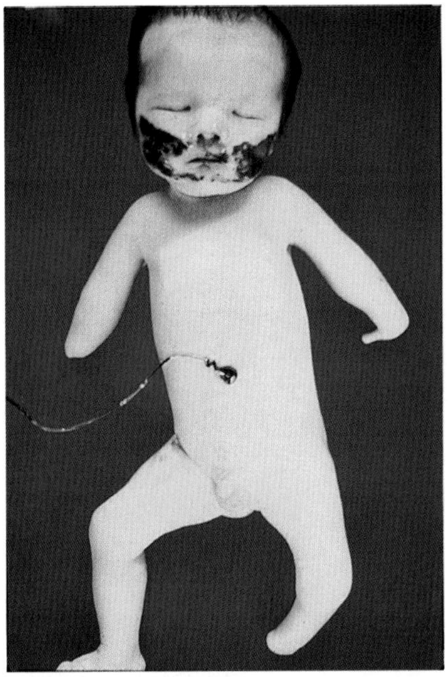

8.2. Hanhart syndrome – defects of upper and lower limbs.

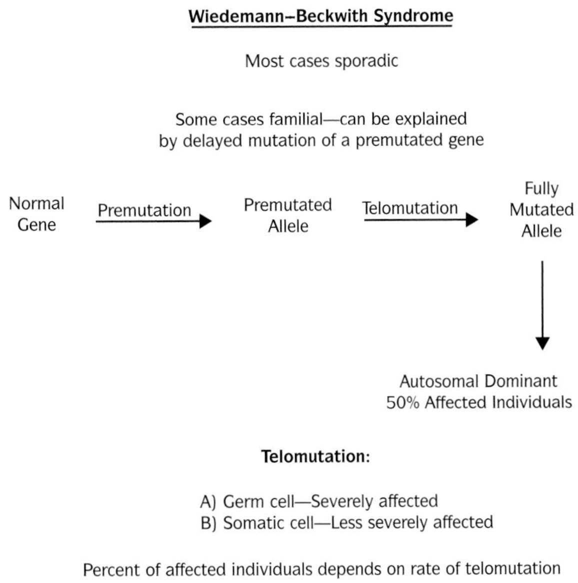
Wiedemann–Beckwith Syndrome
Most cases sporadic
Some cases familial—can be explained by delayed mutation of a premutated gene
Normal Gene
Premutation
Premutated Allele
Telomutation
Fully Mutated Allele
Autosomal Dominant
50% Affected Individuals
Telomutation:
A) Germ cell—Severely affected
B) Somatic cell—Less severely affected
Percent of affected individuals depends on rate of telomutation

8.3. Beckwith-Wiedemann syndrome algorithm.

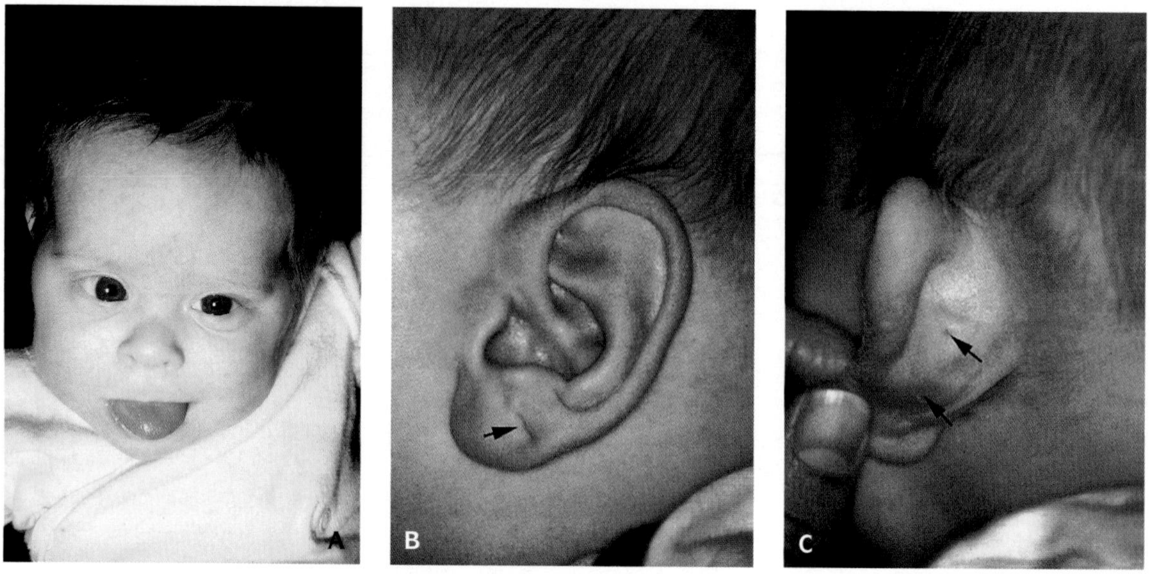

8.4. Beckwith-Wiedemann syndrome. **(A)** Clinical appearance with large protruding tongue. **(B)** Cleft of earlobe (arrow). **(C)** Pits on helix (arrows).

The macroglossia is associated with anterior open bite. Facial hemangiomas, principally in the glabellar area and over the upper eyelids, are seen in over 90% of the patients. They tend to become less prominent during the first year of life. Asymmetric earlobe grooves and pits and circular depressions on the posterior helix are noted in over half the patients. Omphalocele and umbilical hernia or malrotation are present in most cases. Inguinal hernia is common and diaphragmatic eventration occurs in about 30%. Some patients have diastasis recti. Hepatomegaly is common. General visceromegaly (nephromegaly, pancreatomegaly, and hyperplasia of the bladder, uterus, liver, and thymus) is frequent. Clitoromegaly has increased frequency. Cytomegaly of the adrenal glands and dysgenetic renal architecture is usually present. Paternal isodisomy of region 11p15.3–p15.5 leads to a lack of maternal imprinting. Zinc finger motifs within the *WTI* gene have been found.

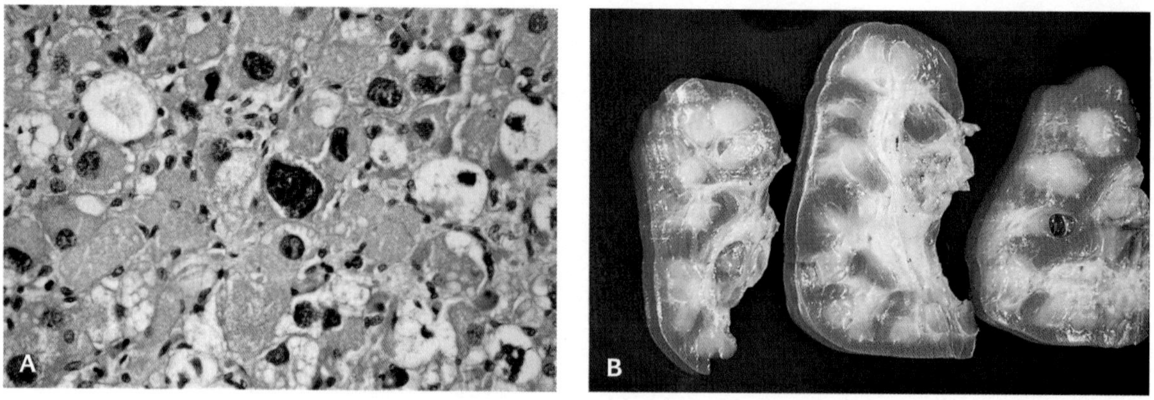

8.5. Beckwith-Wiedemann syndrome. **(A)** Adrenal cytomegaly. **(B)** Cut surface of dysmorphogenetic kidney.

Table 8.2 Clinical manifestations of Beckwith-Wiedemann syndrome

Polyhydramnios	Mental retardaiton
Neonatal hypoglycemia	Prematurity
Large placenta	Nephroblastomatosis
Macroglossia	Cytomegaly of adrenal cortex
Gigantism	Malrotation of intestine
Infants large for gestational age	Seizures
Midface hypoplasia	Nephromegaly
Lobular creases and posterior helical pits	Omphalocele
	Hemihypertrophy
Semilunar dent on helix	Hepatomegaly

Table 8.3 Meckel syndrome

Autosomal recessive
Death in early infancy
Incidence 1 in 13,500–1 in 140,000 births

Table 8.4 Meckel

Microcephaly
Encephalocele
Microphthalmia
Cleft lip/palate
Cystic dysplastic kidneys
Liver fibrosis
Abnormal genitalia
Polydactyly hands/feet

Table 8.5 Meckel syndrome: other manifestations

Cranial rachischisis
Arnold-Chiari malformation
Hydrocephalus
Polymicrogyria
Occular anomalies
Cleft palate
Congenital heart defects
Hypoplasia of the adrenal glands
Pseudohermaphroditism in males

Meckel Syndrome (OMIM *249000)

This is a recessively inherited disorder that usually leads to perinatal death (Figure 8.6). The incidence varies from 1 in 140,000 to 1 in 13,500 (Figures 8.7 to 8.10 and Tables 8.3 to 8.8). The diagnostic triad is occipital encephalocele, polydactyly, and large cystic kidneys. Other malformations are frequently present. There may also be cysts of the liver and pancreas. Maternal and fetal-α-fetoprotein is elevated. Fibrosis and bile duct proliferation resemble congenital hepatic fibrosis. Severe hypoplasia of male genitalia with cryptorchidism, epididymal cysts, and fibrosis of the pancreas are frequent anomalies.

Brachmann-De Lange Syndrome (OMIM 112370)

Major manifestations include mental retardation, hirsutism, and thin,

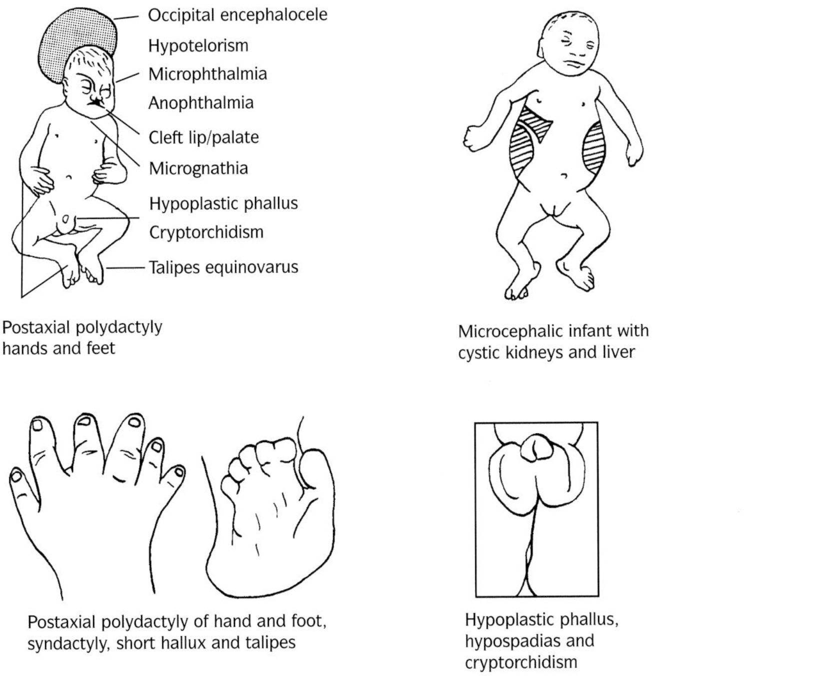

8.6. Meckel syndrome. Clinical manifestations. (From Goodman RM, Gorlin RJ: *The Malformed Infant and Child, An Illustrated Guide*, New York, Oxford University Press, 1985.)

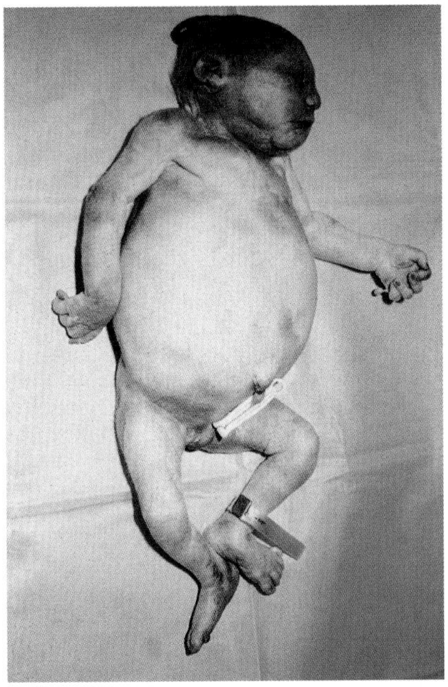

8.7. Infant with Meckel syndrome with occipital encephalocele, polydactyly, and large abdomen due to cystic kidneys.

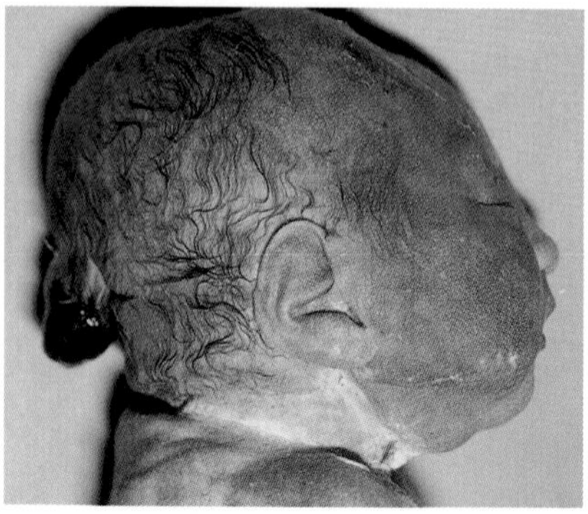

8.8. Meckel syndrome. Close-up view of occipital encephalocele.

Table 8.6 Meckel syndrome: genitourinary anomalies

Agenesis
Atresia
Hypoplasia
Duplication of ureters
Absence or hypoplasia of the urinary bladder

Table 8.7 Meckel syndrome: central nervous system anomalies

Encephalocele
Hydrocephalus
Micropolygyria

downturned vermillion borders (Figures 8.11 and 8.12). Other common anomalies are dental abnormalities, such as late eruption of widely spaced teeth, and male genital abnormalities, such as cryptorchidism and hypospadias, myopia, microcornea, astigmatism, optic atrophy, coloboma of the optic nerve, strabismus, proptosis, choanal atresia, low-set ears, cleft palate, congenital heart defects, hiatal hernia, duplication of the gut, malrotation of the colon, brachyesophagus, pyloric stenosis, inguinal hernia, small labia majora, radial hypoplasia, short first metacarpal, and absent second to third interdigital triradius. A clear genetic cause has not been established, although it may be an autosomal dominant mutation. Although there is some phenotypic overlap of Brachmann-de Lange syndrome and the dup(3q) syndrome, these entities are distinct and distinguishable. Chromosome 9 abnormalities have been implicated as possible causes because of the association with affected children and pregnancy-associated plasma protein A (PAPPA). PAPPA has been reported absent in the maternal serum and placental tissue of affected infants. PAPPA maps to chromosome 9.

Dubowitz Syndrome (OMIM #223370)

This sporadic, possibly autosomal dominant disorder is characterized by low birth weight, postnatal growth retardation, microcephaly, and a distinct facial appearance comprising sparse hair, high sloping forehead, flat supraorbital ridges, relatively high nasal bridge, facial asymmetry, telecanthus, ptosis, blepharophimosis with short palpebral fissures, epicanthal folds, micrognathia, and prominent or low-set ears (Figure 8.13). The lateral portions of the eyebrows may be hypoplastic. Oral manifestations consist of submucous cleft

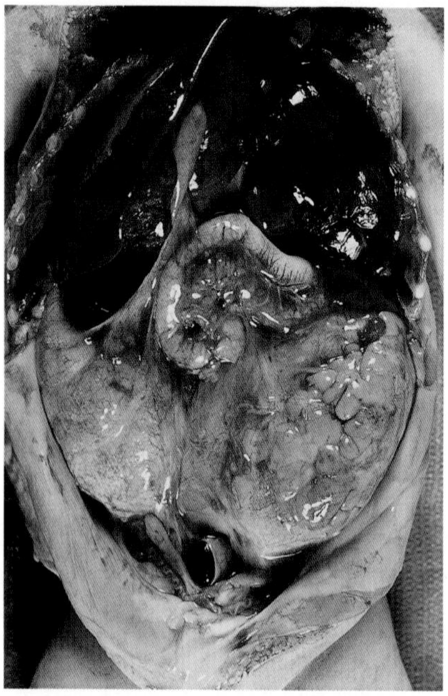

8.9. Meckel syndrome. Opened abdomen showing large cystic kidneys.

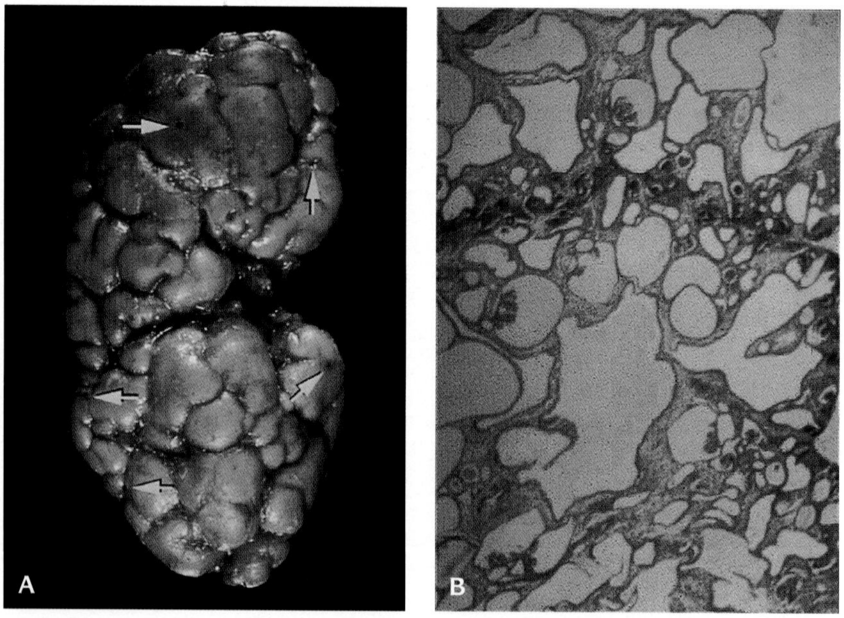

8.10. Meckel syndrome. **(A)** Surface of cystic kidneys (arrows). **(B)** Microscopic appearance of cystic kidney.

Table 8.8 Syndromes with encephalocele

Syndrome	Other features	Genetics	OMIM
Apert	Craniosynostosis, primarily coronal; short skull base; "mitten-like" syndactyly hands and feet; various CNS findings including megalencephaly, heterotopias, gyral anomalies, encephalocele; may have mental retardation	AD	101200
Chromsome abnormalities	Trisomies 13, 18; mosiac trisomy 20; deletion (13q), (2)(q21→q24); monosomy X; duplication (6)(q21→qter), (7)(pter→p11), (8)(q23→qter)	Chromosome Imbalance	
Craniotelencephalic dysplasia	Craniosynostosis; frontal encephalocele at metopic region; microphthalmia; various brain anomalies including septo-optic dysplasia, agenesis of the corpus callosum, lissencephaly, arhinencephaly	AR	218670
Cranium bifidum occultum	Mother with occipital occult cranial defect had child with pedunculated midline occipital encephalocele	Unknown; AD?	123200
Donnai: Meckel-like	Marked hydrocephalus, alobar holoprosencephaly-cebocephaly, anophthalmia, postaxial hexadactyly, cerebellar hypoplasia occipital encephalocele	Unknown	
Dyssegmental dysplasia (Rolland-Desbuquois)	Bones not bowed, ilia and scapulae normal, mild sagittal cleft vertebrae, normal growth plate, occipital defects, live several days to years	AR	224400
Dyssegmental dysplasia (Silverman-Handmaker)	Clefting; encephaloceles; marked micromelia; thick and bowed bones; severe vertebral segmentation defects; small, round, and dense ilia; scapular changes; large calcospherites; stillborn or die within 48 hr	AR	24410
Facio-auriculo-vertebral	Spectrum disorder of first and second arches, usually asymmetric; lower face hypoplasia involving periocular, malar/mandibular, aural anomalies; cardiac and vertebral anomalies similar to VATER with posterior cephalocele	Sporadic; occasionally AR, AD	164210 257700
Fraser: cryptophthalmos	Cutaneous syndactyly of hands and feet, broad nose, depressed tip with groove, coloboma, abnormal ears, cleft lip/palate, laryngeal anomalies, renal agenesis/dysgenesis, abnormal internal/external genitalia, mental retardation	AR	219000
Fried: Meckel-like	Lobar holoprosencephaly, large occipital encephalocele, microcephaly, absence/deformities of left forearm, complex congenital heart defects, absent Müllerian derivatives	Unknown	
Fronto-facio-nasal dysplasia	Cranium bifidum occultum/anterior encephalocele, blepharophimosis, lagophthalmos, S-shaped palpebral fissures, telecanthus, nose hypoplastic/bifid, midface hypoplasia, cleft lip/palate, limbic dermoids, facial tags	AR	229400
Frontonasal dysplasia	Widow's peak, hypertelorism, flat frontonasal encephalocele, broad nose with flat tip and separated nostrils, median cleft lip, mental retardation	Sporadic occasional AD	136760
Keutel: humero-radial synostosis	Humero-radial synostosis, may have hypoplasia of humerus and thumb, minor facial anomalies, hypoplastic ribs, microcephaly, occipital cephalocele rarely	AR	236400
Knoblock: vitreoretinopathy	Severe myopia, progressive retinal detachment leading to blindness, early lens opacities, spontaneous lens dislocation	AR	267750
Laryngeal atresia-hydrops	Syndactyly of all fingers, single palmar creases, toe camptodactyly, flexion anomalies of major joints, encephalocele through parietal bone	Unknown	
Meckel	Microcephaly, encephalocele, microphthalmia, cleft lip/palate, cystic dysplastic kidneys, liver fibrosis/cysts, abnormal genitalia, polydactyly hands/feet	AR	249000

(*continued*)

Table 8.8 (*continued*)

Syndrome	Other features	Genetics	OMIM
Oculo-cerebro-cutaneous	Orbital cysts, microphthalmia, lid coloboma, skin defects, skeletal anomalies, agenesis of the corpus callosum, multiple cysts of brain	Unknown	
Oculo-encephalo-hepato-renal	Epicanthus, nystagmus, ptosis, micrognathia, abnormal external genitalia, syndactyly, postaxial polydactyly, cystic renal dysplasia, cerebellar defects, mental retardation, postnatal growth failure	AR	213010
Pectoralis major-renal anomalies	Posterior encephalocele, absent sternal portion of pectoralis major, Sprengel anomaly, short and webbed neck, fused vertebrae C3-C6, absent right kidney	Unknown	
Phocomelia-encephalocele-urogenital anomalies	Bilateral radial aplasia, absent right thumb, hypoplastic left thumb, fused pelvic kidney, dextroposed heart, hypoplastic lung, thin corpus callosum, large encephalocele from roof of fourth ventricle	Unknown	
Roberts-SC phocomelia	Microbrachycephaly, marked prenatal and postnatal growth failure, mild to severe mental retardation, sparse and silvery hair, cleft lip/palate, thin nares, hypoplastic alae, varying hypomelia, characteristic centromeric puffing, frontal encephalocele and exencephaly rare	AR	268300
Scalp defect-craniostenosis	Left front cranial defect, with tumors of normal scalp, cutis aplasia, sinus tract, distorted internal brain anatomy, bifid nose, no alar or septal cartilage, high palate, small lumbar meningocele, undescended testes	Unknown	
von Voss-Cherstvoy: limb defects-thrombocytopenia	Occipital encephalocele, absent corpus callosum, variable upper limb and digital absence anomalies, hypoplastic thumbs, thrombocytopenia/reduced megakaryocytes, renal agenesis to milder defects, vaginal atresia, other brain anomalies	Unknown	
Walker-Warburg	Type II lissencephaly, cerebellar malformations, vermis hypoplasia retinal dysplasia, microphthalmia, congenital muscular dystrophy, rarely posterior encephalocele	AR	236670
Warfarin embryopathy	Hypoplastic nasal bones, chondrodysplasia calcificans punctata, microphthalmia, cardiac anomalies. CNS damage due to bleeding. Occipital encephalocele may occur.	Coumadin exposure in utero	

Modified from Stevenson RE, Hall JG: In Goodman RM (ed): *Human malformations and related anomalies*, New York, Oxford University Press, 1993.

palate, high arched palate, bifid uvula, delayed dental eruption, and severe dental caries. The voice is usually high-pitched and hoarse. An eczematous skin eruption about the face and limbs has been observed during infancy in some patients. Chronic rhinorrhea and serous otitis media have also been reported. Other findings observed in some patients are diarrhea in infancy, pilonidal dimples, hypospadias, cryptorchidism, preaxial polydactyly, clinodactyly, megalocornea, retinal malformation, vascular abnormalities, migraine headaches, metatarsus varus, pes planus, and pes planovalgus.

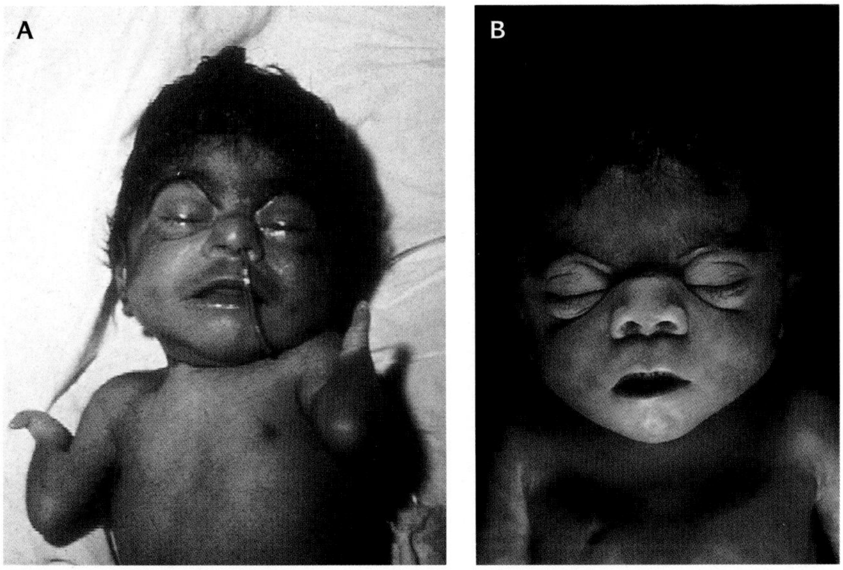

8.11. Brachmann-de Lange syndrome. **(A)** Infant with synophrys and anomalies of upper limbs. **(B)** Infant showing synophrys and hirsutism.

Robinow (Fetal Face) Syndrome (OMIM *180700)

Robinow (fetal face) syndrome is characterized by a fetal appearance of the face, orodental abnormalities, mesomelic dwarfism, and hypoplastic genitalia. At least 85 patients have been reported (Figure 8.14 and Table 8.9). The syndrome is classified into dominant and recessive types. The distinguishing findings in the recessive type (also known as Covesdem syndrome) are severe mesomelic and acromelic dwarfism and multiple rib and vertebral anomalies. Patients with the autosomal recessive (AR) syndrome frequently exhibit radioulnar dislocation and severe hypoplasia of the proximal radius and distal ulna.

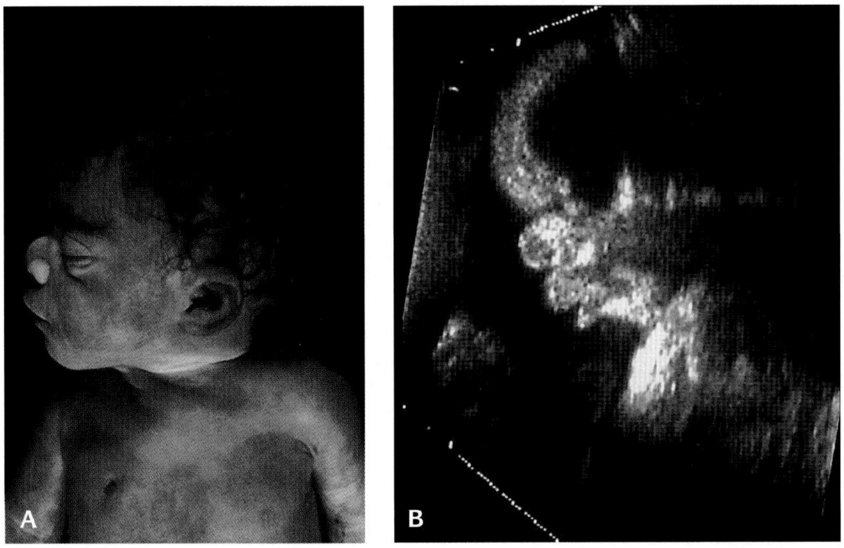

8.12. Brachmann-de Lange syndrome. **(A)** side view of face. **(B)** Ultrasound showing typical signs of the syndrome.

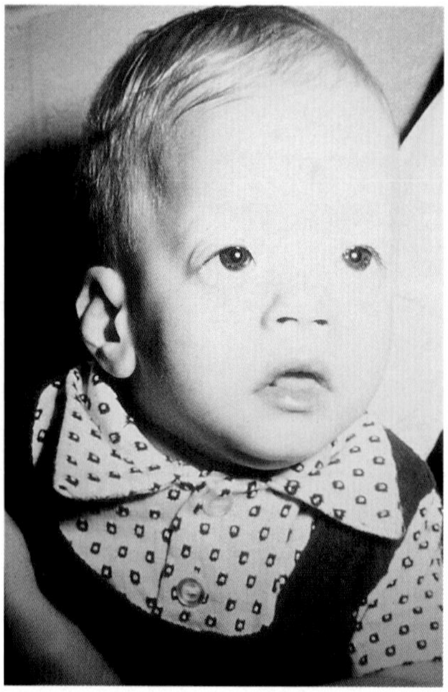

8.13. Infant with Dubowitz syndrome with sparse hair, sloping forehead, low-set ears, and flat supraorbital ridges.

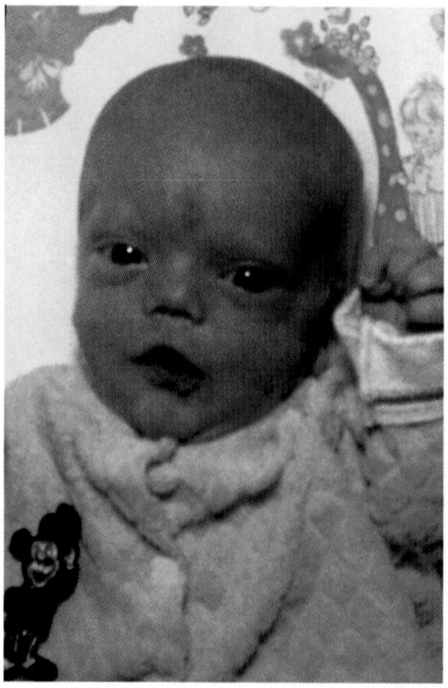

8.14. Infant with Robinow (fetal face) syndrome with large head, bulging forehead, and hypertelorism.

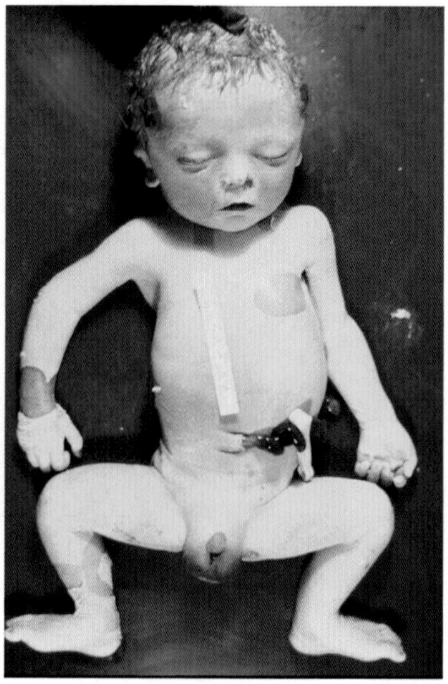

8.15. Infant with Opitz syndrome with hypertelorism, flat bridge of nose, and antimongoloid slant of palpebral fissures.

Table 8.9 Robinow syndrome

1. Fetal face phenotype:
   - Neurocranium disproportionately large leading to bulging forehead
   - Moderate hypertelorism
   - Mid-face hypoplasia
   - Short, upturned nose
   - Wide, triangular mouth with downturned corners (fish-mouth)
2. Forearm brachymelia
3. Mesomelic shortening of lower limbs less marked or absent
4. Genital hypoplasia:
   - Males – penis invisible at birth unless surrounding skin retracted
   - Females – clitoris and labia minora hypoplastic
5. Moderate dwarfing
   - Length usually normal at birth, falls below the 3rd centile before age 2–3 years
6. Other findings

Vertebral or costovertebral anomalies	Mental retardation
Dental malalignment	Rhizomelic shortening, upper extremities
Short hand and/or feet	Umbilical hernia
Clinodactyly	Click-murmur syndrome
Gingival hyperplasia	Delayed eruption of permanent teeth
Cleft lip	Inguinal hernia
Undescended testes (Uni- or bilateral)	Cleft uvula
Hepatosplenomegaly	Absent uvula
Abnormal dermatoglyphics	Macroglossia
Pectus excavatum	Ankyloglossia
Renal abnormalities	Rachischisis
Penile agenesis	

This disorder derives its name from the fact that the facial features are similar to those seen in a fetus of approximately 8 weeks. Facial findings include a disproportionately large neurocranium, bulging forehead, wide palpebral fissure with S-shaped lower lids, hypertelorism, short nose, anteverted nares, flat face, and triangular mouth with downturned angles. Dental malalignment, crowding, gingival hyperplasia, macroglossia, trapezoidal maxillary arch, cleft lip/palate, and minor clefting of the lower lip and tongue have all been reported. Short stature is common because of vertebral and long bone involvement. Scoliosis, fused vertebrae, and hemivertebrae may be observed, while mesomelic brachymelia affects the upper limbs more than the lower. The hands may be short and stubby with hypoplastic nails, while the feet may show bulbous halluces. Clinodactyly with hypoplasia of the middle phalanx of the fifth finger may be present. Varying degrees of genital hypoplasia are seen in males and females.

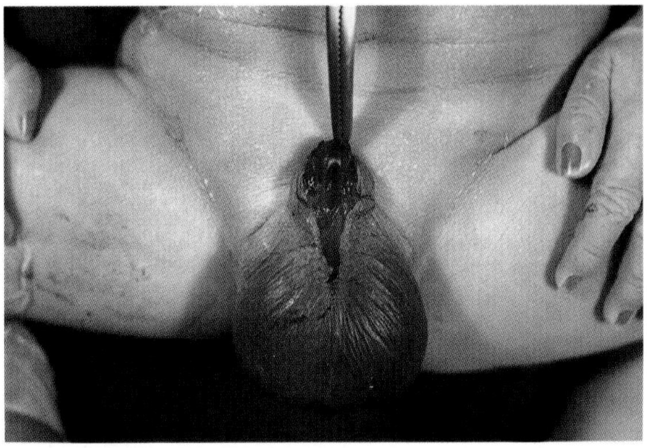

8.16. Opitz syndrome. Hypospadias.

Opitz (GBBB) Syndrome (OMIM *300000)

This is a heterogeneous syndrome due to mutations at 22q11 and at Xp22.3 involving the *MID1* gene (Figures 8.15 to 8.17). One *AD* gene maps near the DiGeorge region but remains uncloned. The *MID1* gene is a ring finger (B-box) gene. Affected males usually have ocular hypertelorism and hypospadias, but heterozygous females have only hypertelorism. The facial appearance is characteristic and consists of hypertelorism, flat bridge of nose, prominence of parietal eminences and occiput with dolichocephaly and large anterior fontanel, small palpebral fissures with mongoloid or antimongoloid slant, epicanthal folds with or without an accessory fold following the upper lid partly to the outer canthus, relative entropion of lower lid, strabismus, anteverted nares, flat and inapparent philtrum, micrognathia, and dysplastic ears with some degree of posterior rotation. Oral anomalies may include a broad or bifid uvula, ankyloglossia or a shortened lingual frenulum, and, rarely, cleft lip/palate. The male genital and anal anomalies when severe are so unusual that they may be diagnostic. The degree of hypospadias varies from mild coronal to a scrotal type with an associated urethral groove. In markedly affected cases the scrotum is cleft and chordee may be so severe as to draw the tip of the glans to the anterior edge of the anus. The testes may be descended and of normal size. Occasionally an imperforate anus with rectourethral fistula has been reported. Bilateral ureteral reflux has been noted. Affected females have normal genitalia. Some infants have stridorous respiration with a hoarse cry.

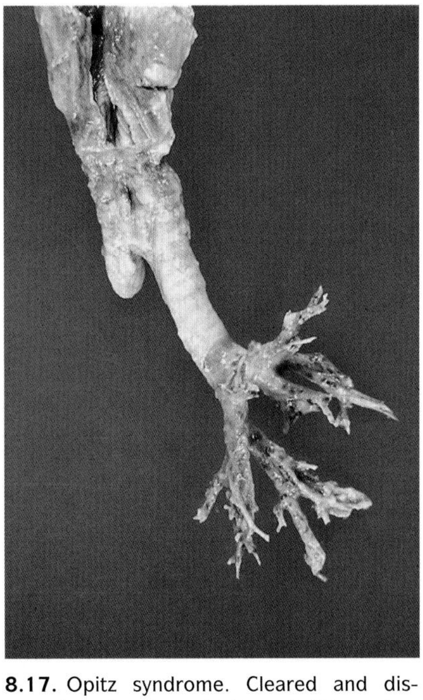

8.17. Opitz syndrome. Cleared and dissected tracheo-bronchial tree. Left bronchus is short. Left lung was absent and there is a short trachea.

Mandibulofacial Dysostosis (Treacher Collins syndrome) (OMIM #154500) – (See Also Craniofacial Chapter)

This autosomal dominant syndrome can be recognized at birth due to a typical facial appearance comprising antimongoloid obliquity of the palpebral fissures,

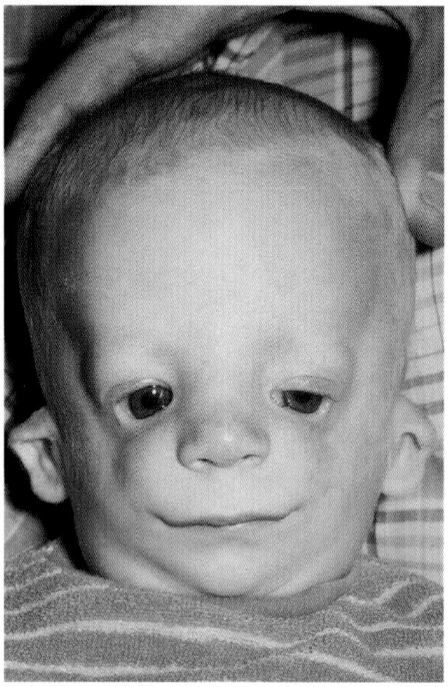

8.18. Treacher-Collins syndrome. The infant has malar hypoplasia, downward slanting eyes with colobomas.

coloboma of the outer third of the lower lid with a deficiency of cilia medial to the coloboma, iridial coloboma, absence of the lower lacrimal, Meibomian glands, microphthalmia, and partial to total absence of the lower eyelashes (Figure 8.18). The nose appears large because of a lack of malar development, while the nares are often narrow and the alar cartilages hypoplastic. The nasofrontal angle is commonly obliterated and the bridge of the nose raised. Choanal atresia has been noted. Micrognathia is almost always present; other oral manifestations include cleft palate (30%), high-arched palate, dental malocclusion, and unilateral or less often bilateral macrostomia. The external ears are frequently small, malformed, low-set or posteriorly angulated. Some patients have an absence of the external auditory canal or ossicle defects associated with conductive deafness. Extra ear tags may be found anywhere between the tragus and angle of the mouth. Other anomalies occasionally are absence of the parotid gland, congenital heart disease, cervical vertebral malformations, congenital defects of the limbs, cryptorchidism, and renal anomalies.

Roberts Syndrome (OMIM *268300)

This autosomal recessive syndrome comprises bilateral cleft lip/palate, tetraphocomelia with reduced number of digits, ocular proptosis with hypertelorism, and growth deficiency (Figure 8.19). Bilateral cleft lip with or without cleft palate is present in almost all patients. Additional findings may include colobomas of the eyelids, shallow orbits, bluish sclerae, cataracts, and corneal opacity. The external ears tend to be dysplastic and rudimentary. Other common craniofacial findings are microbrachycephaly, midfacial capillary

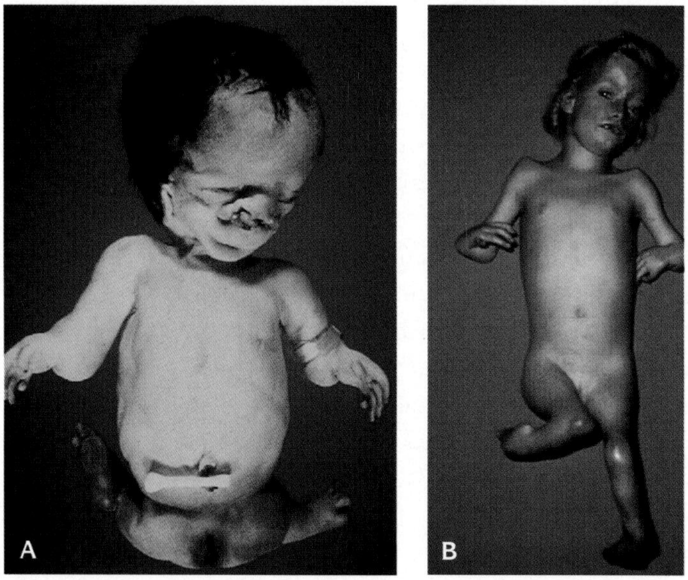

8.19. Roberts syndrome. **(A)** Short limbs, large head, and hair extending on to forehead. **(B)** Short malformed limbs.

hemangioma, thin nares, and sparse, silvery-blond scalp hair. Limb malformations are almost all symmetric aplasias or hypoplasias of all the bones, resulting in shortness of the limbs and sometimes phocomelia. Most commonly absent are the radius alone, radius and ulna, fibula, and marginal digits. In nearly all cases, the number of digits has been reduced more frequently in the hands than in the feet. Malposition of the thumb is a frequent finding. Cutaneous syndactyly is seen in approximately 70% of patients. Low birth weight (less than 2,000 g) and growth deficiency are common. The basic defect is not known. Prophase and metaphase chromosomes in this disorder have shown premature sister-chromatid separation and interphase nuclei have exhibited a striking distortion in their contours.

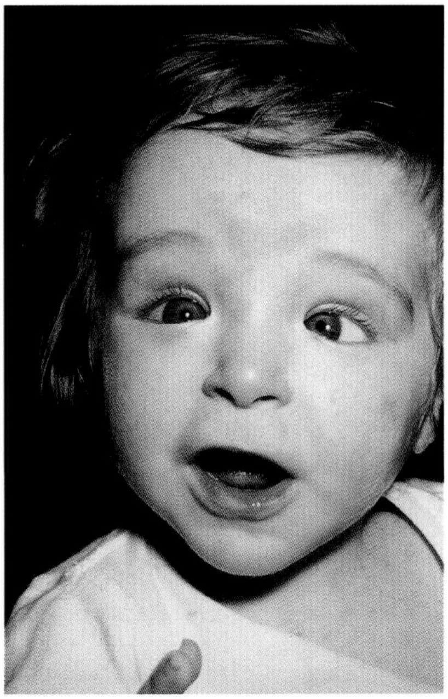

8.20. Rubinstein-Taybi syndrome. This infant has microcephaly with the nasal septum extending onto philtrum, beaked nose, antimongloid slant of the eyes, and short philtrum.

Rubinstein-Taybi Syndrome (OMIM #180849)

This sporadic syndrome is recognizable at birth and is characterized by the presence of distinct facies, mental retardation, and broad thumbs and toes (Figures 8.20 and 8.21). The unusual facial appearance is characterized by microcephaly, prominent forehead, antimongoloid obliquity of the palpebral fissures, epicanthal folds, strabismus, broad nasal bridge, beaked nose with the nasal septum extending below the alae, and mild micrognathia. Other findings may include heavy eyebrows; long eyelashes; ptosis of eyelids; hypertelorism; nasolacrimal duct obstruction; refractive error; minor abnormalities in the shape, position, and degree of rotation of the ears; and nevus flammeus on the forehead. Grimacing or an unusual smile frequently is observed. A high-arched palate and dental malocclusion are frequent, while bifid uvula and tongue, macroglossia,

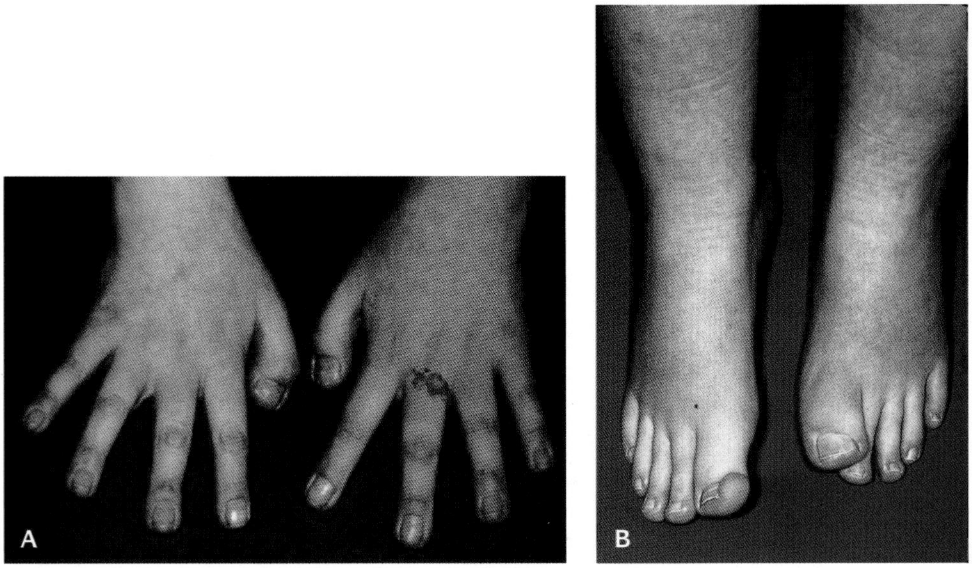

8.21. Rubinstein-Taybi syndrome. Hands showing bulbous tips of fingers **(A)** and toes **(B)**.

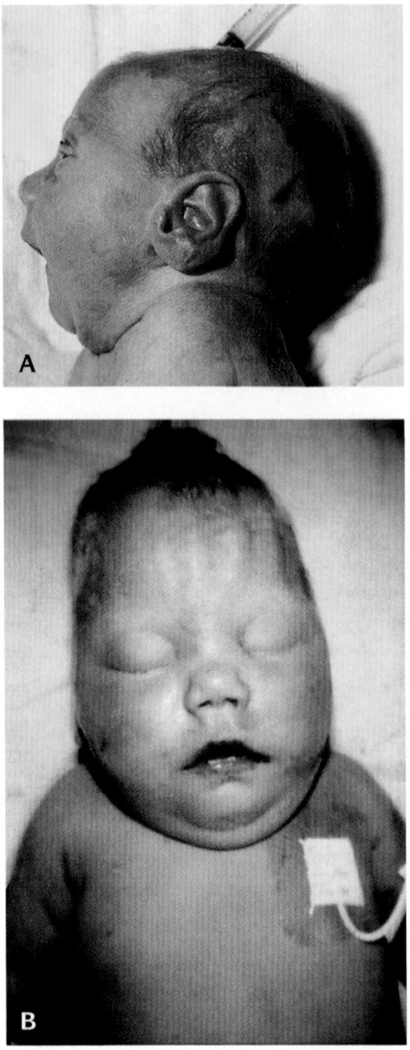

8.22. Smith-Lemli-Opitz syndrome. Infants with micrognathia, microcephaly, and large malformed ear. **(A)** Side view. **(B)** Front view.

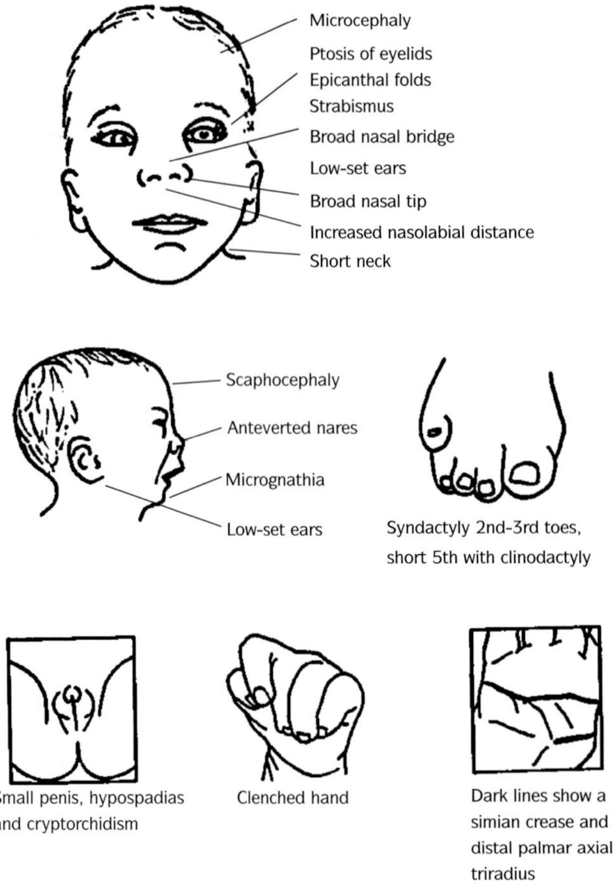

8.23. Smith-Lemli-Opitz syndrome. Clinical manifestations.

short lingual frenulum, and thin upper lip are only rarely observed. Characteristically broad thumbs and halluces are present. In most instances, the terminal phalanges of the fingers are also broad. Angulation deformities of the thumbs and halluces together with abnormally shaped proximal phalanges are common. Clinodactyly of the fifth finger and overlapping of the toes are present in more than 50% of the patients.

Smith-Lemli-Opitz Syndrome (SLO syndrome) (OMIM #270400)

This autosomal recessive disorder is due to a defect of cholesterol synthesis resulting in low to extremely low cholesterol levels and greatly increased plasma concentrations of the immediate precursors of 7-dehydrocholesterol (7DHC) and cholest-5, 7, 24-trien-3β-ol (Figures 8.22 to 8.27 and Table 8.10). Increased expression of low density lipoprotein receptors with elevated bilirubin levels and jaundice is described. The manifestations range from a perinatally lethal form to one of essentially normal growth, multiple minor anomalies, and mild mental retardation.

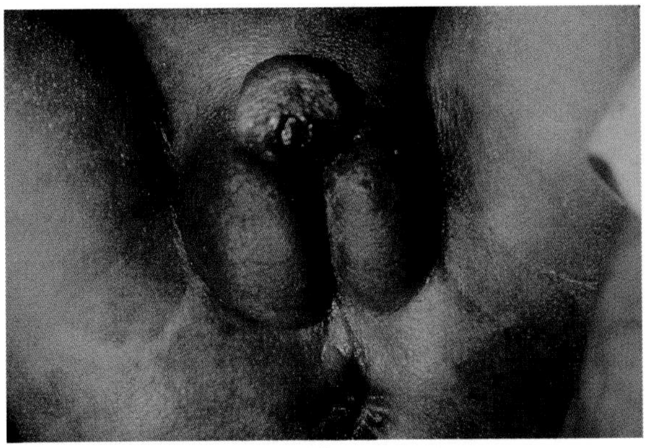

8.24. Smith-Lemli-Opitz syndrome. Ambiguous genitalia in a male infant.

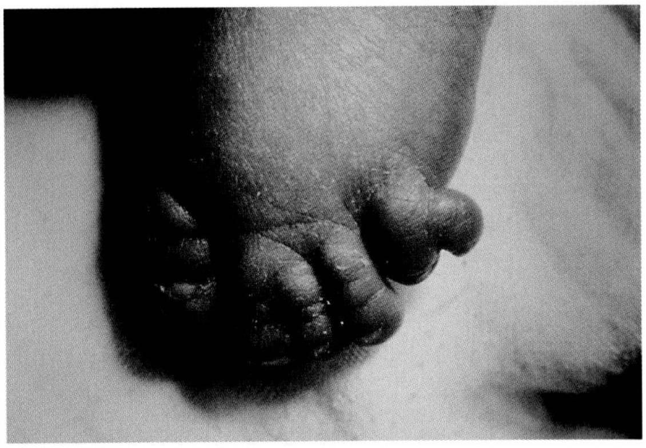

8.25. Smith-Lemli-Opitz syndrome. Syndactyly of 2nd and 3rd toes and polydactyly.

The 7DHCR mutation is cloned and sequenced and the mutations are known. It is recognizable at birth by the following characteristic features: ptosis of eyelids, slanted low-set ears, broad nasal tip with anteverted nares, micrognathia, broad maxillary alveolar ridges, cutaneous syndactyly of the second and third toes, and hypospadias and cryptorchidism. Fetal movements are decreased. Breech presentation is common and birth weight may be less than 2,500 g. The facies may be quite distinct, exhibiting microcephaly, eyelid ptosis, strabismus, epicanthal folds, increased nasolabial distances, upturned nares, broad nasal tip, micrognathia, low-set and/or slanted ears, and short neck. Occasional findings may include congenital cataracts, hypertelorism, mild antimongoloid slant, minor ear anomalies, and plagiocephaly. The maxillary alveolar ridges are broad and the palate may be highly arched. Cleft palate or bifid uvula has been reported in some cases. The hands commonly show a simian crease, camptodactyly, rudimentary postaxial polydactyly, short fingers, clinodactyly, and proximally placed thumbs also have been noted. The feet usually display cutaneous syndactyly between the second and third toes; clinodactyly, hallucal hammer toes, metatarsus adductus, pes equinovarus, and other anomalies are seen in some patients. In males the genitalia can range from normal appearing with small descended testes to severe periscrotal hypospadias with perineal urethral opening, cleft scrotum, and bilateral cryptorchidism. Microencephaly, hypoplasia of the frontal lobes, hypoplasia of cerebellum and brain stem, dilated ventricles, irregular gyral patterns, and irregular neuronal organization are brain abnormalities. Anomalies are rudimentary postaxial hexadactyly, congenital heart defects, and multiple anomalies of renal and spinal cord development. Cystic renal disease, hypoplasia, hydronephrosis, and abnormalities of the ureters are frequent and giant cells in the pancreatic islets are seen. Severe perineoscrotal hypospadias or complete feminization of male genitalia may be seen. The reported higher frequency of males affected than females may be related to a bias in ascertaining the genital anomaly.

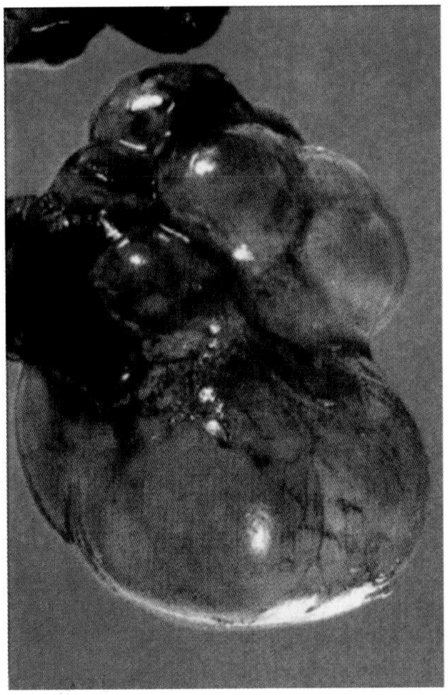

8.26. Smith-Lemli-Opitz syndrome. Large cystic kidney.

Table 8.10 Smith-Lemli-Opitz syndrome autosomal recessive
Abnormalities:
Microcephaly
Mental retardation
Decreased muscle tone
Minor anomalies of face, hand, and feet
Pyloric stenosis
Ptosis
Epicanthal folds
Prominent metopic suture
Capillary Hemangiomata
Syndactyly of 2nd and 3rd toes
Dermatoglyphics – high ridge count
Rudimentary polydactyly
Incomplete development of external genitalia

Leprechaunism (OMIM #246200)

This autosomal recessive disorder is characterized by prenatal and postnatal growth deficiency, retarded osseous maturation and lack of adipose tissue (Figure 8.28). Small and prominent eyes, wide nostrils, thick lips, and large ears impart the typical leprechaun appearance. Failure to thrive, frequent infections, and death in early infancy occur. Islet cell hyperplasia and hyperinsulinism result in hypoglycemia, a large penis, and body and facial hirsutism; motor and mental retardation are usually apparent. Leydig cell hyperplasia in the male and follicular development with cystic ovaries in the female are seen.

Williams Syndrome (OMIM #194050)

Williams syndrome in both familial and sporadic cases is due to a heterozygous deletion at 7q11.23, including the elastin gene (Figure 8.29). The elastin gene deletion can explain the vascular and connective tissue abnormalities but not the hypercalcemia. The syndrome's relationship to vitamin D metabolism is unknown, although hypercalcemia due to hypervitaminosis D appears to be a phenocopy.

Affected infants present with a distinct facial appearance (elfin facies), which becomes more striking with age and includes a depressed nasal bridge, anteverted nares, flat midface with full and dependent checks, long philtrum, thick lips with later drooping of lower lip, wide intercommissural distance, and open mouth. Common eye findings include short palpebral fissures, hypotelorism, epicanthal folds, medial eyebrow flare, strabismus, periorbital fullness, and blue eyes with a stellate iris pattern. Less commonly there may be corneal and/or lenticular opacities. There may be prominence of the ears and thyroid cartilage with age. Various oral anomalies have been described such as hypodontia,

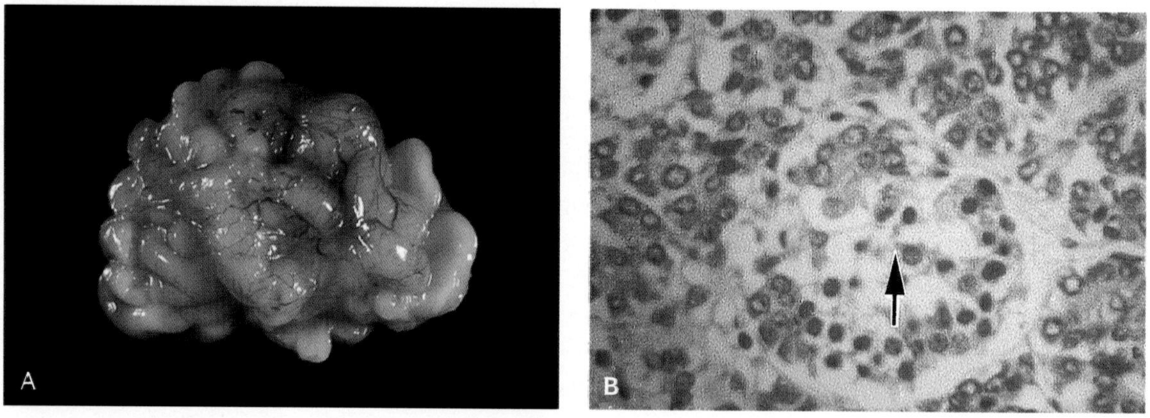

8.27. Smith-Lemli-Opitz syndrome. **(A)** Surface of brain showing very abnormal gyral pattern. **(B)** Smith-Lemli-Opitz syndrome. Microscopic appearance of pancreas showing hyperchromatic islet cells.

microdontia, hypoplasia of the mandible, dental malocclusion, bud-shaped deciduous molars, thickening of the buccal mucous membranes, and prominent and accessory labial frenula. Frequently the voice is hoarse. Numerous cardiovascular findings have been reported particularly supravalvular aortic stenosis, valvular aortic stenosis, aortic hypoplasia, coarctation of the aorta, pulmonary artery stenosis, atrial and ventricular septal defect, anomalous pulmonary venous return, arteriovenous fistula of the lung, interruption of the aortic arch, aplasia of the portal vein, and peripheral artery stenosis. Other features may include craniosynostosis secondary to microcephaly, pectus excavatum, hallux valgus, clinodactyly, hypoplastic deep-set nails, multiple bladder diverticula, small penis, and inguinal and umbilical hernia.

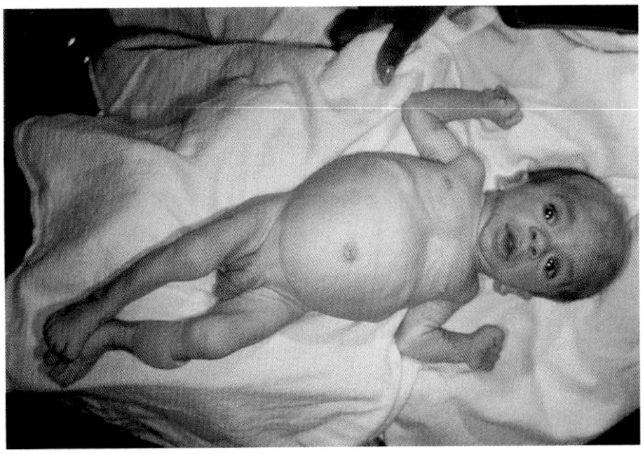

8.28. Leprechaunism. The infant has prominent eyes, thick lips, large ears, a large phallus, a large body, and facial hirsutism. There was hypoglycemia and hyperinsulinemia.

Holt-Oram Syndrome (HOS) (OMIM #142900)

This autosomal dominant syndrome includes skeletal and cardiovascular abnormalities (Figure 8.30). The characteristic findings are a thumb anomaly and/or radial aplasia and atrial septal defect. The thumb may be absent, rudimentary, finger-like, or triphalangeal. Other defects include patent ductus arteriosus, pulmonary hypertension, ventricular septal defect (VSD), and transposition of great vessels. The P-R interval may be prolonged on electrocardiogram.

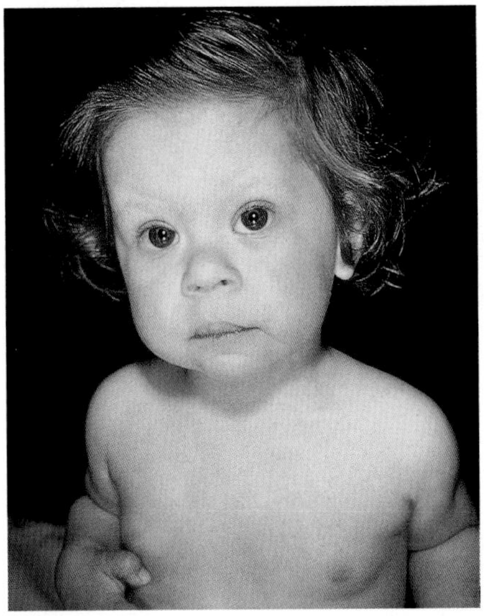

8.29. Williams syndrome. Elfin face with short palpebral fissures, anteverted nares, and everted lips.

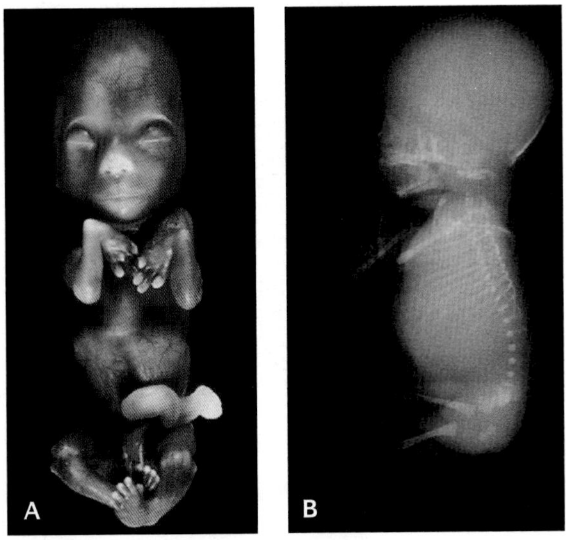

8.30. Holt-Oram syndrome. **(A)** Fetus with radial aplasia. **(B)** X-ray showing radial aplasia. This fetus also had an atrial septal defect.

Like the upper limb malformations, the cardiovascular anomalies are also variable and may be absent in some patients. The cardiac anomaly is usually a secundum-type atrial septal defect, although other cardiac defects may occur.

Thrombocytopenia – Aplasia of Radius (TAR Syndrome) (OMIM *274000)

This autosomal recessive trait includes thrombocytopenia with absence or hypoplasia of megakaryocytes, leukemoid granulocytosis, eosinophilia, anemia and limb defects including absence or hypoplasia of the radius despite the presence of thumbs. These defects are usually bilateral and occur with associated ulnar hypoplasia and defects of the hands, legs, and feet. Abnormalities include a congenital heart defect, spina bifida, brachycephaly, strabismus, micrognathia, syndactyly, short humerus, and dislocation of the hips and less commonly genitourinary anomalies such as unilateral agenesis of the kidney with hypospadias and transposition of the penis and scrotum. Bone marrow shows an absence or decrease in megakaryocytes. Prenatal diagnosis demonstrates the defects of the upper limbs. About 40% die during infancy.

Focal Dermal Hypoplasia (Goltz Syndrome) (OMIM *305600)

This disorder transmitted as an X-linked dominant trait is characterized by atrophy and linear hyperpigmentation of the skin, localized deposits of superficial fat, multiple papillomas of mucous membranes or perioral skin, abnormalities

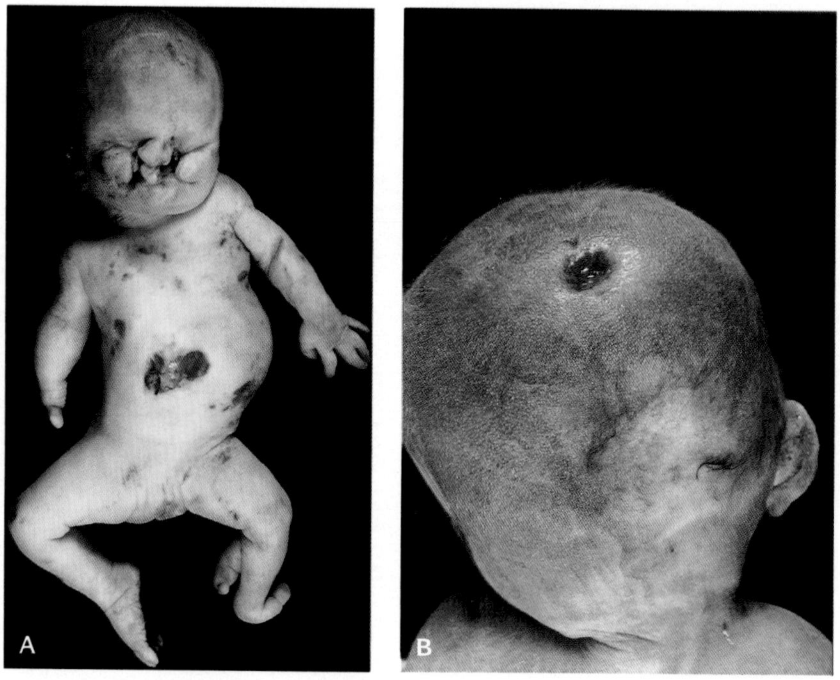

8.31. Goltz syndrome. **(A)** The infant has bilateral facial clefts, anomalies of upper and lower extremities. **(B)** Aplasia of scalp.

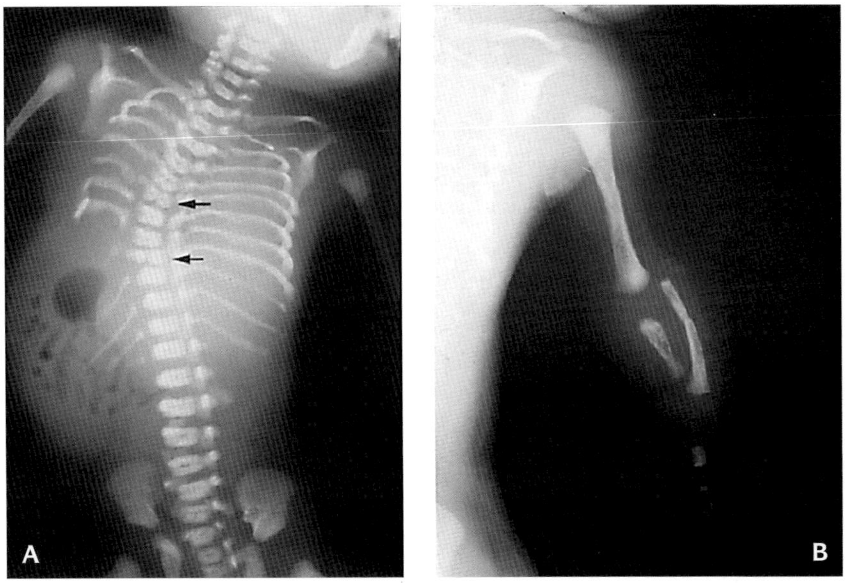

8.32. Goltz syndrome. X-rays **(A)** rib and vertebral anomalies, **(B)** defects of upper limb with short radius and absent metacarpal and phalangeal bones.

of limbs, and anomalies of nails (Figures 8.31 and 8.32). At birth asymmetric skin lesions are usually present in the form of scar-like abnormalities, streaky hyperpigmentation, atrophy, and telangiectasia. Some infants may show isolated areas of total absence of skin. A pathognomonic finding is the presence of soft, yellow, baggy herniations of subcutaneous fat mainly in the regions of the iliac crest, groin, and posterior aspect of thigh. Papillomas frequently develop on the lips, gums, base of tongue, circumoral area, anogenital and inguinal regions, axillae, and around the umbilicus. The scalp hair is usually sparse and brittle, or there may be areas where hair is absent. The nails may be absent, dystrophic, spooned, grooved, or hypopigmented. The most common eye anomalies are chorioretinal and iris colobomata. The external ears may be hypoplastic and deafness has been reported. A frequent hand anomaly is bilateral syndactyly between the third and fourth fingers. Other findings include clinodactyly, polydactyly, oligodactyly, and adactyly. Brachydactyly can be present due to shortened phalanges, metacarpals, or metatarsals. An increase in spontaneous abortions is recognized in the families.

Hydrolethalus Syndrome (See CNS Chapter) (OMIM *236680)

Abnormalities include hydrocephalus, micrognathia, polydactyly, and abnormal lobation of the lungs, as well as microphthalmia, cleft lip or palate, small tongue, anomalous nose, and low-set, malformed ears, and less commonly bilateral pulmonary agenesis (Figures 8.33 and 8.34). The foramen magnum is keyhole-shaped. Renal anomalies include unilateral renal agenesis and hypoplasia or tubular cysts.

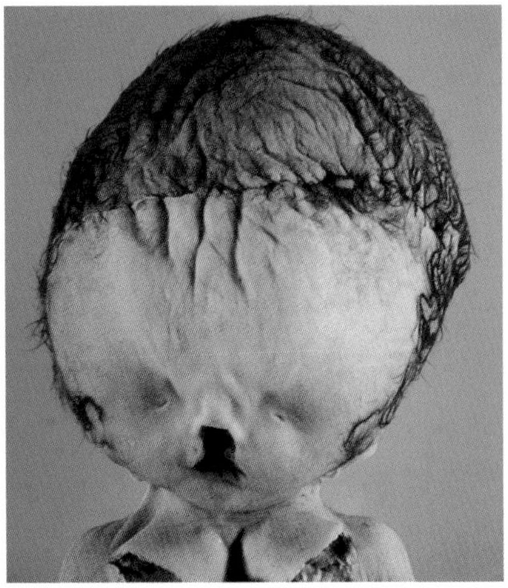

8.33. Hydrolethalus.

Menkes Kinky Hair Syndrome (OMIM #309400)

This is characterized by progressive cerebral deterioration with seizures and twisted fractured hair (pilo torti) (Figure 8.35). A copper deficiency with a defect in intestinal copper absorption results in low serum levels of copper and ceruloplasmin in affected infants. Pudgy cheeks and sparse hair that is stubby and lightly pigmented with twisting and partial breakage with a steel-wool appearance is characteristic.

Skeletal changes include wormian bones of the cranium, metaphyseal widening, particularly of ribs and femora, and lateral spurs. Arteriograms show tortuosity due to deficiency of copper-dependent cross-linking in the internal elastic membrane of the arterial wall. Neurologic deterioration occurs with death in infancy. Torpedo-like swellings of catecholamine-containing axons are seen in the peripheral nerve tracts. Two chromosome breakpoints have been mapped and are contiguous at Xq13. The occipital horn syndrome is a variant of Menkes syndrome. First-trimester prenatal diagnosis has been described with a specific DNA probe.

Seckel Syndrome (OMIM *210600)

Seckel syndrome is a rare autosomal recessive disorder. Severe intrauterine and postnatal growth retardation, microcephaly, and mental retardation characterize this condition (Figure 8.36 and Table 8.11). Craniofacial characteristics include a prominent beaked nose, a sloped forehead, and a receding jaw. Frequently, the ears are low set and the lobules may be hypoplastic with relatively

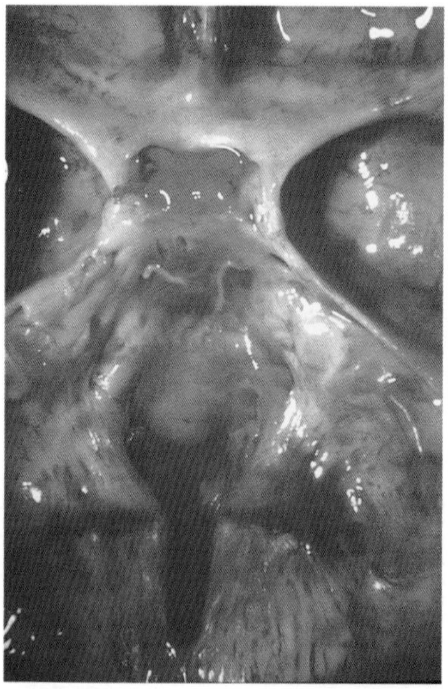

8.34. Hydrolethalus. Keyhole foramen magnum.

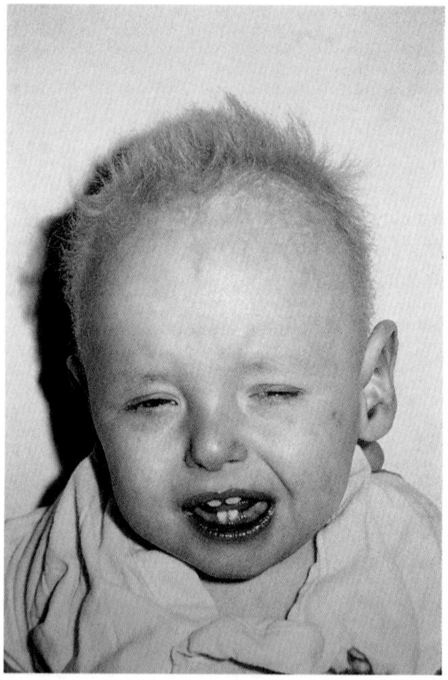

8.35. Menkes kinky hair syndrome. Infant with kinky (steel wool) hair.

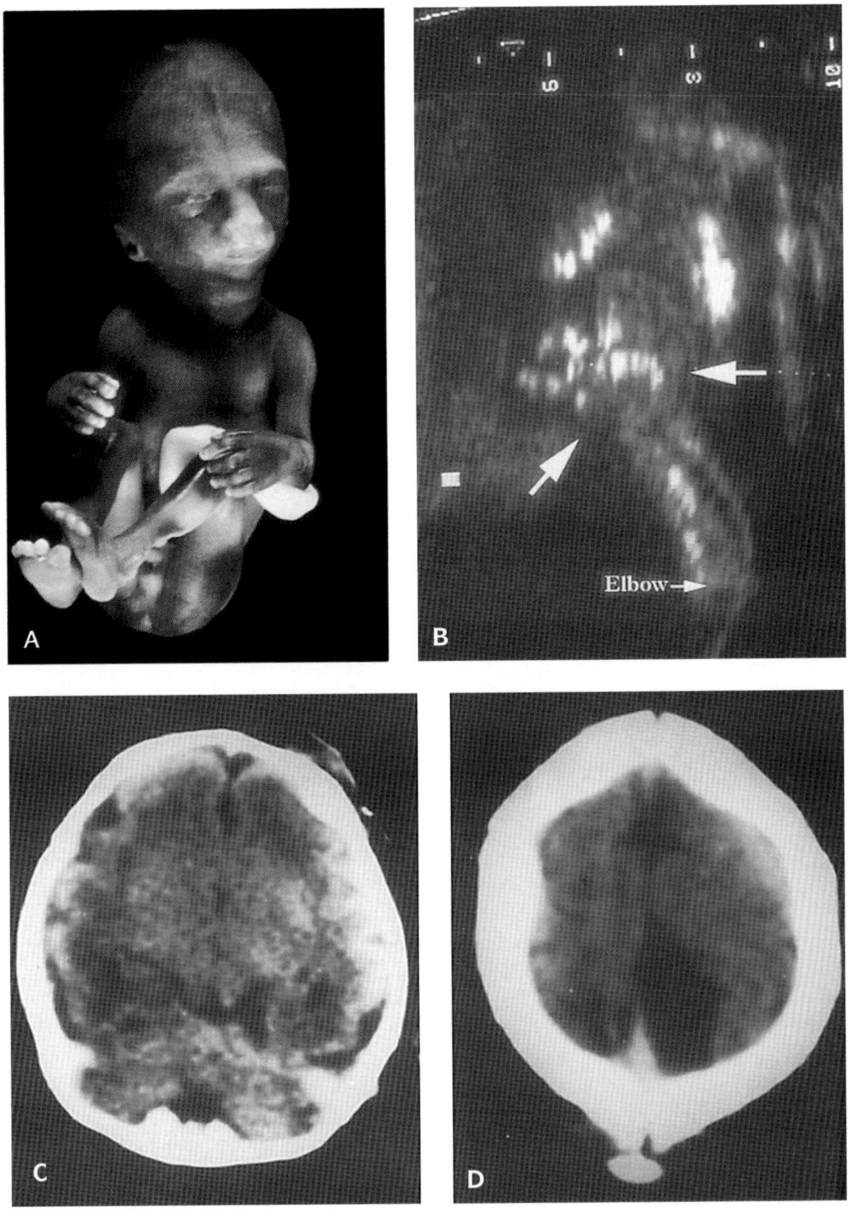

8.36. Seckel syndrome. **(A)** 22-week gestation fetus. **(B)** Ultrasound showing camptodactyly of the second digit (arrow = hand). **(C)** magnetic resonance imaging showing pachygyria and absence of the corpus callosum. **(D)** Cerebral cyst. (Courtesy of Dr. Alan Shanske.)

large eyes with down-slanting palpebral fissures. The palmar dermatoglyphics may be abnormal with or without simian creases.

Characteristic skeletal anomalies include premature closure of the cranial sutures and fifth finger clinodactyly. Dislocation of the radial heads and hips is typical and there is often difficulty with extension of the elbows and knees. Sclerotic areas in the phalanges known as ivory epiphyses are seen. Abnormalities of the central nervous system include complete agyria, overall brain weight markedly decreased, multiple arachnoid cysts, and absent corpus callosum.

Table 8.11 Seckel syndrome

Orofacial anomalies	Pachygyria
Dental abnormalities	Dilated ventricles
Enamel hypoplasia	Urogenital abnormalities
Precocious eruption of teeth	Males
Delayed dental age	Cryptorchidism
Malalignment of teeth	Hypoplasia of testis
High-arched palate	Females
Cleft palate	Clitoromegaly
Craniofacial anomalies	Hypoplasia of labia majora
Microcephaly	Endocrine abnormalities
Receding forehead and chin	Pituitary gland
Prominent nose	Delayed development
Down-slanting palpebral fissures	Decreased adrenocorticotropic hormone production
Ears	Decreased growth hormone production
Low-set	Absence of adenohypophysis
Hypoplastic lobules	Hypophyseal hypoplasia
Skeletal	Precocious puberty
Premature closure of cranial sutures	Adrenal hypoplasia
Fifth finger clinodactyly	Hematopoietic abnormalities
Dislocation of the radial heads	Acute myelogenous leukemia
11 pairs of ribs	Refractory anemia with excess blasts
Disharmonic bone development	Pancytopenia
Hypoplasia of proximal radii and fibulae	Miscellaneous findings
Absence of epiphyseal ossification centers in fingers and toes	Strabismus
Central nervous system	Congenital heart defects
Agyria	Patent ductus arteriosus
Agenesis of the corpus callosum	Atrial septal defects
Arachnoid cysts	Ventricular septal defects
Neuronal heterotopia (cerebral cortex)	Multiple intestinal atresias
Hypoplasia of cerebellar vermis	

The cortical cell layers have irregularly distributed neuroblasts and heterotopic collections of neurons in the white matter polymicrogyria and hypoplasia of the cerebellar vermis, pachygyria, and hydrocephalus may be present. Abnormal dental development with malalignment and crowding of the teeth are described. Serial fetal sonograms may be helpful in making a prenatal diagnosis of Seckel syndrome.

Variants of bird-headed dwarfism are described. Type I osteodysplastic bird-headed dwarfism is distinguished by absence of the acetabula and bowed, broad femora. Agenesis of the corpus callosum and lissencephaly have also been noted. There may also be alopecia. Type II has disproportionately short arms and legs, bone anomalies, and a Seckel-like phenotype.

The etiology of Seckel syndrome remains unclear. These patients have normal karyotypes. The mode of inheritance is thought to be autosomal recessive.

Endocrine abnormalities include hypophyseal hypoplasia, severe testicular atrophy, cryptorchidism, and hypoplasia of the testis and penis. Heart defects may include patent ductus arteriosus, ventricular septal defects, and complex cardiac anomalies. Hematopoietic disorders occur in approximately

20% of patients including acute myeloid leukemia and refractory anemia with excess blasts and pancytopenia.

Zellweger Syndrome (ZS) (OMIM #214100)

This autosomal recessive trait (ZS) is due to a peroxisomal defect. It is lethal in infancy and dominated clinically by severe central nervous system dysfunction. A pear or light-bulb shape of head, large fontanelles, flat occiput, high forehead with shallow supraorbital ridges and flat face, minor ear anomalies, inner epicanthic folds, Brushfield spots of the iris, mild micrognathia, and redundant skin of neck characterize this condition (Figures 8.37 to 8.41 and Table 8.12). Death before 1 year of age usually occurs from respiratory complications. Some atypical cases have hypertonia. Other manifestations are frequent. Stippled calcification of the epiphyses and hepatomegaly and occasional jaundice with increased serum iron content and evidence of tissue siderosis can be seen. Focal lissencephaly with gyral abnormalities, heterotopic cerebral cortex, olivary nuclear dysplasia, defects of the corpus callosum, numerous lipid-laden macrophages and histocytes in cortical and periventricular areas, and dysmyelination. The liver is characterized by micronodular cirrhosis, biliary dysgenesis, and siderosis. The kidneys show cortical cysts, elevated very-long-chain fatty acids, and abnormal bile acids; dicarboxylic aciduria and hypocarnitinemia are helpful in diagnosis.

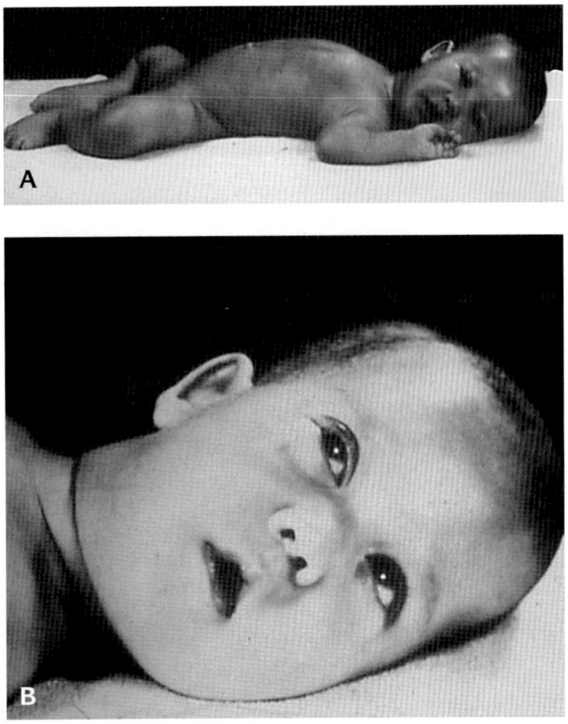

8.37. Zellweger syndrome. **(A)** Infant with hypotonia and **(B)** typical facial appearance.

Persistent fetal lobulations with renal cortical cysts are a consistent finding. They are commonly glomerular in origin and occasionally connect directly to terminal ends of collecting tubules. It is due to defective production of a peroxisomal membrane protein or of a cytochrome *b* oxidase enzyme required for import of peroxisomal proteins into this organelle with the absence of peroxisomes in the liver.

Hyperpipecolic acidemia, hepatic and cerebral glycogen storage, elevated very-long-chain fatty acids, abnormal bile acids, dicarboxylic aciduria, and hypocarnitinemia are biochemical findings.

Prenatal diagnosis of ZS has been established by the observation of an increase in the number of very-long-chain fatty acids, particularly hexacosanoic acids (C26:0 and C26:1), in plasma, cultured skin fibroblasts and amniotic cells, and in a chorionic villus biopsy. There are many complementation groups.

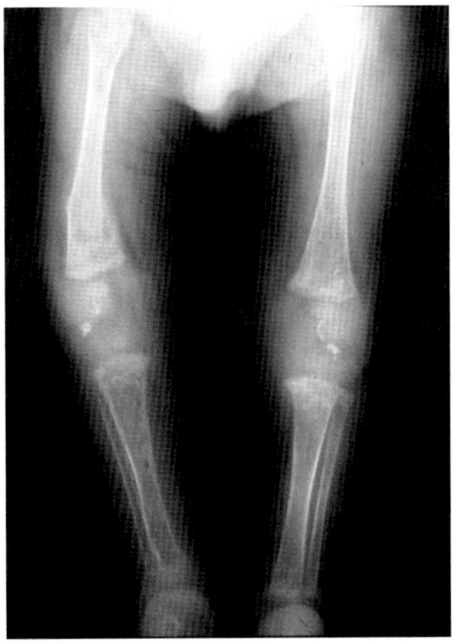

8.38. Zellweger syndrome. X-ray showing stippled calcification of distal femur.

Fryns (anophthalmia-plus) Syndrome (OMIM *229850)

This autosomal recessive multiple congenital anomaly syndrome has a diaphragmatic hernia and distal limb hypoplasia (Figure 8.42). Characteristic features are a broad nasal bridge, microretrognathia, abnormal ears, cleft palate,

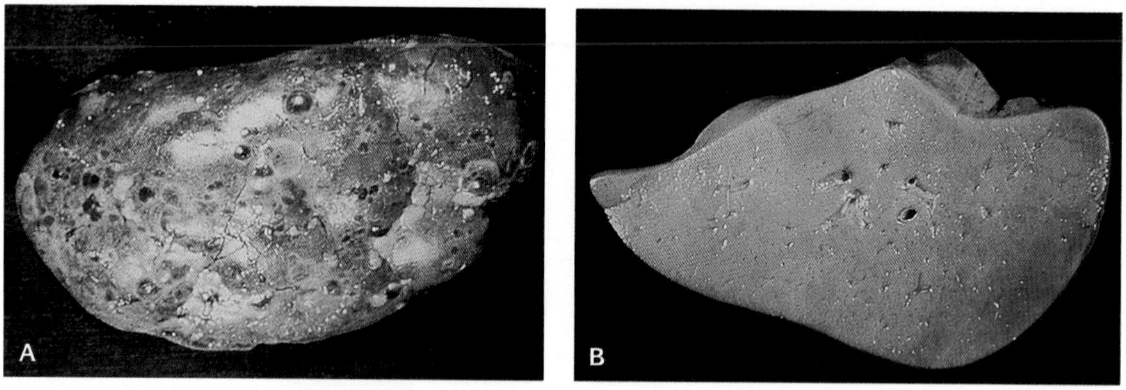

8.39. Zellweger syndrome. **(A)** Capsular surface of cystic kidney. **(B)** Zellweger syndrome. Cut surface of liver showing rust-brown discoloration due to iron accumulation.

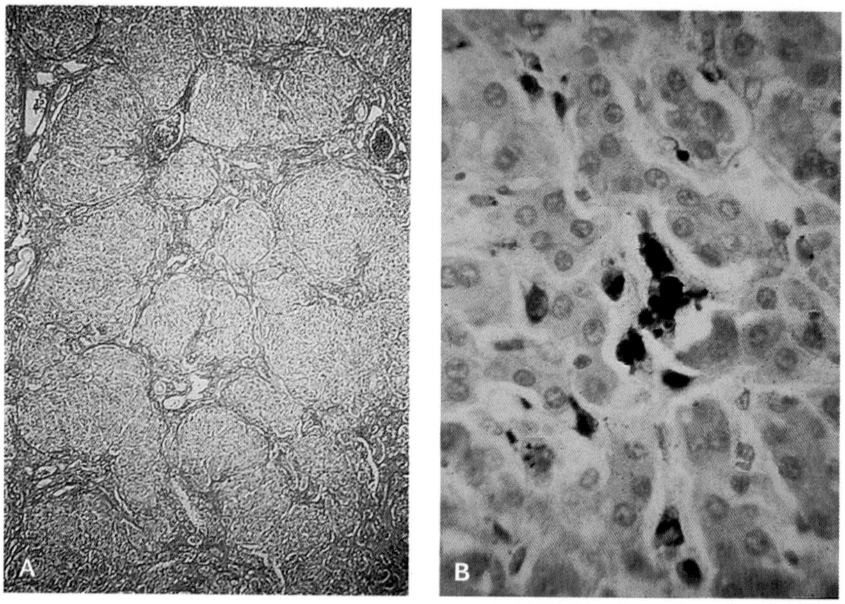

8.40. Zellweger syndrome. Microscopic appearance of liver. **(A)** Showing cirrhosis. **(B)** Iron accumulation in Kupffer cells (Prussian blue stain).

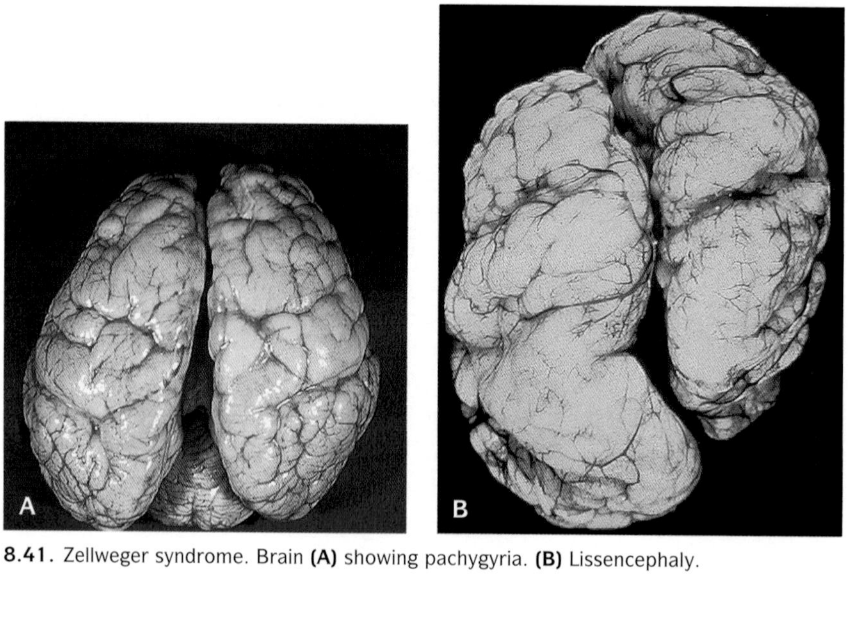

8.41. Zellweger syndrome. Brain **(A)** showing pachygyria. **(B)** Lissencephaly.

Table 8.12 Zellweger syndrome

Craniofacial anomalies	Eyes
Macrocephaly, high forehead, dolichocephaly	Cataracts, prominent Y-suture
Large anterior fontanelle, open metopic suture	Glaucoma
Mongoloid slant of palpebral fissures, hypertelorism, shallow supraorbital ridges, epicanthal folds	Corneal clouding
	Brushfield spots
Highly-arched palate, posterior cleft of palate	Pigmentary retinopathy
Minor anomalies of ears	Optic nerve dysplasia, hypoplasia
Central nervous system	Radiological abnormalities
Hypotonia, rarely hypertonia	Chondrodysplasia calcificans (especially patellae)
Severe mental retardation	Delayed skeletal maturation
Seizures	Bell-shaped thorax
Nystagmus, oculogyric fits	Large fontanelles
Absent neonatal reflexes	Other
Limbs	Cardiac defects
Talipes equinovarus	Jaundice with hepatomegaly
Camptodactyly	Cryptorchidism, clitoromegaly
Contractures	Simian creases
	DiGeorge developmental field defect

facial clefts, digital hypoplasia, urogenital abnormalities, microphthalmia, or anophthalmia, and perinatal mortality; distal limb defects, central nervous system malformations with hydrocephalus, renal cystic dysplasia and cardiac defects are described. Mosaicism for a tandem duplication of 1q24-q31–2 is present. Abnormalities of chromosome 15, 6, and 22 have all been reported in cases of possible Fryns syndrome. It is perinatally lethal.

Batsocas-Papas Syndrome (Popliteal Pterygium syndrome) (119500)

This rare autosomal recessive disorder is a lethal multiple pterygium syndrome

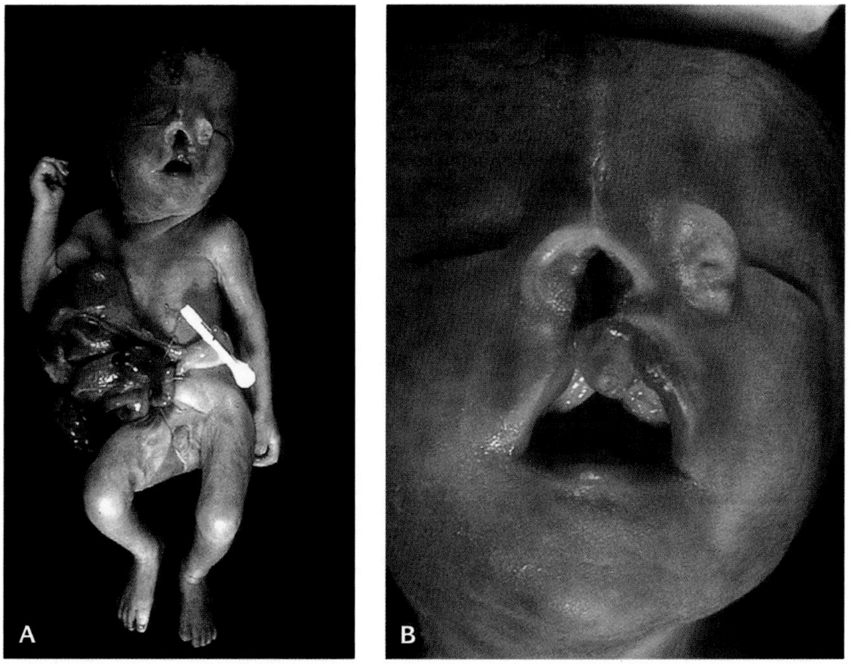

8.42. Fryns syndrome. **(A)** Fetus 32-weeks gestation with facial defects and gastroschisis. **(B)** Facial clefting and duplication of nose.

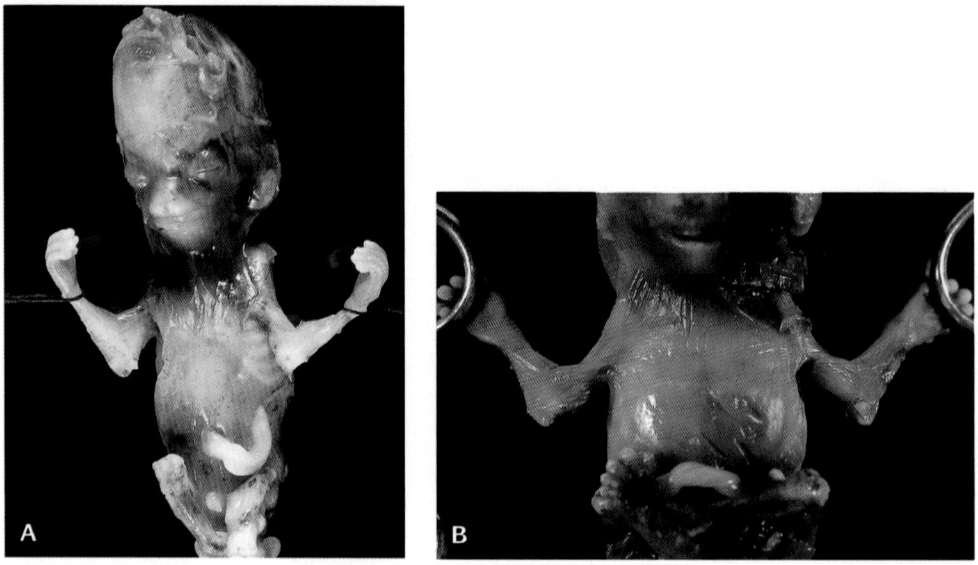

8.43. Batsocas-Papas syndrome. **(A)** Fetus with pterygia at elbows and axilla 15-weeks gestation. **(B)** Fetus, sibling of **(A)** showing similar features. Diaphragmatic hernias were also present.

(Figure 8.43). Microcephaly, digital hypoplasia, and syndactyly occur and bilateral oral and facial clefts, syndactyly of the hands and feet, bilateral aplasia of the thumbs, and phalangeal hypoplasia are described. This is a distinct form of the lethal multiple pterygium syndromes with associated malformations. Most cases of Bartsocas-Papas syndrome are of Mediterranean origin.

REFERENCES

Cohen MM: Craniosynostosis. *The Child With Multiple Birth Defects*, 2nd ed. Oxford, Oxford University Press, 1997, p. 178.

Cohen MM Jr, Neri G, Weksberg R: Overgrowth syndromes. *Oxford Monographs on Medical Genetics No. 41*. Oxford, Oxford University Press, 2002.

Gilbert-Barness E, Opitz JM: Congenital anomalies and malformation syndromes. In Stocker JT and Dehner LP (eds): *Pediatric Pathology*, 2nd ed, vol. 1, Philadelphia, Lippincott, 2001, p. 113.

Gilbert-Barness E, Opitz JM: Congenital anomalies and malformation syndromes. In Wiggleworth JS, Singer DB (eds): *Textbook of Fetal and Perinatal Pathology*, 2nd ed, Boston, Blackwell Scientific, 1998, p. 323.

Goelz SE, Hamilton SR, Vogelstein B: Purification of DNA from formaldehyde fixed and paraffin embedded human tissue. *Biochem Biophys Res Comm* 130:118, 1985.

Kantaputra PN, Gorlin RJ, Ukarapol N, et al.: Robinow (fetal face) syndrome: report of a boy with dominant type and an infant with recessive type. *Am J Med Genet* 84:1, 1999.

Larsen WJ: *Essentials of Human Embryology*. NY, Churchill Livingstone, 1998.

Li M, Squire JA, Weksbeg R: Molecular genetics of Wiedemann-Beckwith syndrome. *Am J Med Genet* 79:253, 1998.

Martínez-Frías ML, Frías JL, Opitz JM: Errors of morphogenesis and developmental field theory. *Am J Med Genet* 76:291, 1998.

Martínez-Frías ML, Urioste M, Bermejo E, Rodríguez-Pinilla E, Félix V, Parisan L, Martínez S, Egües J, Gómez F, Aparicio P, Cucalon F, Arroyo A, Meipp C, Vázquez S, Rodríguez

JI, Rosa A, Garcia J, Jiménez N, Moro C. Primary midline developmental field II. Clinical/epidemiological analysis of alterations of laterality (normal body symmetry and asymmetry). *Am J Med Genet* 56:382, 1995.

Martínez-Frías ML, Frías JL, Vazquez I, Ferandez J: Bartsocas-Papas syndrome: three familial cases from Spain. *Am J Med Genet* 39:34, 1991.

McKusick VA: *Mendelian Inheritance in Man*, 12th ed, Baltimore, Johns Hopkins University Press, 1998.

Moore KL, Persaud TVN: *The Developing Human*, 5th ed, Philadelphia, WB Saunders, 1993.

Ness GC, Borrego O, Gilbert-Barness E: Increased expression of low-density lipoprotein receptors in a Smith-Lemli-Opitz infant with elevated bilirubin levels. *Am J Med Genet* 68:294, 1997.

Opitz JM, Wilson GN: Causes and pathogenesis of birth defects. In Gilbert-Barness E (ed): *Potter's Pathology of the Fetus and Infant*, St. Louis, Mosby-Year Book, 1997, p. 44.

Opitz JM, Wilson GN, Gilbert-Barness: Malformations, malformation syndromes, and deformations. In Gilbert-Barness E (ed): *Potter's Atlas of Fetal and Infant Pathology*, St. Louis, Mosby, 1998, p. 1.

Stevenson RE, Hall JG, Goodman RM: Human Malformations. New York, Oxford University Press, 1993.

Warburg M, Jensen H, Prause JU, Bolund S, et al.: Anophthalmia-microphthalmia-oblique clefting syndrome: confirmation of the Fryns anophthalmia syndrome. *Am J Med Genet* 73:36, 1997.

NINE

Dysplasias

Dysplasias are defects of tissue differentiation or defects of histogenesis. These involve principally connective tissue, bone, blood vessels, skin. Dysplasias are characterized by the abnormal growth of tissues. They are frequently caused by autosomal dominant mutations, rarely by the homozygous state of recessive mutations. Occasionally caused by teratogens, dysplasias are not biochemically defined. They are primarily expressed as extensive, multiple, or generalized abnormalities of one type of tissue.

CONNECTIVE TISSUE DYSPLASIAS

Neurofibromatosis (von Recklinghausen Disease) (OMIM *162200)

Neurofibromatosis is inherited as an autosomal dominant trait; 50% represent a new mutation.

Type I, peripheral neurofibromatosis, affects 1 in 4,000 live births; the gene is on chromosome 17. It is associated with the presence of six or more café-au-lait spots more than 5 mm in diameter in children; neurofibromas and plexiform neurofibromas occur along nerves (Figures 9.1 to 9.7 and Tables 9.1 to 9.3). Hamartomatous lesions include lipomas, angiomas, optic gliomas, iris hamartomas, sphenoid dysplasia, and frequently local overgrowth and

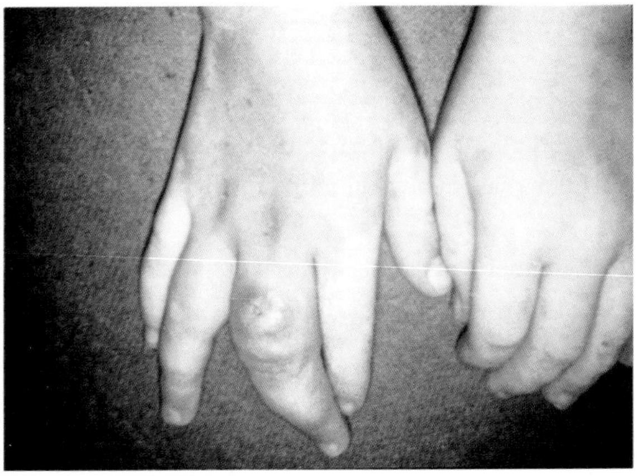

9.1. Hypertrophy of middle finger in neurofibromatosis.

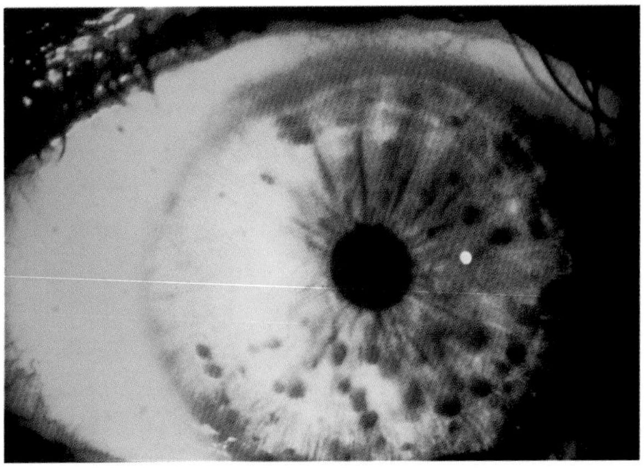

9.2. Lisch nodules of iris of eye in neurofibromatosis.

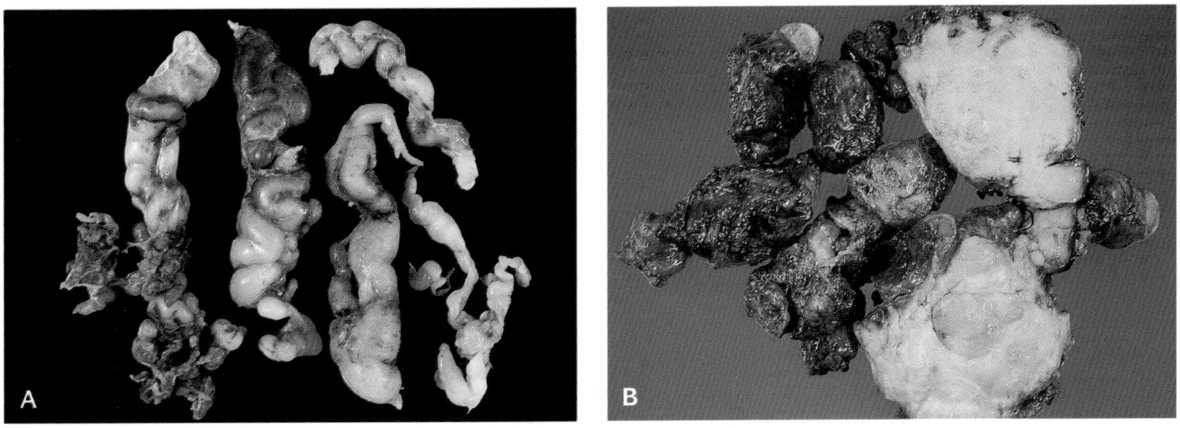

9.3. **(A)** Resected hypertrophied peripheral nerves with multiple nodules of neurofibromas. **(B)** Cut surface of a neurofibroma.

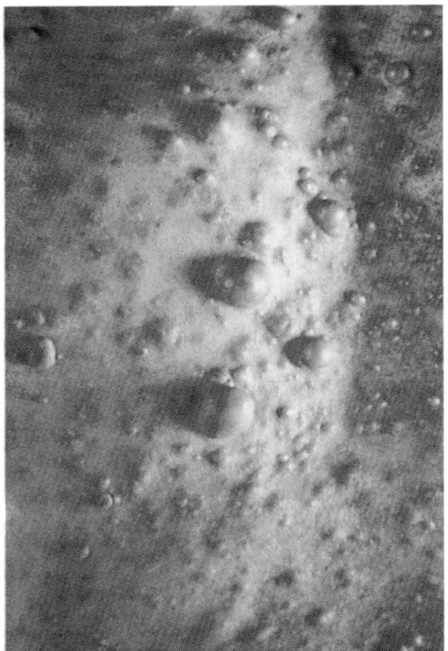

9.4. Multiple neurofibromatosis of skin.

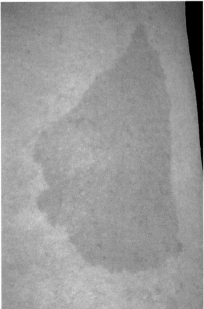

9.5. Café-au-lait lesion in neurofibromatosis (coast of California).

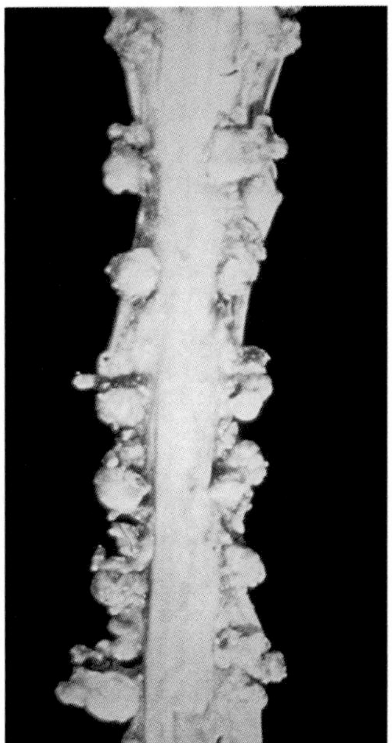

9.6. Spinal cord with multiple neurofibromas of spinal nerves.

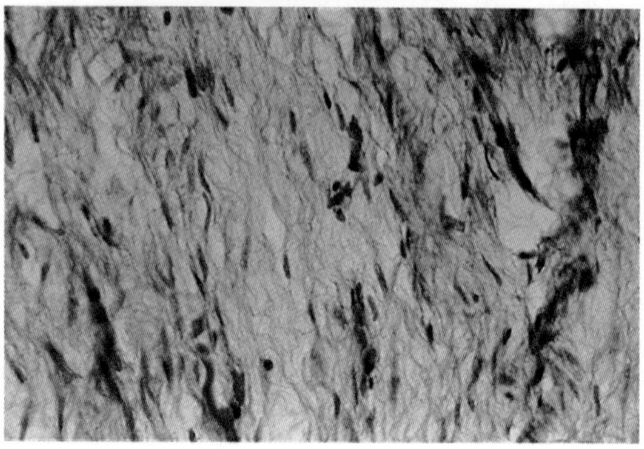

9.7. Neurofibromatosis. Microscopic appearance showing spindle cells in parallel array.

hemihypertrophy. Malignant change occurs in approximately 3–15%. An intestinal form may involve the length of the gastrointestinal tract.

Type 2, central neurofibromatosis, has an incidence of 1 in 50,000. The gene is on chromosome 22. It includes acoustic schwannomas, neurofibromas, meningiomas, gliomas, schwannomas, and lenticular opacity.

Type 3 is the intermediate type with neurofibromas limited to the gastrointestinal tract.

Type 4 is a variant form.

Table 9.1 Types of neurofibromatosis

Name	OMIM	Inheritance pattern	Chromosome localization of gene	Gene	Types of mutation	Comments
Neurofibromatosis, type 1 (NF1)	162200	Autosomal dominant	17q11.2	NF1	Nonsense Deletions Insertions Missense	NF1 most common type NF1 gene product = neurofibromin tumor suppressor gene. There are several partial NF1 gene copies (pseudogenes) on other chromosomes that occurred during evolution
Neurofibromatosis, type 2 (NF2)	101000	Autosomal dominant	22q12.2	NF2	Nonsense Frameshift Missense (rare)	NF2 gene product = merlin tumor suppressor gene
Neurofibromatosis, type 3, Riccardi type	162260	Sporadic	–	–	–	Combined NF1 and NF2 features with some added distinctive findings: neurofibromas of palms and absent Lisch nodules. CNS tumors in 2nd and 3rd decades usually lead to rapid and fatal course
Neurofibromatosis, type 3, Intestinal type	162220	Autosomal dominant	?12	–	–	Neurofibromas limited to intestine
Neurofibromatosis, type 4		Autosomal dominant	–	–	–	Variant form (s) that differ from NF1, NF2, and NF3, Riccardi type
Familial spinal neurofibromatosis	162210	Autosomal dominant	17q11.2	NF1	Frameshift mutation in exon 46	Although spinal neurofibromatosis is a serious complication in 1–2% of NF1 patients and occurs more commonly in NF2, several families have only spinal neurofibromatosis
Duodenal carcinoid syndrome	162240					Combination of duodenal carcinoid tumor, neurofibromatosis, and pheochromocytoma

Source: Cohen MM Jr: Some neoplasms and some hamartomatous syndromes: Genetic considerations. *Int J Oral Maxillofac Surg* 27:363–369, 1998, Munksgaard International Pub Ltd., Copenhagen, Denmark.

Table 9.2 Neurofibromatosis (von Recklinghausen disease)

Peripheral nerves	Automatic nerves	Cranial nerves	Central nervous system
Cutaneous tumors Plexiform neuromas ↓ Hemihypertrophy (digits or limbs) Oral neurofibromas -enlarged lips -macroglossis	Vagal neuromas Intestinal obstruction Glaucoma	Optic gliomas Acoustic neuromas (may be familial) Trigeminal or hypoglossal neuromas	Multiple meningiomas Gliomas Choroid plexus tumors Ependymomas Ganglioneuromas ↓ Mental retardation Epilepsy ↑ Intracranial pressure Proptosis
	↓ Sarcomatous degeneration (5–10%) Fibrosarcomas and myxosarcomas More common in males		

Table 9.3A Clinical manifestations of NF-1

Skin lesions	Vascular dysplasia
Café-au-lait macules (>6 macules >5cm)	Aneurysms
Cutaneous neurofibromas	Megalencephaly
Plexiform neurofibromas	Fibrous dysplasia of bones
Various other hamartomas	Scoliosis
Freckling in intertriginous areas	Short stature
Xanthomatosis	Pseudoarthrosis
Granuloma annulare	Overgrowth of body parts, elephantiasis included
Melanosis of palms, soles, penis	Central nervous system effects
Visceral neurofibromas in gastrointestinal and genitourinary tracts	Learning disabilities
Subcutaneous neurofibromas	Lisch nodules
Pruritus	Pheochromocytoma
Renal artery stenosis	White matter lesion
Moyamoya disease	Malignant degeneration
	Seizures
	Mental retardation

Table 9.3B Clinical manifestations of NF-2

Plaque-like neurofibromas	Nuclear cataracts
Café-au-lait macules (rare)	Dorsal root schwannomas
Lisch nodules (very frequent)	Brain meningiomas
Pigment epithelial and retinal hamartomas	Acoustic neuromas
Cranial nerve schwannomas	Subcapsular lens opacities

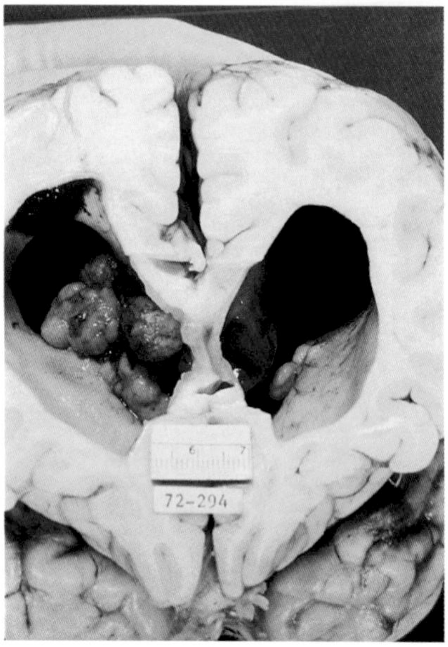

9.8. Coronal section of brain showing subependymal glial nodules in the ventricles, candle guttering.

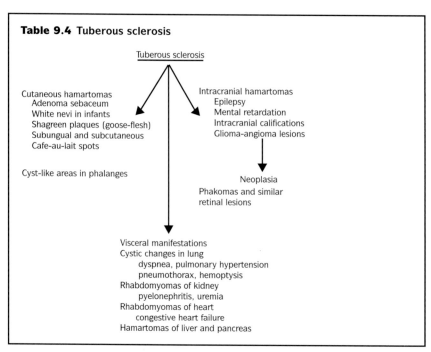

Table 9.4 Tuberous sclerosis

Tuberous sclerosis

- Cutaneous hamartomas
  - Adenoma sebaceum
  - White nevi in infants
  - Shagreen plaques (goose-flesh)
  - Subungual and subcutaneous
  - Cafe-au-lait spots
- Cyst-like areas in phalanges
- Intracranial hamartomas
  - Epilepsy
  - Mental retardation
  - Intracranial calcifications
  - Glioma-angioma lesions
    - Neoplasia
    - Phakomas and similar retinal lesions
- Visceral manifestations
  - Cystic changes in lung
    - dyspnea, pulmonary hypertension
    - pneumothorax, hemoptysis
  - Rhabdomyomas of kidney
    - pyelonephritis, uremia
  - Rhabdomyomas of heart
    - congestive heart failure
  - Hamartomas of liver and pancreas

Tuberous Sclerosis (See Also Renal Chapter) (TS) (OMIM # 191100)

This is an autosomal dominant mutation; approximately 60% are new mutations. Incidence is between 1:10,000 and 1:40,000 (Figures 9.8 to 9.14 and Table 9.4). Two types are TSC1 mapped to 9q34 and TSC2 mapped to 16p13. Hamartin is the gene product of TSC1 and Tuberlin is the gene product of TSC2. The disorder is characterized by seizures, mental retardation, and facial angiofibromas as well as hypomelanotic macules, shagreen patches, fibromas, and café-au-lait spots. Hamartomas involve the heart (rhabdomyoma), kidney (angiomyolipomatosis), lung (lymphangiomatosis), spleen (hemangiomatosis),

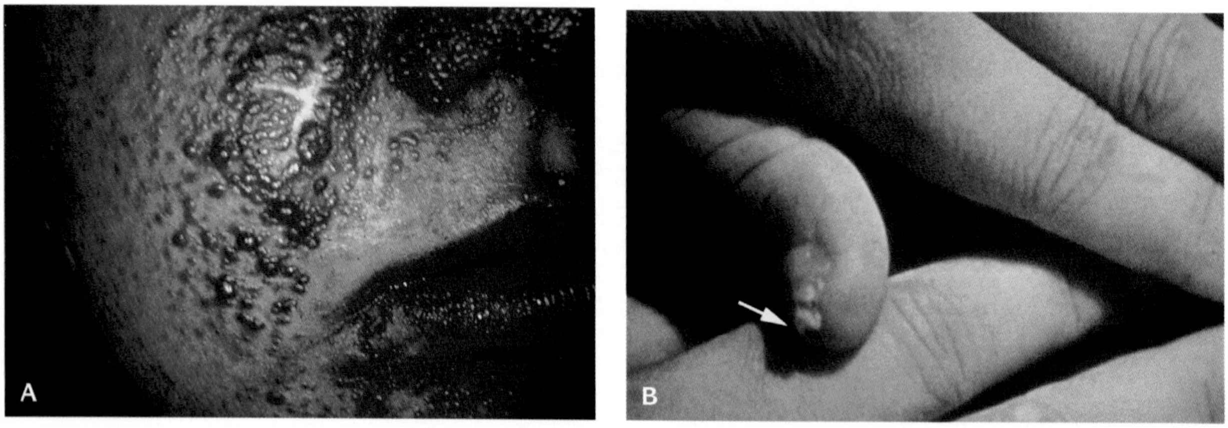

9.9. (A) Angiofibromas of the skin of the face in tuberous sclerosis. **(B)** Subungual nodule (arrow).

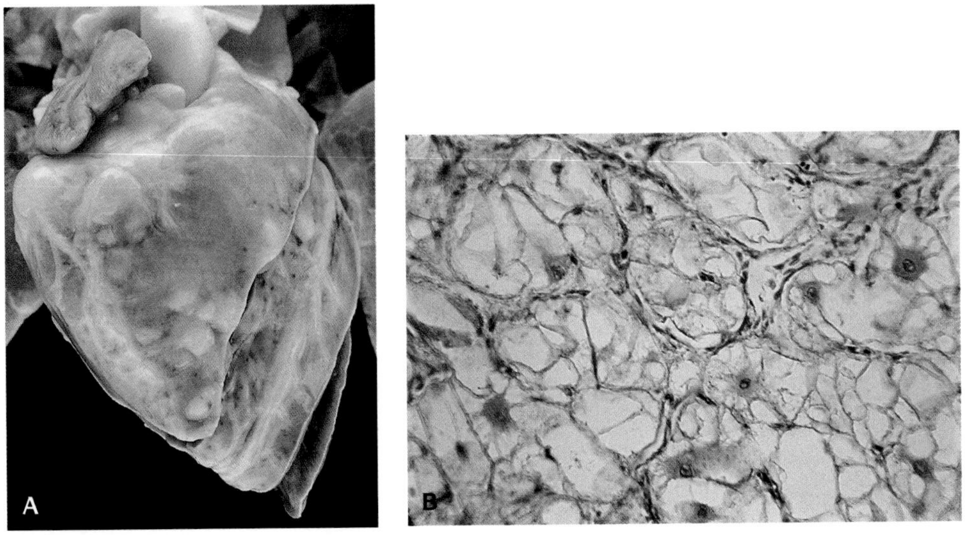

9.10. (A) Rhabdomyomas involving the epicardium of the heart. **(B)** Microscopic appearance showing typical "spider" cells.

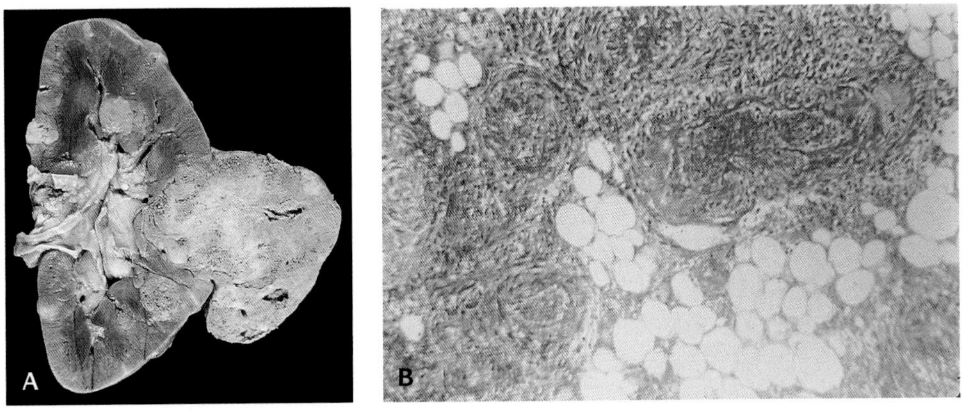

9.11. (A) Angiomyolipomas of kidney in tuberous sclerosis. **(B)** Microscopic appearance showing hamartomatous proliferation of blood vessels, smooth muscle, and adipose tissue.

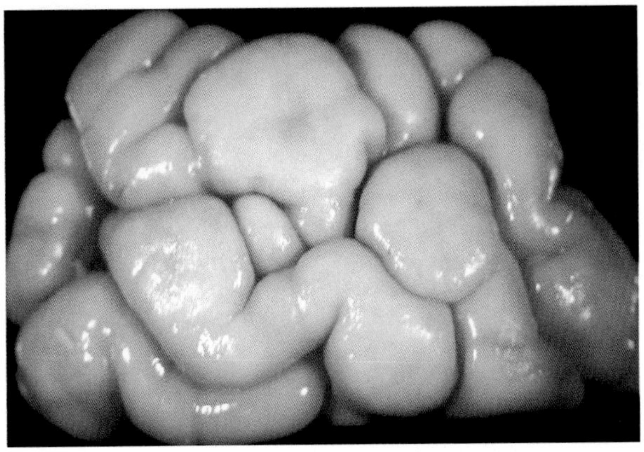

9.12. Pachygyria of the brain in tuberous sclerosis.

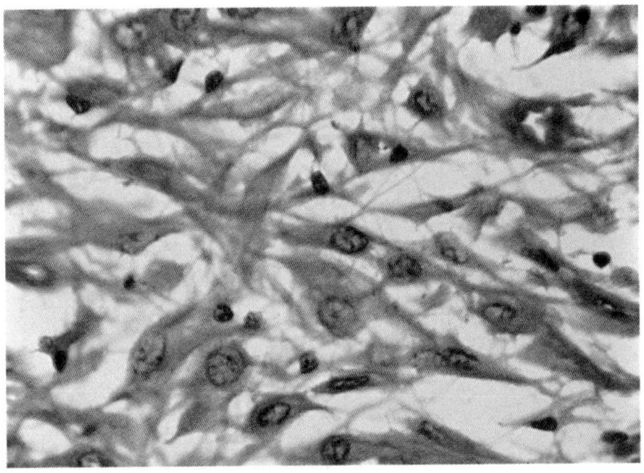

9.13. Microscopic appearance of giant cell astrocytoma in tuberous sclerosis.

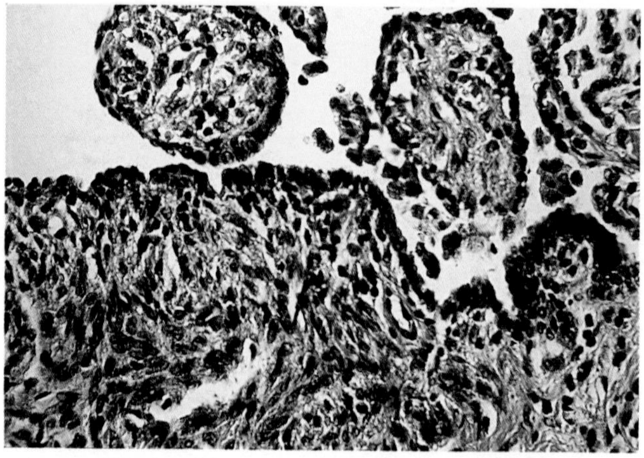

9.14. Leiomyomatosis in the lung in tuberous sclerosis.

liver (hemangiomatosis), and bone (fibrous dysplasia). Cysts occur in the kidneys.

The brain shows pachygyria with cortical tubers. Subependymal glial nodules appear as "candle guttering" along the wall of the lateral ventricles.

von Hippel-Lindau Disease (See Also Renal Chapter) (vHL) (OMIM *193300)

This is an autosomal dominant trait. It is characterized by angiomatosis retinae, keratoangiomas and hemangioblastomas of the cerebellum (Figures 9.15 and 9.16 and Tables 9.5 and 9.6). Hemangiomas may involve the face, adrenal, lung, and liver, and multiple cysts of the pancreas, kidney, and epididymis. Renal cysts are lined by plump clear cells that may proliferate and result in renal cell carcinoma in 25% of cases. The gene has been localized to 3p25–26. The renal cell carcinoma gene has also been mapped to 3p25–26. As

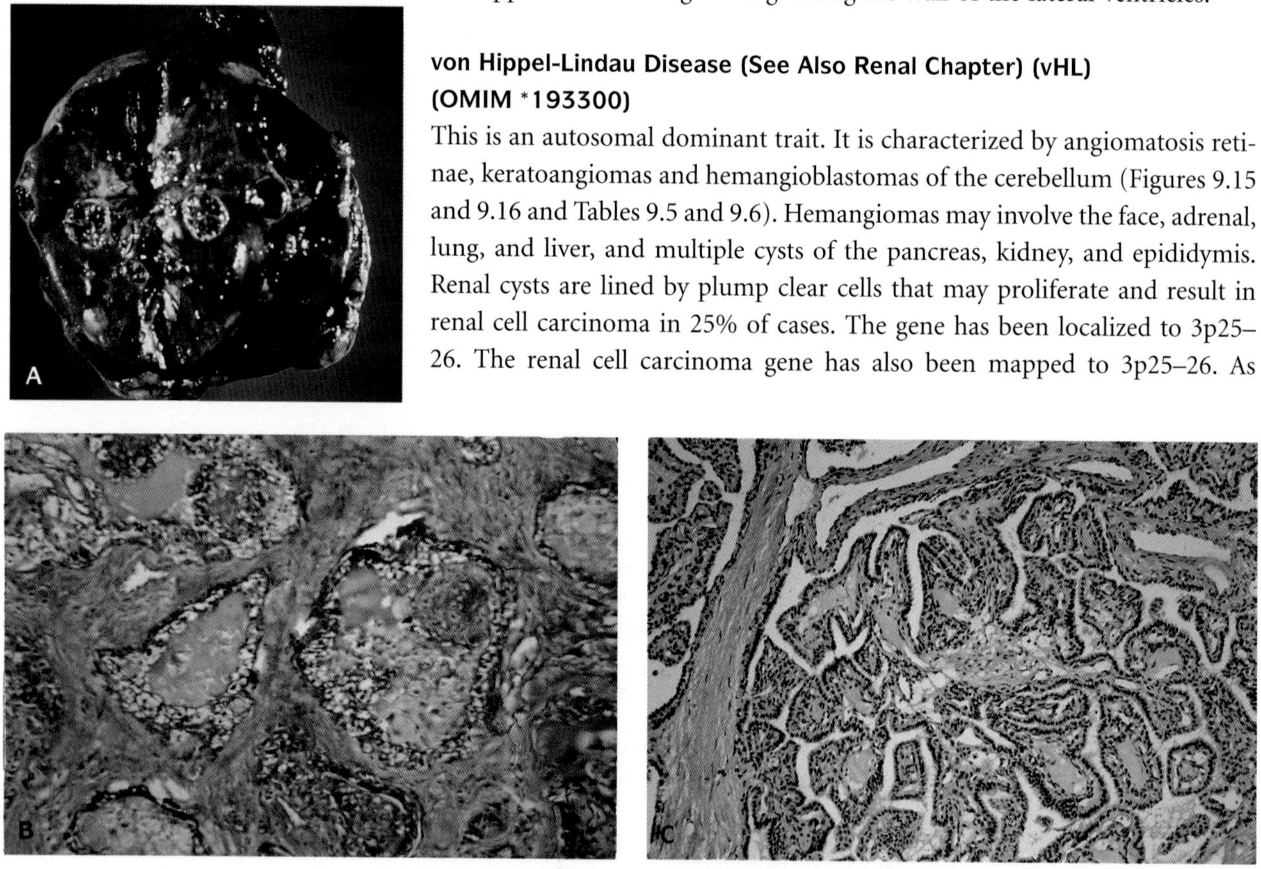

9.15. Renal cysts in von Hippel Lindau disease. (A) Gross appearance. (B) Microscopic appearance. (C) Epididymis with papillary change and cyst formation.

Table 9.5 Inheritance of von Hippel Lindau syndrome

Large germline deletions detectable by:	
	Southern blot analysis in 19%
	pulsed-field gel electrophoresis in 3%
Pheochromocytoma-associated mutations (62%)	
	arginine 238 to tyrosine
	arginine 238 to glycine
Islet tumors result from loss of proximal 3p allele	
Renal cell carcinoma (RCC) is also mapped to 3p26–25	

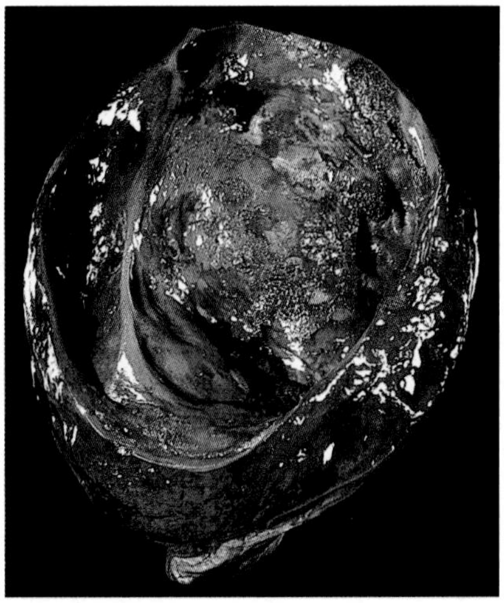

9.16. Pheochromocytoma in von Hippel Lindau disease. Note the thin rim of adrenal at the bottom edge.

Table 9.6 von-Hippel Lindau

Retinae	Hemangioblastoma usually with calcification
Brain	Cerebellar hemangioblastoma
Pancreas	Simple cysts
	Hemangioblastoma
	Papillary cystadenoma
Epididymus	Simple cysts and papillary cystadenomas
Liver	Adenoma
	Simple cysts
	Angiomas
Spleen	Angiomas
Adrenal cortex	Adenomas
Adrenal medulla	Pheochromocytoma
Lung	Cysts
Meninges	Meningiomas
Bones	Cysts
	Angiomas
Bladder	Hemangioblastoma
Skin and mucosa	Nevi
	Angiomas
Omentum	Cysts
Mesocolon	Cysts

many as 75 different mutations within the gene have been described. vHL types 1 (without pheochromocytoma), 2A (with pheochromocytoma), and 2B (with pheochromocytoma and renal cell carcinoma) may be related to Wyburn-Mason syndrome (arteriovenous aneurysm of retina and midbrain with facial nevi or hamartomas). The vHL gene may be a recessive tumor suppressor gene. Loss of heterozygosity (LOH) alone does not appear to be sufficient for hamartomas to develop; LOH has been found not only at 3p26 but also at 5q21, 13q, and 17q.

Marfan Syndrome (OMIM #154700)

Marfan syndrome is an autosomal dominant mutation and is characterized by tall stature with long slender limbs, joint laxity, scoliosis and hypotonia, dislocation of the lens, myopia, retinal detachment and cardiovascular complications

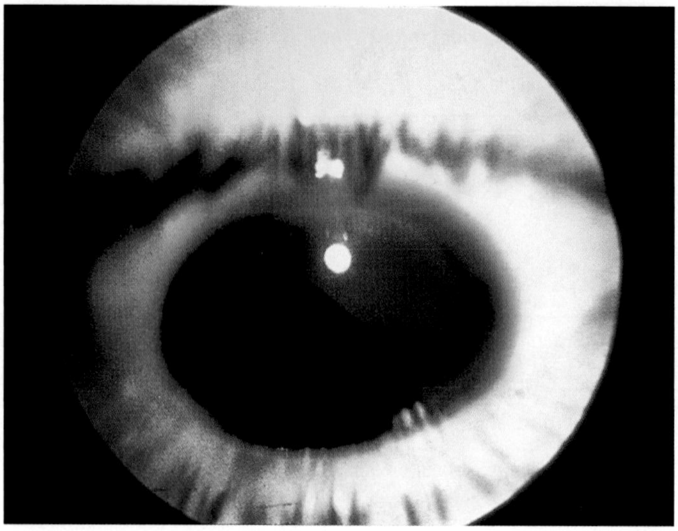

9.17. Dislocation of the lens of the eye in Marfan syndrome.

(Figures 9.17 to 9.19 and Table 9.7). Glucosaminoglycans accumulate in the connective tissue, skin, lung, kidney, cartilage, tendon, muscle, cornea, and ciliary zonule as well as in vascular smooth muscle. The fibrillin gene for Marfan syndrome has been localized to chromosome 15q15-21.3. At least two genes encoding fibrillin collagen have been identified. Many mutations in the fibrillin gene have been reported that, along with compound heterozygotes between them, explain much of the syndrome's great variability. About 25% of affected individuals arise as new mutations. The mean paternal age effect is increased in sporadic cases.

PROTEUS SYNDROME (OMIM 176920)

This is a sporadic overgrowth dysplasia syndrome characterized by lipomatosis, nevi, phakomatosis, Klippel-Trenaunay-Weber-like vascular anomalies, and

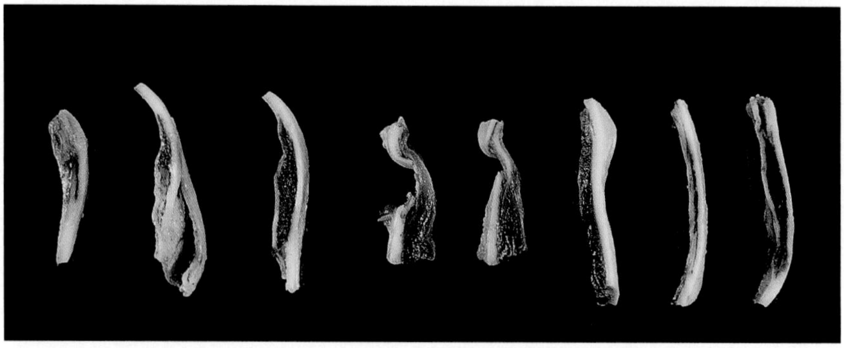

9.18. Strips of a resected aorta showing dissection in Marfan syndrome.

Table 9.7 Marfan syndrome

Clinical manifestations

Tall with marfanoid habitus	Cleft palate sometimes
Ligamentous laxity leading to joint hypermobility	Inguinal hernias
Arachnodactyly	Atrophic striae distensae
Scoliosis	Retinal detachment, glaucoma
Ectopia lentis	Myopia, keratoconus, megalocornea, hypoplasia of iris
Dilatation of the ascending aorta	Spontaneous pneumothorax

Main phenotypic manifestations

Skeletal system
Anterior chest deformity, especially asymmetric pectus excavatum/carinatum
Dolichostenomelia not due to scoliosis
Arachnodactyly
Vertebral column deformity
Scoliosis
Tall stature, especially compared to unaffected parents and sibs
High, narrowly arched palate
Crowding of teeth
Protrusio acetabulae
Abnormal joint mobility
Congenital flexion contractures
Hypermobility

Skin and integument
Striae distensae without obvious cause
Hernia

Cardiovascular system
Dilatation of the ascending aorta*
Aortic dissection*
Aortic regurgitation
Mitral regurgitation
Mitral valve prolapse

Pulmonary system
Spontaneous pneumothorax

Ocular system
Ectopia lentis*
Elongated globe
Retinal detachment
Myopia

Central nervous system
Dural ectasia*
Widening of the lumbosacral canal and neural foramina

Diagnostic criteria

With a first-degree relative with Marfan syndrome
1. Involvement of at least two systems
2. At least one major manifestation (although this requirement is age dependent and occasionally depends on peculiarities of the family's phenotype)

With no first-degree relative affected by Marfan syndrome, the proband must have
1. Involvement of the skeleton
2. Involvement of at least two other systems
3. At least one major manifestation

* Major manifestations

Source: Gilbert-Barness E, Barness LA: *Metabolic Diseases: Foundations of Clinical Management, Genetics and Pathology*, Vol. II, Natick, MA, Eaton Publishing, 2000.

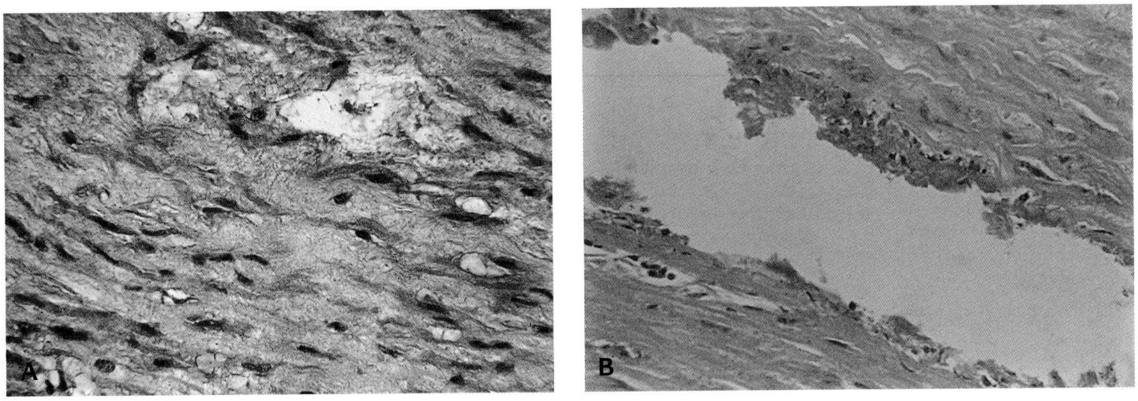

9.19. **(A)** Microscopic appearance of cystic medionecrosis in Marfan syndrome. **(B)** Dissection of aortic wall.

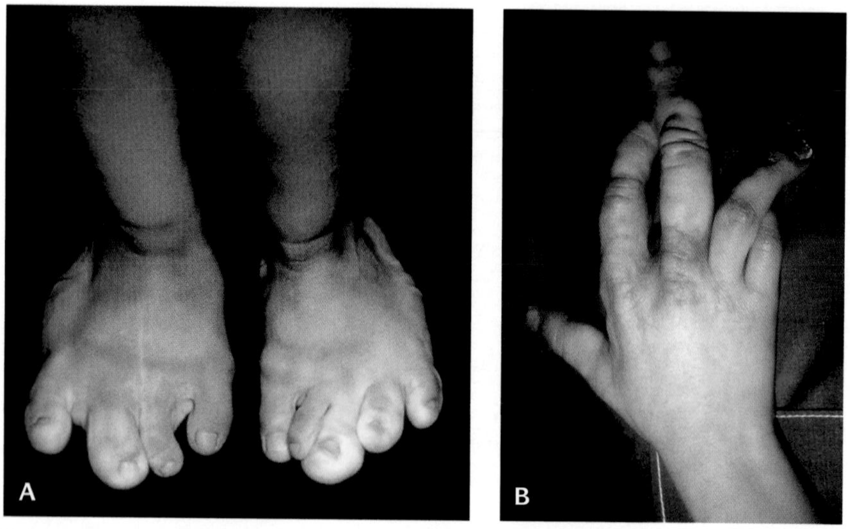

9.20. Proteus syndrome. **(A)** Dorsal surface of feet. **(B)** Overgrowth of fingers.

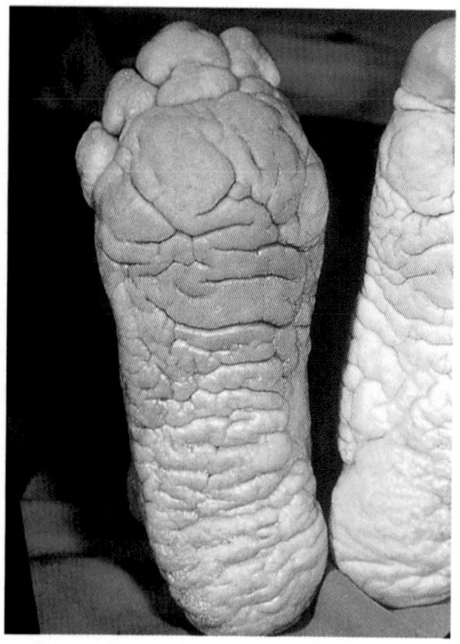

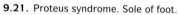

9.21. Proteus syndrome. Sole of foot.

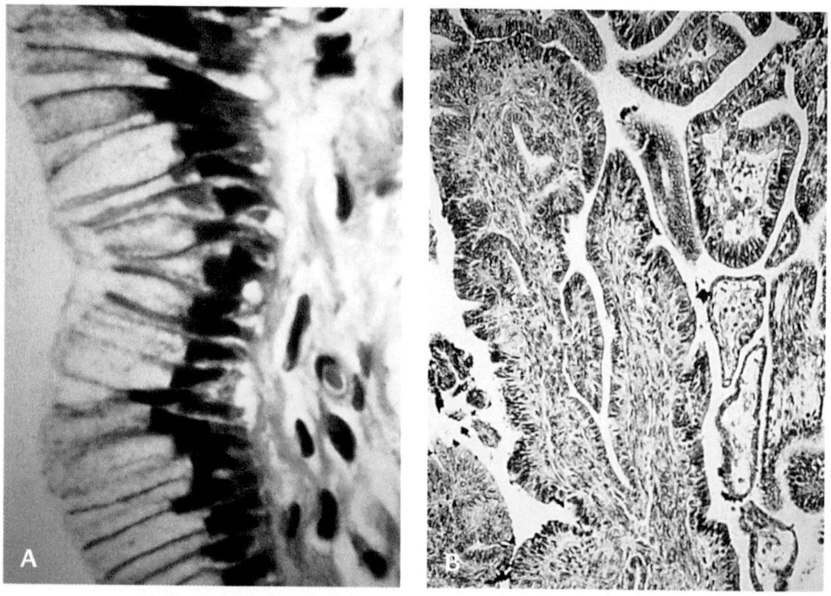

9.22. Ovarian mucinous cystadenoma of ovary **(A)**, microscopic appearance of ovarian papillary cystadenoma **(B)** in Proteus syndrome.

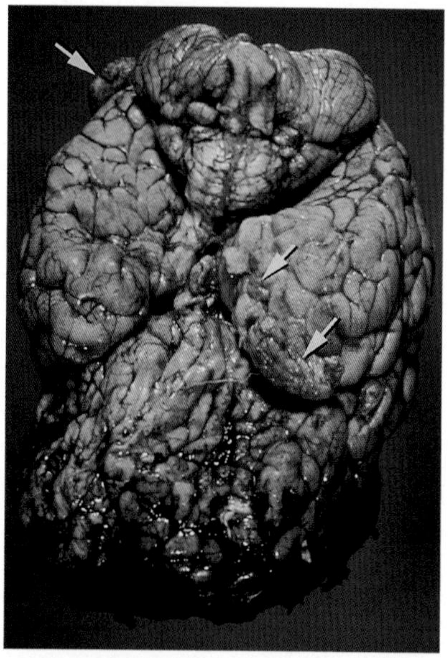

9.23. Meningiomas (arrows) in Proteus syndrome.

Table 9.8 Usual clinical manifestiations of Proteus syndrome

Infants large for gestational age	Palmar and plantar pits
Mental retardation (40%)	Cobblestone-like papules of gums and oral mucosa
Short stature	Partial gigantism of body parts
Hypertrichosis	Multiple facial trichilemmomas
Choristomas	Dentigenous cysts
Macrodactyly	Hamartomatous polyps of colon and other parts of gastrointestinal tract
Seizures	
Kyphoscoliosis	
Hemihypertrophy	

Table 9.9 Possible findings in Proteus syndrome

Skin	Lungs
Connective tissue nevi	Cystic lung alternations (10%)
Epidermal nevi	Progressive diffuse cystic changes
Disproportionate overgrowth	Central nervous system
Limbs	Mental deficiency (20%)
Arms/legs/digits	Seizures (13%)
Skull	Brain malformations
Hyperostoses	Other abnormalities (low frequency)
Vertebrae	Neoplasms
Megaspondylodysplasia (low frequency)	Facial phenotype with seizures and severe mental deficiency (see text)
Viscera	Epibulbar dermoids
Spleen/thymus (low frequency)	Craniosynostosis
Disregulated adipose tissue	Renal anomalies
Lipomas	
Regional absence of fat	
Vascular malformations	
Capillary malformations	
Venous malformations	

Adapted from Cohen MM Jr: Proteus syndrome: clinical evidence for somatic mosaicism and selective review. *Am J Med Genet* 47:645–652.

Table 9.10 Neoplasms in Proteus syndrome

Central nervous system	**Thyroid**
Meningiomas	Goiter
Optic nerve tumor	**Genitourinary**
Salivary gland	Papillary carcinoma of ovary
Pinealomas	Cyst or cystadenoma
Monomorphic adenoma (parotid)	Leiomyoma of uterus
Breast	Yolk sac tumor of testis
Intraductal papillomas and epithelial hyperplasias	Papillary adenoma of appendix testis
Kidney	Mesothelioma of tunica
Papillary adenoma	Vaginitis
	Cystadenoma of epididymis

Table 9.11 Pathologic brain abnormalities in Proteus syndrome

Polymicrogyria
Heterotopias
Asymmetry
Abnormal neuronal migration
Lissencephaly
Pachygyria

the Schimmelpenning-Feurerstein-Mims dysplasia (Figures 9.20 to 9.23 and Tables 9.8 to 9.11). Somatic mutations may be causative. The prevalence is unknown; genes have not been mapped. The hamartomatous growth of most of the lesions in Proteus syndrome and related conditions may be a dysregulation of the paracrine growth of cells and extracellular matrix.

Pallister-Hall Syndrome (Hamartoblastoma Syndrome) (OMIM # 146510)

Pallister-Hall syndrome, often neonatally lethal, consists of hypothalamic hamartoblastoma and postaxial or central polydactyly, associated with a variable array of other malformations, including imperforate anus, laryngeal cleft, abnormal lung lobation, renal agenesis or dysplasia, short fourth metacarpals, nail dysplasia, multiple buccal frenulae, hypoadrenalism, microphallus,

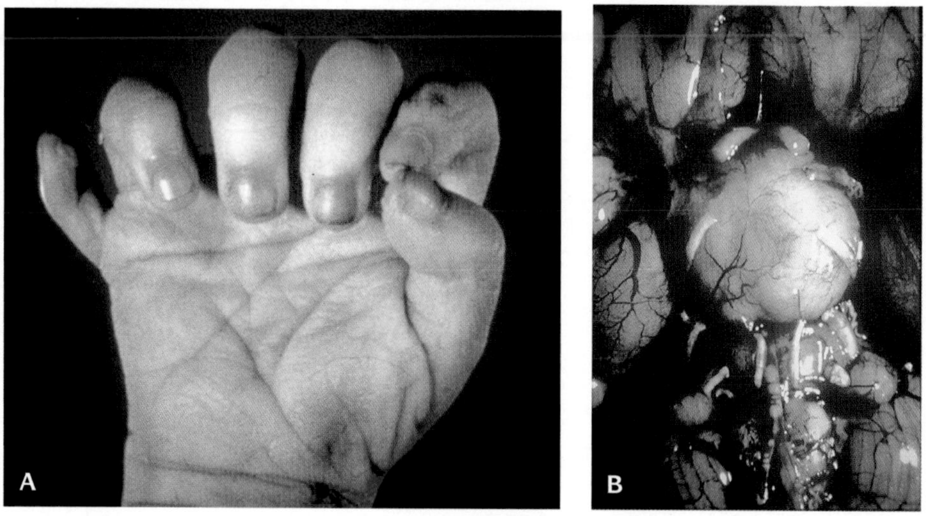

9.24. Pallister-Hall syndrome. **(A)** Postaxial polydactyly. **(B)** Base of brain showing hamartoblastoma.

Table 9.12 Clinical manifestations of Pallister-Hall syndrome

Hypothalamic hamartoblastoma
Multiple buccal frenulae
Postaxial polydactyly
Feeding difficulties
Imperforate anus
Renal agenesis/dysplasia
Intrauterine growth retardation
Congenital heart defects
Cleft lip and palate
Short limbs
Short nose with flattened bridge
Seizures

congenital heart defect, and intrauterine growth retardation (Figure 9.24 and Table 9.12). The radiologic abnormalities in the hand are helpful in differentiating this from other syndromes in which hypothalamic hamartoblastoma occurs. Preaxial oligodactyly has been reported. Most cases are sporadic.

Dysplasia of the hypothalamic plate between 34 and 40 days of gestation appears to be the main pathogenetic event. Gene mapping and linkage of this AD trait have not been accomplished. The gene has been mapped to 7p13.

Gorlin Syndrome (Basal Cell Carcinoma Syndrome [BCNS]) (OMIM #109400)

BCNS has an AD (autosomal dominant) inheritance (approximately 40% of cases represent new mutations) mapped by linkage to 9q22.3–q31 (Figure 9.25 and Table 9.13). There is high penetrance (97%). The prevalence

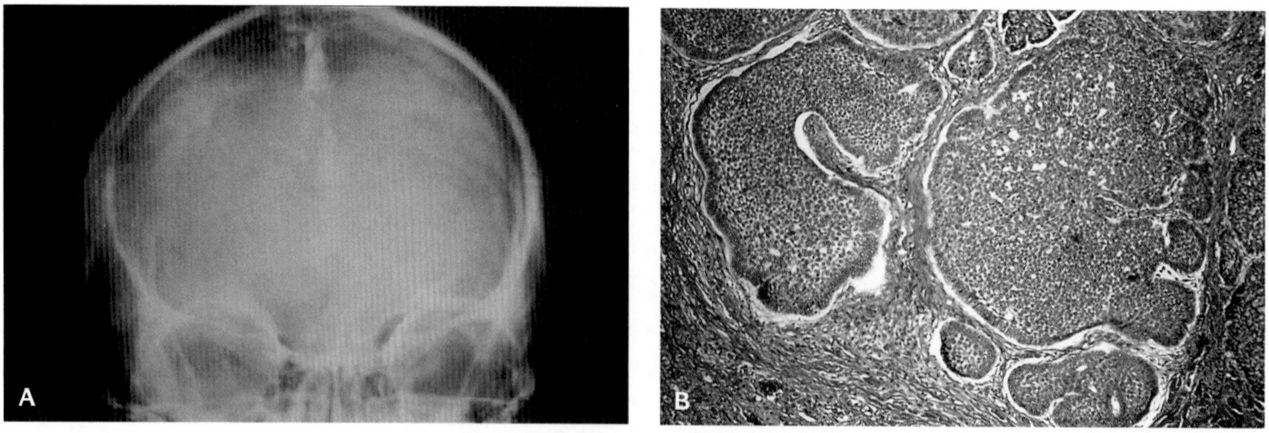

9.25. Gorlin (Basal cell nevus) syndrome. **(A)** X-ray of cranium showing calcification of falx cerebri. **(B)** Microscopic appearance of basal cell carcinoma.

is approximately 1/60:000. BCNS is a mutation in the gene PTC. This autosomal dominant syndrome is characterized by nevoid basal cell carcinomas plus bridging of the sella turcica, characteristic lamellar calcification of the falx cerebri, mild mandibular prognathism, lateral displacement of the inner canthi, frontal and biparietal bossing, odontogenic keratocysts of the jaws, pits on the palms and soles, short fourth metacarpals, kyphoscoliosis, bifid, missing, fused and/or splayed ribs, imperfect segmentation of cervical vertebrae, and ovarian fibromata and lymphomesenteric cysts, which tend to calcify.

Table 9.13 Clinical manifestations of Gorlin (basal cell nevus syndrome)

Multiple basal cell carcinomas
Broad face
Basal cell nevi
Hypertelorism
Palmar and plantar pits
Dystopia canthorum
Odontogenic keratocysts in jaw
Megalencephaly
Costovertebral anomalies
Subcortical cysts
Calcifications of falx cerebri, tentorium cerebelli, and petroclinoid ligaments

Source: Gilbert-Barness E, Barness LA: *Metabolic Diseases: Foundations of Clinical Management, Genetics and Pathology*, Vol. II, Natick, MA, Eaton Publishing, 2000.

EHLERS-DANLOS SYNDROME (MIM *130000, 130010, 130020, *130050, 130060, *130080, 130090, *147900, 225310, 225320, *225350, 225360, *225400, 225410, *304150, *305200)

Many genes have been identified. Ehlers-Danlos syndrome (EDS) is a heterogeneous group of connective tissue disorders. Genetic and biochemical studies define more than 10 types of EDS that include autosomal dominant, autosomal recessive, and X-linked forms (Figure 9.26 and Tables 9.8 to 9.16).

The clinical manifestations include hyperelastic, doughy, soft skin; easy bruising; joint hypermobility; connective tissue fragility; and dystrophic scarring in variable degrees. The hyperelasticity of the skin is attributed to a collagen (enzymatic) defect resulting in a decrease in the amount of elastic tissue and thinning of the dermis. Associated malformations include short stature, ocular defects, and skeletal and cardiac malformations.

The biochemical basis of EDS types I, II, and III is not known. Genetic linkage studies with polymorphic endonuclease restriction sites in COL1A1, COL1A2, and COL2A1 excluded those genes as sites of mutations in some families.

Classic Type, Autosomal Dominant. The major diagnostic criteria for the classic type include skin hyperextensibility, widened atrophic scars (manifestations of tissue fragility), and joint hypermobility. Minor diagnostic criteria

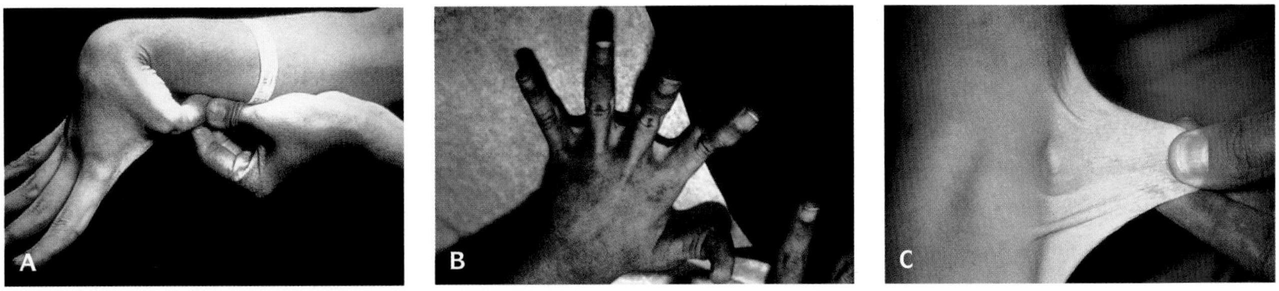

9.26. Ehlers-Danlos syndrome. **(A)** Hyperextensibility of fingers. **(B)** Webbing of fingers. **(C)** Hyperelasticity of skin.

Table 9.14 Ehlers-Danlos syndrome

In Ehlers-Danlos syndrome the following features should be assessed:

- Skin hyperextensibility
- Joint hypermobility
- Easy bruising
- Tissue fragility
- Mitral valve prolapse and proximal aortic dilation
- Chronic joint and limb pain
- Kyphoscoliosis, arthrochalasia, and dermatosparaxis

Table 9.15 Clinical manifestations of Ehlers-Danlos syndrome

Hyperelastic skin
Bowel perforations (vascular or type IV)
Ecchymoses
Atrophic papyraceous scars with redundant skin on hands and feet
Habitual dislocations
Joint hypermobility
Connective tissue fragility
Peripheral neuropathy
Rectal prolapse
Ptosis viscerum
Arthralgias
Arterial rupture (vascular or type IV)
Osteoporosis
Mitral valve prolapse
Joint contractures (vascular or type IV)
Retinal detachment
Short stature
Keratoconus

Source: Gilbert-Barness E, Barness LA: *Metabolic Diseases: Foundations of Clinical Management, Genetics and Pathology*, Vol. II, Natick, MA, Eaton Publishing, 2000.

Table 9.16 Classification of Ehlers-Danlos syndrome

New	Former	OMIM	Inheritance
Classic type	Gravis (EDS type I) Mitis (EDS type II)	130000 130010	AD AD
Hypermobility type	Hypermobile (EDS type III)	130020	AD
Vascular type	Arterial-ecchymotic (EDS type IV)	130050 (225350) (225360)	AD
Kyphoscoliosis type	Ocular-scoliotic (EDS type VI)	225400 (229200)	AR
Arthrochalasia type	Arthrochalasis multiplex congenita (EDS types VIIA and VIIB)	130060	AD
Dermatosparaxis type	Human dermatosparaxis (EDS type VIIC)	225410	AR
Other forms	X-linked EDS (EDS type V)	305200	XL
	Periodontitis type (EDS type VIII)	130080	AD
	Fibronectin-deficient EDS (EDS type X)	225310	?
	Familial hypermobility syndrome (EDS type XI)	147900	AD
	Progeroid EDS	130070	?
	Occipital horn syndrome [allelic to Menkes syndrome (EDS type XI)]	309400	XL

AD, autosomal dominant; AR, autosomal recessive; XL, X-linked; ?, unknown

Source: Gilbert-Barness E, Barness LA: *Metabolic Diseases: Foundations of Clinical Management, Genetics and Pathology*. Eaton Publishing Co., Natick, MA, 2000.

include smooth, velvety skin; molluscoid pseudotumors, subcutaneous spheroids, complications of joint hypermobility (e.g., sprains/dislocations/subluxations, pes planus); surgical complications (postoperative hernias); and a positive family history.

Diagnosis is based on the abnormal electrophoretic mobility of the proα1 (v) or proα 2 (v) chains of collagen type V. In most families genetic linkage studies can be used for prenatal and postnatal diagnosis. Genetic linkage to intragenic markers of the COL5S1 and COL5AZ genes has been excluded in some families. Abnormalities in the collagen fibril structure can be found by electronmicroscopy in many families; a cauliflower deformity of collagen fibrils is characteristic but not specific.

Hypermobility Type, Autosomal Dominant. The major diagnostic criteria for the hypermobility type include skin hyperextensibility and/or smooth, velvety skin, and generalized joint hypermobility. Minor diagnostic criteria include recurring joint dislocations, chronic joint/limb pain, and a positive family history.

Diagnosis is based on the dominant clinical manifestation joint hypermobility. Shoulder, patellar, and temporomandibular joints dislocate frequently. Skin extensibility is variable. Musculoskeletal pain is early in onset, chronic, and possibly debilitating.

Vascular Type, Autosomal Dominant. The major diagnostic criteria for the vascular type include thin, translucent skin; **arterial/intestinal/uterine fragility or rupture**; extensive bruising; and characteristic facial appearance. Minor diagnostic criteria include acrogeria, hypermobility of small joints, tendon and muscle rupture, talipes equinovarus (clubfoot), early-onset varicose veins, arteriovenous carotid-cavernous sinus fistula, pneumothorax/pneumohemothorax, gingival recession, and positive family history or sudden death in a close relative(s).

Arterial rupture is the most common cause of death. Diagnosis involves the demonstration of structurally abnormal collagen type III. Demonstration of a mutation in the COL3A1 gene confirms the diagnosis.

Kyphoscoliosis Type, Autosomal Recessive. The major diagnostic criteria for the kyphoscoliosis type include generalized joint laxity, severe muscle hypotonia at birth, scoliosis at birth (progressive), and scleral fragility and rupture of the ocular globe. Minor diagnostic criteria include tissue fragility, including atrophic scars; easy bruising; arterial rupture; marfanoid habitus, microcornea; radiologically considerable osteopenia; and a positive family history (i.e., affected sibs).

Clinical diagnosis may be based on the presence of three major criteria in an infant. Muscular hypotonia may be pronounced and is manifested as a “floppy infant,” and loss of ambulation may occur in the second or third decade. Scleral fragility may result in rupture of the ocular globe after minor trauma.

The biochemical diagnosis is based on measurement of total urinary hydroxylysyl pyridinoline and lysyl pyridinoline cross links after hydrolysis by high-pressure liquid chromatography. The determination of hydroxylysine is possible from fibroblast cultures and mutation analysis of the gene.

Arthrochalasia Type, Autosomal Dominant. This is caused by mutations resulting in deficient processing of the aminoterminal end of proα1 (type A) or proα 2 (type B) chains of collagen type I that causes skipping of exon 6 in either gene.

The major diagnostic criteria for the arthrochalasis type include severe generalized joint hypermobility with recurrent subluxations and congenital bilateral hip dislocation. Minor diagnostic criteria include skin hyperextensibility; tissue fragility, including atrophic scars; easy bruising; muscle hypotonia; kyphoscoliosis; and radiologically mild osteopenia.

Congenital hip dislocation is present in all cases. Short stature is not present unless complicated by kyphoscoliosis and/or hip dislocation.

Diagnosis is based on the biochemical defect determined by electrophoretic demonstration of pNα1 or pNα 2 chains extracted from dermal collagen or from cultured fibroblasts.

Dermatosparaxis Type. This type is caused by a deficiency of procollagen I N-terminal peptidase caused by homozygosity or compound heterozygosity of mutant alleles (in contrast to the arthrocalasia type caused by mutations involving the substrate sites of procollagen type I chains).

The major diagnostic criteria for the dermatosparaxis type include severe skin fragility and sagging, redundant skin. Minor diagnostic criteria include soft, doughy skin texture; easy bruising; premature rupture of fetal membranes; and large hernias (e.g., umbilical, inguinal).

Skin fragility and bruising are severe. Wound healing is impaired and the scars are not atrophic. Redundancy of the facial skin resembles cutis laxa, although skin fragility and bruising are not seen in cutis laxa.

Other Types of EDS. Other types of EDS are rare. Type IX is X-linked and is now called occipital horn syndrome.

METABOLIC DYSPLASIAS

Beckwith-Wiedemann Syndrome (OMIM *130650) (See Chapter 8) (Table 9.17)

Table 9.17 Clinical manifestations of Beckwith-Wiedemann syndrome

Omphalocele
Hemihypertrophy
Polyhydramnios
Neonatal hypoglycemia
Macroglossia
Wilms tumor
Gigantism
Splenomegaly
Midface hypoplasia
Infants large for gestational age
Hepatomegaly
Mental retardation
Cytomegaly of adrenal cortex
Malrotation of intestine
Seizures
Nephromegaly
Large placenta
Lobular creases and posterior helical pits
Nephroblastomatosis
Prematurity
Semilunar crease on helix

Multiple Endocrine Neoplasia (MEN) (OMIM #171400)

This is an AD trait with clinical penetrance of 60% and subclinical penetrance of 93%. The genes for MEN 2A, MEN, 2B, and familial medullary thyroid carcinoma (MTC) have been mapped to 10q11.2. There is cosegregation or overlap with NF-1 and VHL. MEN 1 is mapped at 11q13. Mutational analysis leads to merging of the phenotypes of MEN 2A, MEN 2B, and familial MTC; MEN 2A is the prototype of the MEN syndromes (Figure 9.27 and Tables 9.18 to 9.22).

Table 9.18 Clinical manifestations of MEN

Medullary thyroid carcinoma
Prominent corneal nerves
Pheochromocytoma
Megacolon/Hirschsprung disease
Parathyroid adenomas
Carcinoidosis
Mucosal neuromas
Zollinger-Ellison syndrome
Intestinal ganglioneuromatosis

Table 9.19 Multiple endocrine neoplasia syndrome1 (MEN 1)

Organ/Pathology	Approximate incidence	Hormones	Symptoms
Parathyroid glands	>90%		
Diffuse or nodular hyperplasia with adenomatosis		Parathyroid hormone	Hyperparathyroidism
Endocrine pancreas/duodenum	50–85%	Multihormonal	
Diffuse microadenomatosis of the pancreas with or without one or several macrotumors (>0.5 cm)			
PP (pancreatic polypeptide)-oma	Most frequent	Pancreatic polypeptide	
Insulinoma	10–30%	Insulin	Hypoglycemia
Vipoma	2–10%	VIP	Verner-Morrison syndrome
Glucagonoma	Rare	Glucagon	Glucagonoma syndrome
Somatostatinoma	30–50%	Somatostatin	Growth hormone inhibition
Gastrinoma of the duodenum	30–65%	Gastrin	Hypergastrinemia, Zollinger-Ellison syndrome
Anterior pituitary			
Inactive or Growth hormone (GH) adenoma	70%	Often inactive, growth hormone	Local symptoms, hypopituitarism, acromegaly
GH adenoma, prolactinoma	25%	Growth hormone, prolactin	Acromegaly, hyperprolactinemia; Cushing disease
Adrenocorticotropic (ACTH) adenoma	Rare	ACTH	
Gastrointestinal and thymic endocrine cells	5%		
Carcinoids			
Adrenal cortex	40%	Hypercorticism	
Nodular hyperplasia, adenoma			
Thyroid gland	20%	Hyperthyroidism, mild	
Follicular adenoma			

Source: Gilbert-Barness E, and Barness, LA: *Metabolic Diseases: Foundations of Clinical Management, Genetics and Pathology*. Eaton Publishing Co., Natick, MA, 2000.

Table 9.20 Multiple endocrine neoplasia syndrome 2A

Organ/Pathology	Approximate incidence	Hormones	Symptoms
Thyroid	>90%	Calcitonin, calcitonin gene related peptide	
Multifocal diffuse and nodular C-cell hyperplasia			
Thyroid medullary carcinoma (bilateral)			Diarrhea, tends to progress
Adrenal medulla	20–40%		
Medullary hyperplasia	85–90%		
Pheochromocytoma	85–90%		Hypertension
Bilateral	70–80%	Epinephrine, norepinephrine	
Extra-adrenal	10–15%		
Parathyroid glands			
Chief-cell hyperplasia	60%	Parathyroid hormone	Hyperparathyroidism, often asymptomatic

Source: Gilbert-Barness E, and Barness, LA: *Metabolic Diseases: Foundations of Clinical Management, Genetics and Pathology*. Eaton Publishing Co., Natick, MA, 2000.

Table 9.21 Multiple endocrine neoplasia syndrome 2B

Organ/Pathology	Approximate incidence	Hormones	Symptoms
Thyroid	>90%		
Multifocal diffuse and nodular C-Cell hyperplasia		Calcitonin, calcitonin gene-related peptide	
Thyroid medullary carcinoma (bilateral)			Diarrhea, tends to develop early and progress rapidly
Adrenal medulla	20–40%		
Medulary hyperplasia	85–90%		
Pheochromocytoma	85–90%		Hypertension
Bilateral	70–80%	Epinephrine, norepinephrine	
Extra-adrenal	10–15%		
Parathyroid glands	Rarely		No hyperparathyroidism detectable
Chief-cell hyperplasia		Parathyroid hormone	
Peripheral neural system	100%		
Marfanoid habitus	100%		
Mucosal neuromas	100%		
Intestinal ganglioneuromatosis	40–50%		Diarrhea or constipation

Table 9.22 Thyroid medullary carcinoma

Features	Sporadic (nonfamilial)	Familial (inherited)
Percentages of cases	80%	20%
Inheritance	Noninherited	Autosomal dominant
Associated lesions	None	MEN 2A MEN 2B Familial non-MEN (Thyroid medullary carcinoma (TPC) alone)
Genetics	No genetic abnormalities	The gene for MEN 2A (and the other forms of MEN) has been mapped to a locus near the centromere of chromosome 10 MEN 2A: women > men; third decade and younger
Sex age (mean age at diagnosis)	Women more than men; fifth to sixth decades	MEN 2B: women > men; second decade and younger Non-MEN: women > men; fifth decade Total thyroidectomy
Treatment	Total thyroidectomy	In decreasing order of survival: non-MEN, MEN 2A, MEN 2B
Prognosis	Indolent course 5-year survival rates of 60% to 80% 10-year survival rates of 40% to 60%	

Source: Gilbert-Barness E, and Barness, LA: *Metabolic Diseases: Foundations of Clinical Management, Genetics and Pathology*. Eaton Publishing Co., Natick, MA, 2000.

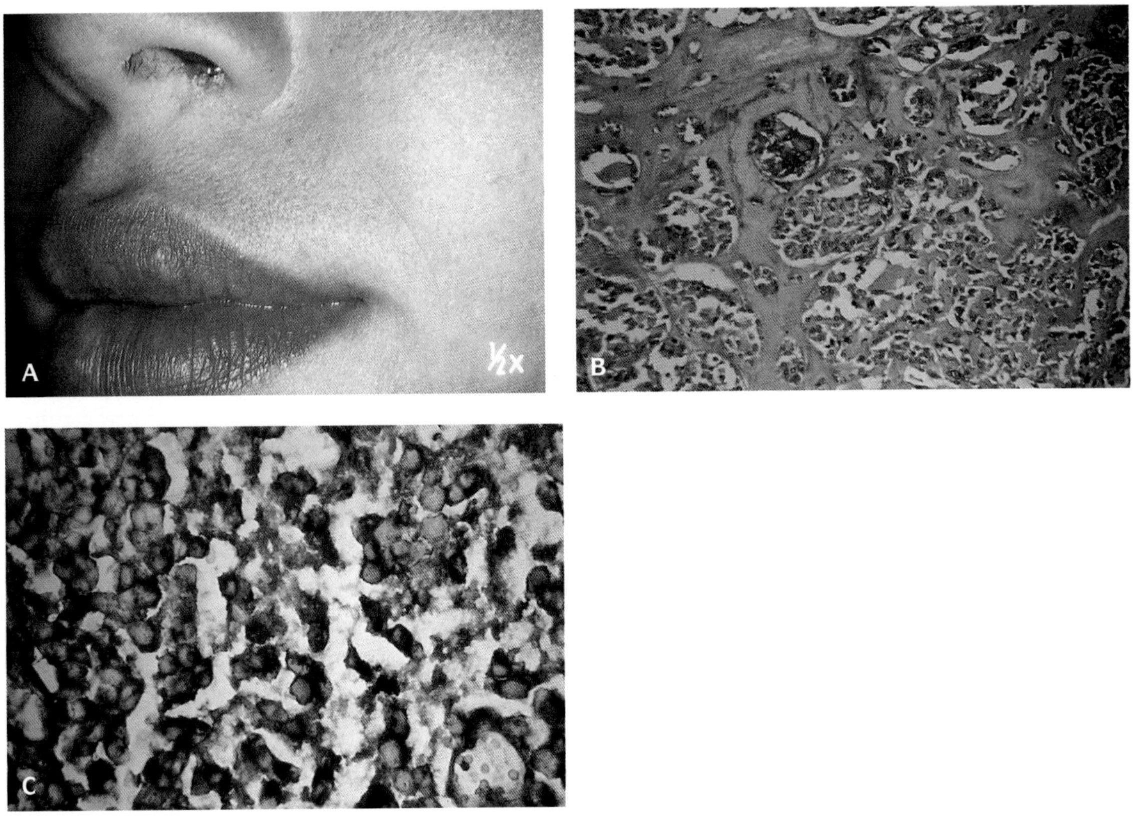

9.27. Multiple endocrine neoplasia (MEN) type 2B. **(A)** Mucosal neuromas of lips. **(B)** Medullary thyroid carcinoma with amyloid stroma. **(C)** Medullary thyroid carcinoma with positive immunostaining for calcitonin.

Mutations affecting different domains of the RET gene account for the phenotypic diversities or pleiotropy (allelic heterogeneity). Mutations resulting in inactivation of the RET gene product account for Hirschsprung disease in a subset of patients with familial Hirschsprung disease.

Multiple Hamartoma (Cowden) Syndrome (OMIM #158350)

The multiple hamartoma syndrome has an AD inheritance with high penetrance (Figure 9.28 and Table 9.23). Lhermitte-Duclos disease is part of the syndrome. There is a male/female ratio of 1/2.5. The prevalence is unknown. The gene locus has been identified at 10q22–q23.

Multiple hamartomatous lesions, especially of the skin, mucous membranes, breast, and thyroid are encountered. Verrucous skin lesions of the face and limbs, cobblestone-like papules of the gingiva and buccal mucosa, and multiple facial trichilemmomas are leading findings. Hamartomatous polyps of the colon and other intestines occur also.

On histologic study, the gums show thick dense bundles of collagen in the submucosa and lamina propria. Lichenoid lesions exhibit lobules of follicular acanthosis (similar to basal cell carcinoma). A central follicular plug is common. The papillomatous lesions are verrucous with marked irregular acanthotic epidermis (with hyperkeratosis and vascular dilatation within the dermis). The

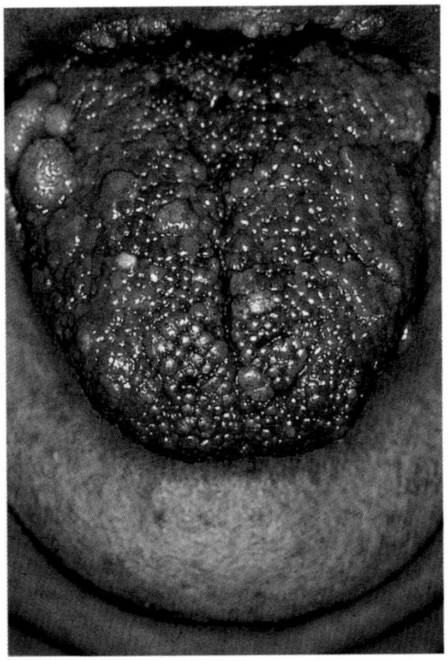

9.28. Cowden syndrome (multiple hamartoma syndrome). Cobblestone-like papules on tongue.

Table 9.23 Clinical manifestations of multiple hamartoma syndrome

Multiple hamartomas of skin, mucous membranes, breast, and thyroid
Palmar and plantar pits
Cobblestone-like papules of gums and oral mucosa
Hypertrichosis
Multiple facial trichilemmomas
Mental retardation (40%)
Hamartomatous polyps of colon and other parts of gastrointestinal tract
Dentigerous cysts

Table 9.24 Examples of metabolic dysplasia syndromes

Mucopolysaccharidoses	Hurler, Hunter, and Morquio diseases
Mucolipidoses, sialidoses	I-cell disease, sialidosis
Glycoprotein degradation diseases	Fucosidosis, aspartylglycosaminuria
Lipid storage disease	Wolman disease
Lipidoses	Farber, Gaucher, and Tay-Sachs diseases
Peroxisomal disorders	Zellweger syndrome, adrenoleukodystrophies
Cholesterol metabolism disorders	Smith-Lemli-Opitz syndrome
Antley-Bixler syndrome	Desmosterolosis
Greenberg dysplasia	CHILD–2 types
Chondrodysplasia punctata XL–2 types	Conradi-Hünermann-Happle syndrome (CDPX2)

acrokeratoses show marked hyperkeratosis, hypergranulosis, and acanthosis of the epidermis, underlying a sharply circumscribed hyperkeratotic mass.

METABOLIC DYSPLASIA SYNDROMES (SEE CHAPTER 24)

Metabolic Dysplasias

There are a number of metabolic disorders that result in malformations. These metabolic dysplasias include Zellweger syndrome, Smith-Lemli-Opitz syndrome, acid mucopolysaccharidoses conditions, and glutaric acidemias (Table 9.24).

REFERENCES

Beighton P: *McKusick's Heritable Disorders of Connective Tissue*, 5th ed. St. Louis, Mosby Publishers, 1993.

Cohen MM Jr: *The Child with Multiple Birth Defects*. Oxford, Oxford University Press, 1997.

Cohen MM Jr, Neri G, Weksberg R: *Overgrowth Syndromes*. Oxford, Oxford University Press, 2002.

Gilbert-Barness E, ed: *Potter's Pathology of the Fetus and Infant*. St. Louis, Mosby Publishers, 1997.

Gilbert-Barness E, ed: *Potter's Atlas of Fetal and Infant Pathology*. St. Louis, Mosby Publishers, 1998.

Gilbert-Barness E, Barness LA: *Metabolic Diseases: Foundations of Clinical Management, Genetics and Pathology*. Natick, Massachusetts, Eaton Publishing Co., 2000.

Goelz SE, Hamilton ST, Vogelstein B: Purification of DNA from formaldehyde fixed and paraffin embedded human tissue. *Biochem Biophys Res Commun* 130:118, 1985.

Kousseff BG: The phakomatoses as paracrine growth disorders/ paracrinopathies. *Clin Genet* 37:97, 1990.

McKusick VA: *Mendelian Inheritance in Man: A Catalog of Human Genes and Genetic Disorders*, 12th ed. Johns Hopkins University Press, Baltimore, 1998.

Opitz JM, Wilson GN: Causes and pathogenesis of birth defects. In Gilbert-Barness E (ed): *Potter's Pathology of the Fetus and Infant*, St. Louis, Mosby Publishers, 1997.

Opitz JM, Gilbert-Barness E, Ackerman J, Lowichik A. Cholesterol and development: The RSH ("Smith-Lemli-Opitz) syndrome and related conditions. *Ped Path Mole Med* 21:153, 2002.

TEN

Disruptions and Amnion Rupture Sequence

Disruption is defined as a morphologic or structural anomaly of an organ, part of an organ, or a larger region of the body resulting from the extrinsic breakdown of, or interference with, an originally normal conceptus or developmental process. Disruptions tend to be sporadic occurrences (Figure 10.1 and Tables 10.1 to 10.6).

TYPES OF DISRUPTIONS AFFECTING MORPHOGENESIS OF THE DEVELOPING EMBRYO AND FETUS

- Radiation
- Hyperthermia
- Infection
- Teratogenic drugs
- Metabolic
- Vascular
- Amnion disruption

TERATOGENIC DISRUPTIONS

Growth and development of the embryo can be adversely affected by a wide variety of environmental agents (teratogens). Teratogens include intrauterine

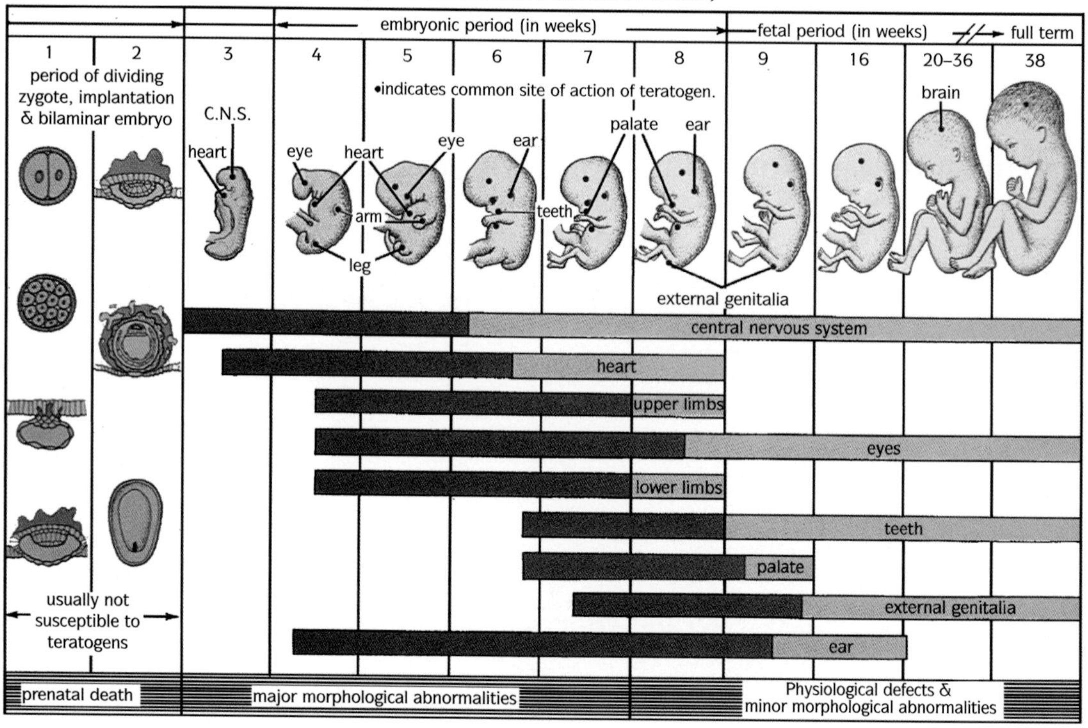

10.1. Critical periods in human development and the site of action of teratogens. (Courtesy of Dr. Keith L. Moore and WB Saunders Pub.)

Table 10.1 Time of action of human teratogens

Teratogen	Gestational age (days)	Malformation
Rubella virus	0–60 0–129+	Cataract or heart defect more likely Deafness
Thalidomide	21–40	Reduction defects of extremities
Hyperthermia	18–30	Anencephaly
Male hormones (androgens, tumors)	Before 90 After 90	Clitoral hypertrophy and labial fusion only Clitoral hypertrophy
Coumadin anticoagulants	Before 100 After 100	Hypoplasia of nose and stippling of epiphyses Possible mental retardation
Diethylstilbestrol	After 14 After 98 After 126	Vaginal adenosis (50%) Vaginal adenosis (30%) Vaginal adenosis (10%)
Radioiodine therapy	After 65–70	Fetal thyroid aplasia
Goitrogens and iodides	After 180	Fetal goiter
Tetracycline	After 120 After 250	Dental enamel staining of primary teeth Staining of crowns of permanent teeth

Table 10.2 Disruption: examples

Ischemic disruptions – porencephalic cysts or ileal atresia
Radiation disruption
Infectious disruptions – caused by viruses and toxoplasmosis
Amniotic adhesions – the ADAM complex (amniotic deformities adhesions mutilations)
Caused by teratogenic drugs
  Thalidomide Embryopathy
  Warfarin embryopathy, etc.

Table 10.3 Human teratogens 1991: agents proved or virtually certain to be teratogenic

Environmental exposures

Alcohol	Fetal alcohol syndrome
Cocaine	Placental abruption, ? vascular based fetal anomalies
Cytomegalovirus	CNS, other
Lead	CNS
Mercury	Fetal minimata disease
Radiation	CNS, eye, pregnancy loss
high doses only	
Rubella	Rubella syndrome
Smoking	Intrauterine growth retardation, pregnancy loss
Syphilis	Congenital syphilis
Toxoplasmosis	CNS, eye, other
Varicella [chickenpox]	Limb, skin, cataracts

Maternal factors

Hyperphenylalaninemia (including phenylketonuria)
Maternal diabetes mellitus
Maternal myotonic dystrophy
Rh incompatibility

Prescribed drugs

Accutane [isotretinoin] anti-acne	Isotretinoin embryopathy
Aminopterin [and other anti-folates] anti-cancer	Aminopterin syndrome
Curare [chronic use only] in treatment of tetanus	Arthrogryposis
Diazepam [valium] sedative-muscle relaxant	Clefts
Diethylstilbesterol no longer used	Vaginal clear cell carcinoma etc.
Hydantoins (dilantin) anti-seizure	Fetal hydantoin effects
Iodine	Thyroid abnormalities
Lithium antidepressant	Cardiac malformations
Propylthiouracil for hyperthyroidism	Thyroid abnormalities
Progestins, synthetic	Masculinization
Streptomycin antibiotic	Hearing loss
Testosterone	Masculinization
Tetracycline antibiotic	Enamel abnormalities
Thalidomide (no longer in general use)	Thalidomide syndrome
Trimethadione anti-seizure	Trimethadione syndrome
Valproic acid (anti-seizure)	Fetal valproate syndrome
Warfarin anticoagulant	Warfarin embryopathy

Table 10.4 Teratogenic disruptions

The first two weeks of development is an all-or-none phenemonon – death or survival of the embryo.
The next 45 days are especially dangerous for the embryo for this is the critical period of embryogenesis and organogenesis.

Table 10.5 Teratogenic agents: infections

Rubella virus
Cytomegalovirus
Herpes simplex virus I and II
Toxoplasmosis
Venezuelan equine encephalitis virus
Syphilis

Table 10.6 Radiation teratogenicity

Growth retardation
Microcephaly (small head)
Mental retardation
Structural eye abnormalities

infections, various chemical agents and medications, and maternal metabolic disorders.

The first two weeks of life – that is, the time before organogenesis – appears to be a relatively safe time for the embryo regarding teratogenic exposure. The next 45 days, however, are especially dangerous for it is during this period that most organs develop. After an organ has developed, unless there is disruption, the teratogen cannot cause a malformation. The same teratogen can cause different defects at different times of exposure.

Most teratogens produce a characteristic, clinically recognizable, pattern of abnormalities.

RADIATION EMBRYOPATHY

In utero radiation is associated with microcephaly, mental retardation, and stunted growth, especially in infants exposed between the 8th and 15th weeks of gestation, and there is an increased incidence of leukemia.

HYPERTHERMIC EMBRYOPATHY

Hyperthermia, a body temperature of at least 38.9°C, is an antimitotic teratogen when the fetus is exposed to a high temperature between the 4th and 16th week of gestation (Figure 10.2 and Table 10.7). Severe mental retardation, seizures, hypotonia, microphthalmia, midface hypoplasia, and mild digital abnormalities can result. Exposure at 21–28 days, neural tube defects (including

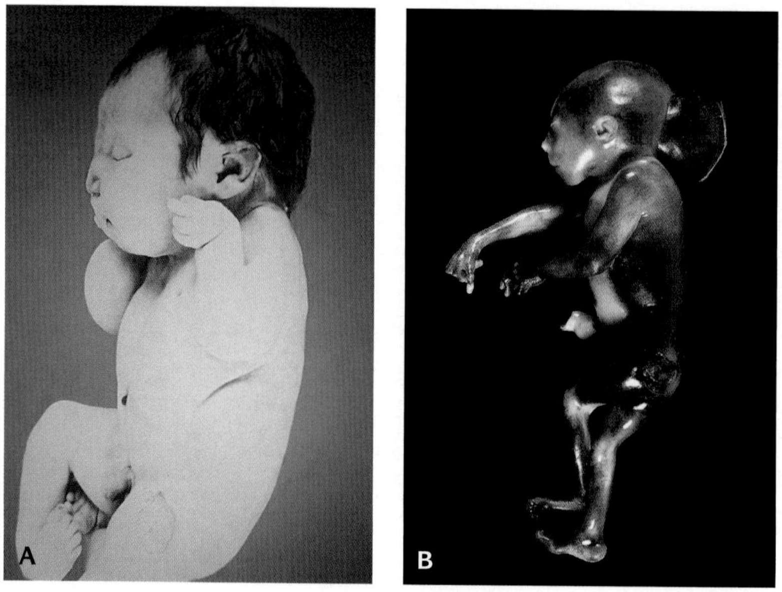

10.2. **(A)** Infant with hyperthermic embryopathy. **(B)** Fetus with encephalocele.

anencephaly, myelomeningocele, and occipital encephalocele) may occur. Exposure between the 7th and 16th week of gestation may result in neurogenic arthrogryposis. Exposure during the latter half of gestation does not increase the likely occurrence of anomalies.

Table 10.7 Hyperthermic embryopathy

Hyperthermia is a body temperature of at least 38.9°C.
Exposure during the time of neural tube development (21–28 days), may result in:
- neural tube defects
- anencephaly
- myelomeningocele
- occipital encephalocele

Exposure from weeks 7 to 16 may result in arthrogryposis.

TORCH INFECTIONS

Rubella Embryopathy

Rubella contracted before the 11th week of gestation has a complication rate of close to 100% – principally congenital heart disease, particularly patent ductus arteriosis, and sensorineural hearing loss (Figures 10.3 and 10.4 and Table 10.8). About 35% of those infected during the 13th to 16th week have complications (primarily hearing loss). After the 17th week, the embryo appears to be unaffected.

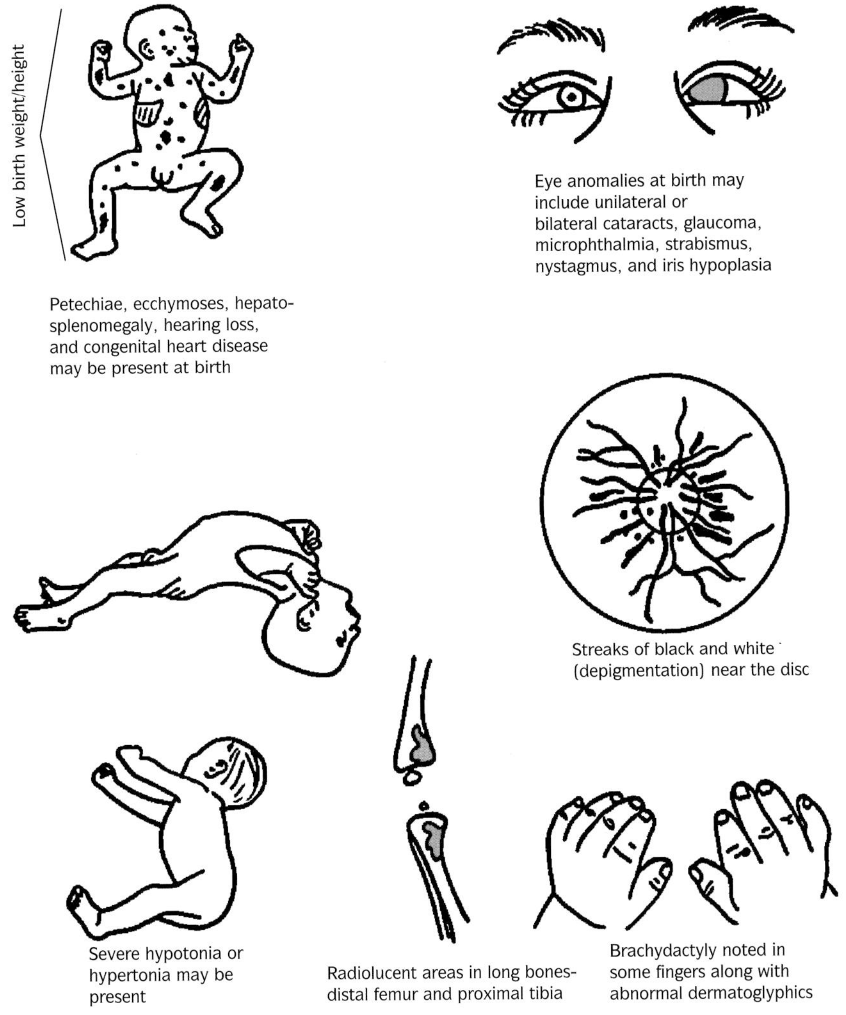
Low birth weight/height
Eye anomalies at birth may include unilateral or bilateral cataracts, glaucoma, microphthalmia, strabismus, nystagmus, and iris hypoplasia
Petechiae, ecchymoses, hepato-splenomegaly, hearing loss, and congenital heart disease may be present at birth
Streaks of black and white (depigmentation) near the disc
Severe hypotonia or hypertonia may be present
Radiolucent areas in long bones-distal femur and proximal tibia
Brachydactyly noted in some fingers along with abnormal dermatoglyphics

10.3. Fetal rubella syndrome.

Table 10.8 Congenital rubella

Defects	Conceptional weeks
Cataracts	2–7
Heart disease	1–8
Deafness	1–17
Mental retardation	2–5

Viremia occurs 6–7 days before appearance of rash.

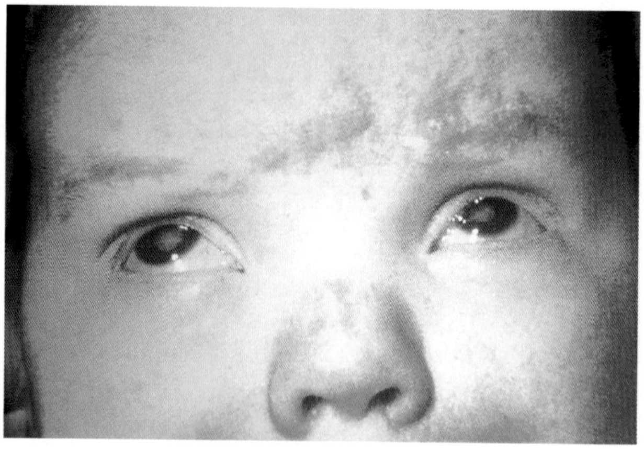

10.4. Rubella embryopathy infant with cataracts.

Cytomegalovirus

Cytomegalovirus (CMV) is the most common cause of congenital infections, occurring in 0.5–2.5% of all live births. Intrauterine growth retardation, meningoencephalitis, pneumonitis, and hepatitis can be seen (Figures 10.5 and 10.6). Because CMV causes cellular necrosis, infections such as

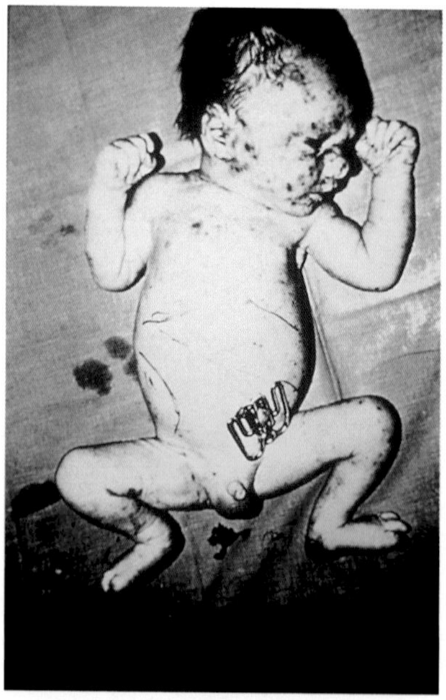

10.5. Infant with congenital cytomegalovirus infection with hepatosplenomegaly and multiple petechial hemorrhages.

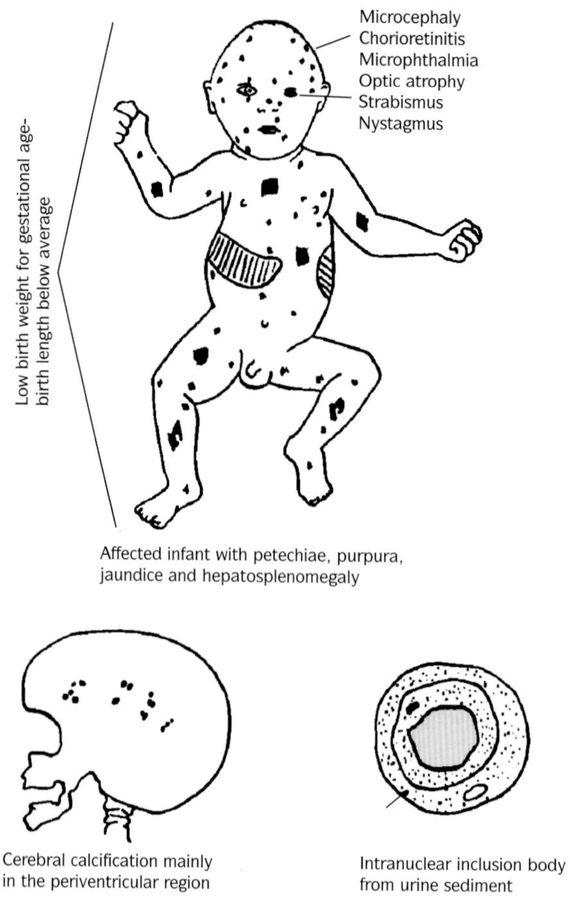

10.6. Fetal cytomegalovirus syndrome.

necrotizing meningoencephalitis eventuate in microcephaly, periventricular calcifications, mental retardation, seizures, sensorineural hearing loss, and motor deficits. Obstructive hydrocephalus may occur. CMV infections of the eye result in chorioretinitis and optic atrophy. Hepatosplenomegaly, thrombocytopenia, and hemolytic anemia may also be seen.

Herpes Virus

Herpes virus infection is usually acquired by the fetus or newborn during delivery from a mother with genital herpes (herpes virus type 2) (Figures 10.7 and 10.8). Disruptive lesions with necrosis occur principally in the brain, liver, and adrenal glands.

Varicella Embryopathy

There is a 5–10% rate of fetal damage with infection with the varicella/zoster virus during pregnancy. In maternal varicella, risk to fetus is low. There is no increased frequency of spontaneously aborted fetuses. (Figure 10.9 and Table 10.9). Varicella embryopathy consists of cortical atrophy, mental deficiency, limb hypoplasia, skin scarring, eye defects, and retarded growth.

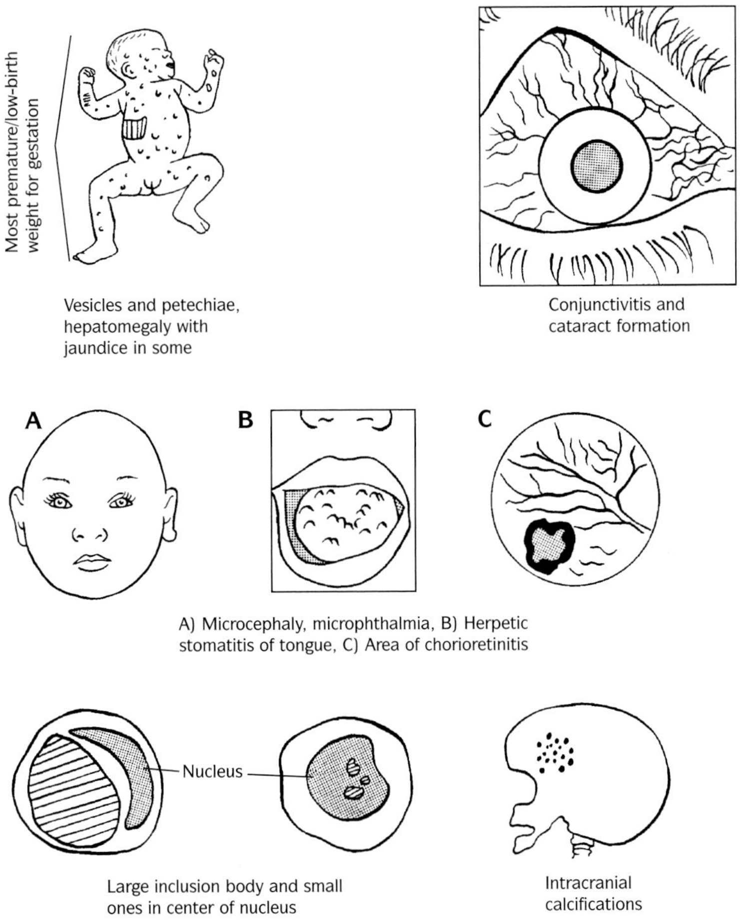

10.7. Herpes simplex virus infection. (From Goodman RM, Gorlin RJ: *The Malformed Infant and Child, An Illustrated Guide*, New York, Oxford University Press, 1985.)

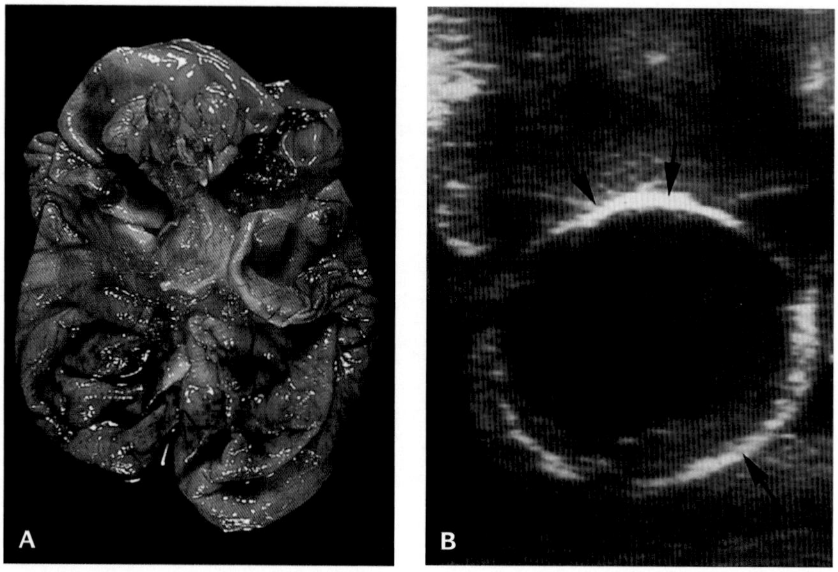

10.8. (A) Herpes virus type 2 infection. Hydranencephaly with disruption of the cerebral cortices leaving an empty sac. **(B)** Ultrasound of hydranencephaly showing almost complete absence of brain substance (empty skull). (Arrows – skull bone.)

The most frequent findings have been limb hypoplasia and paralysis, cutaneous scars with dermatome distribution, hydrocephaly, microcephaly, chorioretinitis, anisocoria, nystagmus, cataracts, microphthalmia, and Horner syndrome.

The risk to the fetus of maternal varicella is low. There appears to be no increased frequency of spontaneously aborted fetuses.

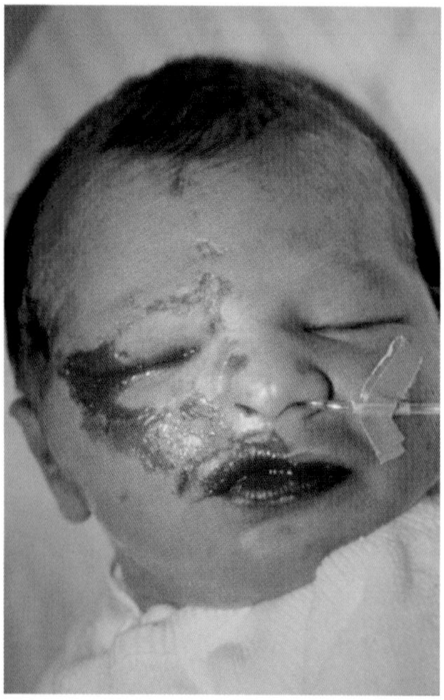

10.9. Varicella embryopathy. Note extensive cutaneous facial scarring. The infant also had an inability to swallow. (From Unger-Köppel J, Kilcher P, Tönz O: Helv *Paediatr Acta* 40:339, 1985.)

Toxoplasmosis

Hydrocephalus (5%) and microcephaly (5%) may result from chronic destructive meningoencephalitis and, as in the case of CMV, chorioretinitis may progress to loss of vision (Figure 10.10). Cerebral calcifications may be seen in about 10%. Hydranencephaly may result from any intrauterine infection including the TORCH infections.

Table 10.9 Varicella embryopathy

Varicella embryopathy consists of:	Most frequent findings:
• cortical atrophy	• cutaneous scars with dermatome distribution
• mental deficiency	• hydrocephaly
• limb hypoplasia	• microcephaly
• skin scarring	• chorioretinitis
• eye defects	• anisocoria
• retarded growth	• nystagmus
	• cataracts
	• microphthalmia
	• Horner syndrome

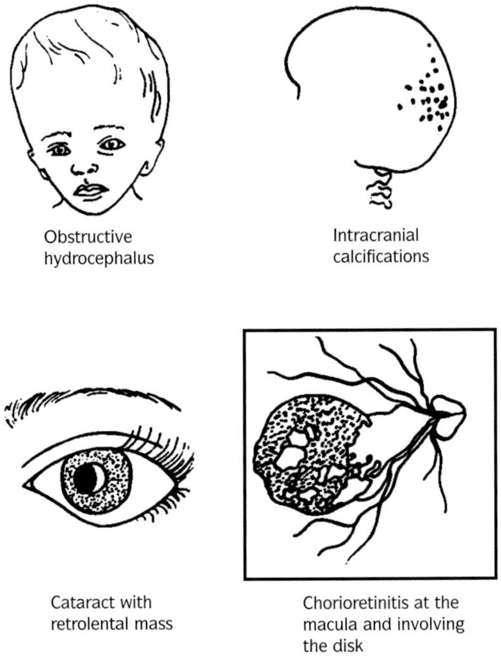

10.10. Fetal toxoplasmosis embryopathy.

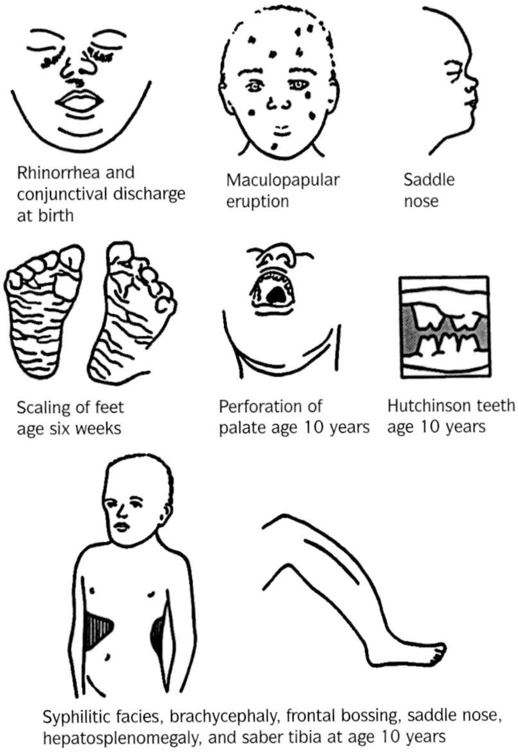

10.11. Fetal syphilis syndrome.

Congenital Syphilis (See Infection Chapter)

See Figures 10.11 and 10.12.

DRUGS AS CAUSES FOR DISRUPTION

Diethylstilbestrol Embryopathy (DES)

Exposure to DES during the 4th to the 12th week of gestation is teratogenic. While vaginal adenosis has been found in 60–75% of females exposed to DES before the 9th week of gestation, the frequency of mesonephric adenocarcinoma is very low, 1/10,000.

Males may have micropenis, hypospadias, cryptorchidism, small testes with indurated capsule, epididymal cysts, and impaired sperm production.

Thalidomide Embryopathy

Most notable defects are limb defects which range from triphalangeal thumb to phocomelia (principally of the upper limbs) (Figure 10.13 and Table 10.10). The most critical period for amelia is from the 27th to the 30th day of development. Triphalangeal thumb (digitalization) occurs most frequently if the drug is given at 32–36 days of development.

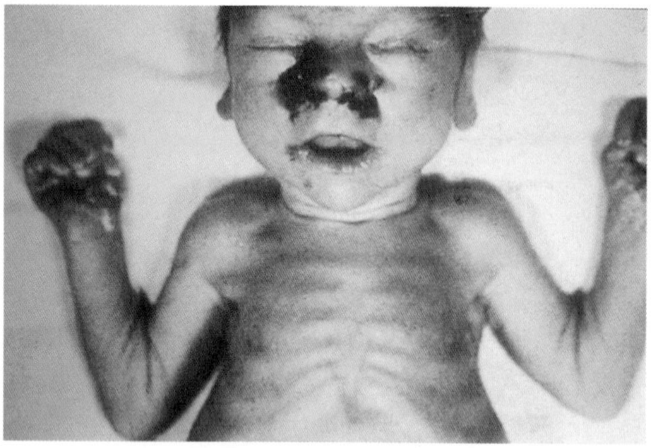

10.12. Infant with congenital syphilis with snuffles.

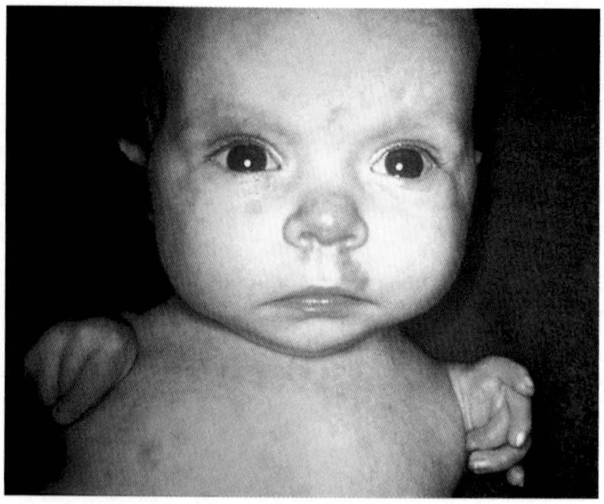

10.13. Thalidomide embryopathy with phocomelia.

Table 10.10 Thalidomide embryopathy

- Skeletal defects
  - Absent radii
  - Hand
    - Limited extension
    - Club hand
    - Hypoplastic or fused phalanges
    - Finger syndactyly
    - Carpal hypoplasia or fusion
    - Radial deviation
  - Ulna
    - Short and malformed
    - Unilaterally absent
    - Bilaterally absent
  - Humerus
    - Hypoplastic
    - Absent
  - Shoulder girdle
    - Abnormally formed with absent glenoid fossa and acromion process
    - Hypoplastic scapula and clavicle
- Hips
  - Unilaterally or bilaterally dislocated
- Legs
  - Coxa valga
  - Femoral torsion
  - Tibial torsion
    - Bilateral
    - Unilateral
  - Stiff Knee
  - Abnormal tibiofibular joint
  - Dislocated patella(e)
- Feet
  - Overriding fifth toe
  - Calcaneovalgus deformity
  - Other foot deformity
- Ribs
  - Asymmetric first rib
  - Cervical rib
- Spine
  - Cervical spina bifida
  - Fused cervical spine
- Mandibular hypoplasia
- Maxillary hypoplasia
- Cardiac anomalies
  - Tetralogy of Fallot
  - Atrial septal defect
  - Patent foramen ovale
  - Dextrocardia
  - Congestive heart failure leading to death
  - Systolic murmur
  - Cardiomegaly
  - Suspected congenital heart disease
- Other abnormalities
  - Apparently low-set ears and malformations extending to microtia
  - Urogenital anomalies
  - Micrognathia
  - Meckel diverticulum
  - Uterine anomalies

Source: Gilbert-Barness E, Opitz JM: Congenital anomalies and malformation syndromes. In Wigglesworth JS, Singer DB (eds): *Textbook of Fetal and Perinatal Pathology,* Oxford, Blackwell Scientific Publications, 1991, p 388.

Table 10.11 Fetal alcohol syndrome (FAS)

Incidence – 1.9 per 1,000 live births
Incidence of less severe clinical manifestations – 1 per 300 live births
1,200 children with FAS are born every year in USA
Neuropathologic lesions:
- Decreased brain weight
- Heterotopic neurons in the cerebral and cerebellar white matter
- Agenesis of the corpus callosum
- Deformity or agenesis of the cerebellar vermis
- Fusion and decreased volume of the thalami
- Abnormalities of dentate gyrus and inferior olive
- Syringomyelia

In vitro studies demonstrate that ethanol causes:
- Adverse effects on neuronal proliferation
- Migration
- Morphologic differentiation

Table 10.12 Pathogenic mechanisms of fetal alcohol syndrome

Maternal nutritional deficiencies
Conversion of ethanol to acetaldehyde
Fetal hypoxic ischemia
Impairment of retinoic acid synthesis
Disruption of neurotransmitters and second messengers
Impairment of neuronal growth and differentiation
Disruption of excitotoxic activity
Disruption of white matter development
Disruption of ganglioside production
Genetic disregulation of cellular adhesion
Suppression of Msx2 expression

Alcohol Embryopathy

Fetal alcohol syndrome (FAS) is the most common recognizable and preventable cause of mental and growth retardation in children (Figures 10.14 to 10.17 and Tables 10.11 to 10.16). A less severe manifestation has been termed fetal alcohol effect (FAE). Up to one-half of FAS infants are born to women who drink 2 oz or more of absolute alcohol per day. Infants of moderate drinkers – i.e., those who drink from 1 to 2 oz. of absolute alcohol per day – may have functional and growth disturbances without other morphologic changes (FAE).

Anticonvulsant Embryopathy

Anticonvulsants (hydantoin, phenytoin, carbamazepine, valproic acid, and

Table 10.13 Fetal alcohol syndrome features and effects

Growth		Performance		Craniofacial	
Prenatal and postnatal growth deficiency	>80%	Developmental delay/mental retardation	>80%	Microcephaly	>80%
Decreased adipose tissue	50–80%	Hyperactivity	50–80%	Short palpebral fissures	50–80%
		Hypotonia, poor coordination	50–80%	Ptosis	26–50%
		Fine motor dysfunction		Retrognathia in infancy	>80%
		Speech problems		Maxillary hypoplasia	50–80%
		Behavioral/psychosocial problems		Hypoplastic philtrum	>80%
				Thin vermillion of upper lip	>80%
				Short upturned nose	50–80%
				Micrognathia in adolescence	50–80%

Cardiac		Other			
Ventricular septal defects	<26%	Cleft lip and/or cleft palate	26%	Microophthalmia, blepharophimosis	26%
Atrial septal defects	26–50%	Myopia	<26%	Small teeth with faulty enamel	<26%
Tetralogy of Fallot, great vessel anomalies	<26%	Strabismus	26–50%	Hypospadias, small rotated kidneys, hydronephrosis	<26%
		Epicanthal folds	26–50%	Hirsutism in infancy	26%
		Hearing loss, protuberant ears		Hernias of diaphragm, umbilicus or inguinal	<26%
		Abnormal thoracic cage			
		Strawberry hemangiomata	26–50%		
		Hypoplastic labia majora	26–50%		

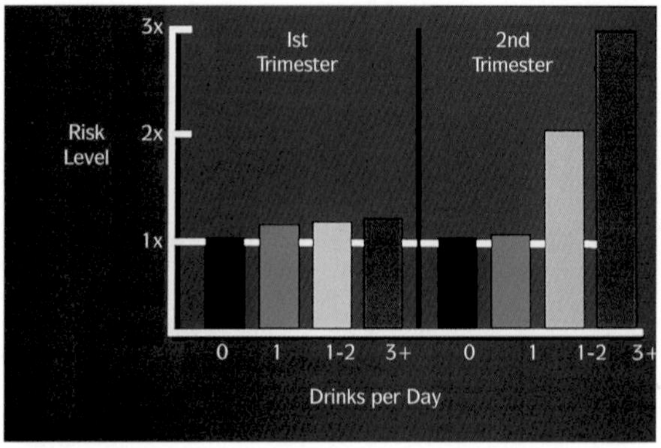

10.14. Relative risk of miscarriage associated with maternal drinking.

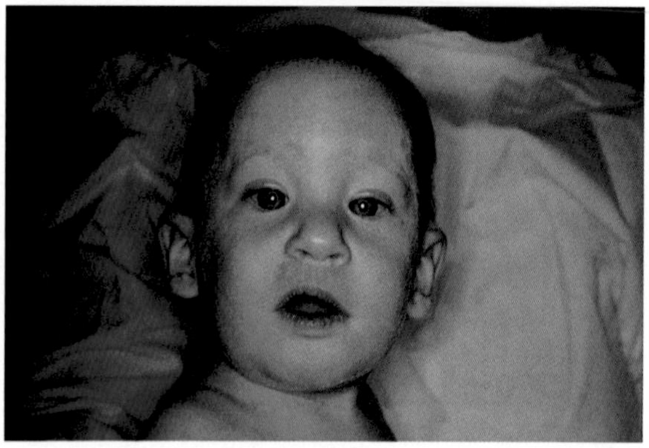

10.15. Infant with fetal alcohol syndrome. Microcephaly, long philtrum, and thin upper lip.

phenobarbital), often used in combination, are mildly teratogenic (Figures 10.18 to 10.21 and Tables 10.17 and 10.18). Polytherapy presents a greater risk for major malformations than monotherapy, but the relative risks of monotherapy versus polytherapy remain unresolved.

Angiotensin-Converting Enzyme (ACE) Inhibitors

These drugs may cause spontaneous abortion and other defects, particularly renal tubular dysgenesis resulting in oligohydramnios. Intrauterine and neonatal death, neonatal respiratory distress, limb and CNS defects, calvarial hypoplasia, and patent ductus arteriosus can be caused by these drugs.

Vitamin A Congener (Isotretinoin, Etretinate) Embryopathy

Current data indicate that use of isotretinoin or etretinate at 0.4–1.5 mg/kg/

Table 10.14 Impact of drinking in pregnancy

Estimated cost of care (extrapolated from N.Y. State study and modified to account for inflation)
- United States – around 4 billion dollars per year
- Wisconsin – around 90 million dollars per year

Table 10.15 Fetal alcohol syndrome

Short palpebral fissures
Hypoplastic philtrum
Thin upper vermilion border
Micrognathia

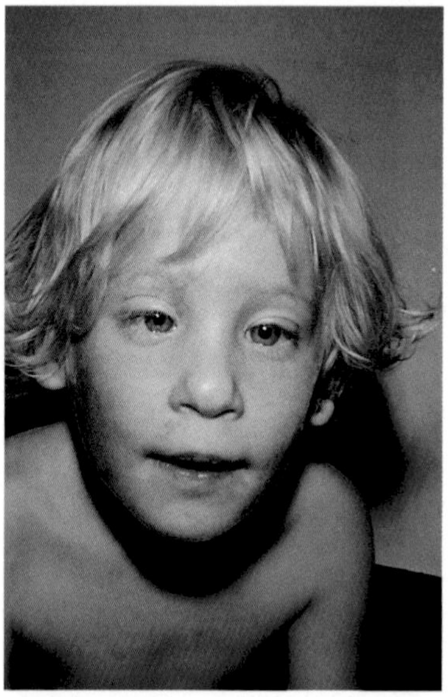

10.16. Child with characteristic features of fetal alcohol syndrome.

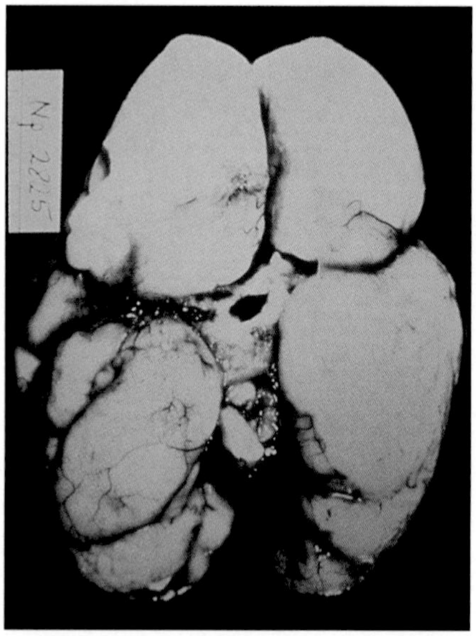

10.17. Brain in fetal alcohol syndrome. There is partial lissencephaly.

Table 10.16 Fetal alcohol syndrome

	Percent abnormalities 0 25 50 75 100%	Percent
Performance	Perinatal growth deficiency	100
	Postnatal growth deficiency	100
	Developmental delay	100
Craniofacies	Microcephaly	91
	Short palpebral fissures	100
	Epicanthal folds	36
	Maxillary hypoplasia	64
	Cleft palate	18
	Micrognathia	27
Limbs	Joint abnormalities	73
	Altered palmar crease pattern	73
Other	Cardiac anomalies	70
	Anomalous external genitalia	36
	Capillary hemangiomata	36
	Fine-motor dysfunction	80

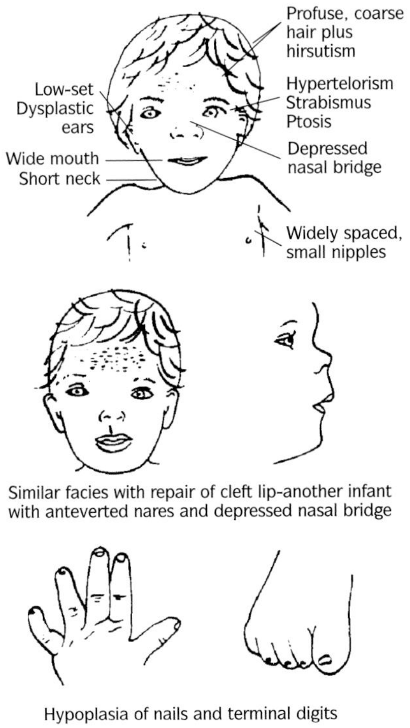

10.18. Fetal hydantoin syndrome.

day of vitamin A at 0.2–1.5 mg/kg/day (greater than 15,0000 units/day) during pregnancy may be associated with a significant increase in risk for serious congenital anomalies in the fetus (Tables 10.19 and 10.20). If exposure takes place within the first 10 weeks after conception, at least 35% of pregnancies result in malformed infants or in spontaneous abortions. The use of topical Retin A has not been implicated as a teratogen.

Manifestations of Isotretinoin Embryopathy

- Abnormal neural crest development
- Migration and excess cell death
- Craniofacial anomalies include:
  - profound mental retardation
  - microcephaly with serious developmental central nervous system
  - anomalies hydrocephalus and posterior fossa cysts.
- Dysmorphic facial features include:
  - facial asymmetry with midface hypoplasia
  - metopic synostosis
  - microphthalmia
  - oculomotor palsies
  - cleft palate
  - microtia/anotia
  - anomalies of the external, middle, and inner ear.
- Other:
  - cardiovascular anomalies
  - thymic hypoplasia
  - genitourinary anomalies (hypoplastic kidneys and hydroureter)

Table 10.17 Anticonvulsants: Embryopathy

Dilantin
Valproic acid
  Facial dysmorphism
  Microcephaly
  Cardiac defects
  Neural tube defects
Trimethadione
  Facial dysmorphism
  Growth retardation
  Mental retardation
  Cleft palate
  Cardiac defects

Table 10.18 Features of fetal anticonvulsant syndromes

Associated more with one particular anticonvulsant than with others:
  Spina bifida (valproic acid)
  Distal digital hypoplasia (phenytoin)
  Nail hypoplasia (phenytoin)
  Tracheomalacia (valproic acid)
  Talipes equinovarus (valproic acid)

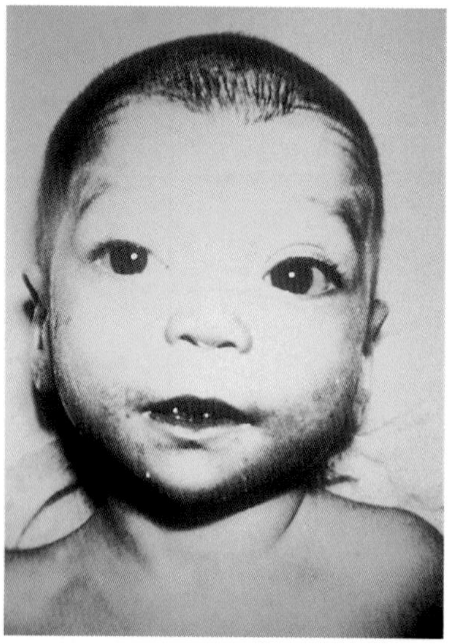

10.19. Infant with hydantoin syndrome. Note hypertelorism.

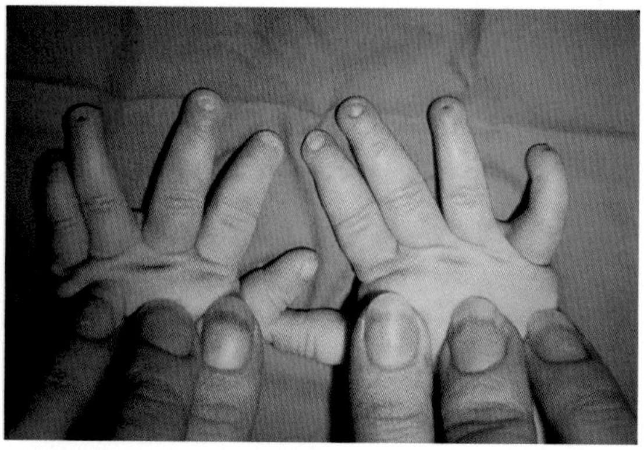

10.20. Hands of infant with hydantoin syndrome showing brachysyndactyly.

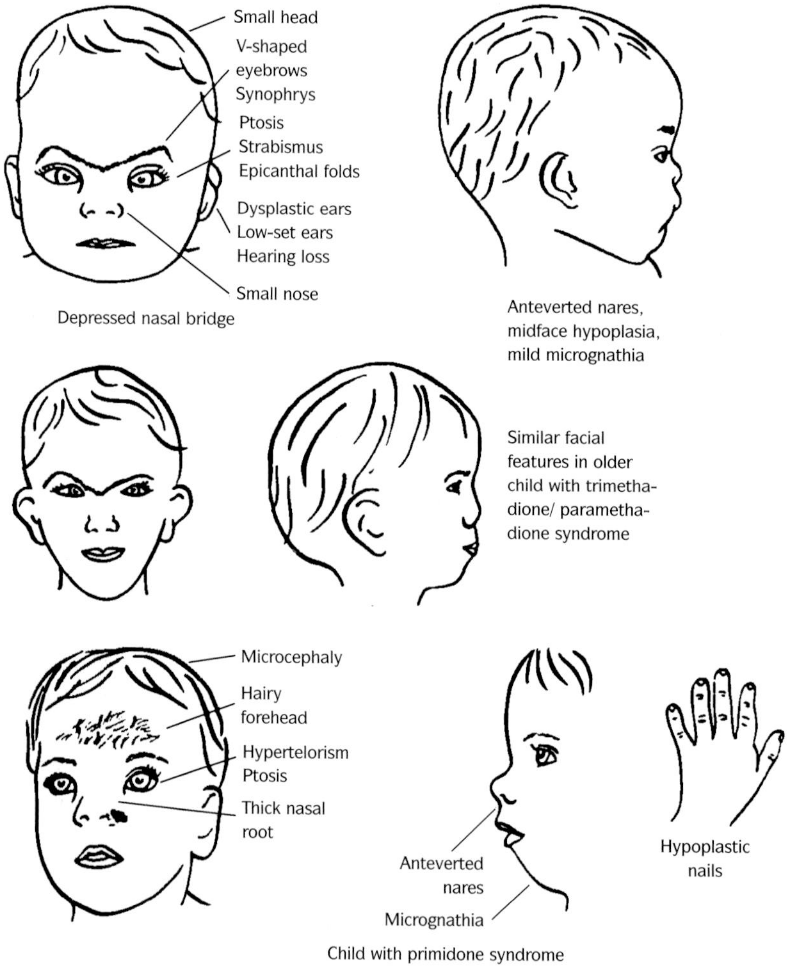

10.21. Fetal trimethadione, paramethadione, and primidone syndromes.

Table 10.19 Vitamins – teratogenic effects

Vitamin A toxicity
- Absence or hypoplastic ears
- CNS anomalies – hydrocephalus
- Cortical blindness
- Congenital heart defects

Vitamin D excess
- Facial dysmorphism
- Infantile hypercalcemia
- Intrauterine growth retardation
- Postnatal growth retardation
- Mental retardation
- Cardiac anomalies
- Calcium deposits in cornea

Vitamin K deficiency
- Chondrodysplasia punctata
- Bleeding

Table 10.20 **Isotretinoin embryopathy manifestations**

Abnormal neural crest development Migration and excess cell death Other anomalies: • Cardiovascular • Thymic hypoplasia • Genitourinary anomalies (hypoplastic kidneys and hydroureter)	Craniofacial anomalies: • Profound mental retardation • Microcephaly with serious developmental CNS anomalies • Hydrocephaly • Posterior fossa cysts	Dysmorphic facial features: • Facial asymmetry with midface hypoplasia • Metopic synostosis • Microphthalmia • Oculomotor palsies • Cleft palate • Microtia/anotia • Anomalies of the external and inner ears

Warfarin Embryopathy

When exposed during the first trimester (6–9 weeks), the embryo may rarely (about 4%) exhibit premature calcification of nasal cartilages with subsequent small nose (10%), and choanal atresia (Figures 10.22 to 10.24 and Table 10.21). About 30% exhibit prenatal growth deficiency.

Warfarin prevents the reduction of vitamin K with consequent gamma carboxyglutamation of osteocalcin that is deposited in fetal cartilage.

Table 10.21 **Warfarin embryopathy**

Short stature
Facial dysmorphism
Chondrodysplasia punctata

Exposure – 8–14 weeks gestation:
- 25% risk
- Choanal stenosis
- Calcific stippling
- Brachydactyly and small nails
- Optic atrophy
- CNS abnormalities

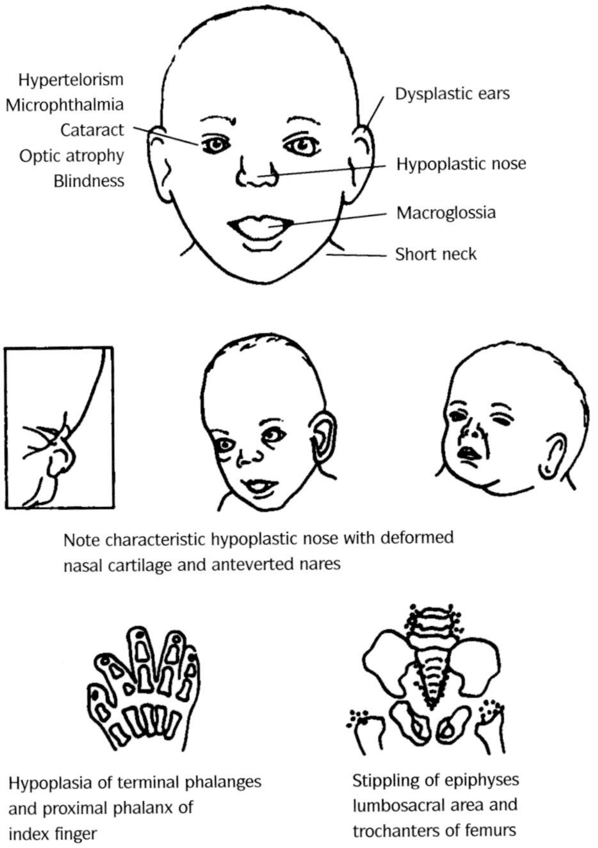

10.22. Warfarin embryopathy.

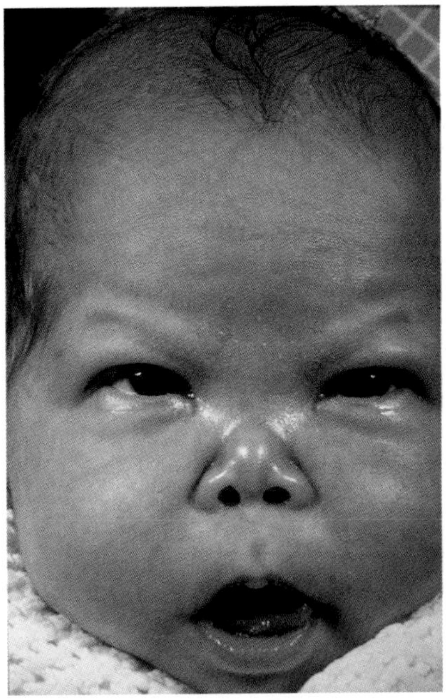

10.23. Infant with Warfarin embryopathy. Depressed nasal bridge and hypoplasia of nose.

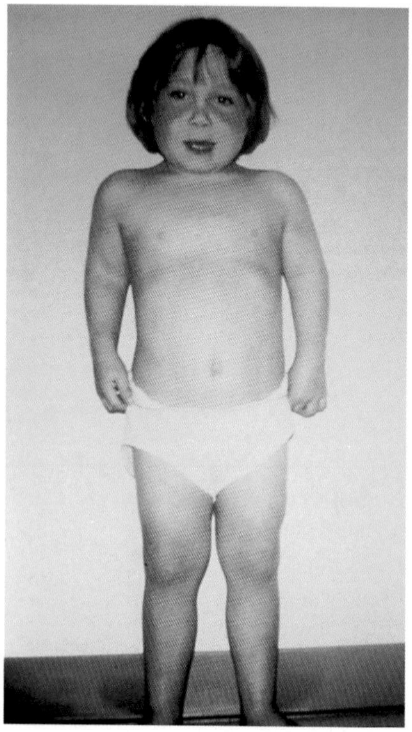

10.24. Warfarin embryopathy. Note short extremities.

Folate Antagonist (aminopterin, methotrexate) Embryopathy

The compounds, aminopterin and its methylated derivative, methotrexate, are currently used as chemotherapeutic agents and in the treatment of psoriasis and some connective tissue disorders including rheumatoid arthritis and systemic lupus erythematosus (Figures 10.25 to 10.29 and Tables 10.22 to 10.26).

The susceptible period appears to be during the 8th and 9th weeks of gestation.

Manifestations

- Growth deficiency of prenatal onset may be present.
- Craniofacial abnormalities include:
  - hydrocephalus
  - abnormal calvaria with widely patent cranial sutures
  - craniolacunae
  - abnormal skull shape
  - craniosynostosis
  - neural tube defects
- Dysmorphic facial features include:
  - hypertelorism
  - dysmorphic pinnae

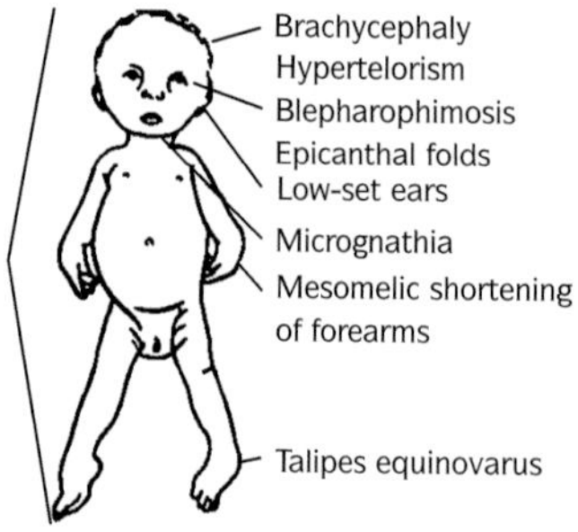

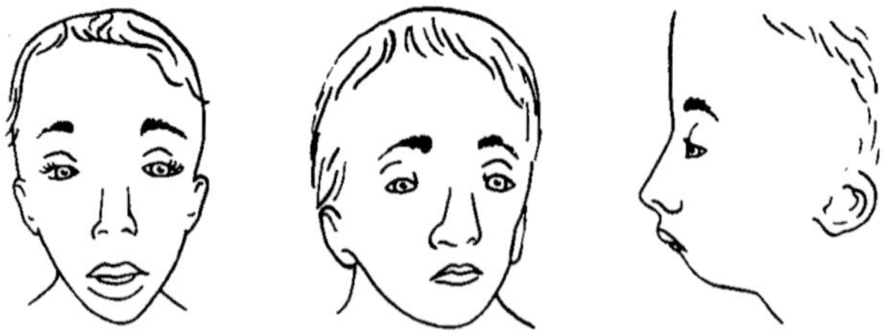

Shallow supraorbital ridges, sparse eyebrows laterally,
blepharophimosis, prominent nose, low-set ears, micrognathia

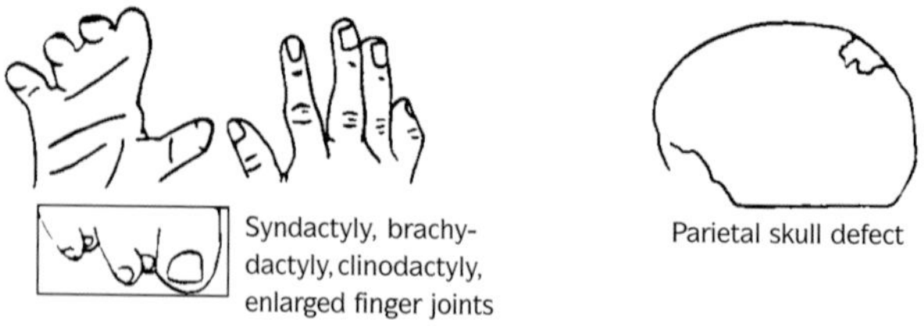

10.25. Folic acid antagonists embryopathy.

Table 10.22 Folic acid deficiency

Neural tube defects (NTD) – anencephaly
70% NTD due to folic acid deficiency
Prevention – 0.4 mg of folic acid daily preconceptional

Table 10.23 Developmental processes requiring folic acid

DNA replication
Cell turnover
Methylation
Gene regulation
5,10-methylenetetrahydrofolate reductase activity
Others

Table 10.24 Preconception folic acid supplementation

Congenital heart defects, particularly defects of the outflow tract (conotruncal) – reduced by 30–50%
Congenital obstructive urinary tract anomalies – reduced by 78–85%
Orofacial Clefts – reduced by 25–65%
Congenital hypertrophic pyloric stenosis – reduced by 76%
Congenital limb defects – reduced by 30–81%

Table 10.25 Food sources of folic acid

Per Serving: Excellent = more than 0.10mg; Good = 0.05–0.1 mg; Fair = 0.015–0.05 mg; Poor = less than 0.015

Breads and cereals
- Fortified breakfast cereals – excellent
- Whole grain bread, fortified white bread, whole grain pasta, brown rice, oats, bran – fair
- Unfortified breakfast cereals, white rice, white pasta, white bread – poor

Vegetables
- Asparagus, beets, brussel sprouts, kale, romaine lettuce, spinach, turnip greens – excellent
- Avocados, bean sprouts, broccoli, cabbage, cauliflower, green beans, iceberg lettuce, okra, peas, parsnips – good
- Most fresh and cooked vegetables – fair

Fruits
- Orange juice, grapefruit juice – good
- Most fresh fruits – fair

Meats and meat alternatives
- Liver (not recommended for pregnant women), cooked black – eyed beans, kidney beans, cooked lima beans – excellent
- Kidney, beef extracts, roasted peanuts, almonds, cashew nuts, cooked soy beans, chickpeas, white beans – good
- Eggs, salmon, beef, most other nuts – fair

Milk and soy products
- Milk, yogurt, cheese – fair

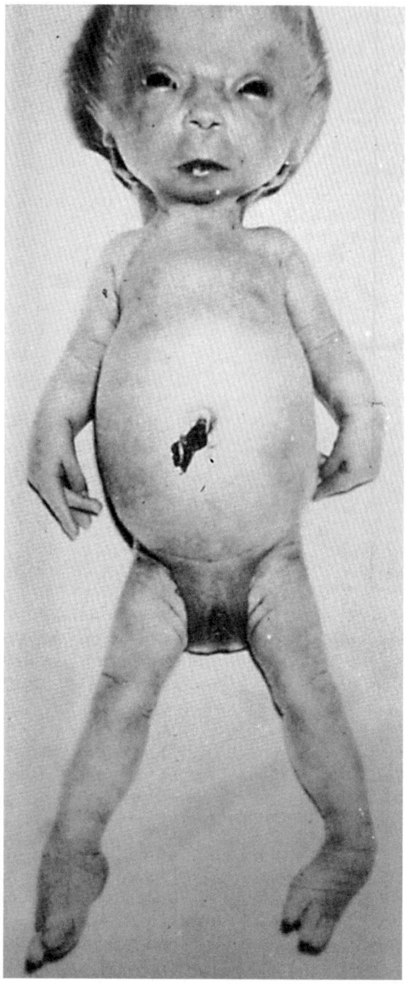

10.26. Infant with aminopterin embryopathy.

- large nose
- striking micrognathia
- cleft palate

Other skeletal defects include:
- absence or hypoplasia of digits
- stenotic changes in long bones
- rib anomalies
- syndactyly and talipes equinovarus

Table 10.26 Folic acid antagonists

Aminopterin
Methotrexate
- Intrauterine growth retardation
- Abortion
- Anencephaly, CNS malformations
- Skeletal malformations

TETRACYCLINE EMBRYOPATHY

Discoloration of the teeth depends upon dose, time, length of administration, and the homologue of the tetracycline employed (Figure 10.28 and Table 10.27). Oxytetracycline stains to a lesser degree than tetracycline.

Table 10.27 Tetracycline embryopathy

Discoloration of the teeth
Deciduous teeth have a yellow to brownish discoloration

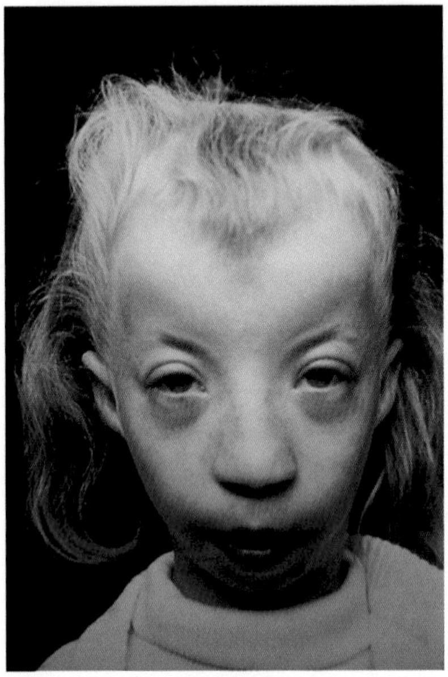

10.27. Child with aminopterin embryopathy. Note widow's peak, hypoplastic eyebrows, large nose, small chin.

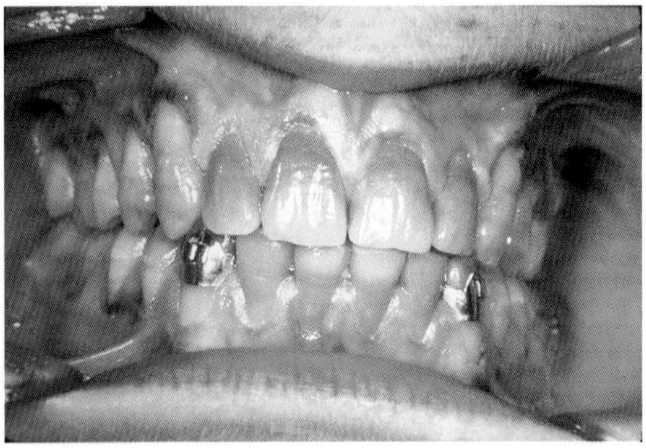

10.28. Staining of permanent teeth due to maternal tetracycline.

The deciduous teeth present a yellow to brownish discoloration of the crown located primarily near the gingival third of the incisors and the occlusal and incisal third of the molars and canines, respectively. In premature infants, a larger surface is stained, and enamel hypoplasia is often found. The bright yellow color, which is striking upon eruption of deciduous teeth, becomes brown after exposure to light. As the teeth become brown, fluorescence under ultraviolet light progressively declines.

LYSERGIC ACID DIETHYLAMIDE (LSD)

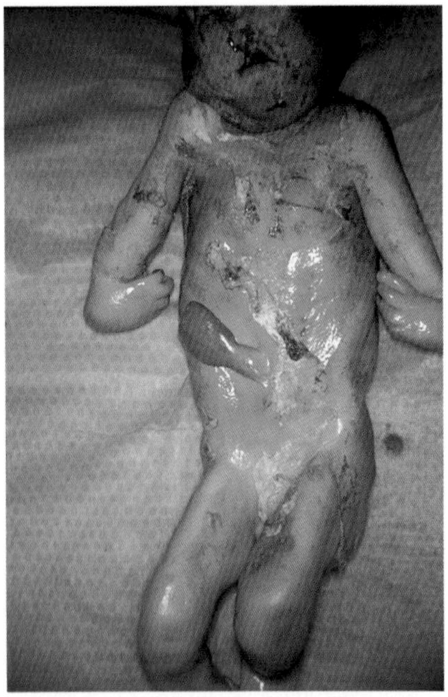

10.29. Limb reduction defects after lysergic acid diethylamide (LSD) exposure during the first trimester of pregnancy.

LSD has been associated with limb defects particularly radial aplasia (Figure 10.29 and Table 10.28).

SYNTHETIC PROGESTIN EMBRYOPATHY

Ambiguous genitalia on the female may result from maternal progesterone therapy (Table 10.29). An increase in the expected frequency of cardiovascular defects and hypospadias has also been reported but is not well documented.

SYMPATHOMIMETICS

These drugs taken during the first trimester of pregnancy have been associated with gastroschisis, limb defects, and minor anomalies, including inguinal hernia and clubfoot (Figure 10.30). First branchial arch developmental field defect (otocephaly) has been related to the use of sympathomimetic drugs and theophylline.

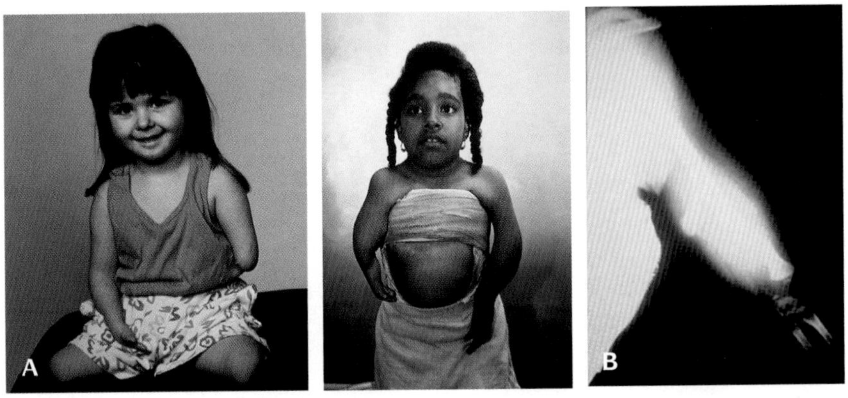

10.30. **(A)** and **(B)** Limb defects following exposure to sympathomimetic drugs during pregnancy. **(C)** X-ray showing fusion of humerus and ulna with bony spur and absence of radius (oligoectosyndactyly). The mother was exposed to high doses of Primatene (ephedrine, theophylline, phenobarbital) throughout pregnancy.

Table 10.28 Lysergic acid diethylamide

LSD has been associated with: *Limb defects* and particularly *radial aplasia*.

Table 10.29A Diethylstilbestrol (DES)

Females – Vaginal adenosis
Males – Reproductive anomalies
– Testicular germ cell tumor

Table 10.29B Synthetic progestin embryopathy

- Females – Enlargement of clitoris
- Males – Hypospadias

Maternal Phenylketonuria Embryopathy

Individuals with phenylketonuria, when placed on a phenylalanine-free diet, lead a reasonably normal life (Table 10.30). However, females with the disorder who are not diet protected during their pregnancy nearly always give birth to infants with intrauterine and postnatal growth retardation, microcephaly, mental retardation, congenital heart anomalies, dislocated hips, and other defects. The anomalies in the fetus have been attributed to the maternal metabolic disturbances. When maternal phenylalanine exceeds 20 mg per deciliter, 95% of their infants have mental retardation, 73% have microcephaly, 40% have intrauterine growth retardation, and 12% cardiac anomalies. About 25% of pregnancies are spontaneously aborted.

Toluene Embryopathy

Toluene embryopathy is a consequence of solvent abuse (spray paint, lacquer or glue sniffing) (Figure 10.31 and Tables 10.31 and 10.32).

Toluene easily crosses the placenta, producing changes in infants very reminiscent of those seen in fetal alcohol embryopathy. Both toluene and alcohol embryopathy probably result from a common insult to the mesoderm ventral to the forebrain.

Table 10.30 Maternal phenylketonuria embryopathy

When the mother is not diet protected during pregnancy, infants may have:
- Intrauterine and postnatal growth retardation
- Microcephaly
- Mental retardation
- Congenital heart anomalies
- Dislocated hips
- Other defects

When maternal phenylalanine exceeds 20 mg/dl, infants have:
- 95% – mental retardation
- 40% – intrauterine growth retardation
- 12% – cardiac anomalies
- 25% – spontaneous abortion
- 73% – microcephaly

Table 10.31 Toluene embryopathy

Crosses the placenta and causes:
- Changes similar to fetal alcohol embryopathy
- Insult to mesoderm ventral to the forebrain

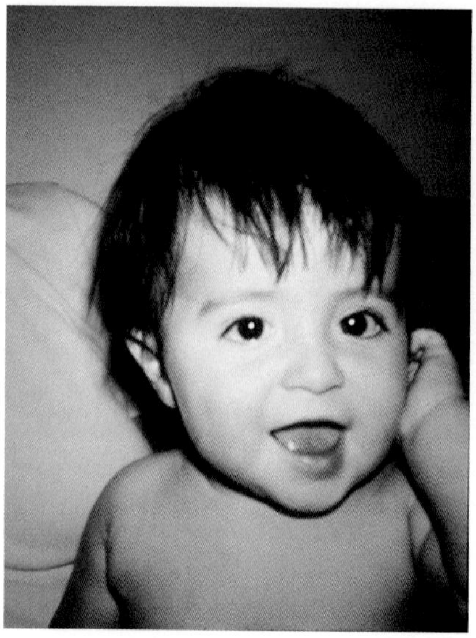

10.31. Child with toluene embryopathy. Note microcephaly, midfacial hypoplasia, small palpebral fissures.

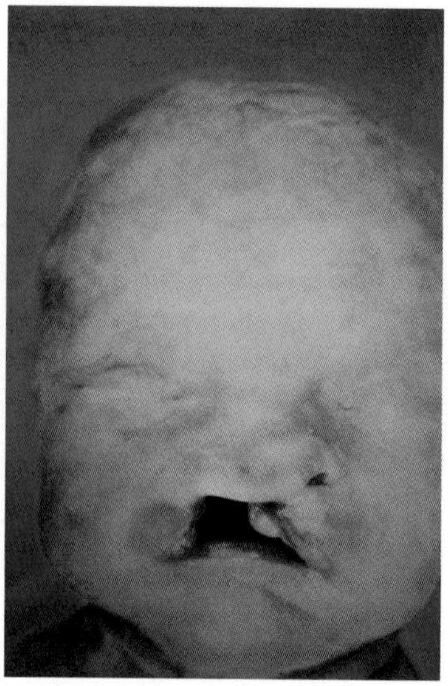

10.32. Infant stillborn with cleft lip, and palate due to maternal prednisone. There was also an atrioventricular septal defect.

PREDNISONE

Given in high doses, prednisone administered during the first trimester may result in cleft lip/palate and/or cardiac defects, particularly endocardial cushion defects (Figure 10.32).

OPIATES

Opiates include heroin and methadone. Intrauterine exposure may result in effects on the fetus (Tables 10.33 and 10.34).

Table 10.32 Effects of toluene embryopathy

	Incidence (%)		Incidence (%)
Prematurity	40	Small nose	35
Pre- and postnatal growth deficiency	50	Downturned corners of mouth	33
Prenatal microcephaly	30	Large anterior fontanel	20
Developmental delay	80	Nail hypoplasia	40
Micrognathia	65	Altered palmar creases	35
Midfacial hypoplasia	65	Blunt fingertips	50
Small palpebral fissures	65	Clinodactyly	20
Dysmorphic pinnae	60	Hypotonia or hypertonia	35
Narrow bifrontal diameter	50	Hemangiomata	30
Abnormal scalp hair pattern	45	Hydronephrosis	25
Thin upper lip and smooth philtrum	35		

Table 10.33 Intrauterine exposure to opiates

Prevalence	Pathogenic mechanisms of neurologic toxicity
2–3% in all USA births	Disruption of the sensitivity of the *locus ceruleus*
6,000–10,000 births each year are to mothers addicted to heroin or methadone	Dysfunction of second messengers
	Abnormal expression of early immediate genes
Clinical manifestations	
Newborns	Infants and children
Low birth weight	Growth retardation
Intrauterine growth retardation	Microcephaly
Microcephaly	Sudden infant death syndrome
Abstinence syndrome	Psychomotor and cognitive deficit
Seizures	Learning disabilities
	Behavior abnormalities

COCAINE EMBRYOPATHY

Cocaine has been hypothesized to cause disruption of embryonic and fetal vasculature, especially in the second and third trimesters (Table 10.35). Structural anomalies reported in infants exposed in utero to cocaine that are consistent with vascular disruption are nonduodenal intestinal atresia or infarction, unilateral terminal transverse limb reduction defects, atypical ectrodactyly, asymmetric radial ray anomalies, single forearm bone and digit, aplasia cutis congenita, unilateral renal agenesis (URA), urinary obstruction sequence (UOS), cerebral infarctions and hemorrhage, and placental infarctions and abruptions.

The most likely mechanism for cocaine causing vascular disruption is alteration of blood flow at the uterine-placental unit by a direct effect on the embryonic-fetal vasculature with increase in blood pressure, and/or the effects of toxic oxygen-free radicals.

MARIJUANA EXPOSURE

The active ingredient of marijuana is 8,9-tetrahydoconnabinol that crosses the placenta easily. Its effects are shown in Table 10.36.

Table 10.34 Intrauterine exposure to opiates (IEO): abstinence syndrome

Present in 50–80% of IEO fetuses

Symptoms:
- Irritability
- Gastrointestinal dysfunction
- Respiratory distress
- Autonomic changes

Neurologic signs:
- Hypertonia
- Tremor
- Hyperreflexia
- Sleep anomalies
- Difficulties with feeding
- Seizures

Table 10.35 Cocaine embryopathy

Structural anomalies:
- Intestinal atresia or infarction
- Unilateral terminal transverse limb reduction defects
- Atypical ectrodactyly
- Asymmetric radial ray anomalies
- Single forearm bone and digit
- Aplasia cutis congenita
- Unilateral renal agenesis
- Cerebral infarctions and hemorrhage
- Placental infarctions and abruptions

Table 10.36 Intrauterine exposure to marijuana

Prevalence	Clinical manifestations	
Most widely used illicit drug in the United States	Newborns	Infants and children
66 million Americans have admitted to trying it at least once	Intrauterine growth retardation	Psychomotor developmental delay
Use of marijuana during pregnancy – 14–27%	Dysmorphic features – Similar to FAS	Diminished abstract and visual reasoning
	Decreased response to light or increased response to surprise stimuli	Sleep abnormalities

DIABETIC EMBRYOPATHY

Infants born to insulin-dependent diabetic mothers (IDM) have a two- to threefold increased risk of congenital malformations and spontaneous abortion (Tables 10.37 and 10.38 and Figures 10.33 to 10.36).

Most frequently noted are anomalies of the cardiovascular, genitourinary, and central nervous systems. In addition, infants with caudal dysplasia, femoral hypoplasia, and unusual facies are born more frequently to diabetic mothers. The most severe degree of malformation is sirenomelia. The injuries to the fetus occur before the 7th week of gestation.

HEAVY METALS

Heavy metals including lithium, methyl mercury, and lead can result in malformations (Table 10.39).

VASCULAR DISRUPTIONS

A vascular disruption is a structural abnormality resulting from damage to or interruption of normal embryonic or fetal development of the arteries, veins, or capillaries.

Alteration in blood flow to the uterine-placental unit, from either chronic or acute reduction of uterine blood supply, affects the developing embryo and fetus (Tables 10.40 and 10.41). Acute reduction in blood flows may occur after

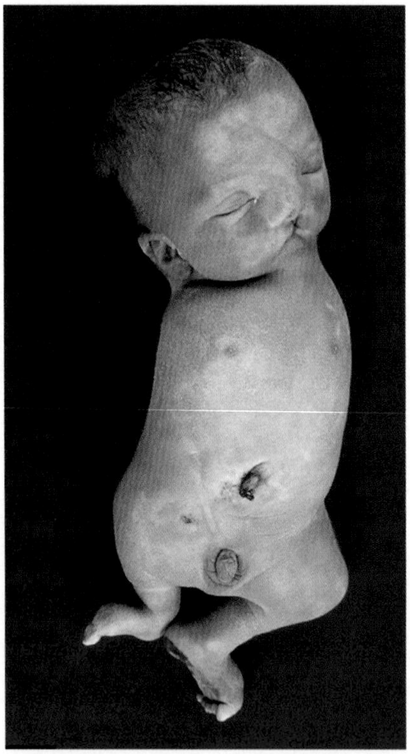

10.33. Infant of diabetic mother with amelia of upper limbs, cleft lip, and caudal dysplasia.

Table 10.37 Maternal diabetes

Hemoglobin AIC	>11.5 mg–66% malformations
	< 9.5 mg% – no malformations
Hyperinsulinism in utero	macrosomia visceromegaly
Congenital malformations:	caudal regression
	CV defects
	CNS defects
	Skeletal defects
	Renal defects

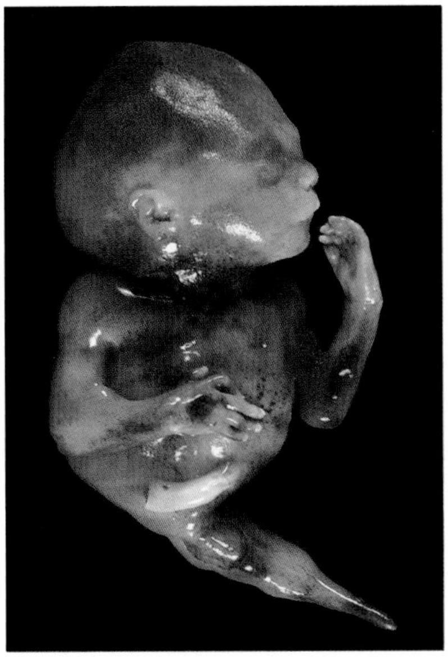

10.34. Infant of diabetic mother with sirenomelia.

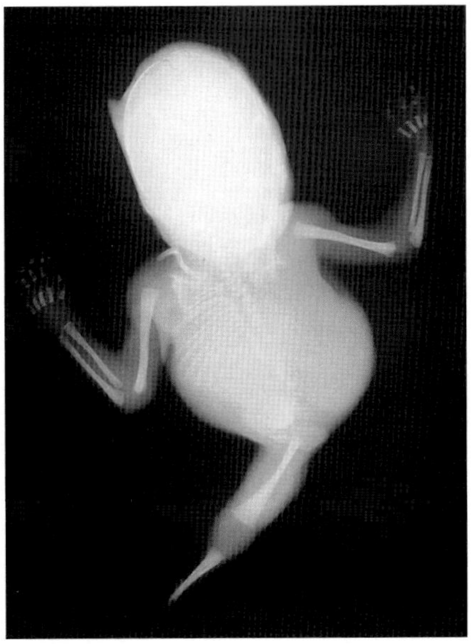

10.35. Infant of diabetic mother x-ray of sirenomelia.

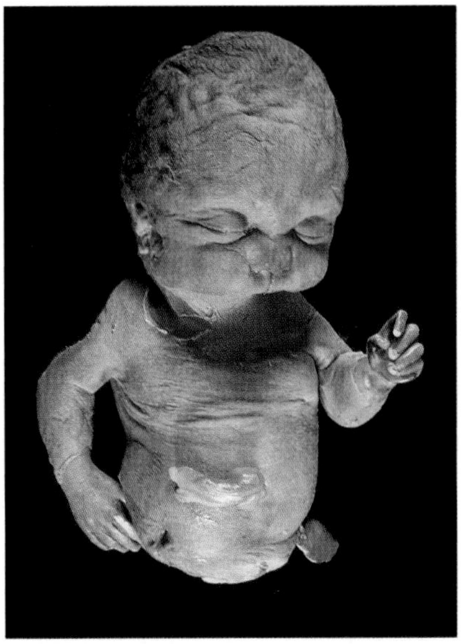

10.36. Infant of diabetic mother with complete absence of lower half of abdomen and lower extremities.

Table 10.38 Major congenital anomalies in offspring of diabetic mothers

Central nervous system	Cardiovascular system	Other abnormalities
Holoprosencephaly	Transposition of the great vessels	Hypoplastic lungs
Anencephaly	Ventricular septal defect	Omphalocele
Occipital encephalocele	Pulmonary stenosis	Unilateral renal agenesis
Arhinencephaly	Hypoplastic left heart	Caudal regression
	Ebstein malformation	Amelia of upper limbs
	Atrial septal defect	Bilateral auricular atresia
	Tetralogy of Fallot	Cleft lip
	Mitral valve atresia	

Table 10.39 Heavy metals

Lithium	heart defects – Ebstein anomaly
Methyl mercury	Minimata disease cerebral palsy microcephaly
Lead	abortion stillbirth minor malformations

maternal trauma, hypotension, sympathetic nerve stimulation, and clamping of uterine vessels.

Encephaloclastic Lesions

Encephaloclastic lesions can result from insults during the fetal period, at birth, or postnatally. They result from necrotic softening and destruction of the brain. They usually communicate with the ventricular or subarachnoid space, or both.

Multicystic encephalomalacia has been reported in twins and is thought to result in multiple emboli occluding cerebral vessels resulting in "Swiss cheese brain."

Clinical and experimental evidence supports vascular disruption in the pathogenesis of some cases of **hydranencephaly**, although many result from intrauterine infection.

Table 10.40 Mechanisms of vascular disruption of normally developing tissues

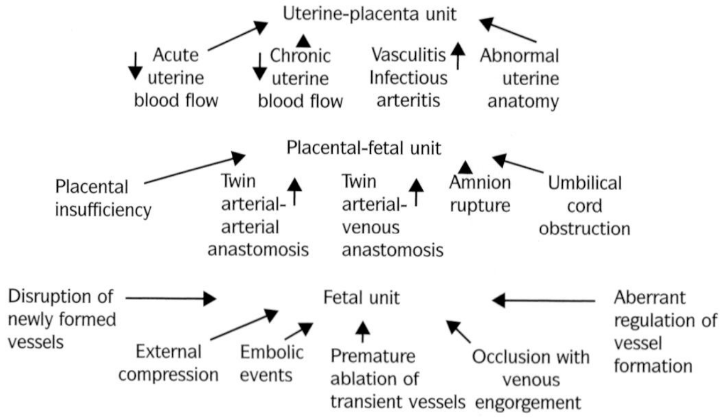

Table 10.41 Result of vascular disruption in the embryo and fetus

Mechanism	Examples of resultant structural anomalies
Disruption of embryonic capillary plexus	Early amnion disruption sequence Limb body wall complex Oromandibular hypogenesis syndrome
Persistence of embryonic vessels	Structural anomalies of limbs, e.g., radial aplasia, tibial aplasia, clubfoot, fibular aplasia
Premature ablation of embryonic vessels	Subclavian artery supply disruption sequence (Poland, Möbius, Klippel-Feil sequences) Horseshoe kidney
Failure of maturation of vessels	Capillary hemangiomas Arteriovenous fistulas Berry aneurysms
Occlusion (external compression) of vessels	Amniotic band syndrome Anomalies associated with fibroids, tubal pregnancies, and bicornate uterus
Occlusion (emboli, thrombosis) of vessels	Twin anomalies Comparable anomalies in singletons
Altered hemodynamics	Anomalies associated with cocaine use

Limb Reduction Defects

Limb reduction defects are multifactorial in nature. Isolated limb anomalies, especially terminal transverse defects that are sporadic, may be due to vascular disruption.

Transverse limb defects, absent limbs, and limb girdles may result from extensive involvement by a hematoma or disruption during early limb bud formation. This has occurred after chorionic villus sampling.

Limb/Body Wall Defect (LBWD)

Limb/body wall defect is a body wall defect with evisceration of thoracic and/or abdominal organs associated with other congenital anomalies, including in some cases limb deficiencies. The LBWD is different from gastroschisis, which is usually a small body wall defect lateral to the umbilical cord, which is not covered by any membrane and, in most cases, is an isolated defect.

The limb body wall malformation complex results from a malfunction in the ectodermal placodes.

The amnio-ectodermal transition zone plays an important role in the formation of the ventral body wall. A surface ectoderm placode is at the transition zone, depositing mesectodermal cells that will form the mesodermal structures of the body wall (e.g., muscles, connective tissue, vessels).

Placodes are specialized parts of the surface ectoderm that add cells to the mesodermal compartment. They are involved in the formation of many organs and structures, including the neural tube, nose, branchial arches, ventral body wall, and limbs. When these ectodermal placodes do not function correctly, the mesoderm remains underdeveloped and severe malformations may be expected.

In secondary abdominoschisis the body wall placode is deficient in depositing mesoectodermal cells after the amnioectodermal transition zone has attached to the connecting stalk, and the body cavity has separated from the extraembryonic coelom. The body wall remains very thin and eventually ruptures because of the increase of the abdominal and/or the thoracic organs. The margins of such a body wall defect are smooth and show a transition from skin into the mesothelium of the body cavity. This is a gastroschisis.

Small developmental defects in the mesodermal compartment can easily result in severe limb malformations due to abnormal function of the limb bud placodes.

Constrictive amniotic bands, amniotic adhesions, and LBWD are discrete but often combined disruption sequences with important pathogenetic overlap.

Four groups of LBWD:

1. Body stalk anomalies. This is characterized by severe clefts of the abdominal wall with absence of, or very small, umbilical cord, or it is continuous with the placenta.
2. Body wall defects without amniotic bands.
3. Body wall defects produced by amniotic bands.
4. Gastroschisis.

Diagnosis of LBWD is based on the presence of two of three of the following characteristics: exencephaly or encephalocele with facial clefts; thoracoschisis (upper body wall deficiency), abdominoschisis (lower body wall deficiency), or thoracoabdominoschisis; and limb defects. Classically, pleurosomas refers to body wall and upper limb defects, and cyllosomas to body wall deficiency and lower limb defects.

Ninety-five percent of fetuses with LBWD have associated internal structural anomalies.

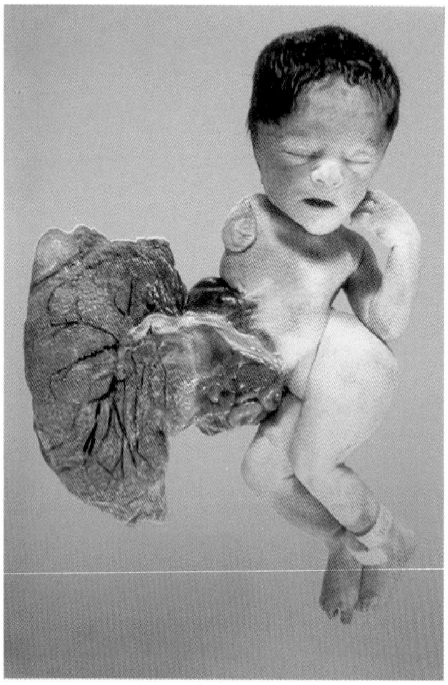

10.37. Newborn infant with short umbilical cord, gastroschisis, and pleurosomas.

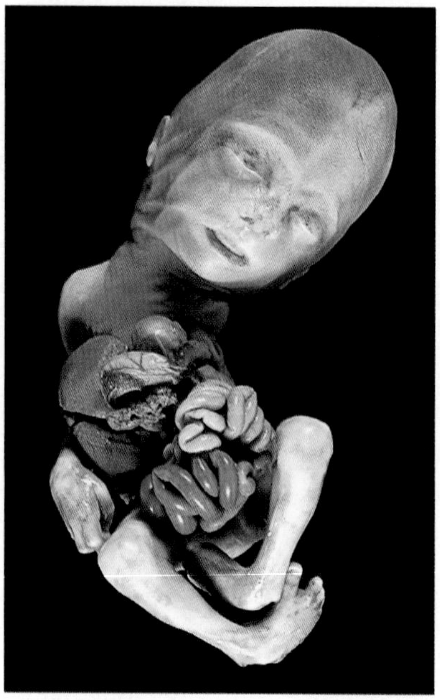

10.38. Fetus with thoraco-abdominal body wall defect.

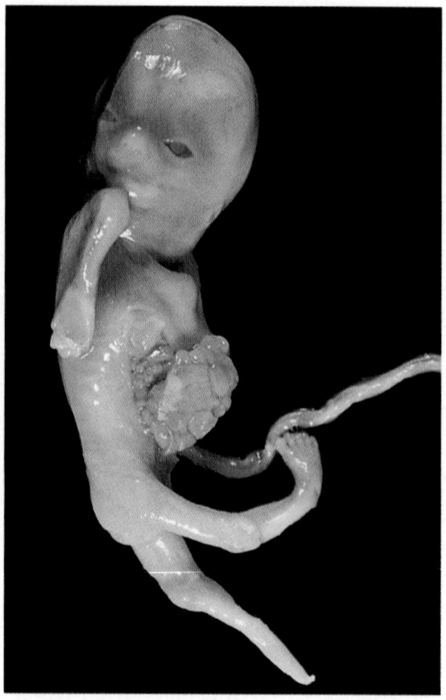

10.39. Fetus with abdominal wall defect and cyllosomas.

In 72% of fetuses, the internal anomalies are recognized to be secondary to vascular disruption.

Ultrasonography

- Cloacal exstrophy – absent bladder, lumbo-sacral neural tube, single umbilical artery.
- Pentalogy of Cantrell – (often in trisomy 13, trisomy 18, Turner syndrome) omphalocele, ectopia cordis, diaphragmatic hernia, pericardial defect, structural cardiac anomalies.

Gastroschisis

Gastroschisis is an abdominal wall defect lateral to the umbilical cord (more commonly on the left) (Figures 10.37 to 10.39). It is distinguished from an omphalocele by the absence of a membranous sac. The extrusion of abdominal organs is into the amniotic cavity rather than the extracoelomic space, as occurs in a body wall defect. Gastroschisis appears to result from premature ablation and/or disruption of the embryonic omphalomesenteric artery. The resultant abdominal wall defect leads to extrusion of abdominal contents into the amniotic cavity.

Associated structural anomalies in the gastrointestinal tract are present in 40–50% of cases. Frequent associated anomalies include nonduodenal intestinal atresia or stenosis, atresia of the appendix, atresia of the gallbladder, absence of one kidney, hydronephrosis and hydroureters, and porencephaly.

Pentalogy of Cantrell

Pentalogy of Cantrell (Figure 10.40) is characterized by:

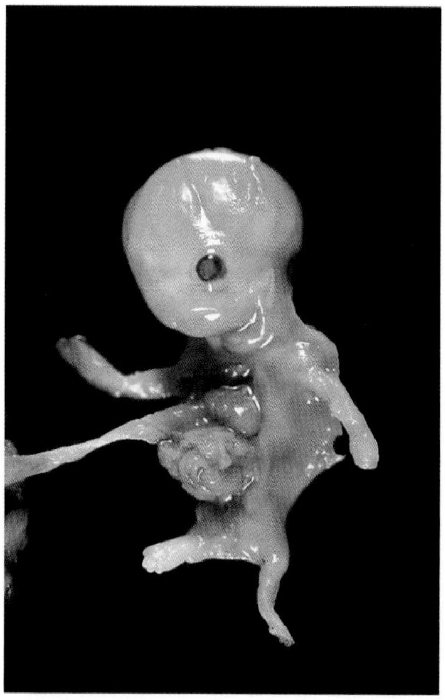

10.40. Pentalogy of Cantrell. Fetus with thoraco-abdominal wall defect, ectopia cordis with cardiac defects, defect of sternum and diaphragm.

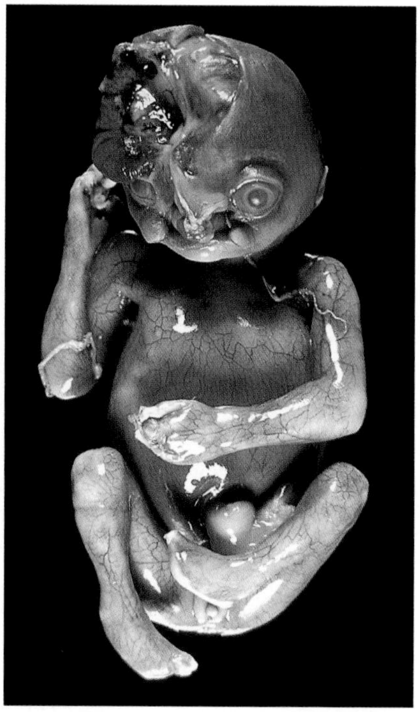

10.41. Fetus with amniotic bands resulting in disruption of head, fingers, and toes.

1. Anterior abdominal wall defect.
2. Diaphragmatic defect.
3. Absent lower sternum.
4. Absent pericardium.
5. Ectopia cordis with congenital cardiac defects.

Twins (See Twin Chapter)

Vascular disruption in twins may result from:

1. Emboli from the placenta to both monogygotis twins, causing death of one twin and structural anomalies from embolic infarction in the surviving twin.
2. Thromboplastin from the demised co-twin causing disseminated intravascular coagulation and structural anomalies in the surviving twin (Swiss cheese brain).
3. Altered fetal hemodynamics with transient hypotension or hypertension.
4. Altered growth and anomalies from embryonic hypoperfusion.
5. Disparate placental blood flow (maternal-placental unit) resulting in altered growth and anomalies from hypo- to hyperperfusion.

Amnion Disruption Sequence (ADS)

There are three types of lesions: (1) constrictive tissue bands, (2) amniotic adhesions, and (3) more complex anomaly patterns, designated as limb-body wall complex (LBWC) (Figures 10.41 to 10.50 and Tables 10.42 to 10.45).

Table 10.42 Results of amnion rupture

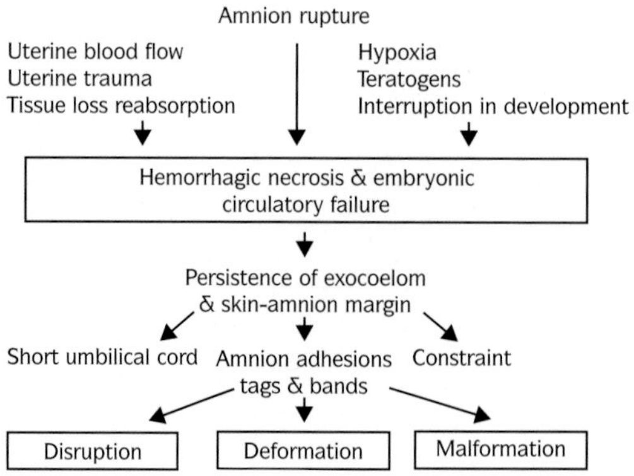

Table 10.43 Amnion rupture

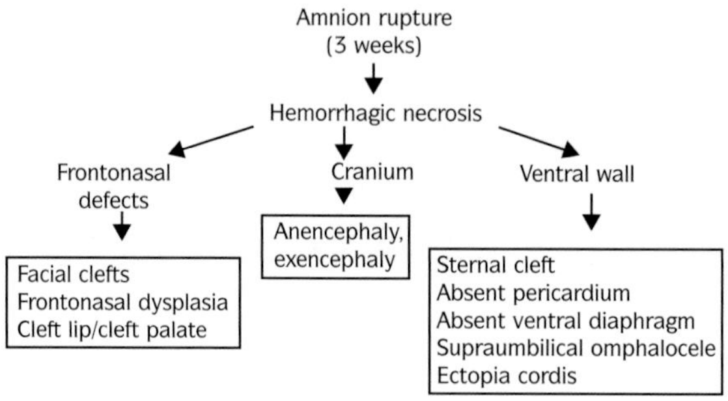

Table 10.44 Classification of disorders within amnion disruption sequence

Group	Disruption complex	Prognosis
Group I: Early embryonic period		
1. Before 4 weeks gestation	i. Anencephaly with amnionic bands	Neonatal lethal
	ii. Craniofacial clefts with ectopia cordis	Almost always lethal Usually neonatal lethal
	iii. Limb body wall complex	Variable; amenable to plastic surgery
2. 3–6 weeks gestation	iv. Unusual facial clefting	Variable intellectual impairment; dependent on degree of brain malformation
	v. Encephalocele/pseudoencephalocele	
Group II: Midembryonic period (4–7 weeks)	i. CL/CP ± limb defect ± CHD ± associated internal anomalies	Usually good but dependent on associated anomalies
	ii. Limb reduction defect ± associated anomalies ± constriction bands	Good but dependent on associated anomalies
Group III: Late embryonic to early fetal period (7–12 weeks)	i. Pierre Robin sequence secondary to transient oligohydramnios	Good
	ii. Oligohydramnios sequence from persistent oligohydramnios	Dependent on degree of pulmonary hypoplasia
Group IV: Late embryonic to fetal period (9 weeks on)	i. Limb entanglement in amnion Limb amputation Constriction bands Distal lymphedema	Good

CL/CP, cleft lip and/or palate   CHD, congenital heart defect

Table 10.45 Temporal relationship of abnormalities in early amnion rupture – ADAM complex

Fetal timing	Craniofacial	Limbs	Other
before 4 weeks	Anencephaly Facial distortion, proboscis Unusual facial clefting Eye defects Encephalocele, meningocele		Placenta attached to head and/or abdomen Short umbilical cord
4–7 weeks	Cleft lip Choanal atresia	Limb deficiency Polydactyly Syndactyly	Abdominal wall defects Thoracic wall defects Scoliosis
7–12 weeks and onward	Cleft palate Micrognathia Ear deformities Craniostenosis	Amniotic bands Amputation Hypoplasia Pseudosyndactyly Distal lymphedema Foot deformities Dislocation of hip	Short umbilical cord Omphalocele
Later	Oligohydramnios deformation sequence		

Constrictive bands, are caused by primary amnion rupture with subsequent entanglement of fetal parts (mostly limbs) by shriveled amniotic strands. Adhesive bands are the result of a broad fusion between disrupted fetal parts (mostly cephalic) and an intact amniotic membrane. Most of the craniofacial defects (encephaloceles and/or facial clefts) occurring in these fetuses are not caused by constrictive amniotic bands but are the result of a vascular disruption sequence with or without cephalo-amniotic adhesion.

A spectrum of structural anomalies is seen in **amnion disruption sequence.** The type of anomalies depends on the stage of embryonic development and the severity of the disruptive event.

The amniotic membrane sometimes may become attached to areas of cell death or imperfect histogenesis in the fetus; in this way, amniotic bands can be formed secondary to the malformations.

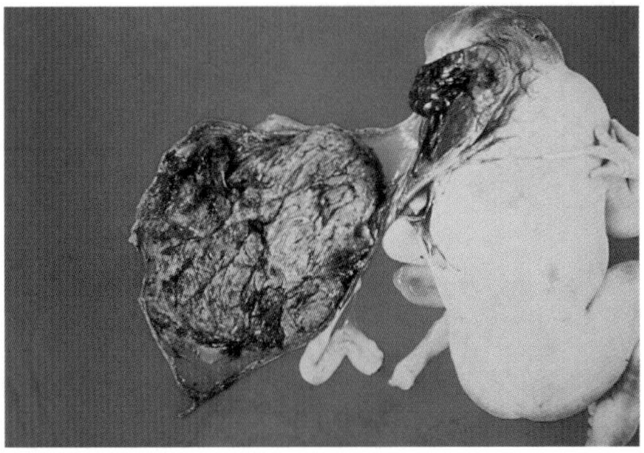

10.42. Amniotic bands attached to fetus resulting in anencephaly. A finger is attenuated and attached by amniotic bands to placenta.

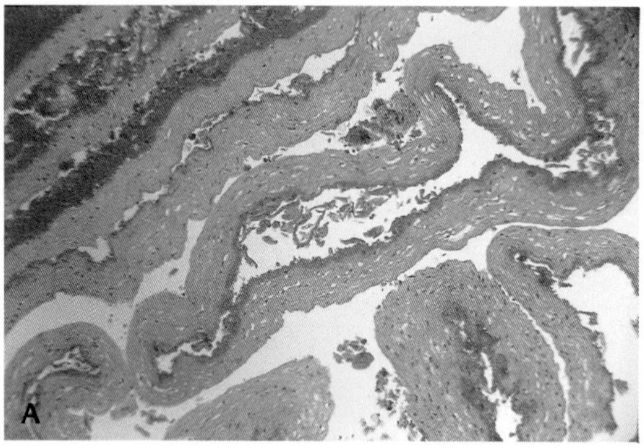

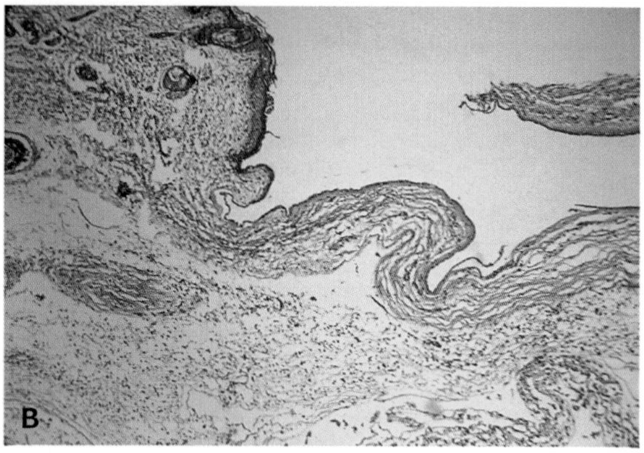

10.43. Microscopic appearance. **(A)** Amniotic bands with attached fragments of fetal keratin. **(B)** An amniotic band with fetal skin (left), keratin (right).

Structures that have been mistaken for amniotic bands fall into two categories: macerated sheets of epidermis or strands of hyalinized fibrous tissue that are the residua of localized areas of defective tissue.

In **chorionic villus sampling (CVS)** when performed earlier than 10 weeks (70 days) of gestation (8 weeks postconception), transverse limb reduction defects, ring constrictions, and oromandibular hypogenesis spectrum have been reported (Figure 10.51 and Table 10.46). These anomalies most likely result from vascular disruption but amnion rupture may also occur in some cases.

Oligohydramnios disruption sequence is a well-documented complication of amniocentesis and CVS.

In ADS, structural anomalies result from (1) disruption of existing and developing tissues due to damage of developing vasculature or mechanical disruption of the embryo and fetus; (2) deformations secondary to *in utero* constraint if there is persistent oligohydramnios from fluid leakage; and (3)

Table 10.46 **Chorionic villus sampling**

Before 70 days may cause:
- Transverse limb defects
- Oromandibular hypogenesis

Rate of fetal loss – 2.3–2.5%
Between 9 and 12 weeks gestation
Results available in 24–48 hours
Useful for DNA or enzymatic analysis
Amniotic fluid necessary for α-fetoprotein concentration

Table 10.47 **Factors influencing the linear growth of umbilical cord**

1. Tensile forces placed upon the umbilical cord.
2. Fluid space in amniotic cavity.
3. Intrauterine movement of early embryo.

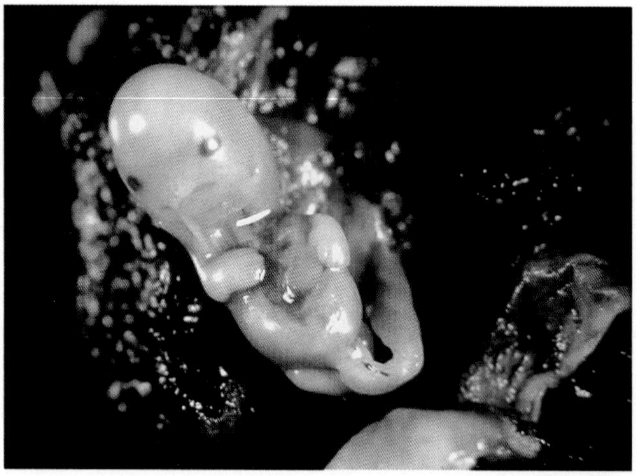

10.44. Embryo 6 weeks gestation with amniotic band attached to lip.

Table 10.48 Short umbilical cord

Reduced fetal activity	Etiology
Anencephaly	Reduced fetal activity
Neuromuscular disorders	Amniotic-deformity-adhesion-mutilation sequence (ADAM)
Multiple joint contractures	Limb body wall defect – cyllosomas/ pleurosomas
Arthrogryposis	Acephalus-acardia
Severe limb deficiences	Primary defect of umbilical cord formation
Pena-Shokair syndrome	Schisis association and sirenomelia
Maternal uterine malformation	
Neu-Laxova syndrome	
Trisomy 21 and other chromosome defects	

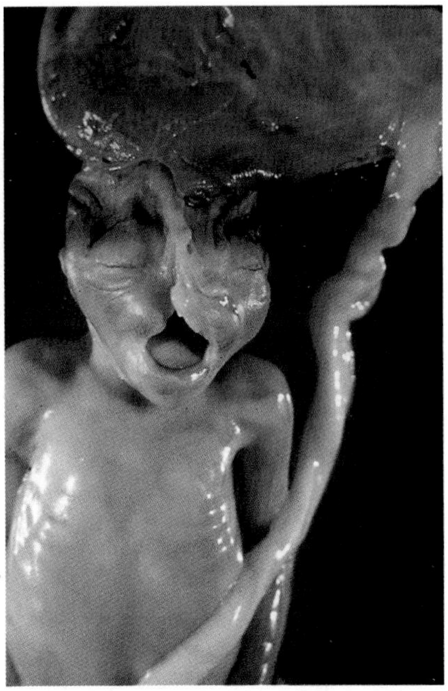

10.45. Amniotic bands attached to placenta and fetal head resulting in cleft of face and lip.

the fetus becoming entangled in the amnion either at the time of the initial amnion rupture or with subsequent activity.

Short Umbilical Cord

A short umbilical cord is frequently associated with underlying major structural anomalies in the fetus (Figures 10.52 and 10.53 and Tables 10.47 to 10.51). Multiple congenital anomalies are frequently associated with a short umbilical cord (SUC), in particular if there are lateral body wall defects, severe CNS abnormalities, or amniotic bands. The length of the umbilical cord is determined by fetal activity and the tension placed on the cord during growth. Structural malformations that limit movement are more likely to have a SUC. A short umbilical cord may be related to omphalocele where traction on a short cord precludes the return of the abdominal contents to the coelomic cavity.

Neonatal Gangrene

Neonatal gangrene of a limb at the time of birth is rare; most arterial thromboses in infants occur postnatally as a complication of umbilical artery catheters.

Table 10.49 Short umbilical cord associated malformations

Period of development	Defect → malformations	Reason
1. *Intrauterine constraint*		
(A) Before 5–6 wks gestation	(1) Lateral body wall defect + ipsilateral lower limb defect (2) Lateral body wall defect + ipsilateral upper limb defect (3) Amniotic bands (4) Adams syndrome	Limitation of early movement Tethering and adherence aberrant tissue
(B) Second trimester	Renal agenesis, oligohydraminos	Limitation of movement
2. *Structural limb defect*	Werdnig-Hoffman disease Amelia secondary to thalidomide Arthrogryposis Pena Shokair syndrome Acardia acephalus	Structural and functional limitation of movements
3. *Neurological defects*		Lack of intrauterine movements

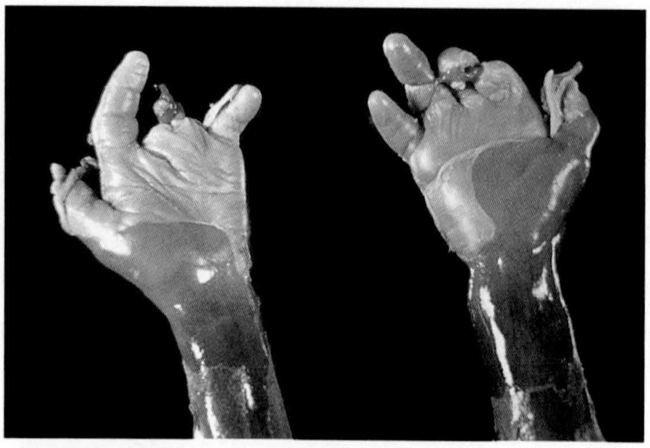

10.46. Amniotic bands on hands of fetus causing amputations.

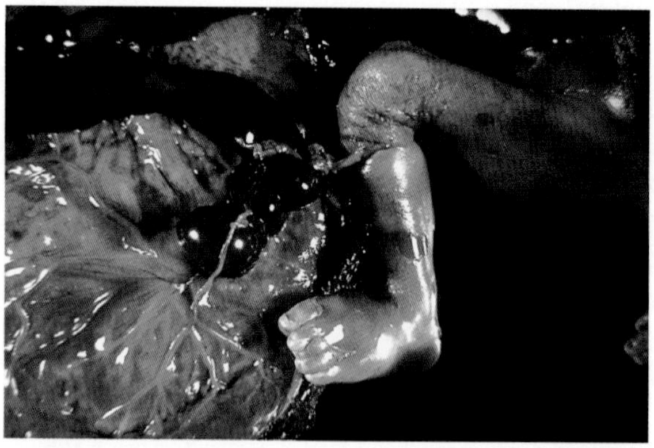

10.47. Amniotic bands causing constriction of leg and umbilical cord.

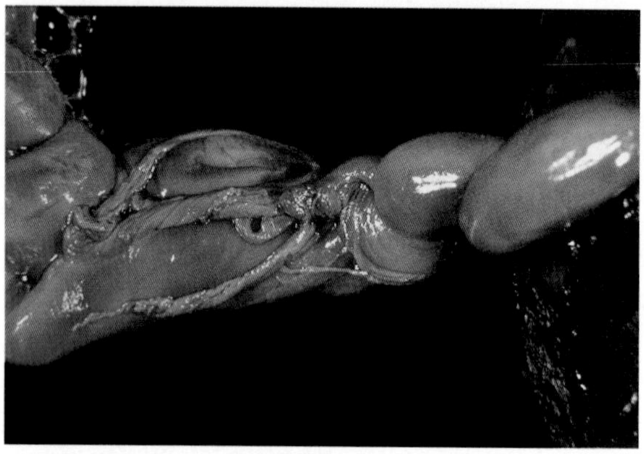

10.48. Amniotic bands constricting umbilical cord.

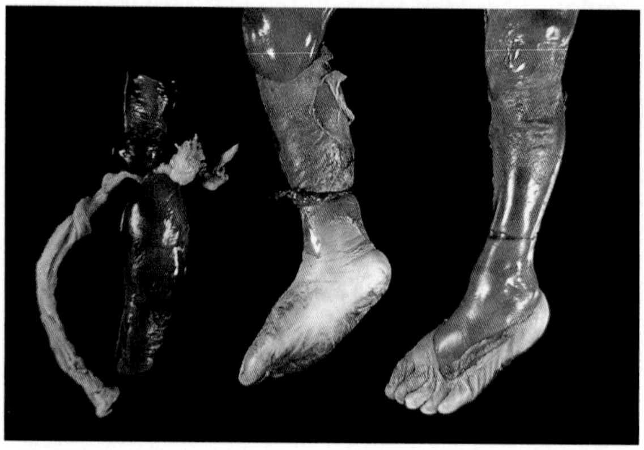

10.49. Amniotic bands attached to legs and constricting umbilical cord.

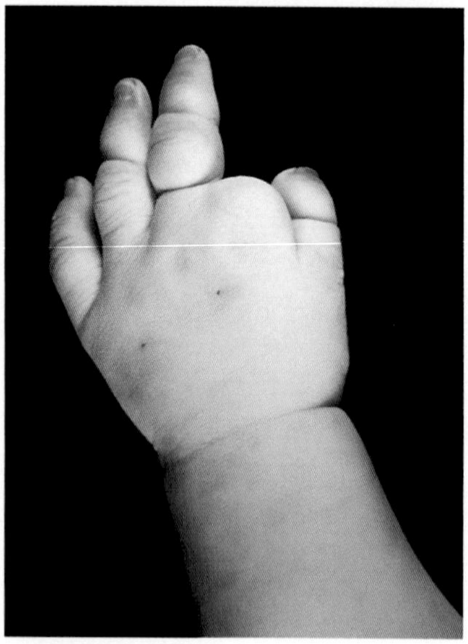

10.50. Amputation of second finger with constriction bands on first, third, and fourth fingers.

Table 10.50 Short umbilical cord (SUC) syndrome

Group	Anomalies
Group I: SUC + amnion bands	ADAM sequence Variable clefts Variable amputations
Group II: SUC + abdominal wall defect	Severe SUC (<10 cm) Abdominal wall defect Bent fetal body axis (pleurosomas, cyllosomas) Missing extremity
Group III: SUC + severe midline field schisis defect	Midline developmental field schisis defect with omphalocele, CL/CP, ectopia cordis, bladder exstrophy, neural tube defect
Group IV: SUC + acephalus-acardia	
Group V: SUC + fetal hypokinesia	Arthrogryposis Extremity defect
Group VI: SUC primary defect	Abdominal wall defect Omphalocele

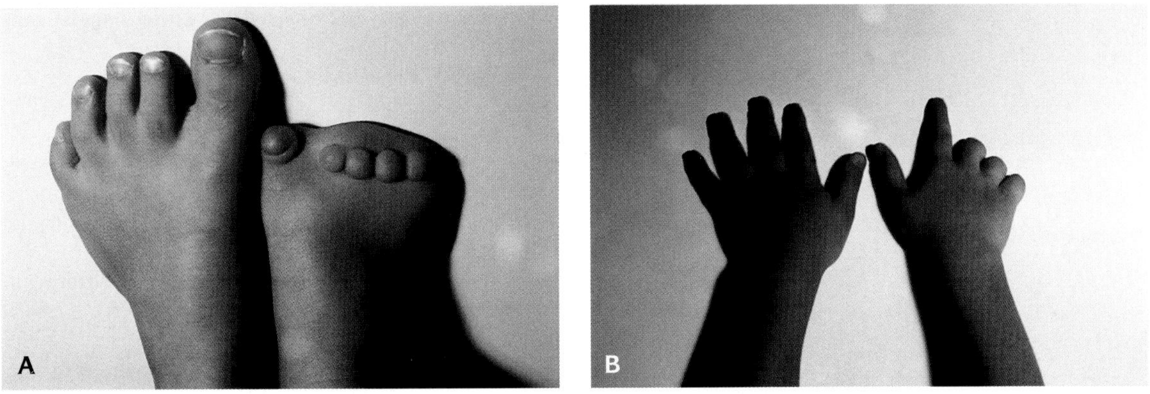

10.51. Transverse digital reduction defects of **(A)** right toes **(B)** fingers.

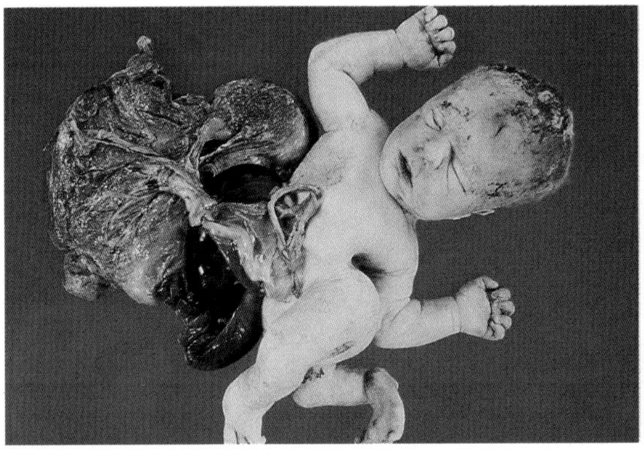

10.52. Infant with short umbilical cord with omphalocele.

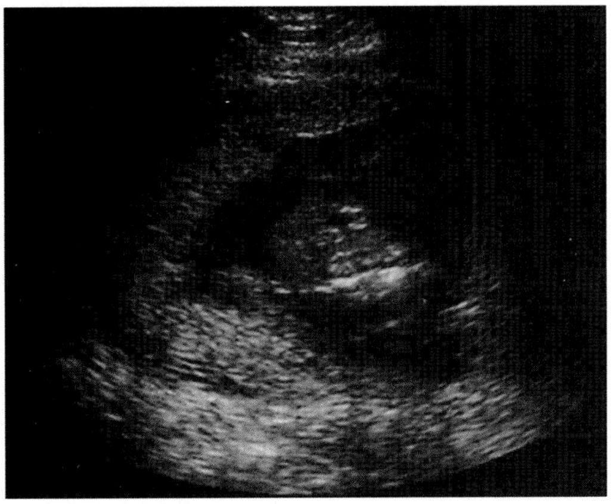

10.53. Ultrasound of fetus with short umbilical cord.

Table 10.51 Short umbilical cord early amnion rupture

Effects on fetus:
- Malformations – interruption of normal morphogenesis
- Deformations – distortion of established structures
- Mutilation of structures already formed
- Entanglement of fetus by amniotic bands
- Decreased fetal movement and prevention of return of bowel to abdominal wall
- Umbilical cord constriction → intrauterine death
- Decreased fetal movement → short cord

Venous thrombosis and thromboembolism is more common in infants of diabetic mothers than arterial thrombosis and may contribute to embolic occlusion of the femoral or brachial artery. The most likely cause of arterial as well as venous thrombosis in IDM is a hypercoagulable state associated with poorly controlled maternal diabetes.

REFERENCES

Arnold GL, Kirby RS, Langendoerer S, Wilkins-Haug L: Toluene embryopathy: clinical delineation and developmental follow-up. *Pediatrics* 93:216, 1994.

Balducci J, Rodis JF, Rosengren S, et al.: Pregnancy outcome following first-trimester varicella infection. *Obstet Gynecol* 79:5, 1992.

Beceerra JE, Khoury MJ, Cordero JF, et al.: Diabetes mellitus during pregnancy and the risk for specific birth defects: a population based case-control study. *Pediatrics* 85:1, 1990.

Brent RL: Radiation teratogenesis. *Teratology* 21:281, 1980.

Chiappinelli JA, Walton RE: Tooth discoloration resulting from long term tetracycline therapy. *Quintessence Int* 23:539, 1992.

Firth HV, Boyd PA, Chamberlain PF, et al.: Analysis of limb reduction defects in babies exposed to chorionic villus sampling. *Lancet* 343:1069, 1994.

Fisch RO, Tagatz G, Stassart JP: Gestational carrier – a reproductive haven for offspring of mothers with phenylketonuria (PKU): an alternative therapy for maternal PKU. *J Inherit Metab Dis* 16:957, 1993.

Geiger JM, Baudin M, Saurat JH: Teratogenic risk with etretinate and acitretin treatment. *Dermato* 198:109, 1994.

Gilbert-Barness E. Chapter 10, Part II – Vascular disruptions. In Gilbert-Barness E (ed): *Potter's Pathology of the Fetus and Infant*, Philadelphia, Mosby, 1996.

Gilbert-Barness E: Chapter 10, Part I – Teratogenic disruptions. In Gilbert-Barness E (ed): *Potter's Pathology of the Fetus and Infant*, Philadelphia, Mosby, 1996.

Hartwig NG, Vermeij-Keers CHR, DeVries HE, et al.: Limb body wall malformation complex: an embryologic etiology? *Hum Pathol* 20:1071, 1989.

Hersh JH: Toluene embryopathy: two new cases. *J Med Genet* 26:333, 1989.

Hoyme HE, Jones KL, Dixon DS, et al.: Prenatal cocaine exposure and fetal vascular disruption. *Pediatrics* 85:743, 1990.

Hunter AGW: Brain. In Stevenson RE, Hall JG, Goodman RM (eds): *Human Malformations and Related Anomalies*, vol. II, New York, Oxford University Press, 1993, p. 74.

Jones KL, Johnson KA, Chambers CD: Offspring of women infected with varicella during pregnancy: a prospective study. *Teratology* 49:29, 1994.

Kurosawa K, Imaizumi K, Masuno M, et al.: Epidemiology of limb-body wall complex in Japan. *Am J Med Genet* 51:143, 1994.

Luebke HJ, Reiser CA, Pauli RM: Fetal disruptions: assessment of frequency, heterogeneity, and embryologic mechanisms in a population referred to a community-based stillbirth assessment program. *Am J Med Genet* 36:56, 1990.

Majewski F: Alcohol embryopathy: experience in 200 patients. *Dev Brain Dysfunct* 6:248, 1993.

Martinez-Frias ML: Epidemiological analysis of outcomes of pregnancy in diabetic mothers: identification of the most characteristic and most frequent congenital anomalies. *Am J Med Genet* 51:108, 1994.

Moerman P, Fryns J-P, Vandenberghe K, et al.: Constrictive amniotic bands, amniotic adhesions and limb-body wall complex: Discrete disruption sequences with etiopathogenetic overlap. *Am J Med Genet* 42:470, 1992.

Moore KL: *The Developing Human*, 3rd ed. Philadelphia, Saunders, 1982.

Olney RS, Khoury MJ, Alo CJ, et al.: Increased risk for transverse digital deficiency after chorionic villus sampling: results of United States multistate case-control study, 1988–1992. *Teratology* 10:55, 1974.

Sheffield LJ, Halliday JL, Jensen F: Maxillonasal dysplasia (Binder syndrome) and chondrodysplasia punctata. *J Med Genet* 28:503, 1991.

Smits-Van Prooije AE, Vermeij-Keers Chr, Poelmann RE, et al.: The formation of mesoderm and mesectoderm in 5- to 41-somite stage rat embryos cultured in vitro, using WGA-Au as a marker. *Anat Embryol* 177:245, 1988.

Stevenson RE, Jones KL, Phelan MC, et al.: Vascular steal: the pathogenetic mechanism producing sirenomelia and associated defects of the viscera and soft tissues. *Pediatrics* 78:451, 1986.

Streeter GL: Focal deficiencies in fetal tissues and their relation to intrauterine amputation. *Contrib Embryo Carnegie Inst* 22:1, 1930.

Van Allen MI: Structural anomalies resulting from vascular disruption. *Pediatr Clin North Am* 39:255, 1992.

Van Allen MI: Vascular disruptions. In Gilbert-Barness E (ed): *Potter's Pathology of the Fetus and Infant*, St. Louis, Mosby Year-Book Publishers, 1996.
Van Allen MI, Curry C, Gallagher L: Limb body wall complex: J. Pathogenesis. *Am J Med Genet* 28:529, 1987.
Van Allen MI, Johnson JM, Toi A, et al.: Occurrence of vascular disruption in 250 fetuses with structural anomalies identified by ultrasound. *Proc Greenwood Genetics Center* 11:70, 1992.
Vermeij-Keers Chr, Mazzola RF, Van der Meulen JC, et al.: Cerebro-craniofacial and craniofacial malformations: an embryological analysis. *Cleft Palate J* 20:128, 1983.
Wong V, Cheng CH, Chan KC: Fetal and neonatal outcome of exposure to anticoagulants during pregnancy. *Am J Med Genet* 45:17, 1993.

ELEVEN

Intrauterine Growth Retardation

Estimation of fetal maturity is the most accurate method of estimating gestation age by ultrasonographic measurements of crown–rump length during the first trimester. From the first trimester through 34 weeks, the biparietal diameter is accurate to within 10 days. Other measurements used in the 2nd and 3rd trimesters include fetal abdominal diameter and femur length.

Low birth weight (LBW) is a worldwide problem usually defined as birth weight <2,500 g, irrespective of gestational age. It is associated with increased perinatal morbidity and is used as a marker of increased neonatal risk. It is not an ideal marker of fetal growth and development and combines both prematurity and various degrees of growth retardation. Morbidity is associated with LBW and growth retardation. Twenty-one million LBW infants are born each year internationally, 90% in developing countries.

Insulin growth factor (IGF) II is essential for organogenesis and early fetal growth. IGF-I is essential for late fetal growth. IGF-I is low in intrauterine growth retardation (IUGR) infants.

Proportion of LBWs varies by type of society:

- 3–12% rates of LBW infants occur in developed countries, 60% premature, 40% growth retarded
- 12–40% rates of LBW in developing countries, 20% premature, 80% growth retarded

There is a high rate of perinatal morbidity in growth-retarded infants:

- perinatal depression is 3 times more likely
- hypoglycemia is 4–6 times more likely
- hypothermia is 5 times more likely
- meconium aspiration is 13 times more likely
- fetal distress in labor is 6 times more likely

Proportion of LBW varies by gestational age:

- 90% of infants at 32–33 weeks gestation
- 50% of infants at 34–35 weeks gestation
- 10% of infants at 37–38 weeks gestation

Degrees of growth retardation increase as gestational age increases. Disproportion between developmental age is established by crown–rump length or hand and foot length and brain maturation (chronologic appearance of various gyri and sulci) in an otherwise normally developed fetus confirms the diagnosis of intrauterine growth retardation. In growth-retarded fetuses, the brain development is significantly advanced for the established developmental age.

Table 11.1 Mechanism of asymmetric growth restriction

Redistribution of fetal blood flow, maintaining perfusion of the head, heart, and adrenal glands

Particularly severe insults may cause asymmetric growth retardation to progress to symmetric growth retardation, as redistribution of blood flow fails to maintain growth of the head

PATTERNS OF GROWTH

Two overlapping periods of fetal cellular activity, cellular hyperplasia and cellular hypertrophy, result in three phases of fetal growth and development.

1. First phase, occurring from 4 to 20 weeks gestation, is characterized by proportional increases in fetal weight, protein content, and DNA content (cellular hyperplasia).
2. Second phase, occurring from 20 to 28 weeks gestation, is characterized by increases in protein and weight and lesser increases in fetal DNA content (hyperplasia and concomitant hypertrophy).
3. Third phase, occurring from 28 weeks to term, is characterized by continued increases in fetal protein and weight but no increase in DNA content (hypertrophy).

Table 11.2 Fetal growth retardation

Characteristics	
Symmetrical:	*Asymmetric:*
early onset	late onset
constitutional	environmental
reduced growth potential	late growth arrest
organ weight ratios normal	brain relatively large

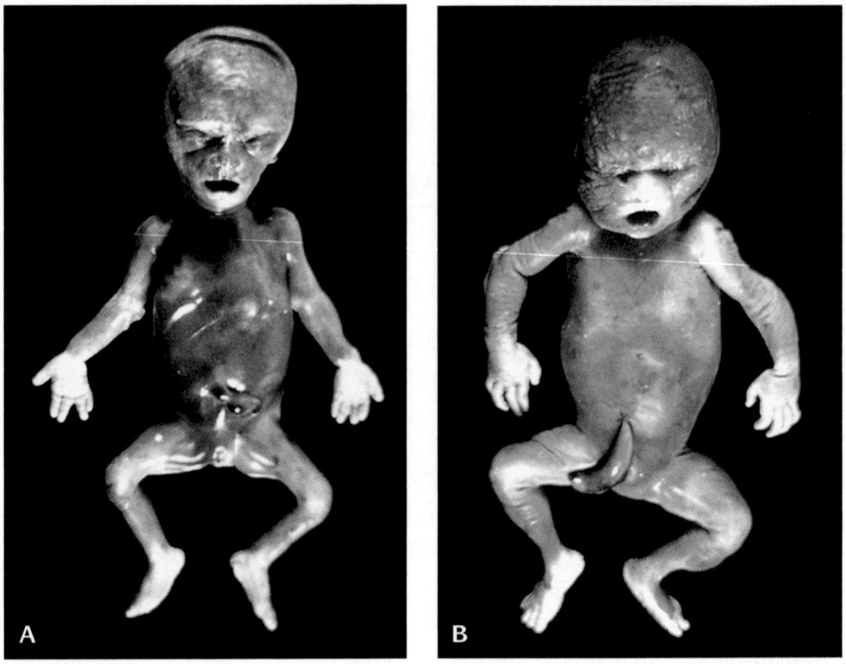

11.1. Symmetric growth retardation **(A)** compared with a normal **(B)** fetus at 26 weeks gestation.

There are two types of IUGR; symmetric (proportionate) (Figure 11.1) and asymmetric (disproportionate) (Figure 11.2). In the symmetric type, the head is reduced in size to the same extent as the body; in the asymmetric type, the head is normal in size and only the body is small. Symmetric growth retardation is seen early in development; asymmetric growth retardation usually is not manifested until after 20 weeks gestation.

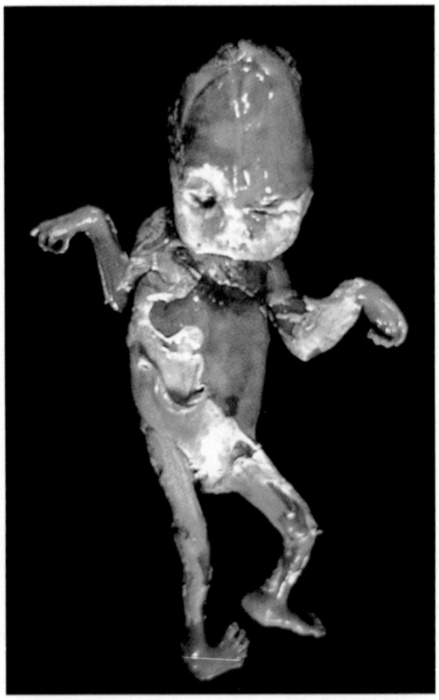

11.2. Asymmetric growth retardation in a fetus due to chronic hypoxemia with reduced uteroplacental blood flow. The body is growth retarded but the head is of normal size.

Timing of the insult to the fetus predisposes to the type of growth retardation: early insults usually result in symmetric growth retardation, probably by restricting fetal cellular hyperplasia. Third trimester insults that restrict cellular hypertrophy usually result in asymmetric growth retardation. Uteroplacental insufficiency and other similar insults result in stresses on the fetus that cause the fetus to redistribute blood flow, maintaining perfusion of the head, heart, and adrenal glands. Particularly severe insults to the fetus may cause asymmetric growth retardation to progress to symmetric growth retardation, as redistribution of blood flow fails to maintain growth of the head.

Potential causes of growth retardation:

- Incorrect dates by mother
- Hereditary predisposition: Mothers with prior IUGR infants are at increased risk for future IUGR infants. This effect may extend to grandchildren in some cases.
- Mothers with prior IUGR infants are at increased risk for future IUGR infants.
- Racial predisposition
- Primiparity

Table 11.3 Fetal growth retardation

Causes

Early fetal infection:
- rubella
- CMV
- toxoplasmosis
- malaria
- syphilis

Chromosome abnormalities:
- trisomy 13, 18, 21
- triploidy
- sex chromosome abnormalities

Metabolic abnormalties:
- agenesis of pancreas/absent inlets of Langerhans
- gangliosidosis
- I cell disease
- hypophosphatasia
- Menkes syndrome

Reduced uteroplacental perfusion:
- pre-eclampsia
- maternal hypertension
- diabetes mellitus
- maternal smoking

Undernutrition:
- evidence of malnutrition
- adolescent mother
- chronic infection
- alcholism; drug ingestion
- maternal PKU

- Genetic syndromes
- Chromosomal abnormalities
- Early onset infections
- Maternal diseases affecting the vascular system
- Cyanotic heart disease
- Renal disease, chronic (without hypertension)
- Thyrotoxicosis
- Collagen vascular disease (polymyositis/dermatomyositis, lupus erythomatosus)
- Multiple gestation
- Hypertension
- Advanced stage diabetes
- Pregnancy-induced hypertensive disorders
- Substrate availability (caloric deprivation and high altitude low O_2 produce decreased fetal size)

Toxic effects-drugs and chemicals:

- Folic acid antagonists such as methotrexate
- Chemotherapeutic agents
- Anti-epileptics such as phenytoin or trimethadione

Table 11.4 Effects of maternal cigarette smoking

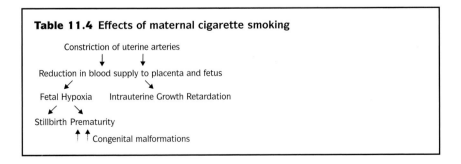

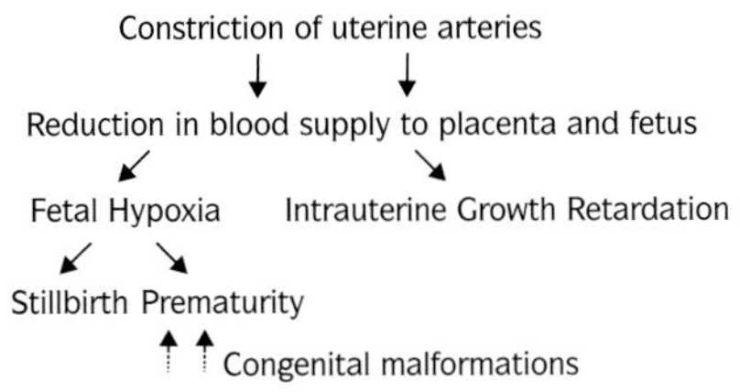

- Warfarin
- Substance abuse (ethanol, tobacco, illicit drugs)

Many drugs and chemicals taken by the mother during pregnancy produce IUGR; these include heavy smoking and chronic alcoholism. Some drugs that are teratogens may cause IUGR; for example, acutane. Drugs that are teratogens usually produce symmetric growth retardation.

- Systemic steroid usage
- Heavy metals such as lead and mercury
- Organic solvents
- Insecticide exposure

FETAL FACTORS CAUSING IUGR

Aneuploidy has been reported to occur in approximately 20% of growth retarded fetuses (Snijders et al. 1993). It results in symmetric growth retardation. First trimester growth retardation – Although first trimester sonography is generally held out as a "gold" standard for estimation of gestational age, it has recently been noted both that approximately 10% of gestations with certain menstrual dates and 28 day cycles will show a dates/sonographic variation of more than 7 days (Giersson et al. 1991), and that certain karyotypic abnormalities will predispose to early onset growth retardation. Chromosome abnormalities often cause symmetric growth retardation.

1. Autosomal trisomies
   a. Trisomy 13
   b. Trisomy 18
   c. Trisomy 21
2. Triploidy
3. Monosomy X
4. Extra-sex (X) chromosomes (47 XXY, etc.)
   a. average birthweight decreases by 300 gm per each additional X chromosome
5. Autosomal deletion syndromes
   a. 5p- (cri du chat)
   b. 5q-
   c. 4p-
   d. 4q-
   e. 18p-
   f. 18q-
   g. others

Kuhn (1995) evaluated 170 aneuploid fetuses relative to these norms, and found that fetuses with trisomy 18 ($n = 32$) were significantly shorter for gestational age, while those with trisomy 21 ($n = 72$), trisomy 13 ($n = 11$), Turner syndrome ($n = 5$), and sex chromosome disorders ($n = 12$) were unaffected. The tendency for decreased crown–rump length in trisomy 18 fetuses and the absence of such a predisposition in other aneuploid fetuses has been reported by several other authors (Lynch et al. 1989; Drugan et al. 1992; Wald et al. 1993; Snijders and Nicolaides 1996).

Although dating gestational age by early sonography will tend to miss trisomy 18 fetuses, many such fetuses also will be noted to have increased nuchal "lucency" in the first trimester and subsequently will be found to have other anomalies if evaluated later in pregnancy.

Second- and third-trimester growth retardation – Aneuploidy was noted in 19% ($n = 89$) of 458 fetuses evaluated for growth retardation (<5% for gestation age) at gestational ages ranging from 7 to 40 weeks. Before 26 weeks triploidy was most common, while in later gestation fetuses trisomy 18 occurred most often (Snijders RJ, Sherrod C, et al. 1993).

Frequency of anomalies detected vary with gestational age:

Gestational age	Number	Aneuploidy (all) % (n)	Triploidy % (n)	Trisomy 18 %(n)
18–25	132	38% (50)	22% (29)	5% (7)
26–33	208	10% (21)	3% (7)	4% (9)

Increased maternal age is associated with increased likelihood of aneuploidy in growth retarded fetuses:

Maternal age	Number	Aneuploidy (all) % (n)	Triploidy % (n)	Trisomy 18 % (n)
16–19	28	8% (2)	4% (1)	4% (1)
20–23	90	22% (16)	9% (8)	7% (6)
24–27	110	25% (22)	8% (9)	5% (6)
28–31	108	26% (22)	11% (12)	6% (7)
32–35	79	23% (15)	6% (5)	9% (5)
36–39	32	23% (6)	3% (1)	9% (3)
40–43	11	55% (6)	0	40% (4)

Intrauterine growth retardation with normal umbilical arterial Doppler findings increases the likelihood of a genetic cause for the growth abnormality (Snijders et al. 1993).

- Aneuploidy in 19% of the IUGR study population
- 12% aneuploidy in those with abnormal Doppler findings
- 8% aneuploidy in those with oligohydramnios
- 40% aneuploidy in those with normal Doppler findings
- 44% aneuploidy in those with normal or increased amniotic fluid

Other factors causing IUGR

- Open neural tube defects
- Renal agenesis
- Osteochondrodystrophies
- Single umbilical artery

Infections in the fetus associated with IUGR:

1. Bacterial infections:
   - Listeria
   - malaria
   - syphilis
   - toxoplasmosis
   - tuberculosis
2. Viral infections:
   - cytomegalovirus
   - rubella
   - herpes
   - AIDS

MULTIPLE GESTATION

Twins and higher-order multiple gestation infants are at increased risk of growth retardation. These infants have increased rates of LBW for gestational age and increased rates of asymmetric growth restriction (abnormally lean body morphology).

Twins have distinct patterns of growth. Growth patterns generally overlap singletons until 32 weeks gestation. Twins do not maintain singleton average birthweight growth in the last 6–8 weeks of pregnancy. The value of separate growth tables for twins is controversial. Discordance of more than 20–25% in birthweight relative to the larger twin is associated with IUGR and increased perinatal morbidity.

Gestational Age Assessment

It is necessary to properly assign percentile rankings of fetal weight by gestational age. Dubowitz scoring of infants often varies 1 or 2 weeks from menstrual dating but is unavailable until after delivery of the infant. Obstetric dating often is inaccurate. Fifteen percent of patients with proper dating criteria have sonographic dating findings that differ by more than 2 weeks from menstrual dating determinations.

Prenatal Sonographic Estimation of Fetal Weight

- Accuracy limited to ±15%
- Should be used with caution

- Accuracy less at extremes of estimated weight
- Decreased accuracy if fetal positioning precludes accurate measurements of oligohydramnios if present.

Types of Markers of Neonatal Growth and Development

1. Absolute measurements
   a. Example: LBW
   b. Prematurity and growth retardation may be classified together into the same marker.
2. Birthweight relative to gestational age, gender, ethnicity, etc.
   a. Examples: small for gestational age (LBW percentile for gestational age); low fetal growth ratio (observed birthweight/adjusted birthweight)
   b. Gestational age is not always accurately documented.
3. Body symmetry relative to gestational age
   a. Examples: ponderal index, weight/length ratio, body mass index, mid-arm circumference/head circumference ratio.
   b. Require gestational age and another body measurement, such as length or mid-arm circumference.
   c. Identify abnormal growth patterns independent of absolute birthweight.
   d. Identify groups of infants with otherwise normal birthweights who are at increased risk for perinatal mortality and morbidity, 6- to 10-fold increases in rates of hypoglycemia, perinatal depression, meconium aspiration, and prolonged hospitalization.
   e. May be better correlates of perinatal morbidity than birthweight for gestational age.

Indices of Growth Retardation

Small for gestational age (low percentile birthweight for gestational age). Most commonly used method of neonatal and fetal assessment is birthweight < 10% for gestational age usually used in the United States and birthweight standard deviation (S.D.) (birthweight < 2.5%) often used in Europe. Sensitivity and specificity can be adjusted by choice of percentile range for population screening versus more specific categorization of growth retarded infants.

Fetal Growth Ratio (FGR)

- FGR < 0.90 occurs in 18% of patients
- FGR < 0.85 occurs in 9.0% of patients
- FGR < 0.80 occurs in 4.3% of patients
- FGR < 0.75 occurs in 1.7% of patients

Ponderal Index

Ponderal index = birthweight in g/length in $cm^3 \times 100$. Low ponderal index is a marker of asymmetric growth restriction and is associated with increased perinatal morbidity (normal 2.0–3.0).

Weight/Length Ratio

Weight/length = birthweight in g/length in cm. Weight/length ratio $< 5\%$ or 10%, asymmetric growth restriction, is associated with increased perinatal morbidity.

Body Mass Index

Body mass index = birthweight in g/length in cm^2. Body mass index has not been extensively evaluated as a marker of neonatal status.

Amniotic Fluid Volume

Two common methods of assessment:

1. Single pocket technique:
    a. Presence of at least one 2×2 cm (or one 1×1 cm) pocket of amniotic fluid indicates adequate amniotic fluid volume.
2. Amniotic fluid index:
    a. Deepest vertical amniotic fluid pocket in each of four uterine quadrants is measured
    b. Need for pocket to be completely free of umbilical cord
    c. Values vary with gestational age
    d. Values less than 5–6 cm quadrants indicate oligohydramnios at term
    e. Values in excess of 25 cm quadrants indicate polyhydramnios. If present, evaluation of maternal and fetal correlates of polyhydramnios is indicated.

Markers for Abnormal Fetal Growth in Multiple Gestation

- Discordance in estimated sonographic fetal weights of 20–25% using the larger twin as the index case.
- Intratwin pair difference in biparietal diameter > 5 mm. Intratwin pair differences in abdominal circumference > 20 mm.
- Intratwin pair difference in abdominal circumference and/or femur length with the abdominal circumference.

Sonographic (Antenatal) Markers of Abnormal Fetal Growth

Head circumference: abdominal circumference ratio

- useful to detect asymmetric growth restrictions, due to head sparing effect active in most cases of growth retardation rate
- values vary by gestational age

Femur length/abdomen circumference ratio

- minimal variation during pregnancy: 0.22 ± .015 (mean ± 11 SD)
- altered if skeletal dysplasia present

Doppler Sonography

Systolic/diastolic flow velocity ratios correlate with placental resistance

a. decrease over the course of pregnancy
b. increased values for gestational age indicate increased placental resistance
c. absent or reversed end diastolic flow is often associated with imminent fetal compromise; reverse flow has occasionally been noted to resolve
d. fetuses with estimated fetal weights in the growth-retarded range and normal Doppler flow indices are at increased risk of aneuploidy

REFERENCES

Divon M (ed): *Abnormal Fetal Growth*, New York, Elsevier, 1991.
Dorovini-Zis K, Dolman CL: Gestational development of the brain. *Arch Pathol Lab Med* 101:192, 1977.
Drugan A, Johnson MP, Isada NB, et al.: The smaller than expected first trimester fetus is at increased risk for chromosome anomalies. *Am J Obstet Gynecol* 167:1525, 1992.
Giersson RT, Busby E: Certain dates may not provide a reliable estimate of gestational age. *Br J Obstet Gynaecol* 98:108, 1991.
Goldstein, I, Lockwood C, Hubbins JC: Ultrasound assessment of fetal intestinal development in the evaluation of gastational age. *Obstet Gynecol*, 70:682, 1987.
Goldstein, et al.: *Obstet Gynecol*, 70:641, 1987.
Gross TL, Sokol RJ (eds): *Intrauterine Growth Retardation – A Practical Approach.* Chicago, Year Book Medical Publishers, 1989.
Kalousek D, Gilbert-Barness E: Causes of stillbirth and neonatal death. In Gilbert-Barness E (ed): *Potter's Pathology of the Fetus and Infant*, Philadelphia, Mosby Year Book, 1997.
Kalousek D: The role of confined placental mosaicism in placental function and human development. *Growth Genet Horm* 4:1, 1988.
Kuhn P: Fetal nuchal edema in the 11th and 14th week of pregnancy–indication of trisomy? *Schweiz Med Wochenschr* 125:2494, 1995.
Kurjak A, Beazley JM (eds): *Fetal Growth Retardation: Diagnosis and Treatment*, Boca Raton, FL, CRC Press, 1989.
Lynch L, Berkowitz GS, Chitkara U, et al.: Ultrasound detection of Down syndrome: it is really possible? *Obstet Gynecol* 73:267, 1989.
Moller JH: Incidence of cardiac malformations. In Moller Jr and Neal WA (eds): *Fetal, Neonatal, and Infant Cardiac Disease*, East Norwalk, Appleton and Lange, 1990.
Nicolaides KH, Salvesen DR, Snijders RJ, et al.: Strawberry-shaped skull in fetal Trisomy 18. *Fetal Diagn Ther* 7:132, 1992.
Pandya PP, Kondylios A, Hilbert, et al.: Chromosmal defects and outcomes in 1015 fetuses with increased nuchal transluceancy. *Ultrasound Obstet Gynecol*, 5:15, 1995.
Silverman NH, Schmidt KG: Ultrasound evaluation of the fetal heart. In Callen PW (eds): *Ultrasonography in Obstetrics and Gynecology*, Philadelphia, WB Saunders, 1994.
Snijders RJ, Abbas A, Melby O, et al.: Fetal plasma erythropoietin concentration in severe growth retardation. *Am J Obstet Gynecol* 168:615, 1993.
Snijders RJ, Sherrod C. Godsen CM, et al.: Fetal growth retardation: associated malformations and chromosomal abnormalities. *Am J Obstet Gynecol* 168:547, 1993.

Snijders RJM, Nicolaides KH: *Ultrasound Markers for fetal Chromosomal Defects.* London, U.K. Parthenon Pub. Group, 1996.

Vorherr H: Factors influencing fetal growth. *Am J Obstet Gynecol* 142:577, 1982.

Wald NJ, Smith D, Kennard A, et al.: Biparietal diameter and crown-rump length in fetuses with Down's syndrome: implications for antenatal serum screening for Down's syndrome. *Br J Obstet Gynaecol* 100:430, 1993.

Warshaw J: Perspectives of intrauterine growth retardation. *Growth Genet Horm* 2:1, 1986.

Wigglesworth J, Singer D: *Textbook of Fetal and Neonatal Pathology*, 2nd ed, London, Blackwell Scientific Publications, 1998.

TWELVE

Fetal Hydrops and Cystic Hygroma

Minor hydrops is common, particularly in premature infants. **Severe hydrops** is generalized edema of 7.5 mm subcutaneous edema in a third-trimester fetus with an effusion of at least one body cavity, usually accompanied by polyhydramnios and edema of the placenta.

POLYHYDRAMNIOS

Amniotic fluid volume is approximately 800 mL at term. The volume is increased by fetal urine and is simultaneously removed by fetal swallowing. Fetal anomalies that interfere with swallowing are associated with polyhydramnios, while a decrease of fetal renal function and production of urine result in oligohydramnios. The volume of amniotic fluid falls rapidly after 40 weeks gestation to about 400 mL at 42 weeks and 200 mL at 44 weeks. Polyhydramnios is the presence of an excess of 1,500 mL of amniotic fluid at term and is present in up to 1% of pregnancies.

Causes of polyhydramnios

I. Maternal
   A. Diabetes and gestational diabetes

II. Fetal anomalies
   A. Anencephaly
   B. Esophageal atresia

Table 12.1 Laboratory studies for fetal hydrops

Mother	Ultrasonography
Fetal hemoglobin (Kleihauer-Betke test)	Severity of hydrops and polyhydramnios
Alphafetoprotein	Multiple pregnancy
ABO, rhesus, and other blood groups	Fetal heart rate/rhythm
Hemolysins, hemagglutinins	Fetal anomaly
Serological tests for syphilis	heart
Glucose tolerance test	other
Antinuclear factor	Placenta
Autoantibodies	thickness/abnormality
	biopsy virus culture

C. Small intestinal obstruction
D. Diaphragmatic hernia
E. Central nervous system malformations
F. Chromosomal defects

III. Placenta
A. Chorangioma

FETAL HYDROPS (FH)

Hydrops fetalis (HF) has a mortality rate in excess of 90% (Tables 12.1 to 12.5).

Intrauterine diagnosis of hydrops by ultrasound may allow successful treatment and reversal in selected cases, but the majority die without an established causative diagnosis.

Conditions associated with fetal hydrops:

I. Hypoproteinemia
A. Congenital nephrotic syndrome
B. Finnish type congenital nephrotic syndrome
C. Defect of hepatic protein synthesis

Table 12.2 Laboratory studies in hydropic infant

At birth	
Full blood count	Viral antibodies
Blood group and antibodies	Karyotype
Hemoglobin electrophoresis	Echocardiogram
Clotting screen	Radiological examination
Red cell enzymes	Ultrasound examination
	heart
	abdomen
Liver function tests	Effusions
	culture
	biochemical analysis
TORCH screen	Examination of placenta

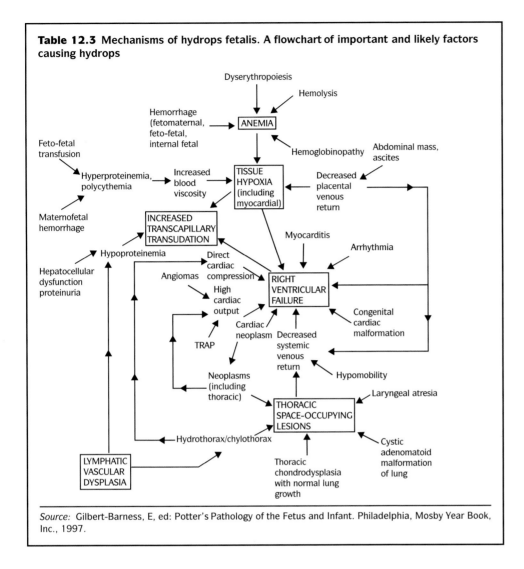

Table 12.3 Mechanisms of hydrops fetalis. A flowchart of important and likely factors causing hydrops

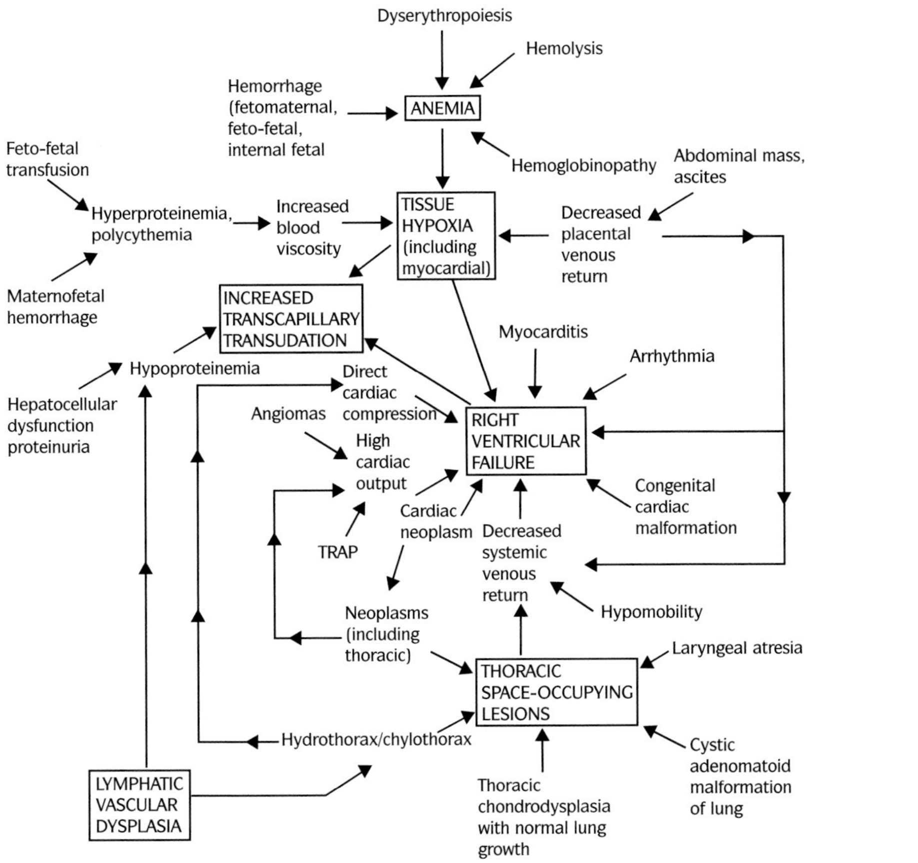

Source: Gilbert-Barness, E, ed: Potter's Pathology of the Fetus and Infant. Philadelphia, Mosby Year Book, Inc., 1997.

II. Obstructed venous return
  A. Congenital neoplasms with obstruction at level of:
    1. Umbilical vein
    2. Ductus venosus
    3. Inferior vena cava
  B. Tumors:
    1. Neuroblastoma Stage IV S
    2. Large ovarian cysts
    3. Retroperitoneal fibrosis
    4. Vena caval thrombosis
    5. Congenital cystic adenomatoid malformation of lung

III. Cardiac failure
  A. Intrauterine fetal tachycardia
  B. Low output cardiac failure with complete heart block

Table 12.4 Placentomegaly, immune hemolytic anemia

Rh isoimmunization
Fetal-maternal ABO blood group incompatiblity
Kell antigen isoimmunization
Other antigens – rare

Table 12.5 Fetomaternal hemorrhage

- Minor – 75% of all pregnancies
- Massive
  - Fetal death
  - Fetal distress
  - Hypovolemic shock
  - Anemia

  Fetal hydrops

  Placental hydropic changes

Diagnosis Kleihauer-Betke acid elution test

If 2% of maternal red blood cells are fetal

- Size of hemorrhage is 90 mL (significant)
- (normal term infant blood volume 240 mL)

C. Cardiac defects
1. Narrowing or closure of foramen ovale
2. Endocardial fibroelastosis
3. Hypoplastic left heart complex
4. Cardiac tumor – tuberous sclerosis
5. High output cardiac failure – large arteriovenous fistula

IV. Anemia
A. Blood group isoimmunization
1. Erythroblastosis fetalis
B. Hemolytic anemia due to red cell enzyme defects
C. Homozygous $\alpha 1$ thalassemia
D. Hemorrhage – twin-to-twin transfusion
E. Fetomaternal hemorrhage
F. Infantile Gaucher disease

Frequency of causes of fetal hydrops:

Idiopathic	20%
Fetomaternal hemorrhage	15%
Congenital malformations	12%
Metabolic disease	10%
Twin-to-twin transfusion	10%
Isoimmunization	5%
Congenital infections	6%
Congenital nephrotic syndrome	5%
Cardiac malformation	5%
Obstructed venous return	5%
High-output failure	3%
Cardiac tumor	2%
$\alpha 1$ thalassemia	2%

IMMUNOLOGIC HYDROPS

Immunologic hydrops is caused by isoimmunization due to blood group incompatibility between mother and fetus (Figures 12.1 to 12.6). Since the advent of Rhogam the incidence of Rh immunization has dramatically decreased. This occurs when the mother is Rh negative and the infant is Rh positive. Rh-negative cells from the mother mixed with Rh-positive cells of the fetus stimulate the production of antibodies in the maternal circulation that enter the fetal circulation and cause hemolysis of fetal red blood cells. The more common blood group antigens causing immunologic hydrops are Kell and Duffy.

In nonimmunologic hydrops not due to isoimmunization, the following changes occur: extreme pleural and peritoneal effusions with compression of

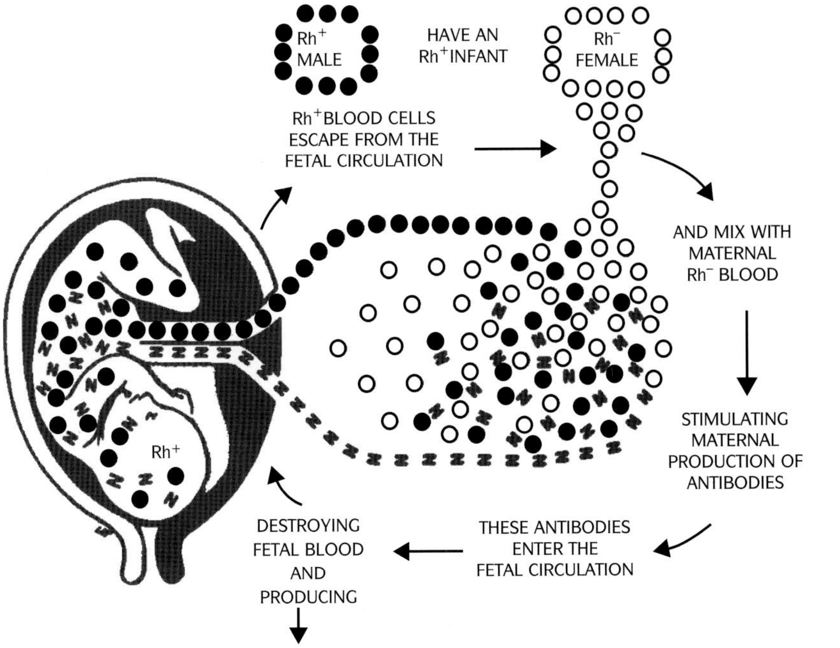

12.1. Mechanism of blood group incompatibility between mother and fetus in immunologic hydrops.

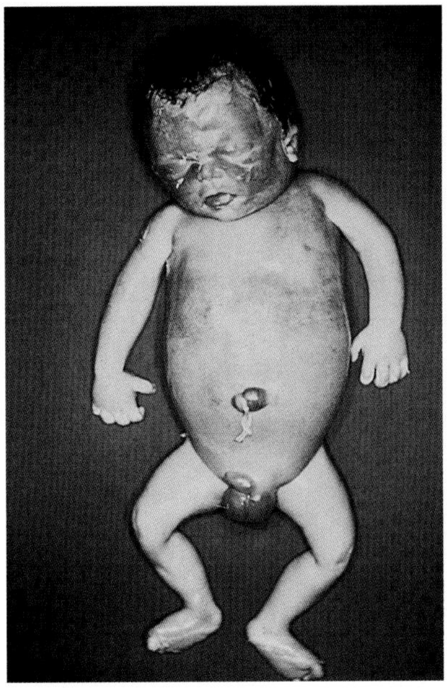

12.2. Infant with hydrops due to erythroblastosis fetalis in Rh incompatibility. (Table 12.1.)

abdominal and thoracic viscera, absence of hepatosplenomegaly, and absence of widespread erythropoiesis.

Conditions associated with nonimmunologic hydrops fetalis:

I. Idiopathic

II. Fetal

A. Severe chronic anemia in utero
1. Fetal–maternal transfusion
2. Twin-to-twin transfusion

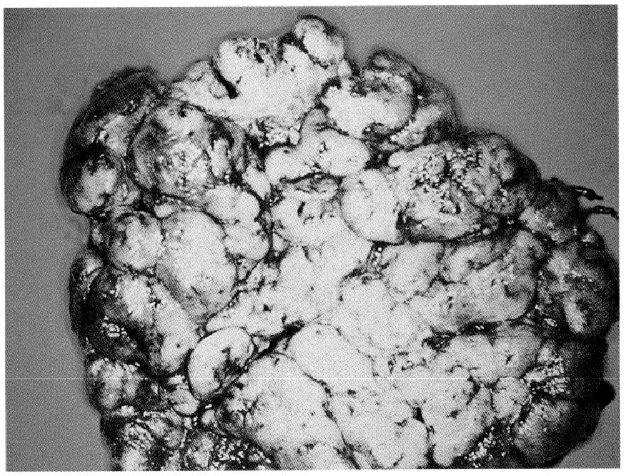

12.3. Placenta in erythroblastosis fetalis is large, pale, and bulky.

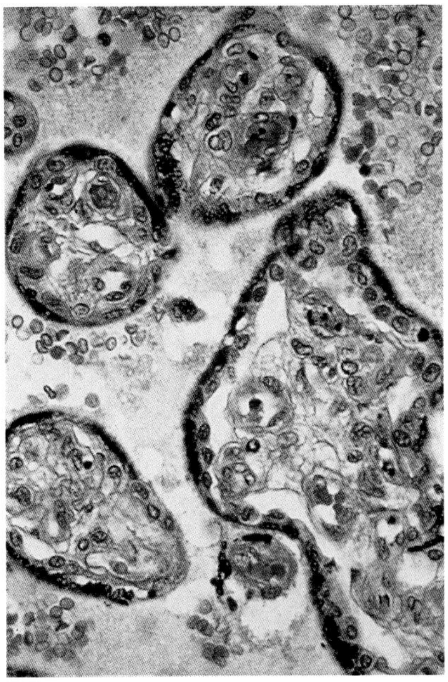

12.4. Microscopic appearance of placenta in erythroblastosis fetalis showing retention of cytotrophoblasts and nucleated red blood cells.

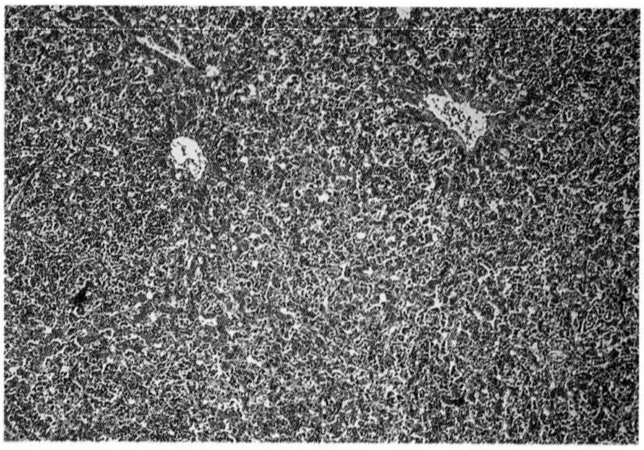

12.5. Microscopic appearance of liver in erythroblastosis fetalis showing excessive extramedullary hematopoiesis.

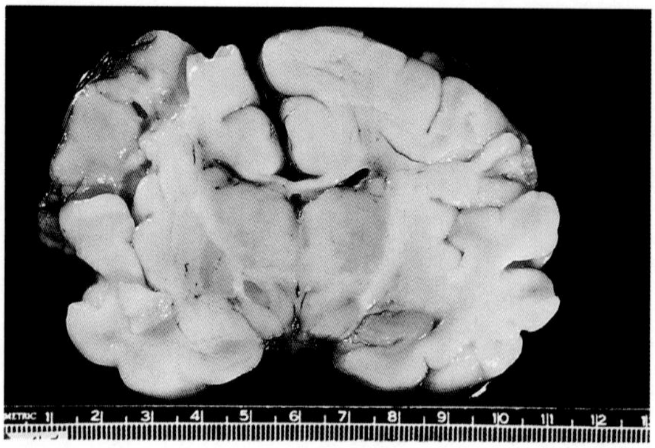

12.6. Coronal section of the brain with kernicterus showing yellow bilirubin staining of the basal ganglia due to erythroblastosis fetalis. The bilirubin level was 35 mg/dL.

  3. Homozygous α-thalassemia
  4. Parvovirus infection
  5. Intrafetal hemorrhage

B. Cardiovascular
  1. Severe congenital heart disease
  2. Large atrioventricular (A-V) malformation
  3. Premature closure of foramen ovale
  4. Cardiopulmonary hypoplasia with bilateral hydrothorax
  5. Premature closure of ductus arteriosus with hypoplasia of lungs
  6. Fetal arrhythmias
  7. Myocarditis
  8. Cardiomyopathy

C. Pulmonary
  1. Cystic adenomatoid malformation of the lung
  2. Pulmonary hypoplasia
  3. Pulmonary lymphangiectasia
  4. Pulmonary sequestration
  5. Bronchogenic cysts
  6. Laryngeal abrasion
  7. Diaphragmatic lesion

D. Hepatic
  1. Congenital hepatitis

E. Renal
  1. Congenital nephrosis
  2. Renal vein thrombosis
  3. Recessive polycystic renal disease
  4. Urethral obstruction

F. Developmental/genetic disorders
  1. Skeletal dysplasias (lethal congenital short-limb dwarfisms)
  2. Multiple congenital abnormalities

G. Infections (intrauterine)
   1. Syphilis
   2. Toxoplasmosis
   3. Cytomegalovirus
   4. Coxsackie B virus pancarditis
   5. Chagas disease
   6. Leptospirosis
   7. Listeria
H. Chromosomal defects
   1. 45X
   2. Trisomy 21
   3. Trisomy 18
   4. Trisomy 13
   5. Triploidy
   6. Tetraploidy
I. Miscellaneous conditions
   1. Fetal neuroblastomatosis
   2. Hemangioendothelioma
   3. Tuberous sclerosis
   4. Storage diseases
   5. Dysmaturity
   6. Small bowel volvulus

III. Placental
   A. Chorionic vein thrombosis
   B. Umbilical vein thrombosis
   C. Angiomyxoma of umbilical cord
   D. Aneurysm of umbilical cord
   E. Chorangioma of placenta

IV. Maternal conditions
   A. Maternal diabetes mellitus
   B. Maternal nephritis

V. Metabolic causes of hydrops fetalis (Table 12.6)
   A. Gaucher disease
   B. GM1 gangliosidosis
   C. β-Glucuronidase deficiency
   D. Morquio syndrome
   E. Neuraminidase deficiency
   F. Myotonic dystrophy
   G. Perinatal iron storage syndrome
   H. Carnitine deficiency
   I. I cell disease
   J. Sialidosis
   K. Salla disease
   L. Wolman disease

Table 12.6 Lysosomal storage disorders associated with hydrops fetalis

Disorders	Abnormality
Mucopolysaccharidosis VII (MPS VII)	β-Glucuronidase deficiency
Mucopolysaccharidosis IVA (MPS IVA)	*N*-acetylgalactosamine-6-sulfatase (galactose-6-sulfatase) deficiency
Type 2 Gaucher disease	Glucocerebrosidase (acid β-glucosidase) deficiency
Sialidosis	Neuraminidase (sialidase) deficiency
GM1 gangliosidosis	β-galactosidase deficiency
Galactosialidosis	Protective protein deficiency
Niemann-Pick disease type C	NPC-1 protein deficiency
Disseminated lipogranulomatosis (Farber disease)	Acid ceramidase deficiency
Infantile free sialic acid storage disease	Defective carrier-mediated transport of sialic acid
Mucolipidosis II (I-cell disease)	*N*-acetylglucosamine-1-phosphotransferase deficiency

FETAL ASCITES

In **urinary ascites**, bladder outlet or ureteric obstruction causes urine to leak into the retroperitoneum (urinoma) and peritoneal cavity (Figure 12.7). Some cases of prune belly syndrome result from transmission of urinary ascites after obstruction has destroyed renal function. Chylous ascites is caused by localized intra-abdominal lymphatic vascular dysplasia. Intestinal perforation may be secondary to intestinal atresia, volvulus, or meconium ileus. Meconium in the peritoneum stimulates a peritoneal exudate.

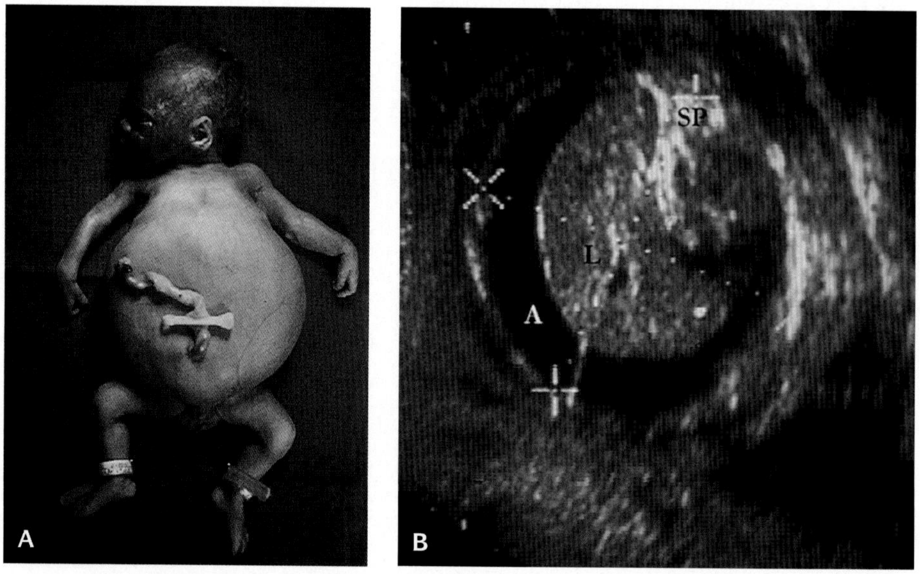

12.7. (A) Fetal ascites in mucolipidosis II (I cell disease). **(B)** Ultrasound showing marked ascites in fetus at 31 weeks gestation. (A, ascites; L, liver; SP, spine.)

Infectious causes include syphilis, toxoplasmosis and cytomegalovirus. In some of these cases, ascites is caused by portal hypertension secondary to hepatitis and/or cirrhosis.

Genetic metabolic causes include sialidosis, GM1 gangliosidosis, α_1-antitrypsin deficiency, infantile Gaucher disease, generalized *N*-acetylneuraminic acid storage, and Niemann-Pick disease type C and neonatal type A.

Causes of fetal ascites:

A. Visceral abnormalities
   1. Lower urinary tract obstruction
      a. Posterior urethral valves
   2. Liver disease – α_1-antitrypsin deficiency
   3. Extrahepatic biliary atresia
   4. Prenatal intussusception
   5. Intestinal atresias
   6. Cardiovascular malformations
      a. Hypoplastic left heart complex
   7. Pulmonary sequestration
      a. Congenital cystic adenomatoid malformations
      b. Sacral agenesis
B. Infections
   1. Syphilis
   2. Toxoplasmosis
   3. Cytomegalovirus
C. Genetic disorders
   1. Lysosomal storage diseases
      a. Niemann-Pick disease
      b. GM1 gangliosidosis
      c. Mucolipidosis II (I cell disease)
      d. Gaucher disease

FETAL HYDROTHORAX

Caused by localized pleural lymphatic malconnection or by local intrathoracic lesions – e.g., congenital cystic adenomatoid malformation of lung (Figure 12.8). Prenatal management requires diagnosis of the cause. In the absence of an obvious intrathoracic lesion as the likely cause, a diagnosis of lymphatic pleural effusion (fetal chylothorax) is likely.

CHYLOTHORAX

The pleural fluid is rich in lymphocytes, and this confirms the diagnosis of chylothorax. Pleural fluid can also be used for cytogenetic studies. Cases of chylothorax have pulmonary lymphangiectasia.

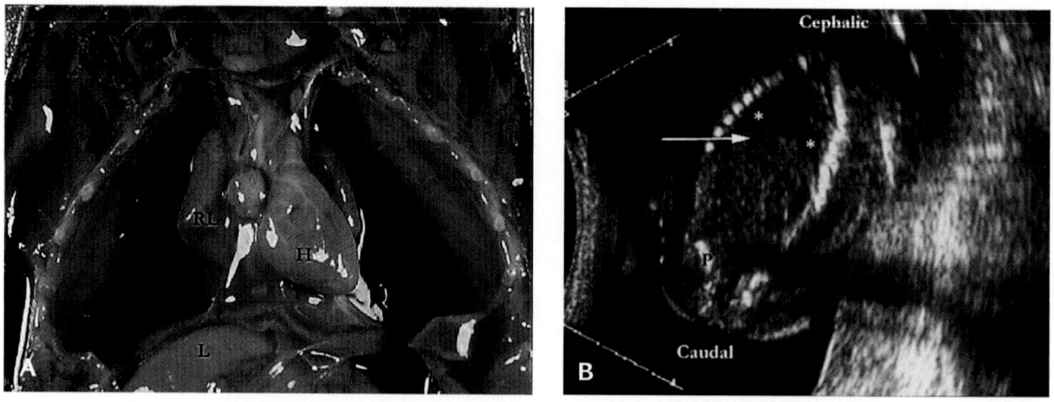

12.8. **(A)** Cardiopulmonary hypoplasia due to bilateral hydrothorax. (RL, right lung; H, heart; L, liver.) **(B)** Ultrasound of bilateral hydrothorax. (∗ = Pleural cavities; arrow = diaphragm.)

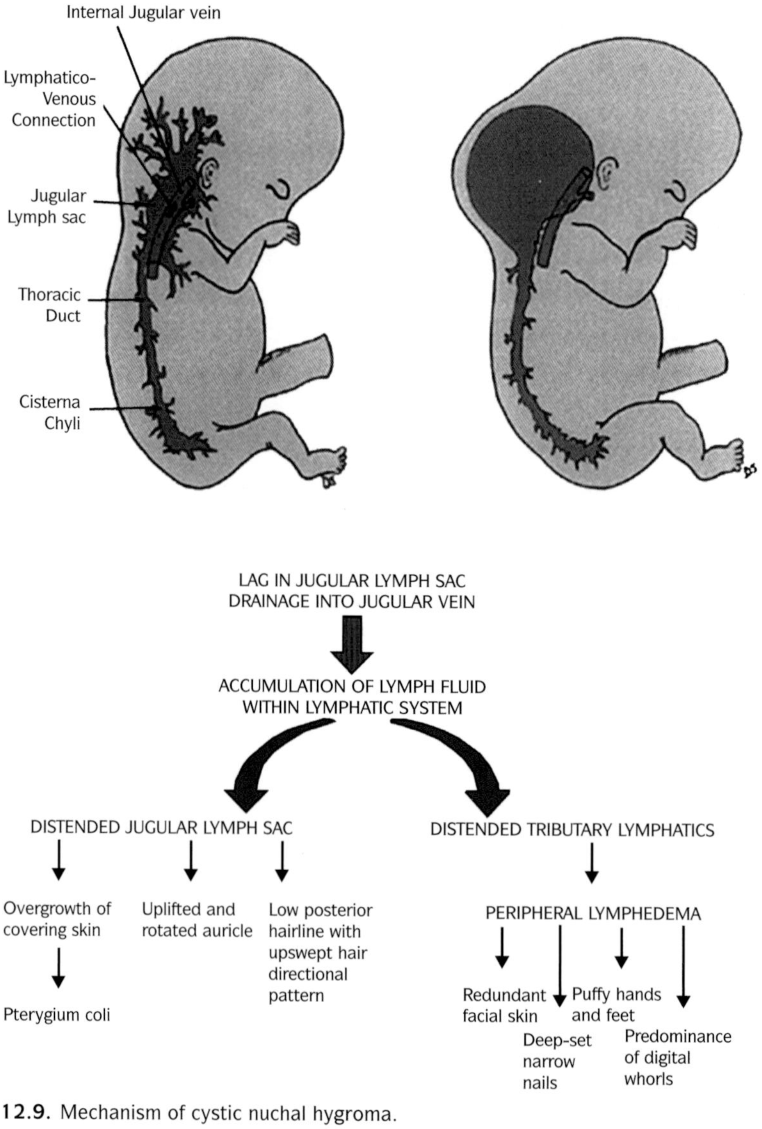

12.9. Mechanism of cystic nuchal hygroma.

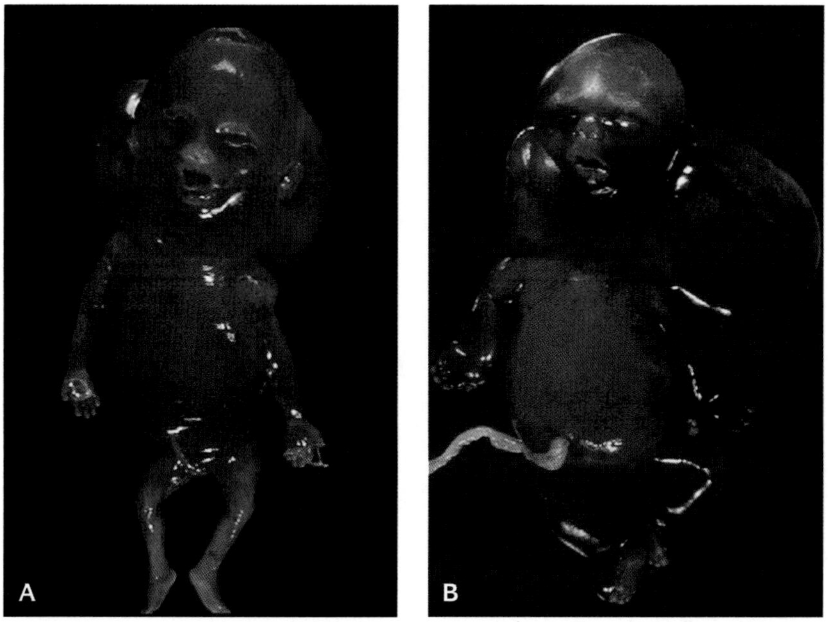

12.10. **(A)** Fetus with cystic hygromas in trisomy 21. **(B)** Fetus with cystic hygromas in monosomy X.

Fetal pericardial effusions are usually components of hydrops fetalis (HF), but local causes include isolated chylopericardium and effusions secondary to mediastinal teratoma and other tumors.

CYSTIC HYGROMA (CH)

An abnormal development of lymphatic vessels results in accumulation of pooled lymph fluid in and around the tissues of the neck, in regions where the principal lymphaticovenous connections normally form (Figures 12.9 to 12.12 and Table 12.7).

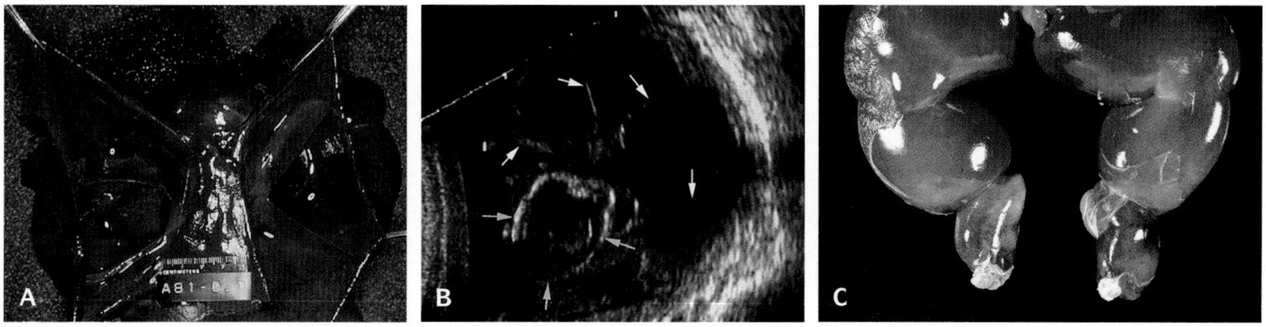

12.11. **(A)** Gross appearance of opened multiloculated cystic hygromas in monosomy X. **(B)** Ultrasound of multiloculated cystic hygromas in monosomy X. **(C)** Typical appearance of the feet (and hands) in monosomy X.

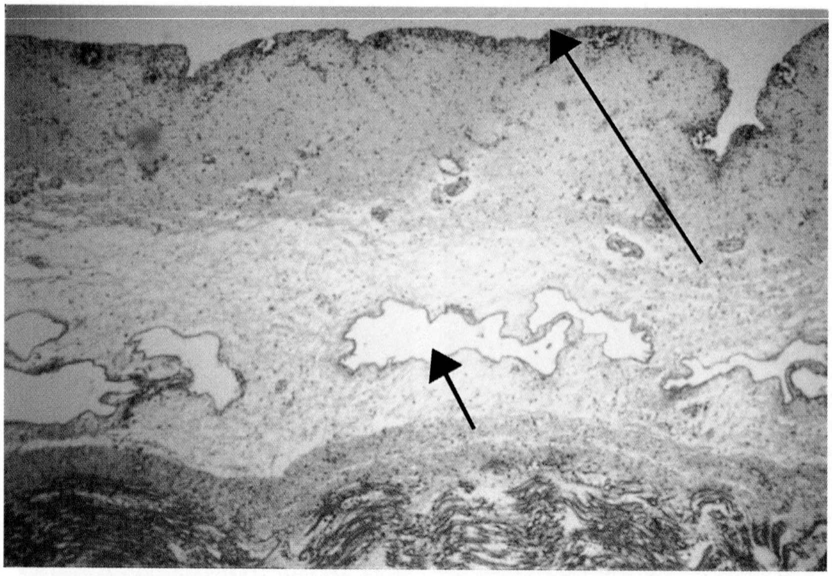

12.12. Microscopic appearance of cystic hygromas with lymphatic lining of cyst (long arrow) with dilated lymphatics in subcutaneous tissue (short arrow). (Table 12.7.)

Sixty percent of CH fetuses are chromosomally abnormal; 45,X, trisomy 21, 18, and 13 are the most frequent.

Euploid cases are usually unilocular and commonly resolve spontaneously – i.e., they represent delayed rather than completely failed lymphaticovenous connection. Delayed cases usually have residual neck webbing and may have flow-type congenital cardiac defects. Unilocular CH is usually euploid and has a better prognosis than multilocular CH.

45,X fetuses typically have very large hygromas that are multiloculated, with generalized brawny lymphedema of the subcutaneous tissues constricted at the wrists and ankles. Tubular hypoplasia of the aortic arch may be caused by the pressure of pleural and pericardial lymph accumulations of the developing

Table 12.7 Fetal cystic hygroma

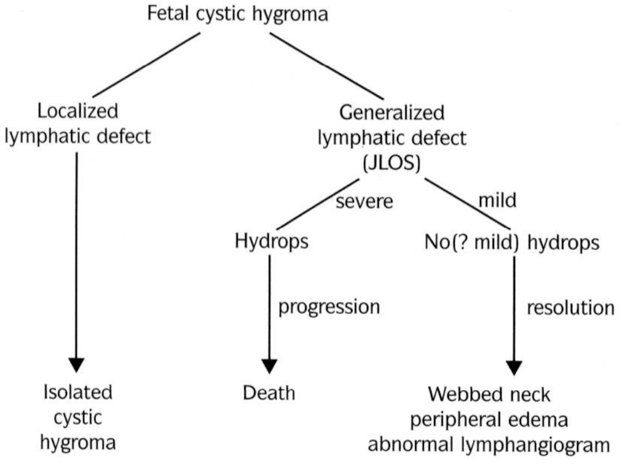

heart. Peripheral lymphatics are absent. Other CH fetuses usually have dilated peripheral lymphatic vessels.

For prenatal diagnosis, fluid aspirated from CH can be used for rapid chromosome analysis because it is rich in lymphocytes.

CYSTIC HYGROMA AND NUCHAL THICKENING

In the first trimester, nuchal translucency is associated with aneuploidy

Nuchal thickness	Odds ratio (trisomy 21)	Odds ratio (trisomy 18)
≥3 mm	3.2	3.1
≥4 mm	19.8	14.0
≥5 mm	28.6	27.8
≥6 mm	21.7	69.2

(From Pandya PP, Kondylios A, Hilbert et al.: Chromosomal defects and outcome in 1015 fetuses with increased nuchal translucency. *Ultrasound Obstet Genecol* 1995:15.)

- Width of 6 mm or more suggest possible Down syndrome in second-trimester fetuses
- Increased nuchal lucency in twin fetuses is associated with aneuploidy
- In chromosomally normal infants, consider other potential causes:
  - toxoplasmosis
  - parvovirus
  - coxsackie virus B

Cystic hygroma ultrasonography:

- The most common neck mass
- Results from failure of the neck lymphatics fail to connect with the venous system due to either abnormal embryonic sequestration of lymphoatic tissue or abnormal budding of the lymphatic epithelium between six and nine weeks of gestation
- Occurs in approximately 1/6,000 pregnancies
- Generally bilateral, asymmetric, thin-walled, multiseptate cystic masses located posterior and lateral to the high cervical vertebrae, often with located posterior and lateral to the high cervical vertebrae, often with hydrops as well. In severe hydrops, skin thickening may be in excess of 3–5 mm. The skull and spine should appear normal and without defect.
- High association with aneuploidy (monosomy, trisomy 21, trisomy 18)
- Septations within the hydroma are associated with chromosomal defects and with increased risk for cephalocele
- Spontaneous resolution may occur

REFERENCES

Boyd PA, Keeling JW: Fetal hydrops. *J Med Genet* 29:91, 1992.

Hansmann M, Gembruch U, Bald R: New therapeutic aspects of nonimmune hydrops based on 402 prenatally diagnosed cases. *Fetal Ther* 4:29, 1989.

Machin G: Cystic hygroma, hydrops and fetal ascites. In Gilbert-Barness E (ed): *Potter's Pathology of the Fetus and Infant*, Philadelphia, Mosby, 1997, p. 388.

Machin GA: Hydrops revisited: literature review of 1414 cases published in the 1980s. *Am J Med Genet* 34:366, 1989.

Pandya PP, Kondylios A, Hilbert, et al.: Chromosomal defects and outcome in 1015 fetuses with increased nuchal translucency. *Ultrasound Obstet Gynecol* 1995:15.

Salzman DH, Frigoletto FD, Harlow BL, et al.: Sonographic evaluation of hydrops fetalis. *Obstet Gynecol* 74:106, 1989.

Santolaya J, Alley D, Jaffe R, Warsof SL: Antenatal classification of hydrops fetalis. *Obstet Gynecol* 79:256, 1992.

THIRTEEN

Central Nervous System Defects

Central nervous system (CNS) defects are the most common developmental defects both at birth and in spontaneously aborted conceptuses. The incidence is from 1 to 65 per 1,000 births.

The incidence of neural tube defects in embryos from spontaneous abortions is about 10 times higher than in newborns. In aborted embryos, CNS defects are usually components of chromosomal syndromes that are lethal early in development and thus are seen less commonly in aborted fetuses that have fewer chromosome anomalies. Most fetal specimens with CNS defects, therefore, are obtained from terminated pregnancies after prenatal detection of an isolated CNS defect.

NEURAL TUBE FORMATION

Neurulation occurs between days 20 and 30 of embryonic development (Stages 9–12) (Figures 13.1 to 13.3 and Table 13.1). Failure of the neural folds to fuse during this period results in a permanent open neural tube defect. Five sites of closure have been proposed. However, careful study of a series of staged human embryos has shown only two de novo sites of fusion: in the rhomboencephalon that proceeds rostrally and caudally, and in the prosencephalon that fuses caudally. It is debated whether failure of closure is due to a deficiency in the

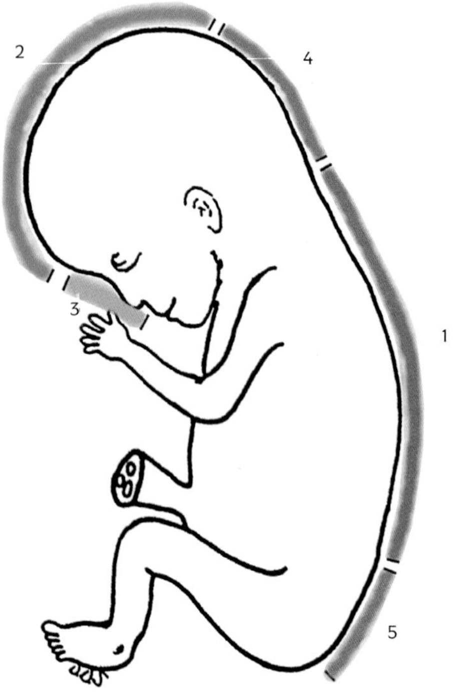

Zipper	Susceptible To	Result
● 1	Folic Acid Deficiency	Spina Bifida
● 2	Hyperthermia and Folic Acid Deficiency	Anencephaly
● 3	Rarely Fails to Close	Midline Facial Cleft
● 4	Hyperthermia	Encephalocele
● 5	Valproic Acid Toxicity	Sacral Meningocele

13.1. Initial proposed sites of closure of the neural tube. Now two sites proposed in the rhombencephalon and the prosencephalon.

axial cephalic mesoderm or in the neuroepithelium itself, but in either case the result is an eversion of the cephalic neural tube and absence of the cranium in anencephaly.

The first sign of neurulation is the appearance of the neural plate in Stage 8. The neural folding process begins at Stage 9. Fusion of the neural folds occurs during Stage 10. The initial site of fusion is at the level of the third to fourth somite, which corresponds to the future rhombencephalon. After this initial fusion occurs, there are the openings between rostral and caudal neural folds, the *anterior and posterior neuropores.* Closure of the anterior neuropore is completed during Stage 11, and primary neurulation is completed during Stage 12. The final site of closure in primary neurulation is at or around the future midlumbar level.

The spinal cord subsequently lengthens and the spinal column develops further segmentation. When primary neurulation has been completed, additional lengthening must take place by a different process. The overall process of elongation of the caudal neural tube through the formation of a lumen is called *canalization.* It occurs during Stages 13–20, when the notochord and the caudal end of the neural tube merge as an undifferentiated mass of cells. Through vacuolization and lumen formation, this cellular mass differentiates to form and connect additional spinal and vertebral segments.

After neural tube closure, there is rapid neural tissue proliferation and differentiation. At the end of the 4th week, Stage 12, the primary brain vesicles have formed. These consist of the forebrain (prosencephalon), midbrain (mesencephalon), and hindbrain (rhombencephalon). In the 5th week (Stages 13–15), the forebrain evaginates laterally. The forebrain consists of two parts, the lateral evaginations that become the cerebral hemispheres, and the area posterior to these evaginations that becomes the thalami and adjacent structures. The anterior part of the forebrain is called the telencephalon, the posterior part the diencephalon. The olfactory bulbs arise from the lateral wall of the telencephalon; the optic bulbs from the lateral sides of the diencephalon. As these telencephalic vesicles grow, the original wide connection with the diencephalic cavity narrows and the foramen of Monro and the third ventricle are formed.

The choroid plexuses, which produce cerebrospinal fluid (CSF), begin to differentiate during the 7th and 8th week in the telencephalic vesicles and the roof of the third and the fourth ventricles. In the midfetal period, the foramina of Magendie and Luschka are formed in the fourth ventricle, and CSF is able to flow into the subarachnoid space. Absorption of CSF is mainly through the arachnoid villi, which project into the dural sinuses. Cysts of the fetal choroid plexus in the posterior horn of the lateral ventricle have been noted by ultrasound at 16–20 weeks gestation. They usually disappear a few weeks later and are considered normal variants.

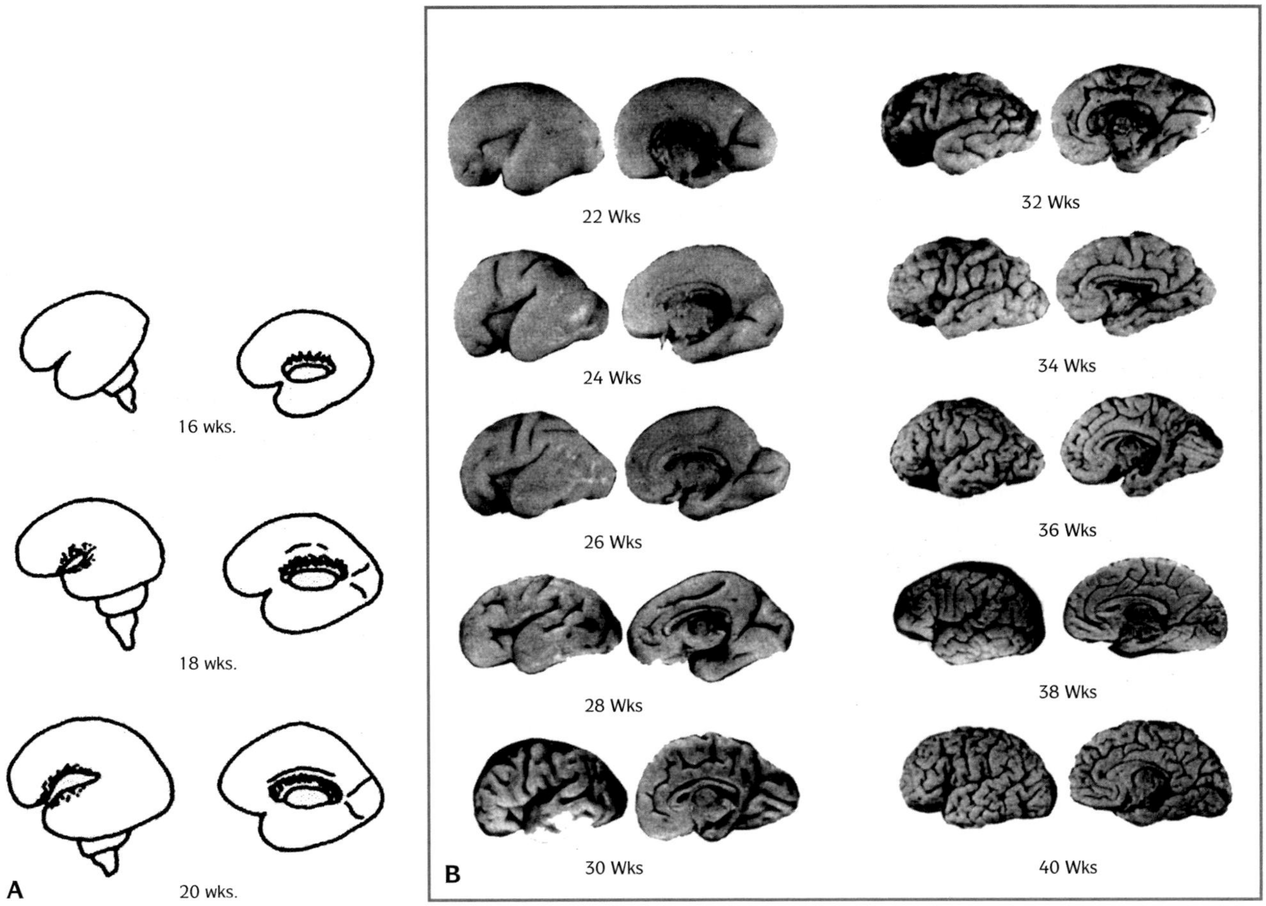

13.2. (A) and **(B)** Development of the fetal brain.

There are many different types of CNS defects and many different causes of these defects. Defects may be caused by chromosome abnormalities, a single gene mutation, a combination of genetic predisposition and environmental factors (multifactorial inheritance), or environmental factors alone.

In embryos with CNS defects, 80% have an abnormal karyotype. The most common chromosome abnormalities associated with a CNS defect in the embryo are triploidy, 45,X, and trisomy 13. In embryos and fetuses with CNS defects, 40% have chromosome abnormalities.

Many gene mutations affect the development of the CNS. Hydrocephalus can be produced by an autosomal dominant, autosomal recessive, or an X-linked gene. Holoprosencephaly may be caused by a gene mutation inherited as a dominant trait with reduced penetrance. The CNS defects that show an autosomal recessive inheritance includes microcephaly, encephalocele in the Meckel-Gruber syndrome, aplasia of the cerebellar vermis, and neuronal migration defect in Zellweger syndrome.

One of the environmental factors involved in neural tube defects may be a vitamin deficiency, particularly of folic acid, and multivitamin or folic acid supplements have been recommended as a preventive measure.

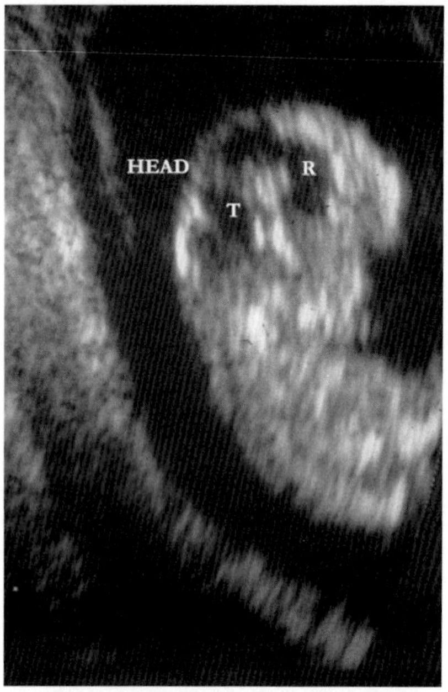

13.3. Ultrasound of a 5-week embryo showing the developing brain (R = rhombencephalon, T = telencephalon).

Alcohol and valproic acid are well known teratogens that cause CNS defects. Maternal diabetes mellitus, chronic heart disease, and chronic lung disease are also associated with an increased incidence of CNS abnormalities.

ANENCEPHALY

Anencephaly is the absence of most of the brain and most or all of the cranial vault (Figures 13.4 to 13.6). It can be divided into cases in which the defect is localized to the cranium (*meroacrania*) and cases in which the defect ends through the foramen magnum (*holoacrania*). If the vertebral column is included in the defect, the condition is called *holoacrania with rachischisis* or *craniorachischisis.*

The incidence of anencephaly in the newborn is from 0.6 to 3.5 per 1,000 births.

The recurrence risk for multifactorial anencephaly, or spina bifida cystica, is around 4%. It varies from about 2% in British Columbia to 10% in Northern Ireland.

The sequence of pathogenetic events seems to be that the neural tissue continues to proliferate and forms enough brain tissue to induce eye development. The exposed brain tissue still may be intact in early embryos; this condition is

Table 13.1 Causes of neural tube defects

Chromosome abnormalities
13 trisomy
18 trisomy
Triploidy
Other abnormalities, such as unbalanced translocation and ring chromosome
Multifactorial
Anencephaly
Meningomyelocele
Meningocele
Encephalocele
Single mutant genes
Meckel syndrome-autosomal recessive
Median-cleft face syndrome-autosomal dominant (may include anterior encephalocele)
Robert syndrome-autosomal recessive (may include anterior encephalocele)
Syndrome of anterior sacral meningomyelocele and anal stenosis-dominant, autosomal or X-linked
Jarco-Levin syndrome-autosomal recessive (may include meningomyelocele)
Syndrome of occipital encephalocelė, myopia and retinal dysplasia
Anterior encephalocele among Bantus and Thais
Syndrome of craniofacial and limb defects secondary to amniotic bands
Cloacal exstrophy
Sacrococcygeal teratoma may include meningomyelocele
Teratogens
Folic acid deficiency
Valproic acid (phenotype includes spina bifida)
Aminopterin/amethopterin (anencephaly and encephalocele)
Thalidomide (rarely anencephaly and meningomyelocele)
Infant of diabetic mother (anencephaly more frequent than spina bifida)

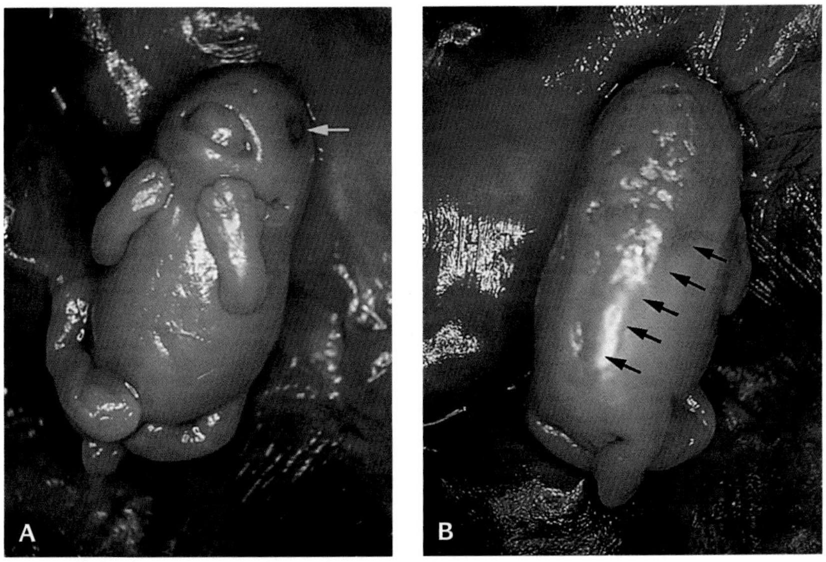

13.4. Anencephaly and complete rachischisis (arrows in B) in an embryo of 52 days. **(A)** Anterior view (arrow, eye). **(B)** Posterior view.

called *exencephaly*. Subsequently, this brain tissue degenerates, leaving a mass of thin-walled vascular structures and degenerated neural tissue (*area cerebrovasculosa*) over the brain stem structures.

ANENCEPHALY WITHOUT RACHISCHISIS

The anencephalic newborn has a unique appearance. The vault of the skull is missing and the brain tissue has degenerated into a spongy mass. Most of the bones at the base of the skull are abnormal. A typical head and facies include low-set ears with overfolded helices, proptosis, and large cheeks, nose, mouth, and tongue. The palate is often highly arched with deep grooves on both sides of the raphe. Other defects may involve a short neck, vertebral abnormalities, a shortened thorax, a large thymus, pulmonary hypoplasia, and deformations of the limbs such as clubfeet (talipes).

The pituitary fossa is usually flattened; and the optic nerves are usually small or absent. The internal organs show variable defects. Hypoplasia of the adrenal cortex is a constant finding from 16 weeks of development. It is due to hypoplasia of the fetal zone caused by the absence of the hypothalamus and the consequent abnormal regulatory function of the pituitary gland. Additional major abnormalities occur in 20–30% of anencephalic fetuses.

Facial clefting and renal defects are most common. Renal defects consist of hydronephrosis, polycystic kidney, unilateral and bilateral agenesis, and unilateral hypoplasia. Skeletal defects include club hands and abnormal thumbs. Esophageal atresia and intestinal malrotation are among the gastrointestinal defects. Heart defects vary from simple septal defects to complex transpositions. Hypospadias and a hypoplastic penis are among the genital defects.

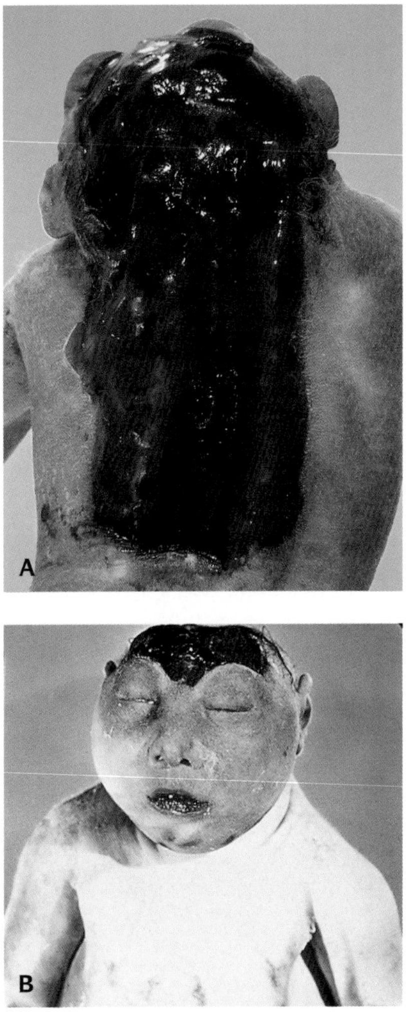

13.5. Anencephaly with complete rachischisis in an 18-week-gestation fetus. **(A)** Posterior view. **(B)** Anterior view.

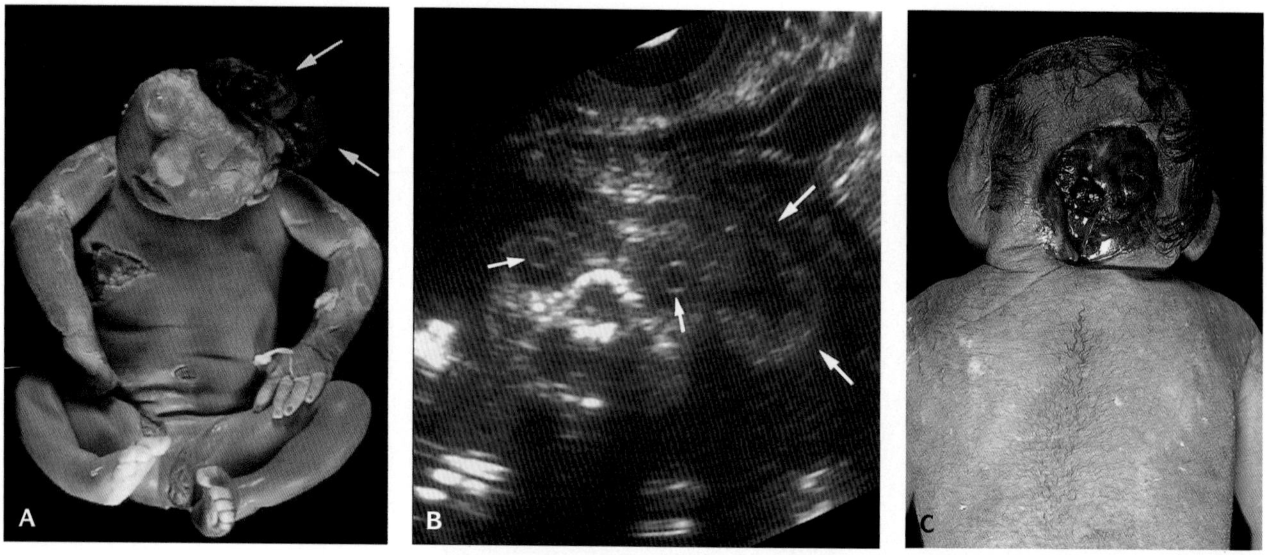

13.6. **(A)** Anencephaly at 27-weeks gestation with a "beret" of brain tissue (yellow arrows) present. **(B)** Ultrasound showing the "beret" of brain (large arrows) adjacent to the orbit (small arrows) on the right. **(C)** Cranio-occipital rachischisis in a stillborn fetus at 28 weeks gestation.

ANENCEPHALY WITH SPINAL RACHISCHISIS

Vertebral defects, pulmonary hypoplasia, and clubfeet are more common in anencephaly with spinal rachischisis than in anencephaly alone. Usually the neck and thorax are shortened due to vertebral defects, and there may be scoliosis, which reduces the volume of the thorax and the abdomen. Major defects in anencephaly with rachischisis are:

- renal defects – 17%
- cleft lip/palate – 10%
- gastrointestinal defects – 9%
- spleen abnormalities – 2%
- omphalocele – 5%
- diaphragmatic defect – 5%
- heart defects – 4%

Rarely, anencephaly with spinal rachischisis is accompanied by cyclopia, proboscis, microphthalmia, a single nostril, and other features of holoprosencephaly.

INIENCEPHALY

In iniencephaly, the head is extremely retroflexed and the neck is absent. The face skin is continuous with the chest skin, and the posterior scalp is directly connected to the skin of the back (Figure 13.7). There may be a large encephalocele protruding from the open foramen magnum. There is often cleavage of the

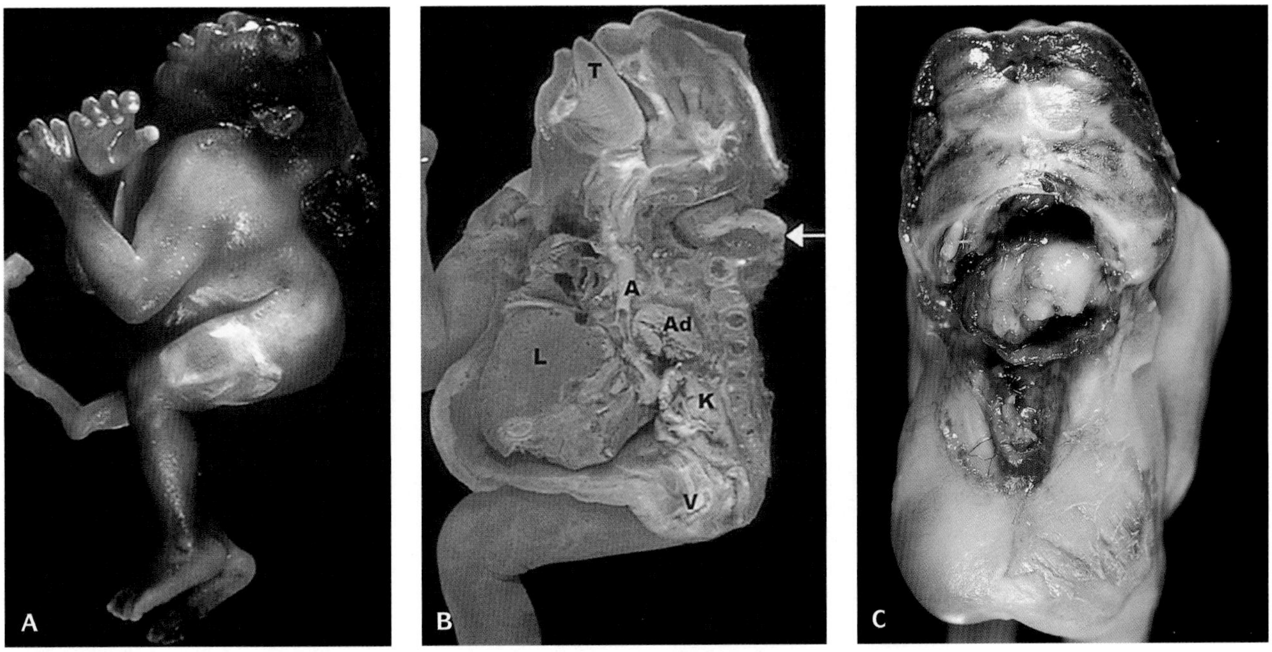

13.7. Iniencephaly. **(A)** Lateral view. **(B)** Midsagittal section view. (T, tongue; A, aorta; L, liver; Ad, adrenal; K, kidney; V, vagina; arrow, brain tissue.) **(C)** Posterior view.

occipital region of the skull, and the occipital bone is found with the cervical vertebrae. The cervical vertebrae are always abnormal (abnormalities of shape and fusion), and the other vertebrae are often also abnormal. The skin of the neck and back is usually hirsute.

Iniencephaly has been regarded as an extreme form of the Klippel-Feil syndrome.

Iniencephaly is associated with additional malformations in 84% of cases. CNS abnormalities include anencephaly, hydrocephaly, and myelocele. There may be face abnormalities such as cyclopia, an absent mandible, and a cleft lip and palate. Renal malformations – for example, a horseshoe, ectopic, or polycystic kidney – are common. Cardiovascular and gastrointestinal malformations are also frequent, as is a diaphragmatic hernia. It is more common in females.

MYELOCELE

A defect due to the failure of the spinal neural tube to close, in which the neural tissue is exposed at the surface, is called a *myelocele*, or *rachischisis* (Figure 13.8). If the neural tissue is enclosed in a sac covered with arachnoid and dura, it is called a *myelomeningocele* or a *meningomyelocele*. If the sac contains only arachnoid and dura, it is called a *meningocele*. The most usual locations are lumbar or lumbosacral. About 50% of all CNS defects are myeloceles.

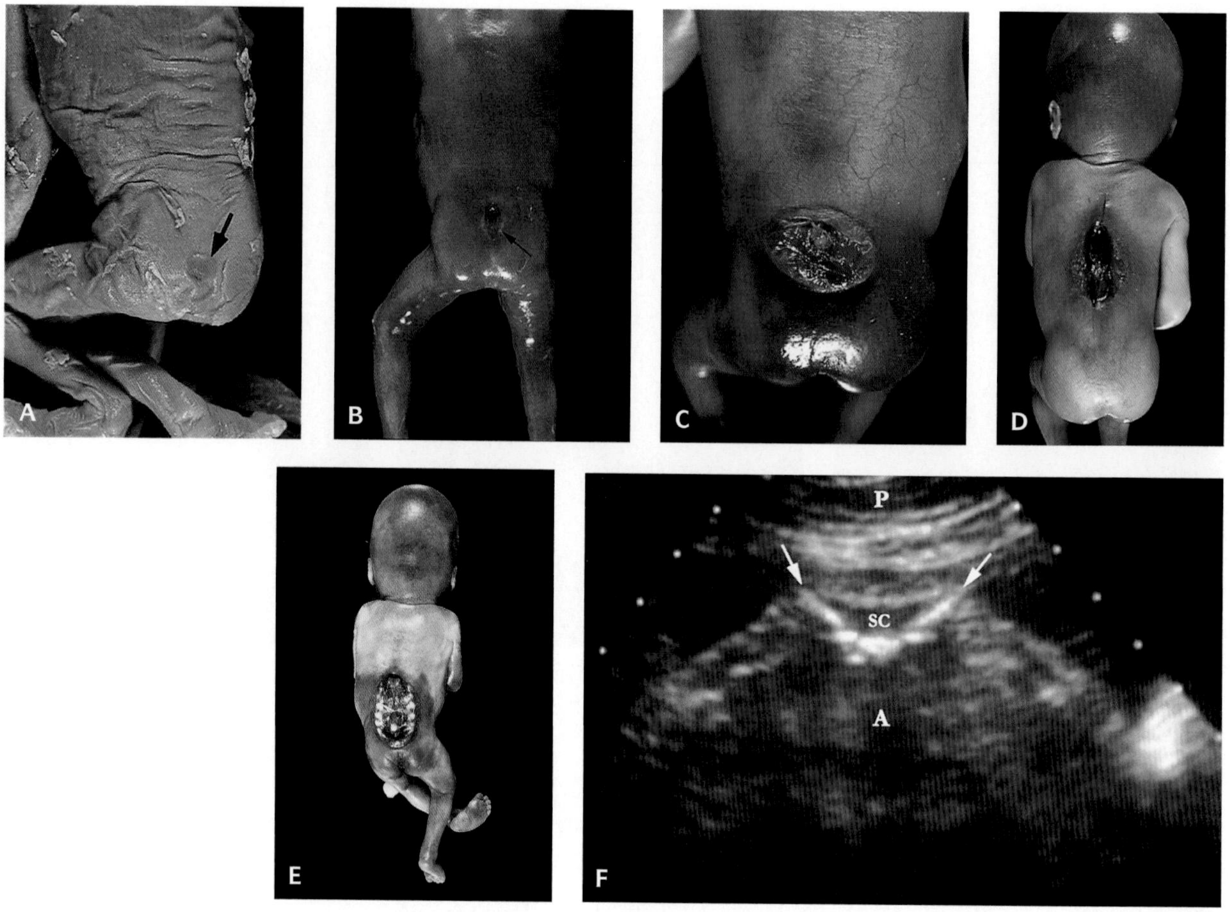

13.8. **(A)** Spina bifida occulta (arrow). **(B)** Meningomyelocele (arrow) in 14-week fetus. **(C)** Ruptured meningomyelocele in 20-week fetus. **(D)** Thoracolumbar open neural tube defect. **(E)** Long lumbosacral neural tube defect. **(F)** Ultrasound of a meningomyelocele. The vertebral bones are splayed (arrows) posteriorly (P). (SC, spinal canal; A, anterior.)

In embryos, myelocele has been found in triploidy and trisomy 16. In older conceptuses, myelocele and meningomyelocele have been associated with trisomy 13 and trisomy 18.

From 10% to 20% of infants with myelocele have additional major defects. In live-born infants, associated defects occur in approximately 10%, including:

- cleft lip and/or palate
- rib fusion
- accessory spleen
- aortic coarctation
- short esophagus
- imperforate anus with lesions below T_{11}
- unilateral renal agenesis
- ventricular septal defect
- pelvic bone ossification defects in lesions at or above T_{11}
- renal agenesis
- duplicated ureter

Of fetuses with midspine defects, 30% have associated abnormalities such as an accessory spleen, a horseshoe kidney, Meckel diverticulum, and malrotation

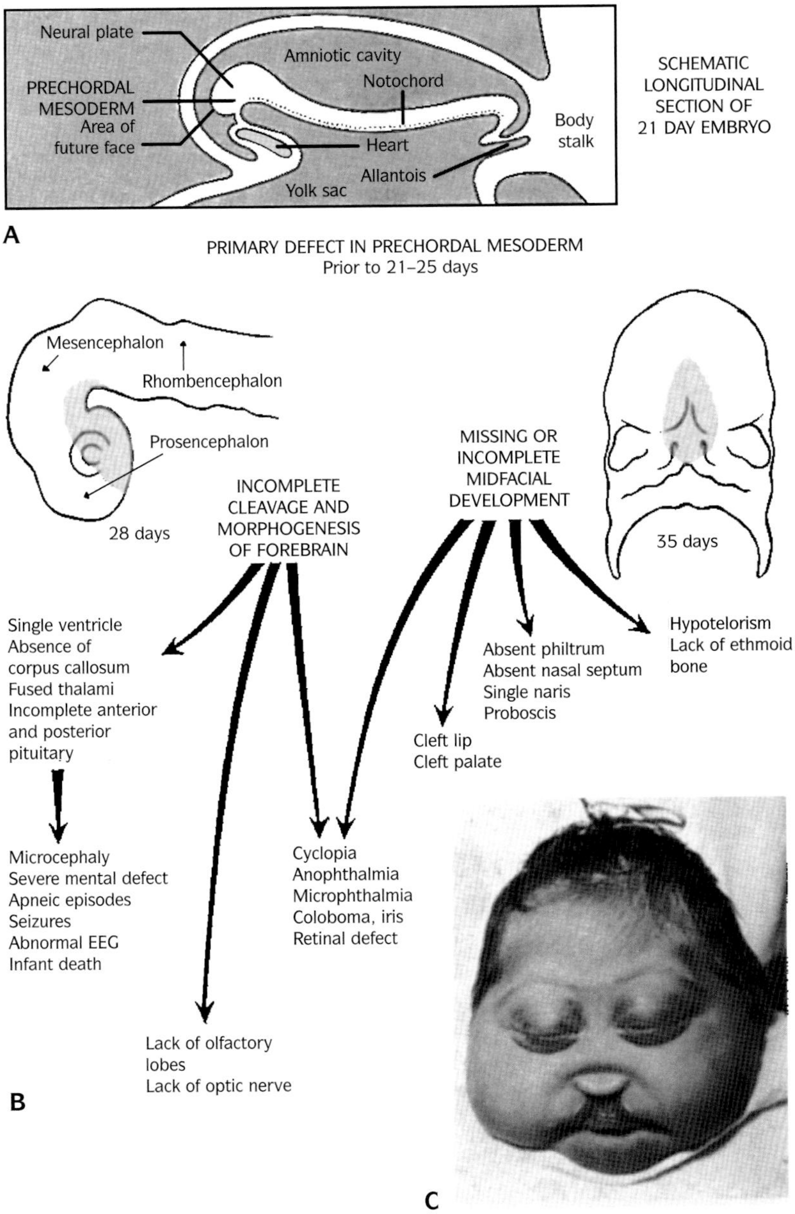

13.9. Pathogenesis of holoprosencephaly. (From Jones KL: *Smith's Recognizable Patterns of Malformation Syndromes*, 6th ed, Philadelphia, Saunders, 1997.)

of the intestine. Cases with lower spine defects usually are not associated with other abnormalities.

HOLOPROSENCEPHALY (SEE ALSO CHROMOSOME CHAPTER)

Holoprosencephaly is the most common major developmental defect of the forebrain in humans (Figures 13.9 to 13.12 and Tables 13.1 to 13.5). The incidence of holoprosencephaly in newborns is between 0.02% and 0.006%. In

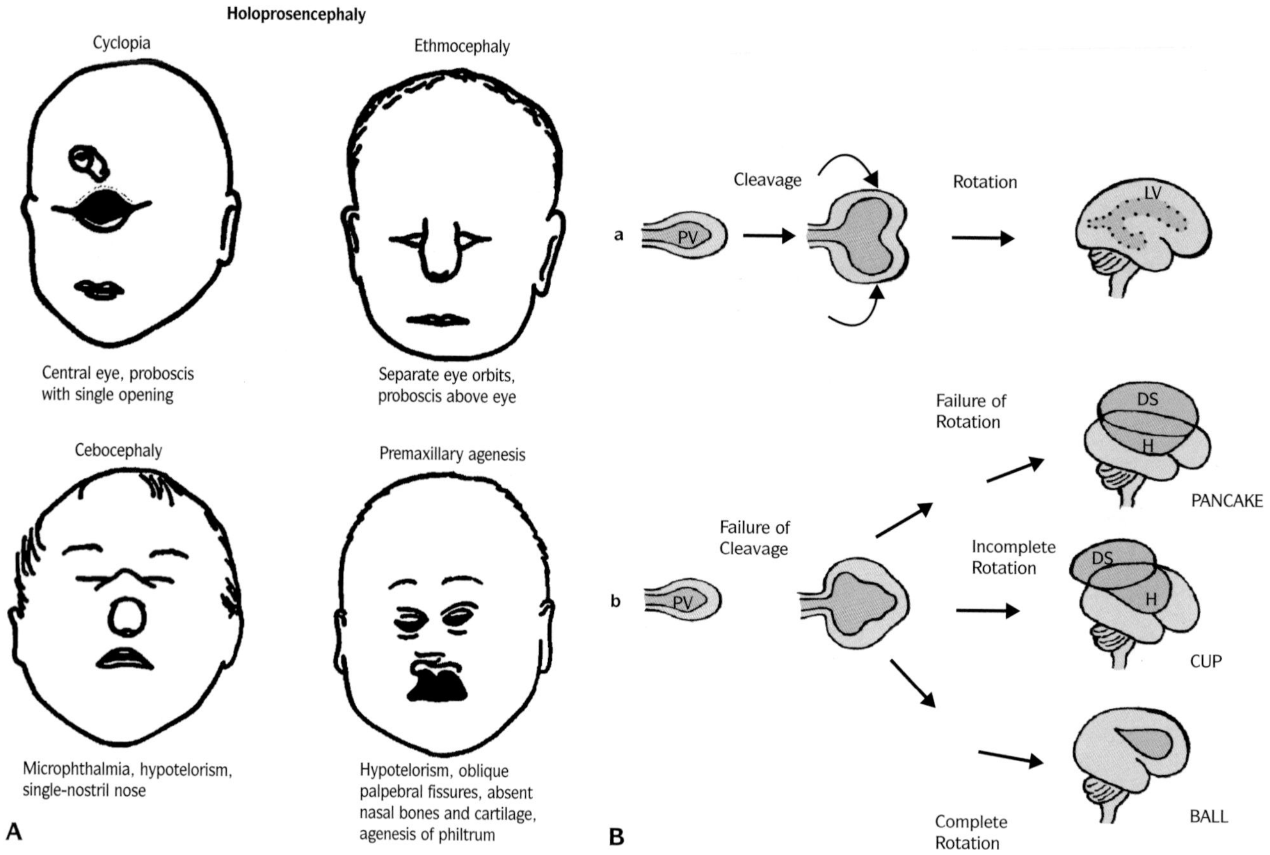

13.10. **(A)** Spectrum of holoprosencephaly drawing. **(B)** Development of normal (**a**) and holoprosencephalic brain (**b**). The primitive prosencephalon undergoes cleavage then the two hemispheres rotate medially to form the interhemispheric fissure. From the primitive ventricular cavity (PV), two separated lateral ventricles (LV) are formed (**a**), (**b**). In alobar holoprosencephaly, failure of cleavage results in a single ventricular cavity (H). The degree of subsequent inward rotation of the cortex determines the morphologic type. Failure of rotation results in the pancake type, in which the membranous diencephalic roof bulges to form the so-called dorsal sac (DS). In the intermediate form-cup type, the cortex rolls over to partially cover the diencephalic roof. In the ball type, full rotation has occurred, and the single ventricle is completely covered.

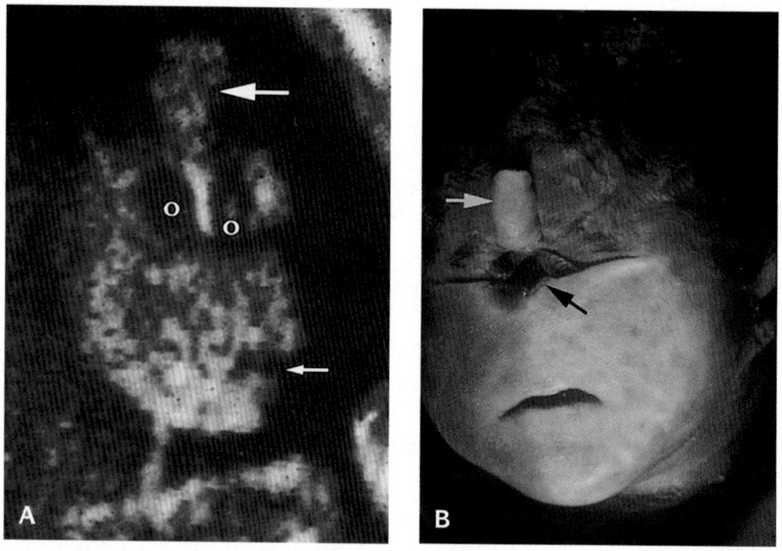

13.11. **(A)** Ultrasound of cebocephaly with hypotelorism (large arrow, proboscis; O, orbits; small arrow, mouth). **(B)** Cyclopia (black arrow) with a proboscis (yellow arrow).

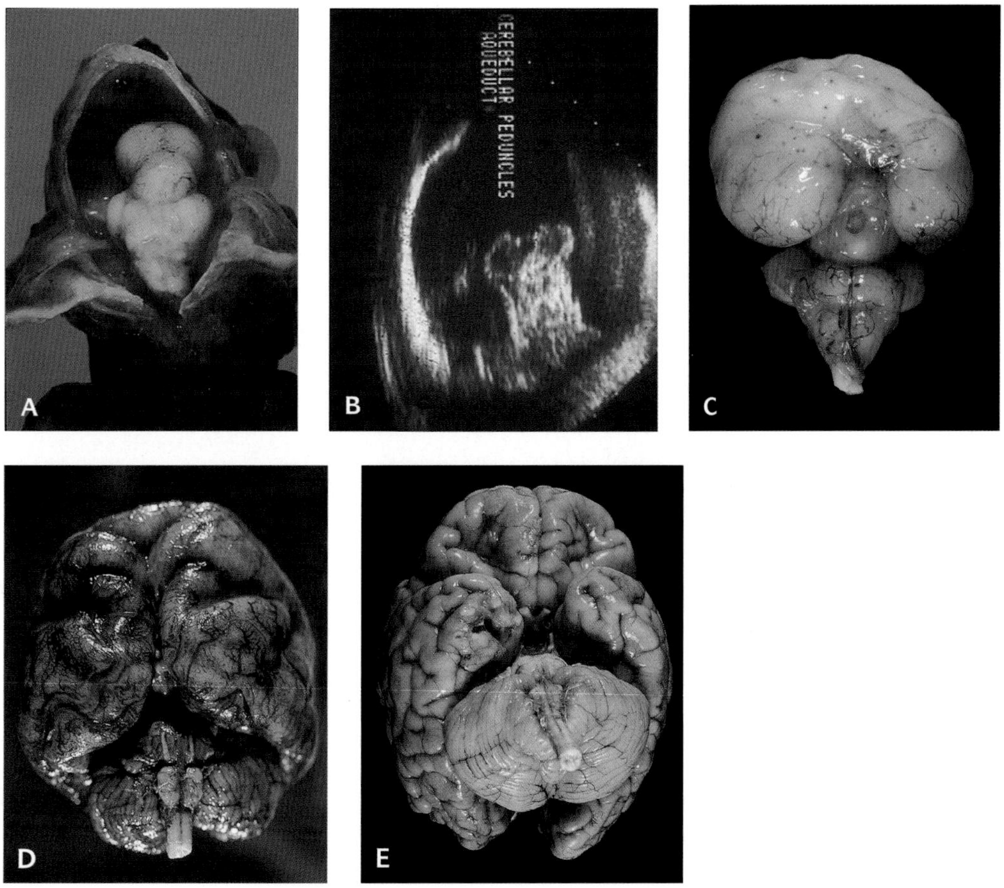

13.12. Holoprosencephaly **(A)**. Aprosencephaly **(B)**. Ultrasound of aprosencephaly **(C)**. Alobar **(D)**, lobar **(E)**, arhinencephaly (absent olfactory bulbs and tracts).

embryos, it is higher, around 0.4%; thus, most holoprosencephalic conceptuses are eliminated before birth.

The prechordal mesenchyme induces the development of the anterior brain (prosencephalon) and there is an intimate relationship between midface development and the development of the optic and olfactory bulbs and the growth of the cerebral hemispheres.

Many different chromosome abnormalities have been reported with holoprosencephaly, the most common being trisomy 13 or (del)13q. Other chromosome abnormalities observed in holoprosencephaly include duplications and deletions of chromosome 18, trisomy 21, and triploidy. Holoprosencephaly may be caused by an autosomal recessive gene or by a dominant mutation.

The least severe form of holoprosencephaly is arrhinencephaly with absence of the olfactory bulbs and tracts. The most severe end of the spectrum is aprosencephaly (atelencephaly) when the brain consists of a brainstem and cerebellum with absence of the structures derived from the prosencephalon/telencephalon. In addition, holoprosencephaly may be alobar,

Table 13.2 Monogenic syndromes with holoprosencephaly

Condition	Inheritance	Frequency of holoprosencephaly	Other features
Autosomal recessive holoprosencephaly	AR	Always present	Severity of facial dysmorphism varies. Variation within families
Autosomal dominant holoprosencephaly	AD	Present, variable expression	Wide spectrum of facial anomaly, variation within families, attributed to incomplete penetrance
Meckel syndrome	AR	Occasional	± median/lateral cleft lip; occipital encephalocele most common of wide spectrum of CNS anomalies. Cystic dysplastic kidney and hepatic ductal plate abnormally consistently present, polydactyly, frequent congenital heart defects, genital anomalies, other anomalies
Martin syndrome	AD	Inconsistent	+ median cleft lip; microcephaly, mental deficiency, ocular hypotelorism, down-slanting palpebral fissures, cleft lip, large ears, clubfoot, spinal anomalies
Velocardiofacial syndrome	AD	Occasional	+ median cleft lip; long face, narrow palpebral fissures, prominent nose with square nasal root and narrow alar base, long philtrum, cleft or submucous cleft palate, small ears, cardiac anomalies
Grote syndrome	AR	Always present	Hydrocephaly, octodactyly, absent tibiae, cardiac malformations
Steinfield syndrome	AD (probable)	Always present	Median cleft lip, short forearms, absent thumbs, cardiac defects, renal anomalies, absent gallbladder
Holoprosencephaly-fetal akinesia syndrome	X-linked	Always present	Microcephaly, sloping forehead, flattened nasal tip, micrognathia, multiple contractures, talipes equinovarus

Adapted from Cohen MM Jr: Perspectives on holoprosencephaly: Epidemiology, genetics and syndromology. *Teratology* 40:211, 1989.
AR, autosomal recessive inheritance; AD, autosomal dominant inheritance.

Table 13.3 Holoprosencephaly

Developmental field:
- Midline facial structures and prosencephalon in same developmental field
- Mesoderm migrates anterior to notochord at third week of gestation
- Responsible for the induction and differentiation of midline facial structures and forebrain

Table 13.4 Isolated absence of the olfactory bulbs and tracts: single gene defects

Condition	Features	Inheritance
Kallman syndrome, type I	Hypogonadotropic hypogonadism, mental deficiency, ocular hypotelorism, unilateral renal agenesis, other anomalies X-linked or sex-linked autosomal dominant	AD
Isolated anosmia type II		AD
Anosmia/radiohumeral synostosis		AD
Kallman syndrome type II	Hypogonadotropic hypogonadism, other anomalies, diabetes mellitus or hearing defect Hypogonadotropic hypogonadism, alopecia, conductive deafness, dysplastic ears	AR
OFD V1	Cleft-lip palate, lingual nodule, growth and psychomotor retardation duplicated halluces, supernumerary fingers, congenital heart defect, cryptorchidism	AR
Campomelic dysplasia	Absent corpus callosum, hydrocephaly, absent left hemidiaphragm, ventricular septal defect, absent fifth fingernail	AR
Isolated anosmia type I	Hypogonadotrophic hypogonadism, mental deficiency, congenital ichthyosis	XLR

Modified from Cohen, MM Jr. 1989b, with permission of the publisher Alan R Liss and of the author.
AD, autosomal dominant; AR, autosomal recessive; XLR, X-linked recessive.

Table 13.5 Facial defects in holoprosencephaly

Type of face	Facial features	Cranium-brain
Cyclopia	Single eye or partially divided eye in single orbit Arhinia with proboscis	Microcephaly Alobar holoprosencephaly
Ethmocephaly	Extreme hypotelorism Arhinia with proboscis	Microcephaly Alobar holoprosencephaly
Cebocephaly	Orbital hypotelorism Proboscis-like nose but no median cleft of lip	Microcephaly Usually alobar holoprosencephaly
With median cleft lip	Orbital hypotelorism Flat nose	Sometimes trigonocephaly Usually alobar holoprosencephaly
With median philtrum-premaxilla anlage	Orbital hypotelorism Bilateral cleft lip with median process philtrum-premaxilla anlage Flat nose	Sometimes trigonocephaly Semilobar or lobar holoprosencephaly

Modified from DeMyer et al.: *Pediatrics* 34:256, 1964.

semilobar, or lobar with varying degrees of failure of clefting of the prosencephalon.

Teratogens that have an effect during early gastrulation may cause holoprosencephaly. About 1–2% of newborn infants of mothers with diabetes develop holoprosencephaly. Diabetic embryopathy is the result of any interference with the glycolytic pathway leading to a decreased rate of glycolysis and conversion of glucose to pyruvate. Maternal alcohol consumption during early pregnancy has been associated with holoprosencephaly in the offspring. Retinoic acid embryopathy, isotretinoin, and etretinate produce their main effects by acting on neural crest cells. Holoprosencephaly also can be caused by mutated genes and teratogens involving the sonic hedgehog signaling network and cholesterol biosynthesis as in the Smith-Lemli-Opitz (SLO) syndrome. Currently four genes have been identified that include sonic hedgehog (SHH) an chromosome 7q36, Z1C2, S1X3, and TG-interacting factor (TGIF).

Teratogenic causes of holoprosencephaly include maternal diabetes, ethyl alcohol, retinoic acid, mutated genes, and teratogens involving the sonic hedgehog signaling network and cholesterol biosynthesis, cholesterol trafficing, sterol adducts, target issue response, and sterol sensing domain.

Holoprosencephaly is known to be etiologically heterogeneous and may be caused in some cases by an autosomal recessive gene in the homozygous state, in other cases by trisomy 13, and in still other cases by maternal diabetes. The pathogenesis may also be heterogeneous. It may be based on an insult to the prechordal mesoderm, a slightly later insult to the neural plate, or an insult producing decreased cellular proliferation of all three germ layers simultaneously.

ENCEPHALOCELE

In encephalocele, the intracranial contents protrude through a bony defect of the skull (Figure 13.13 and Table 13.6). When brain tissue is in the herniated sac, it is called an *encephalocele.* The incidence is 0.3 to 0.6 in 1,000 live births. It may be associated with maternal rubella, hyperthermia, and diabetes.

In occipital encephalocele, the bony defect may include the foramen magnum and the posterior arch of the atlas. The brainstem is often abnormal and the spinal cord may show developmental defects. Occipital encephalocele is common in iniencephaly and in the Meckel syndrome.

Encephalocele also may occur in the parietal and anterior regions. Parietal encephaloceles are usually midline, and the associated abnormalities may be an absent corpus callosum, a Dandy-Walker defect, or other brain malformations. An anterior encephalocele may be visible or externally invisible, and the amount of brain tissue present within the sac varies greatly. With all types of encephaloceles, there may be an associated microcrania or a hydrocephalus.

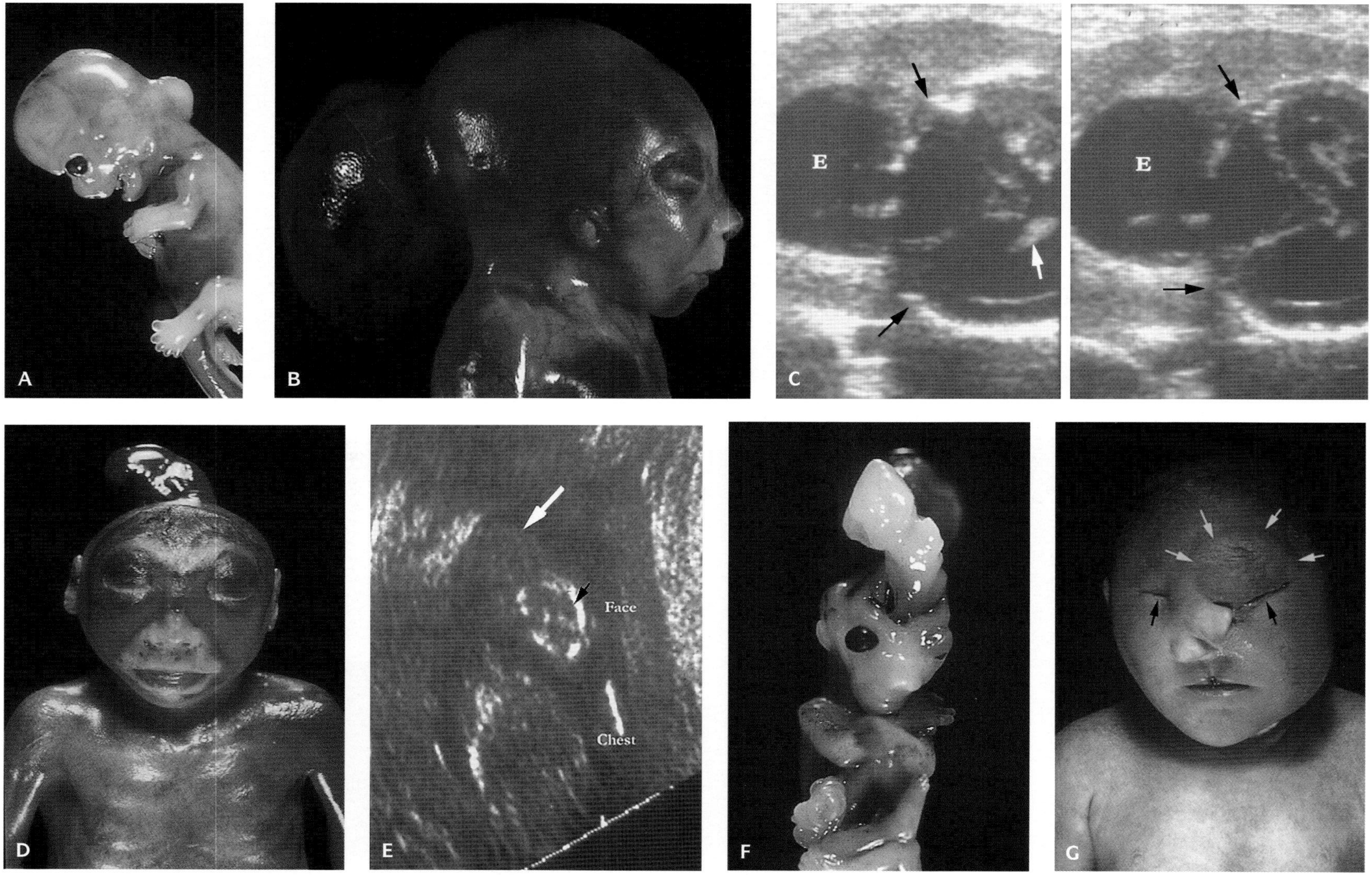

13.13. Encephaloceles. **(A)** Occipital encephalocele in a 58-day gestation fetus. **(B)** Occipital encephalocele in a 22-week fetus. **(C)** Ultrasound of occipital encephalocele. (Black arrows, edge of skull bone defect; white arrow, choriod plexus.) **(D)** Large parietal encephalocele. **(E)** Ultrasound of parietal encephalocele (white arrow) (black arrow, skull bone). **(F)** Frontal encephalocele in 12-week fetus. **(G)** Orbital encephalocele (yellow arrows) in a 32-week fetus (black arrows, orbits).

Table 13.6 Syndromes with encephaloceles (see also Chapter 8)

Syndrome	Manifestation
Amniotic band	Multiple encephaloceles (predominantly anterior), constriction and amputation of digits or limbs, polydactyly, syndactyly, facial disruptions, cleft lip/palate
Walker-Warburg (HARD- or Chemke, or cerebrooculodysplasia)	Occipital encephaloceles, hydrocephaly, cerebellar dysgenesis, agyria, retinal dysplasia, cataracts, congenital muscular dystrophy
Chromosomal defects	Triploidy, trisomy 14, trisomy 13, mosaic trisomy 20, deletion of 13q, duplications 6, 7, 8, 45 X
Cryptophthalmos (Fraser)	Occipital encephalocele, one or both eyes covered by skin, syndactyly of hands and/or feet
Dyssegmental dwarfism	Occipital encephalocele, narrow chest, reduced joint mobility, abnormal vertebrae, short bent limbs
Frontonasal dysplasia	Frontal encephalocele, hypertelorism, anterior cranium bifidum occultum, widely set nostrils
Knoblock	Occipital encephalocele, vitroretinal degeneration, meningocele
Meckel	Occipital encephalocele, polydactyly, polycystic kidneys, holoprosencephaly, microphthalmia, hepatic bile duct proliferation
Van Voss	Occipital encephalocele, phocomelia, urogenital anomalies, absent corpus callosum
Warfarin	Occipital encephalocele, limb shortening, hydrocephaly, nasal hypoplasia
Associations	Absent corpus callosum, cleft lip/palate, craniostenosis, Dandy-Walker malformation, Arnold-Chiari malformation, ectrodactyly, hemifacial microsomia, iniencephaly, Klippel-Feil syndrome, meningomyelocele

Adapted from Cohen MM Jr, Lemire RJ: Syndromes with encephaloceles. 25:161, 1982.

Other associated defects may be meningomyelocele, cleft palate, or congenital heart disease.

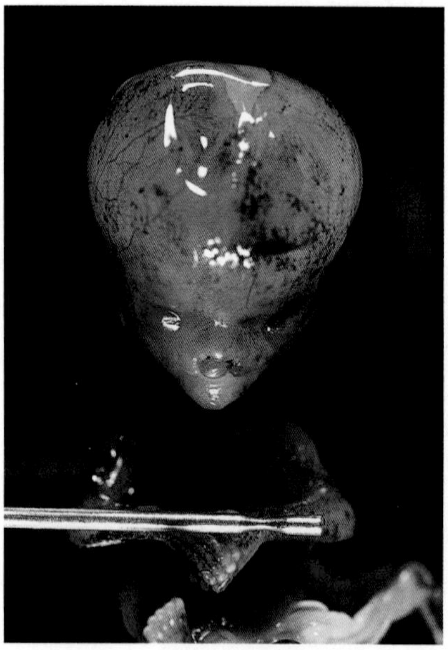

13.14. Hydrocephalus in a ruptured ectopic pregnancy at 10-weeks gestation.

HYDROCEPHALUS

Hydrocephalus is an increase in the amount of intraventricular cerebrospinal fluid (CSF). It is usually due to an obstruction. The incidence varies from 0.3 to 2.5 per 1,000 live births (Figures 13.14 and 13.15 and Table 13.7).

Ex vacuo hydrocephalus, due to a loss of brain tissue, has not been described in previable fetuses.

Obstruction may be at the aqueduct of Sylvius that is narrowed or malformed. There may be malformations of the hindbrain such as the Arnold-Chiari malformation, in which the cerebellar vermis protrudes through the foramen magnum and the medulla is displaced past the foramen magnum to obstruct CSF flow. This malformation is commonly seen with myelocele and has been detected as early as the 10th week of gestation. Dandy-Walker malformation consists of hypoplastic or absent cerebellar vermis, enlarged fourth ventricle widely separating the cerebral hemispheres, and the foramina of Magendie and Luschka absent from the abnormal roof of the ventricle.

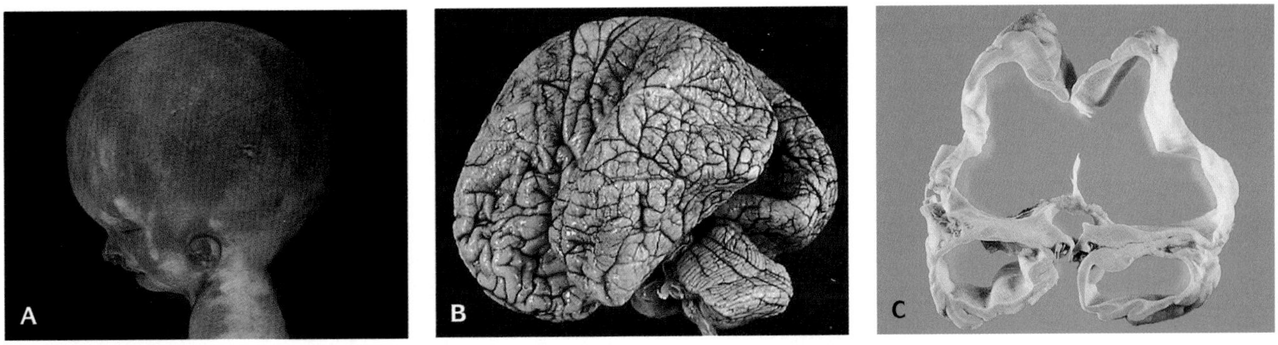

13.15. X-linked hydrocephalus. **(A)** A 30-week fetus with large hydrocephalic head. **(B)** The brain shows micropolygyria. **(C)** Cross section of hydrocephalic brain.

Hydrocephalus can develop early in the second trimester of pregnancy or it may not develop until after birth. It may be associated with a variety of infections or mutant genes. An X-linked recessive aqueductal stenosis occurs in about 2% of cases in which there are no other abnormalities. Hydrocephalus also may be inherited as a dominant or a multifactorial condition. It also may be part of syndromes such as achondroplasia, osteogenesis imperfecta, Hurler syndrome, or, rarely, tuberous sclerosis.

Table 13.7 Systemic anomalies that may be associated with hydrocephalic fetuses

Anomaly
Trisomy 18
Trisomy 21
Complete atrioventricular canal
Pulmonary atresia with intact ventricular septum
Duodenal atresia
Obstructive uropathy
Unilateral renal agenesis and rectovesical fistula
Thanatophoric dysplasia

Modified from Pilu et al.: *Ultrasound Med Biol* 12:319, 1986.

ARNOLD-CHIARI MALFORMATION

Type I is ectopia of the cerebellar tonsils; the anomaly usually is an isolated feature (Figures 13.16 and 13.17).

Type II is characterized by spinal myelomeningocele associated with cerebellar hypoplasia and displacement of the tonsils and of the elongated distal brainstem through the enlarged foramen magnum.

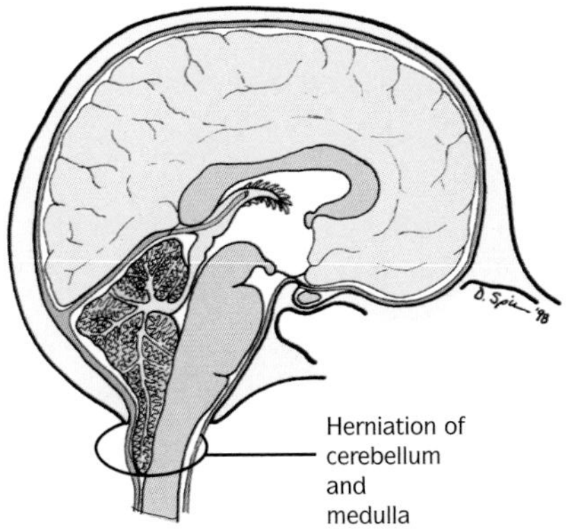

13.16. Arnold Chiari malformation.

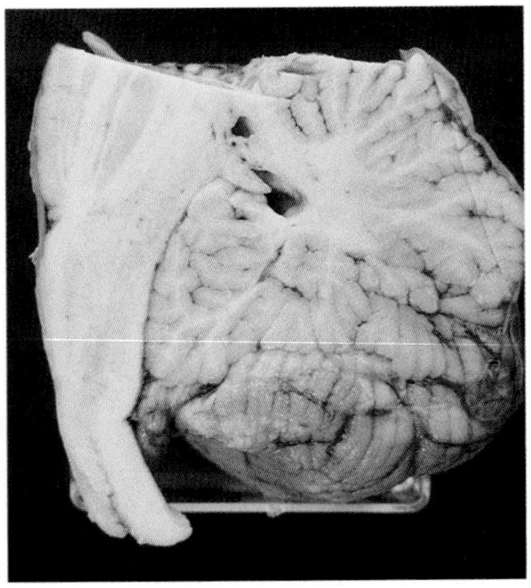

13.17. Beak-like deformity of quadrigeminal plate. Arnold-Chiari malformation type 1.

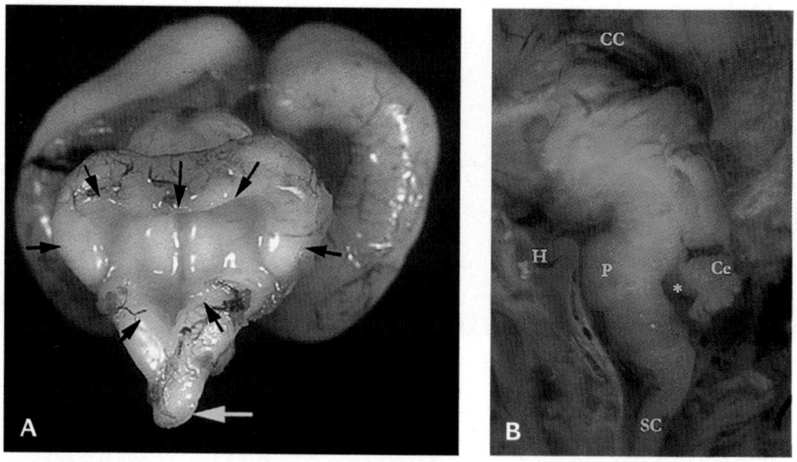

13.18. Dandy-Walker malformation. **(A)** There is a large posterior fossa cyst (black arrows) with absence of the cerebellar vermis (yellow arrow, cut edge of cervical spinal cord). **(B)** A midsagittal cross section of the brain with a posterior fossa cyst (*) and hypoplastic cerebellum (Ce) (CC, corpus callosum; H, hypophysis; P, pons, SC, spinal cord).

Type III is herniation of the cerebellum through a cervical spina bifida with a defect of the basal occipital bone.

Type IV is cerebellar hypoplasia.

DANDY-WALKER MALFORMATION (DWM)

DWM includes dilation of the fourth ventricle, described as a posterior fossa cyst and hypoplasia or absent vermis (Figures 13.18 to 13.20 and Table 13.8). The membrane of the pseudocyst, composed of dysplastic ependyma and

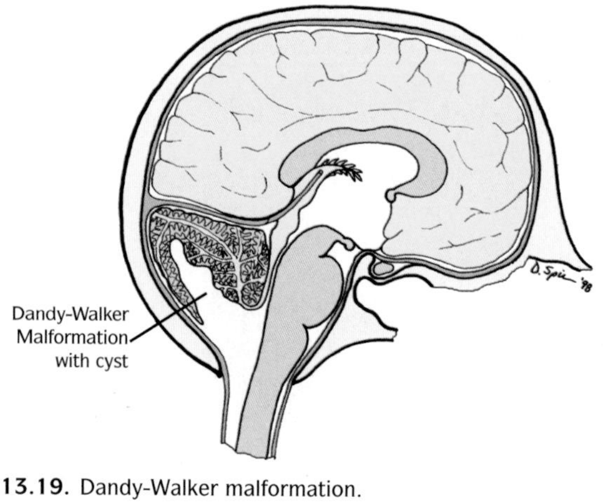

13.19. Dandy-Walker malformation.

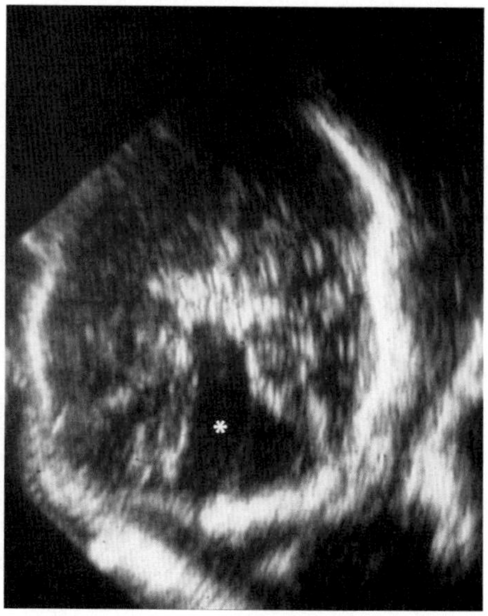

13.20. Ultrasound of Dandy-Walker malformation (*).

Table 13.8 Association of other abnormalities with Dandy-Walker syndrome

Chromosomal	Genetic defects	Multifactorial	Environmental	Sporadic
45, X	Warburg (AR)	Congenital heart disease	Rubella	Holoprosencephaly
6p−	Aase-Smith (arthrogryposis) (AD)	Neural tube defects	Coumadin	Cornelia de Lange
9q+	Ruvalcaba syndrome	Cleft lip/plate	Alcohol	Goldenhar
dup 5p	Coffin-Siris syndrome (AR)		CMV	Kidney abnormalities
dup 8p dup 8q	Oral-facial digital syndrome, type II (AR)		Diabetes	Facial hemangiomas
Trisomy 9	Meckel syndrome (AR)		Isotretinoin	Klippel-Feil
Triploidy	Aicardi syndrome (XL)			Polysyndactyly
dup 17q	Joubert-Boltshauser syndrome (AR) X-linked cerebellar hypoplasia (XL) Ellis van Creveld (AR) Fraser cryptophthalmos (AR)			

AD, autosomal dominant; AR, autosomal recessive; XL, X-linked.

meninges with ectopic cerebellar tissue, is continuous with the lining of the fourth ventricle. Hydrocephalus is usually associated with DWM, a prominent occiput, and an enlarged posterior fossa.

DWM is frequently associated with other CNS and/or extra-CNS abnormalities including defects of the corpus callosum, polymicrogyria, heterotopias, and malformed or ectopic inferior olives, also with Meckel and fetal alcohol syndromes.

POLYMICROGYRIA

Polymicrogyria may be either focal or diffuse and is characterized by excessive folding of all layers of the cortex (Figure 13.21). The two major types of polymicrogyria are four layered and unlayered.

Four-layered polymicrogyria is thought to follow a laminar necrosis secondary to intrauterine hypoxic-ischemic injury.

Unlayered polymicrogyria is most common in severely malformed brains. The festoon-like cortical plate forms deep indentations into the white matter.

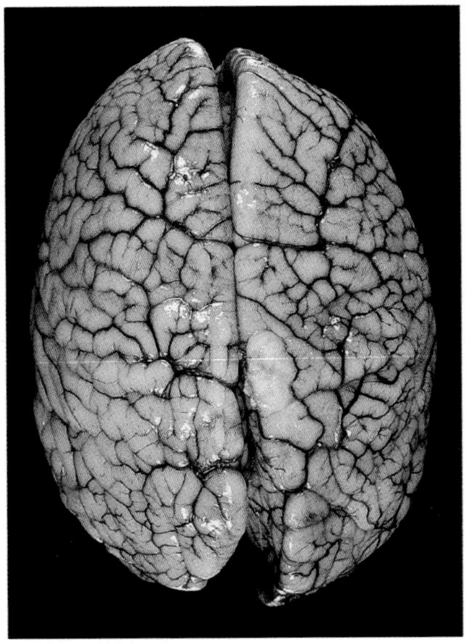

13.21. Polymicrogyria.

LISSENCEPHALY

The smooth brain of lissencephaly resembles the brain at 28 weeks gestation (Table 13.9 and Figure 13.22). It has been described in at least 10 malformation syndromes.

Table 13.9 Malformation syndromes associated with lissencephaly*

Malformation syndrome	Inheritance	Gene location
Classical lissencephaly syndromes		
Baraitser-Winter syndrome	Unk	Unmapped
Isolated lissencephaly sequence, X-linked	XL	Xq22.3–q23
Isolated lissencephaly sequence, 17-linked	AD	17p13.3
Isolated lissencephaly sequence, other	AD	Unmapped
Miller-Dieker syndrome	AD	17p13.3
Subcortical band heterotopia, X-linked	XL	Xq22.3–q23
Subcortical band heterotopia, other	Unk	Unmapped
Cobblestone lissencephaly syndromes		
Cobblestone lissencephaly only syndrome	AR	Unmapped
Fukuyama congenital muscular dystrophy	AR	9q31
Muscle-eye-brain-disease	AR	1p13.2–p13.4
Walker-Warburg syndrome	AR	Unmapped
Other lissencephaly syndromes		
Lissencephaly with cerebellar hypoplasia	AR	Unmapped
Winter-Tsukahara syndrome	AR	Unmapped

* From Dobyns WB, Berry-Krause E, Havernick NJ, et al.: X-linked lissencephaly with absent corpus callosum and ambiguous genitalia. *Am J Med Genet* 86:331, 1999.

LISSENCEPHALY TYPE I

Type I Miller-Dieker syndrome (MDS) is due to deletion of the short arm of chromosome 17. It consists of reversal of the normal gray-white matter ratio with a four-layered cortex. It is characterized by minor facial anomalies, occasional hirsutism, clouding of cornea, polydactyly, and severe brain anomalies. Interstitial deletion of 17p close to the region in the Smith-Magenis syndrome. The incidence is 1:100,000 live births.

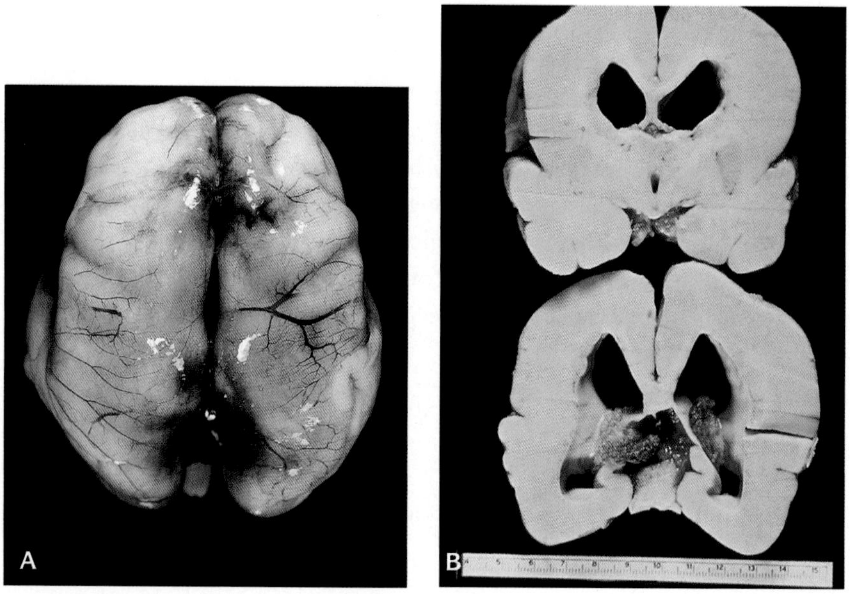

13.22. (A) Lissencephaly type I in Miller-Dieker syndrome. The brain is smooth. **(B)** Lissencephaly type II in Walker-Warburg syndrome.

LISSENCEPHALY TYPE II

In lissencephaly type II (Walker-Warburg syndrome) there is cortical dysplasia that is characterized by obliteration of the arachnoid spaces with ectopic neurons and glial cells and a chaotic cortex. Ectopic cells extend into the subarachnoid space through multiple pial-glial gaps and results in a thick and milky appearance of the meninges and hydrocephalus. The entire cortex is malformed.

Eye anomalies include microphthalmia with optic chiasm hypoplasia, coloboma, cataract, and abnormal anterior chamber and retinal dysplasia.

Testicular dysplasia and genital malformations have always been found in males.

LISSENCEPHALY TYPE III

In lissencephaly type III, there is association with micrencephaly and agyria/pachygyria, loss of neurons, immature lamination, focal areas of unlayered polymicrogyria, foci of calcification, and pseudocyst formations. The brainstem, cerebellum, and medulla are hypoplastic with a poor neuronal population and absence of pyramidal tracts.

In fetal akinesia and arthrogryposis described under various eponyms of Pena-Shokeir type II, cerebrooculofacioskeletal (COFS), and Neu-Laxova syndromes, type III lissencephaly may represent a distinct clinicopathologic sequence.

X-LINKED LISSENCEPHALY (XLIS)

An X-linked form of lissencephaly has been described with absent corpus callosum and ambiguous genitalia that is associated with XLIS (DCX) gene.

MICROCEPHALY

Microcephaly is a small head, while micrencephaly is a small brain. Microcephaly is a head circumference below 3 SD (Figures 13.23 and 13.24 and Table 13.10). In newborns, isolated microcephaly is present in about 1 in 6,200 to 1 in 40,000 live births. In embryos with chromosome abnormalities such as trisomy 9, 13, 14, 18, 22, microcephaly is common. Microcephaly is rare in spontaneously aborted, chromosomally normal fetuses. Ultrasound intrauterine diagnosis of fetal microcephaly can be made.

Primary microcephaly may be recessive, dominant, or X-linked. One hundred distinct familial syndromes with microcephaly have been documented. Twenty to 30% are estimated to be genetic. It is a common feature in chromosomal disorders.

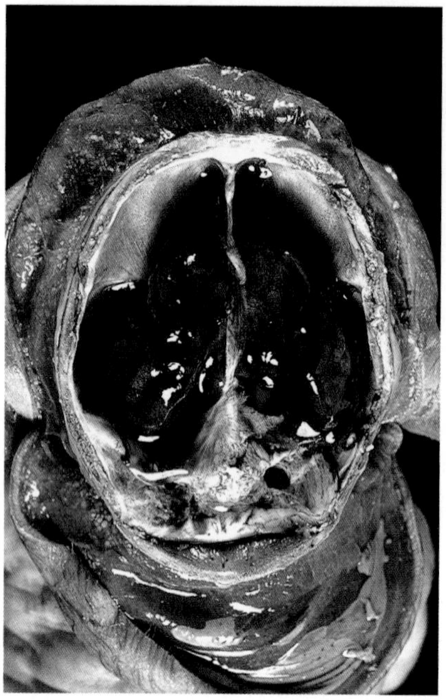

13.23. Micrencephaly. The brain is extremely small (weight 13 g).

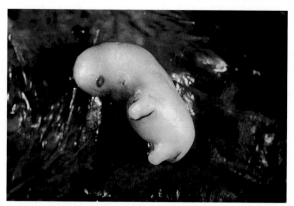

13.24. Embryo of 41 days with microcephaly.

Secondary, acquired microcephaly may be due to maternal/fetal infections, CNS circulatory impairment, intoxication, or radiation. In intrauterine malnutrition with growth retardation, the brain is less affected than the other organs.

Isolated Microcephaly (IMC)

Most cases of IMC have autosomal recessive inheritance. However, cases of autosomal dominant and X-linked inheritance have been reported.

MICROGYRIA

In microgyria small gyri appear increased in number. It is found in Arnold-Chiari type II but the underlying cortex is rarely abnormal.

Ulegyria consists of small and shrunken gyri, most pronounced at their base, with enlarged sulci and is a sequel of hypoxic-ischemic accident.

PACHYGYRIA

Pachygyria is characterized by large and broad gyri. Agyria and pachygyria may coexist in different parts of the same brain and overlie an abnormal cortical

Table 13.10 Classification of microcephaly

Microcephaly	Chromosomal abnormalities	Genetic	Environmental
Without associated malformations		Primary microcephaly Paine syndrome Alpers disease	Radiation exposure, malnutrition, trauma, hypoxia
Without associated malformations	Trisomy 9, 13, 18, 21, 22 Abnormalities of chromosomes 1–5, 7–15, 22	Many syndromes	Infections; prenatal exposure to alcohol drugs or chemicals, maternal phenylketonuria

Adapted from Ross J, Frias J: Microcephaly. In Vinken P, Bruyn G (eds): *Congenital Malformations of the Brain and Skull, Handbook of Clinical Neurology*, Amsterdam, Elsevier, 1977, p. 507.

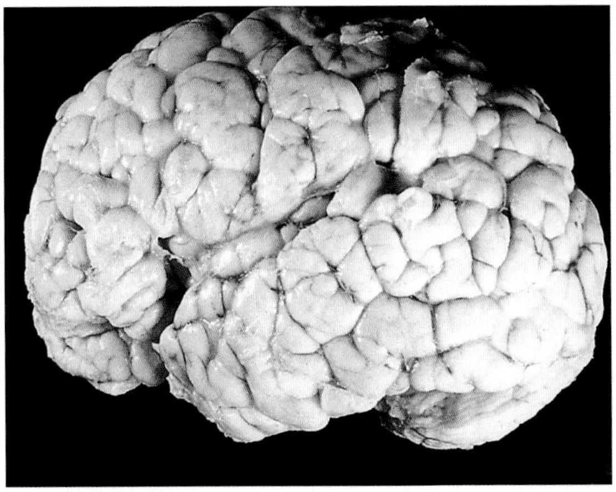

13.25. Brain with pachygyria in child with tuberous sclerosis.

plate (Figure 13.25). Pachygyria is a feature of tuberous sclerosis, Zellweger syndrome, and of many malformation syndromes.

THANATOPHORIC DYSPLASIA WITH CLOVERLEAF SKULL

Megalencephaly is always associated with abnormal surface configuration of prominent temporal lobes. On coronal sections, the brain shows a trilobed shape with a poorly outlined hippocampal gyrus. The corpus callosum and brainstem are hypoplastic with fused inferior colliculi. The cerebellum is small. There is an abnormal pattern of the hippocampus and an unlayered polymicrogyria.

MECKEL SYNDROME

Meckel syndrome, an autosomal recessive disorder, includes a distinctive triad. Occipital encephalocele, polydactyly, and large cystic dysplastic kidneys. There are abnormal gyri, and underlying polymicrogyria and heterotopias, cerebellar hypoplasia and vermian hypoplasia. Dandy-Walker malformation may be present.

HYDROLETHALUS SYNDROME

Hydrolethalus syndrome is a familial lethal syndrome with severe hydrocephalus and polyhydramnios characterized by peculiar facial dysmorphia with cleft lip/palate, micrognathia, and polydactyly (Figure 13.26). A midline defect of the occipital bone, posterior to the foramen magnum results in a keyhole appearance. Most cases have been described in abortuses or stillborn infants.

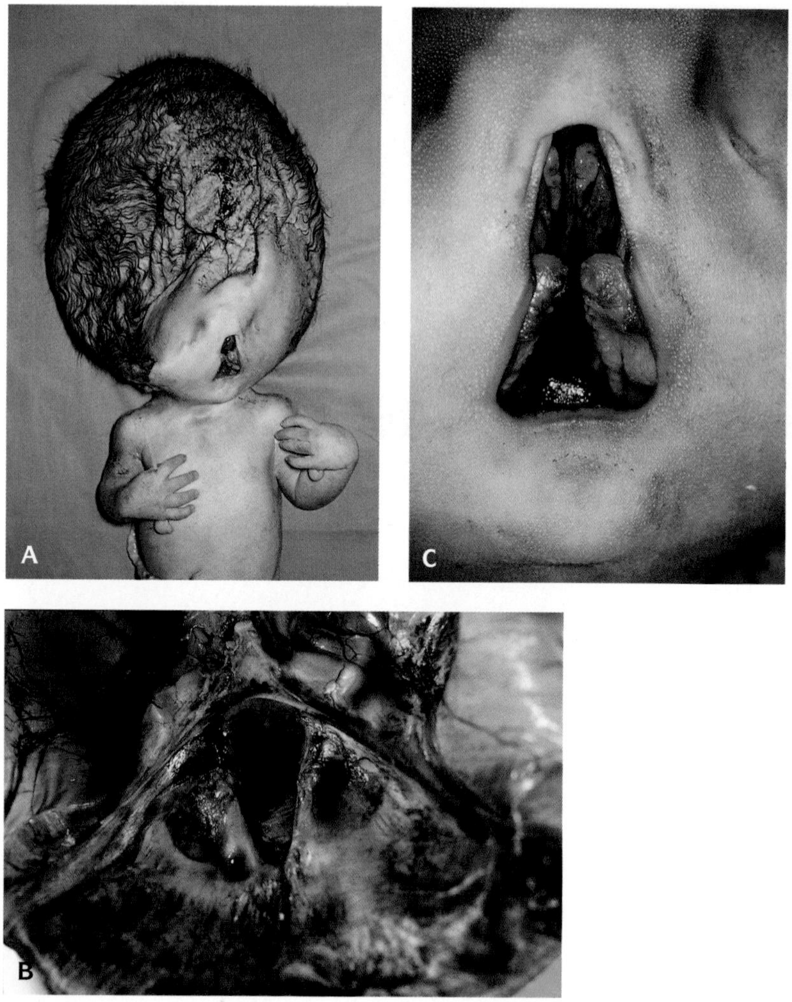

13.26. Hydrolethalus. **(A)** Appearance of newborn infant. **(B)** Base of skull with keyhole foramen magnum. **(C)** Midline facial cleft with clefting of palate.

SCHIZENCEPHALY

This is a term that has been used for a bilateral clefting defect that may be due to a developmental defect of the cerebrum during the first two months of gestation or more commonly to a vascular disruptive event involving the middle cerebral arteries between 31 and 35 weeks gestation (Figure 13.27). If the lesions do not cause a cavity and the insult occurs before migration is complete, bilateral clefting results (schizencephaly).

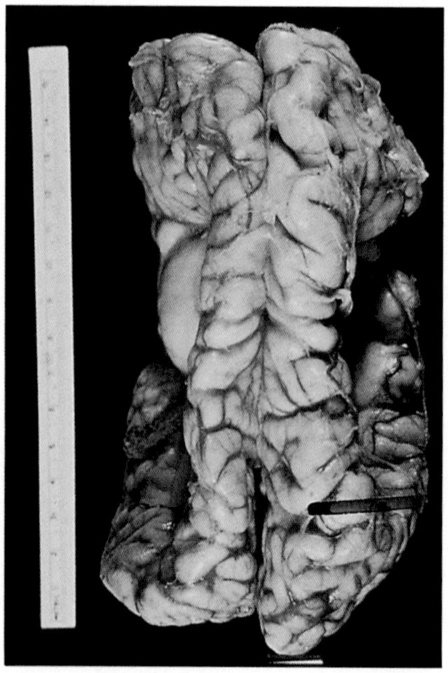

13.27. Schizencephaly. There is bilateral clefting malformation of the cortex due to vascular disruption.

ABSENCE OF CORPUS CALLOSUM

There are multiple causes for conditions and syndromes associated with agenesis (Figure 13.28 and Table 13.11).

Table 13.11 Syndromes with agenesis of the corpus callosum

Syndrome	Genetics
Acrocallosal	AR
Aicardi	XLD, male lethal
Alcohol, prenatal	In utero exposure
Andermann; mental retardation-neuropathy	AR
Apert	AD
Basal cell nevus	AD
Brumback: microcephaly	Unknown
Buntinx: ocular anomalies-polydactly	Unknown
Cerebro-facio-thoracic dysplasia	Unknown
Cao: microcephaly	AR
Chromosomal aberrations	Chromosomal imbalance
Cleft lip/palate-ectrodactyly	Uncertain
Coffin-Siris	AR?
Corpus callosum agenesis, isolated	AR, XLR, AD
Crane: skeletal dysostosis-clefting	AR
Craniotelencephalic dysplasia	AR
Da Silva: mental retardation-microcephaly	AR
Dwarfism-microcephaly	AR
Dellman: focal dermal defects	Unknown
Ectodermal dysplasia-hypothyroidism	Unknown
Edwards: microphthalmia	Uncertain, possible AD
FC	XLR
Fine	Unknown
Focal dermal hypoplasia	XLD, male lethal
Frontonasal dysplasia	Most sporadic; some AD
Frontonasal dysplasia-polydactyly	Unknown
G	AD
Goldenhar	Sporadic, some AD
Hydrolethalus	AR
Iris dysplasia-hypertelorism	AD
Kallmann	AD, AR, XLSD
Leigh	AR
Leprechaunism	AR
L'Hermitte: oxycephaly-mental retardation	AR
Lujan: marfanoid	XLR
Marshall-Smith	Unknown
Meckel	AR
Moerman	Unknown
Neu-Laxova	AR
Neuroepithelial cysts-absent corpus callosum	Unknown
Neurofibromatosis	AD
Nonketotic hyperglycinemia	AR
Oculo-pituitary	Unknown
Oral-facial-digital	XLD, male lethal
Rubinstein-Taybi	Uncertain; AD?
Say: cloverleaf skull-skeletal anomalies	Unknown
Shapira: hypothermia	Most sporadic; AR
Siber: microphthalmia	XLR
Smith: hypopituitarism	Unknown
Smith-Lemli-Opitz type II	AR
Thanatophoric dysplasia	AD; most new mutations?
Toriello	AR
Tuberous sclerosis	AD
Van Biervliet: thoracic dystrophy	AR
Vici: immunodeficiency-cataracts	XLR or AR
Walker-Warburg	AR
Young: macrocephaly	AR
Zellweger	AR
Zimmer: tetra-amelia	AR or ?XLR

AR, autosomal recessive; XLD, X-linked dominant; AD, autosomal dominant; XLR, X-linked recessive.

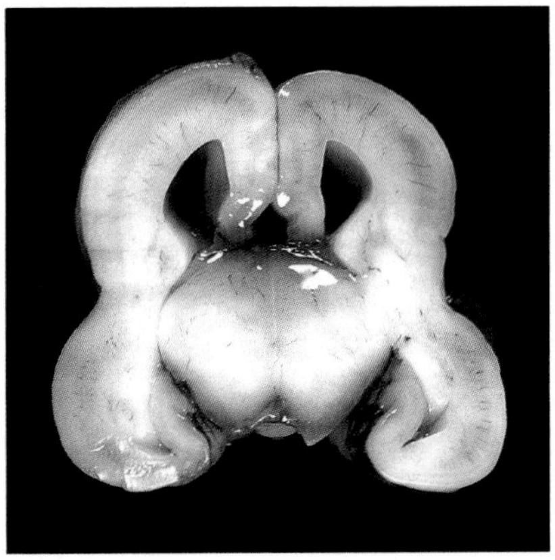

13.28. Cross section of brain with absence of corpus callosum.

ULTRASONOGRAPHY

The cerebral ventricles:

- Verify scanning planes, and determine if either ventricle is enlarged.
- Associated abnormalities are found in 70–85% of fetuses with ventriculomegaly.
- Other CNS abnormalities are seen in 50–60%.
- Extra-CNS anomalies seen include cardiac, thoracic, renal, facial, ventral wall abnormalities, and abnormalities of the extremities.
- Infants with ventriculomegaly have karyotypic abnormalities (2% in isolated ventriculomegaly and in 17% if ventriculomegaly and one or more other findings are present).
- Ventriculomegaly occurs in 9–18% of trisomy 21, 18, 31, and triploid infants, and is associated with various abnormalities.

Syndromic associations with ventriculomegaly:

- Neural tube defects (spina bifida, Arnold-Chiari II malformation)
- CNS anomalies (Dandy-Walker malformation, agenesis of the corpus callosum, lissencephaly)
- Aqueductal stenosis (X-linked recessive, autosomal, sporadic, postinflammatory)
- Aneuploidy (trisomy 13, trisomy 18, trisomy 21, fragile X, triploidy)
- Obstructed flow (postinfectious, postinflammatory, posthemorrhagic)
- Inherited syndromes (Meckel, Apert, nasal-facial-digital, Robert, Walker-Warburg)
- Chondrodystrophies (achondroplasia, osteogenesis imperfecta, thanatophoric dysplasia)

Caution: Toxoplasmosis sometimes presents with ventriculomegaly and is sometimes treatable in utero with salvage of fetal neurologic prognosis.

Ventricle/hemisphere ratios vary by gestational age:

	16 wks	**18 wks**	**20 wks**	**22 wks-term**
	2 S.D.	2 S.D.	2 S.D.	2 S.D.
V/H Ratio	0.45–0.69	0.40–0.52	0.29–0.56	0.22–0.37

(Johnson ML, et al. *Semin Perinatol* 7:83, 1983).

Absolute size can be assessed:

- Transverse diameters in excess of 1.1 cm likely reflect hydrocephaly (Pretorius DL. *Am. J. Neurol. Radiol* 1985;6:23–7).
- The transverse ventricular atrial diameter rarely exceeds 8 or 10 mm from 15 to 35 weeks gestation.
- Dangling choroid plexus is strongly suggestive of ventriculomegaly.
- Determine whether the choroid plexuses appear homogenous or there are cystic regions.

- The choroid plexus fill ventricles until 16–18 weeks gestation, gradually fill less, and never "dangle."
- Choroid plexus cysts, single or multiple, unilateral or bilateral, may be a normal variant, but often indicate increased risk of aneuploidy, especially if any other sonographic abnormalities are noted. They are often an indication for fetal karyotypic analysis.

Cerebral abnormalities: Cephalocele (encephaloceles, meningoceles)

- A protrusion of cerebral structures outside the cranium which occurs in 1:2,000 live births. It results from failure of closure of the rostral end of the neural tube during the fourth week of gestation.
- It is usually located in the midline anteriorly or posteriorly, and often is accompanied by hydrocephalus (60–80% of posterior lesions and 20% of anterior lesions). Spina bifida is present in 15% of cases, and a "lemon sign" deformity may also be present. If only meningeal structures protrude, it is termed a meningocoele, while if encephalon is involved, the anomaly is termed an encephalocele.
- Frontal cephaloceles may be missed by usual scanning planes, and occipital cephaloceles are often only seen when the cerebellum is visualized with a standard cisterna magna view.
- Caution: temporal bulging of cranial structures in the cloverleaf skull in thanatophoric dysplasia has been falsely diagnosed as an encephalocele
- Cephaloceles are often seen in autosomal recessive conditions such as Meckel, Robert, Chemke Knoblock, and cryptophthalmus syndromes, and in dyssegmental dwarfism. Anterior cephalocoeles occur more often in oriental patients (75%), while occipital lesions predominate in the Western world.
- Amniotic band syndrome may result in cephalocoeles in atypical and asymmetric locations.
- Prognosis depends on the presence and quantity of brain outside the cranium. Almost 50% of infants with isolated meningocoeles have normal development after surgical repair of their defects, while fetuses with large amounts of brain protruding out of the skull have a very poor prognosis.
- Delivery by cesarean section should be considered for anomalies sufficiently large and solid enough to cause dystocia, when indications relating to maternal health or another (twin) fetus are present, or if an isolated cephalocoele is present and it is felt that minimization of birth trauma may improve neonatal outcome.

Choroid plexus cysts:

- Cysts greater than 2 or 5 mm may occur alone or in multiples, unilaterally or bilaterally, and are seen in 1% of pregnancies between 16 and 24 weeks gestation
- 90% resolve by 26–28 weeks gestation.
- Resolution of cysts DOES NOT correlate with normal fetal karyotype.

- Aneuploid karyotypes have been reported in 8% of infants with choroid cysts (1% aneuploidy in cases of isolated cysts, 46% aneuploidy if other anomalies are present).
- Forty-seven percent of trisomy 18 infants have cysts, while lower rates of cysts are seen in trisomy 21 (8%) and trisomy 13 (2%) infants.
- Counseling for choroid cysts varies by correction for maternal age and fetal wastage tendencies with trisomy 18 and the ability to accurately detect other sonographic findings. As the most common additional findings in trisomy 18, ventricular septal defects and abnormalities of the extremities, may be subtle and difficult to detect, proper risk assessment for risk of trisomy 18 may depend to a certain degree on the skill of the sonographer and advantageous fetal positioning.
  - Among all fetuses with choroid cysts at 20 weeks gestation, the risk of a trisomy 18 fetus is approximately 1:98.
  - If NO other anomalies other than choroid cyst are present on prenatal sonographic evaluation at 20 weeks, the risk of trisomy 18 is greater than 1:300 only in women aged 37.5 years of age or older.
  - If one or more other findings are present in addition to choroid cysts at 20 weeks gestation, all fetuses have a risk exceeding 1:98, regardless of maternal age.

Holoprosencephaly: A group of disorders that result from abnormal differentiation of the prosencephalon (forebrain) into the cerebral hemispheres and lateral ventricles is present in 1:5,000 to 1:16,000 liveborns and in up to 0.4% of conceptuses.

- Three common types – alobar, semilobar, and lobar
- Holoprosencephaly is characteristically present with hydrocephaly, severe distortions of the overall cerebral sonographic architecture, and often with facial abnormalities.

Conditions associated with holoprosencephaly:

- Aneuploidy (trisomy 13, trisomy 18, triploidy, 13q-, 18p-, others) in up to 50% of cases
- Pallister-Hall syndrome
- Kallman syndrome
- Meckel syndrome
- Vasadi syndrome
- Campomelic dysplasia
- Maternal diabetes (200-fold increased risk in infants of diabetes mothers)
- The prognosis is very poor for alobar and semilobar holoprosencephaly, as most infants die at birth or within one year of life.
- With isolated holoprosencephaly 4% are aneuploid; if other abnormalities are present 39% are aneuploid.

- There is a 39% incidence of holoprosencephaly in trisomy 13 infants and 3% incidence of holoprosencephaly in trisomy 18 infants
- If a prior infant had holoprosencephaly unrelated to karyotypic abnormalities, the estimated recurrence rate is 6%, although some families appear to exhibit either autosomal recessive (25% recurrence) or dominant (50%) inheritance.

Dandy-Walker malformations:

- This cerebral malformation is characterized by partial or complete absence of the cerebellar vermis and cystic dilation of the fourth ventricle, often in association with hydrocephalus.
- The Dandy-Walker anomaly is associated with a variety of underlying conditions:
  - Autosomal recessive conditions such as Aicardi, Meckel, Walker-Warburg syndrome
  - Aneuploidy (trisomy 18)
  - Infection (toxoplasmosis, cytomegalovirus, rubella)
  - Maternal disease (diabetes)
  - Toxic exposure (coumadin, ethanol)
- Agenesis of the corpus callosum
- Porencephaly/schizencepahly

The skull:

1. Lemon sign – Frontal narrowing of the skull is often seen in fetuses with open neural tube defects. Careful evaluation for open neural tube disorders is recommended.
2. Brachycephaly – Fetuses with excessively round skull morphology are at increased risk of trisomy 21. Twenty percent of trisomy 21 infants have frontothalamic/BPD ratios less than the 5th percentile. Due to the decreased growth of the frontal lobes.
3. Microcephaly – this occurs in 1/1,000 births and is often a consequence of chromosomal abnormalities, genetic syndromes, *in utero* infection, teratogen exposure, and radiation. It has been diagnosed for BPDs < 1% for gestational age, for head circumference/femur length ratios < 2.5% for gestation, and for head circumferences < 5th centile for gestation in infants with otherwise normal growth of the abdomen and femur. It may not become apparent until the third trimester. Twenty percent of microcephalic fetuses have karyotypic abnormalities; trisomy 13 is the most common.
4. Strawberry skull – Hypoplasia of the facial bones may result in proportionately narrowed anterior skull dimensions, leaving a strawberry-shaped appearance. Of 54 infants with these findings, 80 percent had karyotypic abnormalities, most often trisomy 18.

Posterior fossa and nuchal fold region:

1. Imaging characteristics
   a. Obtained at a 30–45° from that used for the BPD view
   b. Image should include a bilobed or dumbbell-shaped cerebellar structure, cisterna magna, and posterior nuchal region
2. Characteristics to evaluate
   a. Cisterna magna depth averages 5 mm (1–10 mm) over gestational age ranges of 15–36 weeks.

      Suboptimal views (improper angle relative to the axis of the cerebellum) may yield abnormal depths of up to 13 mm but should not be higher
   b. Cerebellum, cerebellar vermis
   c. Nuchal fold

      This measurement is somewhat poorly reproducible due to high dependence on angle of imaging relative to the axis of the cerebellum

Narrow or absent cisterna magna:

- Decreased or absent cisterna magna (widths < 3 or 4 mm) suggests the possible presence of open neural tube defect (ONTD)
- Additional finding of a fused, splayed banana-shaped cerebellum (banana sign) increases risk for ONTD
- With open neural tube abnormalities cerebellar abnormalities are present in 95%. Banana cerebellar deformities are present in 70% of infants before 24 weeks gestation but in only 17% of infants at later gestational ages. Additionally, the cerebellum cannot be visualized in an additional 27% of infants before 24 weeks and is absent in 74% of infants at later gestational ages.

Enlarged cisterna magna:

- May (in rare cases) be a normal variant
- May be caused by improper measurement due to excessive angulation
- The cerebellar vermis is sometimes obscured by inadequate imaging planes
- Increased risk for Arnold Chiari malformations, Dandy-Walker malformation (see above), and trisomy 18
- Forty percent incidence of karyotypic abnormalities (most with trisomy 18)
- Posterior fossa cysts are present in 10% of trisomy 18 infants, 15% of trisomy 13, and 1% of trisomy 21, and in 6% of triploidy

Encephalocoele:

- Posterior encephalocoeles sometimes present as masses in the posterior neck
- They should be distinguished from cystic hygroma and meningocele in the neck.

- Small posterior encephalocoeles may not be evident except in the standard cisterna magna view.

REFERENCES

Ahdab-Barmada M, Claassen D: A distinct triad of malformations of the central nervous system in the Meckel-Gruber syndrome. *J Neuropath Exp Neurol* 49:610, 1990.

Barr M Jr., Cohen MM Jr: *Holoprosencephaly Survival and Performance*, New York, Wiley-Liss, 1999.

Camera G, Lituania M, Cohen MM Jr: Holoprosencephaly and primary craniosynostosis: the Genoa syndrome. *Am J Med Genet* 47:1161, 1993.

Cohen MM: Perspectives on holoprosencephaly: Part III. Spectra, distinctions, continuities and discontinuities. *Am J Med Genet* 34:271, 1989.

Cohen MM Jr: Perspectives on holoprosencephaly: Part I. Epidemiology, genetics and syndromology. *Teratology* 40(3):211, 1989.

Cohen MM Jr, Sulik KK: Perspectives on holoprosencephaly: Part III. Central nervous system, craniofracial anatomy, syndrome commentary, diagnostic approach, and experimental studies. *J Craniofac Genet Dev Biol* 12(4):196, 1992.

Cohen MMJr, Shiota K: Teratogenesis of holoprosencephaly. *Am J Med Genet* 109:1, 2002.

Delezoide AL, Narcy F, Larroche JC: Cerebral midline developmental anomalies: spectrum and associated features. *Gen Counsel* 1:187, 1991.

de Vries LS, Larroche JC, Leven MI: Germinal matrix haemorrhage and intraventricular haemorrhage. In Levene MI, Bennet MJ, Punt J (eds): *Fetal and Neonatal Neurology and Neurosurgery*, New York, Churchill Livingstone, 1988.

Dobyns WB, Pagon RA, Armstrong D, et al.: Diagnostic criteria for Walker-Warburg syndrome. *Am J Med Genet* 32:195, 1989.

Dobyns WB, Berry-Kravis E, Havernick NJ, et al.: X-linked lissencephaly with absent corpus callosum and ambiguous genitalia. *Am J Med Genet* 86:331, 1999.

Fitzsimmons J, Wilson D, Pascoe-Mason J, et al.: Choroid plexus cysts in fetus with trisomy 18. *Obstet Gynecol* 73:257, 1989.

Golden JA, Chernoff GF: Multiple sites of anterior neural tube closure in humans: evidence from anterior neural tube defects (anencephaly). *Pediatrics* 95:506, 1995.

Hamilton RL, Grafe MR: Complete absence of the cerebellum: a report of two cases. *Acta Neuropath* 88:258, 1994.

Heussler HS, Suri M, Young ID, Muenke M: Extreme variability of expression of a Sonic Hedgehog mutation: attention difficulties and holoprosencephaly. *Arch Dis Child* 86:293, 2002.

Jeanty P, Kepple P, Poussis D, et al.: In utero detection of cardiac failure from an aneurysm of the vein of Galen. *Am J Obstet Gynecol* 163:50, 1990.

Kashimi AH, Hutchins GM: Meningeal-cutaneous relationships in anencephaly: evidence for primary mesenchymal abnormality. *Hum Patol* 32:553, 2001.

Kelley RL, Roessler E, Hennekam RC, et al.: Holoprosencephaly in RSH/Smith-Lemi-Opitz syndrome: does abnormal cholesterol metabolism affect the function of Sonic Hedgehog? *Am J Med Genet* 66:478, 1996.

Kjaer I, Keeling JW, Gream N: Cranial base and vertebral column in human anencephalic fetuses. *J Craniofac Genet Dev Biol* 14:235, 1994.

Larroche JC, Nesmann C: Focal cerebral anomalies and retinal dysplasia in a 20-24-week-old fetus. *Brain Dev* 15:51, 1993.

Larroche JC, Encha-Razav F, DeVries L: Central nervous system. In Gilbert EB (ed): *Potter's Pathology of the Fetus and Infant*, St. Louis, Mosby, 1997.

Larroche JCL: Perinatal brain damage. In Adams JH, Corsellis JAN, Duchen LW (eds): *Greenfield's Neuropathology*, 4th ed, London, Edward Arnold, 1984.

Lasjaunias P: Arteriovenous malformations in infancy: aneurysmal malformation of the vein of Galen. *Rev Neuroradiol (Ital)* 4:399, 1991.

Leech RW, Shuman RM: Holoprosencephaly and related midline cerebral anomalies: a review. *J Child Neurol* 1:3, 1986.
Levene MI, Lilford RJ, Benett JM, Punt J: *Fetal and Neonatal Neurology and Neurosurgery*, 2nd ed, London, Churchill Livingstone, 1995.
Mann LI: Pregnancy events and brain damage. *Am J Obstet Gynecol* 155:6, 1986.
Muenke M, Cohen MM Jr: Genetic approaches to understanding brain development: holoprosencephaly as a model. *Ment Retarda Dev Disabil Res Re* 6:15, 2000.
Muenke M, Beachy PA: Genetics of ventral forebrain development and holoprosencephaly. *Curr Opin Genet Dev* 10:262, 2000.
Norman MG, McGillivary BC, Kalousek DK, et al.: *Congenial Malformations of the Brain*, New York, Oxford University Press, 1995.
On-Line Mendelian Inheritance in Man OMIM (http://www3.ncbi.nlm.nih.gov/omim/).
O'Rahilly R, Muller F: The two sites of the neural folds and the two neuropores in human embryo. *Teratology* 65:162, 2002.
Philip AGS: The changing face of neonatal infection: experience at a regional medical center. *Pediatr Infect Dis J* 13:1098, 1994.
Rorke BL: A perspective: the role of disordered genetic control of neurogenesis in the pathogenesis of migration disorders. *J Neuropath Exp Neurol* 53:105, 1994.
Roume J, Larroche JC, Razavi F, et al.: Fetal hydrocephalus. Clinical significance of associated anomalies and genetic counseling: a pathological approach. *Gen Counsel* 1:185, 1991.
Seller MJ: Sex, neural tube defects, and multisite closure of the human neural tube. *Am J Med Genet* 58:332, 1995.
Squier M, Keeling JW: The incidence of prenatal brain injury. *Neuropath Appl Neurobiol* 17:29, 1991.
Squier MW: Development of the cortical dysplasia of type II lissencephaly. *Neuropathol Appl Neurobiol* 19:209, 1993.
Sung In Kyung, Vo B, Oh W: Growth and neurodevelopmental outcome of very low birth weight infants with intrauterine growth retardation: comparison with control group subjects matched by birth weight and gestational age. *J Pediatr* 123:618, 1993.
Van Allen MI, Kalousek DK, Chernoff GF, et al.: Evidence for multi-site closure of the neural tube in humans. *Am J Med Gen* 47:723, 1993.
Volpe JJ: *Neurology of the Newborn*, 3rd ed, Philadelphia, WB Saunders, 1995.
Wallis D, Muenke M. Mutations in holoprosencephaly. *Hum Mutat* 16:99, 2000.

FOURTEEN

Craniofacial Defects

The source of developmental anomalies lies within deviations from the normal pathways of embryogenesis.

Early stages of embryonic development can be studied by identification of developmental genes and their products, using in situ hybridization and immunochemistry and computerized three-dimensional reconstruction of aborted sectioned human embryos.

OROFACIAL CLEFTS

The most frequent craniofacial anomalies are clefts of the upper lip and palate that can now be diagnosed prenatally.

Cleft Lip

Clefts of the lip and palate are among the most common congenital anomalies, occurring in ±1.7 per 1,000 births in Asians, approximately 1 per 1,000 Caucasian births, and approximately 1 per 2,500 births in those of African lineage (Figures 14.1 to 14.5 and Tables 14.1 and 14.2). The frequency of cleft lip/palate is highest in Native Americans, occurring in over 3.6 per 1,000 births and showing a 2:1 female-to-male frequency. Unilateral cleft lips are more frequent on

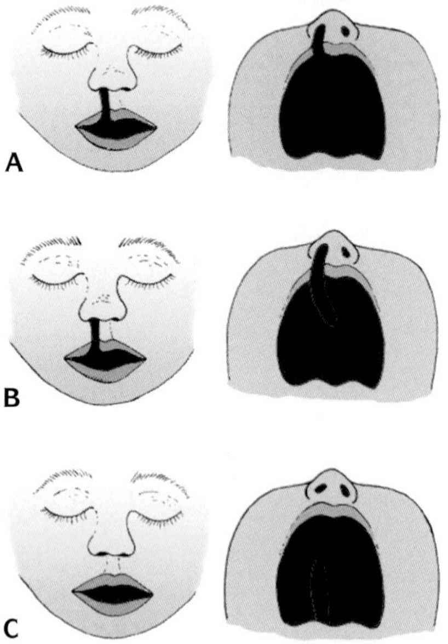

14.1. Illustrations of various types of cleft lip and cleft palate. **(A)** Unilateral cleft lip. **(B)** Unilateral cleft lip and palate. **(C)** Isolated cleft palate.

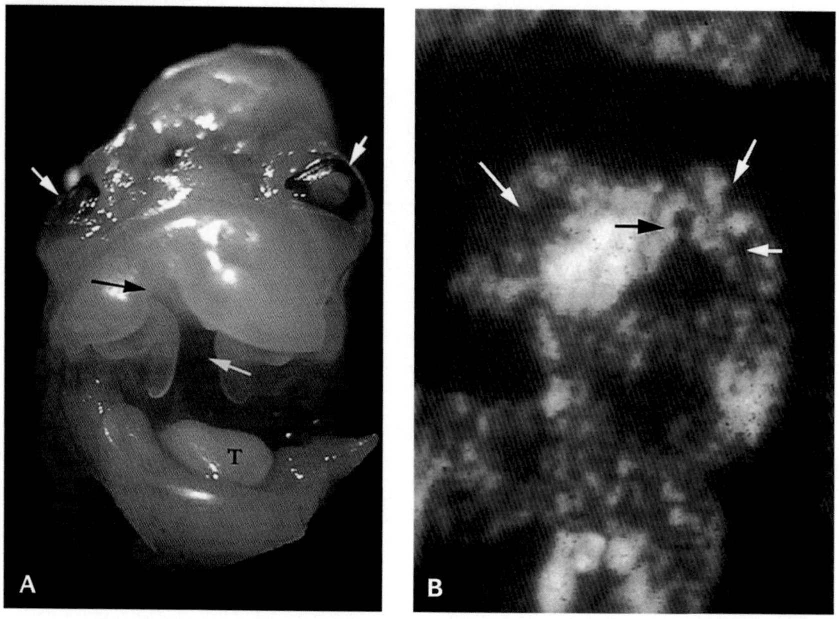

14.2. (A) An 8-week embryo with a median cleft lip and palate (white arrows, eyes; black arrows, cleft lip; yellow arrow, cleft palate; T, tongue). **(B)** Ultrasound of a cleft (black arrow) similar to that shown in **(A)** (white arrows, eyes; gray arrow, intact nostril).

the left than the right and are least frequent bilaterally in the respective ratios of 6:3:1. Isolated cleft palate is distinguished from combined cleft lip and palate; the former occurs about twice as frequently as the combination. Some 20–50% of cleft palates are associated with other anomalies. About 5% of facial clefting is syndromic, with over 250 cleft-associated syndromes.

Pathology of Cleft Lip. If the embryo is examined shortly after Carnegie Stage 18 and autolysis is severe, the newly fused tissue may degenerate and an artifactual cleft may appear. Thus, cleft lip cannot be diagnosed in a severely autolyzed embryo.

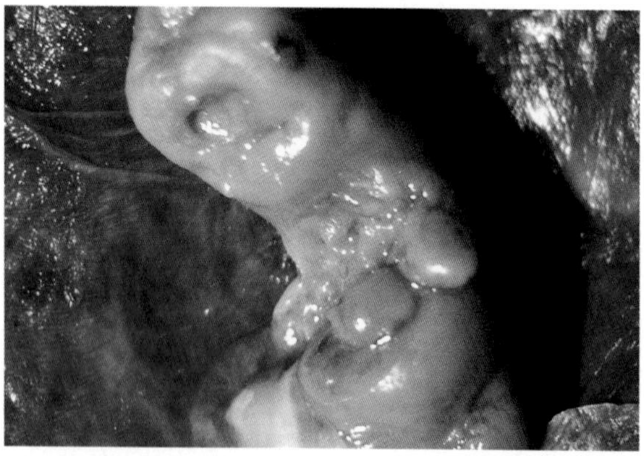

14.3. Eight week embryo with midline facial defect and thoracic wall defect with ectopia cordis.

Morphologically, lateral, median, and irregular facial clefts are readily distinguished. Lateral clefts may be unilateral or bilateral. The clefting caused by amniotic bands is usually bizarre and may involve the oral, nasal, and orbital cavities.

Cleft palate can be diagnosed only after the embryonic period, because the hard palate starts closing after the 8th week of development. The posterior soft palate closes after the 9th week, and the uvula remains bifid until the 10th week of development. The degree of clefting can vary from a notch to a full-thickness cleft.

Because cleft palate can occur as an isolated defect, it is always important to examine the palate.

Table 14.1 Syndromes with cleft lip/palate

OMIM #	Syndrome	Inheritance	Manifestations
*268300	Roberts	AR	Tetraphocomelia, enlarged penis/clitoris
*207410	Antley-Bixler	AR	Microtia, ectopic kidneys, heart defect
	Bowen-Armstrong	AR	Toe syndactyly, ankyloblepharon filiforme, hyperpigmented areas
218090	Crane-Heise	AR	Low-set ears, absent cervical vertebrae and clavicle, finger and toe syndactyly
	Juberg-Hayward	AR	Microcephaly, hypoplastic distally placed thumbs, short radii
*249000	Meckel	AR	Polydactyly, polycystic kidney, encephalocele
	Michel	AR	Blepharophimosis, ocular chamber defect, short fifth fingers
*277170	Varadi-Papp	AR	Polydactyly, arhinencephaly, heart defect
	Clefting/ ankyloblepharon	AD	Ankyloblepharon filiforme
*129900	Ectrodactyly-ectodermal dysplasia	AD	Hand and foot ectrodactyly
	Martin	AD	Microcephaly, hypotelorism, absent premaxilla, spinal anomalies
#119500	Popliteal pterygium	AD	Popliteal pterygia, hypoplastic digits
	Rapp-Hodgkin	AD	Dystrophic nails, thin wirey hair
#119300	van der Woude	AD	Lip pits
	Clefting/ectropion	UG	Ectropion lower eyelids, limb reduction defects
	Golz	X-linked dominant male lethal	Focal dermal hypoplasia, syndactyly, dental anomalies, facial clefts
	Amniotic Bands	SP	Multiple disruptions including facial clefts
*229850	Fryns	AR	Anophthalmia, microphthalmia craniofacial anomalies, facial clefting

AR, autosomal recessive; AD, autosomal dominant; UG, unknown genesis, SP, sporadic; XLD, X-linked dominant OMIM – Online Mendelian inheritance in man.
* before an entry number means the phenotype determined by the gene at the given locus is separate from those represented by other asterisked entries and the mode of inheritance of the phenotype has been proved. No asterisk before an entry number means the mode of inheritance has not been proved, although it is suspected, or the separateness of this locus from that of another entry is unclear.
# symbol before an entry number means the phenotype can be caused by mutation in any of two or more genes.

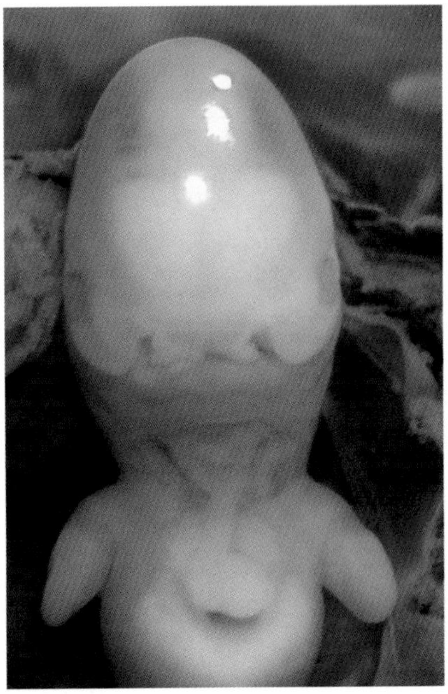

14.4. Spontaneous abortion in a 9-week fetus with triploidy with bilateral cleft lip.

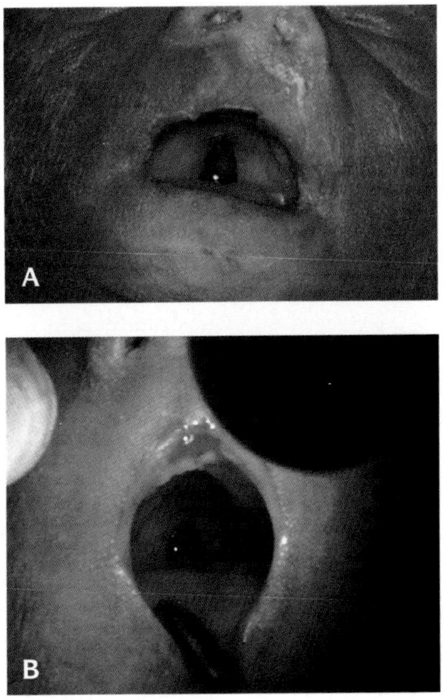

14.5. **(A)** Cleft hard palate in a 34-week gestation stillborn fetus. **(B)** Cleft soft palate in a 28-week gestation stillborn fetus.

Table 14.2 Syndromes in which cleft palate alone is common

OMIM #	Syndrome	Inheritance	Additional manifestations
#114290	Campomelia	AR	Bowing of femora and tibiae
	de la Chapelle	AR	Micromelia, short curved radius and ulna
	Christian	AR	Craniosynostosis, arthrogryposes
#162100	Cleft palate/brachial plexus neuritis	AR	Facial asymmetry, deep-set eyes, hypotelorism, recurrent brachial plexus neuritis
	Cleft palate/connective tissue dysplasia	AR	(? X-linked), cervical fusions, dislocated radial heads, clinodactyly
	Cleft palate/stapes fixation	AR	Skeletal anomalies, stapes fixation
#222600	Diastrophic dysplasia	AR	Contractures, hitchhiker's thumb, deformed ear
*223370	Dubowitz	AD	Microcephaly, blepharophimosis, eczema, vertebral anomalies
	Lowry-Miller	AR	Persistent truncus arteriosus, abnormal right pulmonary artery
#263520	Majewski	AR	Short narrow thorax, polydactyly of hands and feet
	Micrognathic dwarfism	AR	Micromelia, cleft vertebrae
	Multiple pterygia	AR	Multiple pterygia
	Palant	AR	Microcephaly, bulbous nasal tip, toe clinodactyly
268650	Rüdiger	AR	Hand flexion contracture, small fingers and fingernails
	Wallace	AR	Short limbs, hydrocephalus
	Weaver-Williams	AR	Midface hypoplasia, bone hypoplasia, delayed osseous maturation
	Abruzzo-Erickson	AD	(? X-linked dominant) Coloboma, large ears, hypospadias
#101200	Apert	AD	Craniosynostosis, midface deficiency, hand and foot syndactyly
117650	Cerebrocosto-mandibular	AD	Robin anomaly, upper thoracic deformity
	Cleft palate/lateral synechiae	AD	Lateral synechiae
129830	Ectrodactyly cleft palate	AD	Ectrodactyly, syndactyly, hands and feet
	Gordon	AD	Camptodactyly, clubfoot
#156550	Kniest dysplasia	AD	Dwarfism, kyphoscoliosis, tibial bowing
	Wildervanck	AD	Cervical fusion
	Orofaciodigital	XL	Bifid tongue, dystopia canthorum, brachydactyly
#311200	Otopalatodigital I	XL	Frontal prominence, short terminal phalanges and nails, curved toes
	Otopalatodigital II	XL	Microstomia, flexed overlapping fingers, hypertelorism
	Persistent left superior vena cava	XL	Persistent left superior vena cava, ASD
	Femoral-facial syndrome	UG	Short nose, short/absent femurs and fibulas
*148900	Klippel-Feil	UG	Fusion of cervical vertebrae
	de Lange	AD	Microbrachycephaly, confluent eyebrows, limb anomalies

AR, autosomal recessive; AD, autosomal dominant; XL, X-Linked; UG, unknown genesis; OMIM, online mendelian inheritance in man.
* before an entry number means the phenotype determined by the gene at the given locus is separate from those represented by other asterisked entries and that the mode of inheritance of the phenotype has been proved.
No asterisk before an entry number means the mode of inheritance has not been proved, although it is suspected, or that the separateness of this locus from that of another entry is unclear.
symbol before an entry number means the phenotype can be caused by a mutation in any of two or more genes.

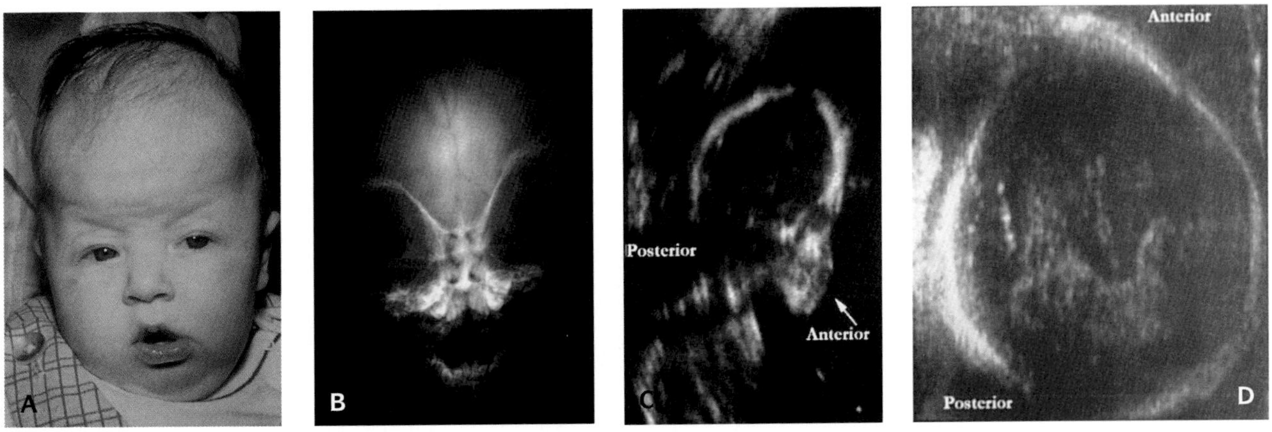

14.6. **(A)** Craniosynostosis-nonsyndromal of the sagittal suture resulting in turricephaly (oxycephaly). **(B)** X-ray of cranium showing sagittal craniosynostosis. **(C)** Sagittal ultrasound of the head with oxycephaly. Note the reduction in the occipitofrontal diameter. **(D)** Ultrasound showing trigonocephaly resulting from premature closure of the metopic or frontal suture. Note the triangular or egg-shaped skull.

Skull Malformations

The skull develops from paraxial mesoderm and neural crest ectomesenchyme that are reflected in different pathological lesions related to each embryonic tissue. Mesodermal lesions are largely confined to endochondrally derived bones (the cartilaginous basicranium), while neurocristopathies are reflected in membrane-derived calvarial bones. The viscerocranium, derived from the pharyngeal arch apparatus, forms the face, jaws, ear ossicles, and hyoid and thyroid skeletons.

Anomalies of the skull may be sporadic, syndromal, autosomal, recessive or dominant.

Craniosynostoses. A number of syndromal and nonsyndromal premature fusions of various sutures of the skull lead to distortions of skull shape (Figures 14.6 and 14.7 and Tables 14.3 and 14.4).

Non-syndromal craniosynostosis is causally heterogeneous and pathogenetically variable. It may be caused in some cases by an autosomal dominant gene, in other cases by hyperthyroidism. The pathogenesis in these cases are variable; there may be a defect in the mesenchymal blastema, accelerated osseous maturation, or lack of growth stretch across the sutures. Growth stretch across the sutures, which results from brain growth itself, keeps the sutures patent. Without significant brain growth, as in microcephaly, the sutures lack growth stretch and may close prematurely. In some cases, there may be a common pathogenesis; microcephaly and low-pressure shunting for hydrocephalus both may occur with craniosynostosis secondary to lack of growth stretch across the sutures.

The severity of deformation is proportional to the extent of the sutures involved; the range includes a mild viable trigonocephaly with early closure

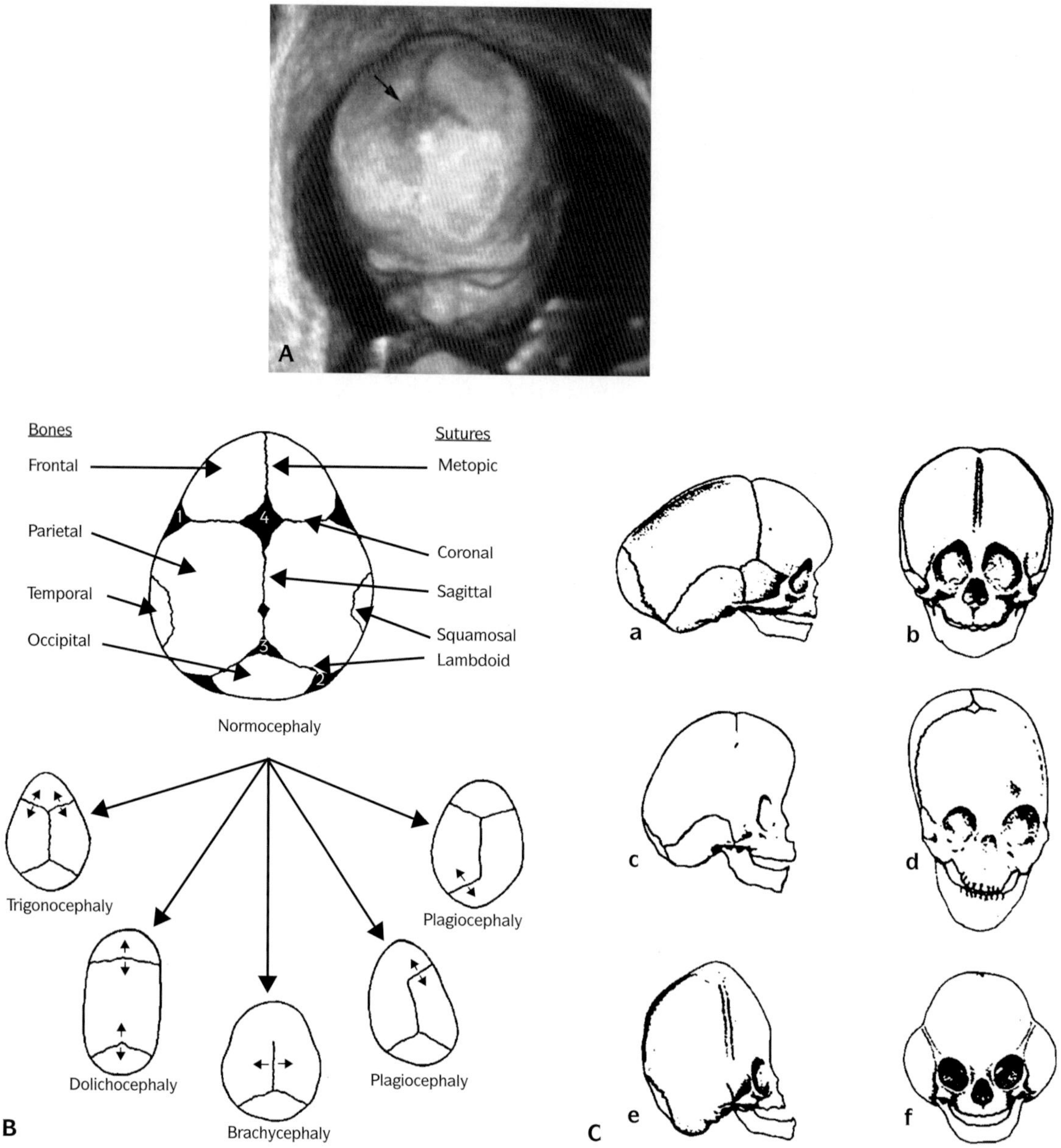

14.7. **(A)** Three-dimensional ultrasound of a fetus at 30 weeks gestation with normal sutures and anterior fontanelle (arrow). **(B)** Illustrations of normocephaly and different types of craniosynostosis. **(C)** Common types of craniosynostosis. **(a)** Scaphocephaly. **(b)** Trigonocephaly. **(c)** Turricephaly. **(d)** Frontal plagiocephaly. **(e)** Oxycephaly. **(f)** Cloverleaf skull.

of the metopic suture to the most deformed lethal cloverleaf skull resulting from multiple premature sutural synostoses. Coronal suture fusion results in a heightened, wide, and basally short skull (brachycephaly); sagittal suture fusion results in an elongated skull (dolicocephaly); unilateral coronal or lambdoidal suture fusion results in a twisted skull (plagiocephaly); fusion of the coronal and sagittal sutures leads to a tower-like skull (turricephaly); fusion of all sutures

Table 14.3 Some conditions with known causes of craniosynostosis

		OMIM
Chromosomal syndromes		
Monogenic	Autosomal dominant simple craniosynostosis*	
	Apert syndrome	101200
	Crouzon syndrome	123500
	Pfeiffer syndrome	101600
	Jackson-Weiss syndrome	123150
	Boston type craniosynostosis	604757
	Saethre-Chotzen syndrome*	101400
	Greig cephalopolysyndactyly*	175700
Metabolic disorders	Hyperthyroidism	
	Rickets	
Mucopolysaccharidoses	Hurler syndrome	
	Morquio syndrome	
	β-Glucuronidase deficiency	
Hematologic disorders	Thalassemias	301040
	Sickle cell anemia	603903
	Congenital hemolytic icterus	
	Polycythemia vera	263300
Teratogens	Aminopterin	
	Diphenylhydantoin	
	Retinoic acid	
	Valproic acid	
Malformations	Microcephaly	
	Encephalocele	
	Shunted hydrocephalus	
	Holoprosencephaly	

OMIM, online mendelian inheritance in man.
* before an entry number means the phenotype determined by the gene at the given locus is separate from those represented by other asterisked entries and the mode of inheritance of the phenotype has been proved.
No asterisk before an entry number means the mode of inheritance has not been proved, although it is suspected, or the separateness of this locus from that of another entry is unclear.

produces a tall, pointed skull (acrocephaly or oxycephaly). Craniosynostoses may extend down to the cranial base and affect facial growth. Maxillary and orbital hypoplasia with exorbitism and midface retrusion are then present, constituting a combined craniofacial dysostosis.

Craniosynostosis may occur alone or together with other anomalies constituting various syndromes. Although most cases of simple craniosynostosis are sporadic, familial instances have been observed; autosomal dominant inheritance has been identified most frequently. Some pedigrees have synostosis of a single suture such as the coronal, sagittal, or metopic. However, different sutures may be fused in affected relatives of the same family.

Acrocephalosyndactyly Syndromes. Apert syndrome is autosomal dominant. It constitutes the combination of craniosynostosis especially coronal sutures,

Table 14.4 Craniosynostosis syndromes

OMIM	Syndrome	Phenotype	Chromosome localization	Gene
101200	Apert syndrome	Craniosynostosis, symmetric syndactyly of hands and feet, and other anomalies	10q25.3–q26	FGFR2
123500	Crouzon syndrome	Craniosynostosis, midface deficiency, ocular proptosis	10q25.3–q26	FGFR2
101600	Pfeiffer syndrome	Craniosynostosis, broad thumbs broad great toes, other anomalies	8q11.2–p12 10q25.3–q26	FGFR1 FGFR2
123150	Jackson-Weiss syndrome	Tarsal/metatarsal coalitions and, variably, craniosynostosis and broad great toes	10q25.3–q26	FGFR2
123790	Beare-Stevenson cutis gyrata syndrome	Cloverleaf or crouzonoid skull, cutis gyrata, furrowed palms and soles, cutaneous/mucosal tags, prominent umbilical stump	10q25.3–q26	FGFR2
187600	Thanatophoric dysplasia	Type I (curved humeri and femora; may have cloverleaf skull) Type II (straight humeri and femora; cloverleaf skull more commonly found)	4p16	FGFR3
	Crouzon syndrome with acanthosis nigricans	Craniofacial dysostosis acanthosis nigricans	4p16	FGFR3
604757	Craniosynostosis, Boston type	Fronto-orbital recession or frontal bossing or turribrachycephaly or cloverleaf skull	5qter	MSX2
600593	Craniosynostosis Adelaide type	Craniosynostosis, short stature, mental deficiency, hypoplastic middle and terminal phalanges in fingers	4p16	FGFR3
101400	Saethre-Chotzen syndrome	Craniosynostosis, characteristic facial appearance, brachydactyly other anomalies	7p21	MSX1
175700	Greig cephalopoly-syndactyly	Hypertelorism, polydactyly, Craniosynostosis in 5%	7p13	GLI3

OMIM, online mendelian inheritance in man.

flat facies, shallow orbits, hypertelorism and syndactyly of fingers creating a "mitten hand" and toes (Table 14.5 and Figures 14.8 and 14.9). It is due to mutations of the fibroblast growth factor receptor 2 (FGFR2) gene on chromosome band 10q25–26 operating on calvarial sutures and autopods during embryogenesis.

Crouzon syndrome is autosomal dominant (Figures 14.10 and 14.11). It is due to an FGFR2 mutation on chromosome 10q25–q26. It is characterized by premature craniosynostosis, midface hypoplasia with shallow orbits, and ocular proptosis. Premature and progressive craniosynostosis usually begins during the first year of life and is usually complete by age 2–3 years. Midface hypoplasia with relative mandibular prognathism, drooping lower lip, and short upper lip are hallmarks. Narrow high-arched palate due to lateral palatal

Table 14.5 Acrocephalosyndactyly syndromes

Apert (type I)	Saethre-Chotzen (type III)	Carpenter	Kleeblattschädel (cloverleaf skull)*
Anomalous tracheal cartilages	Brachycephaly with high forehead	Acrocephaly	Absent external auditory canals*
Bicornuate uterus	Broad thumbs and great toes	Associated hernia*	Antimongoloid obliquity
Cystic kidneys	Cutaneous syndactyly	Congenital heart disease	Truncus arteriosus*
Cutaneous syndactyly of all toes with or without syndactyly	Cryptorchidism*	Hypogenitalism	Atrial septal defect*
Downslanted palpebral fissures	Deafness*	Mental retardation	Beak-like nose
Ectopic anus	Facial asymmetry	Mild obesity	Bicuspid aortic valve*
Flat face	Hypertelorism	Preaxial polydactyly and syndactyly of the toes	Corneal ulceration and clouding
Hypertelorism	Large fontanels	Postminimal polydactyly of the hands*	Hydrocephalus
Irregular thumb and toe	Maxillary hypoplasia	Postminimal polydactyly of the hands*	Iris coloboma*
Maxillary hypoplasia	Mental deficiency*		Maxillary hypoplasia
Mental retardation or normal intelligence	Ptosis of eyelids		Mental retardation
Pulmonary aplasia	Renal anomalies*		Obstructed nasolacrimal duct*
Pulmonary stenosis and other cardiac malformations	Shallow orbits		Ocular hypertelorism
Pyloric stenosis	Single upper palmar crease		Omphalocele*
Shallow orbits	Small ears		Patent ductus arteriosus*
Short anterior-posterior skull diameter with high, full forehead and flat occiput	Small stature		Psychomotor retardation
Supraorbital horizontal groove	Synostosis of coronal sutures		Relative mandibular prognathism
Synostosis of the radius and humerus	Vertebral anomalies*		

* Not a causally specific sydrome but symptom complex.

swellings, crowding of upper teeth due to hypoplastic maxilla, and open bite are present. Exophthalmos is a constant finding, which is secondary to shallow orbits. Ectropion, exposure conjunctivitis or keratitis, poor vision, optic atrophy, hypertelorism, and nystagmus are noted. Atretic auditory canals and malformed ear ossicles are associated with conductive hearing loss.

Kleeblattschädel (Cloverleaf Skull). Cloverleaf skull may be an isolated anomaly or may occur in association with bony ankylosis of the limbs,

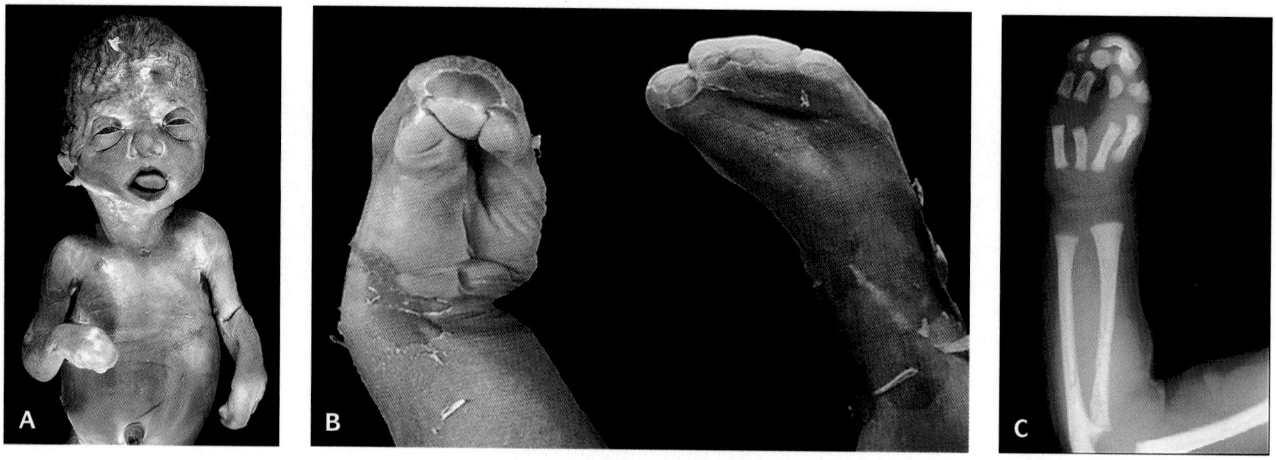

14.8. Apert syndrome. **(A)** Craniosynostosis, bulging forehead, depressed nasal bridge, downslanting palpebral fissures and syndactyly with mitten hands. **(B)** Hand (mitten hand) and foot. **(C)** X-ray of hand.

thanatophoric dysplasia, or a variety of craniosynostotic disorders such as Crouzon syndrome, Apert syndrome, Carpenter syndrome, and Pfeiffer syndrome (Figure 14.12). Cloverleaf skull is trilobular because of multiple premature sutural synostoses. Maxillary hypoplasia and relative mandibular prognathism are frequently encountered. The nasal bridge is depressed and the nose may be beak-like. Severe proptosis, ocular hypertelorism, and antimongoloid obliquity are commonly observed. The eyelids may fail to close, leading to corneal ulceration and clouding. Hydrocephalus, and psychomotor, and mental retardation have been noted. Natal teeth have been observed in several cases as well as oblique facial clefts. It is due to FGFR2, while those with the milder form generally map to FGFR1.

Pfeiffer syndrome (Figures 14.13 and 14.14) is an autosomal dominant mutation. It is due to a FGFR2 mutation on chromosome 10q25–q26. The disorder is recognized at birth and consists of craniosynostosis resulting in turribrachycephaly, broad thumbs and great toes, and variable partial cutaneous soft tissue syndactyly of the hands and feet. Additional craniofacial features include depressed nasal bridge, hypertelorism, antimongoloid slant to the palpebral fissures, proptosis, strabismus, maxillary hypoplasia with relative mandibular prognathism, facial asymmetry in some patients, low-set ears, and occasionally a cloverleaf skull deformity. Malocclusion and crowding of the teeth and, rarely, other features including bifid uvula as well as broad thumbs and great toes usually show varus deformity.

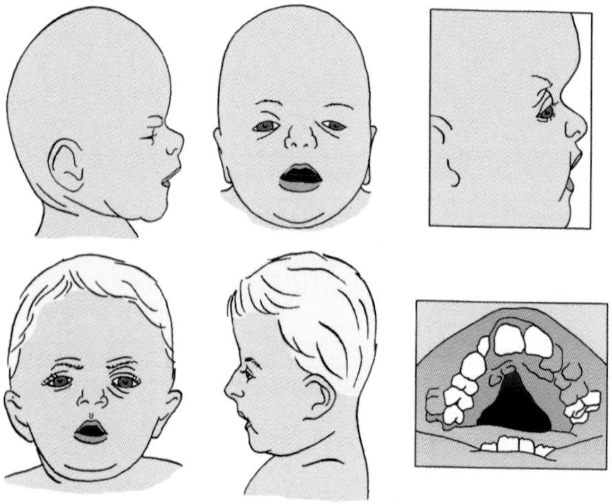

Turribrachycephaly with high, steep, flat frontal bones, small pinched nose, strabismus, proptosis of eyes, downward slant of fissures, flat midface, narrow, high arched palate with malocclusion

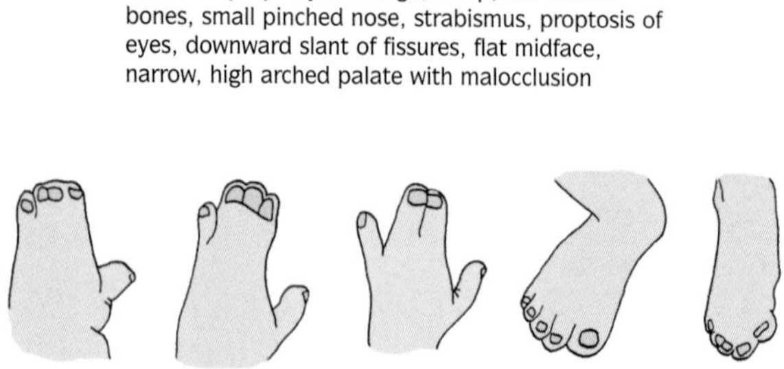

Varying degrees of syndactyly of fingers and toes

14.9. Features of Apert syndrome.

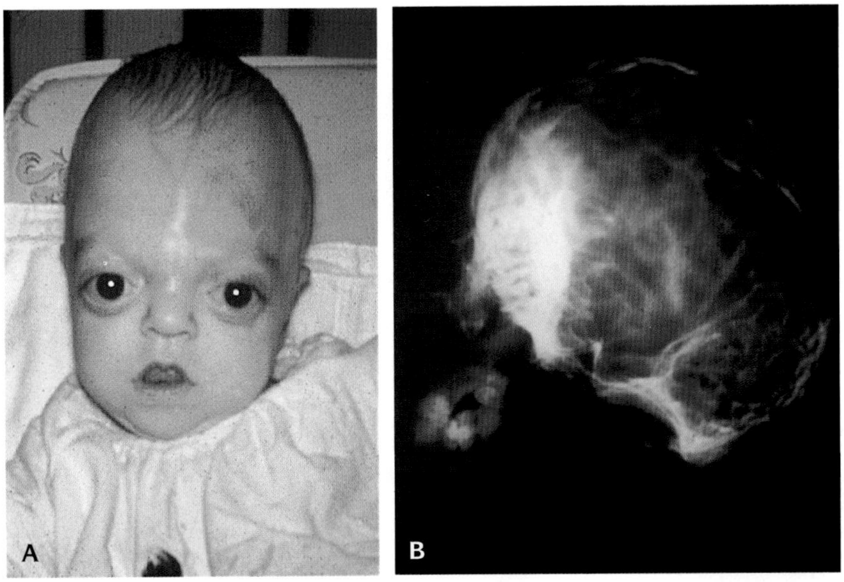

14.10. **(A)** Child with Crouzon syndrome. **(B)** Radiograph of skull of infant revealing craniosynostosis and characteristic increased digital markings on the calvaria.

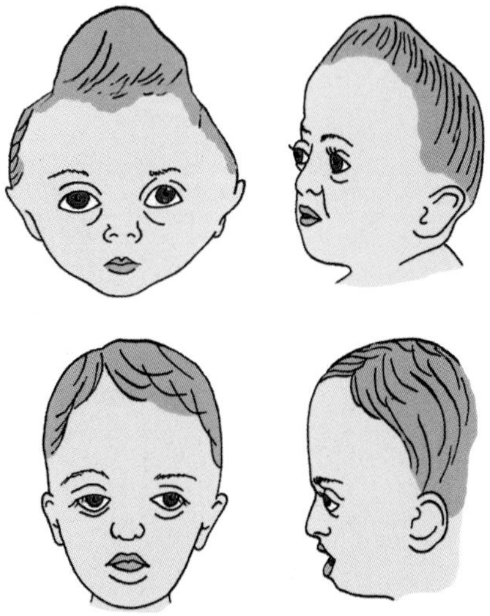

14.11. Features of Crouzon syndrome. Variable cranial form with exophthalmos, divergent strabismus, hypertelorism, short upper lip, relative prognathism and midfacial hypoplasia with beak-like nose.

Carpenter syndrome Asymmetric premature synostosis of all cranial sutures produces a distorted calvaria (Figures 14.15 and 14.16). The nasal bridge is often flat and there may be dystopia canthorum. The hands are short with stubby fingers and with syndactyly most marked between the third and fourth fingers. Several fingers have a single flexion crease. Congenital heart disease, most often ventricular and/or atrial septal defect, omphalocele, undescended testes, and variable mental retardation may be present.

Saethre-Chotzen syndrome Altered facial features may be present at birth (Figures 14.17 and 14.18). The ears may be dysplastic. There is brachycephaly with high forehead, synostosis of coronal sutures, maxillary hypoplasia, shallow orbits, hypertelorism, ptosis of eyelids, large fontanels, and cutaneous

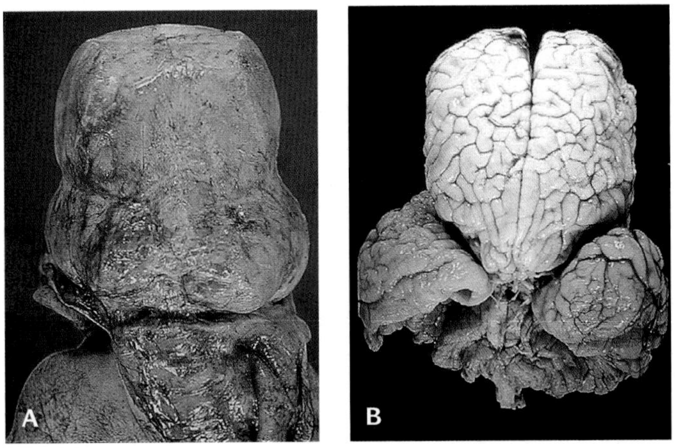

14.12. **(A)** Twenty-six week gestation infant with cloverleaf skull after reflection of scalp. **(B)** Brain showing cloverleaf appearance with bulging temporal lobes.

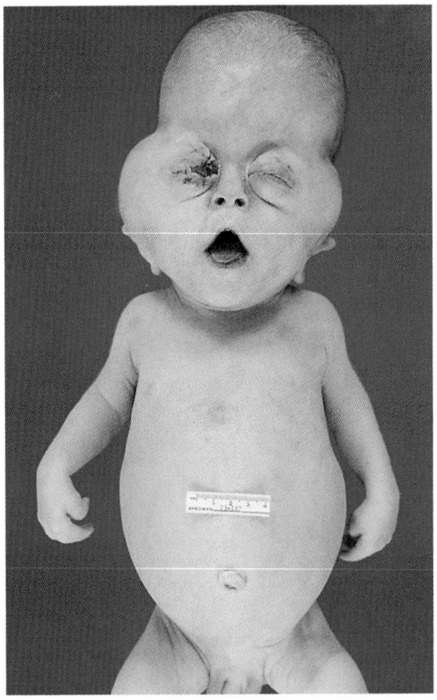

14.13. Pfeiffer syndrome with cloverleaf skull.

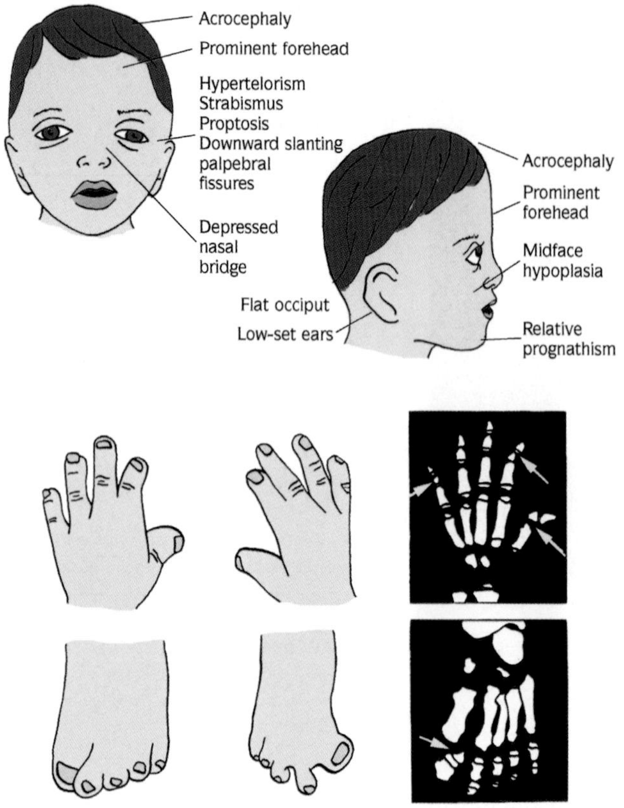

Broad distal phalanges of thumb and hallux with medial deviation, partial syndactyly fingers 2–3, toes 2–4, small middle phalanges of finger (arrows), and delta proximal phalanx of thumb and hallux (arrows)

14.14. Features of Pfeiffer syndrome.

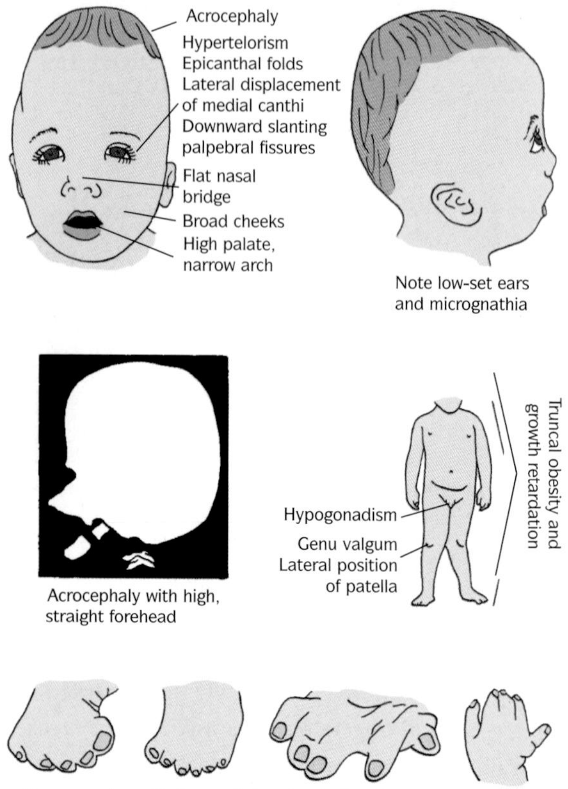

Pes varus, broad hallux, polydactyly, syndactyly and brachydactyly

14.15. Features of Carpenter syndrome. Acrocephaly, hypertelorism, and high, straight forehead.

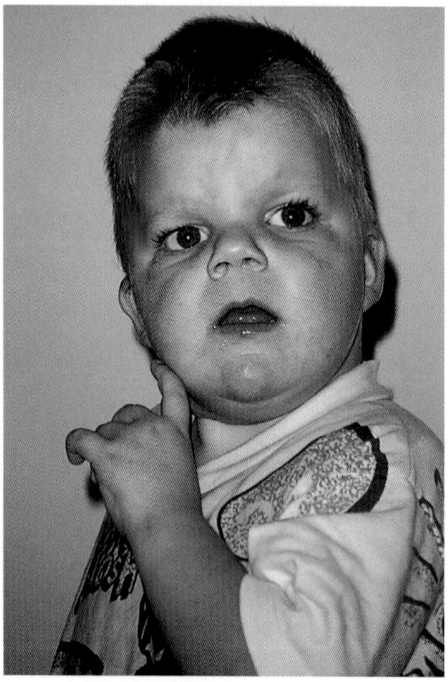

14.16. Carpenter syndrome.

syndactyly (most commonly of second and third fingers or third and fourth toes). Brachydactyly, including short fourth metacarpals, bifid terminal hallucal phalanx, radioulnar synostosis, and fifth finger clinodactyly may be present. These anomalies may be seen by ultrasound prenatally and are clearly visible in the neonate. Occasionally, mental deficiency, small stature, deafness, vertebral anomalies, cryptorchidism, and renal anomalies may occur.

Goldenhar Syndrome. Goldenhar syndrome, comprising the microtia-auriculo-faciovertebral complex, first and second branchial arch syndrome, oculoauriculo-vertebral dysplasia, and hemifacial microsomia, represents defects in morphogenesis of the first and second branchial arches (Figures 14.19 and 14.20 and Table 14.6). Most cases occur sporadically. Facial anomalies include hypoplasia of the malar, maxillary, or mandibular regions (especially the ramus and condyle of the mandible and temporomandibular joint), macrostomia, and hypoplasia of facial muscles. Microtia, accessory preauricular tags and pits, middle ear anomalies with various degrees of deafness, decreased

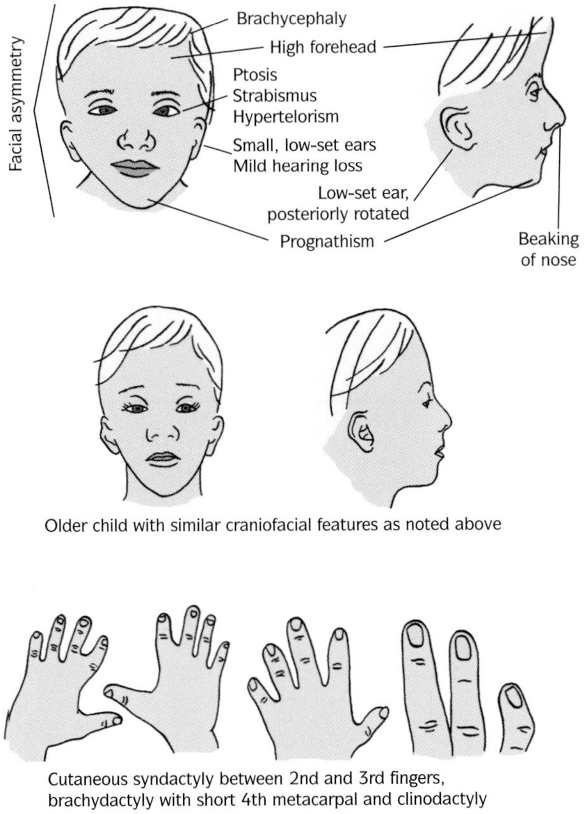

14.17. Features of Saethre-Chotzen syndrome.

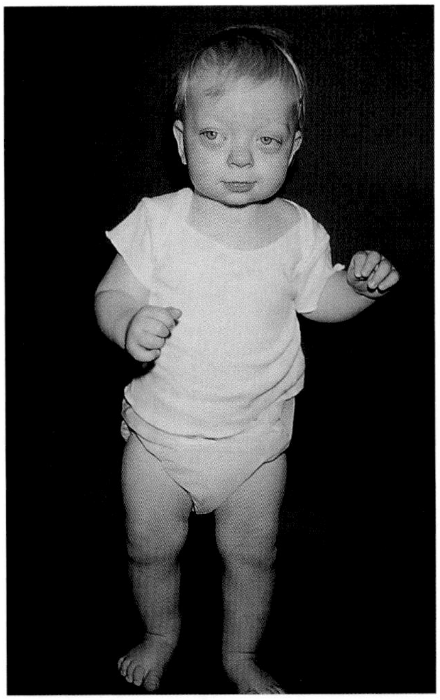

14.18. Saethre-Chotzen. Infant with hypertelorism, high forehead, beak nose, and syndactyly of second and third fingers.

secretion of saliva, anomalies of the tongue and soft palate, and hemivertebrae also occur frequently. It is mostly sporadic, rarely dominantly inherited.

Hydrocephalus (See CNS Chapter). Cerebral fluid accumulation in the ventricles of the brain usually due to obstruction of flow of cerebrospinal fluid results in its distortion, either as an isolated phenomenon or secondary to a neural

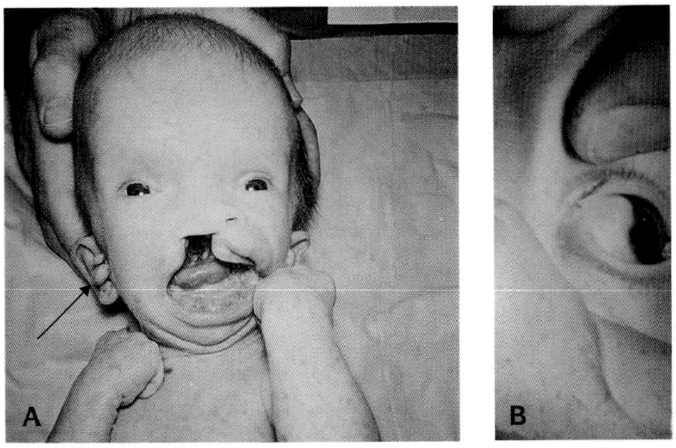

14.19. (A) Infant with Goldenhar syndrome. Facial asymmetry, prominent forehead, downward slanting of eyes, and a preauricular appendage (arrow). **(B)** Epibulbar dermoid.

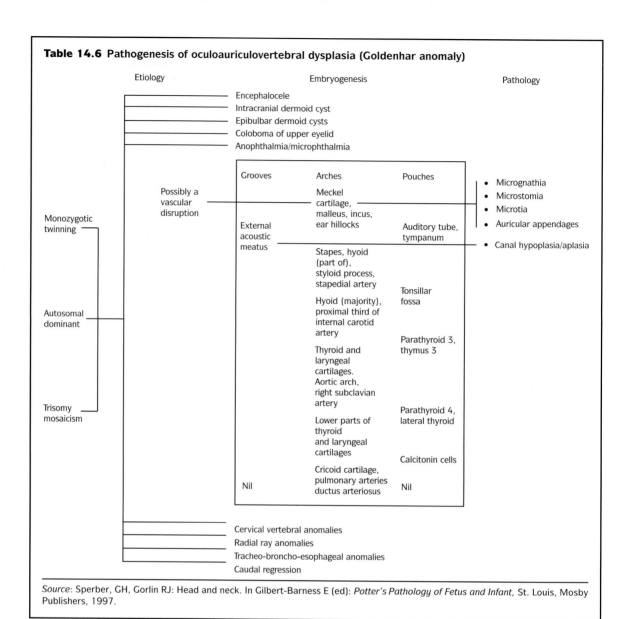

Table 14.6 Pathogenesis of oculoauriculovertebral dysplasia (Goldenhar anomaly)

Etiology		Embryogenesis			Pathology
Monozygotic twinning; Autosomal dominant; Trisomy mosaicism		Encephalocele			
		Intracranial dermoid cyst			
		Epibulbar dermoid cysts			
		Coloboma of upper eyelid			
		Anophthalmia/microphthalmia			
		Grooves	**Arches**	**Pouches**	
	Possibly a vascular disruption		Meckel cartilage, malleus, incus, ear hillocks		• Micrognathia • Microstomia • Microtia • Auricular appendages
		External acoustic meatus		Auditory tube, tympanum	• Canal hypoplasia/aplasia
			Stapes, hyoid (part of), styloid process, stapedial artery	Tonsillar fossa	
			Hyoid (majority), proximal third of internal carotid artery	Parathyroid 3, thymus 3	
			Thyroid and laryngeal cartilages. Aortic arch, right subclavian artery	Parathyroid 4, lateral thyroid	
			Lower parts of thyroid and laryngeal cartilages	Calcitonin cells	
		Nil	Cricoid cartilage, pulmonary arteries ductus arteriosus	Nil	
		Cervical vertebral anomalies			
		Radial ray anomalies			
		Tracheo-broncho-esophageal anomalies			
		Caudal regression			

Source: Sperber, GH, Gorlin RJ: Head and neck. In Gilbert-Barness E (ed): *Potter's Pathology of Fetus and Infant,* St. Louis, Mosby Publishers, 1997.

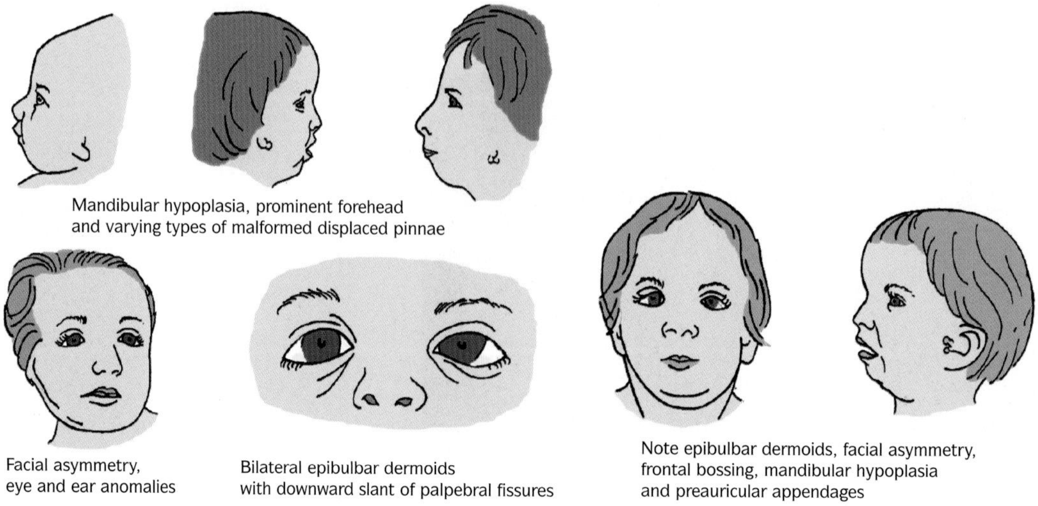

Mandibular hypoplasia, prominent forehead
and varying types of malformed displaced pinnae
Facial asymmetry,
eye and ear anomalies
Bilateral epibulbar dermoids
with downward slant of palpebral fissures
Note epibulbar dermoids, facial asymmetry,
frontal bossing, mandibular hypoplasia
and preauricular appendages

14.20. Features of Goldenhar (oculoauriculovertebral dysplasia) syndrome.

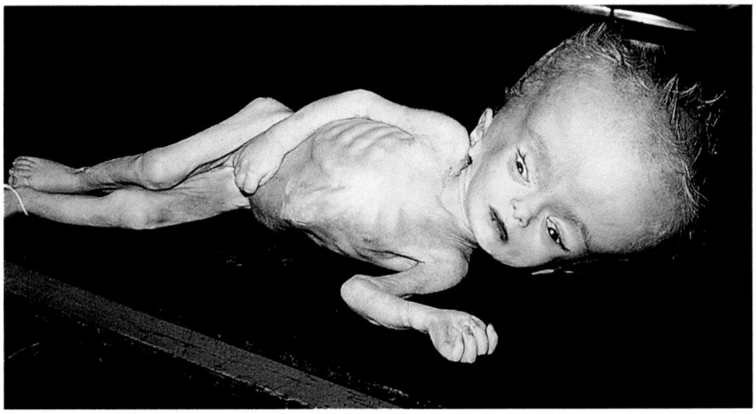

14.21. Infant with extreme hydrocephalus.

tube defect (Figure 14.21). It may be due to aqueductal stenosis which may be an X-linked trait.

Cleidocranial dysplasia – This is an autosomal dominant mutation with marked variability. There are absent clavicles, a hypoplastic mandible (Figure 14.22A). Deciduous teeth, and supernumerary teeth have distorted shapes (Figure 14.22B).

An intramembranous bone defect results in lesions of the skull calvaria, viscerocranium (face), and clavicles. It has been identified in a mouse homolog.

Mandibulofacial Dysostosis (Treacher Collins Syndrome)

This syndrome can be recognized at birth due to a typical facial appearance (Figures 14.23 and 14.24 and Table 14.7). The eyes may show several anomalies which include the following: antimongoloid obliquity of the palpebral fissures, coloboma of the outer third of the lower lid with a deficiency of cilia medial to the coloboma, iridial coloboma, absence of the lower lacrimal pits, Meibomian glands and intermarginal strip, and microphthalmia. The nose appears large due to a lack of malar development, while the nares are often narrow and the

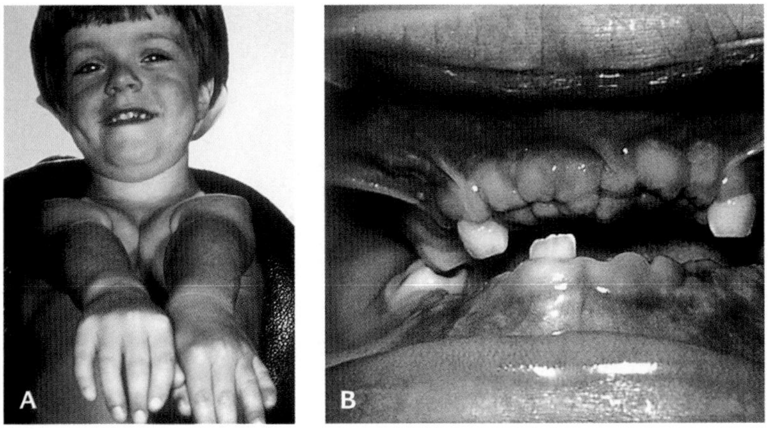

14.22. Cleidocranial dysplasia. **(A)** Absent clavicles, hypoplastic mandible, and zygomas characterize cleidocranial dysplasia. **(B)** Prolonged retention of deciduous teeth and supernumerary teeth with distorted shapes and delayed eruption.

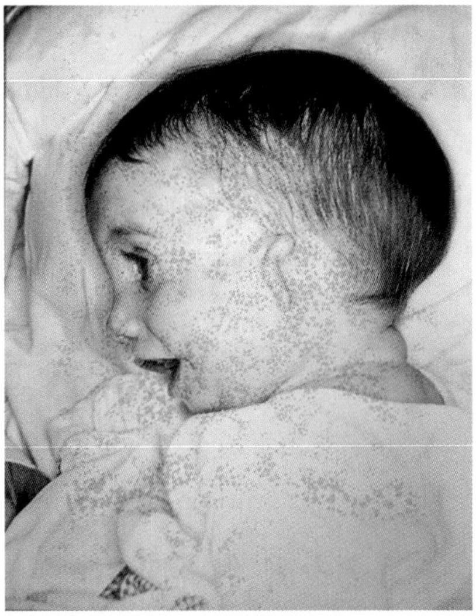

14.23. Treacher Collins syndrome: hypoplastic zygoma, mandibular condyle and ramus, receding chin, and malformed pinna.

Table 14.7 Mandibulofacial dysostosis (Treacher-Collins syndrome)

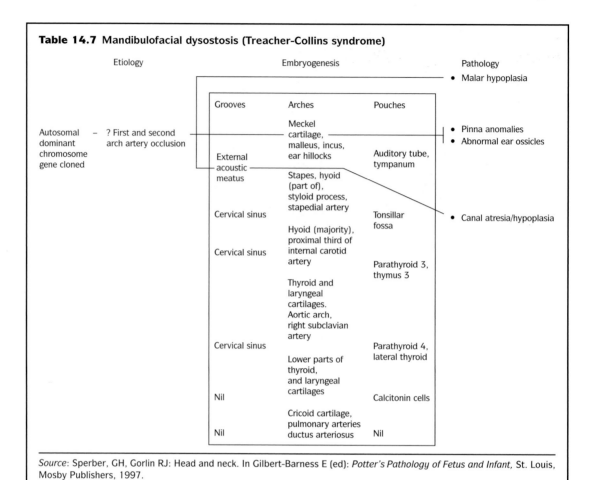

Etiology		Embryogenesis: Grooves	Embryogenesis: Arches	Embryogenesis: Pouches	Pathology
Autosomal dominant chromosome gene cloned –	? First and second arch artery occlusion	External acoustic meatus	Meckel cartilage, malleus, incus, ear hillocks	Auditory tube, tympanum	• Malar hypoplasia • Pinna anomalies • Abnormal ear ossicles • Canal atresia/hypoplasia
		Cervical sinus	Stapes, hyoid (part of), styloid process, stapedial artery	Tonsillar fossa	
		Cervical sinus	Hyoid (majority), proximal third of internal carotid artery	Parathyroid 3, thymus 3	
		Cervical sinus	Thyroid and laryngeal cartilages. Aortic arch, right subclavian artery	Parathyroid 4, lateral thyroid	
		Nil	Lower parts of thyroid, and laryngeal cartilages	Calcitonin cells	
		Nil	Cricoid cartilage, pulmonary arteries ductus arteriosus	Nil	

Source: Sperber, GH, Gorlin RJ: Head and neck. In Gilbert-Barness E (ed): *Potter's Pathology of Fetus and Infant,* St. Louis, Mosby Publishers, 1997.

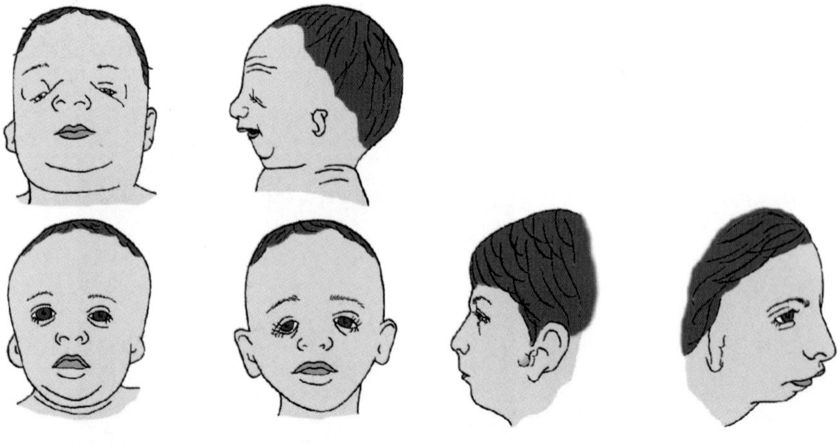

Degrees of lateral downward slant of palpebral fissures, coloboma of outer portion lower lids, malformed ears and facial asymmetry

Malformed ears, ear tags, micrognathia, large appearing nose with narrow nares

14.24. Treacher Collins (mandibulofacial dysostosis) syndrome.

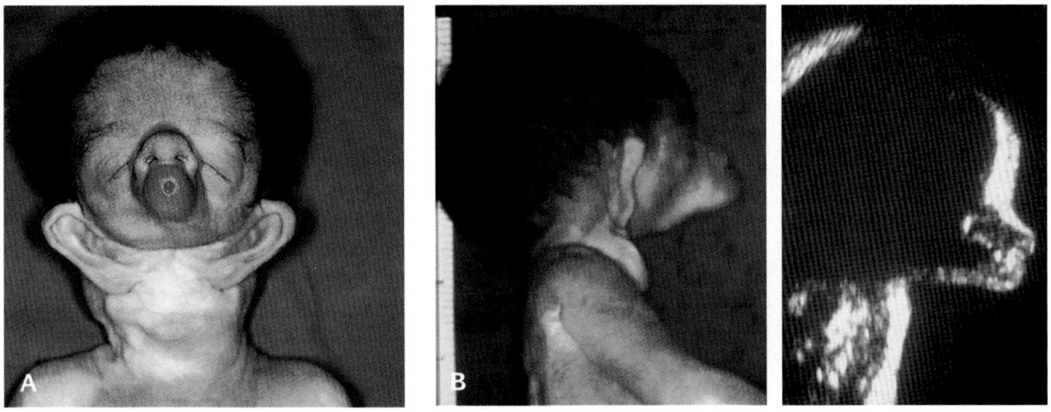

14.25. Otocephaly. **(A)** Absent mandible and ears approximate in the midline and the mouth is a pinpoint blind orifice. **(B)** Side view of same infant (left) and ultrasound (right).

alar cartilages hypoplastic. The nasofrontal angle is commonly obliterated and the bridge of the nose raised. Choanal atresia has been noted. Micrognathia is almost always present; other oral manifestations include cleft palate (30%), high-arched palate, dental malocclusion, and unilateral or less often bilateral macrostomia. The external ears are frequently deformed, crumpled forward, or misplaced. Some patients have an absence of the external auditory canal or ossicle defects associated with conductive deafness. Extra ear tags and blind fistulas may be found anywhere between the tragus and angle of the mouth; occasionally, other anomalies are absence of the parotid gland, congenital heart disease, cervical vertebral malformations, congenital defects of the extremities, cryptorchidism, and renal anomalies.

Agnathia, Otocephaly

A major lower-facial developmental field defect incurs the derivatives of the first and second pharyngeal arches (Figure 14.25).

Holoprosencephaly (See Chromosome Chapter)

A spectrum of malformations of the face reflects an underlying incomplete division of the prosencephalon (holoprosencephaly). The most severe manifestation of the condition is cyclopia, within which a range of expressions appear. Holoprosencephaly is a component part of trisomy 13 syndrome and other chromosomal defects and may be seen in diabetic embryopathy. It may be sporadic, autosomal dominant, or autosomal recessive.

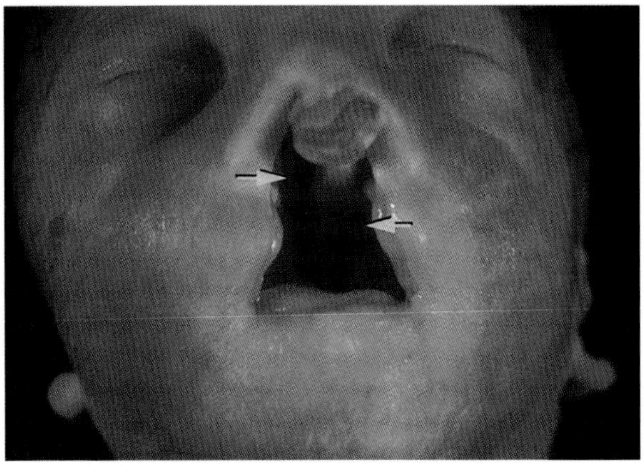

14.26. Bilateral clefting of the face with rudimentary premaxilla and bilateral cleft lip and palate (arrows).

Orofacial Clefts. The most frequent craniofacial anomalies are clefts of the upper lip and palate that can now be diagnosed prenatally (Figures 14.26 to 14.32). Clefts may involve the facial structures and extend into the orbits.

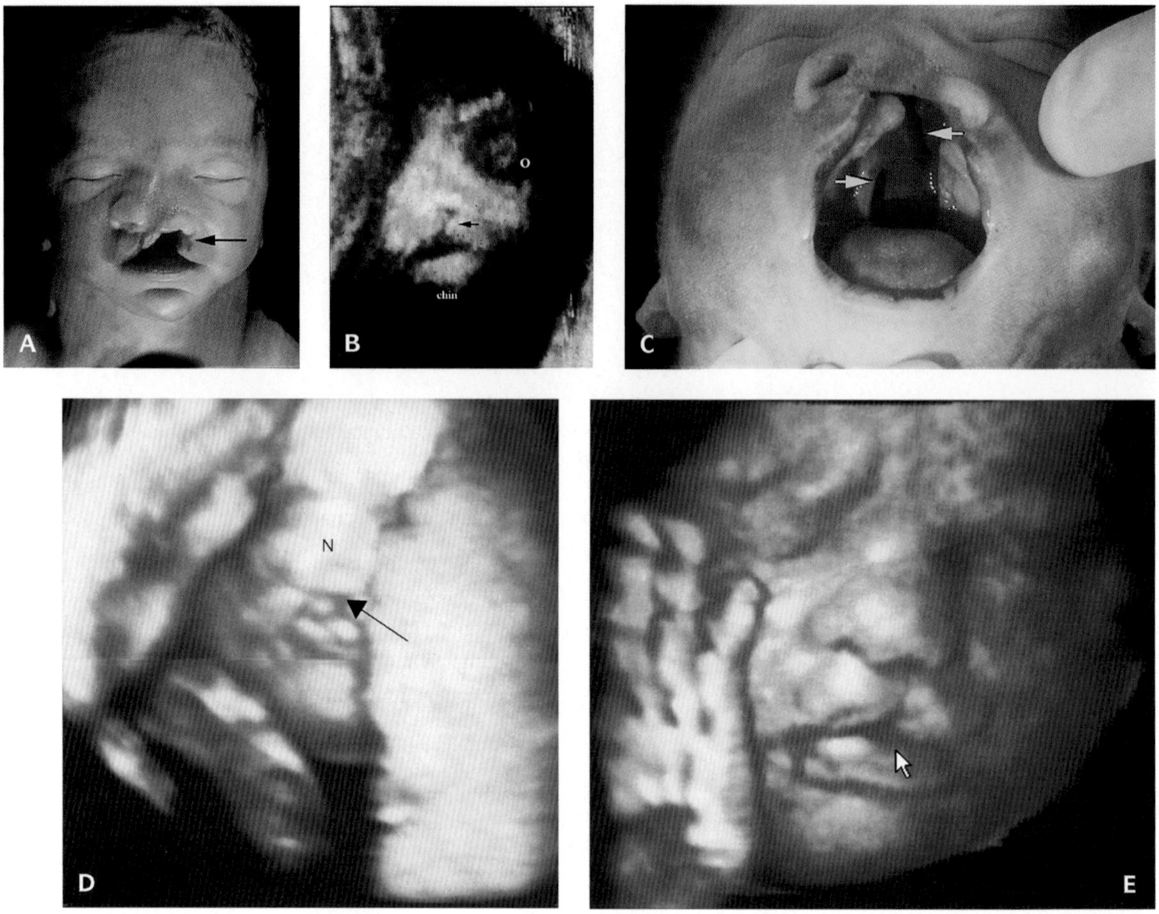

14.27. **(A)** Clefting of the face with extension to left nostril (arrow). Right single nostril deviated. **(B)** Ultrasound with clefting of the lip and nostril (arrow) (O, orbit). **(C)** Open mouth with two palatal clefts (arrows). **(D)** Three-dimensional ultrasound of a cleft lip (arrow) extending into the nostril in a fetus at 31 weeks gestation (N, nose; C, chin). **(E)** Three-dimensional ultrasound of a unilateral cleft lip (arrow) in a fetus at 30 weeks gestation.

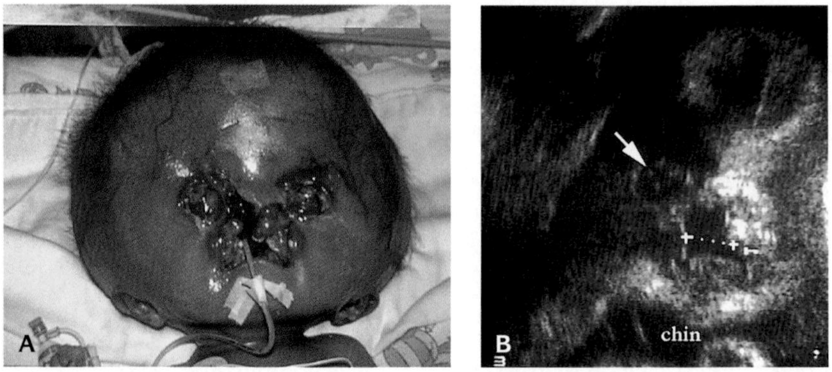

14.28. **(A)** Hydrocephalus and clefts extending from angles of the mouth to inner canthi of the eyes. **(B)** Ultrasound showing the cleft (crosses and dots) (arrow, orbit).

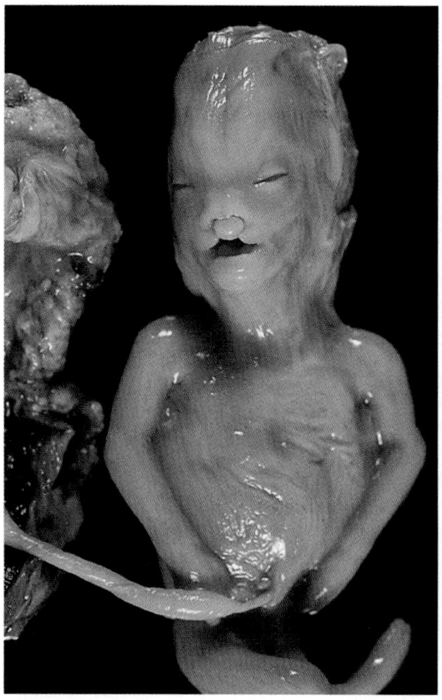

14.29. Bilateral clefts with residual premaxilla in trisomy 21.

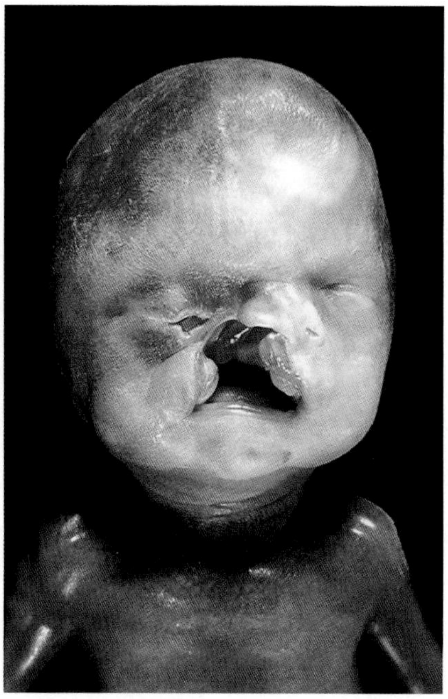

14.30. Oblique clefting of the face due to swallowed amniotic bands with microphthalmia.

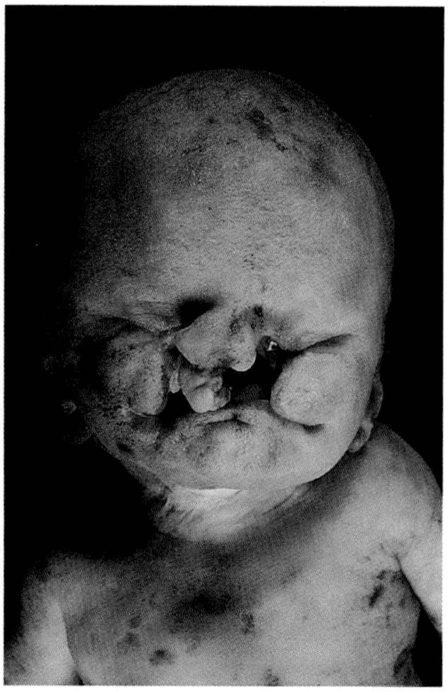

14.31. Clefting of face and cutis aplasia in Golz syndrome. Bilateral clefts of face. Cleft on right to outer and inner canthi and lateral cleft at angle of mouth. On left, cleft extends to inner canthus and left nostril and lateral cleft at angle of mouth.

Ear Anomalies

The external ear may display a wide spectrum of anomalies from complete absence to multiple tags (Figures 14.33 and 14.34). Ear anomalies may be a component part of malformation syndromes or sequences such as the DiGeorge sequence. Low-set ears are present when the helix meets the cranium. At the level below that of a horizontal plane with the corners of the orbit. Slanted ears occur when the angle of the slope of the auricle exceeds 15° from the

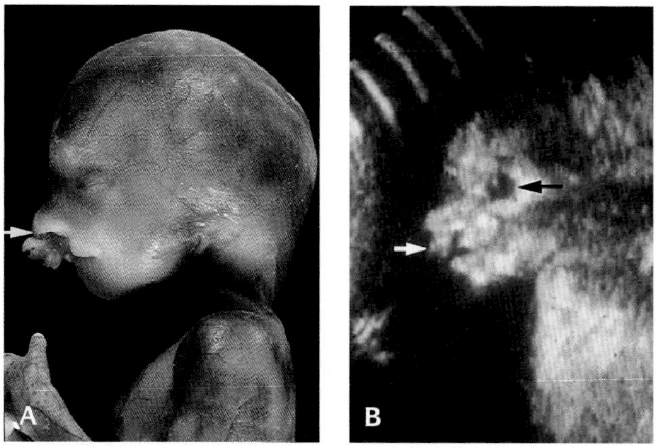

14.32. **(A)** Fetus 22 weeks gestation. Bilateral clefting of face with rudimentary premaxilla (yellow arrow) and microtia. **(B)** Ultrasound of a fetus at 24 weeks gestation, showing rudimentary premaxilla (white arrow) (black arrow, orbit).

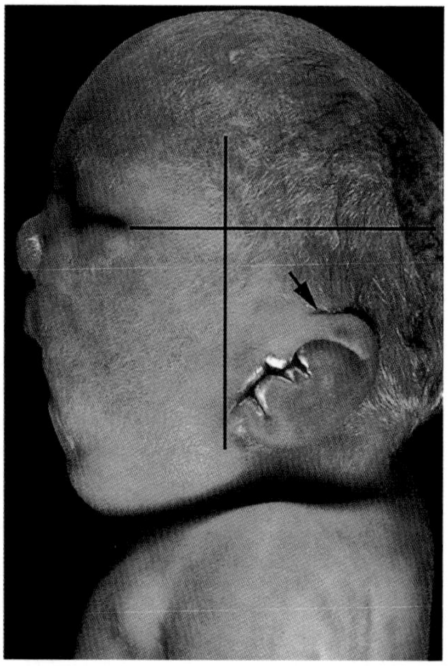

14.33. Low-set postaxially rotated ear (arrow). The normal position should be with the upper border of the pinna at the horizontal line.

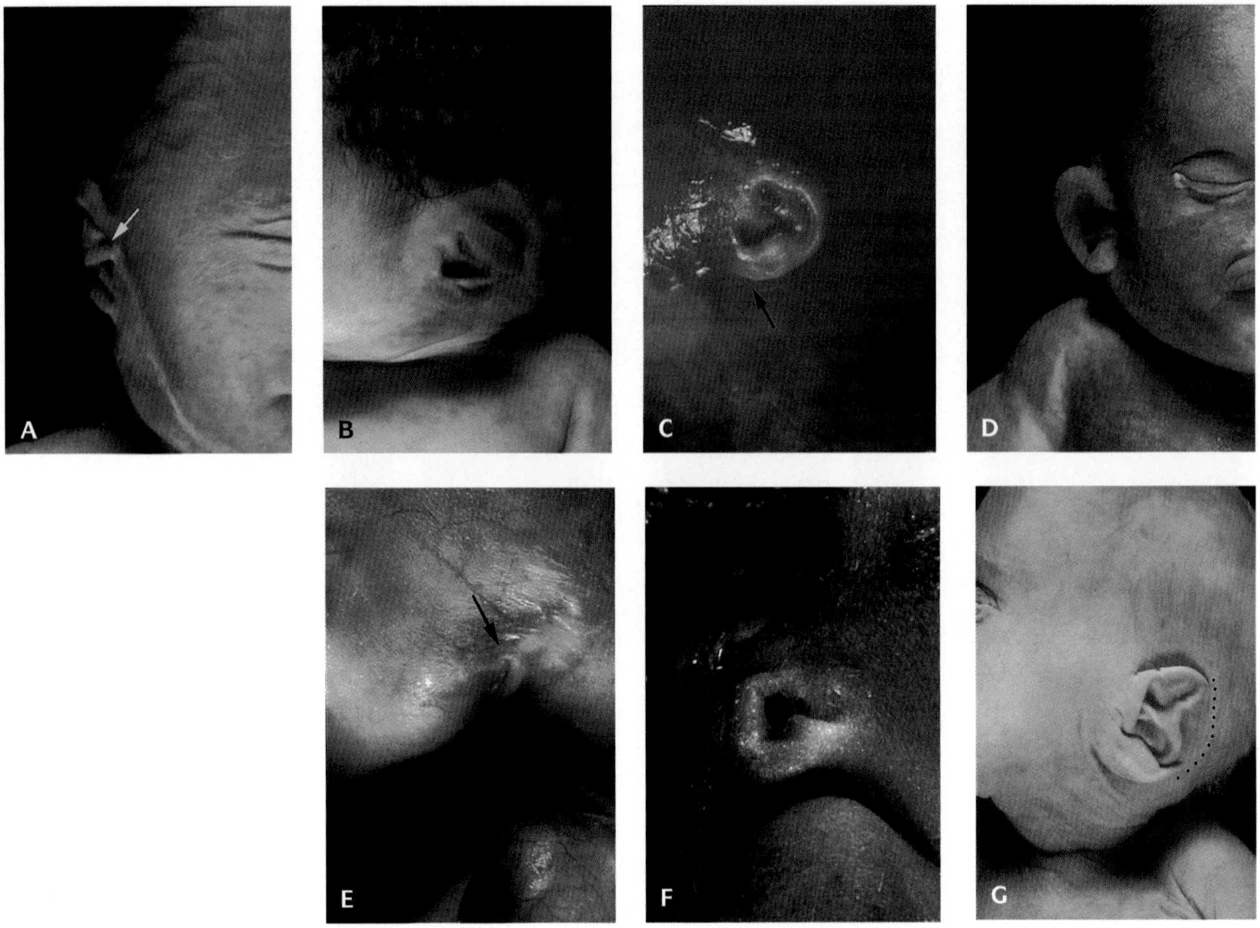

14.34. Abnormal ears: **(A)** Preauricular tag-frequently contains core of cartilage- represents an accessory auricular hillock. **(B)** Incomplete helix development may be a normal variation. **(C)** Lack of lobulus in fetus with trisomy 21. **(D)** Protruding ear due to lack of the posterior auricular muscle. **(E)** Microtia may be seen in Goldenhar syndrome or as an isolated defect. Low-set ear with postaxial rotation and lack of folding of the helix. Helix meets the cranium (arrow) at a level below the horizontal plane with the corner of orbit. **(F)** Cup-shaped "primitive" ear in an anencephalic infant. **(G)** Flattened ear due to oligohydramnios with midportion of helix (dots) compressed on to the calvarium.

perpendicular. It is important to appreciate that in utero constraint deformation of the head may temporarily distort the usual landmarks.

Dental Abnormalities. These may occur in a number of malformation syndromes. In ectodermal dysplasia the teeth are peg-shaped. Erupted teeth may be present in the newborn. A single central incisor is a manifestation of holoprosencephaly.

Facial Clefts Ultrasonography

- Non-syndromic facial clefting occurs in 1/800 births.
- Increased rates noted in Asians and Native Americans, uncommon in blacks.

- More common in increasing maternal age.
- 60–80% of clefts occur in male fetuses.
- If one first degree relative is affected, 4% recurrence risk is present.
- Frequencies of chromosomal abnormalities vary by timing of evaluation.
  - Postnatal surveys find 1% aneuploidy in newborns with facial clefts.
  - Prenatal studies have found 40% aneuploidy (usually either trisomy 13 or 18)
  - Clefting is found in 40% of trisomy 13, 10% of trisomy 18, and in 1–2% of trisomy 21 and in triploid infants.

REFERENCES

Cohen MM Jr: Craniofacial disorders caused by mutations in homebox genes MSX1 and MSX2. *J Craniofac Genet Dev Biol* 20:19, 2000.

Cohen MM Jr, McLean RE: *Craniosynostosis: Diagnosis, Evaluation and Management*, 2nd ed, New York, Oxford University Press, 2000.

Cohen MM Jr: Molecular biology of craniosynostosis with special emphasis on fibroblast growth factor receptors. In Cohen MM Jr, Baum BJ (eds): *Studies in Stomatology and Craniofacial Biology*, Amsterdam, IOS Press, 1997.

Cohen MM Jr: *The Child with Multiple Birth Defects*, 2nd ed, New York, Oxford University Press, 1997.

Cohen MM Jr: Transforming growth factors and their receptors: role in sutural biology and craniosynostosis. *J Bone Mineral Res* 12(3):322, 1997.

Cohen MM Jr. Perspectives on craniofacial asymmetry V. The craniosynostoses. *Int J Oral Maxillofac Surg*, 24:191, 1995.

Gilbert-Barness E, Opitz JM: Congenital anomalies and malformation syndromes. In Stocker JT, Dehner LP (eds): *Pediatric Pathology*, Philadelphia, JB Lippincott Co, 1992, pp. 113.

Goodman RM, Gorlin RJ, eds: *The Malformed Infant and Child: An Illustrated Guide*, New York, Oxford University Press, 1983.

Gorlin RJ: Developmental and genetic aspects of cleft lip and palate. In Moller KT, Starr CD (eds): *Cleft Palate: Interdisciplinary Treatment*, Austin, Pro Ed Publishers, 1993, p. 25.

Gorlin RJ, Cervenka J, Pruzansky S: Facial clefting and its syndromes. *Birth Defects* 7:3, 1971.

Gorlin RJ, Cohen MM Jr, Hennekam RCM: *Syndromes of Head and Neck*, 4th ed, New York, Oxford University Press, 2001.

Gorlin RJ, Cohen MM Jr: The orofacial region. In Wigglesworth JS, Singer DB (eds): *Textbook of Fetal and Perinatal Pathology*, 2nd ed, Malden, Blackwell Science, 1998, pp. 732–778.

Norman MG, McGillivray BC, Kalousek DK, Hill A, Poskitt KJ: *Congenital Malformations of the Brain-Pathological, Embryological, Clinical, Radiological and Genetic Aspects*, New York, Oxford University Press, 1995.

On-Line Mendelian Inheritance in Man. OMIM (http://www3.ncbi.nlm.nih.gov/omim/).

Shprintzen RJ, Siegel-Sadowitz VL, Amato J, Goldberg F: Anomalies associated with cleft lip, cleft palate or both. *Am J Med Genet* 20:585, 1985.

Sperber GH: Head and neck. I. Craniofacial abnormalities. In Gilbert-Barness E (ed): *Potter's Pathology of the Fetus and Infant*, St. Louis, Mosby-Year Book, 1997.

FIFTEEN

Skeletal Abnormalities

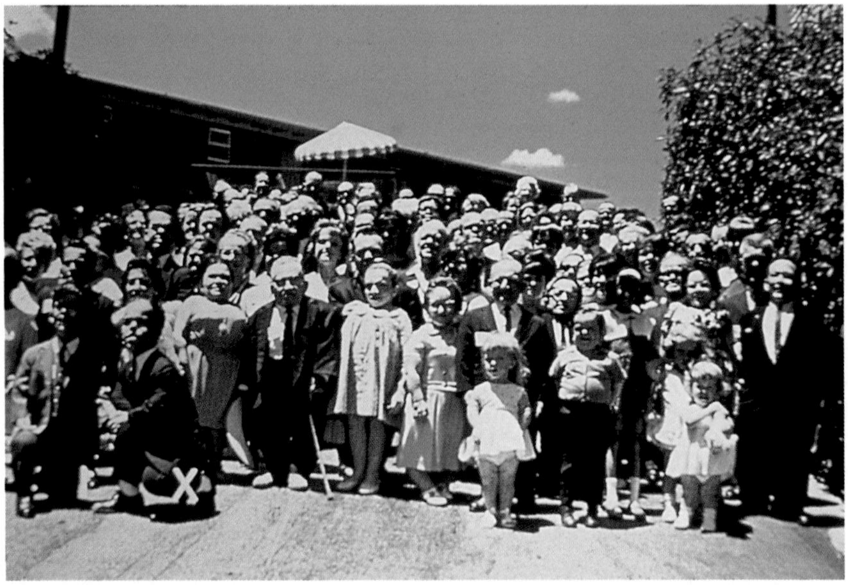

The "Little People of America" representing over 50 types of dwarfism.

OSTEOCHONDRODYSPLASIAS

Bone is formed from collagen. Bone dysplasias predominantly involve one type of collagen (Figure 15.1). Terms used in the description of bone dysplasias according to the defect in collagen are shown in Table 15.1.

Table 15.1 Molecular defects in the chondrodysplasias

Gene	Disorder
Structural proteins of cartilage	
COL2A1	Langer Saldino (achondrogenesis II) Hypochondrogenesis SED SEMD Kneist dysplasia
COL9A2	MED
COL10A1	MD Schmid
COL11A2	Stickler syndrome OSMED
COMP	Pseudoachondroplasia MED
Inborn errors of cartilage metabolism	
DTST	Achondrogenesis IB Atelosteogenesis II Diastrophic dysplasia
ARSE	Chondrodysplasia punctata XR
Lysosomal enzymes	Mucopolysaccharidoses
Local regulators of cartilage growth	
FGFR3	Achondroplasia Hypochondroplasia Thantophoric I and II
PTH-PTHRP	Metaphyseal dysplasia, type Jansen
Systemic defects influencing cartilage development	
Peroxisomal defects	Rhizomelic chondrodysplasia punctata
ADA deficiency	Combined immunodeficiency
Gene identified, mechanism unknown	
SOX9	Campomelic dysplasia
EXT1	Multiple exostoses 1
Gene mapped, not yet identified	
	Cleidocranial dysplasia Ellis van Creveld Trichorhinophalangeal 1 and 2 Pycnodysostosis Multiple exostoses 2 and 3

ADA, adenine desminase; ARSE, arylsulfatase; DTST, diastrophic dysplasia sulfate transporter; FGFR3, fibroblast growth factor receptor 3; MD Shmid, metaphyseal dysplasia-Schmid dysplasia; MED, multiple epiphyseal dysplasia; OSMED, osteospondylomegaepiphyseal dysplasia; PTH-PTHRP, parathyroid hormone-parathyroid hormone related peptide; SED, spondyloepiphyseal dysplasia; SEMD, spondyloepimetaphyseal dysplasia.

Source: Rimoin DL: Molecular defects in chondrodysplasias. *Am J Med Genet* 63:100, 1996.

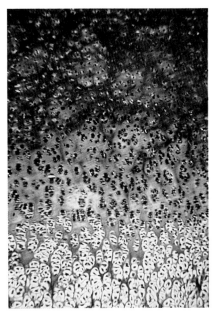

15.1. Normal endochondral ossification (distal femur of a neonate) note the regular columnization of chondrocytes in the physeal growth zone and the straight cartilage-bone junction.

Table 15.2 Generalized osteochondroplasias from the revised international classification,[1] encompassing those disorders that are perinatally lethal and/or amenable to prenatal diagnosis

	Recurrence	Frequency
1. Achondroplasia group		
Thanatophoric dysplasia	AD	1/6400–1/15,300
Thanatophoric dysplasia, straight femur/cloverleaf skull type	AD	Low
Achondroplasia	AD	1/20,000–1/25,000
Hypochondroplasia	AD	1/300,000
2. Achondrogenesis		
Type Ia	AR	Low
Type Ib	AR	
3. Spondylodysplastic group (perinatally lethal)		
San Diego type	Sp	
Torrance type	Sp	Low
Luton type	Sp	
4. Metatropic dysplasia group		
Fibrochondrogenesis	AR	Very low
Schneckenbecken dysplasia	AD	Very low
Metatropic dysplasia	AD	Relatively low
5. Short rib dysplasia group (with/without polydactyly)		
SR(P) type I Saldino–Noonan	AR	Low
SR(P) type II Majewski	AR	Low
SR(P) type III Verma–Naumoff	AR	Very low
SR(P) type IV Beemer–Langer	AR	Very low
Asphyxiating thoracic dysplasia	AR	
Ellis–van Creveld dysplasia	AR	Low except USA Amish
6. Atelosteogenesis/diastrophic dysplasia group		
Boomerang dysplasia	Sp	
Atelosteogenesis type 1	Sp	Low
Atelosteogenesis type 2 (de la Chapelle)	AR	Low
Omodysplasia (Maroteaux)	AD	
Omodysplasia II (Borochowitz)	AR	
Otopalato-digital syndrome type 2	XLR	
Diastrophic dysplasia	AR	Low
Pseudodiastrophic dysplasia	AR	Very Low
7. Kniest–Stickler dysplasia group		
Dyssegmental dysplasia – Silverman–Handmaker type	AR	
Dyssegmental dysplasia – Rolland–Desbuquois type	AR	
Kniest dysplasia	AD	Low
Otospondylomegaepiphyseal dysplasia	AR	
Stickler dysplasia	AD	
8. Spondyloepiphyseal dysplasia congenita group		
Langer–Saldino dysplasia (Anchondrogenesis type II)	AD	Low
Hypochondrogenesis	AD	
Spondyloepiphyseal dysplasia congenita	AD	Not rare
13. Chondrodysplasia punctata (stippled epiphyses) group		
Rhizomelic type	AR	Very low
Conradi–Hünermann type	XLD	Low
X-linked recessive type	XLR	Low
MT-type	Sp	
Other including CHILD syndrome; Zellweger syndrome; warfarin embryopathy, chromosomal abnormalities; fetal alcohol syndrome		
19. Bent bone dysplasia group		
Campomelic dysplasia	AR	Low
Kyphomelic dysplasia	AR	
Stüve–Wiedemann dysplasia	AR	

	Recurrence	Frequency
22. Dysplasias with decreased bone density		
Osteogenesis imperfecta (several types)	AD	1/23,000
	AR	
Osteoporosis with pseudoglioma	AR	
Idiopathic juvenile osteoporosis	Sp	
Bruck syndrome	AR	
Homocystinuria	AR	
Singleton–Merten syndrome	Sp	
Geroderma osteodysplastica	AR	
Menkes syndrome	XLR	
23. Dysplasias with defective mineralization		
Hypophosphatasia (several types)	AD	Low
	AR	Low
Hypophosphataemic rickets	XR	1/25,000
Pseudodeficiency rickets, (several types)	AR	
Neonatal hyperparathyroidism	AR	

[1] Spranger J: International classification of osteochondroplasias. *Eur J Pediatr* 151:407, 1992.
AR, autosomal recessive; AD, autosomal dominant; Sp, sporadic; XLR, X-linked recessive.

Source: Keeling JW: *Fetal Pathology*. New York, Churchill Livingstone, 1994.

The normal growth plate or physis consists of four zones:

1. resting cartilage;
2. proliferative cartilage;
3. hypertrophic cartilage;
4. zone of provisional calcification.

The revised international classification of osteochondrodysplasias encompasses those disorders that are perinatally lethal and/or amenable to prenatal diagnosis (Table 15.2). Prenatal diagnosis has been made in most of the lethal forms of ostechondrodysplasia (Table 15.3). The osteochondrodysplasias include the infant or fetus with dwarfism. Most are lethal. For most convenience in diagnosis they can be divided into the following groups:

- Osteochondrodysplasias with platyspondyly
- Osteochondrodysplasias with short trunk
- Short rib osteochondrodysplasias
- Osteochondrodysplasias with defective bone density
- Miscellaneous group

Osteochondrodysplasias with Platyspondyly (Table 15.4)

Although the trunk of the infants in this group is not significantly short, the vertebral bodies in the radiograph are markedly flattened. Histopathologically the physeal growth zones are usually disorganized and may be retarded, but the resting cartilage is mostly unremarkable.

15.3 Prenatal diagnosis of bone dysplasias

Disorder	Inheritance	Features
Thanatophoric dysplasia	Sporadic	Polyhydramnios, very short limbs, bowed femurs, prominent forehead narrow thorax
Thanatophoric dysplasia with cloverleaf skull	AR	Cloverleaf skull, straight, very short femurs
Achondrogenesis (several types)	AR	Decreased ossification, extreme shortening of limbs
Osteogenesis imperfecta		
I	AD	Usually normal
IIA	AD	IUGR, micromelia, angulation plus bowing
IIIB	AR	Normal bone echogenicity
IIC	AR	Moderate shortening, normal echogenicity
III	AR	Short femurs, decreased echogenicity
IV	AD	Few (no) findings, normal echogenicity
V	AD	Increased alkaline phosphatase during callus formation. No mutation in collagen type 1 genes
VI	?AD	Increased alkaline phosphatase without rickets. No genetic mutation identified. Type I collagen protein analysis normal
Asphyxiating thoracic dystrophy (Jeune)*	AR	Mild rhizomelic shortening, narrow thorax, renal dysplasia
Diastrophic dysplasia*	AR	Severe micromelia, bowing, "hitchhiker" thumb, severe clubbed feet
Spondylo–epiphyseal dysplasia*		Short thorax, short limbs, bowing, abnormal vertebrae, decreased ossification
Congenita	AD	
Tarda	AD	
Achondroplasia*		
Heterozygous	AD	Fall-off long-bone growth >26 weeks, disproportionately (but normal) larger head
Homozygous*	AD	Fall-off long-bone growth <20 weeks, similar to thanatophoric dysplasia
Chondrodysplasia punctata		
Rhizomelic	AR	Micromelia plus contractures; abnormal vertebral bodies, stippling
Conradi-Hunermann	XLD	Punctate calcification, asymmetric long bone shortening, ichthyosiform rash, cataracts
Other		
XLR type	XLR	Similar to Conradi-Hunermann, mental retardation
Tibiametacarpal type	AD	Punctate calcification; sacral, tarsal, and carpal length of long bones variable
Short-rib polydactyly syndromes	AR	Severe micromelia, narrow thorax, polydactyly; oligopolyhydramnios, fetal hydrops (some), cystic renal changes

* Patients at risk for spinal cord compression or other forms of airway compromise.

Osteochondrodysplasias with Significant Platyspondyly (Table 15.4)

- Thanatophoric dysplasia classical
  - Torrance type
  - San Diego type
- Thanatophoric dysplasia with cloverleaf skull
- Achondroplasia, heterozygous and homozygous
- Metatropic dysplasia

Table 15.4 Osteochondrodysplasia with platyspondyly

	Radiography					Physis		Clinical	
			Limb bones						
	Platyspondyly	Large head	Short	Shape	Abnorm Ilia	Disorganization	Retardation	Prognosis	Genetics
TD	+++	+	+++	curved femora (telephone receiver-like)	+	+++	+++	lethal (most common form of lethal osteochondro-dysplasia	AD
TDCS	+++	+ (trilobed)	+++	straight femora	+	+++	+++	lethal	AD
SD									
San Diego	++++	+	++++	very short, broad femora (Ragged metaphyseal margins)	+	+++	+++	lethal	SP
Torrance	++++	+	++++	very short, broad femora (Ragged metaphyseal margins)	+	–	–	lethal	SP
Luton	+++	+	+++	mild metaphyseal irregularity	+	+ (focal)	focal fibrosis	lethal	SP
AP									
Heterozygous	++	+	++	slightly curved femora	+	–	+	compatible with life	AD
Homozygous	+++	+	+++	slightly curved femora	+	+++	+++	lethal	AD
MD	+++	–	+	huge metaphysis (halberd shape)	+	(small hyper-trophic cells)	– –	compatible with life	AD, AR AD, AR
OD	++++	+	++++	very short bones of hands and feet	+	+	–	die within 4.5 years	AR

+, mild; ++, moderate; +++, severe; 4, extreme; AD, autosomal dominant; AR, autosomal dominant; AR, autosomal recessive; SP, sporadic; TD, thanatophoric dysplasia; TDCS, thanatophoric dysplasia with cloverleaf skull; SD, spondylodysplastic chondrodysplasia; AP, achondroplasia; MD, metatropic dysplasia; OD, opsismodysplasia.

Table 15.5 Chondrodysplasias with significant platyspondyly

	Thanatophoric dysplasia	Thanatophoric dysplasia with cloverleaf skull
Genetics	Sporadic	AR
Prognosis	Perinatal death	Perinatal death
Large head	+	+ trilobed
Platyspondyly	+++	+++
Tubular bones	Telephone receiver-like femora	Straight femora
Disorganization	+++	+++ increased number of ossified cartilage canals
Retardation	+++	+++

Thanatophoric dwarfism

Clinical features
- Genetics – sporadic
- Head – large with depressed nasal bridge
- Spine – severe platyspondyly with markedly widened disc spaces
- Long bones – curved with telephone-receiver-like femora

Pathology
- Narrow growth plate
- Lack of columnization
- Marked disturbance of endochondral ossification
- Bone deposited directly on cartilage

By ultrasound examination many affected fetuses may be identified during the second trimester of pregnancy often between 12 and 16 weeks gestation.

At autopsy, Faxitron X-ray examination using fine grain mammography film as well as careful histological examination of bones always including the growth plate of the ribs, vertebral bodies, and long bones is important. Visceral anomalies may contribute to the distinction between specific syndromes.

Thanatophoric dysplasia (Table 15.5) is the most common form of lethal osteochondrodysplasia with an incidence of 1/6,400–1/15,300 births (Figures 15.2 and 15.3). It is a new dominant mutation; however, gonadal mosaicism may result in variable expression and reduced penetrance with a small risk of recurrence. Monitoring by careful ultrasonography in subsequent pregnancies is recommended. The San Diego, Torrance, and Lutow types of platyspondylic lethal skeletal dysplasia are usually considered variants of thanatophoric dysplasia. Microscopically the zone of resting cartilage is hypercellular in the Torrance and Lutow types with normal columnation of chondrocytes in the Torrance and disorganized columns in the Lutow type. Enlarged chondrocytes in normal numbers are present in the resting zone in the San Diego type, but columnation of chondrocytes in the growth plate is poor.

Table 15.6 Homozygous achondroplasia

Pathologic features
- Narrow zone but hypercellular proliferative cartilage
- Narrow zone of hypertrophic cartilage
- Lack of columnization
- Lack of chondrocytic columns opening into metaphysis
- PAS-positive granules in chondrocytes in hypertrophic zone

Radiological features
- Small chondrocranium
- Small foramen magnum
- Platyspondyiy of vertebrae
- Metaphyseal flaring of tubular bones

Achondroplasia (Table 15.6) the heterozygous form is not lethal and is the commonest form of dwarfism – the usual circus dwarf. This is a dominant trait

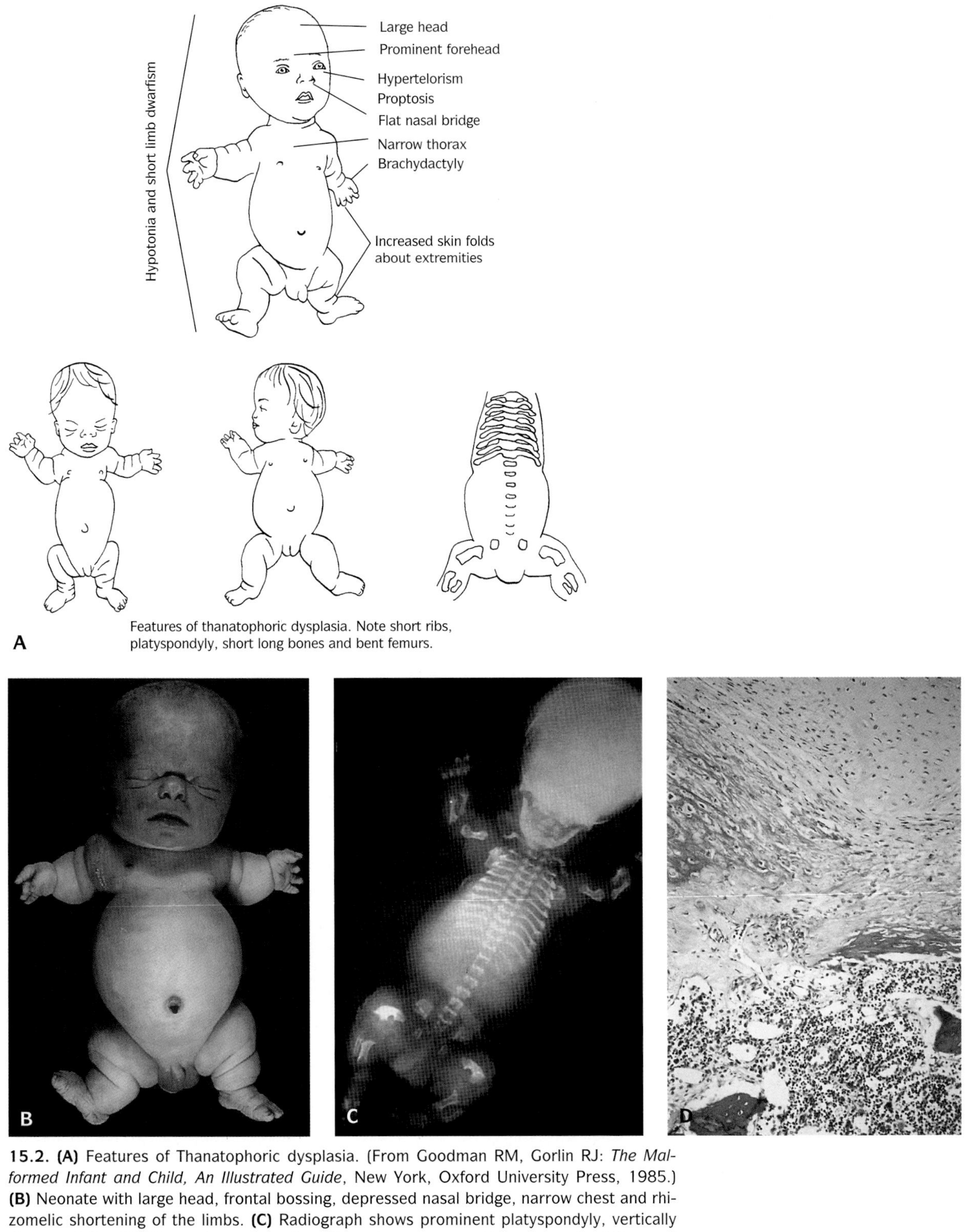

15.2. (A) Features of Thanatophoric dysplasia. (From Goodman RM, Gorlin RJ: *The Malformed Infant and Child, An Illustrated Guide*, New York, Oxford University Press, 1985.) **(B)** Neonate with large head, frontal bossing, depressed nasal bridge, narrow chest and rhizomelic shortening of the limbs. **(C)** Radiograph shows prominent platyspondyly, vertically shortened ilia. **(D)** Photomicrograph of cartilage shows nonspecific severe retardation and disorganization of physeal growth zone with a horizontally oriented band of fibrosis at the physis.

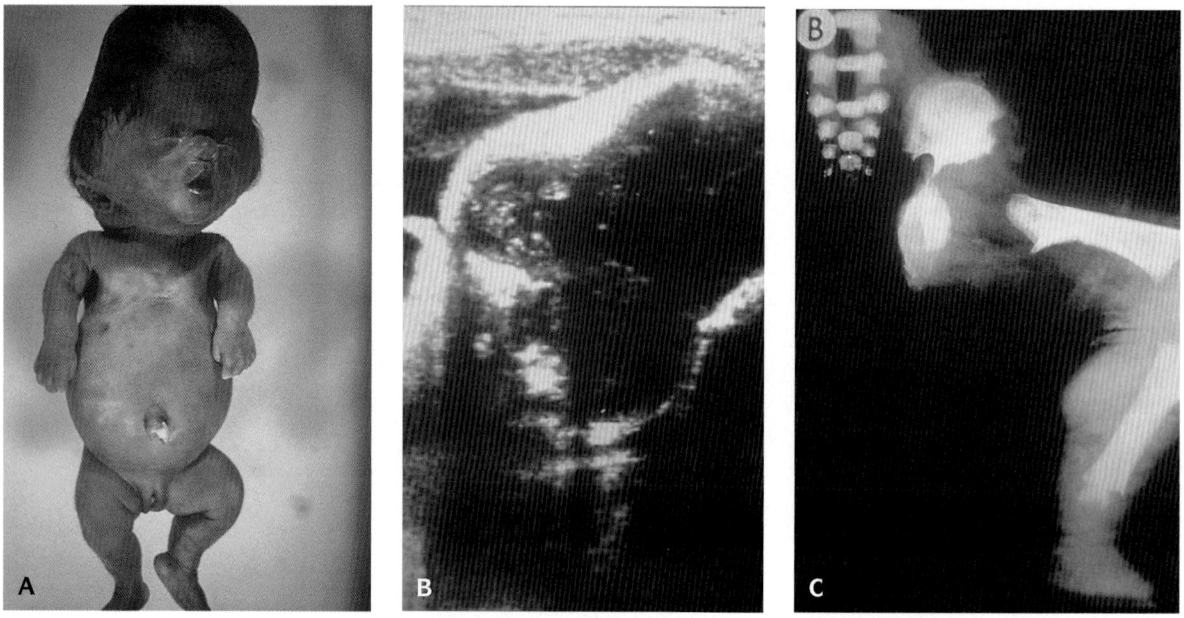

15.3. Thanatophoric dysplasia with cloverleaf skull. **(A)** Newborn with large cloverleaf trilobed skull with rhizomelic shortening of limbs. **(B)** Ultrasound showing cloverleaf skull. **(C)** X-ray. The femur is straight (right).

(Figure 15.4). The homozygous form where both parents are achondroplasics is lethal. It can be detected by ultrasound examination.

Metatropic dysplasia (Table 15.7 and Figure 15.5). Three genetic forms exist: autosomal recessive nonlethal type, dominant nonlethal type, and lethal type with possibly autosomal recessive inheritance. The trunk and limbs are short with bulbous enlargement of the joints and frequently a coccygeal tail. Platyspondyly is more severe than thanatophoric dysplasia and the ribs are short with flared and cupped anterior ends.

Schneckenbecken (snail pelvis), an autosomal recessive condition, is characterized by a snail-like pelvis and short limbs. There is hypercellularity of the resting and proliferating cartilage, the lacunar spaces are inapparent, and the intercellular matrix is relatively inapparent. Reduced columnation and hypervascularity are seen in the proliferating cartilage.

SHORT TRUNK OSTEOCHONDRODYSPLASIAS (TABLE 15.8)

This group of disorders has varying degrees of similarity clinically, radiologically, and even pathologically. The trunk of the affected infant is short. Radiologically, the vertebral bodies show variable abnormalities, ranging from their complete absence to vertebrae that are small, oval, or variable in size. Histopathologically, the cartilage may display significantly abnormal matrix or periodic acid-Schiff (PAS)–positive diastase-resistant chondrocytic inclusions.

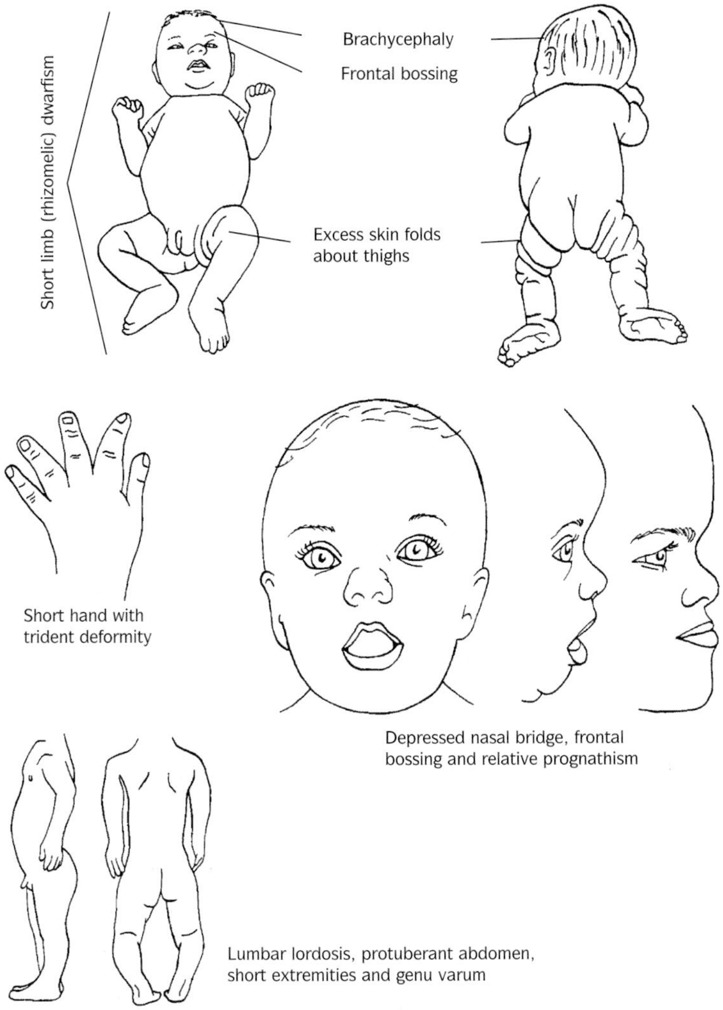

A

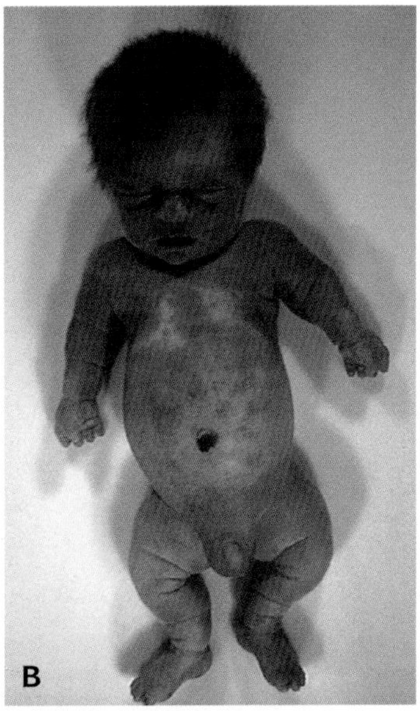
B

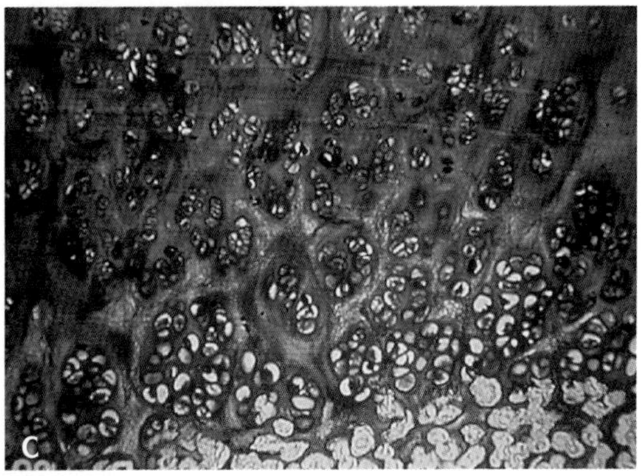
C

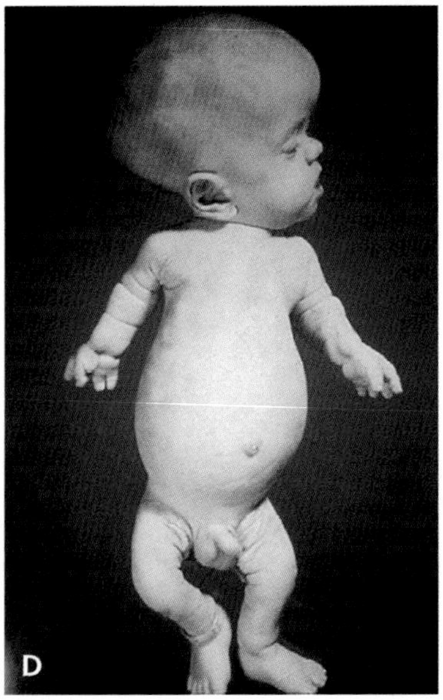
D

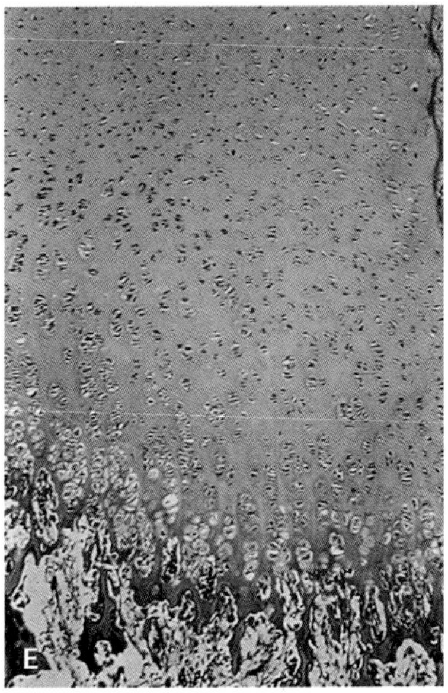
E

15.4. Achondroplasia. **(A)** (From Goodman RM, Gorlin RJ: *The Malformed Infant and Child, An Illustrated Guide*, New York, Oxford University Press, 1985.) **(B)** Newborn with homozygous achondroplasia died shortly after birth. Both parents were also achondroplastic. **(C)** Physeal growth zone of a homozygous achondroplastic with hypercellular proliferative zone and lack of regular columnization (the growth plate in heterozygous achondroplasia shows retardation but no disorganization. **(D)** Newborn with heterozygous (dominant) achondroplasia. One parent was achondroplastic. **(E)** Histologically normal but short growth plate.

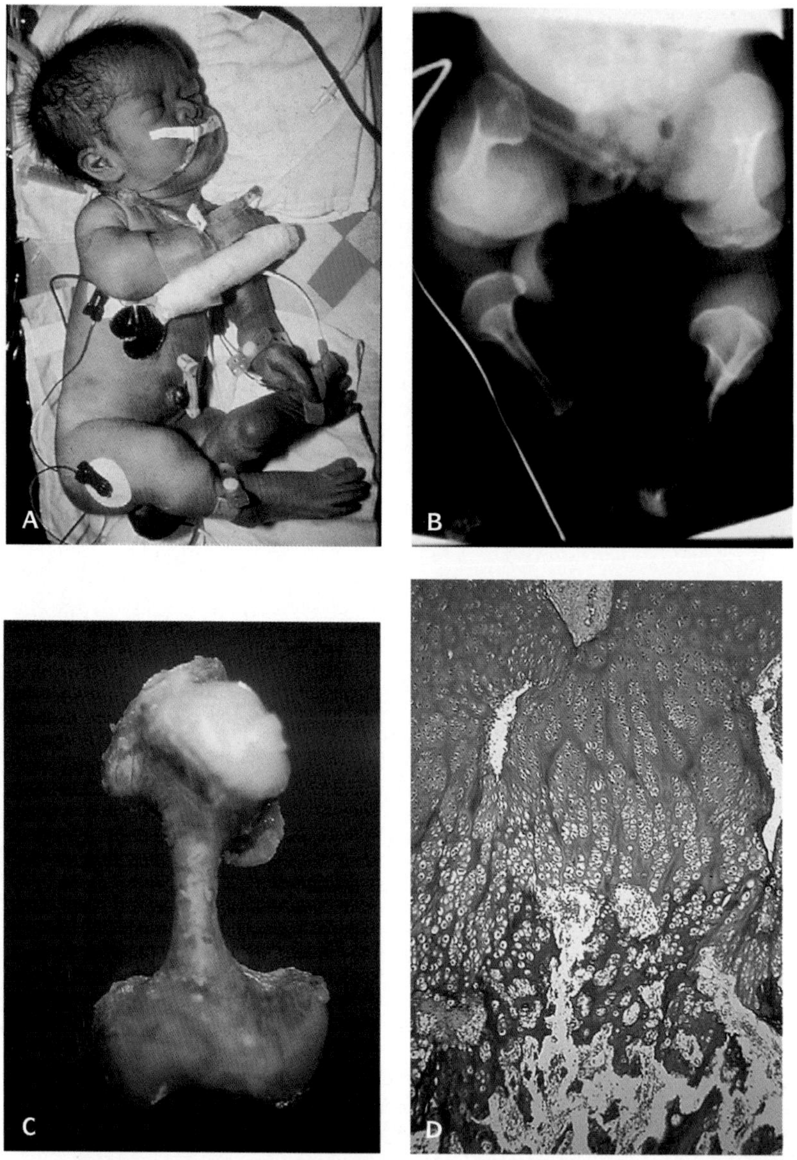

15.5. Metatropic dysplasia. **(A)** Newborn with bulbous enlargement of joints. **(B)** Radiograph shows barbell-like huge metaphyses, severe platyspondyly, and halberd-like ilia. **(C)** Bulbous ends of femora. **(D)** Photomicrograph of the physeal growth zone with irregular vascular penetration of the cartilage and horizontal bars of bone on cartilage. (Courtesy of Dr. Henry Kraus.)

Table 15.7 Metatropic dysplasia

Skeletal abnormalities:
- Small stature, platyspondyly with progressive kyphosis and scoliosis
- Narrow thorax with short ribs
- Short limbs with metaphyseal flaring and epiphyseal irregularity

Table 15.8 Short trunk osteochondrodysplasias

	Radiography				Histopathology	Clinical	
	Short limb	Vertebral body	Metaphysis	Physeal abnormality	Resting cartilage	Prognosis	Genetics
Achondrogenesis IA	++++	Absent	Spikes	+	Chondrocytic inclusions (PAS positive)	Lethal	AR
Achondrogenesis IB	++++	Absent	Spikes	+++	Perichondrocytic collagen rings, matrix deficiency	Lethal	AR
Achondrogenesis II	++++	Absent and small oval	Cupping	+++	Matrix deficiency	Lethal	AD
Hypochondrogenesis	+++	Small oval	Large	+++	Matrix deficiency, focal	Lethal	AD
Spondyloepiphyseal dysplasia congenita	++	Small oval	Slightly increased	+	Chondrocytic inclusions (PAS positive)	Compatible with life	AD
Kniest dysplasia	++	Small oval	Large	+	Chondrocytic inclusions, focal matrix degeneration (PAS positive)	Compatible with life	AD
Dyssegmental dysplasia HS type	++	Irregular segment	Large (campomelia)	+++	Puddle-like spaces	Lethal	AR
Dyssegmental dysplasia RD type	++	Irregular segment (lateral)	Large	–	Foamy Kniest-like degeneration	Lethal (survive beyond neonatal period)	AR
Atelosteogenesis	+++	Absent and small oval	Small distally (club-shaped)	++	Giant cells	Lethal	SP
Boomerang dysplasia	++++	Absent and small oval	Absent or misshapen (boomerang)	+++	Irregularly distributed cells with giant cells	Lethal	SP
Fibrochondrogenesis	+++	Small pear-shaped	Large with spikes	+++	Dysplastic chondrocytes and interwoven fibrous septa	Lethal	AR
Schneckenbecken dysplasia	++++	Flat (AP)	Flared and irregular	++	Hypercellular, lacunar spaces, absent large central nuclei	Lethal	AR

+, mild; ++, moderate; +++, severe; ++++, extreme: (AP), anteroposterior view; (lateral), lateral view; AR, autosomal recessive; AD, autosomal dominant; SP, sporodic.

Source: Gilbert-Barness E, Barness LA: *Metabolic Diseases: Foundations of Clinical Management, Genetics and Pathology*, Natick, Massachusetts, Eaton Publishing, 2000.

Table 15.9 Achondrogenesis: features

Clinical	Radiological	Pathological
Autosomal recessive Death in utero or shortly after birth Hydropic appearance – large head, short trunk and prominent abdomen Micromelia	Vertebral bodies absent or severely retarded ossification In type I, ribs thinner with multiple fractures, tubular bones more severely shortened and bowed	Minimal zone of proliferative cartilage. Lack of columnization. Irregular physeal-metaphyseal junction. Lack of advancing cartilage columns in metaphysis. Paucity of osteoblasts and osteoclasts. Intranuclear inclusions in resting cartilage (type 2). Deficient cartilagenous matrix (type 2).

Achondrogenesis (Table 15.9)

These forms of lethal osteochondrodystrophies represent the most severe forms and are recessively inherited with very short limbs and trunk, large head and protuberant abdomen (Figures 15.6 and 15.7). Types IA (Houston and Harris) and IB have poor cranial ossification and spinal ossification is absent in type IA and incomplete in type IB. An occipital encephalocele has been associated with type 1A and the infant frequently is born prematurely and with fetal hydrops. The growth plate in type 1A is hypercellular and the enlarged chondrocytes have inclusions within a cytoplasmic vacuole that is periodic acid-Schiff (PAS) positive.

Type II has been reclassified as Langer-Saldino dysplasia and forms a spectrum of severity with **congenital spondyloepiphyseal dysplasia** (SED congenita)(Table 15.10 and Figure 15.8) and **hypochondrogenesis** being least and less severe respectively.

Kniest Dysplasia (Table 15.11)

This is an autosomal dominant condition. Limb bones are barbell shaped with large metaphyses (Figure 15.9). Prominent eyes, cleft palate, hearing loss, myopia, and coronal clefting of the lumbar vertebrae are characteristic. Histopathologically, Swiss cheese-like myxoid degeneration is present in the resting cartilage and there are PAS-positive cytoplasmic inclusions.

Table 15.10 Spondyloepiphyseal dysplasia (SED) congenita: features

Clinical	Radiological	Pathologic
Large head Flat face Short neck Short trunk Protuberant abdomen Moderately short limbs Compatible with life	Small oval vertebral bodies Vertically shortened reniform ilia Mildly dysplastic limb bones	Slightly to moderately disorganized physes Chondrocytic inclusions

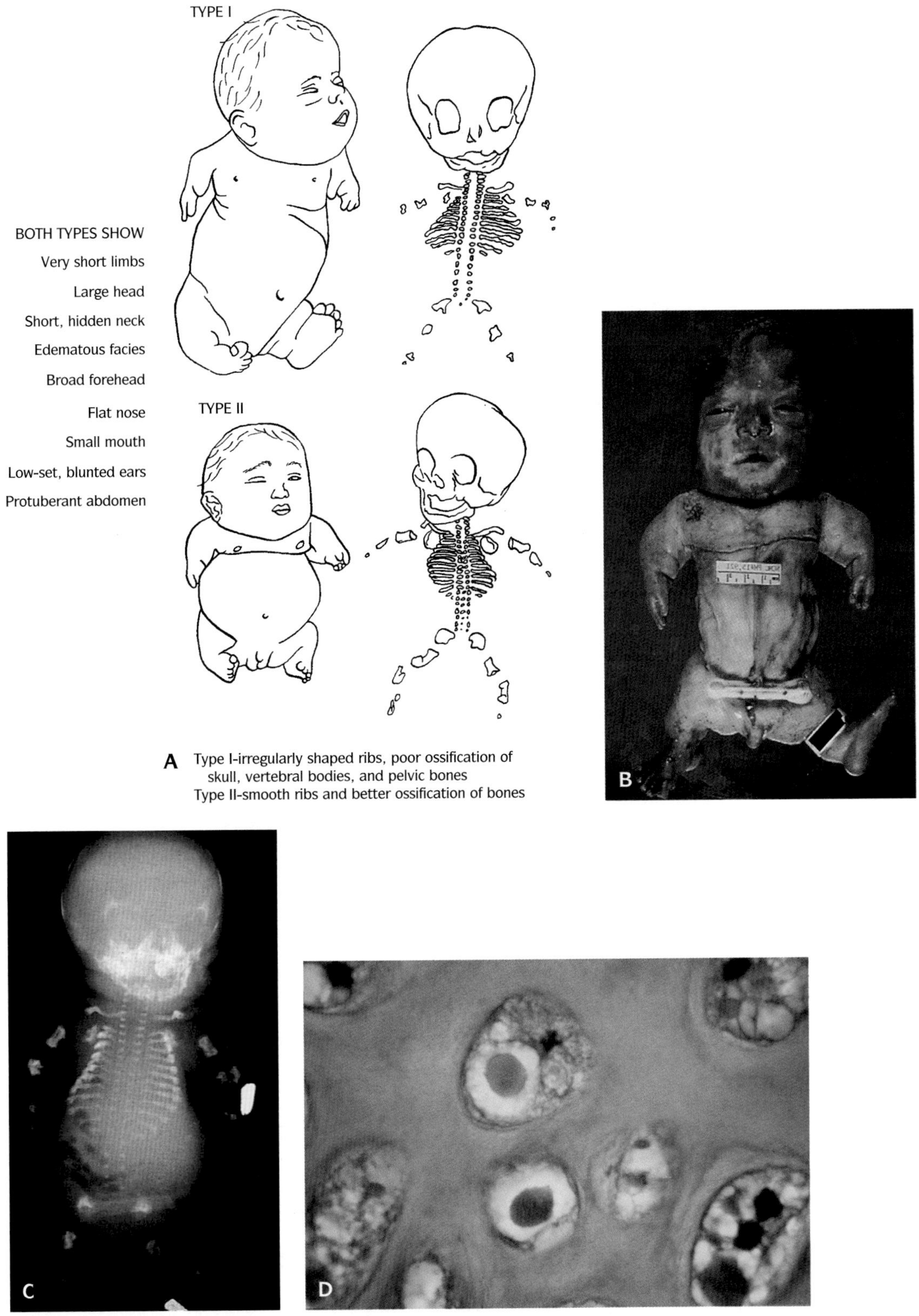

15.6. Achondrogenesis. **(A)** (From Goodman RM, Gorlin RJ: *The Malformed Infant and Child, An Illustrated Guide*, New York, Oxford University Press, 1985.) **(B)** Type IA newborn with extremely short limbs, short trunk, and large head. **(C)** Radiograph of a newborn shows absence of vertebral bodies, ischial and pubic bones, and calvarium. The ribs are irregular in thickness due to multiple fractures. **(D)** Resting cartilage of type IA shows severe retardation and disorganization and large chondrocytic inclusions, which are within vacuoles.

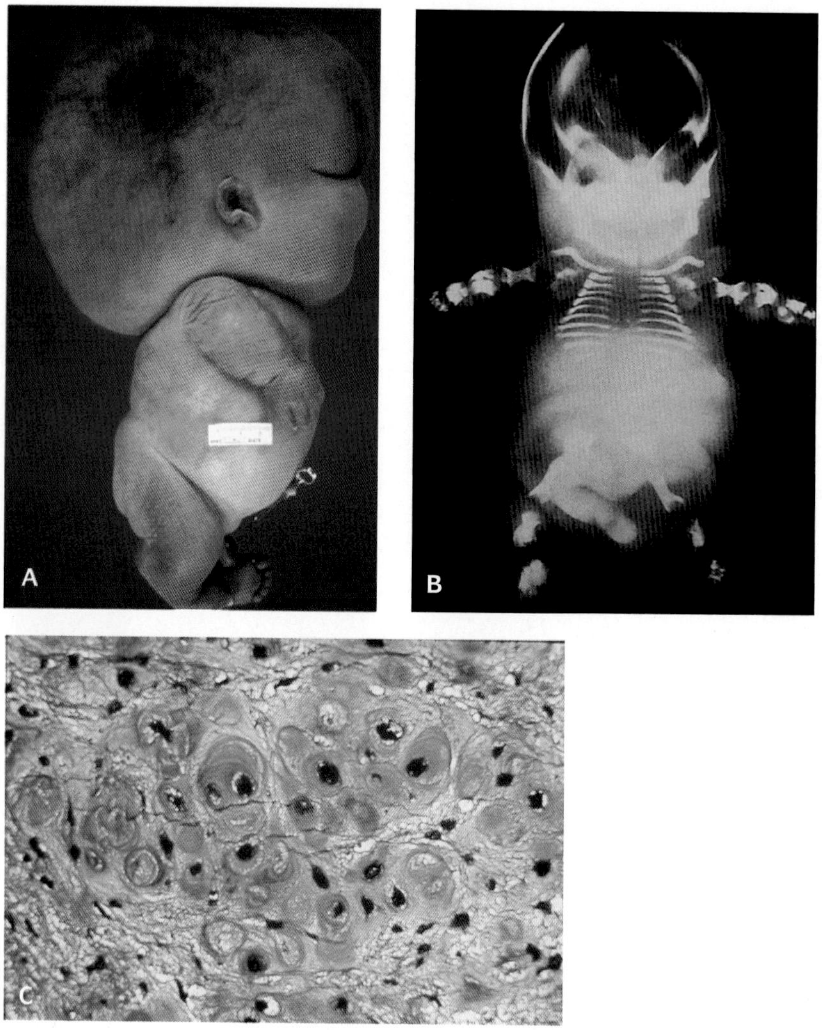

15.7. Achondrogenesis type II. **(A)** Newborn with extremely short limbs, short trunk, and large head. **(B)** Radiograph of a small fetus with absence of vertebral bodies, and ischial and pubic bones. The limb bones are short but better developed than those of type I. The calvarium is well ossified. **(C)** Photomicrograph of resting cartilage shows deficiency of matrix, large chondrocytic lacunae, and large cartilage canals.

Fibrochondrogenesis

The face is round with protuberant eyes, hypertelorism, flat nasal bridge, anteverted nostrils, microstomia, and small dysplastic ears. It is neonatally lethal.

The genetics is autosomal recessive.

Radiologically there are broad limbs with large metaphyses, which are slightly irregular; short ribs and pyriform vertebral bodies on lateral view; and abnormal pelvic bones.

Pathologic changes include interwoven thin fibrous septae encircling clusters of spindle-shaped chondrocytes of the physis.

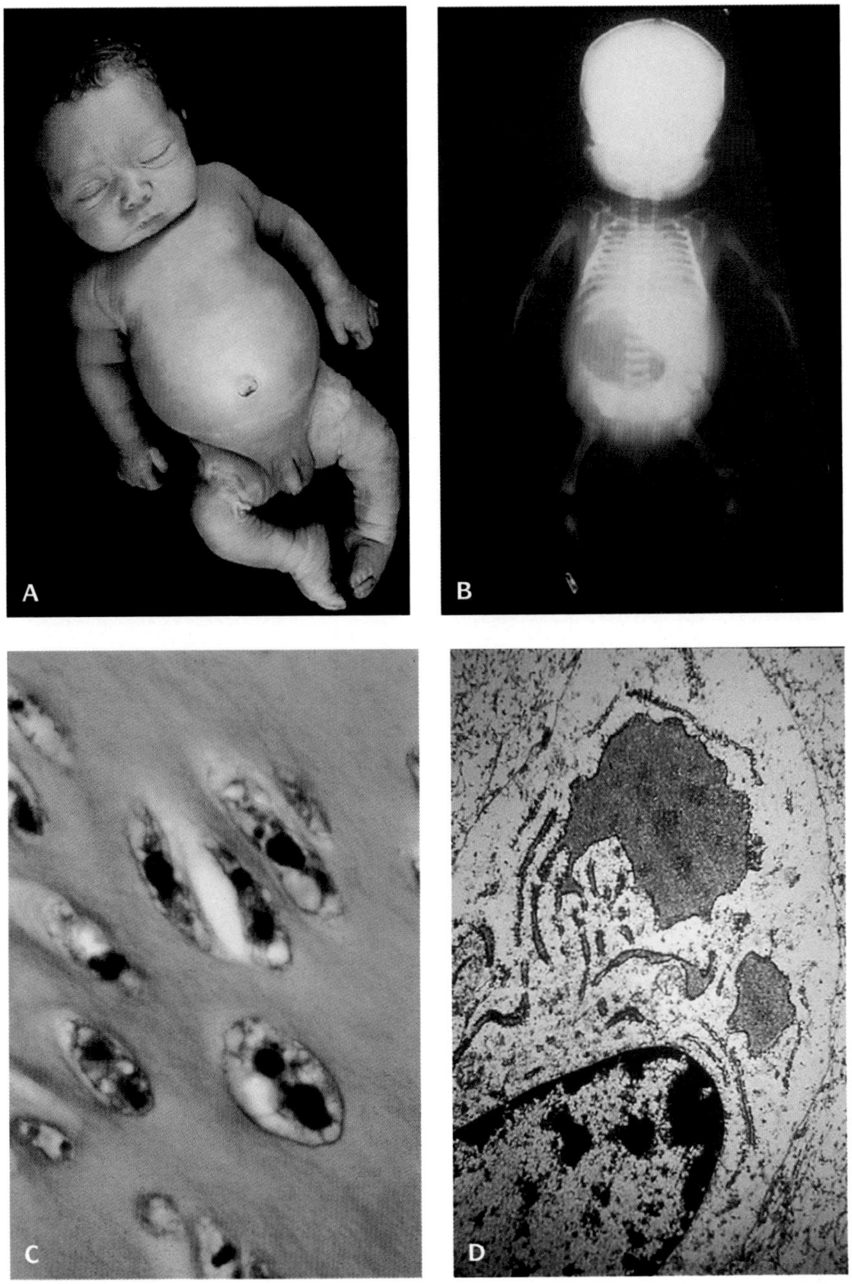

15.8. Spondyloepiphyseal dysplasia congenita. **(A)** Newborn with moderately shortened limbs, short trunk and large head. **(B)** Radiograph showing small oval vertebral bodies, reniform ilia, and slightly dysplastic limb bones. **(C)** Several chondrocytes contain varying sized cytoplasmic inclusions. **(D)** Electronmicrograph of a chondrocyte with dilated cisternae of rough endoplasmic reticulum. The largest cisterna with finely granular material corresponds to an inclusion in **(C)**.

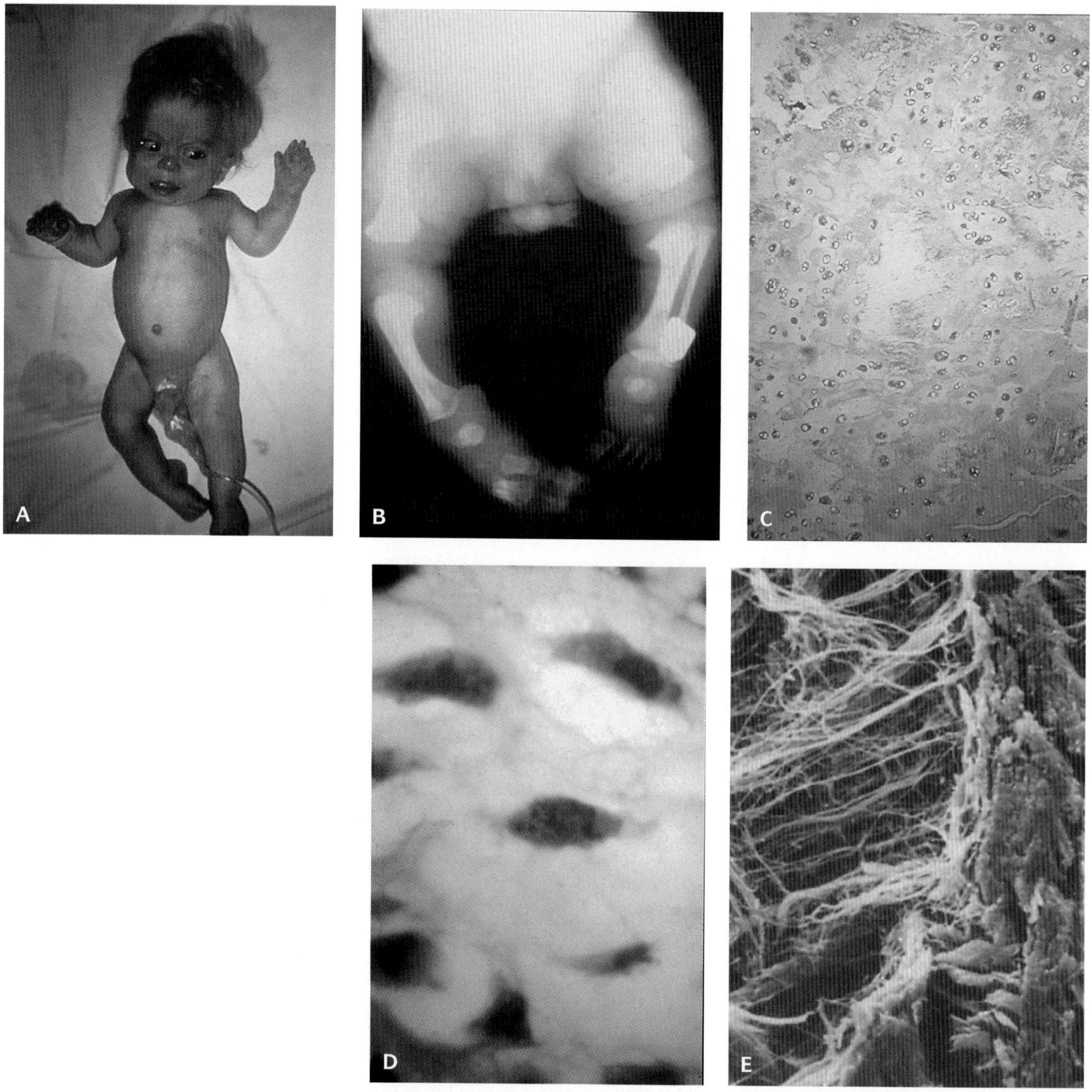

15.9. Kniest dysplasia (KD). **(A)** Infant with severe KD. **(B)** Radiograph of a neonate with markedly enlarged metaphyses of limb bones. **(C)** The cartilage is hypercellular and poorly stained with large cystic spaces. **(D)** Many resting chondrocytes contain cytoplasmic inclusions. **(E)** Scanning electronmicrograph shows web-like cartilage fibrils.

Table 15.11 Kniest dysplasia – severe form: features

Clinical	X-ray
Short-limbed dwarfism.	Bowing of extremities.
Micrognathia.	Short broad tubular bones, metaphyseal widening.
Neonatal respiratory distress.	Coronal clefts of vertebral bodies.
Cleft palate.	Short ribs with flared anterior ends.
Dislocation of lens.	

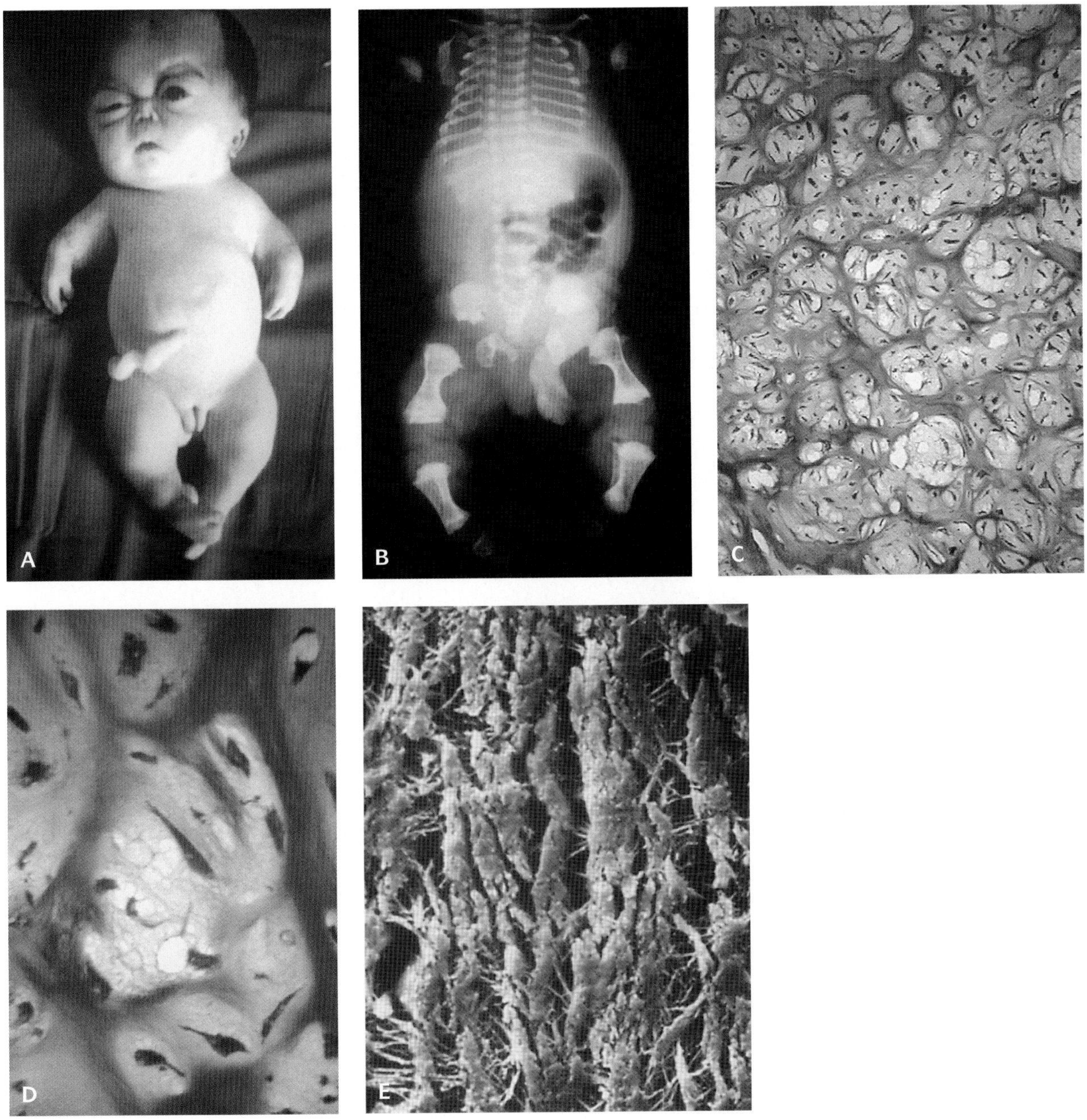

15.10. Fibrochondrogenesis. **(A)** Newborn with short limbs, large head with prominent eyes. **(B)** Radiograph of a neonate with small vertebral bodies, battle-axe-like ilia and barbell-like limb bones. **(C)** Resting cartilage with interwoven fibrous septa and clusters of dysplastic chondrocytes. **(D)** High-power view of spindle-shaped chondrocytes. **(E)** Scanning electron-micrograph showing loosely woven collagen fibrils due to the presence of fibrocytes.

Asphyxiating Thoracic Dysplasia (ATD) (Jeune) (Table 15.12)

This is an autosomal recessive disorder. Infants have a severely narrowed chest with mild shortening of the limbs, polydactyly, congenital heart disease, and abnormal nails and teeth (Figure 15.11). Death occurs shortly after birth due to respiratory failure because of the narrow chest. Mild cystic renal dysplasia

Table 15.12 Asphyxiating thoracic dystrophy (Jeune syndrome)

Autosomal recessive
Severe respiratory distress
Small thoracic cage – short ribs
Protruberant abdomen
Short limbs
Cystic dysplasia kidneys

X-rays
- Chest cage narrow
- Telescoped costo-chondral junction
- Short ribs
- Trident pelvis

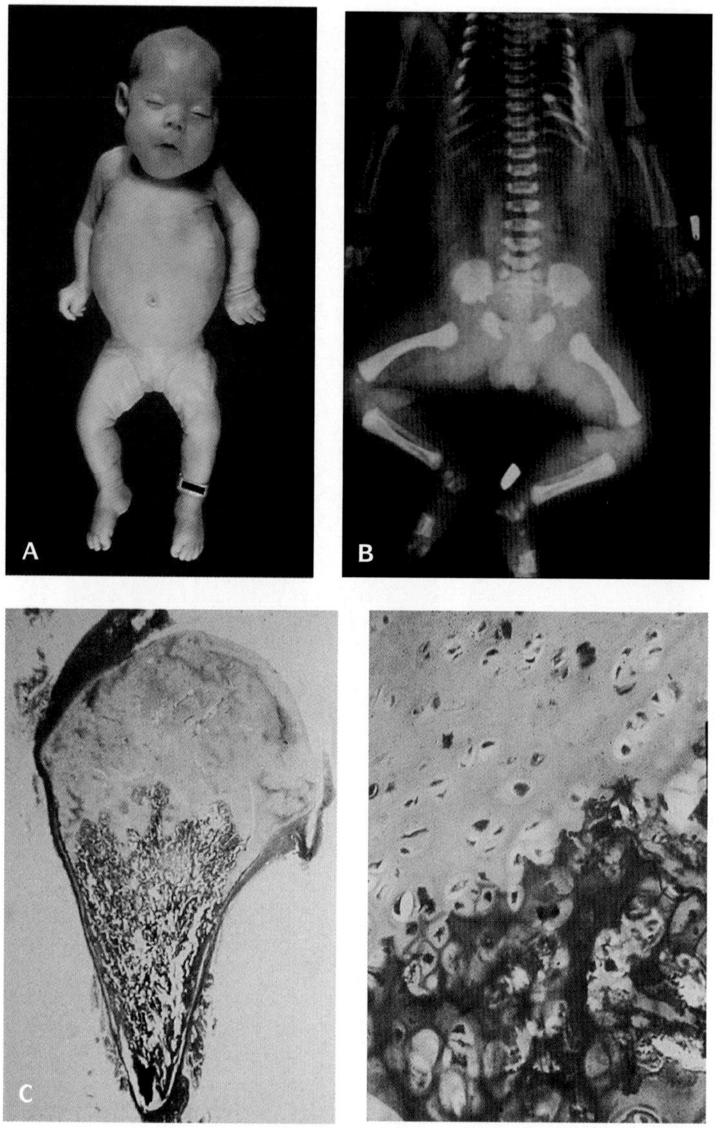

15.11. Asphyxiating thoracic dysplasia, type I. **(A)** Neonate with narrow chest and mild acromelic shortening of the limbs. **(B)** Radiograph of the neonate shows severe shortening of the ribs. The vertebral bodies are unremarkable. **(C)** Growth plate is irregular and disorganized with defective endochondral ossification. Left, low power; right, high power.

and hypoplasia are commonly present. Radiologically, the ribs are very short and the ilia are vertically shortened. Two types have been described: type II is less severe than type I.

Chondroectodermal Dysplasia

The appearance is similar to ATD (Figure 15.12). Postaxial polydactyly and ectodermal dysplasia are present; however, some cases are without polydactyly. There is a short and bound down upper lip. About 50–60% of cases have a congenital heart defect (CHD). There appears to be a better prognosis when a CHD is absent.

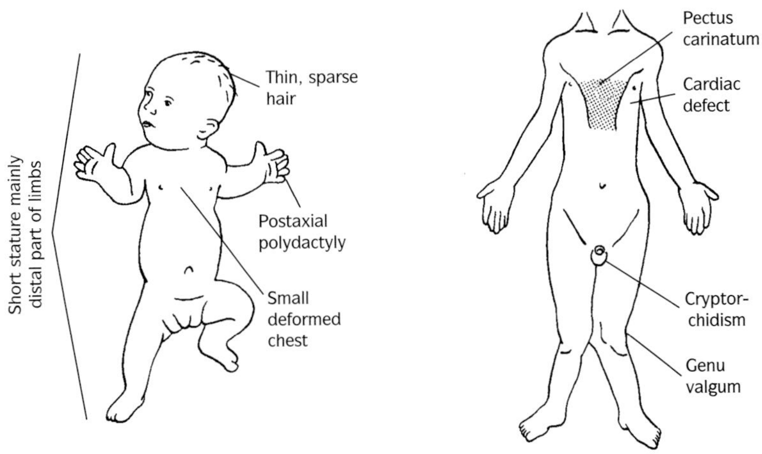

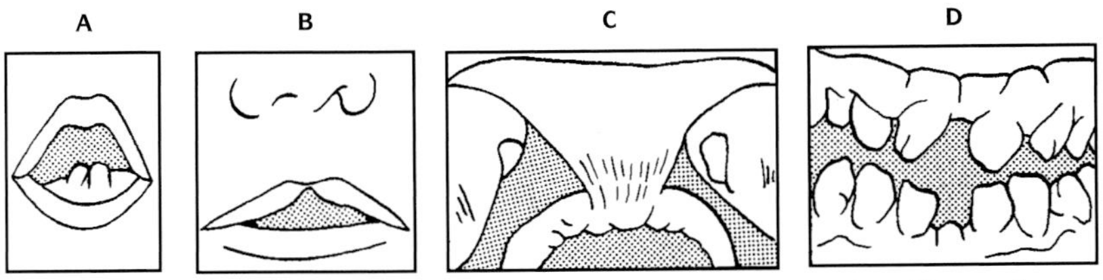

(A) Neonatal teeth, (B) short upper lip with midline defect, (C) upper lip bound by frenulum, (D) malformed, absent and irregularly spaced teeth

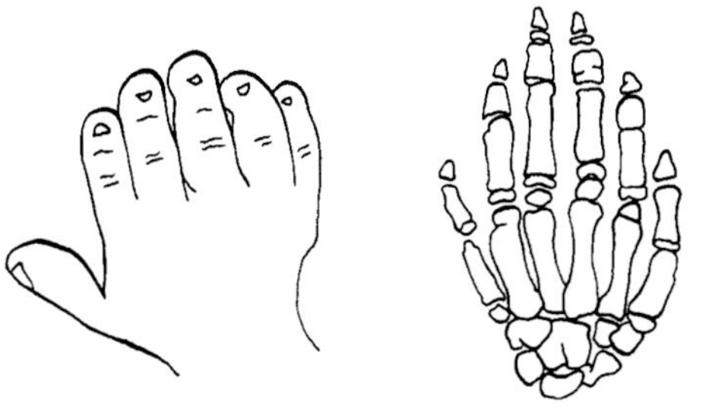

Postaxial polydactyly, hypoplastic nails, malformed middle phalanges and 5th metacarpal, fusion of capitate and hamate

A

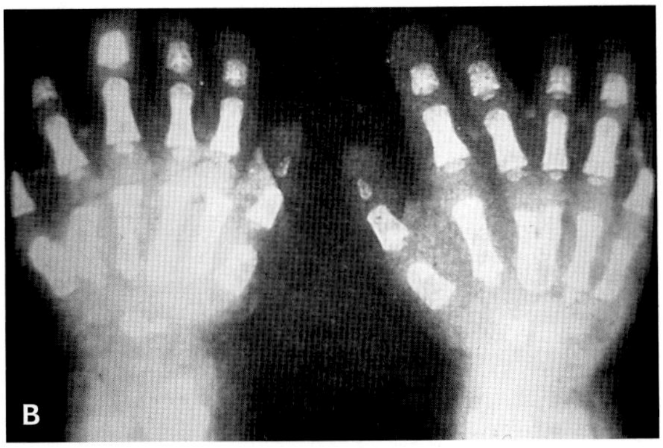

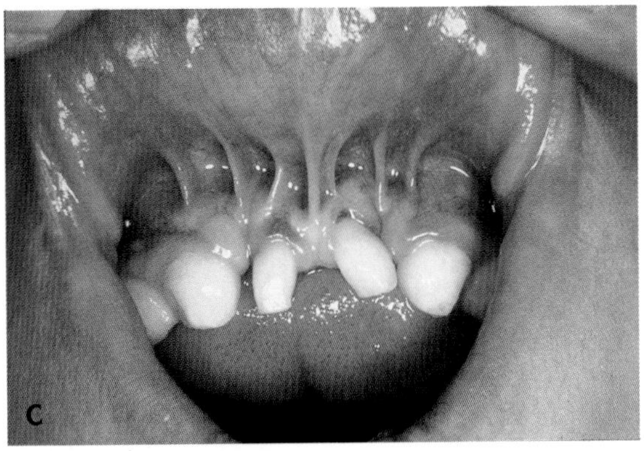

15.12. Ellis-van Creveld (chondroectodermal) dysplasia. **(A)** (From Goodman RM, Gorlin RJ: *The Malformed Infant and Child, An Illustrated Guide*. New York, Oxford University Press, 1985.) **(B)** Radiograph showing polydactyly with fusion of third and fourth metacarpals (right). **(C)** Peg-shaped teeth.

Table 15.13 Short-rib polydactyly dysplasia

	Radiology						Histopathology	Clinical	
	Short ribs	Polydactyly	Short limbs	Vert bod	Ilia	Irreg metaph	Physes	Prognosis	Genetics
Asphyxiating thoracic dystrophy									
Type 1	+++	rare	+	norm	abnorm	+	focal absence	resp and renal insuff	AR
Type 2	+++	rare	+	norm	abnorm	–	abnorm, diff	resp and renal insuff	AR
Ellis van Creveld dysplasia	++	constant	+	norm	abnorm	–	retarded, norm columnization	compatible with life without CHD	AR
Short rib polydactyly dysplasia									
Type I	++++	common	+++	abnorm	abnorm	+++	abnorm, diff	lethal	AR
Type II	++++	common	+++	norm	norm	–	abnorm, diff	lethal	AR
Type III	++++	common	+++	abnorm	abnorm	+++	abnorm, diff	lethal	AR
Type IV	++++	rare	+++	abnorm	abnorm	–	abnorm, diff	lethal	AR

+, mild; ++, moderate; +++, severe; ++++, extreme; vert bod, vertebral bodies; irreg metaph, irregular metaphyseal borders; norm, normal; abnorm, abnormal; diff, diffuse; resp, respiratory; insuff, insufficiency; CHD, congenital heart disease; AR, autosomal recessive.

Source: Gilbert-Barness, E (ed): *Potter's Pathology of the Fetus and Infant*, Philadelphia, Mosby Year Book, 1997.

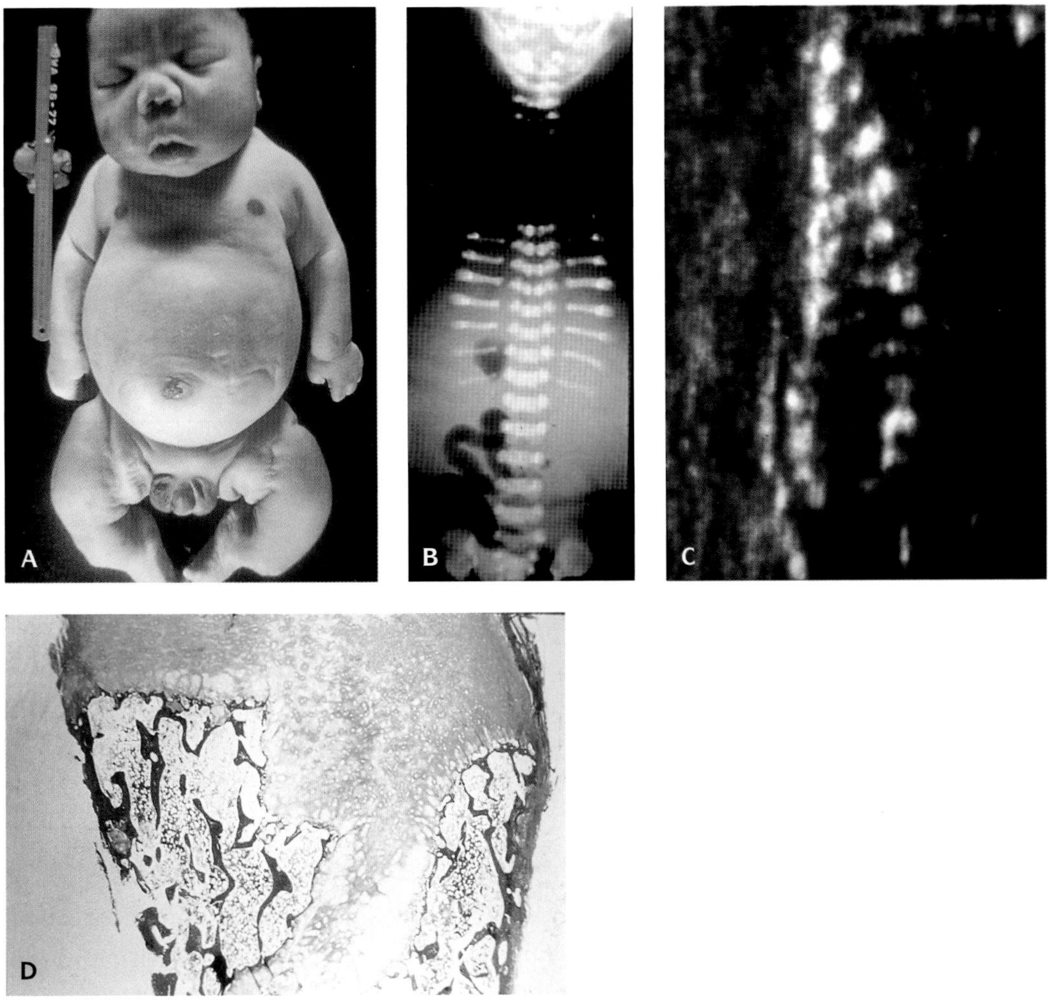

15.13. Short rib polydactyly (SRP) dysplasia, type I. **(A)** Newborn with short limbs, narrow chest, and polydactyly. **(B)** Radiograph of a premature neonate shows extremely shortened ribs. The vertebral bodies, ilia, and limb bones are also severely dysplastic. **(C)** Ultrasound of short ribs. **(D)** Histologic section shows portion of central physeal fibrosis with tongue of fibrosis extending into metaphysis at center. It is surrounded by markedly deranged physeal chondrocytes.

The genetics is autosomal recessive. Radiological changes similar to those in ATD are present with polydactyly.

Short-Rib Polydactyly Syndromes (Table 15.13)

These disorders are characterized by a narrow thorax due to short ribs, usually polydactyly and short limbs with an abnormal growth plate. They are autosomal recessive disorders.

The short-rib polydactyly dysplasias types I–IV have been classified as Saldino-Noonan (type I), Majewski (type II), Verma-Naumoff (type III), and Beemer-Langer (type IV) (Table 15.14 and Figure 15.13).

Table 15.14 Short-rib polydactyly syndrome: features

Clinical (Saldino-Noonan type I)	Pathological (Saldino-Noonan type I)
Autosomal recessive, Hydropic appearance at birth, Short-limb type of dwarfism, Postaxial polydactyly; brachydactyly, Narrow thorax, protuberant abdomen, Death in utero or shortly after birth, Multiple internal malformations, including cardiovascular (mostly transposition of the great vessels), hypoplastic lungs, anal atresia, and abnormalities of the genital organs.	Thin zone of proliferating cartilage Lack of columnization Small irregular areas of calcifying cartilage Tongues of cartilage extend into metaphysis Disarray of osteoid Cystic dysplastic kidneys Hypoplastic lungs Visceral malformations

OSTEOCHONDRODYSPLASIAS WITH ABNORMAL BONE DENSITY

These include the following:

- Osteogenesis imperfecta (OI)
- Hypophosphatasia
- Osteopetrosis (OP)
- Pyknodysostoses (PD)
- Dominant osteosclerosis, type Stanescu (OS)
- Infantile cortical hyperostosis (ICH)

Osteogenesis Imperfecta (OI) (Tables 15.15 and 15.16)

This condition is an autosomal dominantly inherited defect of collagen characterized by osteopenia, multiple fractures, blue or white sclerae, and Wormian bones of the calvaria. Six types have been delineated with subtypes. Type I,

Table 15.15 Classification of osteogenesis imperfecta

Type	Fragility of bone	Sclerae	Bowing	Deafness	Genetics	Abnormality
IA	+	Blue	–	+	AD	Reduced synthesis of pro αI(1) low type 1 collagen Short o2 chain
IB	+	Blue	–	+	AD	
II	++	Blue			AR	Abnormal pro αI(I) collagen chains
IIA					AD	
IIB					AR	
IIC					AR	Structurally abnormal, mannose-rich pro αI(I) chain
III	++	Blue-White	+	?	AR AD	Nonfunctional α2 gene; type 1 – (αI(I)), trimer; defective α2 chain Normal type I collagen production; defective cross-links
IVA	+	White	±	–	AD	Low α(I) chain, low type I total collagen
IVB	+	White	±	–	AD	Normal αI(I) chain, normal type collagen

Subclassifications of types I, II, and IV are distinguished radiologically.

Source: Gilbert-Barness, E, ed: *Potter's Pathology of the Fetus and Infant*. Philadelphia, Mosby Year Book, 1997.

Table 15.16 Osteogenesis imperfecta type 2: features

Clinical	Radiological	Pathological
Short limb dwarfism Large head, wide fontanels Poorly ossified or unossified calvarium (caput membranaceum) Hypotonia, hyperlaxity of ligaments Prominent eyeballs, blue sclerae Small nose, depressed nasal bridge	Caput membranaceum – multiple wormian bones Generalized osteoporosis, multiple fractures, and callus formation Thick, short shafts of long bones Rarely survive – cystic changes long bones Genetic transmission – ? new dominant mutation	Cartilage, columnization, and vascularization normal. Cartilaginous columns invested with PAS-positive and argyrophilic material resembling precollagen. Normal calcification of chondroid columns. Scanty or absent osteoid. Scanty osseous trabeculae thin and spidery. Excessive callus formation at fracture sites.

the most common type with four subtypes, is characterized by recurrent fractures during childhood; type II has fractures in utero; type III is the most severe nonlethal form, frequently with intrauterine fractures; type IV is moderately severe, with fractures and bowing of long bones after birth; type V, with vertebral compression fractures, and type VI, with usually anterior dislocation of the radial head, are rare forms.

Type II (OI Congenita, OI Fetalis, Vrolik Disease)

This is lethal and is the type most commonly seen in the newborn. It is due to a new autosomal dominant mutation with an abnormality in secretion of type I procollagen (Figure 15.14). The clinical features include:

- Multiple fractures in utero, particularly of the long bones and ribs
- Hyperlaxity of joints
- Defective ossification of the calvaria with small islands in the center of each bone (Wormian bones)
- Excessive callus formation at site of fractures
- Deep blue sclerae
- Skeletal X-rays characteristically with beaded ribs and crumpled long bones

CNS Abnormalities in Type II Osteogenesis Imperfecta

Type I collagen promotes neurogenic maturation both in vitro and in vivo in osteogenesis imperfecta; type IIA brains show migrational defects with coexisting periventricular leukomalacia (PVL) and gliosis. In type IIB, the brain has white matter gliosis, PVL, and perivascular calcifications. In type IIC the brain shows hippocampal malrotation agyria, abnormal neuronal lamination, diffuse hemorrhage, and PVL. Collagen mutations appear to negatively affect CNS development.

Pathology

The collagen defect results in a defect of production of osteoid and results in calcification directly in cartilage with severe deficiency of ossification. Abnormal bony spicules in the cortex are composed of primitive woven bone and excessive fibrosis and callus formation at fracture sites.

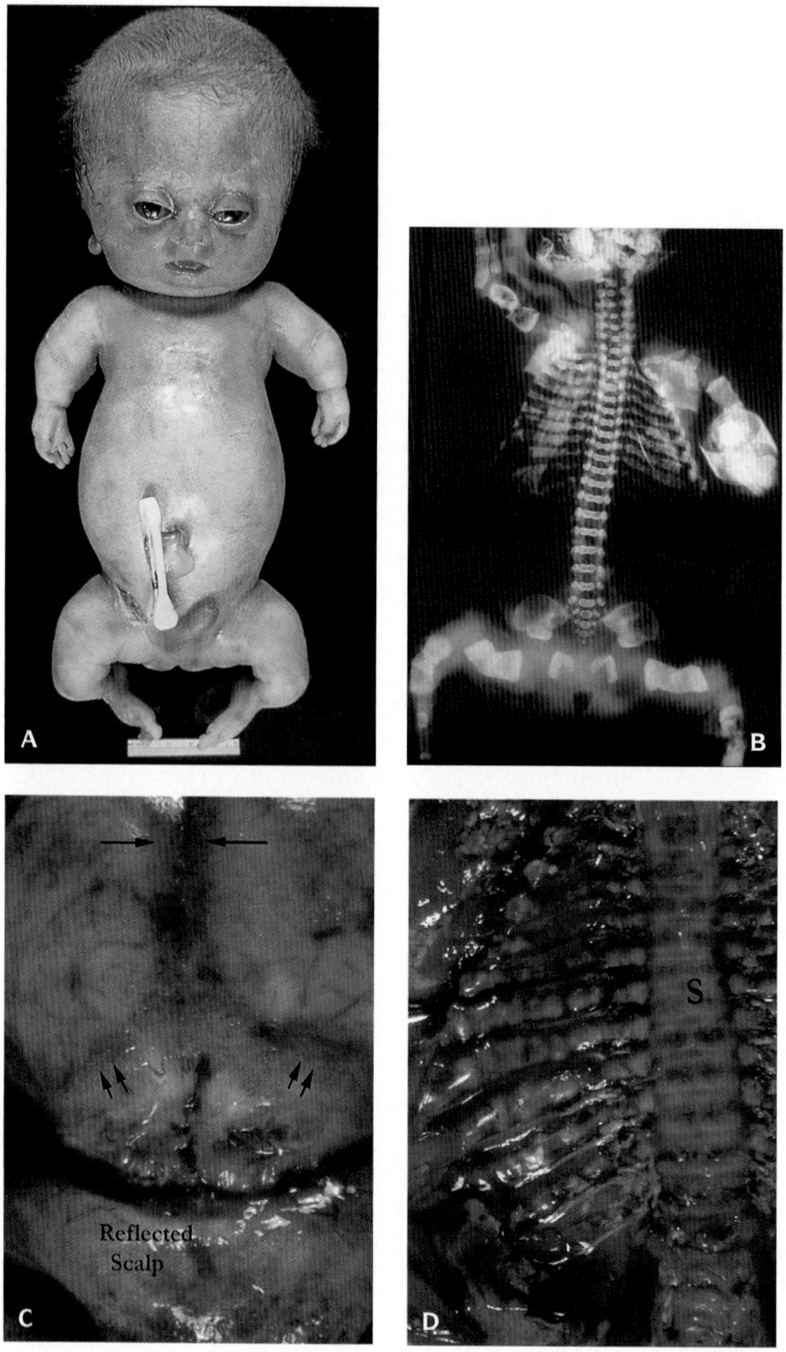

15.14. Osteogenesis imperfecta. **(A)** Type II neonate with short distorted limbs due to multiple fractures. **(B)** Radiograph of type IIA after exhumation. The bones are well preserved and show innumerable fractures involving all tubular bones and ribs. **(C)** The calvarium is parchment-like with poorly ossified small foci of defective bone (Wormian bones) and visable brain beneath (single arrows, sagittal sinus; double arrows, tentorium). **(D)** Multiple rib fractures. (S, spine.)

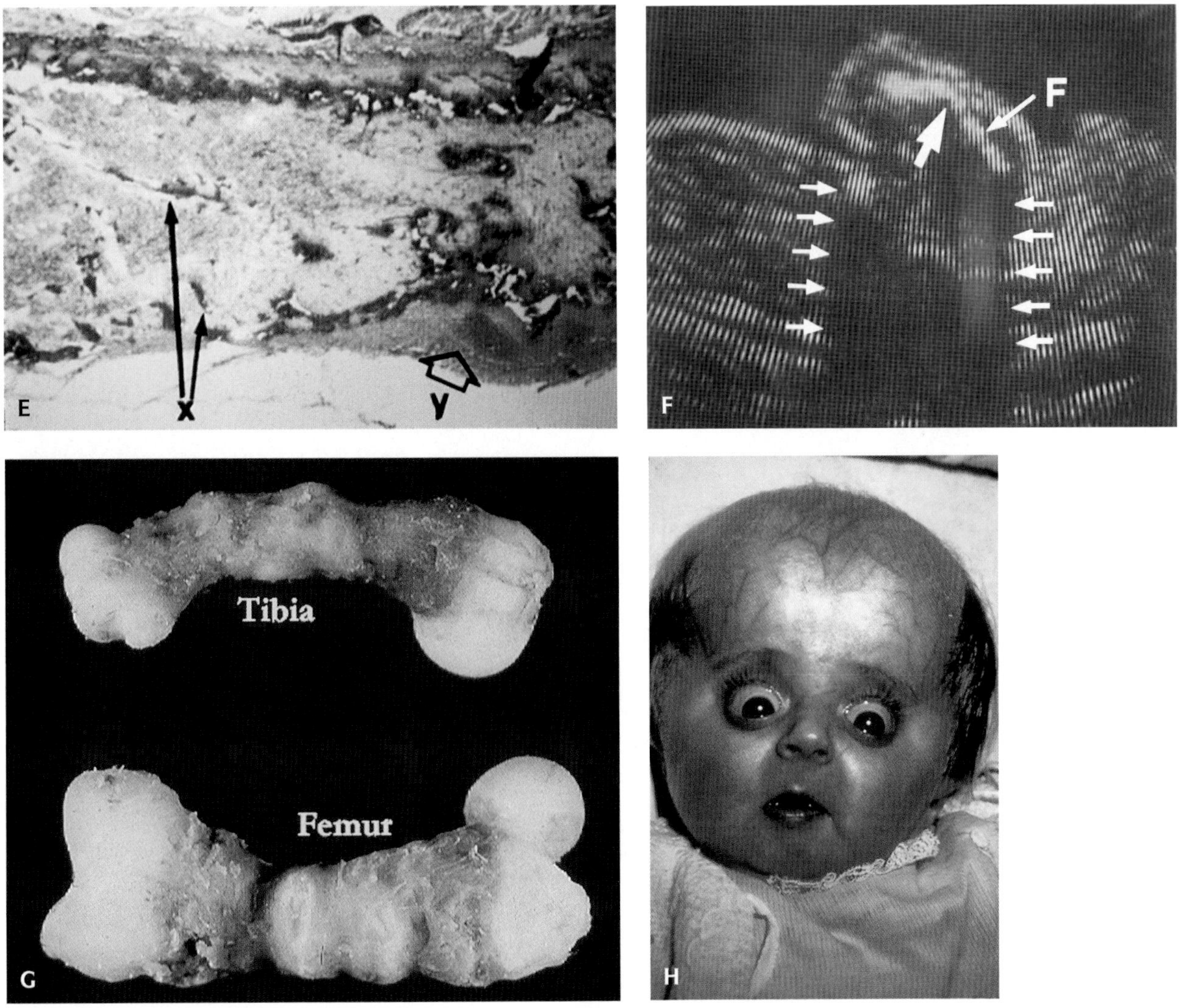

15.14. (*continued*) **(E)** Microscopic section of calvarium with scattered areas (arrows) of calcification but no ossification. **(F)** Ultrasound showing femoral (F) fracture (arrow). **(G)** Tibia and femur with multiple fractures. **(H)** Infant with type III osteogenesis imperfecta with globular skull and blue sclerae.

Prenatal diagnosis is by chorionic villus sampling between 9 and 16 weeks gestation, by serum DNA testing, and by level II ultrasound at 15 weeks gestation.

Hypophosphatasia (Congenital Lethal Type) (Table 15.17)

This disorder is due to defective bone mineralization with deficiency of serum alkaline phosphatase activity in bone/liver/kidney (Figure 5.15). Phosphoethanolamine and inorganic pyrophosphate in the blood and urine are increased. The condition is autosomal recessive due to a point mutation with a small deletion in the alkaline phosphatase gene and in RNA. The gene is located at the distal end of the short arm of chromosome 1.

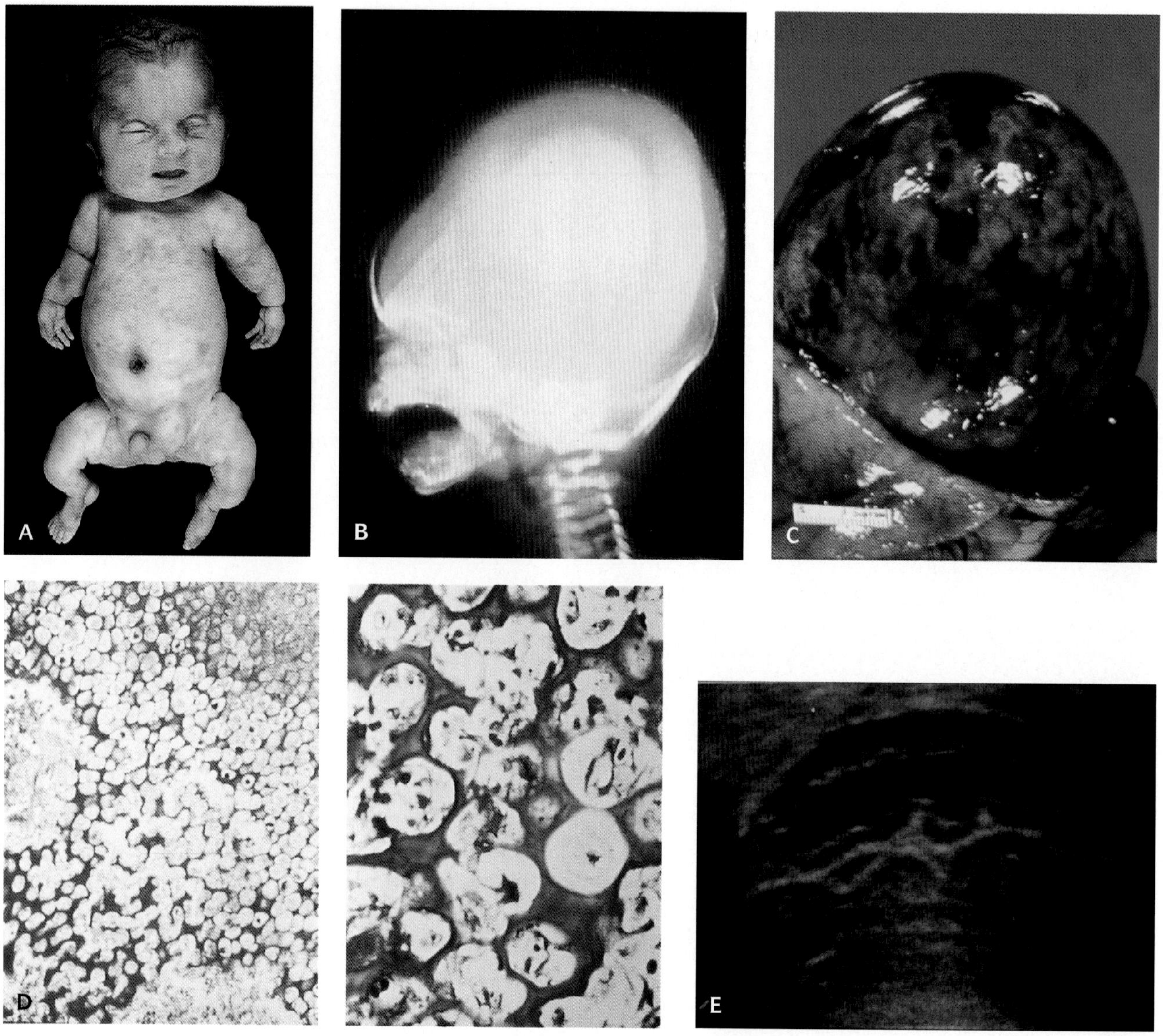

15.15. Hypophosphatasia, congenital lethal type. **(A)** Neonate with short limbs and multiple fractures. **(B)** Radiograph of head shows absence of bone. **(C)** Scalp reflected shows boneless skull. **(D)** Photomicrograph of metaphysis shows unmineralized broad columns of cartilage covered by poorly mineralized osteoid seams. The physeal growth zone is disorganized (left). Cartilage cells are large vacuolated with abundant unossified matrix (right). **(E)** Ultrasound showing demineralized skull.

Clinical features of infantile hypophosphatasia include the following:

- Head of the neonate small, globular, and soft
- Metaphyseal bulging
- Limbs disproportionately shortened
- Hypercalcemia
- Long bones soft and subject to fractures
- Serum phosphorus normal

Table 15.17 Hypophosphatasia (congenital lethal form): features

Clinical	X-ray	Pathological
Autosomal recessive Globular "boneless" skull Soft skeleton Severe deformities and shortening of extremities Blue sclerae Low alkaline phosphatase in serum, bone, and other tissues High urinary excretion of ethanolamine and inorganic pyrophosphate Hypercalcemia	Absent ossification of calvarium and vertebrae Healing fractures with deformities Short, thin ribs and tubular bones	Resting cartilage at growing ends of long bones normal Proliferating cartilage widened Irregularity of cartilage cell columns Failure of calcification of lytic cartilage Osteoid abundant – failure of mineralization Osteoblasts and osteoclasts normal in number and morphology

- Low serum alkaline phosphatase level
- Elevated urinary phosphoethanolamine levels.

Radiology

- Calvarium is poorly ossified.
- Metaphyseal cuppings are irregular.
- Long bones and ribs are thin.
- There are multiple fractures.

Pathology

- Broad columns of unmineralized cartilage covered by poorly mineralized osteoid seams.

Physeal growth zone in the neonatal period is widened and thickened, hypercellular, and disorderly arranged; alkaline phosphatase in this area is markedly reduced.

MISCELLANEOUS GROUP OF OSTEOCHONDRODYSPLASIAS

A miscellaneous group of osteochondrodysplasias are enumerated in Table 15.18.

Chondrodysplasia Punctata (Table 15.19 and 15.20)

- Rhizomelic type – stippled epiphyses (symmetric spine spared); myxoid and cystic degeneration of subarticular cartilage with calcification; autosomal recessive (AR) (Figure 15.16). Two missense mutations in the PEX 7 gene on chromosome 4 (4p16–p14) are the genetic defects.
- Conradi-Hünermann type – stippled epiphyses (extensive and asymmetric); calcification adjacent to the physis; myxoid degeneration in the physis and adjacent resting cartilage; X-linked dominant (XLD). Abnormal cholesterol biosynthesis. A candidate gene for sterol-δ-8-isomerase on Xp11.22–p11.23.

Table 15.18 Miscellaneous osteochondrodysplasias

	Radiography	Histopathology of cartilage	Genetics
Chondodysplasia punctata			
Rhizomelic type	Stippled epiphyses (symmetric spine spared)	Myxoid and cystic degeneration of subarticular cartilage with calcification	AR
Conradi-Hünerman type	Stippled epiphyses (extensive and asymmetric)	Calcification adjacent to the physis. Myxoid degeneration in the physis and adjacent resting cartilage	XLD
X-linked recessive type	Stippled epiphyses (multiple epiphyses, para vertebral and laryngotracheal)	ND	XLR
MT type	Stippled epiphyses (sacral, tarsal and carpal regions)	ND	SP
Campomelic dysplasia	Curved tibiae, fibulae and/or femora	Unremarkable	AR
Kyphomelic dysplasia	Curved short femora	ND	AR
Diastrophic dysplasia	"Hitchhiker" thumbs and great toes	Matrix deficiency with myxoid and microcytic degeneration, especially in subarticular region	AR
Larsen syndrome	Multiple joint dislocations	Unremarkable	AD, AR
Desbuquois syndrome	Multiple joint dislocations	Narrow disorganized physeal growth zone, the cells in ovoid groups. Small hyperplastic cells. Resting chondrocytes increased and large	

AR, autosomal recessive; AD, autosomal dominant; XLD, X-linked dominant; XLR, X-linked recessive; ND, not described.

Source: Gilbert-Barness E, ed: *Potter's Pathology of the Fetus and Infant*. Philadelphia, Mosby Year Book, 1997.

Table 15.19 Chondrodysplasia punctata, rhizomelic form: features

Clinical	Radiological
Autosomal recessive	Coronal cleft of vertebral bodies
Shortness of stature with proximal shortening of extremities	Symmetric shortening, metaphyseal splaying, and calcific stippling of humeri and femora
Chipmunk facies	
Bilateral cataracts	
Icthyosiform rash	
Multiple joint contractures	

Pathological
Degeneration of epiphyseal cartilage
Resorption, vascularization, calcification, and sometimes ossification of epiphyseal cartilage
Disturbance in maturation of cartilage
Lack of columnar alignment
Mucoid degeneration with cyst formation
Tongues of cartilage extending into metaphyses of osseous shaft
Zones of granulation tissue. Sites of reaction to possible metabolic injury
Cancellous bone formed directly on resting cartilage

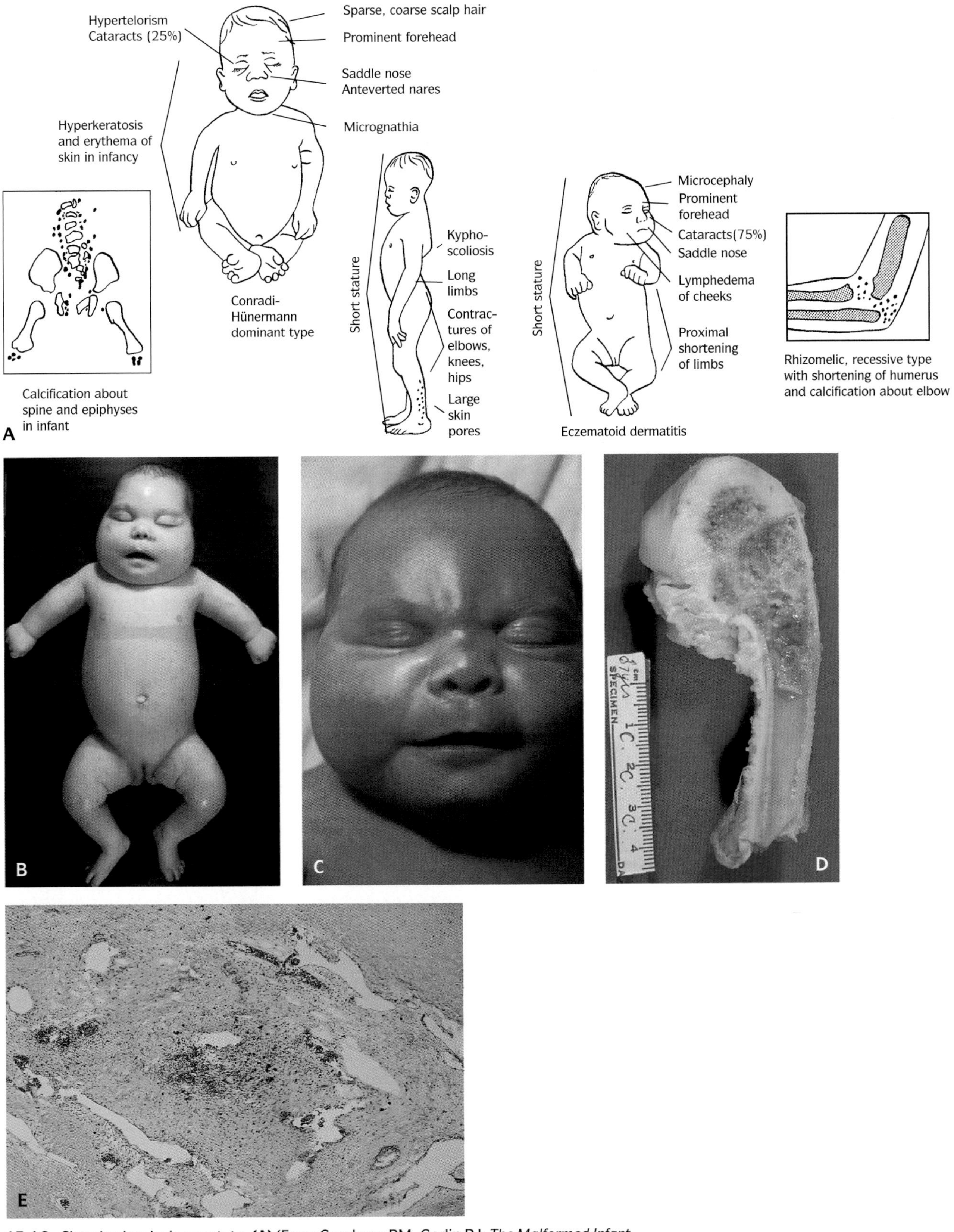

15.16. Chondrodysplasia punctata. **(A)** (From Goodman RM, Gorlin RJ: *The Malformed Infant and Child, An Illustrated Guide*. New York, Oxford University Press, 1985.) **(B)** A neonate with rhizomelic type microcephaly and rhizomelic shortening of extremities. **(C)** Chipmunk-like facies. **(D)** Subarticular myxoid and cystic degeneration of the cartilage in rhizomelic type. **(E)** Microscopic focus of cystic degeneration of cartilage with calcific foci.

Table 15.20 Chondrodysplasia punctata

	Conradi-Hunermann dominant	Rhizomelic type recessive	Dominant sex-linked
Radiology Severe bilateral shortening of femora and/or humeri	Absent	Present	Asymmetric shortening of arms and legs
Severe metaphyseal changes of femora and/or humeri	Absent	Present	Absent
Distribution of lesions	Frequently asymmetric	Mostly symmetric	Asymmetric
Pathology	Calcification in and about cartilage	Subarticular degeneration calcification	?

Campomelic Dysplasia

The features of campomelic dysplasia (Figure 15.17) are summarized in Table 15.22.

OTHER FORMS OF OSTEOCHONDRODYSTROPHIES

- X-linked recessive type of chondrodysplasia punctata – stippled epiphyses (multiple epiphyses, para vertebral and laryngotracheal).
- Campomelic dysplasia – Curved tibiae, fibulae and/or femora; AR (Tables 15.21 and 15.22)
- Kyphomelic dysplasia – curved short femora; AR
- Diastrophic dysplasia – hitchhiker thumbs and great toes; AR (Figures 15.17 and 15.18)
- Larsen syndrome – multiple joint dislocations; autosomal dominant (AD), AR
- Desbuquois syndrome – multiple joint dislocations; narrow disorganized physeal growth zone, the cells in ovoid groups; small hyperplastic cells; resting chondrocytes increased and large; AR

Table 15.21 Conditions associated with epiphyseal calcific stippling

Chromosomal disorders	**Metabolic disorders**
Trisomy 18	Smith-Lemli-Optiz syndrome
Trisomy 21	Cretinism
Lysosomal disorders	**Drug-induced disorders**
Mucopolysaccharidosis	Warfarin embryopathy
Mucolipidosis	Fetal hydantoin syndrome
GM1 gangliosidosis	Alcohol embryopathy
Peroxisomal disorders	**Others**
Chondrodysplasia punctata, rhizomelic type	Chondrodysplasia punctata, other types
Zellweger cerebrohepatorenal syndrome	

Adapted from Wood B, Dimmick JE: Skeletal system. In Dimmick JE, Kalousek DK (eds): *Developmental Pathology of the Embryo and Fetus*, Philadelphia, J.B. Lippincott Company, 1992.

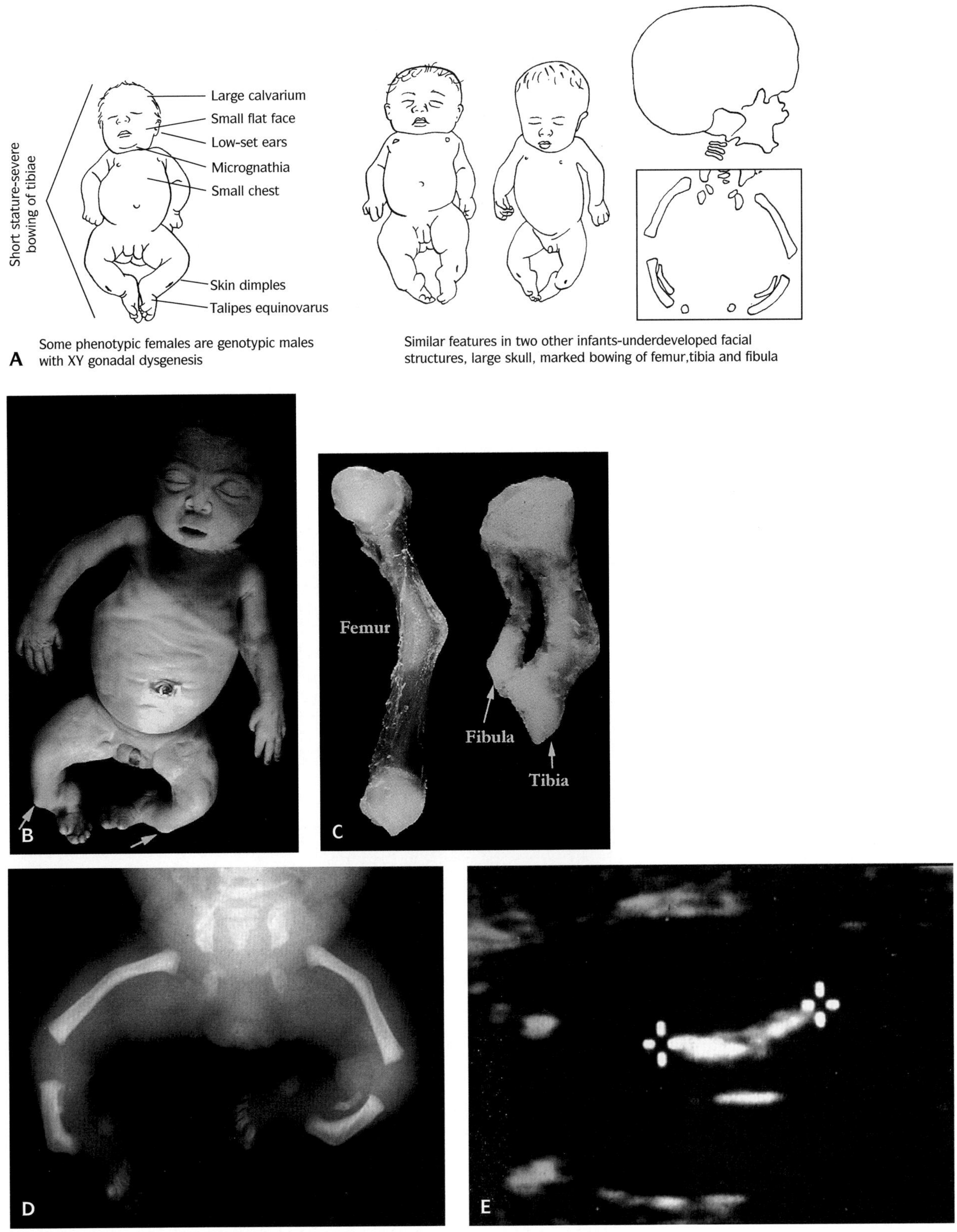

15.17. Campomelic dysplasia. **(A)** (From Goodman RM, Gorlin RJ: *The Malformed Infant and Child, An Illustrated Guide*, New York, Oxford University Press, 1985.) **(B)** Infant shows large head, flat face, low set ears, micrognathia, and bowed legs. A pretibial dimple is visible on the legs (yellow arrows). **(C)** Bent femur, tibia, and fibula. **(D)** Radiograph of the skeletal system with angulation of the femora and bowing of the tibiae and fibulae. **(E)** Ultrasound showing a bent femur.

Table 15.22 Campomelic dysplasia: features

Clinical	Pathological	Radiological
Mesomelic shortening and bowing of limbs Dolichocephaly High forehead Hypertelorism Prominent occiput Micrognathia Short neck Small flared chest Small larynx and narrow trachea	Cartilage including the physis unremarkable Laryngotracheal malacia in fatal cases Large brain with absence of genitalia and gonads	Bone and cartilage histology essentially normal No abnormality of bone matrix or mineralization Abnormal tracheobronchial cartilage

- Atelosteogenesis types I (most severe) and II and omodysplasia phenotypically resemble diastrophic dysplasia.
  - Boomerang dysplasia – a variant of atelosteogenesis/omodysplasia associated with cleft palate and omphalocele. Multinucleated giant chondrocytes present in atelosteogenesis type I and boomerang dysplasia.
  - Piepkorn lethal osteochondrodysplasia is probably a severe form of boomerang dysplasia. Disorganization and shortening in proliferative and hypertrophic zones and reduced cellularity of growth plate within myxoid foci.

A group of unclassified osteochondrodysplasias that are autosomal recessive include the following:

1. **Greenberg dysplasia** fragmented and mottled radiographic appearance of tubular bones, especially at the ends.
2. **Dappled diaphyseal dysplasia** – autosomal recessive.
   - Unique multiple irregular ossification centers of tubular bones.
3. **Glasgow chondrodysplasia** round femoral inferior epiphysis – sublethal.
   - Round inferior epiphyses of femora.
   - Physeal growth zones are retarded and disorganized.
   - Demasked fine fibers are seen in the matrix.
4. **Lethal brittle bone syndrome**, thin bones and multiple fractures (Figure 15.19).
   - Type V collagen defect.
   - **Raine syndrome** – neonatal lethal sclerotic bone dysplasia. Craniofacial anomalies are unique with microcephaly, midface hypoplasia, exophthalmos, small flattened nose, triangular mouth, and micrognathia. X-rays show a generalized increase in bone density with poor corticomedullary demarcation, ragged periosteal thickening, and long tubular bones, especially in the ribs. Pathology shows generalized proliferation of connective tissue – viscera, subcutaneous tissue, and media of vessels and cystic dysplastic kidneys.

Table 15.23 Diastrophic dysplasia

Radiological
Multiple joint dislocations
Abnormal spinal curvatures
Abnormal segmentation of cervical vertebrae
Lack of tapering of proximal and middle phalanges
Pathological
Irregular aggregates of resting chondrocytes with condensed rims of matrix encircling the lacunae.
Cystic degeneration of cartilage with fibrovascular tissue and ossification.
Short physes.

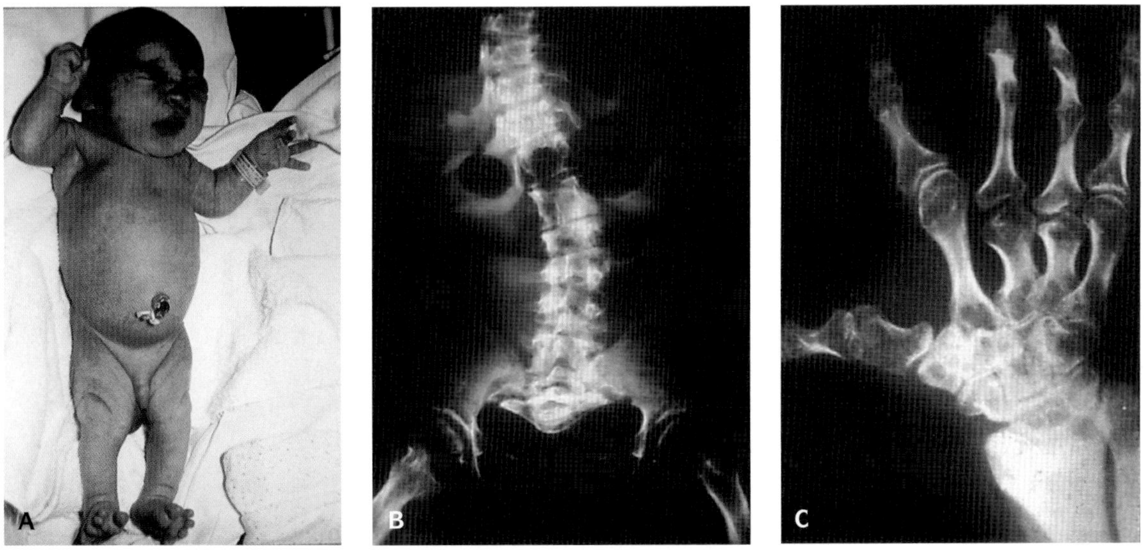

15.18. Diastrophic dysplasia. **(A)** Infant with multiple joint contractures. There is a talipes equinovarus (clubfoot) deformity. **(B)** X-ray showing severe scoliosis. **(C)** Radiograph of hand showing marked distortion of metacarpals and phalanges.

Calcific Stippling of Epiphyses

This is a heterogeneous group of disorders characterized by stippled epiphyseal calcification (Figure 15.20). Rhizomelic and Conradi-Hunermann types of chondrodysplasia punctata were listed in the original International Nomenclature. The subclassification was revised in 1983 and 1992, and the current version includes an X-linked recessive type and tibia-metacarpal (MT) type in addition to the foregoing two types. Many conditions without chondrodysplasia may develop stippled epiphysis.

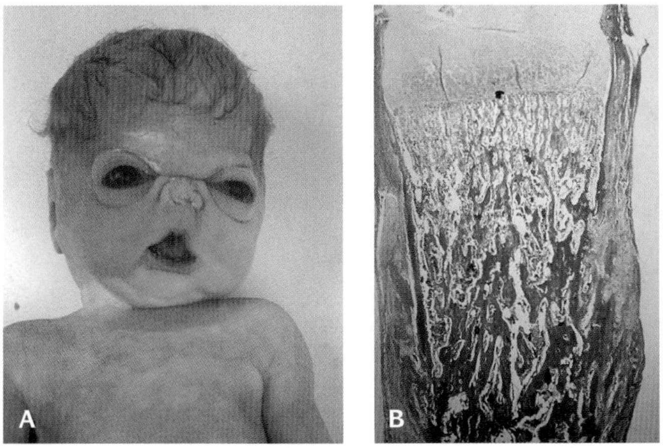

15.19. Raine syndrome. **(A)** Unique facies with mid-face hypoplasia, exophthalmos, triangular mouth and micrognathia. **(B)** Microscopic section shows dense thick bone trabeculae and thickened periosteum. (Courtesy Dr. Alex Kan.)

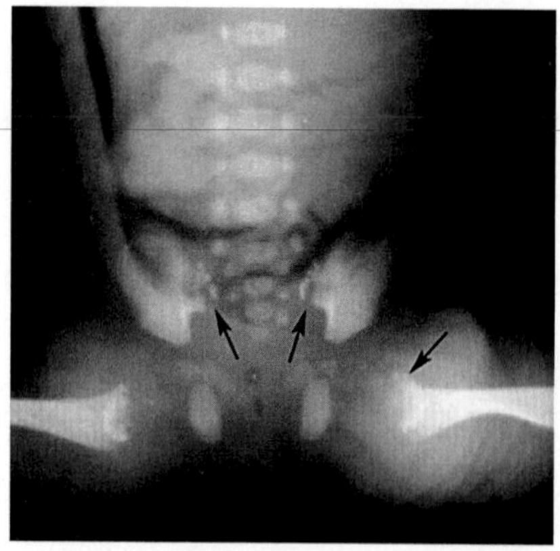

15.20. Stippled calcifications (arrows) of proximal femurs and hips in Warfarin embryopathy.

There are a number of conditions that are characterized by calcific stippling of the epiphysis. These include the following:

- **Chromosomal disorders**
  - Trisomy 18
  - Trisomy 21
- **Lysosomal disorders**
  - Mucopolysaccharidosis
  - Mucolipidosis
  - GM1 gangliosidosis
- **Peroxisomal disorders**
  - Chondrodysplasia punctata, rhizomelic type
  - Zellweger cerebrohepatorenal syndrome
- **Metabolic disorders**
  - Smith-Lemli-Opitz syndrome
  - Cretinism
- **Drug-induced disorders**
  - Warfarin embryopathy
  - Fetal hydantoin syndrome
  - Alcohol embryopathy
- **Bone dysplasias**
  - Chondrodysplasia punctata, all types
- **Others**
  - Neonatal lupus erythematosus
  - Vitamin K deficiency

Limb Reduction Defects (Table 15.24)

Limb reduction defects may be seen in a number of syndromes as in the **thalidomide syndrome, Phocomelia syndrome,** and **Robert syndrome.** Transverse

Table 15.24 Radial hypoplasia/aplasia in conditions diagnosable prenatally

Syndrome	Genetics	Frequency in syndrome	Incidence	Prenatal diagnosis
VATER Association	SP	Always	1/6500	Yes
Radial aplasia/ thrombocytopenia (TAR)	AR	Always	1/500,000–1/1,000,000	Yes
Roberts phocomelia	AR	Common	Rare	Yes
Trisomy 18	SP	Occasional	1/200 conceptuses 1/4,000 LB	Yes
Trisomy 13	SP	Occasional	1/5,000 LB	Yes

VATER, vertebral defects, anal atresia, tracheo-esophageal atresia, radial/renal dysplasia. LB, live births; SP, sporadic; AR, autosomal recessive.

Table 15.25 Association of polydactyly with other anomalies

Anomaly	
Anencephaly	Cleft palate
Spina bifida	Cleft lip
Hydrocephaly	Esophageal atresia
Microcephaly	Duodenal atresia
Anophthalmia	Anal atresia
Microtia	Gut malrotation
Congenital heart disease – conotruncal defects	Intersex
Omphalocele	Hypospadias
Hydronephrosis	Renal agenesis
Diaphragm, defect	Polycystic kidneys
Sirenomelia	Gastroschisis

defects may be the result of **chorionic villus sampling** when performed under 70 days of gestation. They may also be caused by the amnion disruption sequence.

Radial aplasia is characterized by sharp angulation of the wrist and may be seen in **Holt-Oram syndrome** (with atrial septal defect) and **TAR** (thrombocytopenia, absent radius) syndrome as well as the **VATER (VACTERL) complex.** Limb defects may be a component of facial clefting syndromes such as **EEC** (ectodermal dysplasia, ectrodactyly, facial clefting) **complex.** The most severe form of limb defects is seen in the **sirenomelia sequence.**

Syndactyly and polydactyly may be a component manifestation of a malformation syndrome or they may be isolated defects.

Isolated limb defects are not uncommon and appear to be sporadic events; however, their association with other defects and the possibility of an environmental or genetic cause should be investigated.

Polydactyly (Table 15.25) without limb anomalies may occur in a number of malformation syndromes.

Syndactyly (Table 15.26) and other distal limb anomalies may occur in other malformation syndromes including chromosomal defects.

ULTRASONOGRAPHY

Skeletal Anomalies

- Limb shortening is associated with a wide variety of chondrodystrophic syndromes.
  - Syndromic associations with short limbs
    - The strength of the association, usually evaluated by using femur length, appears to depend on the criteria used to define decreased length.

Table 15.26 Polydactyly and syndactyly in syndromes that may be diagnosed prenatally

	Syndrome	Recurrence	Incidence in live births
Polydactyly	Trisomy 13	Low	1/5000
	Meckel Gruber	AR	1/3,000–1/50,000
	Short rib/polydactyly	AR	Low
	Pallister-Hall	SP	Very low
	VATER	Low	1/6,500
	Early amnion rupture sequence	Low	1/3,000 births
	Asphyxiating dystrophy	AR	Low
	9p del	Low	Low
Syndactyly and other distal limb abnormalities	Early amnion rupture sequence	Low	1/3,000 births
	EEC	AD	Low
	Escobar	AR	Rare
	Fraser	AR	Low
	Neu-Laxova	AR	Rare
	Roberts	AR	Rare
	Short rib polydactyly	AR	Low
	Smith-Lemli-Opitz	AR	1/20,000–1/40,000
	Triploidy	Low	2% conceptuses
	Trisomy 21	Low	1/650 births
	Meckel	AR	1/3,000–1/50,000
	TAR	AR	1/500,000–1/1,000,000
	Trisomy 13	Low	1/5,000 LB
	Trisomy 18	Low	1/2,000 conceptuses 1/4,000 LB

EEC, Ectodermal dysplasia, ectrodactyly, facial clefting; TAR, thrombocytopenia aplasia of radius; VATER, vertebral defects, anal atresia, tracheo-esophageal fistula, radial and/or renal dysplasia; SP, sporadic; AR, autosomal recessive; AD, autosomal dominant; LB, live birth.

- Common chondrodystrophic syndromes are as follows:

Syndrome	Rate: livebirths
Thanatophoric dysplasia	1/30,000
Osteogenesis imperfecta	1/55,000
Achondrogenesis (all types)	1/75,000
Chondrodysplasia punctata	1/85,000
Hypophosphatasia (severe)	1/110,000
Campomelic dysplasia	1/150,000

- When diminished fetal measurements are noted, it is important to distinguish them from symmetric growth retardation, as skeletal dysplasias generally are autosomally mediated inherited conditions, while potential causes of severe symmetric growth retardation include early fetal infections, chromosomal abnormalities, and severe uteroplacental insufficiency.
- Morphologically, most skeletal dysplasias do not affect head or abdominal circumstance or fetal foot length.

  - Tables that describe an average long bone length for head circumference or abdominal circumference or biparietal diameter and gestational age assess symmetry and will assist in determining whether long bones are small relative to other body characteristics – as in skeletal dysplasia – or whether body proportions are generally symmetric, indicating symmetric growth retardation.
  - Discriminate between chondrodystrophy and symmetric growth retardation – fetal femur/foot length ratios approximate 1.0 over the course of gestation, and <0.84 occurs in <10% of normal infants. The femur/foot ratio of <0.84 is associated with skeletal dysplasia.
- Methods of assessing long bone length
  - Absolute length for gestational age – shortening as a screening criterion for skeletal dysplasias is <1% or <3–4 SD below the mean.
  - This is clinically efficacious because the degree of shortening of the long bones is usually profound in most skeletal dysplasias.
  - Shortening of the humerus has also been proposed as a screening method for chromosomal aberrations. Shortening of the humerus may be present in up to 60% of trisomy 21 fetuses.
- BPD/Femur length ratio (cutpoint at mean +1.5 SD)

Gestational age	
16 weeks	1.93
18 weeks	1.74
20 weeks	1.58
22 weeks	1.47

Head circumference/femur length ratio (HC/FL):

Gestational age	**Harris Birthright Center >95% HC/FL**
16 weeks	6.52
18 weeks	6.13
20 weeks	5.85
22 weeks	5.66
24 weeks	5.54
26 weeks	5.46
28 weeks	5.41

There appears to be an association between short femur length and chromosomal abnormalities. Trisomy 21 fetuses have IFC/FL ratios > 97/5%. Increased rates of relative shortening of the femur are seen in fetuses with triploidy (60%), Turner syndrome (59%), trisomy 18 (25%), and trisomy 13 (9%).

REFERENCES

Beighton P, Giedion A, Gorlin R et al.: International classification of osteochondrodyslasias. *Am J Med Genet* 44:223, 1992.

Byers P: Osteogenesis imperfecta. In Royce P, Steinmann B (eds): *Connective Tissue and its Heritable Disorders*, New York, Wiley-Liss, 1993.

Diab M, Wu J-J, Shapiro F, Eyre D: Abnormality of type IX collagen in a patient with diastrophic dysplasia. *Am J Med Genet* 49:402, 1994.

Evans JA, Vitez M, Czeizel A: Congenital abnormalities associated with limb deficiency defects: A population study based on cases from the Hungarian Congenital Malformation Registry (1975–1984). *Am J Med Genet* 49:52, 1994.

Foster UG, Baird PA: Congenital defects of the limbs in stillbirths: Data from a population-based study. *Am J Med Genet* 46:479, 1993.

Gilbert E, Opitz JM: Abnormal bone development: histopathology of skeletal dysplasias. In Martini-Neri ME, Neri G, Opitz JM (eds): *Gene Regulation and Fetal Development, BD:OAS*, 30:1, New York, Wiley-Liss, 1996.

Gilbert-Barness E, Langer LO, Opitz JM, et al.: Kniest Dysplasia: Radiologic, histopathological and scanning electronmicroscopic findings. *Am J Med Genet* 63:34, 1996.

Gilbert E, Yang SS, Langer L, Opitz JM, Roskamp JO, Heidelberger KP: Pathologic changes of osteochondrodysplasia in infancy. A review. *Pathol Ann* 22(2):281, 1987.

Gilbert-Barness E, Barness LA. Disorders of collagen metabolism in metabolic diseases. *Foundation of Clinical Management, Genetics and Pathology*, Natick, Massachusetts, Eaton Publishing, 2000.

Hasbacka J, Kaitila I, Sistonen P, de la Chapelle A: Diastrophic dysplasia gene maps to the distal long arm of chromosome 5. *Proc Natl Acad Sci* 87:8056, 1990.

Hill LM, Guzick D, Belfar H, et al.: The current role of sonography in the detection of Down syndrome. *Obstet Gynecol* 74:620, 1989.

Jones KL: *Smith's Recognizable Patterns of Malformations*, 5th ed, Philadelphia, WB Saunders, 1996.

Kan AE, Kozlowski K: New distinct lethal osteosclerotic bone dysplasia (Raine syndrome). *Am J Med Genet* 43:860, 1992.

Le Merrer M, Rousseau F, Legeai-Mallet L, et al.: A gene for achondroplasia-hypochondroplasia maps to chromosome 4p. *Nature Genet* 6:318, 1994.

Pauli RM, Haun JM: Intrauterine effects of coumarin and derivatives. *Dev Brain Dysfunct* 6:229, 1993.

Prockop DJ, Baldwin CT, Constantinou CD: Mutations in type I procollagen genes that cause osteogenesis imperfecta. *Adv Hum Genet* 19:105, 1990.

Qureshi F, Jacques SM, Evans MI, et al.: Skeletal histopathology in fetuses with chondroectodermal dysplasia (Ellis-van Creveld syndrome). *Am J Med Genet* 45:471, 1993.

Qureshi F, Jacques SM, Johnson SF, et al.: Histopathology of fetal diastrophic dysplasia. *Am J Med Genet* 1995.

Rimoin DL, Lachman RS: The chondrodysplasias. In Emery AEH, Rimoin DL (eds): *Principles and Practice of Medical Genetics*, 2nd ed, Edinburgh, Churchill Livingston, 1990.

Shapiro F: Osteopetrosis, current clinical considerations. *Clin Orthop* 294:34, 1993.

Soothill PW, Yuthiwong C, Rees H: Achondrogenesis type 2 diagnosed by transvaginal ultrasound at 12 weeks' gestation. *Prenatal Diagnosis* 13:523, 1993.

Spranger J, Maroteaux P: The lethal osteochondrodysplasias. *Adv Hum Genet* 19:1, 1990.

Spranger J, Winterpacht A, Zabel B: The type II collagenopathies: a spectrum of chondrodysplasia. *Eur J Pediatr* 153:56, 1994.

Temtamy S, McKusick V: Genetics of hand malformations. *BD (OAS)* 14:3, 1978.

Tommerup N, Schempp W, Meinecke P, et al.: Assignment of an autosomal sex reversal locus (SRA1) and campomelic dysplasia (CMPD1) to 17q24.3-q25.1. *Nature Genet* 4:170, 1993.

Urioste M, Martinez-Frias ML, Bermejo E, et al.: Short rib-polydactyly syndrome and pericentric inversion of chromosome 4. *Am J Med Genet* 49:94, 1994.

Ward LM, Rauch F, Travers R, Chabot G, Azouz EM, Lalic L, Roughley RJ, Glorieux FH: Osteogenesis imperfecta type VII: an autosomal recessive form of brittle bone disease. *Bone* 31(1):12, 2002.

Yang SS, Kitchen E, Gilbert E, Rimoin DL: Histopathologic examination in osteochondrodysplasia: time for standardization. *Arch Pathol Lab Invest* 110:10, 1986.

Yang SS: The skeletal system. In Wigglesworth JS, Singer DB (eds): *Textbook of Fetal and Perinatal Pathology*, Oxford, Blackwell Scientific Publications, 1990.

Yang SS: The Skeletal System. In Gilbert-Barness E (ed): *Potter's Pathology of the Fetus, and Infant*, Philadelphia, Mosby Publishers, 1996.

SIXTEEN

Cardiovascular System Defects

PRENATAL DIAGNOSIS

With the advent of ultrasound and its application to the human fetal heart, prenatal diagnosis and management of structural heart disease and cardiac dysrhythmia is possible (Figure 16.1). Congenital heart disease is relatively uncommon in the general population, and not every pregnancy can or should be examined with fetal echocardiography. Only those pregnancies with recognized risk factors for cardiac disease and those with an abnormal four-chamber view on level I obstetrical sonograms should be evaluated.

TECHNIQUE OF FETAL ECHOCARDIOGRAPHY

The fetal heart is most easily examined by ultrasound transabdominally at 18–24 weeks gestation, when a nonfixed fetal position, incompletely calcified bones, and abundant amniotic fluid make cardiac imaging easier (Table 16.1). Transvaginal images show excellent cardiac detail as early as 14 weeks gestation. Transvaginal imaging is invasive, however, and carries a small potential risk; therefore, it should be used when transabdominal imaging is inadequate. Transabdominal ultrasound uses a relatively high-frequency transducer to examine the heart and great vessels segmentally. It uses M-mode, two-dimensional, pulsewave, and color flow Doppler to delineate the cardiac anatomy, fetal hemodynamics, and patency of the fetal circulatory pathways. A normal fetal echocardiogram does not eliminate the potential for congenital heart disease. Lesions that may not be identified prenatally include mild semilunar valve obstruction, atrial septal defect, small ventricular defect, and partial anomalous venous return. In addition, coarctation of the aorta is a significant lesion that is difficult to diagnose.

The early fetal heart can be dissected under a dissecting microscope in the same manner as the heart of an older fetus or a newborn (illustrated in Chapter 3).

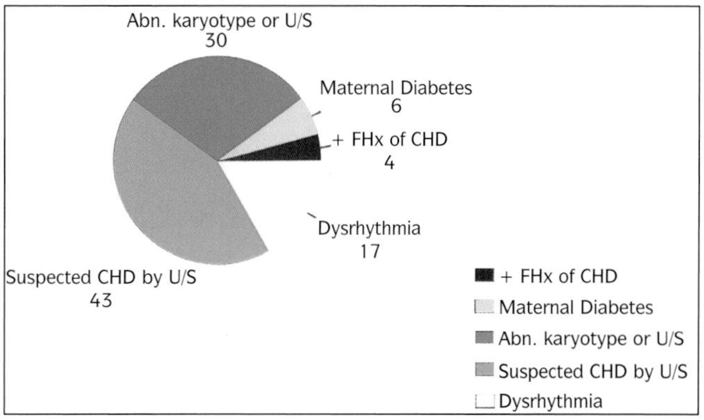

16.1. Percent of total patients with abnormal fetal echocardiograms classified by indication. (From *Pediatric Annals* 27:8, 1998.)

During fetal life, the umbilical vein delivers oxygenated blood from the placenta to the fetal heart and passes through the foramen ovale to the left side. The ductus arteriosus directs blood from the pulmonary artery to the descending aorta.

Prenatal closure of ductus arteriosus or foramen ovale (FO) is incompatible with intrauterine life and results in congestive failure in the fetus and usually stillbirth (Figure 16.2).

INCIDENCE AND ETIOLOGY

Cardiovascular defects occur in 0.8% of live births (Table 16.2). In autopsy studies, the incidence of congenital heart disease in the fetus approaches 30/1,000. In patients with diagnosed intrauterine cardiac malformations, 17.5% do not survive to birth. Of those who do survive to delivery, 30% die before 1 year of life. The echocardiographic exam of the fetal heart is a relatively risk-free procedure and, in the hands of an experienced fetal cardiologist, has a high degree of sensitivity and specificity for the detection of structural heart disease. Causes of cardiovascular diseases include chromosome abnormalities, single gene mutations, and environmental factors – i.e., rubella and multifactorial inheritance (gene–environment interactions). The vast majority of isolated cardiac defects are believed to be multifactorial in which different environmental events are necessary to convert a hereditary predisposition based on the cumulative action of many genes into a final defect.

Most trisomy infants or fetuses have cardiovascular defects, with ventricular septal defect (VSD), atrial septal defect (ASD), pulmonary stenosis, and coarctation of the aorta as the most common. The most common defect in chromosomal disorders is polyvalvular dysplasia in trisomy 18 (Figure 16.3). In trisomy 13, 80% have cardiovascular abnormalities – VSD, patent ductus arteriosus (PDA), ASD, and dextroposition are the most common. Cardiac defects are frequent findings in all chromosome abnormalities, with the exception of sex chromosome duplications including XXY, XXXY, and XXXXY. In

Table 16.1 Indications for fetal echocardiography

Genetic indication
Family history of CHD
Maternal indications:
- Teratogen exposure
- Rubella
- Lithium
- Alcohol
- Anticonvulsants
- Diabetes
- Polyhydramnios/oligohydramnios
- Maternal collagen disease (e.g., lupus erythematosus)

Fetal indications:
- Abnormal chromosomes
- Malformations noted on ultrasound
- Irregular heart rate
- Nonimmune hydrops

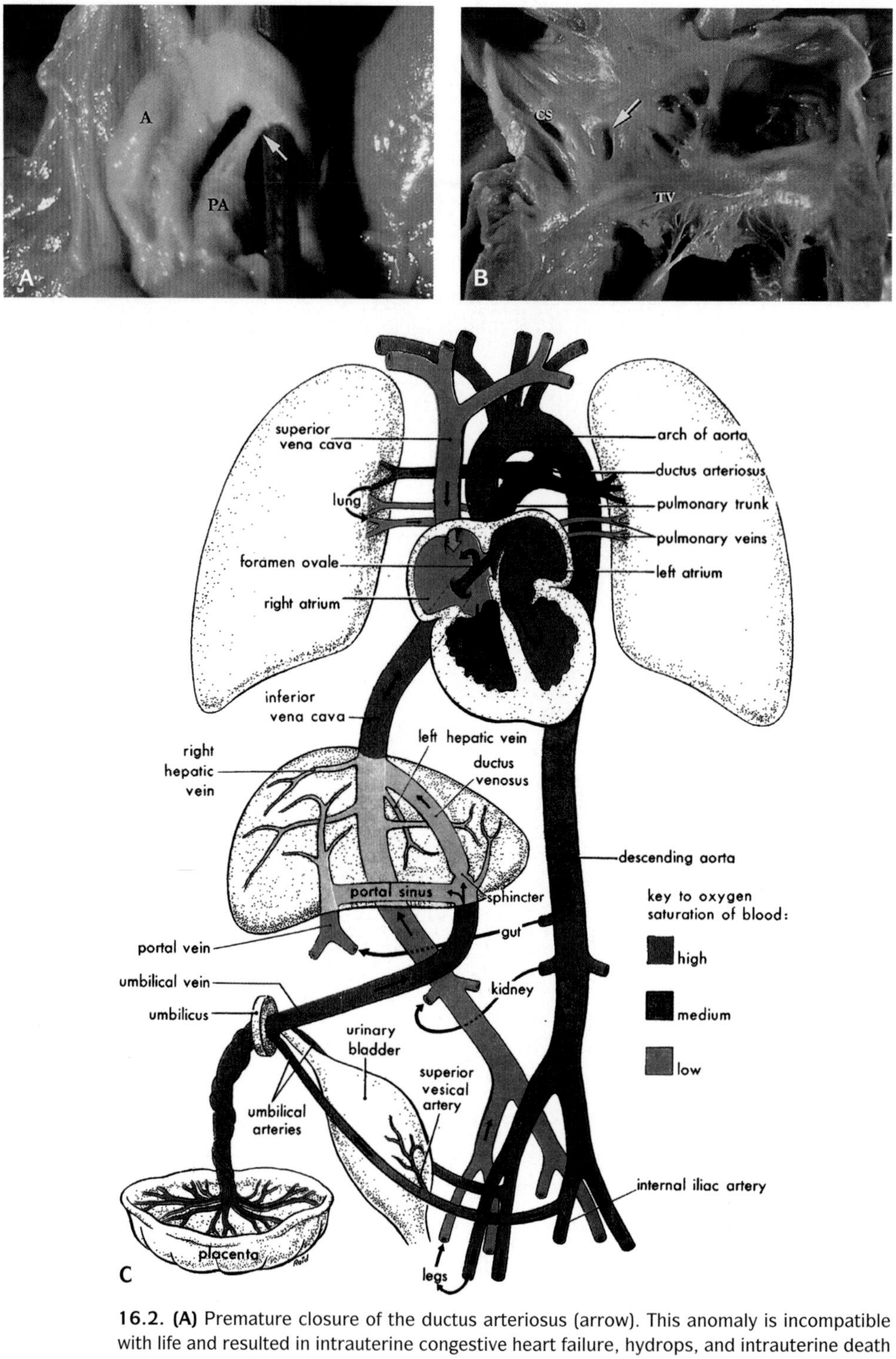

16.2. **(A)** Premature closure of the ductus arteriosus (arrow). This anomaly is incompatible with life and resulted in intrauterine congestive heart failure, hydrops, and intrauterine death in this fetus at 15 weeks gestation. (A, aorta; PA, pulmonary artery.) **(B)** Premature closure of the foramen ovale in a fetus at 30 weeks gestation. The foramen ovale is represented by a slit-like defect (arrow) on the atrial septum that was not probe patent. (CS, coronary sinus; TV, tricuspid valve.) **(C)** A simplified scheme of the fetal circulation. Colors indicate the oxygen saturation of the blood and arrows show the course of the fetal circulation. Organs are not drawn to scale. Observe that there are three shunts that permit most of the blood to bypass the liver and the lungs: 1, the ductus venosus; 2, the foramen ovale; and 3, the ductus arterious. (From Moore KL, Persaud TVN: *The Developing Human*, 5th ed, Philadelphia, WB Saunders, 1993.)

Table 16.2 **Etiology of major cardiovascular malformations**

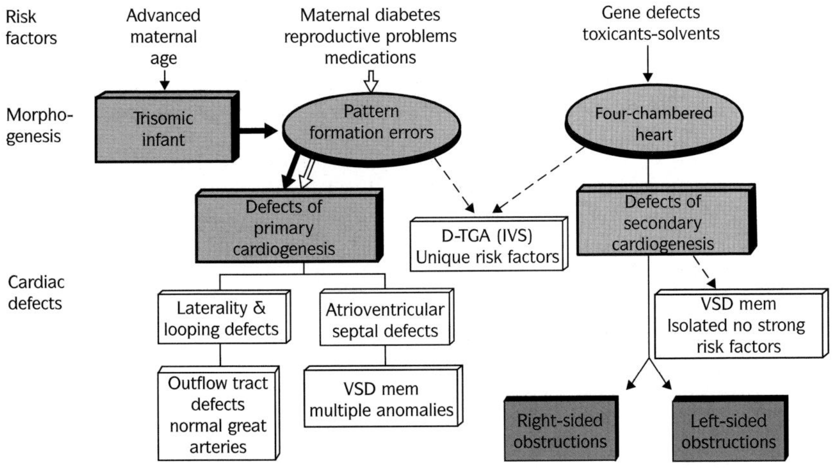

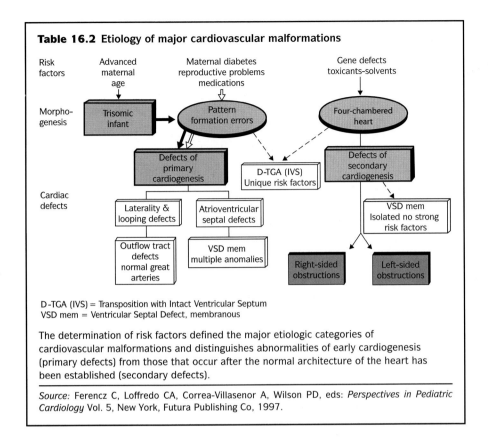

D-TGA (IVS) = Transposition with Intact Ventricular Septum
VSD mem = Ventricular Septal Defect, membranous

The determination of risk factors defined the major etiologic categories of cardiovascular malformations and distinguishes abnormalities of early cardiogenesis (primary defects) from those that occur after the normal architecture of the heart has been established (secondary defects).

Source: Ferencz C, Loffredo CA, Correa-Villasenor A, Wilson PD, eds: *Perspectives in Pediatric Cardiology* Vol. 5, New York, Futura Publishing Co, 1997.

monosomy X (Ulrich-Turner syndrome), preductal coarctation is a common finding.

Syndromes with autosomal dominant inheritance such as Holt-Oram (ASD and VSD) and Marfan syndrome often involve the cardiovascular system. Examples of autosomal recessive syndromes with CHD include Ellis-van Creveld syndrome (ASD or single atrium), Bardet-Biedl syndrome (VSD), thrombocytopenia with absent radius (TAR) [ASD, tetralogy of Fallot (TOF), and dextrocardia], and Smith-Lemli-Opitz (50% have CHD).

In the VATER association (vertebral anomalies, heart defects, anal atresia, tracheo-esophageal fistula, and radial and renal dysplasia) the most frequent heart defects are VSD, ASD, and complex anomalies. In CHARGE syndrome (coloboma, heart disease, choanal atresia, genital, and ear anomalies), the heart defects are usually VSD, ASD, TOF, and double outlet right ventricle (DORV) with an atrioventricular septal defect (AVSD), or a right-sided aortic arch.

Maternal phenylketonuria, diabetes, fetal alcohol syndrome, and rubella are frequently associated with cardiac defects. Other well-recognized environmental causes of cardiovascular abnormalities are hydantoin, isotretinoin (retinoic acid), lithium, thalidomide, and trimethadione.

By ultrasound and fetal echocardiology, isolated major cardiac defects can be diagnosed.

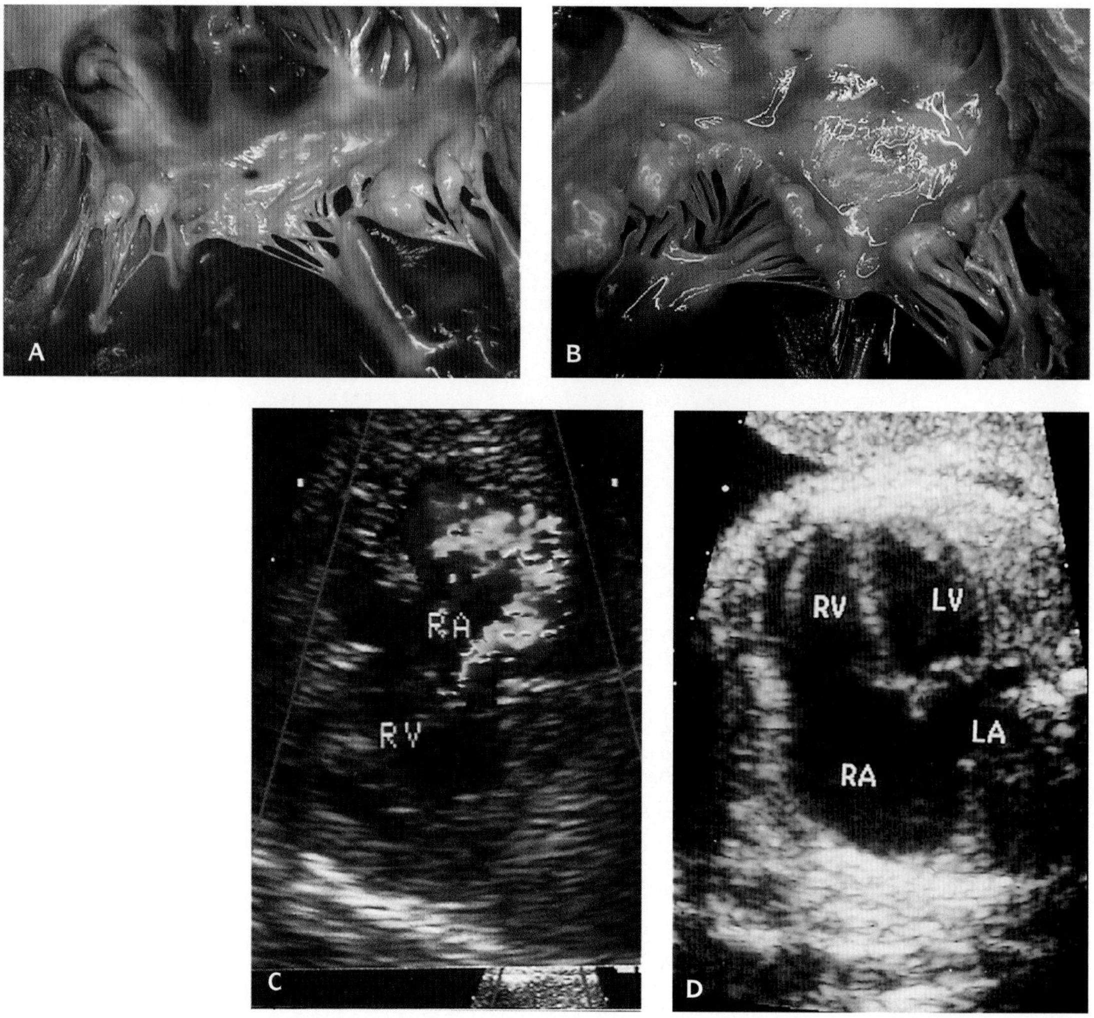

16.3. **(A)** Tricuspid and **(B)** mitral valve dysplasia showing the typical rolled edges and thickened chordae tendinae. **(C)** The degree of tricuspid valve regurgitation (red-yellow area) into the right atrium (RA) is demonstrated with color Doppler imaging. (RV, right ventricle.) (Courtesy of James Huhta, MD, Pediatric Cardiology Associates, Tampa, FL.) **(D)** Ultrasound of a heart at 28 weeks gestation with a dilated right atrium (RA) secondary to tricuspid valve dysplasia. (LA, left atrium; RV, right ventricle; LV, left ventricle.) (Courtesy of Florida Perinatal Associates, Tampa, FL.)

Table 16.3 Chromosomal syndromes with cardiac malformations

Syndrome	Cardiac malformation	Chromosome
Wolf-Hirschhorn	ASD, VSD, PDA, aTOF	4p
Familial TAPVR	TAPVR	4p13–q12
Cri du chat	VSD, ASD, PDA	5p
Holt-Oram	ASD	12q
Noonan	ASD, PS, HCM	12q
Rubinstein-Taybi	ASD, VSDm PDA, CoA	16q
Alagille	Arterial dysplasia	20p

ASD, Atrial septal defect; VSD, ventricular septal defect; PDA, patent ductus arteriosus; TOF, tetralogy of Fallot; TAPVR, total anomalous pulmonary venous return; PS, pulmonic stenosis; HCM, hypertropic cardiomyopathy; CoA, coarctation of the aorta.

Table 16.4 Cardiac malformations in multiple-malformation syndromes*

Name of syndrome	Manifestations	Cardiovascular malformation	OMIM†
Aarskog syndrome	Short stature, ptosis, hypertelorism, widow's peak, "shawl" scrotum, hyperextension of proximal interphalangeal joints	Rare	100050
Achondroplasia	Rhizomelic micromelia (shortness of proximal segments), large head with depressed nasal bridge and prominent forehead	Rare	10080
Acrofacial dysostosis	Antimongoloid palpebral fissures, malar and mandibular hypoplasia, microtia, coloboma of lower lid, cleft palate, underdevelopment of preaxial (in Nager type) or postaxial (in Miller type) structures of upper limbs	Rare	Miller: 26375 Rodriguez: 201170 Catania type: 101805 Palagonia type: 601829
Acrorenal field defect	Underdevelopment of preaxial structures of hands and malformations of kidneys (agenesis, hypoplasia, horseshoe kidney)	Rare	#102520
Alagille syndrome	Hypoplasia of hepatic ducts, butterfly type vertebrae	>50%, mostly peripheral pulmonary artery stenosis	#118450
Apert syndrome	Acrocephaly (shortness of skull in anterior-posterior axis) due to craniosynostosis, almost complete syndactyly of hands and feet	Rare	#101200
BBB syndrome	Hypertelorism, plagiocephaly, hypospadias	25%	#31360
Campomelic syndrome	Micromelia with femoral and tibial bending, sex reversal (female genitalia in 46, XY proband), defects of brain and kidneys	20%	*114290
Cantrell pentalogy	Cleft sternum, supraumbilical defect of abdominal wall, defects of pericardium and anterior diaphragm	Almost constant	*313850
Carnitine deficiency	Progressive generalized myopathy due to abnormal beta oxidation of fatty acids	Frequent cardiomyopathy as a result of primary metabolic defect	#21214
CHARGE association	Coloboma of the eye, heart defects, atresia of choanae, retarded growth, genital, and ear abnormalities	50–70% different forms	302905
Cleft sternum-hemangioma association	Cleft sternum, hemangioma	? Rare	
Cornelia de Lange syndrome	Nanism, mental retardation, microcephaly, synophrys, hirsutism, anteverted nostrils, small hands, underdevelopment of upper limbs	20–30%	112370
Costello syndrome	Short stature, macrocephaly, redundancy of skin on the neck, palms, soles, papillomata around the mouth, nares, anus	20–30% cardiomyopathy	*218040
Cytomegaly	Prenatal hypoplasia, hepatosplenomegaly, thrombocytopenia, intracranial calcifications	Rather common	
DiGeorge syndrome	A- or hypoplasia of thymus, hypocalcemia, hypoparathyroidism, immunodeficiency	Common, >60%	#188400

(*continued*)

Table 16.4 *(continued)*

Name of syndrome	Manifestations	Cardiovascular malformation	OMIM†
Ehlers-Danlos syndrome	Hyperextensibility of joints, hyperlaxity of skin	Rare	
Ellis-Van Creveld syndrome	Short-limbed, dwarfism, postaxial, polydactyly, dysplastic nails, genu valgum	>50%, mostly ASD	#22550
Fanconi anemia	Progressive pancytopenia, hyperpigmentation of skin, a- or hypoplastic thumbs, kidney anomalies	10%	#22765
Fetal alcohol syndrome	Growth and mental deficiency, microcephaly, short palpebral fissures, midface hypoplasia	Common in offspring of mothers with chronic alcoholism	
Frontometaphyseal dysplasia	Hyperostosis, skeletal dysplasia, multiple joint contractures, abnormalities of teeth	15–20%	#30562
Goldenhar syndrome	Epibulbar dermoid, macrostomia, unilateral defects of external and internal ear, deafness, macrostomia, abnormalities of cervical vertebrae	20–40%	*164210
Holt-Oram syndrome	Preaxial hand abnormalities, cardiovascular malformations	Common, mostly ASD	#14290
Holzgreve syndrome	Cleft palate, ankyloglosson, a- or hypoplastia of kidneys, cecum mobile	Common	236110
HOMAGE syndrome	Oligomeganephronia, ambiguous genitalia	Only one family with tetralogy in sibs	
Hydantoin embryopathy	Prenatal hypoplasia, growth deficiency, cleft palate, midface hypoplasia, hypoplastic nails, and distal phalanges	Uncommon	
Hydrocephaly-VACTERL syndrome	Complex of VACTERL-association and hydrocephaly	50%	192350
Ivemark syndrome	Heterotaxia, abnormality of bowel rotation, asplenia with bilateral trilobed lungs, or polysplenia with bilateral bilobed lungs	Common	208530
Kartagener syndrome	Situs inversus, sinusitis, bronchiectasis, immotile spermatozoa	Frequent dextrocardia	#24440
Klippel-Feil syndrome	Fusion of cervical vertebrae, sometimes with involvement of thoracic and lumbar vertebrae, scoliosis, Sprengel deformity, deafness, unilateral renal agenesis, ectopic kidneys	Uncommon	#148900
Larsen syndrome	Multiple joint dislocations, hydrocephaly, prominent forehead, flat face, cleft palate	Common	AR-*245600 AD-*150250
Laurence-Moon-Bardet-Biedl syndrome	Oligophrenia, postaxial polydactyly, obesity, retinitis pigmentosa, hypoplastic genitalia	Rare	#20990
Lazjuk syndrome	Cleft lip and palate, ectrodactyly	Common	*256520
Marden-Walker syndrome	Multiple joint contractures, psychomotor retardation, blepharophimosis, micrognathia	Uncommon	#24780
Meckel syndrome	Occipital encephalocele, cleft lip/palate, polycystic kidneys, postaxial polydactyly, hepatic fibrosis, ambiguous genitalia	10–15%	#24900
Microgastria-limb reduction complex	Underdevelopment of limbs (mostly upper), microgastria, asplenia or hypoplastic spleen, kidney abnormalities, abnormal lung lobation, intestinal malrotation	40%	#156810

Table 16.4 *(continued)*

Name of syndrome	Manifestations	Cardiovascular malformation	OMIM[†]
Noonan syndrome	Short stature, webbed neck, pectus carinatum	75%, mostly valvular pulmonary stenosis	#16395
Opitz-Frias (G syndrome)	Hypospadias, dysphagia, hoarse voice	Uncommon	#14541
Oro-facio-digital syndrome, type I	Multilobulated tongue, hyperplastic frenulum, cleft lip/palate, alopecia, supernumerary teeth, syn- and brachydactyly, polycystic kidneys	Uncommon	#31120
Pena-Shokeir syndrome	Multiple joint ankyloses, camptodactyly, flat face, pulmonary hypoplasia, cystic kidneys, cleft palate, Meckel diverticulum hydroureter	Common	#20815
Peter-plus syndrome	Peters anomaly (mesodermal dysplasia of the anterior eye segment, posterior embryotoxon, corneal opacity, staphyloma, secondary cataracts and glaucoma), rhizomelic micromelia (shortness of proximal segments), narrowing of external auditory canals	Uncommon	604229
Pompe disease	Glycogenesis: absence of α-1,4-glucosidase and secondary accumulation of glycogen in affected tissues	Cardiomyopathy as a result of basic metabolic defect is very common	#23230
Prader-Willi syndrome	Hypogenitalism, obesity, mental retardation, muscular hypotonia	Uncommon	#176270
Prune belly syndrome	Underdevelopment of abdominal musculature (with the wrinkled skin of abdominal wall), defects of urinary tract (dysplastic kidneys, hydro- or megaureter)	Uncommon	
Pseudotrisomy 13	Phenotype similar to trisomy 13 (cleft lip/palate, holoprosencephaly, microcephaly, postaxial polydactyly, abnormal lobation of lungs, anal atresia, renal a- or hypoplasia, ambiguous genitalia) with normal karyotype	Common (50%)	264480
Renal-hepatic-pancreatic dysplasia	Polycystic kidneys, fibrosis of pancreas and liver, secondary hypoplasia of lungs	Uncommon	#26320
Ritscher-Schinzel (3C) syndrome	Dandy-Walker malformation, macrobrachy- and hydrocephaly, brachydactyly, colobomata of iris, webbed neck, facial dysmorphias	Common (80%)	*220210
Roberts syndrome	Tetaphocomelia, microphthalmia, maxillary agenesis, microcephaly, Peters anomaly, cleft lip, polycystic kidneys	Common	#26830
Rubella syndrome	Sensorineural deafness, hepatosplenomegaly, microcephaly, corneal clouding, cataract	Very common, mostly patent ductus arteriosus	
Schnizel-Giedion syndrome	Widely patent sutures and fontanels, hypertrichosis, shortness of forearms and legs, hydronephrosis, cryptorchidism	Common	#26915
Smith-Lemli-Opitz syndrome	Microcephaly, ptosis, epicanthus, cleft palate, postaxial polydactyly, syndactyly two or three toes, pyloric stenosis, hypoplasia or cystic dysplasia of kidneys, hydronephrosis, hypospadias	Common, 40%	#26867, #27040
Spondylocostal dysplasia	Abnormal vertebral segmentation and defects of ribs (without defects of skull or limbs)	Uncommon	#12260
Thomas syndrome	Cleft lip and palate, renal agenesis, or hypoplasia	Constant	236110

(continued)

Table 16.4 *(continued)*

Name of syndrome	Manifestations	Cardiovascular malformation	OMIM†
Townes-Brocks syndrome	Microtia, satyr ear, preaxial polydactyly or triphalangeal thumb, anal atresia or stenosis, horseshoe kidney	15–20% (mostly in sporadic cases)	#10748
VACTERL association	Vertebral dysgenesis, anal atresia, cardiac defects, tracheoesophageal fistula, renal anomalies, limb defects	50–60%	192350
Van der Woude syndrome	Cleft palate, paramedian pits of the lower lips, club foot	Uncommon	#11930
Waardenburg syndrome	Dystopia canthorum, deafness, heterochromic irides, premature graying of hair, syndactyly	Uncommon	#277580
Williams syndrome	Elfin face, full lips, anteverted nares, hypercalcemia, mental retardation	Very common, mostly supravalvular aortic stenosis	#19405

† Online Mendelian inheritance in man. AR, Autosomal recessive. AD, Autosomal dominant.
* before an entry number means the phenotype determined by the gene at the given locus is separate from those represented by other asterisked entries and the mode of inheritance of the phenotype has been proved.
No asterisk before an entry number means the mode of inheritance has not been proved, although suspected, or that the separateness of this locus from that of another entry is unclear.
symbol before an entry number means the phenotype can be caused by mutation in any of two or more genes.
Source: Ferencz C, Loffredo CA, Correa-Villaseñor A, Wilson PD: Perspectives in Pediatric Cardiology; Vol. 5, Genetic and Environmental Risk Factors of Major Cardiovascular Malformations, The Baltimore-Washington Infant Study: 1981–1989. New York, Futura Publ. Co., Inc., 1997.

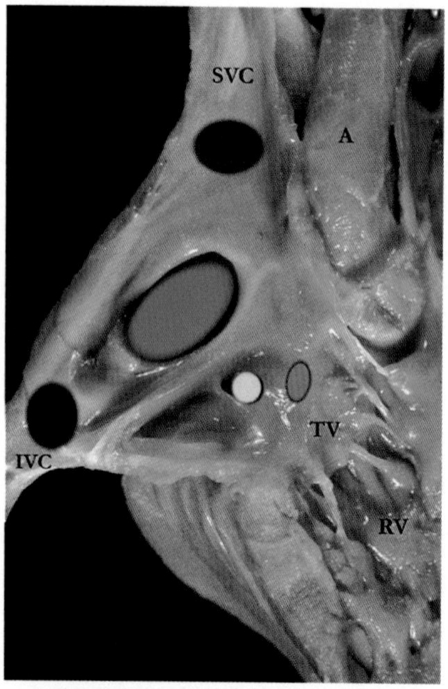

16.4. Atrial septal defect (ASD). Illustration of ASD sites: blue, ostium secundum defect; green, ostium primum defect; red, sinus venosus defects; yellow, defect of the coronary sinus.

CONGENITAL CARDIAC DEFECTS

There are three categories of congenital cardiac defects:

1. arteriovenous shunts
2. venous-arterial shunts
3. obstructive lesions
   a. left-sided obstructions
   b. right-sided obstructions

ARTERIOVENOUS SHUNTS

Atrial Septal Defects (ASD) (Figure 16.4)

- **Ostium secundum defect**, the most common type, appears as multiple perforations or a deficiency of the septum primum (valve of the FO) (Figure 16.5). Mitral valve (MV) prolapse is present in 10–40% of patients with ASD.
- **Isolated ostium primum defects** are rare; they occur most commonly as a component of complete endocardial cushion defects (Figure 16.6).
- **A sinus venosus defect** joins the ostium of the superior vena cava and usually is associated with anomalous pulmonary venous drainage from the right upper pulmonary lobe.

Table 16.5 Selected malformation syndromes with cardiovascular anomalies

OMIM†	Syndrome	Incidence	Percent with cardiac defects	Usual type (s) of cardiac defects
	Chromosome etiology			
190685	Down	1/700	40	AV communis, VSD
	Turner	1/2,500	60	Coarctation of aorta
	Trisomy 18	1/6,000	85	VSD, PDA
	Trisomy 13	1/5,000	80	VSD, ASD
194190	Wolf-Hirschhorn (4p-)	1/50,000	60	VSD, ASD
188400	DiGeorge (22q-)	1/20,000	95	Interrupted aortic arch, conotruncal defects
	Single gene etiology			
14290	Holt-Oram	Unknown	85	ADS, VSD
16395	Noonan	1/2,000	65	PS
192430	Velo-cardio-facial	Unknown	80	VSD, right aortic arch, Tetralogy of Fallot
22550	Ellis-van Creveld	1/150,000	50	ASD, AV communis
154700	Marfan	1/20,000	95	Prolapsed mitral valve, dilated aortic root
	Environmental etiology			
	Alcohol	1/500	25	ASD, VSD
	Retinoic acid	Extremely rare	50	Conotruncal defects, hypoplastic aortic arch, VSD, TGV
	Hydantoin	1/500	2	Valve stenosis, septal defect, PDA
	Valproate	1/1,000	10	VSD, PDA
	Lithium	Extremely rare	<1	Ebstein anomaly
	Rubella	Extremely rare	75	PDA, PPS
	Mumps (?)	Extremely rare	<1	Cardiomegaly
	Unknown etiology			
19405	Williams	1/10,000	100	Supravalvar AS, PPS
	de Lange	1/10,000	25 (?)	VSD, ASD
192350	VACTERL	1/3,500	50	VSD
302905	CHARGE	Unknown	50	Coarctation, PDA, VSD, ASD

ASD, atrial septal defect; VSD, ventricular septal defect; PS, pulmonary valve stenosis; PPS, peripheral pulmonary artery stenosis; TGV, transposition of great arteries; PDA, patent ductus arteriosus.

† Online Mendelian inheritance in man.

Source: Stevenson RE, Hall JG, Goodman RM, eds: *Human Malformations and Related Anomalies*, Vol. II, New York, Oxford University Press, 1993.

- **Complete absence of the atrial septum** results in a **single atrium** (common atrium, cor triloculare biventriculare); it is usually associated with multiple severe cardiac anomalies.

Endocardial Cushion Defects (ECD) (Atrioventricular is Communis, Atrioventricular Canal Defect)

- In **ostium primum ASD** the endocardial cushion fails to close the ostium primum completely. It is associated with a cleft in the anterior MV

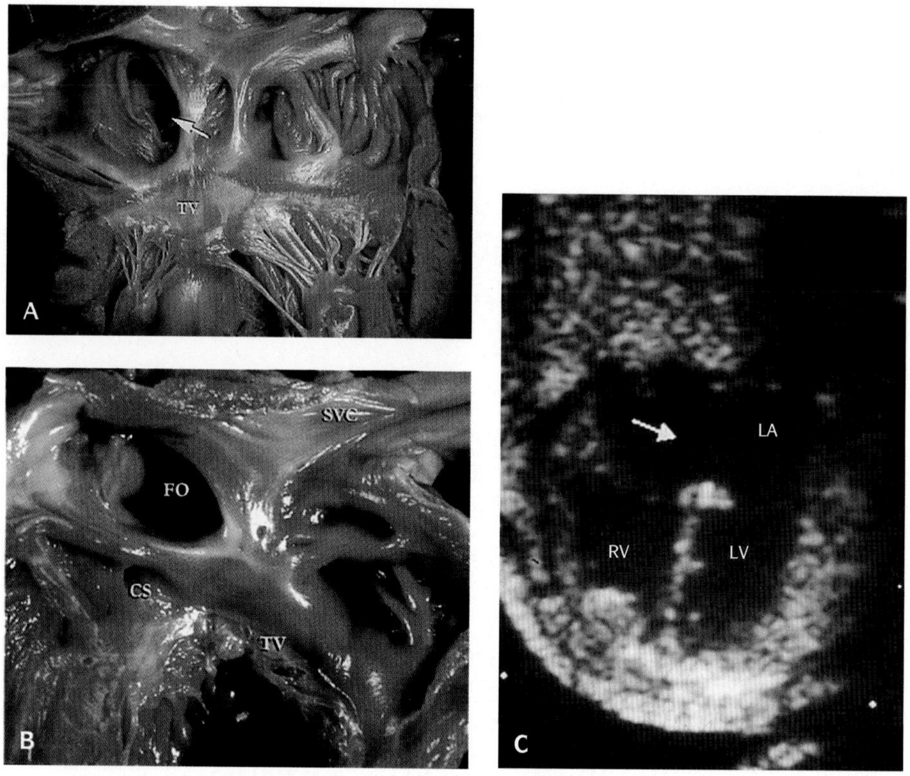

16.5. Ostium secundum ASD. **(A)** The flap valve of the foramen ovale is deficient (arrow). (TV, tricuspid valve.) **(B)** The flap valve of the foramen ovale is absent (FO). (SVC, superior vena cava; TV, tricuspid valve, CS, coronary sinus.) **(C)** Ultrasound of a septum secundum ASD (arrow) at 23 weeks gestation. (RV, right ventricle; LV, left ventricle, LA, left atrium.) (Courtesy of Florida Perinatal Associates, Tampa, FL.)

leaflet, and the two parts have a commisure-like insertion on the ventricular septum.

- In **intermediate atrioventricular septal defect** the MV and the tricuspid valve (TV) have clefts, and the valve commissures are usually inserted into the ventricular septum with fibrous tissue on the right side of the ventricular septum, closing the ring of the TV (Figure 16.7).

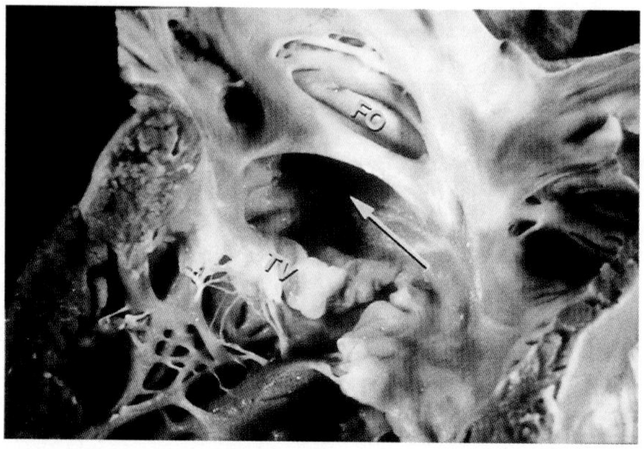

16.6. Ostium primum ASD (arrow). (FO, foramen ovale; TV, tricuspid valve.)

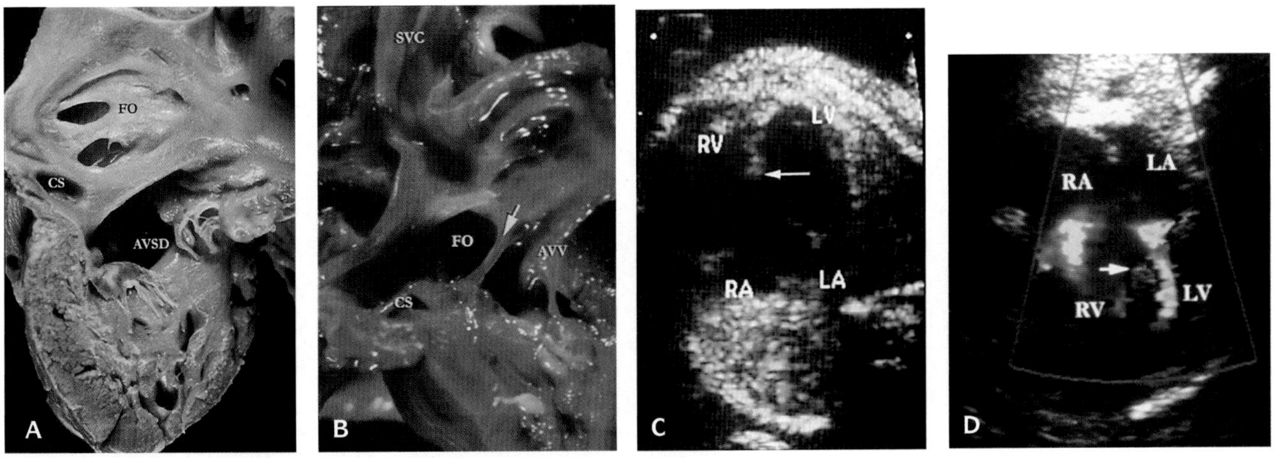

16.7. Atrioventricular septal defect (AVSD). **(A)** The septum secundum (FO) is fenestrated and the apical portion of the ventricular septum is intact. The septum primum and the interventricular septum have failed to fuse (AVSD). (CS, coronary sinus.) **(B)** The septum secundum (FO) is absent and only a thin remnant of the atrial septum remains (arrow) in this heart with an AVSD. (AVV, atrioventricular valve; SVC, superior vena cava, CS, coronary sinus.) **(C)** Ultrasound of an AVSD at 22 weeks gestation. (RA, right atrium; LA, left atrium; RV, right ventricle; LV, left ventricle.) This fetus had trisomy 21. (Courtesy of Florida Perinatal Associates, Tampa, FL.) **(D)** Ultrasound with color Doppler imaging in a heart with a hypoplastic left ventricle (LV), a malaligned AVSD, and a small left-sided inlet. (RA, right atrium; RV, right ventricle; LA, left atrium; arrow, crest of the ventricular septum.) (Courtesy of Dr. James Huhta.)

- There are three types of **complete endocardial cushion** (**AVSD**):
  - Type A – minimal bridging, with attachment to the right medial papillary muscle complex.
  - Type B – moderate bridging, with attachment to an aberrant right apical papillary muscle.
  - Type C – marked bridging, with attachment to the anterolateral papillary muscle of the right ventricle (RV).

A large left-to-right shunt results in severe congestive heart failure and pulmonary hypertensive vascular changes that may appear in the first year of life. Conduction abnormalities with left axis deviation and RV hypertrophy are present. AVSD may accompany other defects, including visceral asymmetry and poly/asplenia syndromes.

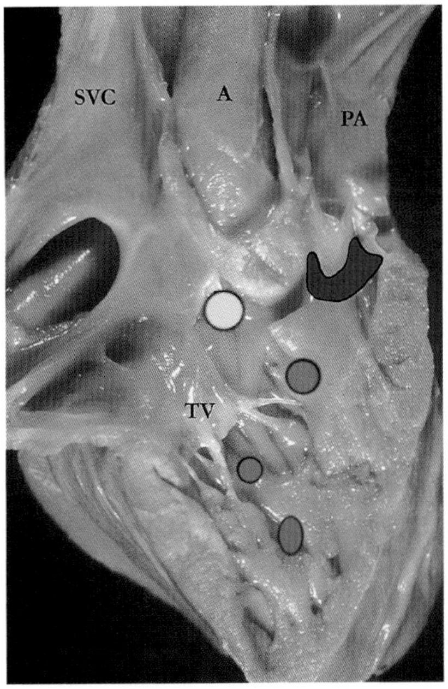

16.8. Types of ventricular septal defect (VSD); yellow, perimembranous VSD; blue, muscular VSDs; red, subarterial (doubly committed) VSD. A portion of the septal leaflet of the tricuspid valve (TV) has been removed. (SVC, superior venan cava; A, aorta; PA, pulmonary artery.)

Ventricular Septal Defects (VSD)

This is the most common congenital cardiac defect and accounts for approximately 30% of all cardiac defects, 80% of which are perimembranous. Eisenmenger complex is a large VSD with shunt reversal from RV to LV, which causes congestive heart failure and cyanosis. The defect may be (Figures 16.8 and 16.9):

1. perimembranous
2. subaortic
3. muscular

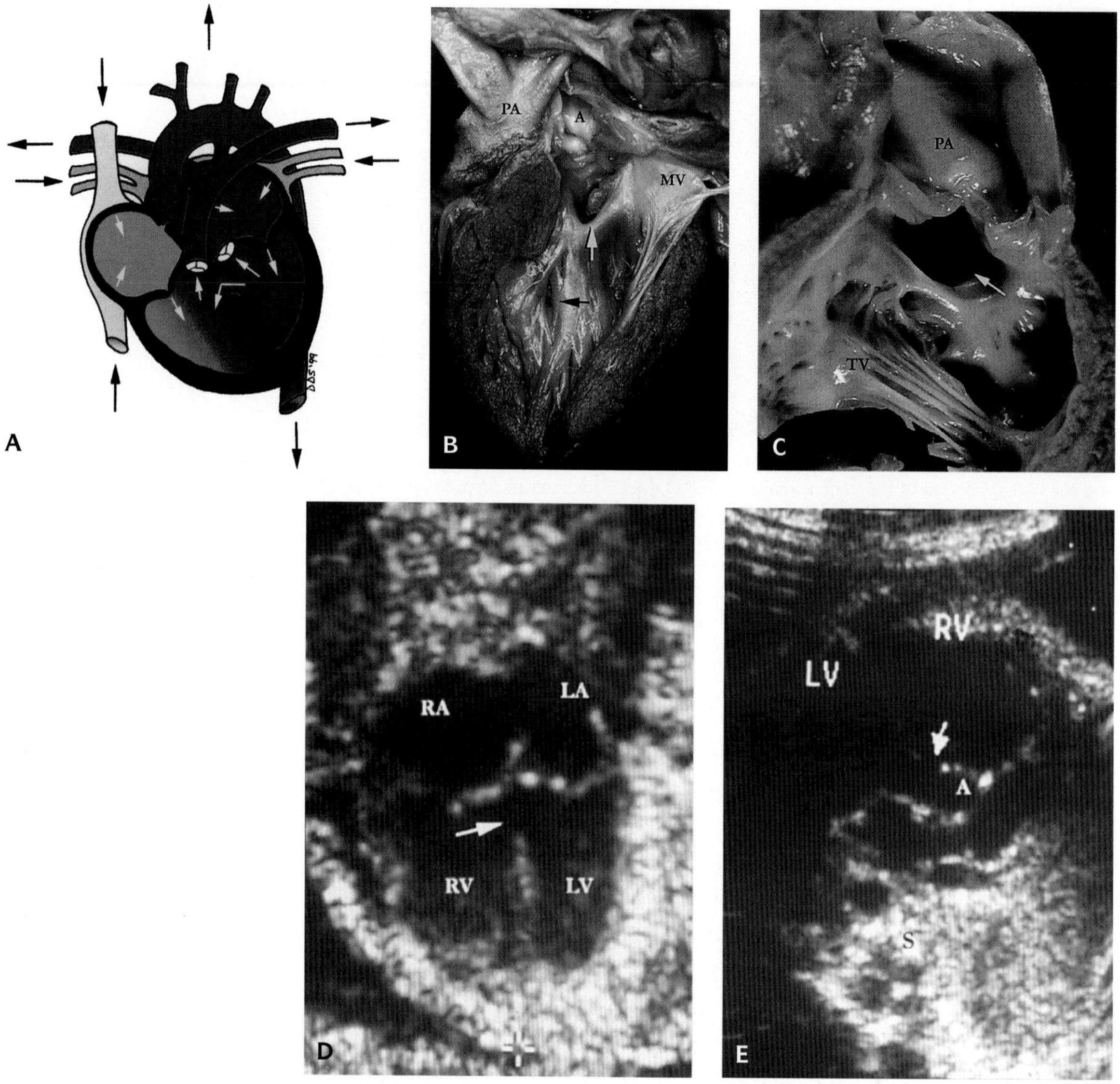

16.9. **(A)** Diagramatic representation of the flow of blood in a heart with a VSD. **(B)** Left ventricular septal surface with a perimembranous (yellow arrow) and a muscular (black arrow) VSD. (PA, pulmonary artery; A, aorta; MV, mitral valve). **(C)** Subarterial VSD (arrow). Note the right ventricular endocardial fibroelastosis. (PA, pulmonary artery; TV, tricuspid valve.) **(D)** Ultrasound of a VSD (arrow) in a four-chamber view of the heart at 23 weeks gestation. Note the normal septum secundum. (RA, right atrium; RV, right ventricle; LA, left atrium; LV, left ventricle.) (Courtesy of Florida Perinatal Associates, Tampa, FL.) **(E)** Ultrasound of the left ventricular outflow tract demonstrating a high perimembranous VSD (arrow) at 33 weeks gestation. (RV, right ventricle; LV, left ventricle; A, aorta, S, spine.) (Courtesy of Florida Perinatal Associates, Tampa, FL.)

Patent Ductus Arteriosus (PDA)

Ductal closure occurs on the aortic side because of the higher oxygen tension in the aorta (Figure 16.10). Physiologic closure is evident by about 16 hours of life; however, anatomic closure may not be complete for 2–3 weeks. Closure often can be induced by administration of prostaglandin inhibitors such as indomethacin.

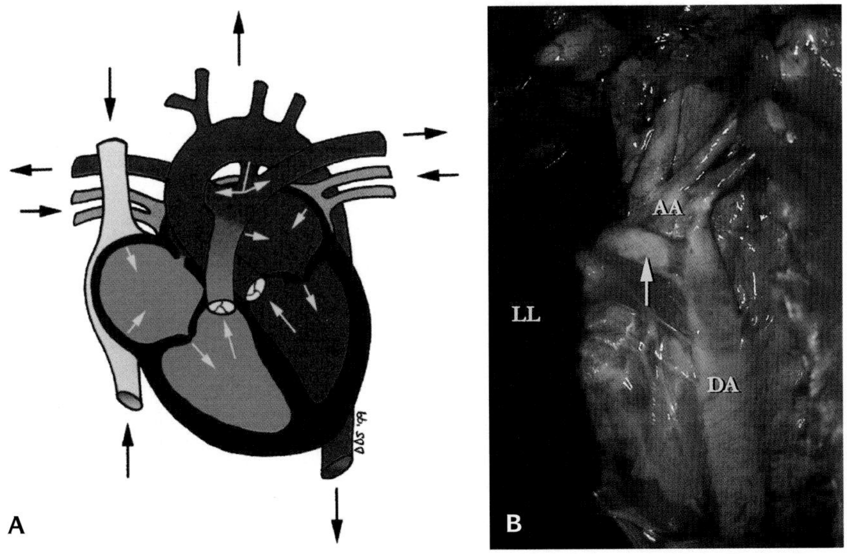

16.10. (A) Diagramatic representation of the flow of blood in a heart with a patent ductus arterious. **(B)** Patent ductus arteriosus (arrow) in an infant born with persistent fetal circulation, viewed from the left posterolateral aspect. The size of the ductus is nearly the same as the descending aorta (DA). (AA, aortic arch; LL, left lung.)

PDA is common in premature infants; patency may remain for some months after birth. In the presence of hypoxia, the DA tends to remain open – a continuous "machinery murmur" is heard over the DA.

VENOUS ARTERIAL SHUNTS

The most common type of a venous arterial shunt is an aortopulmonary window (Figure 16.11). This is usually located immediately superior to the

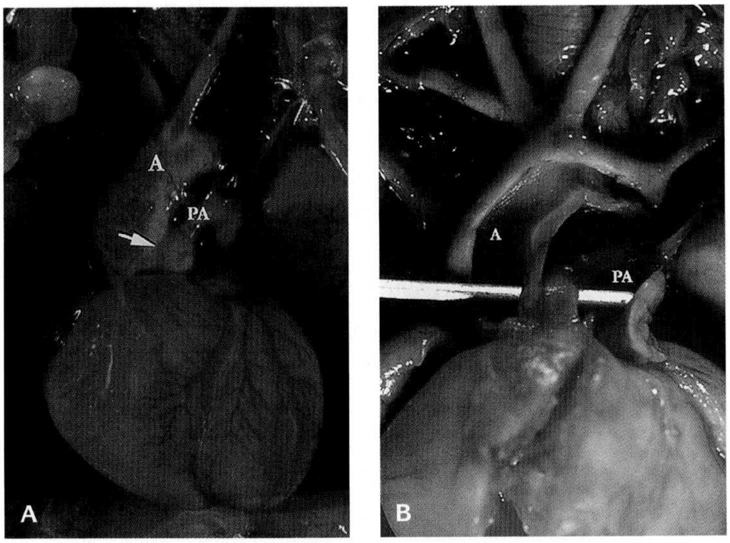

16.11. (A) In situ view of an aorta-pulmonary window (arrow). (A, aorta; PA, pulmonary artery.) **(B)** An opened aorta (A) and pulmonary artery (PA) with a probe passing through the aorta-pulmonary window. The ductus arteriosus is absent.

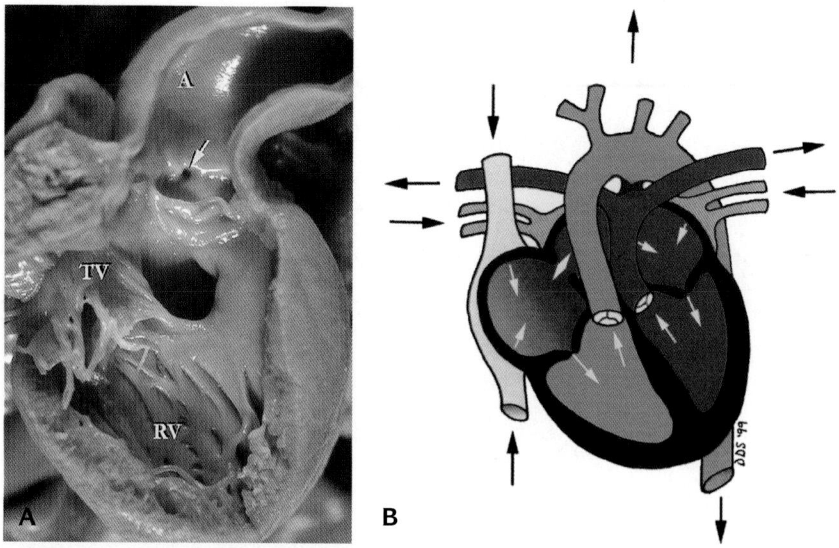

16.12. Transposition of the great arteries (TGA). **(A)** A normally positioned, morphologic right ventricle (RV) with the aorta (A) originating from it. Note the coronary orifice (arrow). The tricuspid valve (TV) is not in fibrous continuity with the aortic valve. A VSD is just beneath the aortic valve. **(B)** Diagrammatic representation of the flow of blood in TGA.

aortic and pulmonic valves and extends into the bifurcation of the pulmonary arteries.

VENOUS ARTERIAL SHUNTS WITH INCREASED PULMONARY BLOOD FLOW

Complete Transposition of Great Vessels (TGA)

Complete TGA accounts for 6% of all CHD (Figure 16.12). The atria may be in the usual or mirror-image position. The coronary arteries arise from the sinuses of the aortic valve and thus receive blood from the RV, resulting in a desaturated blood supply and ischemia of the myocardium. To be compatible with life there must be an exchange of blood between the two circulations, through either a patent foramen ovale, an ASD, a VSD, or a PDA. Severe pulmonary vascular changes occur in 40% of patients by 1 year of age.

Complete transposition may occur with an intact ventricular septum or VSD with pulmonary stenosis (valvular or infundibular). The latter may protect against the development of pulmonary vascular disease.

Corrected Transposition of the Great Vessels

There is no arteriovenous shunt in this defect. This condition is an "inversion" of the ventricles. The aorta is anterior and to the left of the pulmonary artery (PA). The PA connects to a right-sided morphologic LV from which the PA originates (Figure 16.13). The LA connects to a left-sided morphologic RV from which the aorta originates. Corrected transposition usually is asymptomatic

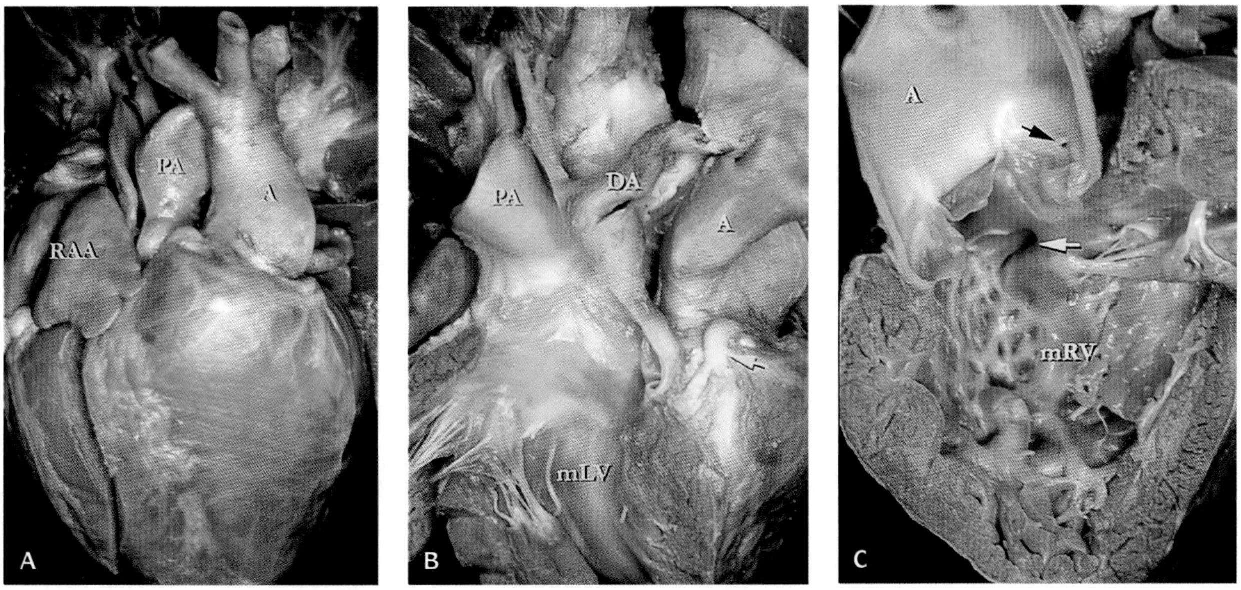

16.13. Congenitally corrected TGA. **(A)** Characteristic outward appearance with the aorta (A) arising anterior and to the left of the pulmonary artery (PA). The pulmonary artery is positioned posterior and to the right. (RAA, right atrial appendage.) **(B)** The pulmonary artery (PA) arises from a morphologic left ventricle (mLV) on the right side of the heart. The pulmonary valve is in fibrous continuity with the mitral valve. (A, aorta; DA, ductus arteriosus; arrow, left anterior descending coronary artery.) **(C)** The aorta (A) arises from a morphologic right ventricle (mRV) on the left side of the heart and is supported by a complete muscular infundibulum. (Black arrow, coronary orifice.) A VSD (yellow arrow) is present.

except when associated with other congenital anomalies (e.g., TV dysplasia, pulmonary outflow obstruction, and VSD).

Truncus Arteriosus (TA)

TA accounts for <1% of CHD (Figure 16.14). A single arterial trunk originates from a single semilunar valve and gives origin to the aorta, one or both pulmonary arteries, and the coronary arteries. The truncal valve has two to five cusps that are often thickened and dysplastic leaflets that may result in stenosis or incompetency and may override a VSD. The truncal valve is always in fibrous continuity with the MV. The coronary arteries have a variable pattern, with a single coronary artery present in almost 20% of cases. Four types have been described:

Type I – single pulmonary trunk and ascending aorta arrising from a common trunk;

Type II – left and right PAs arising close together from the posterior or dorsal wall of the truncus;

Type III – right and left PAs arising independently from either side of the truncus;

Type IV – no PAs identified and there is apparent absence of the sixth arterial arch. The bronchial arteries supply the lungs (this is now considered a variant of pulmonary atresia with VSD).

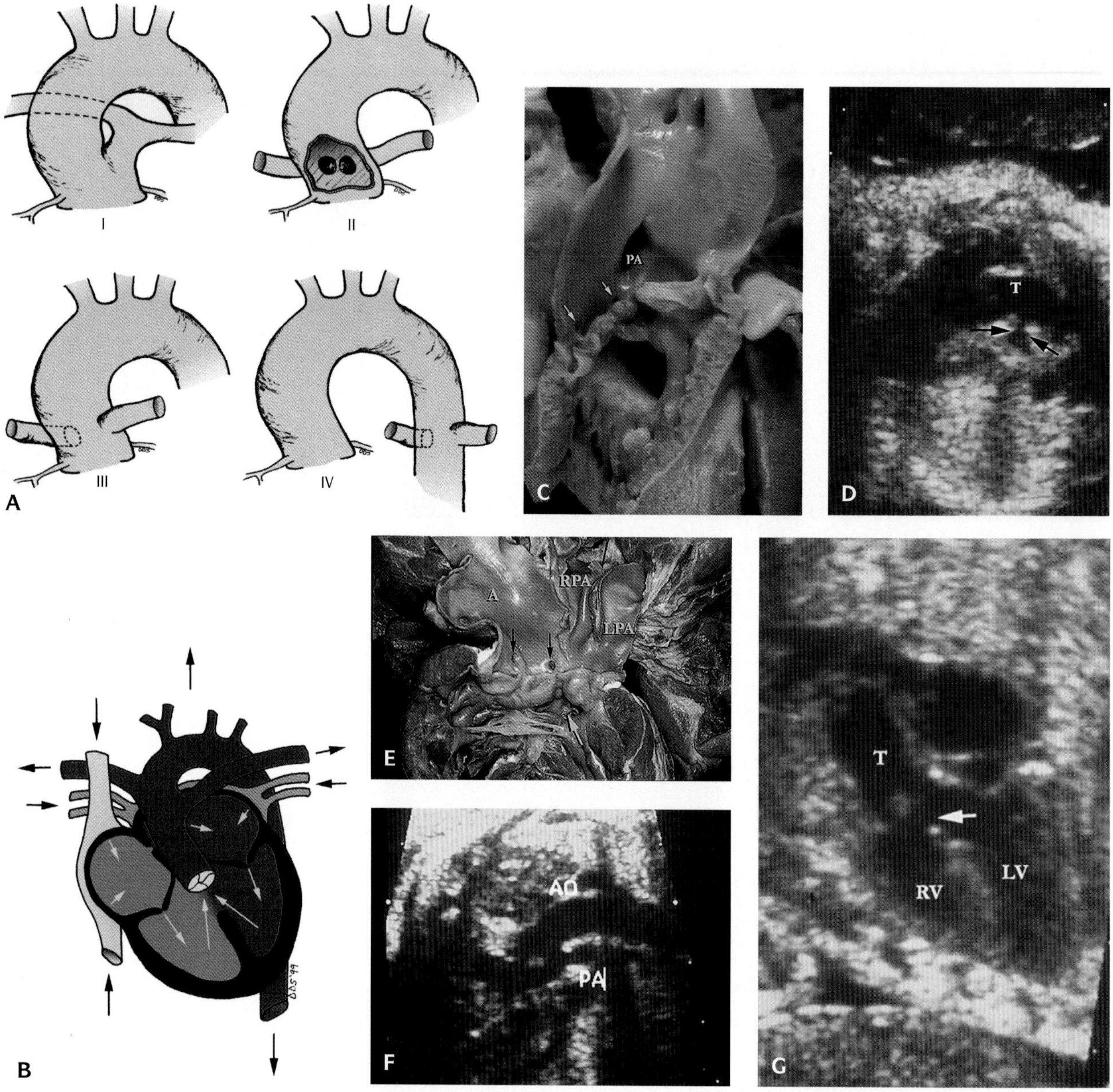

16.14. Truncus arteriosus (TA). **(A)** Illustration of the four types. **(B)** Diagrammatic representation of the flow of blood in a heart with TA. **(C)** Truncus arteriosus type I. The hypoplastic right ventricle is opened, showing a single arterial valve ring composed of three leaflets. (Arrows, coronary orifices.) The pulmonary arterial (PA) component of the common trunk exits posteriorly and divides into the right and left pulmonary arteries. Note the VSD just beneath the valve ring. This heart had tricuspid atresia as well. **(D)** Ultrasound of a truncus arteriosus (T) at 37 weeks gestation with a main pulmonary artery (arrows) branching from it that later branches into right and left pulmonary arteries. (Courtesy of Florida Perinatal Associates, Tampa, FL.) **(E)** Truncus arteriosus type I. The right ventricle is opened and the common trunk is guarded by a thickened valve with three leaflets. Below the valve is a VSD (yellow arrow) and above it are two coronary orifices (black arrows). The pulmonary (RPA, right pulmonary artery; LPA, left pulmonary artery) and aortic (A) portions of the common trunk are easily visualized. **(F)** Ultrasound at 20 weeks gestation showing the aortic (AO) and pulmonary (PA) portions of the truncus branching from a common valve ring. (Courtesy of Florida Perinatal Associates, Tampa, FL.) **(G)** Ultrasound of a truncus arteriosus (T) at 20 weeks gestation with a VSD (arrow) just beneath the valve ring. (RV, right ventricle; LV, left ventricle.) (Courtesy of Florida Perinatal Associates, Tampa, FL.)

Partial Anomalous Pulmonary Venous Connection (PAPVC)

PAPVC occurs when blood from one or more pulmonary veins drains into the systemic venous system (Figure 16.15).

Total Anomalous Pulmonary Venous Connection (TAPVC)

In the supradiaphragmatic form of TAPVC all the pulmonary veins drain into the systemic circulation without obstructing drainage (Figure 16.16). A vertical vein originating from a confluence of pulmonary veins posterior to the LA drains into the innominate vein at its junction with the left subclavian vein or coronary sinus before draining into the RA. Venous drainage may connect on the right to the vena cava or azygous vein or may be infradiaphragmatic into the portal venous system.

When pulmonary veins empty into a common chamber with a muscular shelf or diaphragm separating the pulmonary venous compartment from the atrial chamber (cor triatriatum), this results in pulmonary venous obstruction.

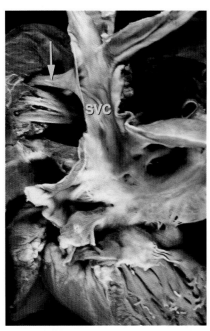

16.15. PAPVC. The upper right pulmonary vein (arrow) drains into the superior vena cava (SVC).

Double Outlet Right Ventricle (DORV)

DORV accounts for 1–3% of CHD (Figure 16.17). A double conus is present and there is discontinuity between the mitral and aortic valves. Pulmonary stenosis occurs in 40–50% of cases. ASD and AVSD may be associated.

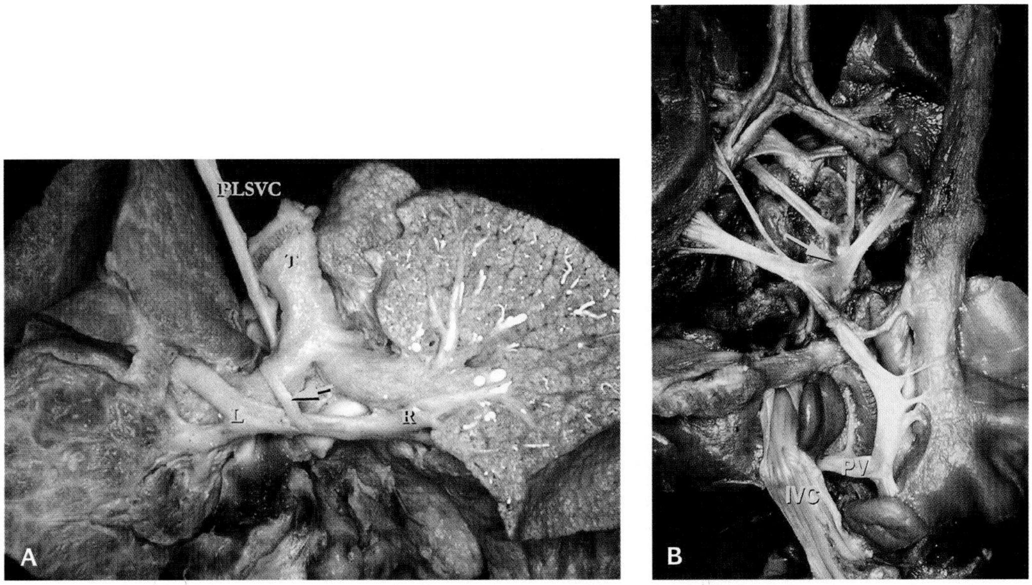

16.16. TAPVC. **(A)** Above the diaphragm. The right (R) and left (L) pulmonary veins form a confluence behind the heart and drain into the persistent left superior vena cava (PLSVC) via a vertical vein (arrow). (T, trachea.) **(B)** Below the diaphragm. The pulmonary veins form a confluence behind the heart (arrow). This single vessel passes through the diaphragm and drains into the portal vein (PV). (IVC, inferior vena cava.) This infant had situs inversus associated with polysplenia and died after attempted surgical correction.

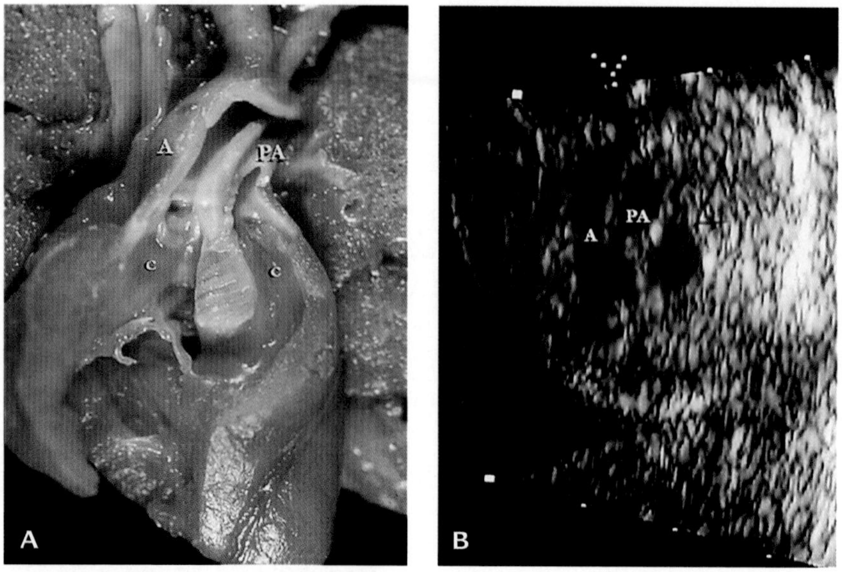

16.17. **(A)** Double outlet right ventricle (DORV) in a fetus at 15 weeks gestation. The aorta (A) and pulmonary artery (PA) exit the heart side by side with the aorta to the right of the pulmonary artery. Both vessels arise from the right ventricle and there is a double conus (C) or infundibulum. There is no fibrous continuity between the aorta and mitral valve. A VSD is usually present. **(B)** Ultrasound showing the characteristic side by side position of the aorta (A) and pulmonary artery (PA) in a DORV at 20 weeks gestation. (Courtesy of Florida Perinatal Associates, Tampa, FL.)

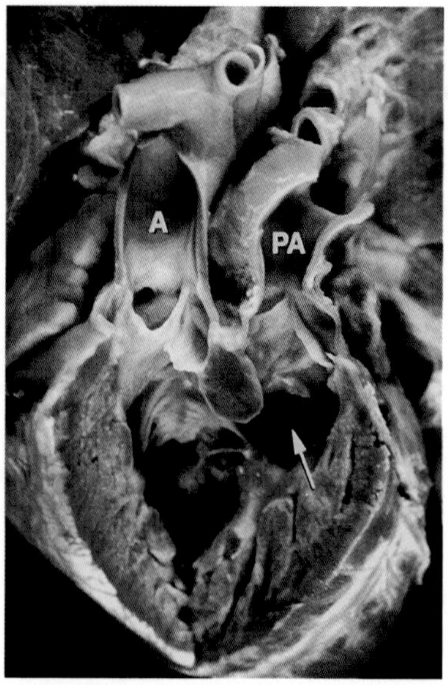

16.18. Taussing-Bing malformation. The aorta (A) lies to the right of the pulmonary artery (PA), which overrides the septum (arrow, VSD).

Taussig-Bing malformation is a variant of DORV in which the VSD is subpulmonic without pulmonary stenosis (Figure 16.18).

EBSTEIN MALFORMATION

This common form of isolated tricuspid stenosis and insufficiency accounts for an incidence of 1% of CHD (Figure 16.19). There is downward displacement of the tricuspid valve and atrialization of the right ventricle. The anomaly may be associated with maternal lithium ingestion during the first trimester of pregnancy.

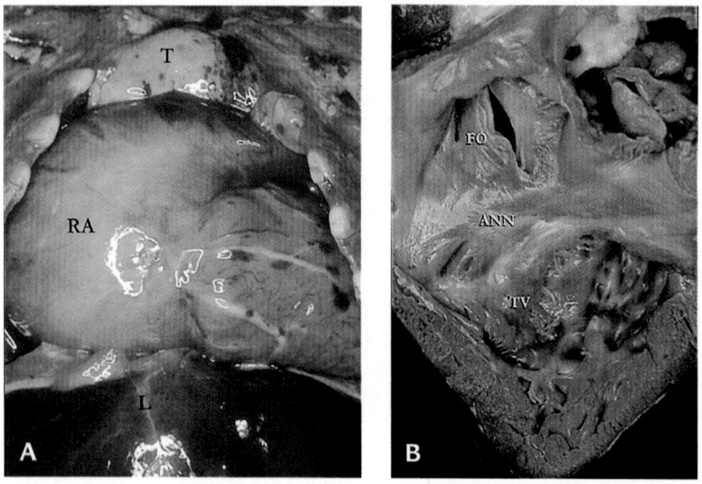

16.19. Ebstein malformation. **(A)** In situ view of a heart with a large, dilated right atrium (RA) secondary to significant tricuspid valve regurgitation. (T, thymus; L, liver.) **(B)** The tricuspid valve (TV) is displaced into the right ventricle. (ANN, normal position of the tricuspid valve annulus; FO, foramen ovale.)

VENOUS-ARTERIAL SHUNTS WITH DECREASED PULMONARY BLOOD FLOW

Tetralogy of Fallot (TOF)

TOF is the most common form of cyanotic CHD, with an incidence of 1 in 4,000 births (Figure 16.20). The components of tetralogy are infundibular pulmonic stenosis, VSD, aortic valve dextroposition, and RV hypertrophy. However, it is the result of a single embryologic defect due

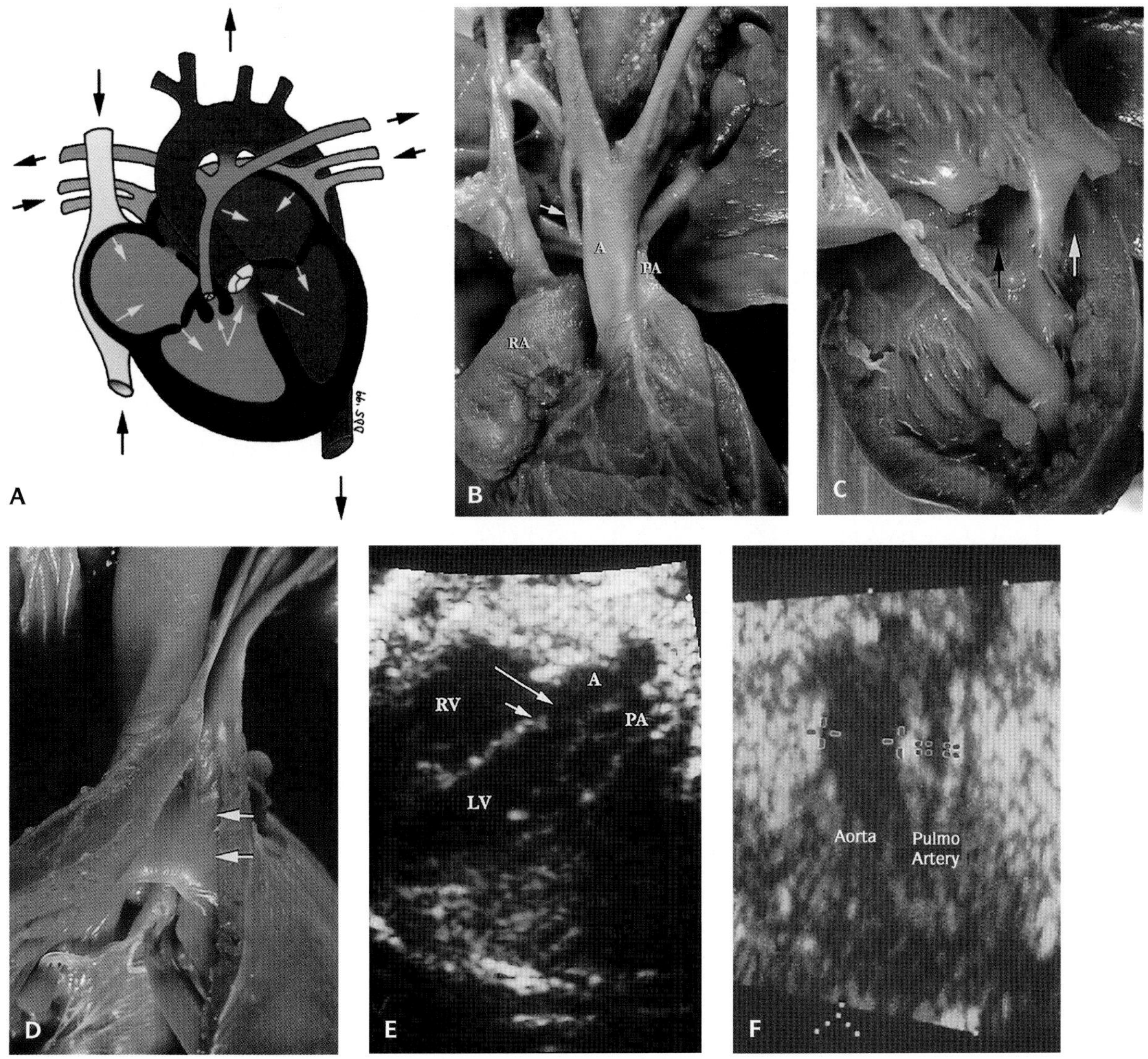

16.20. Tetralogy of Fallot (TOF). **(A)** Diagrammatic representation of the flow of blood in a heart with TOF. **(B)** Anterior, external view. The aorta (A) is large and dextraposed (overriding) and the pulmonary artery (PA) is stenotic. There was a right ductus arteriosus (arrow). (RA, right atrium.) **(C)** Opened right ventricle showing a perimembranous VSD (black arrow) and infundibular stenosis of the pulmonary outflow (yellow arrow). **(D)** Pulmonary infundibular stenosis (arrows). **(E)** Ultrasound of tetralogy of Fallot at 23 weeks gestation showing the aorta (A) overriding the septum (short arrow) with a VSD (long arrow) and a small pulmonary artery (PA). (Courtesy of Florida Perinatal Associates, Tampa, FL.) **(F)** Ultrasound at 23 weeks gestation showing the difference in size between the aorta and pulmonary artery. (Courtesy of Florida Perinatal Associates, Tampa, FL.)

to malalignment with anterior deviation of the conus (infundibular) septum, which creates infundibular narrowing, a perimembranous VSD, and a dextroposition with overriding of the aorta above the VSD. Associated anomalies include ASD (pentalogy of Fallot), right aortic arch, and absence of the DA.

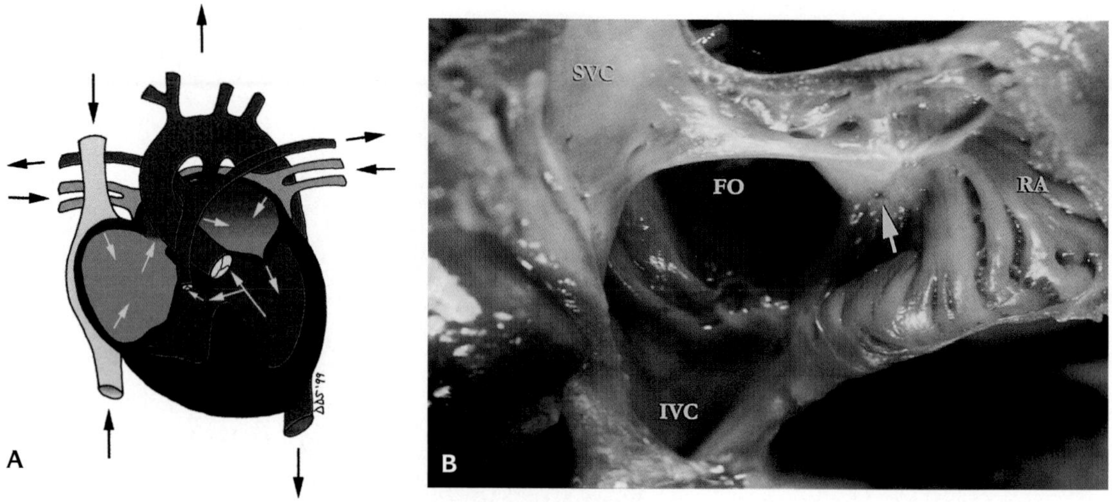

16.21. Tricuspid valve atresia (TVA). **(A)** Diagrammatic representation of the flow of blood in a heart with TVA. **(B)** Opened right atrium in a heart with TVA. The tricuspid valve orifice is nonexistent and is represented by a dimple (arrow) at the base of the atrium. (RA, right atrial appendage; FO, foramen ovale; IVC, inferior vena cava; SVC, superior vena cava.)

A "coeur en sabot" (boot-shaped heart) appearance due to RV hypertrophy and an upward tilting of the LV apex is seen by X-ray. Decreased pulmonary blood flow results in the clear appearance of the chest radiograph because of decreased vascular markings.

Tricuspid Valve Atresia (TVA) (Hypoplastic Right Heart Complex)

TVA accounts for 1–3% of all CHD (Figure 16.21). A hypoplastic RV with marked dilatation of the RA and absence of identifiable valvular tissue is present in 85% of cases (Figure 16.22). The RA becomes enormously dilated and the LV is markedly hypertrophied. The outlet from the RA is through a patent foramen ovale or ASD.

OBSTRUCTIVE LESIONS OF THE RIGHT SIDE OF THE HEART

Pulmonary Stenosis with Intact Ventricular Septum (PS-IVS)

PS-IVS comprises 7% of CHD (Figure 16.23). Obstruction usually is valvular with RV hypertrophy and post-stenotic dilatation of the pulmonary trunk. The valve may be dome shaped with fused cusps and a single central orifice. An ASD or a patent foramen ovale allows shunting of blood to the LA.

Pulmonary Atresia

The valve leaflets usually are fused into a dome, forming a nipple-like projection into the artery (Figure 16.24). The RV may be hypoplastic or normal in size. Cyanosis occurs early because of decreased pulmonary blood flow, which is DA dependent.

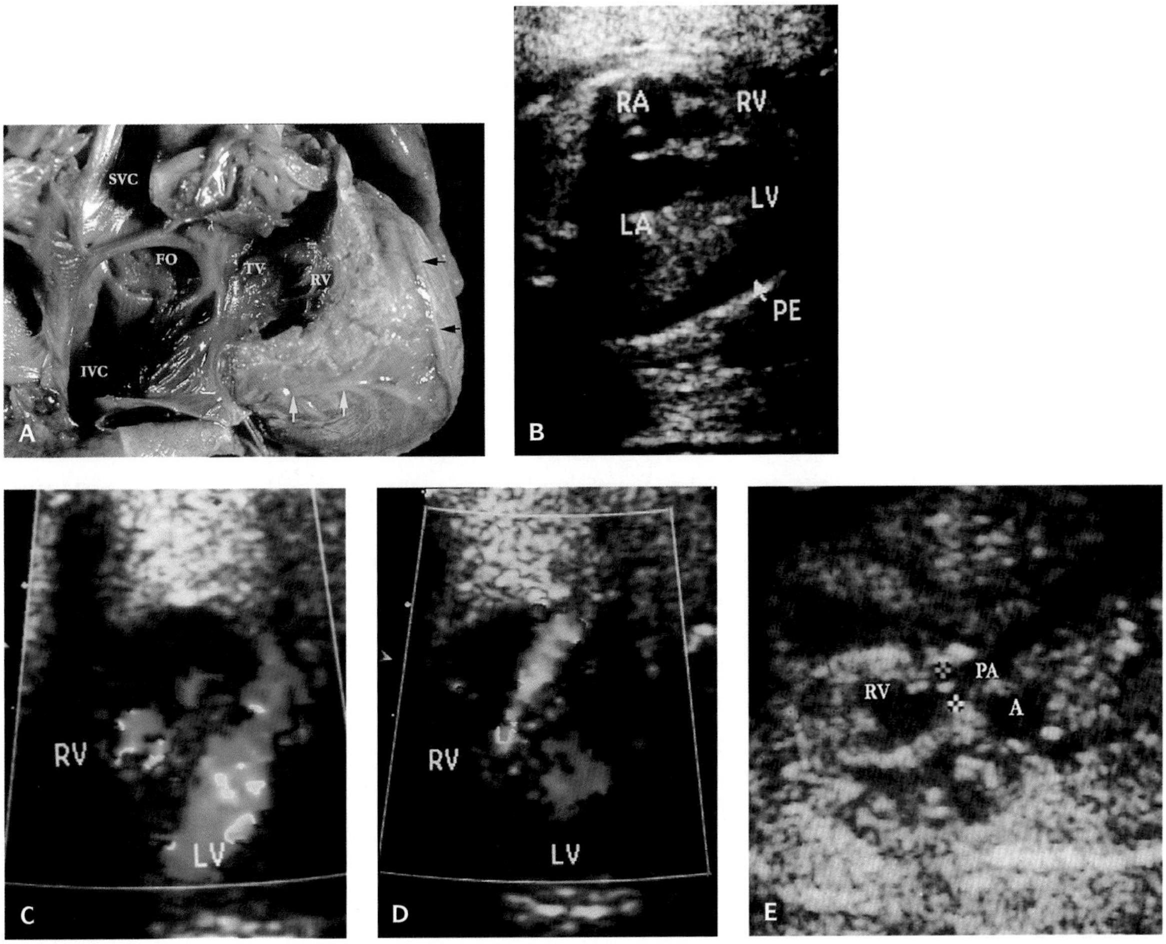

16.22. **(A)** Hypoplastic right ventricle. The small right ventricle (RV) is outlined by the coronary arteries (yellow arrows, posterior descending coronary artery; black arrows, left anterior descending coronary artery.) A thickened tricuspid valve (TV) guards its inlet. (IVC, inferior vena cava; SVC, superior vena cava; FO, foramen ovale.) **(B)** Ultrasound of a heart with a hypoplastic right ventricle showing a small, thick right ventricle (RV). This case exhibited a pleural effusion (PE) and was performed at 22 weeks gestation. (RA, right atrium; LA, left atrium; LV, left ventricle.) (Courtesy of Florida Perinatal Associates, Tampa, FL.) **(C)** Ultrasound with color Doppler imaging showing a small right ventricle (RV) compared with the large left ventricle (LV). (Courtesy of Florida Perinatal Associates, Tampa, FL.) **(D)** Ultrasound with color Doppler imaging showing tricuspid valve regurgitation (red-yellow area) in a heart with hypoplastic right ventricle at twenty weeks gestation. (RV, right ventricle; LV, left ventricle.) (Courtesy of Dr. James Huhta.) **(E)** Ultrasound of a heart with a hypoplastic right ventricle (RV) and pulmonary artery (PA) stenosis. The aorta (A) is shown in cross section. The ultrasound was performed at 22 weeks of gestation. (Courtesy of Florida Perinatal Associates, Tampa, FL.)

OBSTRUCTIVE LESIONS OF THE LEFT SIDE OF THE HEART

Mitral Valve Defect

1. Parachute mitral valve, in which the chordae are inserted into a single papillary muscle group, resulting in a funnel-shaped valve;
2. Shone syndrome, consisting of a parachute mitral valve, a supramitral ring, subaortic stenosis, and coarctation of the aorta.
3. Mitral atresia or severe mitral stenosis.

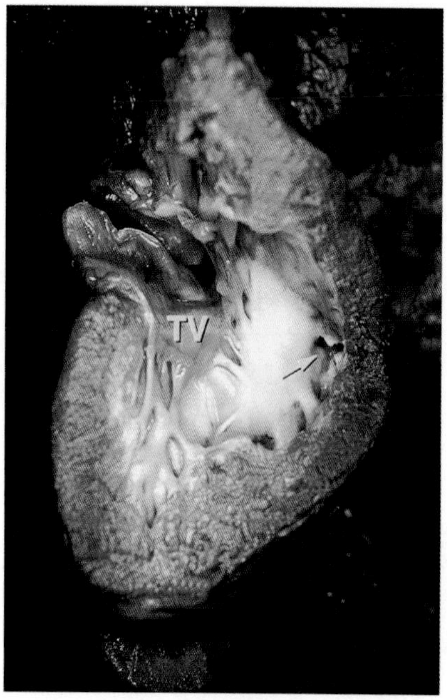

16.23. Pulmonary stenosis (arrow) with an intact ventricular septum. There is hypertrophy and endocardial fibroelastosis of the right ventricle. (TV, tricuspid valve.)

These defects result in an obstruction of blood flow from LA to LV. Pulmonary venous drainage is through a patent FO. Mitral atresia is most commonly associated with aortic atresia and is included in the hypoplastic left heart complex.

Aortic Atresia (AA)

AA has a 2:1 male predominance (Figure 16.25). In isolated AA the mitral valve and LV cavity are hypoplastic. Secondary endocardial fibroelastosis (EFE) and hypertrophy of the LV wall occur.

Aortic Stenosis

There are three types of supravalvular aortic stenosis (SVAS): hourglass deformity, segmental stenosis with diffuse hypoplasia of the ascending aorta, and fibromuscular membrane (Figure 16.26). SVAS may be sporadic. Williams syndrome (WS) is a sporadic disorder (occasionally familial with autosomal dominant transmission) with an incidence of 1 in 20,000 to 1 in 50,000 live births. It is characterized by hypercalcemia in infancy (15%); a dolichocephalic asymmetrical typical face (elfin facies; bitemporal depression; periorbital prominence; epicanthal folds; starburst pattern on blue or green irises; and prominent lips, mouth, and nasal tip with anteverted nostrils), growth retardation; clinodactyly of the fifth fingers; pectus excavatum; valvular aortic and pulmonic stenosis; atrial and ventricular septal defects; hyperacusis and developmental delay in the presence of exceptional linguistic, auditory, and musical abilities; and marked sociability.

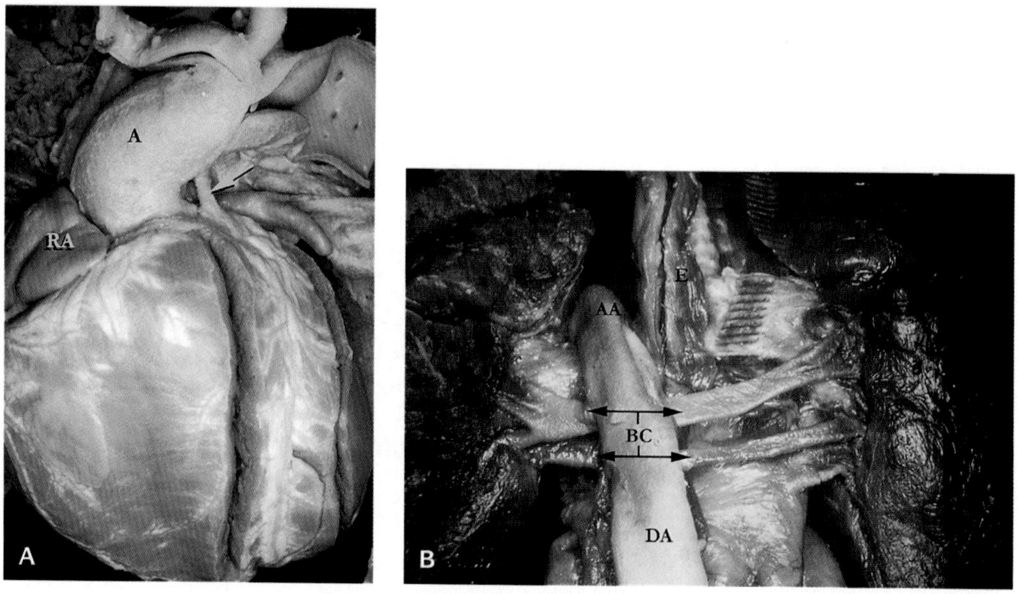

16.24. Pulmonary atresia. **(A)** The pulmonary artery (arrow) is represented by a thin fibrous cord (arrow). (A, aorta; RA, right atrium.) **(B)** Large bronchial collateral vessels (BC) from the descending thoracic aorta (DA) in pulmonary atresia. (AA, aortic arch; E, esophagus.)

This disorder has been associated with loss of one copy of the elastin gene (ELN) containing 34 exons on chromosome 7q11.23 but the cellular mechanisms that lead to the phenotype of WS are as yet undetermined.

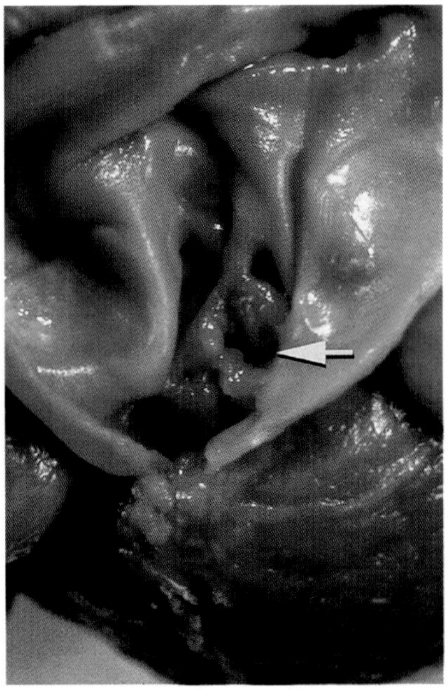

16.25. Aortic stenosis. Thickened leaflets that are fused at the commisures form a dome (arrow).

Subaortic Stenosis (SAS)

There are three types:

1. Dynamic type, hypertrophic cardiomyopathy (HCM).
2. Fixed type, a shelf-like fibrous ridge is on the ventricular septal surface, extending to the ventricular aspect of the anterior mitral leaflet.
3. Tunnel type, a fibromuscular tunnel beneath the aortic valve intervenes between the mitral and aortic valves.

Hypoplastic Left Heart Complex (HLHC)

HLHC takes two forms (Figure 16.27). With mitral atresia, an atrioventricular connection is absent and the LV is a trabecular pouch. With mitral stenosis the ventricular chamber is small and shows considerable endocardial fibroelastosis. There is a rudimentary left ventricle, aortic atresia or stenosis, and hypoplastic or atretic ascending aorta. Blood supply to the lower extremities is through a patent DA. When the DA closes, it is incompatible with life. The infant is pale with absent peripheral pulses. A Norwood procedure (see Table 16.7) has

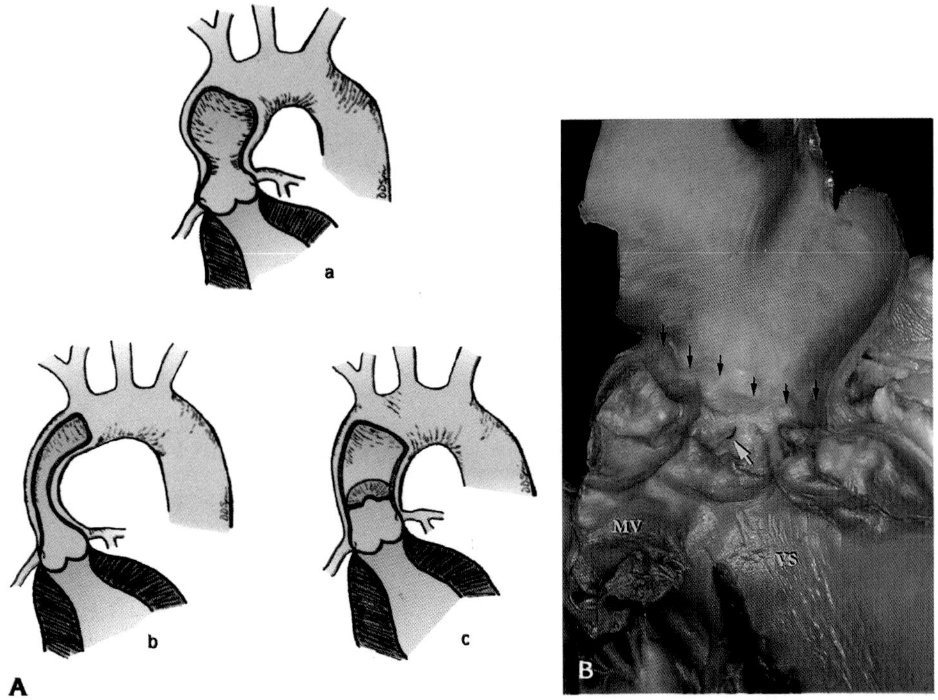

16.26. **(A)** Diagram of SVAS, three types. **(B)** Opened aortic valve with thickened leaflets and a supravalvular ridge (arrows) causing stenosis and an hourglass appearance. (Yellow Arrow, coronary orifice; VS, ventricular septum; MV, mitral valve.)

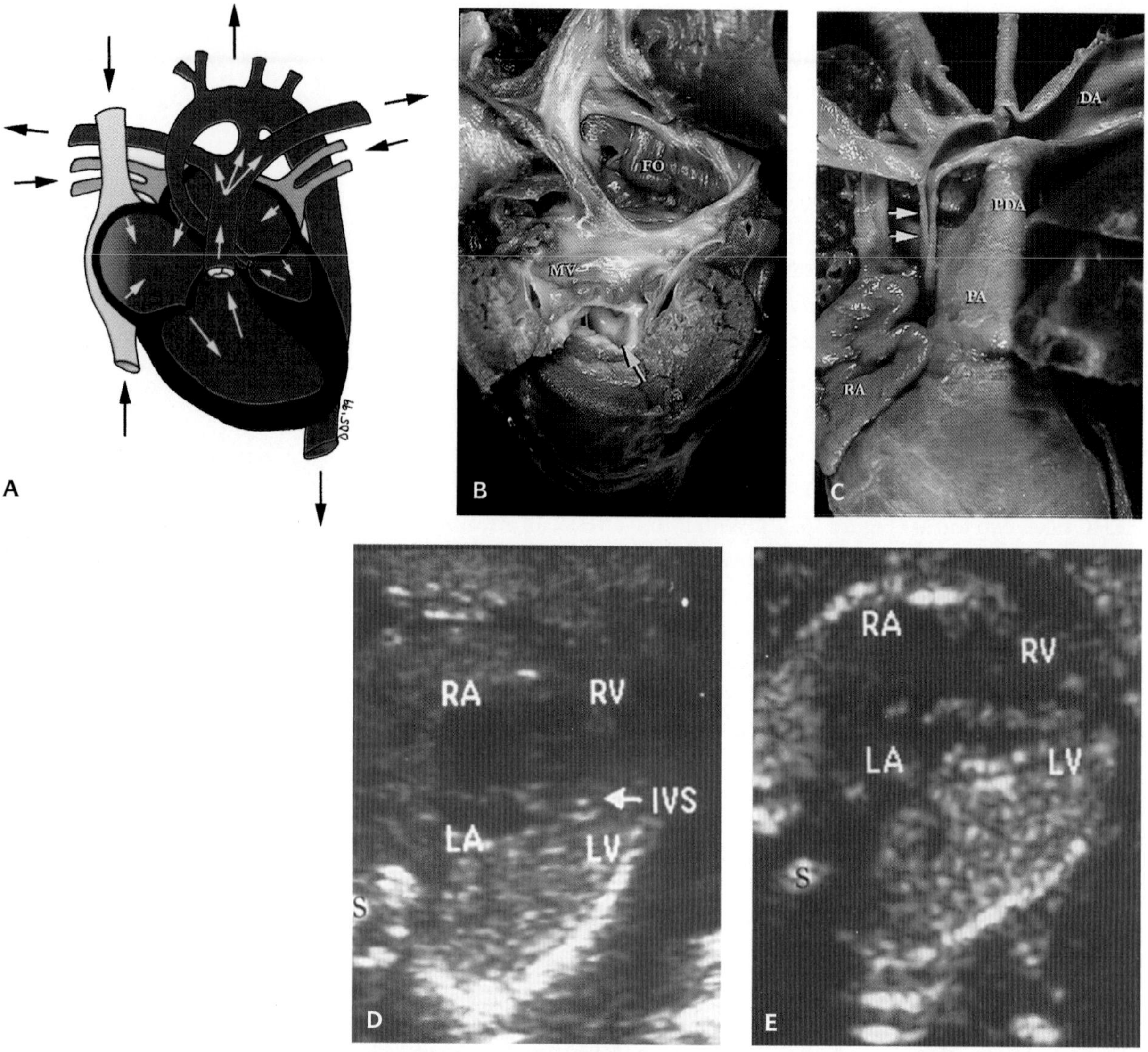

16.27. Hypoplastic left heart (HLH). **(A)** Diagrammatic representation of the flow of blood in a heart with HLH. **(B)** Hypoplastic left ventricle with endocardial fibroelastosis (arrow) and a stenotic mitral valve (MV). (FO, foramen ovale.) **(C)** Typical appearance of the great vessels with a HLH. The ascending aorta is very stenotic (arrows) and the pulmonary artery (PA) and patent ductus arteriosus (PDA) are large. (RA, right atrium; DA, descending aorta.) **(D)** Ultrasound of a hypoplastic left heart at 20 weeks gestation. The right atrium (RA) and right ventricle (RV) are large. The left atrium (LA) and the left ventricle (LV) are very tiny. The interventricular septum (IVS) is identified (arrow). (Courtesy of Florida Perinatal Associates, Tampa, FL.) **(E)** Ultrasound of a heart with a small left ventricle (LV) at 18 weeks gestation that was not diagnosed as being hypoplastic. (RA, right atrium; RV, right ventricle; LA, left atrium.) (Courtesy of Florida Perinatal Associates, Tampa, FL.)

been used with limited success. Transplantation is the only satisfactory form of therapy.

Coarctation of the Aorta

Coarctation may be preductal or ductal (Figure 16.28). In the preductal type there is a tubular hypoplasia of the aortic arch. Symptoms become manifest

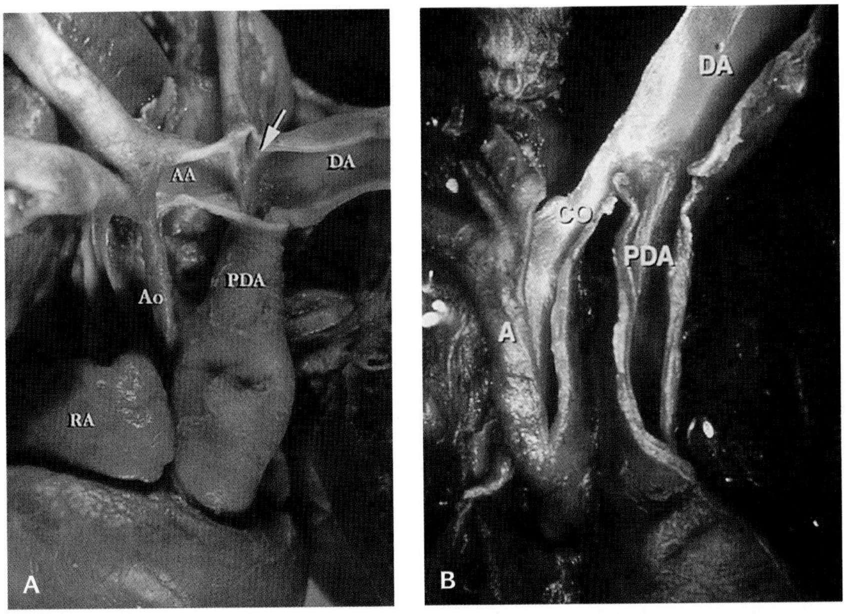

16.28. **(A)** Adult type coarctation of the aorta (arrow). (AA, ascending aorta; AA, aortic arch; DA, descending aorta; PDA, patent ductus arteriosus; RA, right atrium.) **(B)** Infantile (preductal) coarctation (CO) (A, aorta; PDA, patent ductus arterious; DA, descending aorta.)

early in infancy. The ductal type consists of a localized constriction of the aorta in the region of the closure of the ductus arteriosus. Symptoms in this type usually are delayed until adolescence or later.

Interrupted Aortic Arch

This rarely is an isolated lesion (Figure 16.29). Associated malformations include bicuspid aortic valves (5%), PDA (50%), VSD (40–50%), left heart obstruction (24%), subclavian artery anomalies, and TA. Extracardiac anomalies are common.

Anomalous Origin of Left Coronary Artery from Pulmonary Trunk

Most infants become symptomatic in the first months of life, and death ensues if the anomaly is not corrected by surgery. Abundant collateral arteries develop between the right and left coronary arteries, causing shunting of blood from the coronary arterial system to the pulmonary trunk that results in ischemia and/or infarction and sudden death. Ischemic changes and frequently infarction of the LV may occur. Anomalous origin of the right coronary artery usually is asymptomatic.

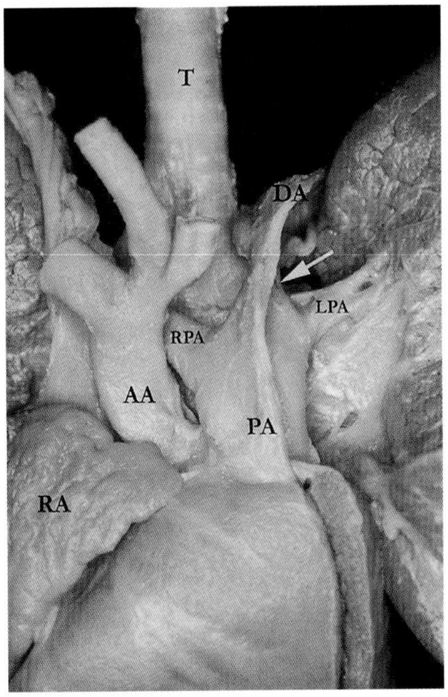

16.29. Interrupted aortic arch. (AA, ascending aorta; PA, main pulmonary artery; arrow, ductus; DA, descending aorta; RPA, right pulmonary artery; LPA, left pulmonary artery; RA, right atrial appendage; T, trachea.)

ABNORMALITIES OF POSITION AND SITUS

Dextroposition describes a heart displaced to the right side of the thorax with a left-sided apex (Figure 16.30). Dextrocardia implies that the heart is located in the right chest with a right-sided apex. This occurs with situs inversus as

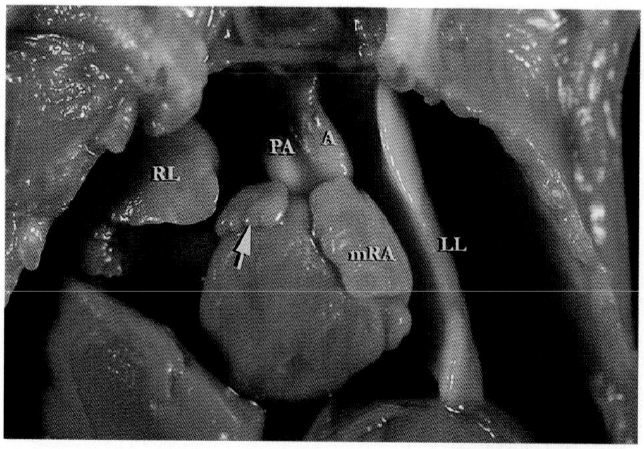

16.30. Dextrocardia in a fetus with situs inversus. Apex of the heart points to the right. (RL, right lung; LL, left lung; PA, pulmonary artery; A, aorta; mRA, left-sided morphologic right atrial appendage; arrow, right-sided morphologic left atrial appendage.)

an isolated finding. Isolated dextrocardia has a high incidence of intra- and extracardiac anomalies.

In asplenia syndrome (right atrial isomerism) bilateral right-sidedness is associated with an absent spleen (Ivemark syndrome) and nucleated red blood cells in the peripheral smear (Figures 16.31 to 16.33). In >50% of cases the liver is symmetric with the gallbladder, stomach, duodenum, and pancreas on the right side, with varying degrees of malrotation of the intestines. The lungs are trilobed with bilateral eparterial bronchi. Severe cardiac defects include bilateral superior venae cavae that drain to the respective atria. Transposition of the great vessels, common atrioventricular valve, and pulmonary stenosis or atresia are common.

In polysplenia (left atrial isomerism) bilateral left-sidedness is associated with multiple spleens located on both sides of the dorsal mesogastrium (Figures 16.34 to 16.37). The abdominal part of the IVC ascends on either the right or left side of the spine and enters the atrium on its corresponding side. Total anomalous pulmonary venous connection (TAPVC) is the rule. In most the IVC connects to the azygos venous system and drains into the SVC. Separate common hepatic veins usually

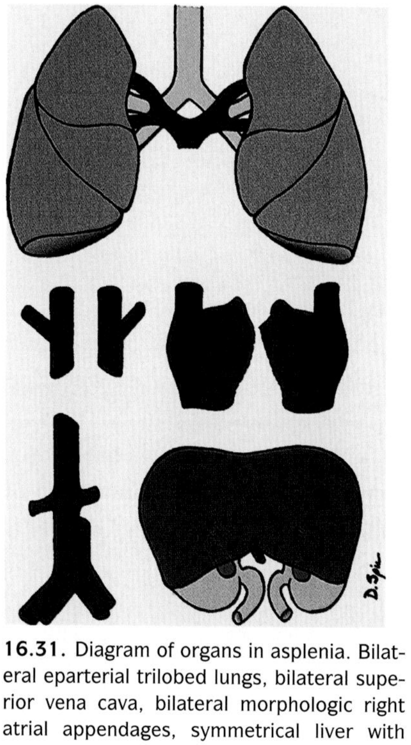

16.31. Diagram of organs in asplenia. Bilateral eparterial trilobed lungs, bilateral superior vena cava, bilateral morphologic right atrial appendages, symmetrical liver with gallbladder and stomach on either side of the abdomen.

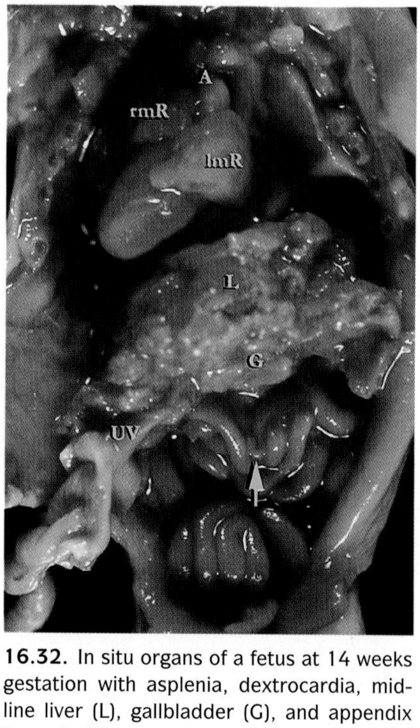

16.32. In situ organs of a fetus at 14 weeks gestation with asplenia, dextrocardia, midline liver (L), gallbladder (G), and appendix (arrow). (A, aorta; rMR, right-sided morphologic right atrial appendage; lMR, left-sided morphologic right atrial appendage; UV, umbilical vein.)

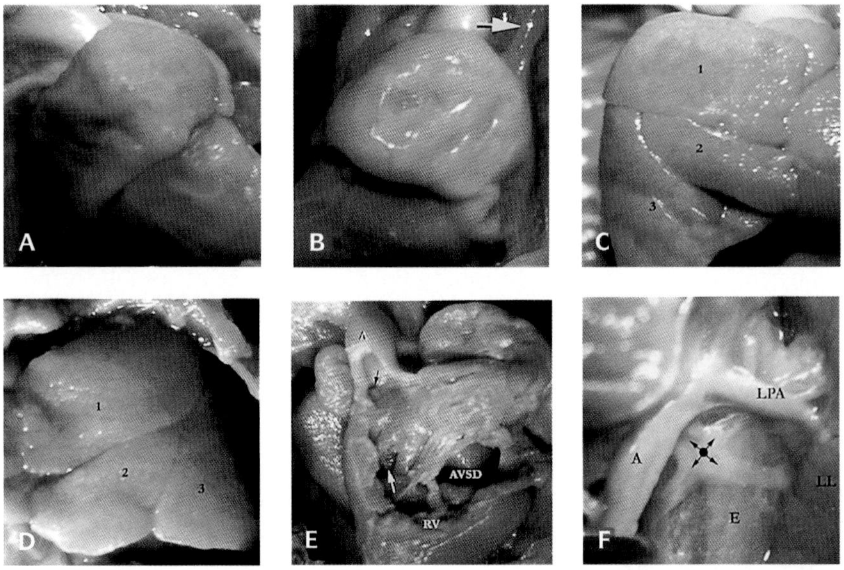

16.33. **(A)** Right-sided morphologic right atrial appendage. **(B)** Left-sided morphologic right atrial appendage (arrow on left-sided superior vena cava) **(C)** and **(D)** Bilateral, eparterial trilobed lungs. **(E)** Double outlet right ventricle with an atrioventricular septal defect (AVSD). (A, aorta; yellow arrow, pulmonary outflow; RV, right ventricle; black arrow, coronary orifice.) **(F)** Total anomalous pulmonary venous connection (arrows). (A, aorta; LPA, left pulmonary artery; LL, left lung; E, esophagus.)

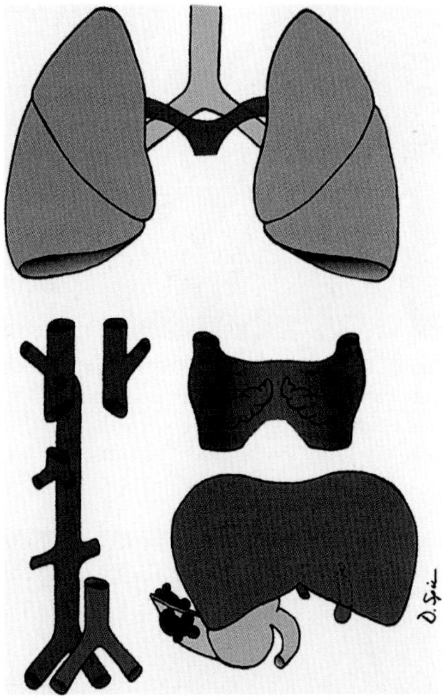

16.34. Diagram of organs in polysplenia. Bilateral, hyparterial, bilobed lungs, bilateral morphologic left atrial appendages, bilateral superior vena cavae, azygos continuation of the inferior vena cava, symmetric liver with left-sided gallbladder, right-sided stomach, and multiple spleens on both sides of the dorsal mesogastrium.

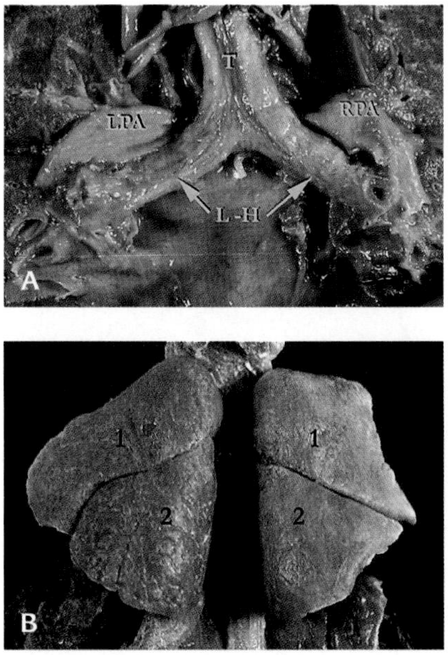

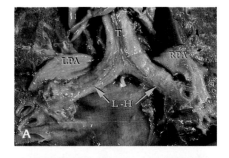

16.35. **(A)** Posterior view of bilateral morphologic left bronchi. Bronchi are long and hyparterial (L-H and arrows). (LPA, left pulmonary artery; RPA, right pulmonary artery; T, trachea.) **(B)** Bilateral bilobed lungs.

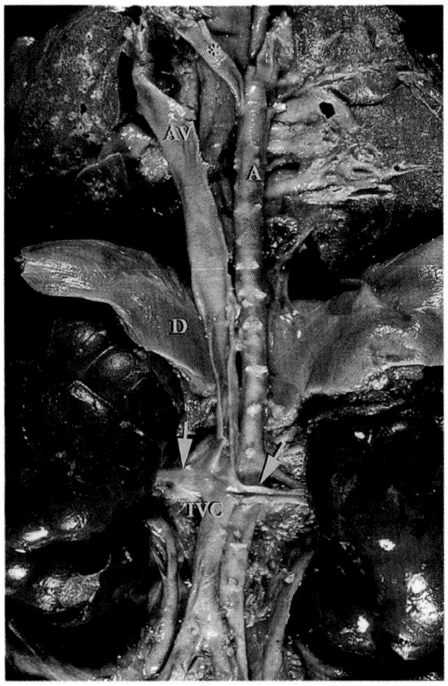

16.36. Azygos (AV) continuation of the inferior vena cava (IVC). Note the renal veins (arrows) posterior to the aorta. (A, aorta, D, diaphragm.)

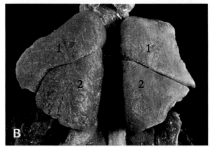

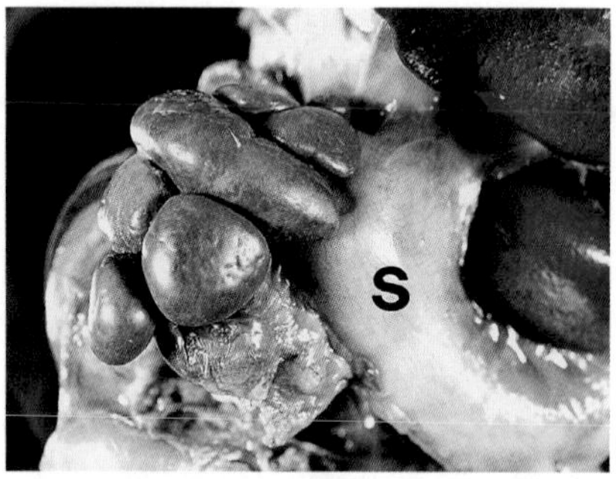

16.37. Polysplenia. Multiple splenic lobules on both sides of the dorsal mesogastrium. (S, right-sided stomach.)

connect the liver to the right of the morphologic LA; a suprahepatic common channel is found in about one-third. Juxtaposition of the abdominal segment of the IVC and the aorta may occur. In some cases, the right and left veins connect to their respective sides of the atria; in others, the right and left pulmonary veins connect to one of the atria. In most, there is an ASD. An ECD is present in approximately 50% of cases. Two ventricles are almost always present, with a high frequency of DORV. PV anomalies are rare. The liver is in its normal location in 25% of cases. In the remainder the major lobe is more commonly found on the left side. The gallbladder is associated with the major lobe, or it may be positioned in the midline or absent. In most patients the stomach, duodenum, and pancreas are on the right side. Malrotation of the intestines is common. The lungs are bilobed with bilateral hyparterial bronchi.

In contradistinction to asplenia, most polysplenia defects are potentially correctable lesions. Polysplenia has been reported with a normal structure of heart.

PERSISTENT LEFT SUPERIOR VENA CAVA (PLSVC)

This can be an isolated condition or associated with poly/asplenia (Figure 16.38). When present it drains into the coronary sinus, which is large and dilated.

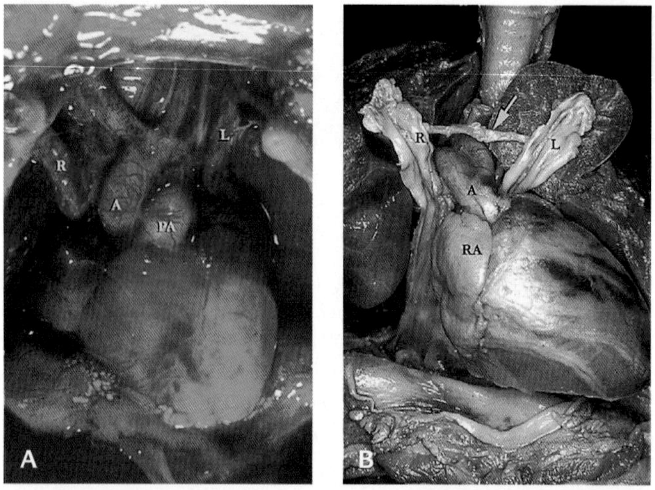

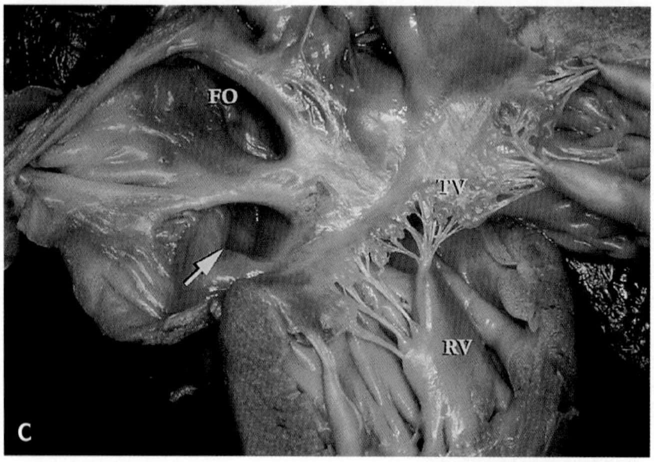

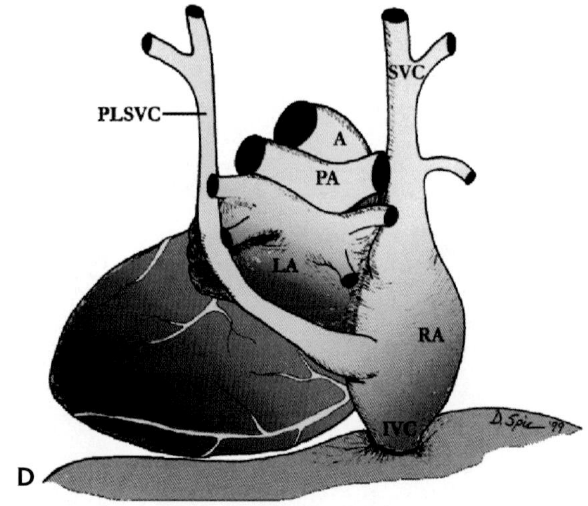

16.38. **(A)** Persistent left superior vena cava (L) with an absent innominate vein. (R, right superior vena cava; A, aorta; P, pulmonary artery.) **(B)** Persistent left superior vena cava (L) with a hypoplastic innominate vein (arrow). (R, right superior vena cava; RA, right atrium.) **(C)** Large coronary sinus (arrow) in a heart with a persistent left superior vena cava. (FO, foramen ovale; TV, tricuspid valve; RV, right ventricle.) **(D)** Illustrations of a posterior view of PLSVC to the coronary sinus.

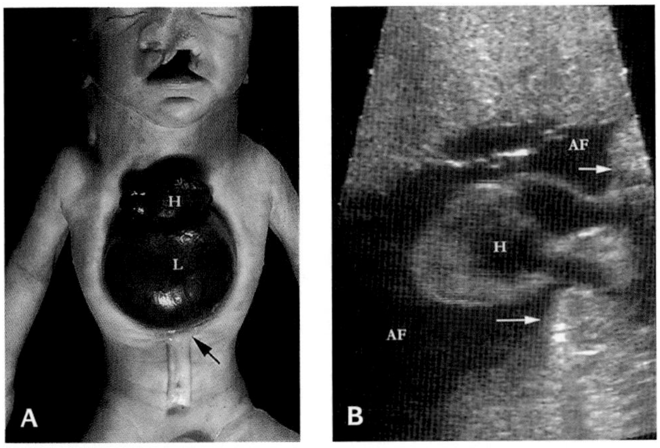

16.39. **(A)** Thoracoabdominal body wall defect. The heart and liver are seen outside the thoracic and abdominal cavities. Midline facial defects are also present. (H, heart; L, liver; Arrow, umbilical cord insertion.) **(B)** Ultrasound at 28 weeks gestation showing ectopia cordis. The heart (H) is outside the chest wall (arrows), surrounded by amniotic fluid (AF). (Courtesy of Florida Perinatal Associates, Tampa, FL.)

ECTOPIA CORDIS

The heart is located partially or totally outside the chest (Figure 16.39). Thoracoabdominal or abdominal ectopia is associated with a defect in the lower sternum, diaphragm, and abdominal wall with omphalocele and heart defects (pentalogy of Cantrell) (Figure 16.2).

VASCULAR RINGS

These include double aortic arch due to persistence of the right 4th branched arch and also an anomalous right subclavian artery vessel coursing behind the trachea and esophagus (Figures 16.3 and 16.40).

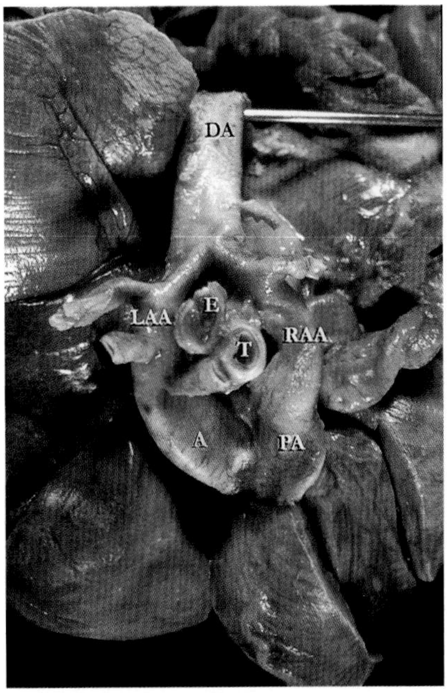

16.40. Vascular ring with double aortic arch (LAA, RAA). (A, ascending aorta; PA, pulmonary artery; T, trachea; E, esophagus; DA, descending aorta.)

ENDOCARDIAL FIBROELASTOSIS (EFE)

The etiology appears to be related to a maternal intrauterine viral infection. Mumps and adenovirus have been usually implicated. It has an incidence of 1 in 6,000 live births. Some cases have been familial. The left ventricular endocardium is greatly thickened by dense plaque-like fibroelastic tissue (Figure 16.41). Secondary EFE is associated with LV outflow obstruction including aortic atresia stenosis and mitral atresia.

CONDUCTION SYSTEM DISORDERS

Histiocytoid (Oncocytic) Cardiomyopathy

Histiocytoid cardiomyopathy is characterized by cardiomegaly, incessant ventricular tachycardia, and frequently sudden death early in life. This lesion has

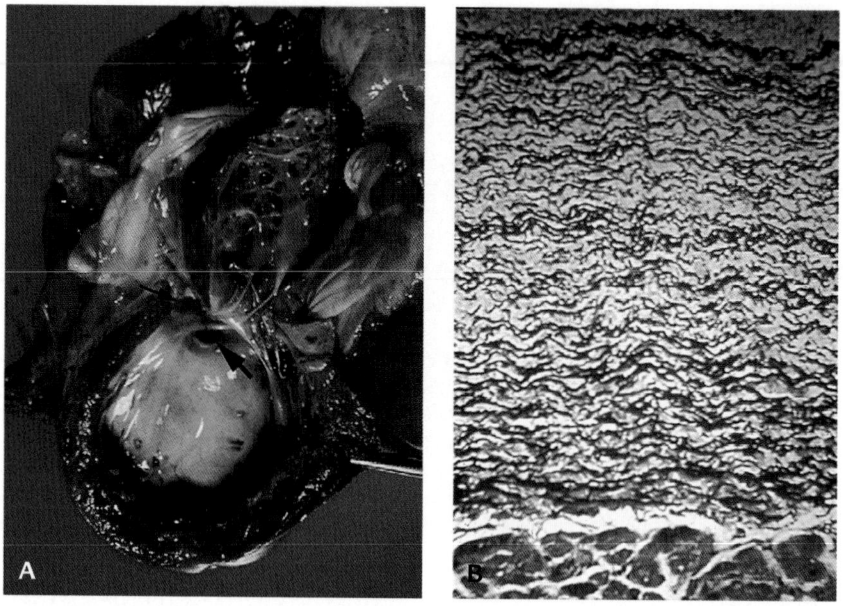

16.41. Endocardial fibroelastosis. **(A)** There is a plaque-like thickening of the left ventricular endocardium. Note the perimembranous VSD (large arrow) (small arrow, coronary orifice). **(B)** Microscopic section showing greatly thickened endocardium by fibroelastic tissue (elastic van Gieson stain).

also been termed isolated cardiac lipidosis, xanthomatous cardiomyopathy, focal myocardial degeneration, multifocal Purkinje cell tumors, arachnocytosis of the heart muscle, and foamy myocardial transformation in infancy. Most cases (90%) present in female infants with intractable ventricular fibrillation or cardiac arrest. The lesion resembles a hamartoma with histiocytoid or granular cell features. It has clearly been defined as a mitochondrial disorder of complex III (reduced coenzyme Q-cytochrome *c* reductase) of the respiratory chain of the cardiac mitochondria. It has been associated with congenital cardiac defects.

An etiology favors either an autosomal recessive gene or an X-linked condition. The female predominance may be explained by gonadal mosaicism for an X-linked gene mutation.

Beneath the endocardial surface of the LV, in the atria, and in all four cardiac valves, are multiple flat to round, smooth, yellow nodules. The nodules are composed of demarcated, large, foamy granular abnormal Purkinje cells in the subendocardium. Glycogen, lipid, and even pigment may be seen in these cells as well as a lymphocytic infiltrate.

Arrhythmogenic Right Ventricular Dysplasia (ARVD)

Arrhythmogenic right ventricular dysplasia is an idiopathic cardiomyopathy characterized pathologically by fatty infiltration of the right ventricular myocardium with ventricular tachycardia often with a left bundle branch block. At least 30% of cases are familial. The gene for this disease has been mapped to

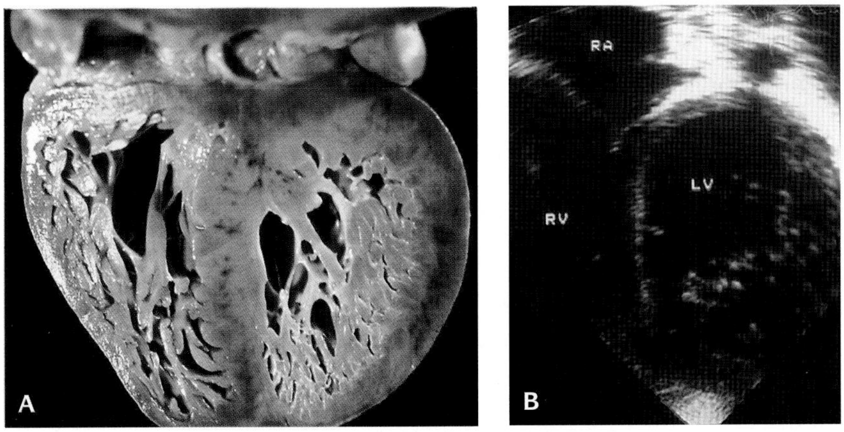

16.42. Noncompaction of the left ventricle **(A)**. **(B)** An echocardiogram shows left ventricular trabeculations with deep intertrabecular recesses involving the apex and free wall. (LV, left ventricle; RV, right ventricle; RA, right atrium.)

chromosome 14q23–q24. There is an autosomal dominant mode of inheritance with variable penetrance and expression.

Noncompaction of Left Ventricle

Isolated noncompaction of the left ventricular myocardium (also known as persistence of spongy myocardium) is a rare form of congenital cardiomyopathy in which the left ventricular wall fails to become flattened and smoother as it normally would during the first 2 months of embryonic development (Figure 16.42). This developmental arrest results in decreased cardiac output with subsequent left ventricular hypertrophy. The aberrant left ventricular trabeculae predispose to abnormal cardiac conduction and potentially fatal cardiac arrhythmias. The interstices within the trabeculated left ventricle predispose to thrombus formation with secondary systemic embolic events. Fibroelastosis of the adjacent ventricular endothelium is a secondary phenomenon resulting from the abnormal blood flow pattern in the left ventricular chamber. A number of mitochondrial disorders may result in cardiomyopathy.

Long QT Syndrome (LQTS)

The LQTS are a heterogeneous group of disorders characterized by prolongation of the corrected QT interval (Qtc) on the surface electrocardiogram, seizures, syncope, and sudden death (Table 16.6). Mortality is presumably due to cerebral hypoperfusion during a malignant ventricular tachycardia known as torsades de pointes.

Seven distinct forms of congenital LQTS have been described. An association between sudden infant death syndrome (SIDS) and the LQTS has been observed. (Table 16.6)

Table 16.6 Genetic defects of long QT syndromes

Type	Inheritance	Chromosome	Gene	Protein	Feature
LQTS1	Autosomal dominant	11p15.5	KVLQT1	K^+channel	Sudden death w/excitement
LQTS2	Autosomal dominant	7q35	HERG	K^+channel	Exacerbated by hypokalemia
LQTS3	Autosomal dominant	3p21	SCN5A	Na^+channel	Resting and exercise bradycardia
LQTS4	Autosomal dominant	4q25–27	?	?	Prominent "U" waves on ECG
LQTS5	Autosomal dominant	?	?	?	?
LQTS6	Autosomal dominant	?	?	K^+channel	?
JERVELL/LANGE-NIELSEN	Autosomal recessive	11p15.5	KVLQT1	K^+channel	Congenital deafness

SURGICAL REPAIR OF CONGENITAL CARDIAC DEFECTS (TABLE 16.7)

ULTRASONOGRAPHY

The common imaging planes are as follows:

1. The standard four-chamber view of the heart is obtained at an approximate 45° angle from the view used to obtain the abdominal circumference view. Two other views are necessary to fully evaluate the heart: the left ventricular outflow view and short axis great vessel views. They are usually obtained by rotating the axis of the transducer from the four-chamber view by 30–45° to the right or left, resulting in imaging planes that transect the scapulla and torso at 30–45° angles from the midsagittal plane. The heart and stomach bubble should have concordant situs.
2. The cardiac axis (the axis of the intraventricular septum) should approximate 45° from the midsagittal plane. Cardiac axis angles greater or less than these values indicate possible cardiac abnormalities or "mass effect" from intrathoracic masses or abnormalities.
3. The intraventricular septum should be intact from the cardiac apex to the crux.
   a. The membranous septal portion of the intraventricular septum, located immediately adjacent to the crux, is anatomically very thin. If imaged in anything other than an ideal imaging plane, it may appear discontinuous (i.e., it may simulate a membranous ventricular septal defect).
      - Further imaging angles and evaluation with color Doppler color flow or pulsed Doppler insonnation usually exclude such false-positive diagnoses.
      - Small ventriculoseptal defects may go undetected, but their clinical significance often is minimal, as the natural course of small defects often is resolution over the first months or years of life.

Table 16.7 Operative procedures for correction of congenital heart defects

Name	Surgical procedure	Objective	Uses	Complications	Diagram
Blalock-Taussig Shunt (Modified)	End to side anastomosis- subclavian artery to ipsilateral PA	Increase pulmonary blood flow Enlarge valve and PAs	TOF PA atresia PA stenosis	Subclavian steal syndrome with brain abscess and infarcts (original procedure) Shunt failure: Anastomosis not expanding with growth, thrombotic occlusion, kinking, or arterial deformities Rare: Pulmonary hypertension, aneurysms	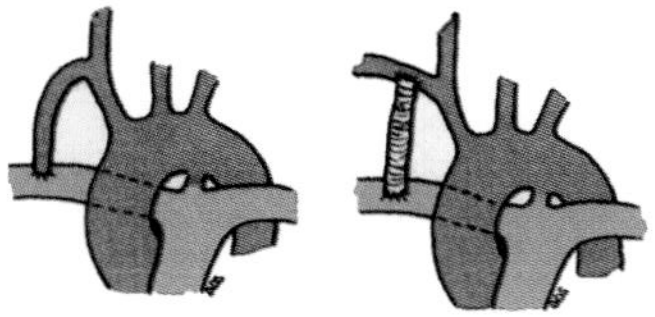
Pott's procedure	Descending thoracic aorta to LPA	Increase pulmonary blood flow	TOF PA atresia PA stenosis	Stenosis or obstruction of RPA anastomosis, excessive PA flow, CHF, PA hypertension, difficult to take down Rare: aneurysm	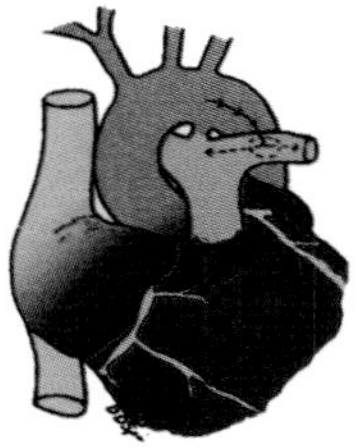
Waterston shunt (modified)	Side to side anastomosis – ascending aorta to RPA (synthetic graft – now more common)	Increase pulmonary blood flow enlarge pulmonary valve annulus and PAs for definitive repair	TOF and L aortic arch	Kinking, distortion, stenosis of PA anastomosis, excessive PA flow, CHF, PA hypertension, obstruction of LPA, false aneurysm of aorta difficult to take down	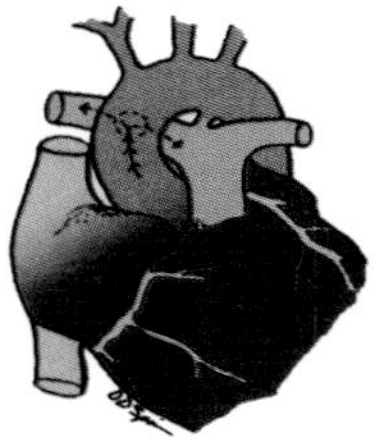
Glenn shunt	SVC to RPA – PA transected (redirectional: pulmonary confluence maintained)	Increase pulmonary blood flow	Tricuspid atresia Univentricular heart with PA stenosis	Abnormal perfusion of R lung, pulmonary arteriovenous fistulas with R to L shunting, SVC syndrome, protein losing enteropathy with intestinal lymphangiectasia, candida sepsis, venous collateral channels	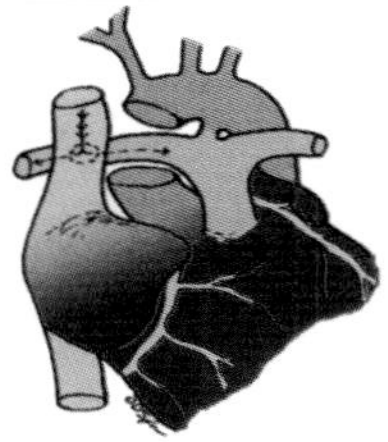

(continued)

Table 16.7 *(continued)*

Name	Surgical procedure	Objective	Uses	Complications	Diagram
Blalock Hanlon	Atrial septectomy – operative	Increase shunting at atrial level	Palliative procedure for: TGA with intact ventricular septum, HLH, tricuspid atresia, failure of a balloon septostomy	Cerebral emboli	
Rashkind	Inflated balloon pulled across FO, tearing the septum – (balloon atrial septostomy)	Increase shunting at the atrial level	Palliative procedure for: TGA with intact ventricular septum, HLH, tricuspid atresia	Failure if FO is stretched, not torn Rare: atrial perforation	
Mustard/ Senning	Atrial switch – removal of atrial septum and create intraatrial baffle with pericardium or dacron	Redirect systemic venous flow to LV and pulmonary venous flow to RV (hemodynamic correction with RV remaining the systemic ventricle)	TGA	Systemic venous obstruction, pulmonary venous obstruction, atrial arrhythmias, eventual RV failure, tricuspid regurgitation, LV outflow obstruction, pulmonary hypertension tricuspid endocarditis	
Transcatheter closure of ASDs, VSDs and PDAs with buttoned devices	Following echocardiogram sizing of the defect, an occluder and counter occluder are inserted through a catheter delivery system	Less invasive, nonoperative repair with decreased hospital stay	Closure of ASD, VSD, and PDA	Device pulling through the defect, dislodging of the implanted device requiring emergency surgery, unsuccessful closure, bradycardia, hypotension, improper implantation	
Rastelli	RV to PA conduit with prosthetic valve, VSD repair so that LV is attached to aorta	Reestablish pulmonary flow and form a LV – aortic connection	TGA, VSD and PA stenosis, PA atresia, TA, DORV, TOF	CHF, conduit obstruction, valve dysfunction, ventricular arrhythmias, heart block	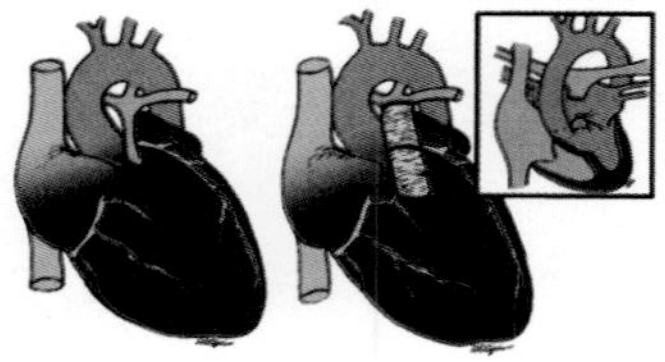

Muller-Dammann	PA banding	Decrease pulmonary blood flow preventing pulmonary hypertension. Prevent massive PA dilatation in TOF with absent pulmonary valve	Large VSD (with or without PDA, coarctations) TGA without subpulmonic stenosis or with large shunts, DORV, TOF with absent pulmonary valve, univentricular heart	Inadequate pulmonary flow leading to cyanosis and polycythemia, distal migration of band, thrombosis, calcification, aneurysm, secondary thickening of pulmonary valve, RV hypertrophy, adhesions may make debanding impossible without arterioplasty	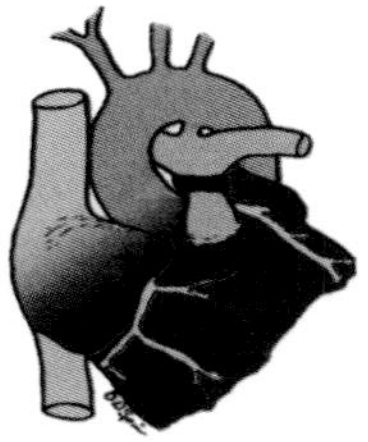
Fontan	Conduit from RA to PA (often using pericardial augmentation). Occasionally from RA to hypoplastic RV (using aortic homograft or conduit). Closure of ASD (tricuspid atresia)	Bypass tricuspid atresia or pulmonary atresia if RV is diminutive	Tricuspid atresia, pulmonary atresia, double inlet ventricle (R AV valve closed mimicking tricuspid atresia)	Mural thrombi in RA, pulmonary thrombosis, stenosis of conduit or homograft, patch dehiscence, LV dysfunction, ascites, edema	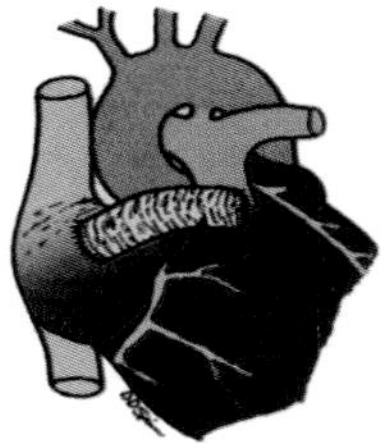
Jatene (great arterial switch)	Transection of PA and aorta reattaching them to form concordant connections; implantation of coronary ostia into pulmonary trunk (neoaorta)	Reestablish ventriculoarterial concordance	TGA	PA stenosis, kinking of coronary artery or ostial stenosis, residual VSD, aortic valvular regurgitation, endocarditis.	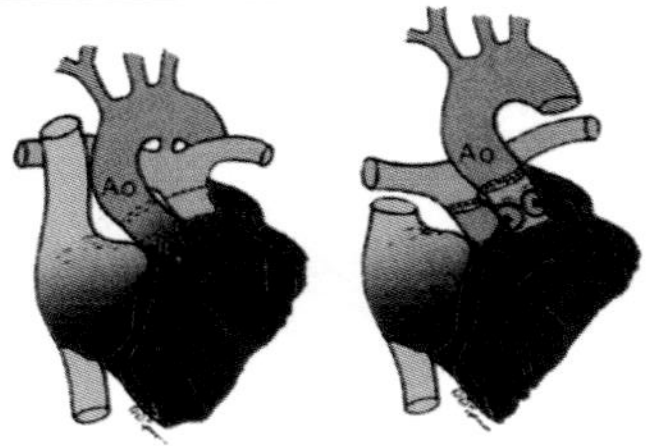
Norwood	An ascending aorta is created from the main PA, RV becomes the systemic ventricle and PAs are supplied via a shunt	To establish adequate systemic and PA blood flow from the larger RV	HLH	Atrial arrhythmias, regulation of pulmonary vascular resistance, regulation of systemic to PA blood flow, aortic arch obstruction	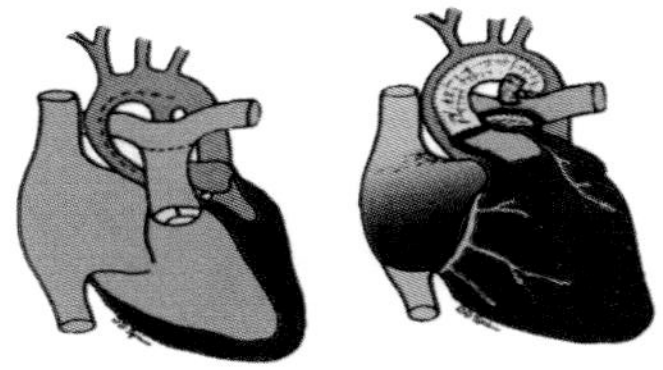
Ross	Transplant of pulmonary valve autograft to aortic position; pulmonary valve replacement	Repair aortic valve disease	Aortic regurgitation	Aortic root dilation	

PA, pulmonary artery; TOF, tetralogy of Fallot; L, left; R, right; CHF, congestive heart failure; SVC, superior vena cava; TGA, transposition of the great arteries; HLH, hypoplastic left heart; FO, foramen ovale; LV, left ventricle; RV, right ventricle; VSD, ventricular septal defect; TA, truncus arteriosus; DORV, double outlet right ventricle; PDA, patent ductus arteriosus; RA, right atrium; RAV, right atrioventricular; ASD, atrial septal defect.

4. Features of the common cardiac imaging views
   a. The four-chamber view
      - Symmetric atria and ventricles, intraatrial and intraventricular septa, the foramen ovale, the flap of the foramen ovale oriented into the left atrium, and the axis is to the left at approximately a 45° angle to the sagittal plane.
      - The left atrium is usually closest to the spine, the tricuspid valve inserts slightly lower on the IVS than the mitral valve, and the heart occupies about one-third of the chest.
      - Helpful for diagnosis of right or left ventricular hypoplasia, ventricular septal defects, tetralogy of Fallot, coarctation of the aorta, Ebstein anomaly, pericardial effusion, dextrocardia, cardiac hypertrophy, situs inversus, ectopia cordis, and single ventricle.
   b. The five-chamber view
      - Modification of the four-chamber imaging plane in which the aortic root origin in the left ventricle is imaged (one chamber) as well as accompanying views of the other four standard chambers giving a "five-chamber view."
      - The ventricular septum should make a smooth transition into the aorta.
   c. The left ventricular outflow tract view
      - Shows left atrium, left ventricle, the mitral valve, and the aorta.
      - Septal defects can be detected in this view.
   d. The right ventricular outflow tract view
      - Shows the right ventricle, the pulmonic valve, the pulmonary artery, and a portion of the ductus arteriosus. The rising aortic arch often is seen in transverse section immediately adjacent to the pulmonary artery.
      - Assists in evaluation for transposition of the great vessels.
   e. The short axis ("hurricane") great vessel view
      - Shows the right cardiac structures (right atrium, tricuspid view, right ventricle, and pulmonic valve) arrayed circumferentially around the aortic root, with the bifurcation of the pulmonary artery into the ductus, and the right pulmonary artery is clearly seen. The aortic root can be viewed as the eye of the hurricane. The triple leaf pattern of the aortic valve (resembling the letter Y or a Mercedes-Benz emblem) often is seen.
      - Helpful to show discrete origin of the major great vessels and assists with evaluation of complex cardiac abnormalities.
   f. Crossing views of the pulmonary artery and aorta
      - The pulmonary artery and right outflow tract often can be shown to cross the aorta and left ventricular outflow tract in a transverse fashion approximately at a 30° angle.
      - This finding generally excludes the possibility of transposition of the great vessels.

g. The aortic arch
   - Begins centrally within the heart, initially crosses from left to right, then curves from right to left, travels somewhat anteriorly to form the transverse arch, and then continues curving interiorly and posteriorly to form the descending aorta.
   - Its shape is often said to resemble a candy cane.
   - Three strap vessels arising from the aortic arch help distinguish the aortic from the ductal arch: the left subclavian artery, the left common carotid artery, and the brachiocephalic trunk.
   - Discontinuities in the arch lead to coarctation
   - Asymmetry in right and left ventricular volumes suggests possible alterations in the relative flow through the pulmonary and systemic circulatory systems, which become more significant after birth.

h. The ductal arch
   - The ductus arteriosus is much more prominent in fetuses than in infants after birth because it is the bridge that allows the normally parallel pulmonary and aortic circulatory systems to develop and function in the absence of significant volume flow through the lungs.
   - The ductus arteriosus is the principle extension of the pulmonary artery that arises from the right ventricle, anterior to the aorta, and curves broadly to join the aorta.
   - The ductal arch has a hockey stick-shaped appearance.
   - Often, the right pulmonary artery and aorta will also be visualized in views of the ductal arch.

i. Risk factors for congenital cardiac anomalies
   - Fetal indicators
     - Heart block – 50% CHD
     - Heart block with maternal connective tissue disorder – 44% CHD
     - Tachyarrhythmia – 0% CHD
   - Associations with congenital cardiac defects
     - Family history
     - One affected sibling – 2% risk, two affected siblings/relatives – 10% risk
     - Parental proband – 9% band
   - Ehlers-Danlos syndrome is associated with aortic and carotid aneurysms
     - Ellis-van Creveld syndrome is associated with single atrium
     - Holt-Oram predisposes to ASD, VSD
     - Kartagener syndrome is associated with dextrocardia
     - Leopard syndrome predisposes to pulmonary stenosis
   - Infectious etiologies
     - Rubella is associated with VSD, PDA, transposition.
     - Other viral illnesses during pregnancy may predispose to CHD

- Metabolic conditions
  - —Diabetes (2% risk) is associated with transposition, VSD, coarctation, and cardiomegaly/myopathy
  - —Fetal alcohol syndrome
  - —SLE is associated with congenital heart block
  - —PKU is associated with tetralogy of Fallot
- Medication/substance exposure
  - —Amphetamine usage is associated with VSD, PDA, transposition
  - —Fetal alcohol syndrome
  - —Hydantoin use is associated with pulmonic stenosis, aortic stenosis, coarctation, and patent ductus arteriosus
  - —Trimethadione use is associated with a 20% risk of transposition, Tetralogy of Fallot, and hypoplastic left heart
  - —Lithium use may be associated with Ebstein anomaly, tricuspid atresia, and atrial septal defect
  - —Sex steroids have a 3% risk of congenital cardiac disease
  - —Thalidomide exposure is associated with tetralogy of Fallot, VSD, ASD, and truncus arteriosus

Other associations with congenital cardiac disease include:

1. Cardiac abnormalities in some studies have found that 30% have chromosomal abnormalities
   a. Isolated cardiac abnormalities are associated with 16% aneuploidy
   b. Two or more detectable abnormalities have a 66% rate of aneuploidy
2. Dysrhythmias – Both bradyarrhythmias and tachyarrhythmias are occasionally noted on auscultation or direct observation of the fetal heart.
   a. Transient bradycardias are often seen as a result of maternal supine positioning during routine sonographic evaluation. They can be avoided by repositioning the patient in a lateral position when symptoms of warmth and faintness develop. These findings are usually a result of the predisposition toward maternal supine hypotension in pregnancy.
   b. Transient bradycardia usually occurs in association with maternal hypotensive symptomatology and resolves without recurrence after positional change. For recurrent or persistent bradycardia, fetal distress should be excluded and further evaluation or consultation should be considered.
   c. Tachyarrhythmias are usually defined as fetal heart rate >180 beats per minute and represent about 15% of fetal cardiac rhythm disturbances.
      - Supraventricular tachycardia is the most common of these, while other potential causes include atrial flutter and atrial fibrillation.
      - The most severe cases result in cardiac failure, hydrops and death. This occurs because as ventricular rate increases, the diastolic filling interval becomes shortened.

- Treatment of tachyarrhythmias centers around assessment of fetal status, correction of the rhythm disturbance by pharmacologic measures (using digoxin, propranolol, verapamil, or other medications), and assessment of the fetal status as measures to control the disturbance are undertaken.

d. Bradyarrhythmias result from several mechanisms, including conduction abnormalities due to structural aberrations of the conduction system, conduction abnormalities as a result of antibodies directed against the conduction system, and, rarely, as a result of fetal distress.
   - 50% have structural abnormalities causing the block. In fetuses with normal appearing anatomy 70% have evidence of maternal collagen vascular disease. Bradycardia associated with maternal collagen vascular disease most often is related to the presence of anti-Rho (anti-Sjogren syndrome A) and infrequently also is present if anti-La (anti-SSB) are detected. With hydrops the mortality is high.

ACKNOWLEDGMENT

We would like to acknowledge the Pathology Department at Children's Hospital of Pittsburgh and the Frank E. Sherman, MD, and Cora C. Lennox, MD, Heart Museum. Many of the photographs within this chapter are taken from the heart specimens in their comprehensive collection.

REFERENCES

Allan LD, Santos R, Pexieder T: Anatomical and echocardiographic correlates of normal cardiac morphology in late first trimester fetus. *Heart* 77:68, 1997.

Anderson RH, Lenox CC, Zuberbuhler JR: The morphology of ventricular septal defects. *Perspect Pediatr Pathol* 8:235, 1984.

Arey JB: *Cardiovascular Pathology in Infants and Children.* Philadelphia, WB Saunders, 1984.

Bamford RN, Roessler E, Burdine RD, Saplakoglu U, dela Cruz J, Splitt M, Goodship JA, Towbin J, Bowers P, Ferrero GB, Marino B, Schier AF, Shen MM, Muenke M, Casey B: Loss-of-function mutations in the EGF-CFC gene CFC1 are associated with human left-right laterality defects. *Nature Genet* 26(3):365, 2000.

Brumund MR, Lutin WA: Advances in antenatal diagnosis and management of the fetus with a heart problem. *Ped Annals* 27:486, 1998.

Casey B: Genetics of human situs abnormalities. *Am J Med Genet* 101(4):356, 2001.

Casey B, Cuneo BF, Vitali C, van Hecke H, Barrish J, Hicks J, Ballabio A, Hoo JJ: Autosomal dominant transmission of familial laterality defects. *Am J Med Genet* 61(4):325, 1996.

Casey B: Two rights make a wrong: human left-right malformations. *Hum Mol Genet* 7(10):1565, 1998.

Clark EB: *Functional Aspects of Cardiac Development*, New York, Raven Press, 1984.

Clark EB: Mechanisms in the pathogenesis of congenital heart defects. In Pierpont MEM, Moller JH (eds): *The Genetics of Cardiovascular Disease*, Boston, Martinus-Nijoff, 1990, p. 3.

Clark EB, Markwald RR, Takao A: *Developmental Mechanisms of Heart Diseases.* New York, Futura Publishing, 1995.

Clark EB, Nakazawa M, Takao A, eds: *Etiology and Morphogenesis of Congenital Heart Disease: Twenty Years of Progress in Genetics and Developmental Biology.* New York, Futura Publishing, 2000.

Cooper MJ, Enderlein MA, Dyson DC, et al.: Fetal echocardiography: Retrospective review of clinical experience and an evaluation of indications. *Obstet Gynecol* 86:577, 1995.

Debich DE, Devine WA, Anderson RH: Polysplenia with normally structured hearts. *Am J Cardiol* 65:1274, 1990.

Digilio MC, Casey B, Toscano A, Calabro R, Pacileo G, Marasini M, Banaudi E, Giannotti A, Dallapiccola B: Marino B. Complete transposition of the great arteries: patterns of congenital heart disease in familial precurrence. *Circulation* 104(23):2809, 2001.

Ferencz C, Loffredo CA, Correa-Villasenor A, Wilson PD, eds: *Perspectives in Pediatric Cardiology, Vol. 5, Genetic and Environmental Risk Factors of Major Cardiovascular Malformations-the Baltimore-Washington Infant Study 1981–1989*, New York, Futura Publishing, 1997.

Friedman AH, Copel JA, Kleinman CS: Fetal echocardiography and fetal cardiology: Indications, diagnosis, and management. *Semin Perinatol* 17:76, 1993.

Gilbert-Barness E, Debich-Spicer D: Cardiovascular system, Part I, Development of the heart and congenital malformations. In *Potter's Pathology of the Fetus and Infant*, Gilbert-Barness E, ed. St. Louis, Mosby-Year Book, 1997.

Gilbert-Barness E, ed.: *Potter's Atlas of Developmental and Infant Pathology*, St. Louis, Mosby Year Book, Inc., 1998.

Gilbert-Barness E, Barness LA: Nonmalformative cardiovascular pathology in infants and children. *Ped Develop Path* 2:499, 1999.

Kalousek DK, Fitch N, Paradice BA: Pathology of embryonic, fetal, and placental development: Cardiovascular system defects. In *Pathology of the Human Embryo and Previable Fetus: An Atlas*, New York, Springer-Verlag, 1990.

Kosaki K, Casey B: Genetics of human left-right axis malformations. *Semin Cell Dev Biol* 9(1):89, 1998.

Landing BH, Hatayama C, Wells TR, et al.: Five syndromes (malformation complexes) of pulmonary symmetry, congenital heart disease, and multiple spleens. *Pediatr Pathol* 2:125, 1984.

Lin AE, Pierpont ME (guest editors): Seminars in medical genetics-heart development and the genetic aspects of cardiovascular malformations. *Am J Med Genet* 97(4):235, 2000.

Maeyama K, Kosaki R, Yoshihashi H, Casey B, Kosaki K: Mutation analysis of left-right axis determining genes in NOD and ICR, strains susceptible to maternal diabetes. *Teratology* 63(3):119, 2001.

Montana E, Khoury MJ, Cragan JD, et al.: Trends and outcome after prenatal diagnosis of congenital cardiac malformations by fetal echocardiography in a well-defined birth population, Atlanta, Georgia, 1990–1994. *Am Coll Cardiol* 28:1805, 1996.

Moss AJ, Adams FH, Emmanouilides GC, ed: *Moss and Adams Heart Disease in Infants, Children and Adolescents: Including the Fetus and Young Adult*, 5th ed, Baltimore, Williams & Wilkins, 1995.

On-Line Mendelian Inheritance in Man OMIM (http://www3.ncbi.nlm.nih.gov/omim/).

Opitz JM, Clark EB: Heart development: an introduction. *Am J Med Genet* 97(4):238, 2000.

Opitz JM, Yost J, Clark EB: Overview: Syndromes, developmental fields, and human cardiovascular malformations. In Clark EB, Nakazawa M, Takan A (ed): *Etiology and Morphogenesis of Congenital Heart Disease: Twenty Years of Progress in Genetics and Developmental Biology*, New York, Futura Publishing, 2000.

Rao PS: Balloon valvuloplasty and angioplasty of stenotic lesions of the heart and great vessels in children. In Barness LA, DeVivo DC, Morrow G III (eds): *Advances in Pediatrics*, vol. 37, St. Louis, Mosby-Year Book, 1990.

Riopel DA: The heart. In Stevenson RE, Hall JG, Goodman RM (eds): *Human Malformations and Related Anomalies*, New York, Oxford University Press, 1993.

Silverman NH, Schmidt KG. Ultrasound evaluation of the fetal heart. In Callen PW (ed): *Ultrasonography in Obstetrics and Gynecology*, Philadelphia, WB Sanders, 1994.
Split MP, Burn J, Goodship J: Connexin43 mutations in sporadic and familial defects of laterality. *N Engl J Med* 333:941, 1995.
Stevenson RE, Hall JG, Goodman RM, eds: *Human Malformations and Related Anomalies*, Vol. II, Chapt 8. New York, Oxford University Press, 1993.

SEVENTEEN

Respiratory System

LUNG MATURITY

1. Amniotic fluid can be tested for phospholipid components of fetal lung surfactant.
2. The lecithin-to-sphingomyelin (L/S) ratio is the most widely used index. An L/S of >2.0 indicates fetal lung maturity in most cases. An L/S of <2 does not reliably exclude lung maturity.
3. The presence of phosphatidylglycerol (PG), a late-appearing surfactant component, has greater positive predictive value than the L/S ratio in determining fetal lung maturity. However, PG has lower sensitivity. A positive PG is helpful when the L/S is marginal.

RESPIRATORY TRACT ABNORMALITIES

Choanal atresia is the failure of communication between the posterior nasal sacs and the oral cavity.
Laryngeal stenosis is a narrowing of the laryngeal cavity (Figure 17.1).
Laryngeal cleft is incomplete formation of the larynx (Figure 17.2).

Tracheoesophageal Fistula

The incidence of tracheoesophageal fistula (TEF) with or without esophageal atresia is 1/1,000 to 1/2,500 births (Figures 17.3 and 17.4 and Table 17.1). TEF is rarely familial and there are at least six anatomic types. More than 85% of all cases are of type 1 esophageal atresia with fistula from the trachea or carina to the lower esophageal segment. Type 2 – esophageal atresia with TEF – is the next most common. The other types are shown in Figure 17.1.

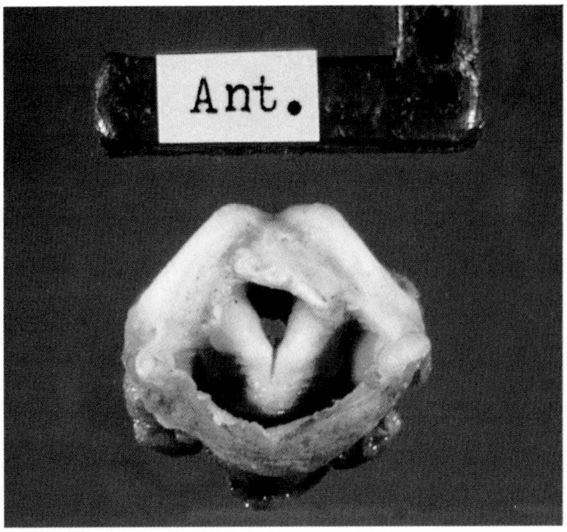

17.1. Laryngeal stenosis with thickened vocal cords.

This anomaly should be considered in the presence of polyhydramnios. Symptoms include mucous secretions at birth, paroxysmal coughing, and choking or cyanosis with feedings, especially with liquids; abdominal distention from air passing through the fistula; and recurrent pneumonia. Esophageal stenosis may coexist. The H-type fistula is relatively rare (approximately 5%). Symptoms of the H-type TEF can resemble those of laryngeal cleft, neuromuscular pharyngolaryngeal dysfunction (as in Opitz syndrome and arthrogryposis), and other respiratory tract disorders. It may not be detected until adult life despite, sometimes, the presence of symptoms from infancy. A parent and child with type 1 TEF have been observed.

The combination of TEF and bronchopulmonary malformations may occur, ranging from lobar hypoplasia and agenesis to unilateral pulmonary hypoplasia or agenesis. Extensive squamous metaplasia of the trachea in patients with TEF with esophageal atresia involves the posterior pars membranacea and sometimes extends to the lateral or anterior walls or to the bronchi. Some studies suggest that this epithelial change may be a primary developmental error related

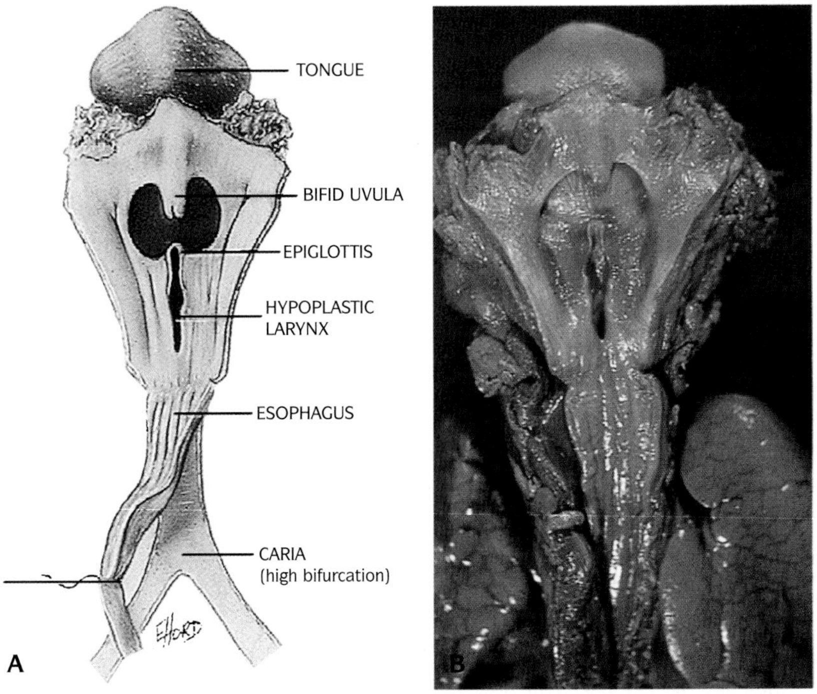

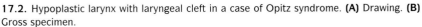

17.2. Hypoplastic larynx with laryngeal cleft in a case of Opitz syndrome. **(A)** Drawing. **(B)** Gross specimen.

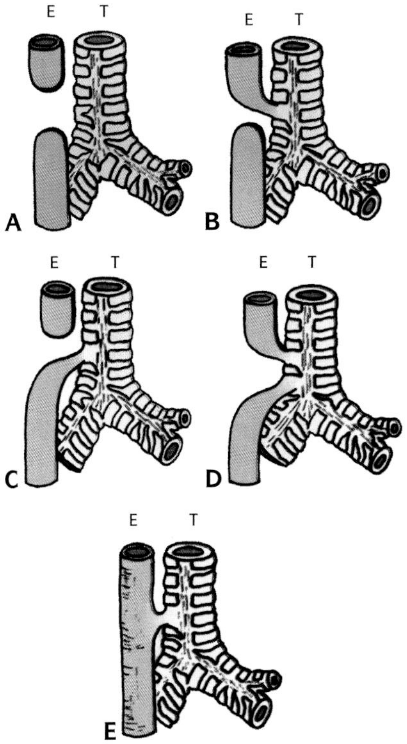

17.3. Types of tracheoesophageal fistula.

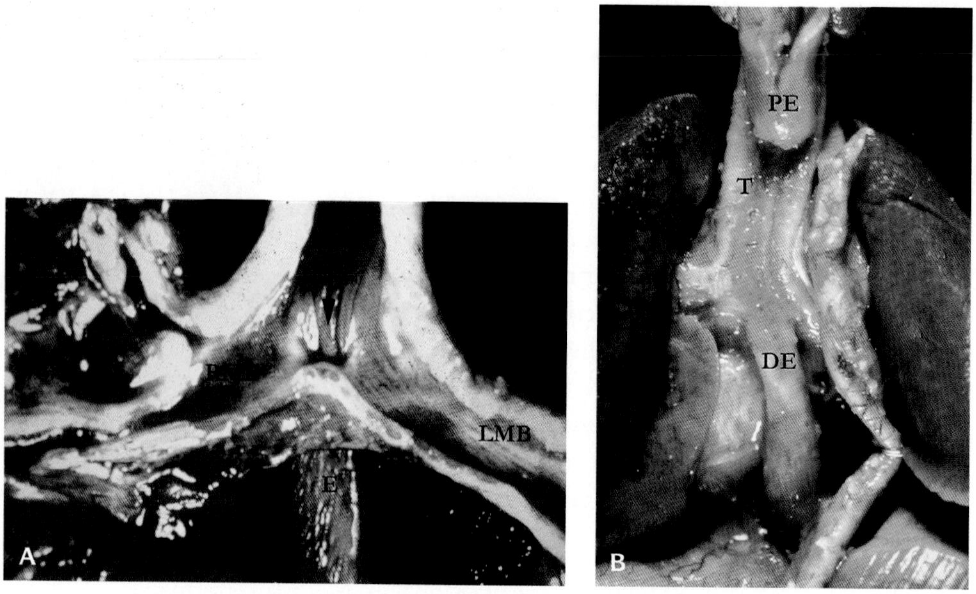

17.4. Tracheoesophageal fistulas. **(A)** Distal esophagus communicates with carina, anterior view. (RMB, right main bronchus; LMB, left main bronchus; Arrow, T-E fistula; E, esophagus.) **(B)** Blind end of proximal esophagus (PE); distal esophagus (DE) communicates with trachea (T).

Table 17.1 Anomalies associated with TEF and esophageal atresia

System	Anomalies
Musculoskeletal	Vertebral defects; rib defects; radial amelia; caudal dysgenesis
Cardiovascular	Ventricular septal defect; patent ductus arteriosus; right aortic arch
Gastrointestinal	Imperforate anus; malrotation; duodenal atresia
Genitourinary	Renal malposition; renal cysts or agenesis; ureteral duplication
Craniofacial	Choanal stenosis; ear malformation; micrognathia
Central nervous	Hydrocephalus
Pulmonary	Congenital cystic adenomatoid malformation; hypoplasia

Table 17.2 Development of the human respiratory tract

Embryonic stage	
24 days	Tracheal bud forms
26–28 days	Stem bronchial buds form
35 days	Lobar bronchi form
Glandular stage	
5–12 weeks	Further bronchial branchings occur
5–16 weeks	Glandular development of lung
15–25/26 weeks	Tracheal glands develop craniocaudally
16 weeks	Terminal bronchioles form
Canalicular stage	
16–24 weeks	Respiratory bronchioles form
Saccular stage	
24–35 weeks	Saccules form
Alveolar stage	
35 weeks to 2 years	Alveoli begin to form

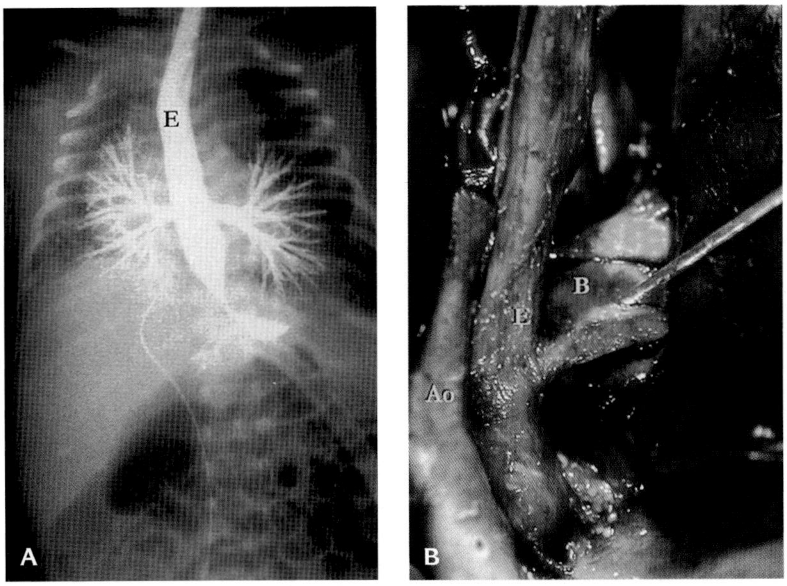

17.5. Tracheal atresia. **(A)** Bronchogram with bronchoesophageal fistula. **(B)** Gross specimen with bronchoesophageal fistula. (B, bronchus; E, esophagus; Ao, aorta.)

to the embryogenesis of the malformation, although it may be exaggerated by infection, gastric acidity, treatment with oxygen, or other factors.

Tracheal Agenesis

Failure of development of the trachea results in a fistula between the esophagus and mainstem bronchus (bronchoesophageal fistula) (Figures 17.5 and 17.6).

Pulmonary Hypoplasia

Pulmonary hypoplasia is best assessed by the lung weight/body weight ratio, or a radial alveolar count. Lung/body weight $\leq$0.12 and a radial alveolar count $\leq$4 are indicative of pulmonary hypoplasia (Table 17.2).

Fetal pulmonary development is divided into the pseudoglandular, canalicular, and terminal sac phases.

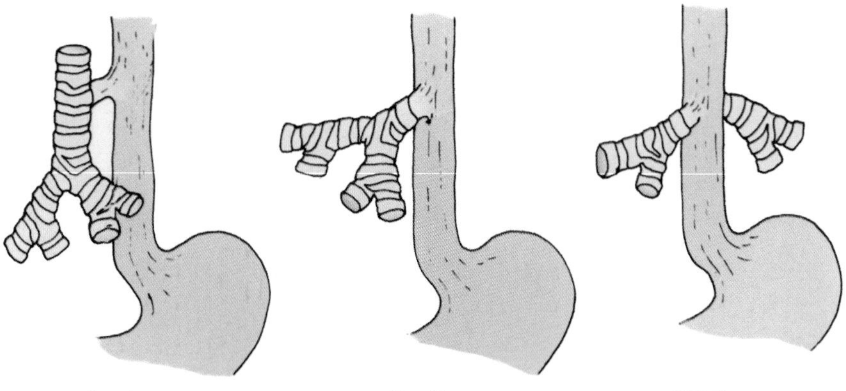

17.6. Types of bronchoesophageal fistulas.

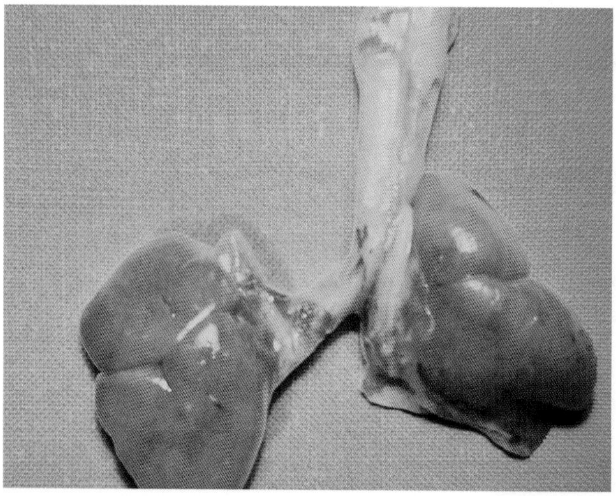

17.7. Hypoplastic lungs in a case of infantile recessive polycystic kidney disease.

Any condition that decreases fetal respiratory movements or reduces the volume of the thorax or the amount of lung liquid will result in poor development of the lungs (Figures 17.7 and 17.8). Restriction of the chest such as skeletal defects as in osteogenesis imperfecta, asphyxiating thoracic dystrophy, and thanatophoric dysplasia prevent normal lung development. Reduction of lung volume occurs in diaphragmatic hernia or infantile polycystic kidneys that compromise the thoracic space and thus the development of the lungs.

The most common cause of pulmonary hypoplasia is oligohydramnios.

In oligohydramnios, the respiratory movements are decreased by external and/or internal compression. The presence of a severe decrease of amniotic fluid leads to a failure to distend the air spaces.

Underdevelopment of the lungs occurs in anencephaly.

Heterotopic brain may be found in the lungs of an anencephalic (Figure 17.9).

Abnormal Pulmonary Fissures and Lobes

Variations in the pattern of bronchial division are common. There may be missing or extra lobes or fissures that are partial divisions of a lobe, medial

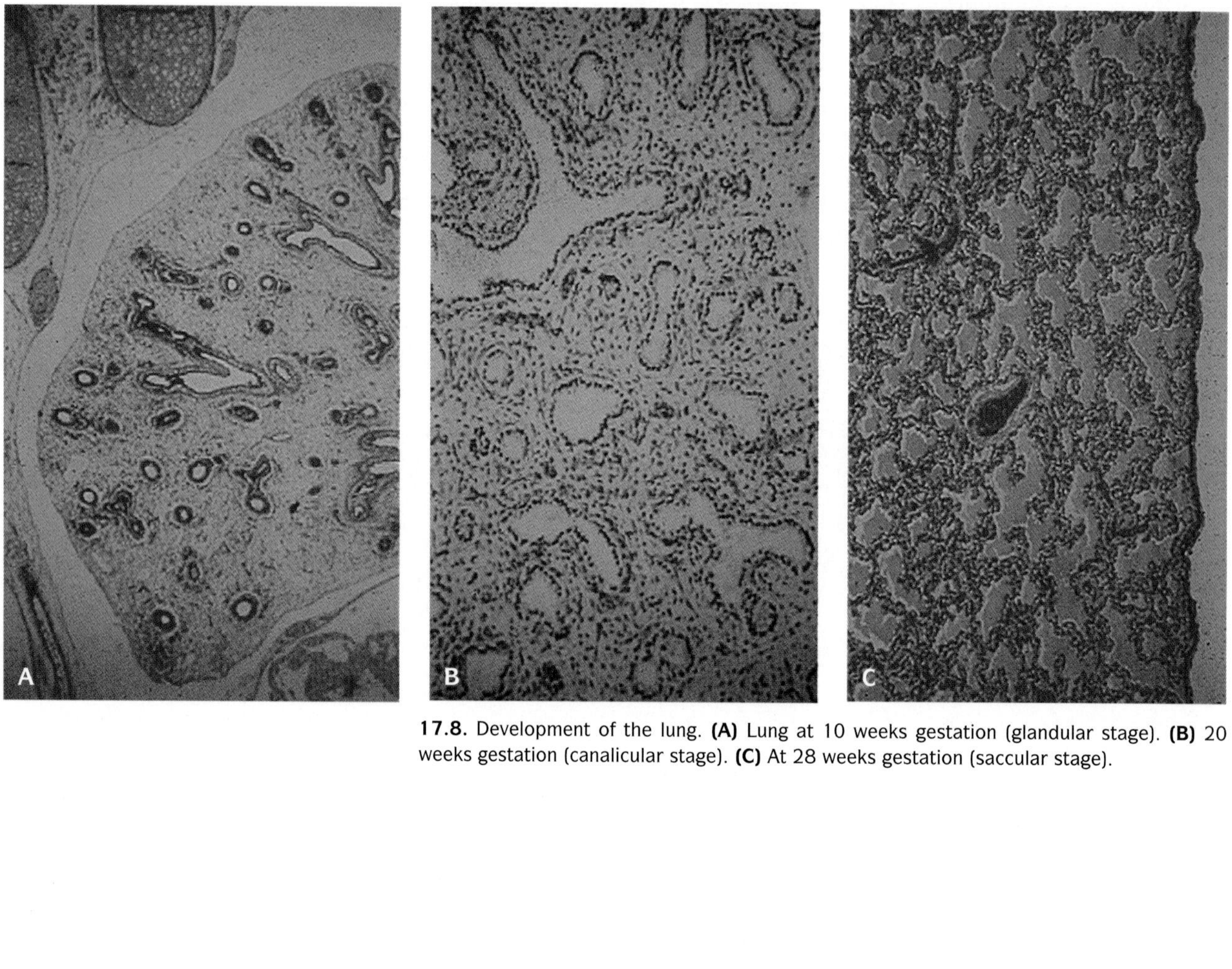

17.8. Development of the lung. **(A)** Lung at 10 weeks gestation (glandular stage). **(B)** 20 weeks gestation (canalicular stage). **(C)** At 28 weeks gestation (saccular stage).

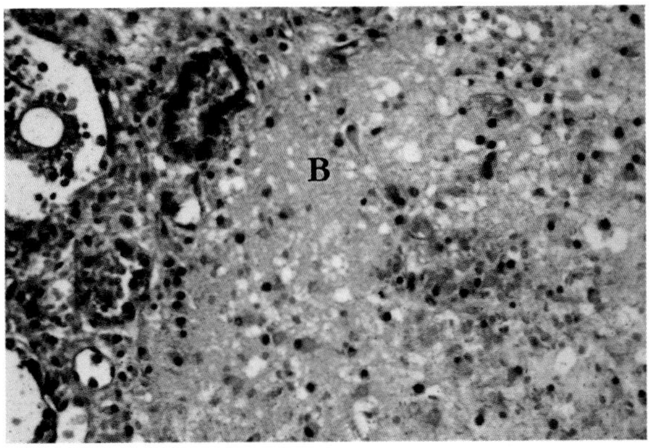

17.9. Heterotopic brain (B) in the lung of an anencephalic.

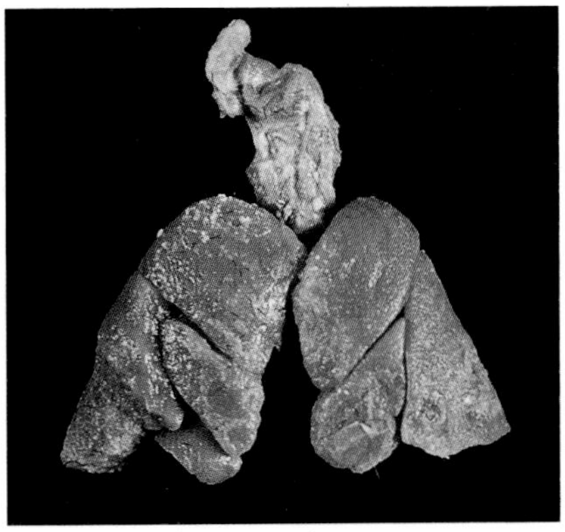

17.10. Symmetrical trilobed lungs in case of asplenia.

accessory left lower lobe, or a lateral accessory right upper lobe (Figure 17.10). The presence of three lobes on each side, or two lobes on each side, is associated with the asplenia/polysplenia syndrome with complex cardiac malformations.

Cystic Adenomatoid Malformation of the Lung

This rare malformation is usually unilateral. Cystic structures arise from an overgrowth of the terminal bronchioles with a reduction in the number of alveoli. It is frequently associated with polyhydramnios and fetal hydrops. Five types have been described: 1) type 0 – acinar dysplasia; 2) type 1 – multiple large cysts or a single dominant cyst; 3) type 2 – multiple, evenly spaced cysts; 4) type 3 – bulky, firm mass; 5) type 4 – peripheral cyst type (Figures 17.11 and 17.12 and Table 17.3).

Cardiac abnormalities, renal agenesis, renal dysplasia, hydrocephalus, jejunal atresia, diaphragmatic hernia, bronchial abnormalities, and prune belly

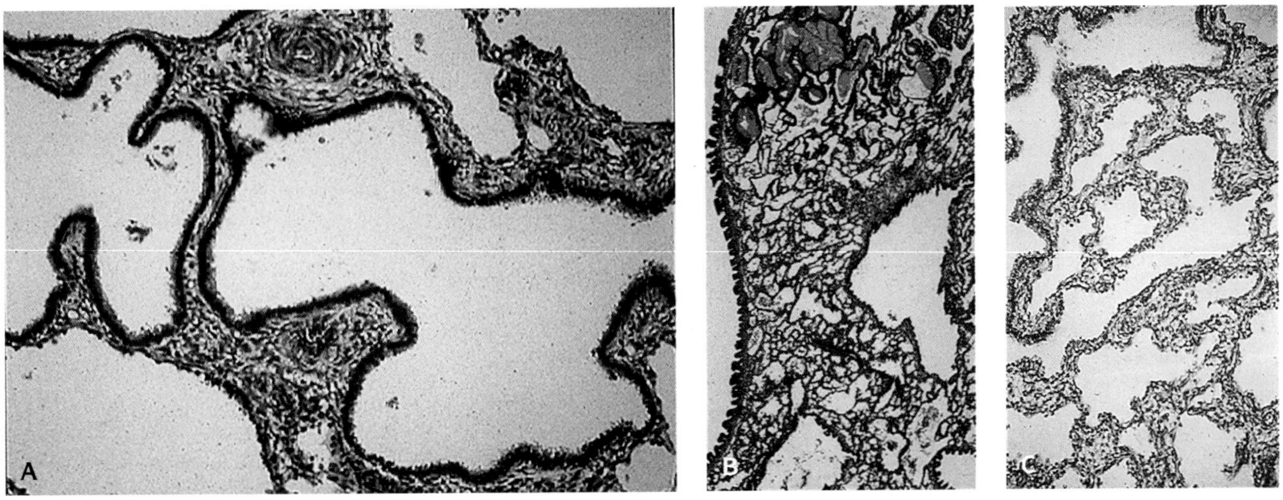

17.11. Microscopic appearance of CCAM. **(A)** Type 1. **(B)** Type 2. **(C)** Type 3.

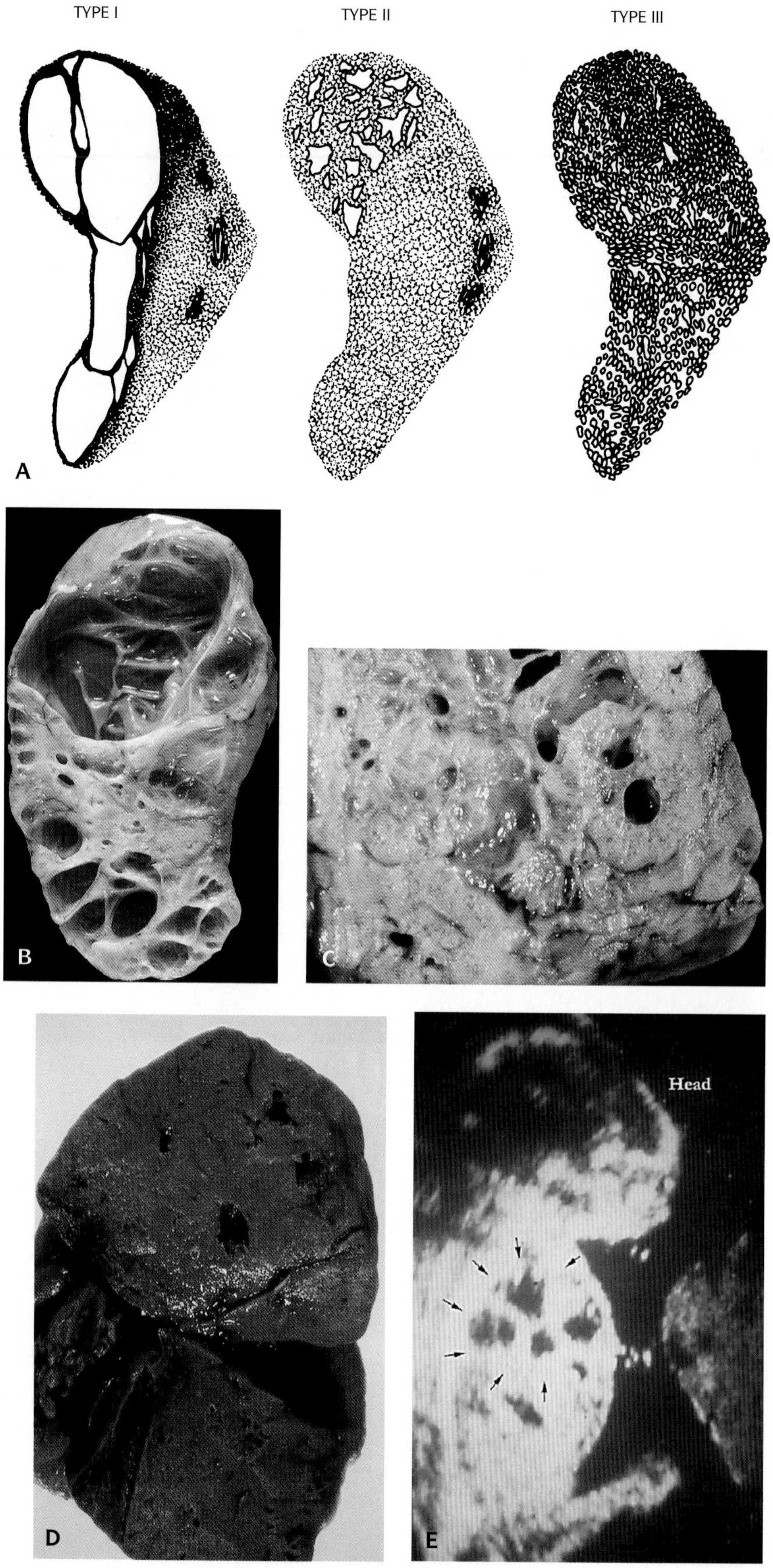

17.12. Congenital cystic adenomatoid malformations (CCAM). **(A)** Diagram of types of CCAM. (Courtesy of Dr. J. Thomas Stocker.) **(B)** Type 1, predominantly cystic. **(C)** Type 2, cystic and solid components. **(D)** Type 3, predominantly solid. **(E)** Ultrasound of CCAM (arrows).

Table 17.3 Pathologic features of congenital cystic adenomatoid malformation

	Type 0 (tracheobronchial)	Type 1 (bronchial/bronchiolar)	Type 2 (bronchiolar)	Type 3 (bronchiolar alveolar)	Type 4 (distal acinar)
Approximate frequency (%)	1–3	>65	20–25	8	2–4
Cyst size (maximum, cm)	0.5 cm	10.0	2.5	2.0	7
Microscopic appearance	Ciliated bronchial-like structures lined by pseudostratified tall columnar epithelium with goblet cells	Multilocular, large cysts Broad fibrous septa Mucogenic cells ciliated pseudostratified tall columnar epithelium	Small, uniform cysts Irregular proliferation of ectatic structures resembling bronchioles	Solid, bulky lesion Irregular curving channels and small air spaces lined by plump cuboidal epithelium	Multilocular, large cysts lined by flattened alveolar lining cells
Muscular wall thickness (mm) of cysts	100–500	100–300	50–100	0–50	25–100
Mucous cells	Present in all cases	Present (33% of cases)	Absent	Absent	Absent
Cartilage	Present in all cases	Present (5–10% cases)	Absent	Absent	Rare
Skeletal muscle	Absent	Absent	Present (5% of cases)	Absent	Absent

Adapted from Gilbert-Barness E. *Potter's Pathology of the Fetus and Infant*. St. Louis, Mosby Publisher, 1997.

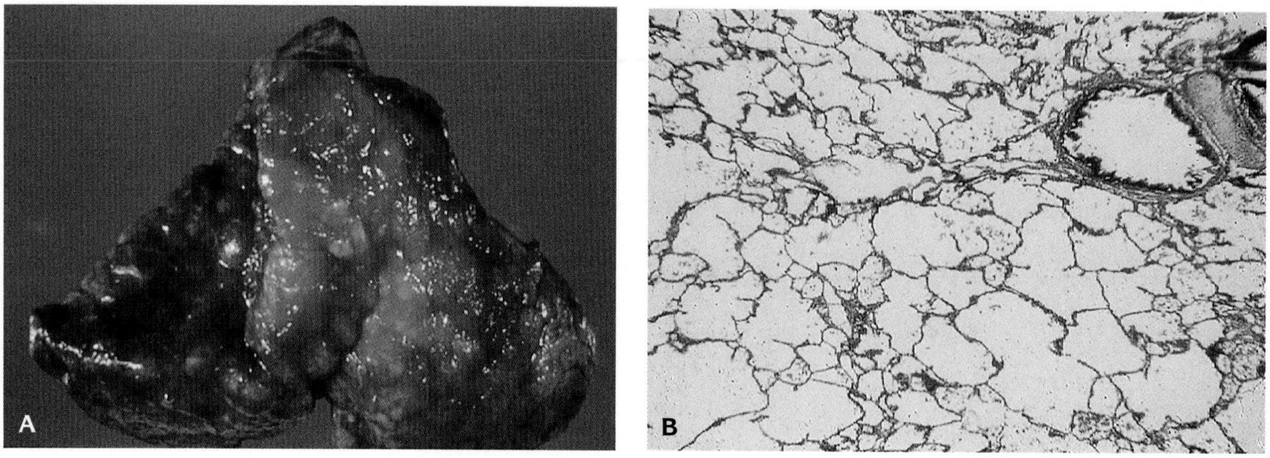

17.13. Congenital lobar emphysema. **(A)** The middle lobe is hyperaerated and emphysematous. **(B)** Microscopic appearance showing hyperdistended alveoli.

syndrome may be associated anomalies. It has been proposed that this malformation be called cystic pulmonary airway malformation (CPAM).

Infantile (Congenital) Lobar Emphysema

Infantile lobar emphysema involves the left upper lobe (50% of cases), right middle lobe (24–30%), and right upper lobe (18–24%). The lower lobes are involved in <5% of cases. The affected lobe is hyperdistended and, characteristically, fails to collapse after sectioning. There is uniform overdistension with alveolar saccules and alveoli often 2–10 times their normal size (Figure 17.13 and Table 17.4). A deficiency of cartilage within the wall of the bronchus appears to be the underlying cause.

Table 17.4 Causes of infantile lobar emphysema

Congenital
Bronchial stenosis
Abnormal origin of bronchus
Tracheal
Eparterial
Obstruction by external mass
Bronchogenic cyst
Bronchogenic atresia
Obstruction by vascular anomaly
Pulmonary artery sling
Patent ductus arteriosus
Anomalous pulmonary venous return
Mediastinal teratoma

Acquired
Aspirated meconium
Granulation tissue
Bronchial mucosal folds
Mucous plug

Congenital Pulmonary Lymphangiectasis (CPL)

If CPL is an isolated lesion, it is a diffuse pulmonary malformation that usually leads rapidly to cyanosis and death. It presents as acute respiratory distress in the first few hours of life; pleural effusion, chylothorax, and maternal polyhydramnios may be present (Figure 17.14). Multiple anomalies are present in >80% of cases. The lungs are bulky and noncompressible, with a delicate network of dilated, fluid-filled lymphatics beneath the pleura. The dilated lymphatics are lined by a thin layer of endothelial cells and may be surrounded by a mild to marked amount of loose connective tissue, often containing extramedullary hematopoiesis.

Pulmonary Sequestration

This rare anomaly consists of the presence of pulmonary tissue that is not attached to the rest of the lung and does not communicate with the trachea (Figure 17.15). It may be intralobar or extralobar pulmonary sequestration. Intralobar sequestration has not been reported among previable fetuses and appears to be usually an acquired condition. If a pleura is not shared, it is

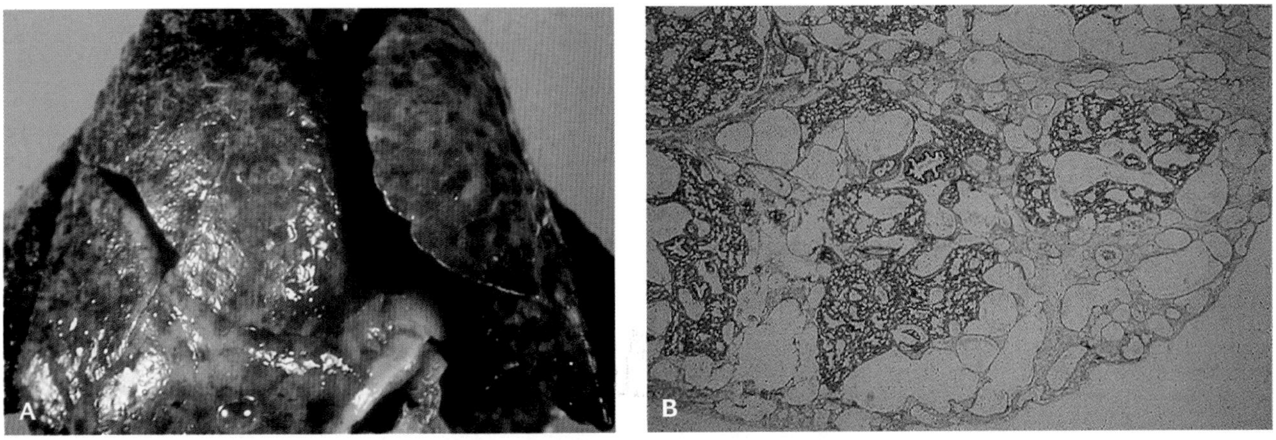

17.14. Congenital pulmonary lymphangiectasia. **(A)** Gross appearance. The pleural surface shows milky white reticular pattern of dilated lymphatics. **(B)** Microscopic appearance showing dilated lymphatics in the interlobular septae.

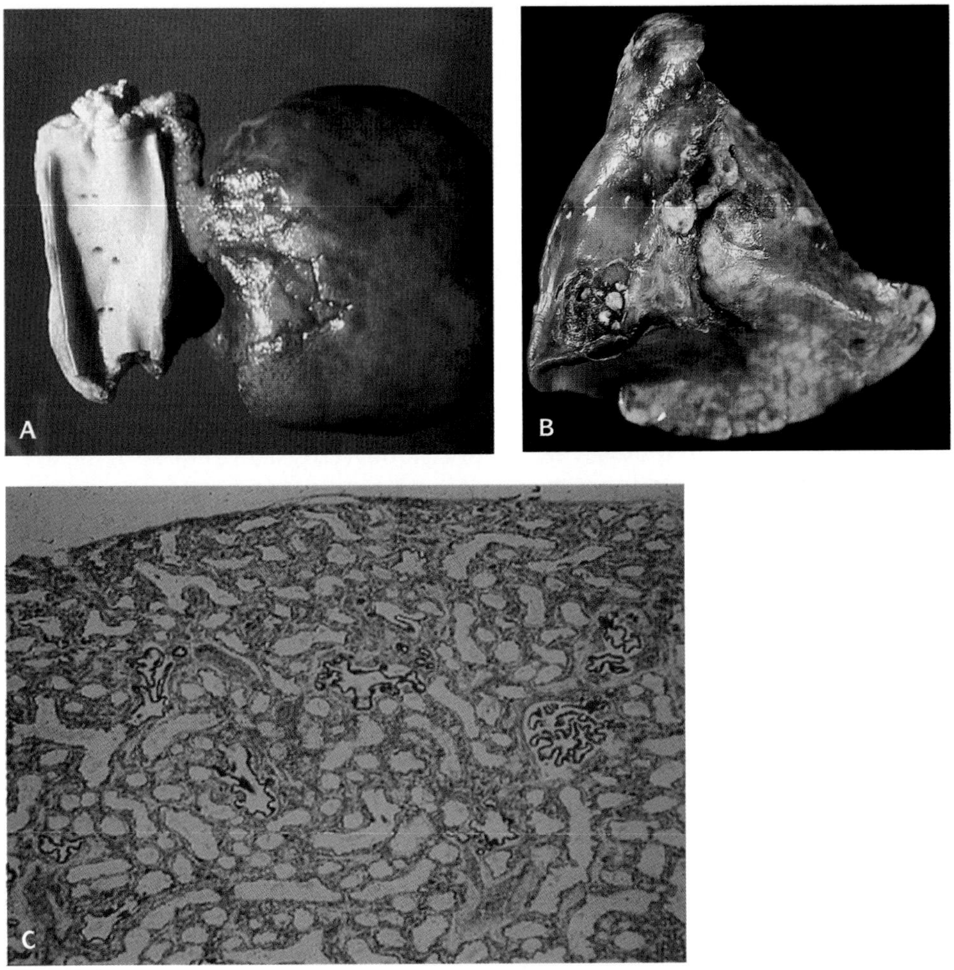

17.15. Pulmonary sequestration. **(A)** Extralobar. The sequestered lobe is firm and atelectatic and has an anomalous vascular supply from the aorta. **(B)** Intralobar. The sequestered lobe is dark purple and atelectatic. **(C)** Microscopic appearance showing poorly expanded and compressed alveoli.

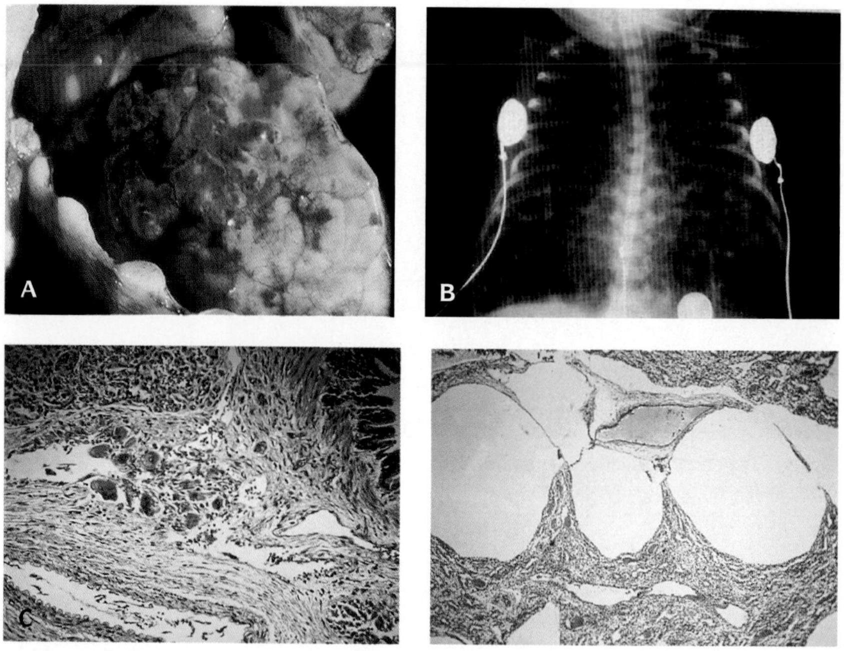

17.16. Pulmonary interstitial emphysema. **(A)** Gross appearance with emphysematous blebs beneath the pleura. **(B)** X-ray. The lungs show a coarse bubbly pattern due to the presence of interstitial air. **(C)** Microscopic appearance with interstitial air (right) and giant cell reaction (left).

an extralobar pulmonary sequestration. It is usually located between the lower lobe and the diaphragm. Associated anomalies are TEF, esophageal defects such as cysts, diverticula, duplications, and bronchogenic and neurogenic cysts.

Pulmonary Interstitial Emphysema

This condition is usually related to vigorous resuscitative efforts in the newborn. Rupture of alveoli allows air to dissect into the interlobar septa to produce pulmonary interstitial emphysema (PIE). Extension of this interstitial air centrally or peripherally can lead to pneumothorax, pneumomediastinum, or pneumopericardium (Figure 17.16).

Capillary Alveolar Dysplasia

This rare condition is characterized by persistent pulmonary hypertension. Pulmonary veins accompany small pulmonary arteries (Figure 17.17). The veins are malpositioned and thick-walled; thus, there is misalignment of the pulmonary veins (pulmonary veins normally are separate from pulmonary arteries and are present in the interlobular septa). Capillaries that normally are very close to the alveolar surface are reduced in number and removed from the alveolar/air interface. The deficiency of capillaries results in pulmonary hypertension and gas exchange is inhibited by reduced numbers of capillaries. Respiratory insufficiency is evident at birth and mortality is very high.

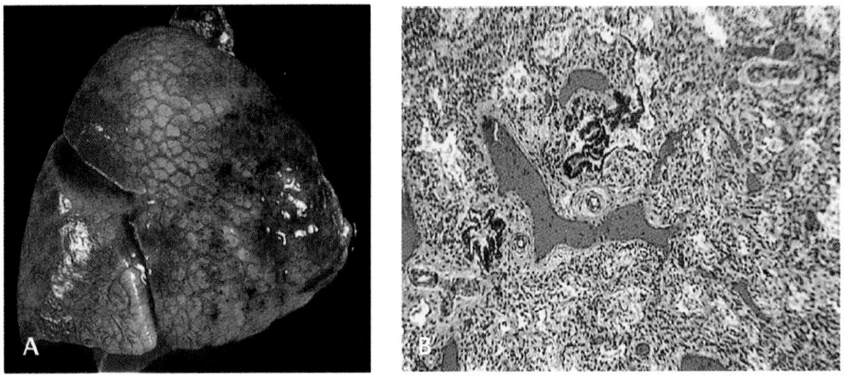

17.17. Capillary alveolar dysplasia. **(A)** Gross appearance of lung. **(B)** Microscopic appearance showing displaced dilated veins in bronchopulmonary space (misaligned pulmonary veins).

Amniotic Fluid and Meconium Aspiration

Aspiration of amniotic fluid or meconium occurs mainly in mature or postmature infants and is not infrequently associated with cerebral hemorrhage, intrauterine pneumonia, congenital cardiac defects, or the administration of drugs to the mother during delivery as well as hypoxia (Figure 17.18).

Cystic Fibrosis (CF) (See Also Chapter 18)

CF is the most common lethal recessive disorder in humans that may be evident soon after birth with hyperplasia of bronchial submucosal glands and inspissation of mucus. Pneumonia, particularly *Pseudomonas* or *Staphylococcus aureus*

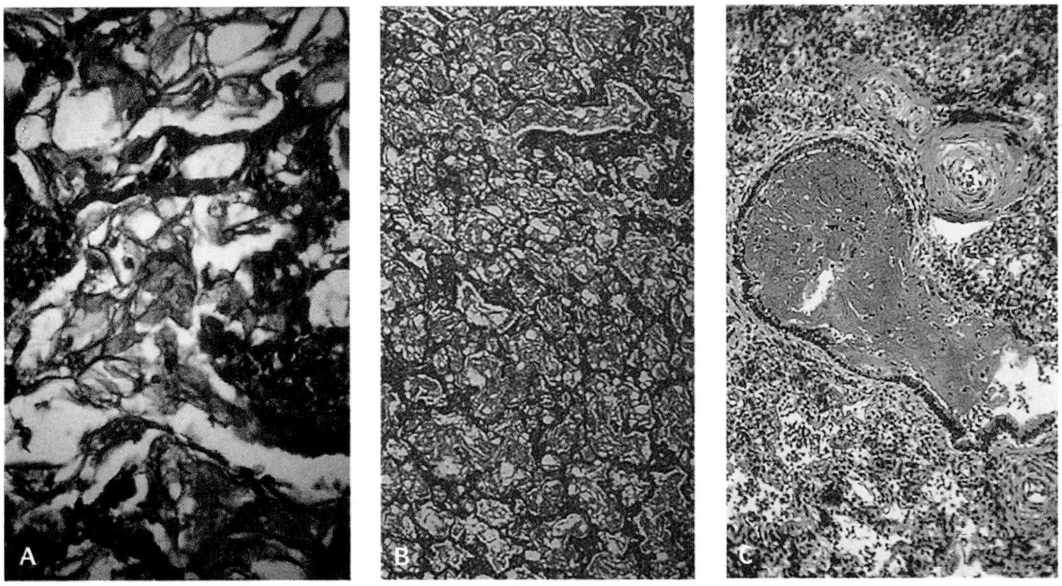

17.18. Amniotic fluid aspiration. **(A)** The alveolar ducts are filled with squames from amniotic fluid (low power). **(B)** High-power view. **(C)** Meconium aspiration. The bronchioles are filled with meconium.

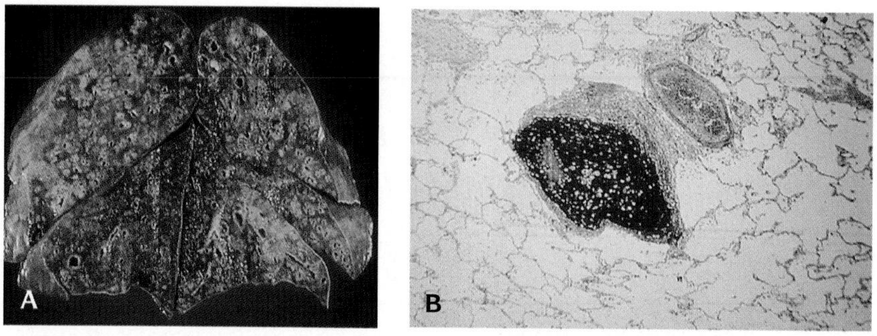

17.19. Cystic fibrosis. **(A)** Cut surface of lungs showing dilatation of bronchi with infection and small abscesses. **(B)** Microscopic section showing mucus plug in bronchiole in a newborn infant.

infection, progresses to bronchiectasis. Other clinical features include exocrine pancreatic insufficiency, neonatal meconium ileus, elevated sweat electrolytes, and male infertility. The sweat test is the usual diagnostic test for CF. The gene responsible for CF is the cystic fibrosis transmembrane conductance regulator (CFTR), which encodes the cyclic adenosine monophosphate (cAMP)-dependent chloride channel. DNA mutation analysis is possible (Figure 17.19). DNA can be isolated and used in a polymerase chain reaction to detect the Δ508, G551D, R553X, and S549N mutations, which account for approximately 80% of all CF mutations. The most common ΔF580 mutation is a 3-base deletion in exon 10 that results in the deletion of the phenylalanine-508 from the final gene product. There are >400 mutations. The incidence is approximately 1/2,500 live births with a carrier rate of 1/25.

Deficiency of Surfactant

Surfactant is a complex mixture of lipids (phospholipids) and proteins including surfactant proteins A, B, C, and D. Deficiency of surfactant is associated with hyaline membrane disease (HMD) in the lungs of newborns (Figure 17.20 and Tables 17.5 to 17.7). It is rarely due to a congenital defect in the production of surfactant protein B. It is most often caused by inadequate production or increased destruction of surfactant in the immature lungs of premature infants. Hyaline membranes can be seen as early as 4–8 hours after birth in premature

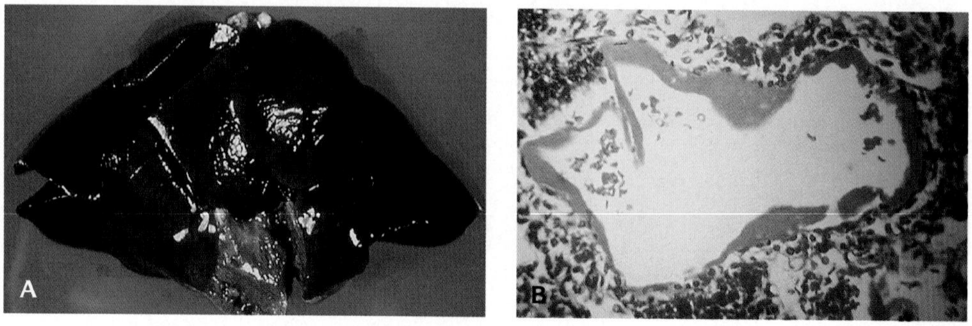

17.20. Hyaline membrane disease. **(A)** Gross appearance. The lungs are firm and dark red. **(B)** Microscopic appearance showing hyaline membranes.

Table 17.5 **Causes of surfactant deficiency in infants and the respiratory distress syndrome**

Pulmonary immaturity	Asphyxia
Immature gestation	Aspiration
Elective cesarean section	Second twin
Maternal diabetes	Maternal hemorrhage
Rh erythroblastosis	Congenital deficiency of surfactant protein B

Table 17.6 **Progression of changes from hyaline membrane disease to bronchopulmonary dysplasia**

Stage	Pathology
Stage 1 (0–4 days)	
Acute-exudative	Hyaline membranes, hyperemia, atelectasis, lymphatic dilation, patchy loss of ciliated cells, and necrosis of bronchiolar mucosa
Stage II (4–10 days)	
Early subacute-reparative	Persisting hyaline membranes, bronchiolar necrosis, eosinophilic exudate into lumen, squamous metaplasia, interstitial edema, and early septal fibrosis
Stage III (10–20 days)	
Late subacute-fibroproliferative	Fewer hyaline membranes, persisting alveolar epithelial injury, bronchial and bronchiolar mucosal metaplasia, irregular aeration with emphysematous and atelectatic alveoli, bronchiolitis obliterans, bronchiolectasis, increasing interstitial fibrosis, perialveolar duct fibrosis, type 2 cell hyperplasia/regeneration, smooth muscle proliferation
Stage IV (>1 month)	
Chronic fibroproliferative	Focally circumscribed groups of emphysematous alveoli; marked separation of capillaries from alveolar epithelia; increased collagen fibers; tortuous, dilated lymphatics; early vascular lesions of pulmonary hypertension; right ventricular hypertrophy; no bronchiolitis or bronchiolectasis; honeycombing

Table 17.7 **Hyaline membrane disease**

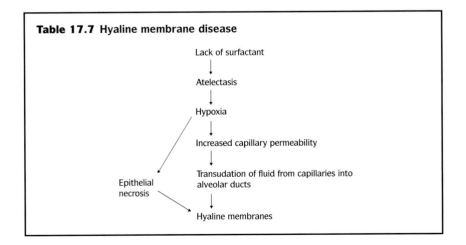

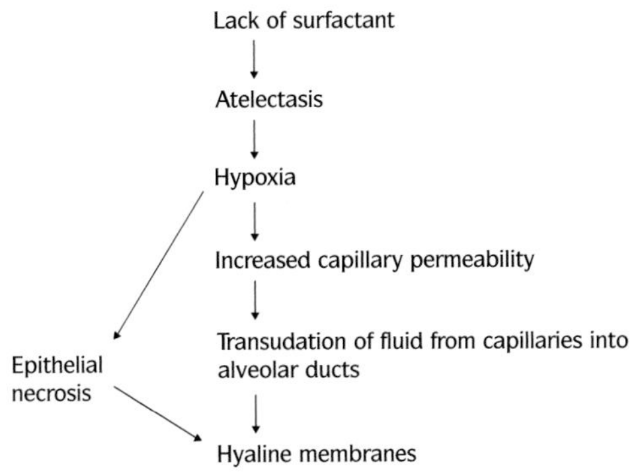

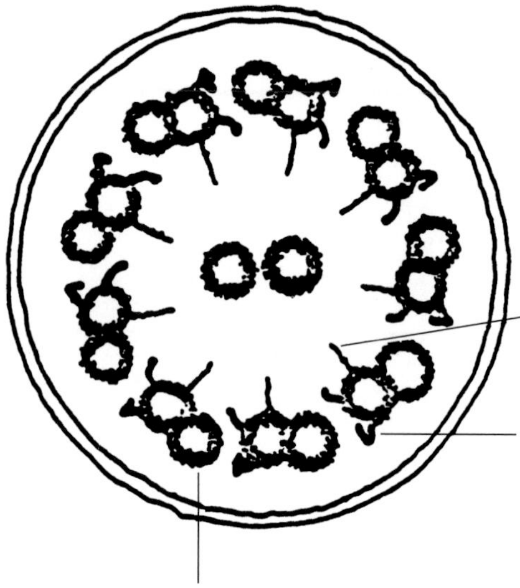

17.21. A normal cilium. In immobile cilia syndrome the dynein arms are absent.

infants dying of respiratory distress syndrome (RDS). The lungs are heavy, atelectatic, firm, and dark red with the consistency of liver.

Bronchopulmonary dysplasia (BPD) is the sequela of HMD in infants treated with mechanical ventilation and high concentrations of oxygen.

Surfactant protein B deficiency is a rare cause of hyaline membrane disease and may be treated with surfactant.

Immotile Cilia Syndrome (ICS) and Kartagener Syndrome (Sinusitis, Bronchiectasis, Situs Inversus)

This disorder is diagnosed by electron microscopy of a biopsy containing the respiratory epithelium such as mucosa of the nasopharynx (Figures 17.21 and 17.22). There is absence of the outer dynein arms of the cilia, rendering the cilia immotile and resulting in a defect of mucociliary transport. Clinical manifestations are chronic rhinitis, sinusitis, otitis, bronchitis, bronchiectasis, frontal headaches, a poor sense of smell, and infertility in males.

Vascular Abnormalities

Pulmonary Hemorrhage. Bleeding into the alveolar spaces and into the interstitium occurs principally in premature infants with birth asphyxia (Figure 17.23). It may occur in stillborn and live-born infants. The lungs are heavy and dark red with multiple anoxic hemorrhage (Tardieu spots).

Pulmonary arteriovenous fistula is one of the manifestations of familial hemorrhagic telangiectasia (Osler-Weber-Rendu disease), accounting for 50–60% of cases of pulmonary arteriovenous fistulas (Figure 17.24). Conversely, 25% of patients with hemorrhagic telangiectasia have pulmonary arteriovenous

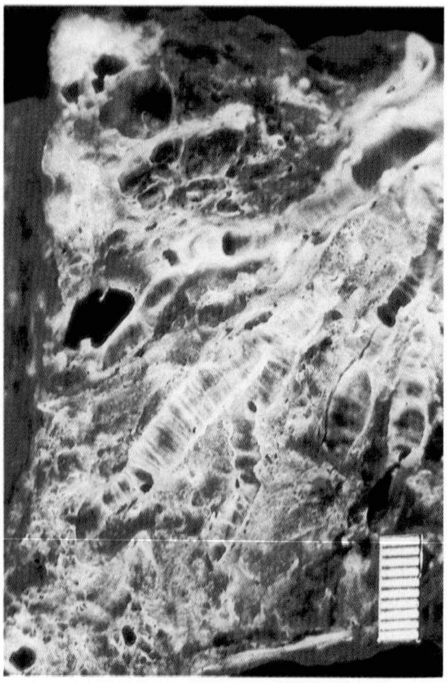

17.22. Cut surface of lung showing widely dilated bronchi in bronchiectasis.

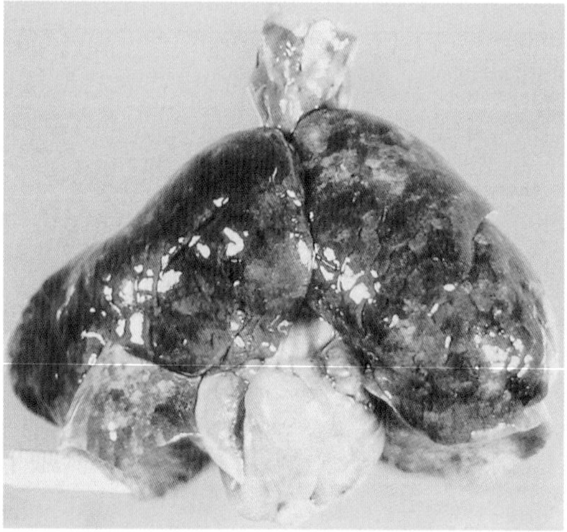

17.23. Multiple pulmonary hemorrhages due to anoxia.

Table 17.8 Grading of pulmonary hypertension

Grade	Histologic changes
Reversible	
1	Medial hypertrophy of arterioles
2	Medial hypertrophy and intimal proliferation of arterioles
3	Intimal and medial fibrosis of medium-sized arteries
Irreversible	
4	Plexiform and aneurysmal changes
5	Angiomatoid lesions
6	Necrotizing arteritis

fistulas. This is an autosomal dominant trait with high penetrance; some evidence indicates that the homozygous form is lethal in early life. It is an abnormal communication between pulmonary arteries and veins and most commonly involves the lower lobes.

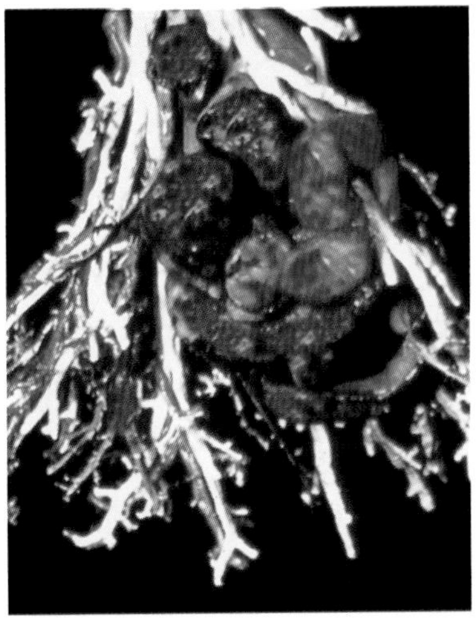

17.24. Arteriovenous malformation in cleared and fixed specimen after gelatin impregnation.

PRIMARY PULMONARY HYPERTENSION (PERSISTENCE OF FETAL CIRCULATION) (PPH)

The small pulmonary arteries resemble fetal vessels. There is marked medial hypertrophy with almost occluded vessels (Figure 17.25 and Table 17.8). Secondary pulmonary hypertension may follow meconium aspiration, thromboemboli of the pulmonary artery, hyaline membrane disease, bronchopulmonary dysplasia, or congenital heart disease with increased pulmonary blood flow. PPH may resolve in the neonatal period or progress to irreversible changes.

Chronic Pneumonitis of Infancy

This rare form of interstitial lung disease is characterized by marked alveolar septal thickening, striking alveolar pneumocyte hyperplasia, and an alveolar exudate containing numerous macrophages (Figure 17.26). Primitive mesenchymal cells predominate within the widened alveolar septa. Inflammatory cells are not seen. It usually occurs in young infants or the newborn. The

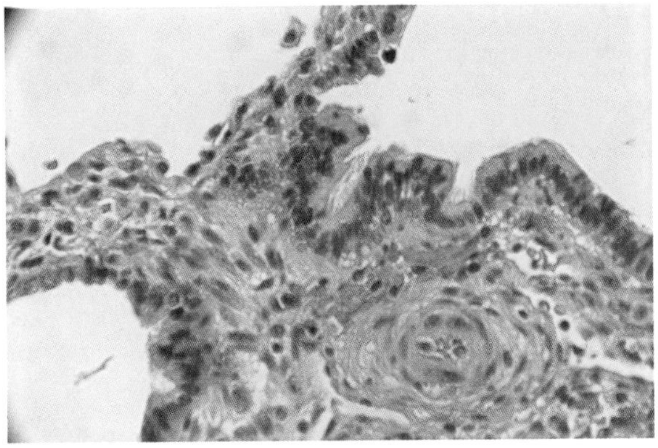

17.25. Microscopic section of newborn lung with primary pulmonary hypertension. The small arteries are thick walled and almost occluded.

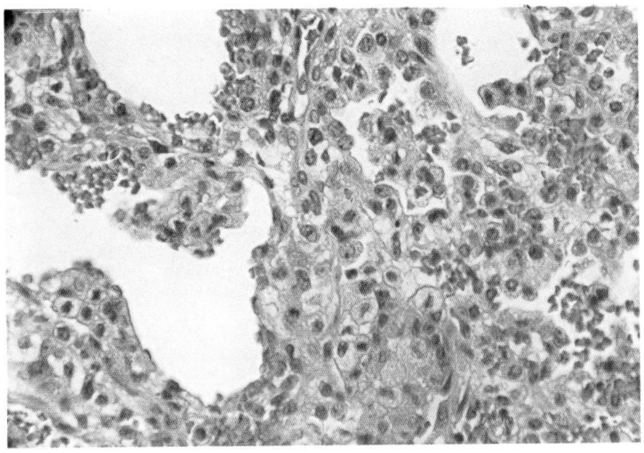

17.26. Chronic interstitial pneumonitis of infancy. Microscopic appearance of lung showing marked alveolar septal thickening. Hyperplastic alveolar lining cells are also present.

infant has respiratory distress, cough, and tachypnea. The etiology is unknown. Prognosis is poor but the infant may respond to steroids and extracorporeal membrane oxygenation (ECMO).

Pneumonia (See Infectious Disease Chapter)

Perinatal pneumonia is usually acquired during delivery and is due to aspiration of infected amniotic fluid from an acute chorioamnionitis; postnatal pneumonia is acquired in the nursery or at home. The organisms commonly involved in ascending infection are those that colonize the maternal vagina, usually β-hemolytic streptococci and Gram-negative bacteria, of which *Clostridium* sp. and *Escherichia coli* are the most common.

Transplacental pneumonias are produced by a variety of infectious agents including TORCH (toxoplasmosis, rubella, cytomegalovirus, and herpes) and *Histoplasma, Treponema pallidum, Mycoplasma, Listeria monocytogenes,* and *Mycobacterium tuberculosis.*

Agents of intrauterine pneumonia arising from vaginal flora and gaining access to the amniotic sac with prolonged rupture of membranes include group B β-hemolytic streptococcus, *Candida albicans, L. monocytogenes,* cytomegalovirus, genital herpes, *S. aureus, Chlamydia trachomatis, Ureaplasma,* and *Mycoplasma pneumoniae.* An intrauterine pulmonary infection is characterized by the presence of peribronchial aggregates of fetal lymphocytes within the airways and should be distinguished from simple aspiration of infected amniotic fluid that contains maternal polymorphonuclear leukocytes.

Viral pneumonia commonly is a cytomegalovirus infection and tiny foci of necrosis with characteristic intranuclear inclusions are present.

DEFECTS OF THE DIAPHRAGM

Pathogenesis of Diaphragmatic Hernia

In the sixth week of development, the abdominal and thoracic cavities are partially separated (Figures 17.27 to 17.29). The septum transversum occupies

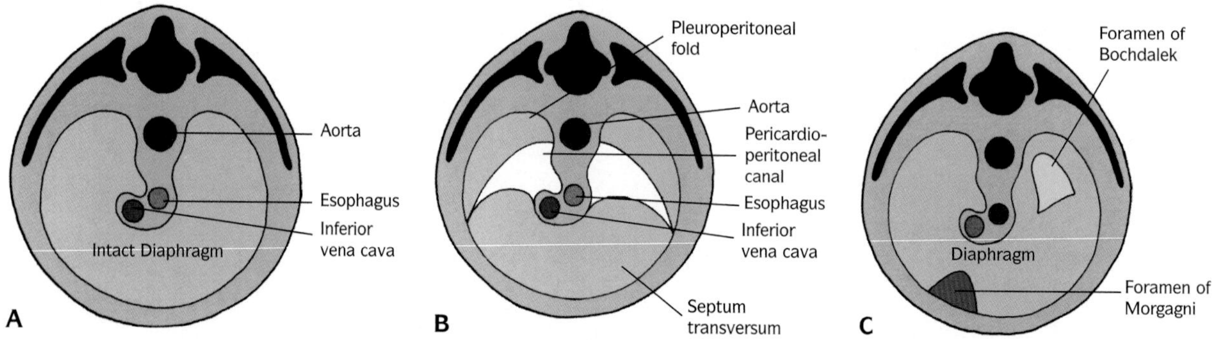

17.27. Types of diaphragmatic defects. **(A)** Normal diaphragm. **(B)** Agenesis of the diaphragm. **(C)** Patent foramen of Bochdalek (yellow). Patent foramen of Morgagni (green).

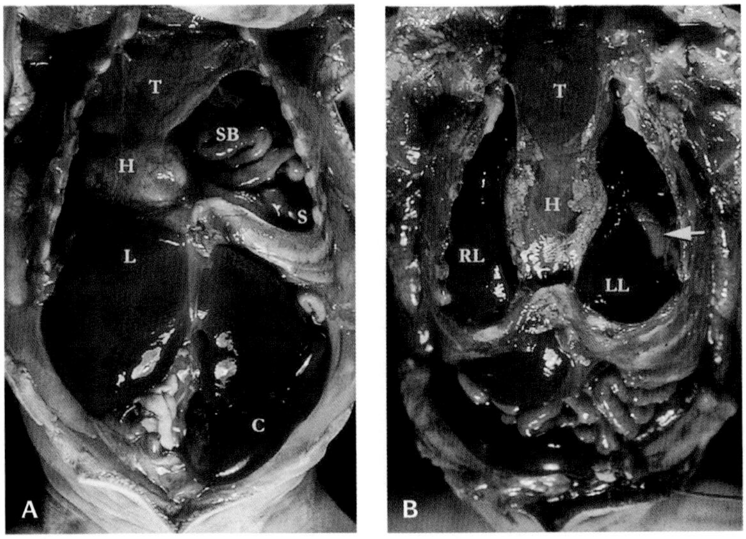

17.28. Diaphragmatic hernia through foramen of Bochdalek. **(A)** Loops of intestine (SB) are present in the left thoracic cavity. (H, Heart; L, Liver; C, Colon; T, Thymus; S, Spleen.) **(B)** Bilateral diaphragmatic hernia. (T, Thymus; H, Heart; RL, right lobe of liver; LL, left lobe of liver; arrow, small bowel.)

the anterior part of the developing diaphragm, the central part of which is composed of the esophageal mesentery, and laterally the pleuroperitoneal folds. The space between the two is called the pericardioperitoneal canal. At this stage, the abdominal and thoracic cavities communicate through these canals. These spaces then become the primitive diaphragm, which is formed by the eighth week of development.

If fusion of the pleuroperitoneal membrane with the esophageal mesentery and the septum transversum is not complete, a defect is created that can allow abdominal contents to extend into the thoracic cavity. This defect is usually unilateral and on the left at the foramen of Bochdalek.

A defect that is in the intersternocostal triangle located between the muscle fibers that come from the xiphoid cartilage and neighboring fibers is called the foramen of Morgagni, and the liver and other abdominal organs many herniate through it.

In diaphragmatic agenesis, one half or both halves of the diaphragm may be absent.

There are some familial cases of diaphragmatic defects or agenesis; a few cases may be autosomal recessive. Diaphragmatic defects may be part of a syndrome, as in Beckwith-Wiedemann, Fryns syndrome, or occasionally, Ivemark or Goltz syndrome.

In Bochdalek hernias, abdominal organs such as the stomach, spleen, and intestine can be seen in the thoracic cavity. These hernias usually occur on the left, and the heart and lungs are compressed toward the right. This results in underdevelopment and hypoplasia of the lung on the left and frequently also on the right side.

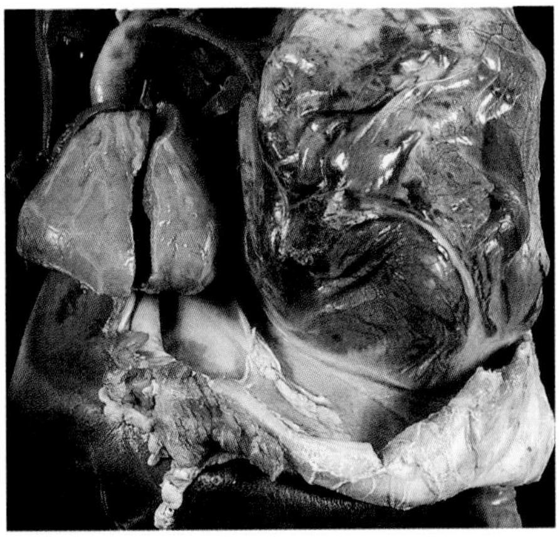

17.29. Eventration of the diaphragm. The diaphragm is extremely thin and the intestinal contents covered by peritoneum have herniated into the right thoracic cavity.

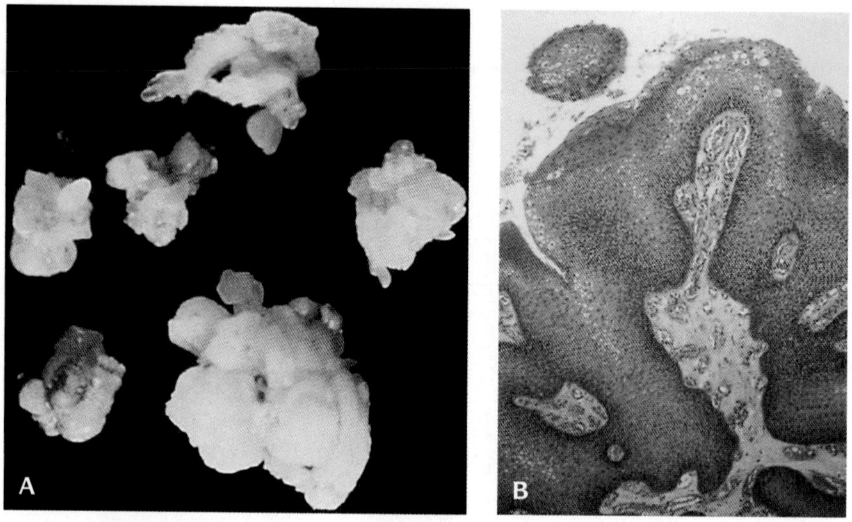

17.30. **(A)** Multiple surgically removed laryngeal papillomas. **(B)** Microscopic section of squamous papilloma with koilocytosis due to human papilloma virus (HPV-6).

In addition, there may be an eventration of the diaphragm due to reduced muscle thickness allowing tenting of the diaphragm into the thoracic cavity. (Fig. 17.29)

The incidence of diaphragmatic hernia is 1/3,000–5,000 and 85–90% are on the left side through the foramen of Bochdalek. About 1–2% are Morgagni hernias, which are usually on the right side, and about 5% represent eventrations of the diaphragm.

Laryngotracheal Papillomatosis

These papillomas may become manifest soon after birth when viral infection of the infant from the maternal vaginal canal has occurred (Figure 17.30). These papillomas most commonly are due to human papilloma virus (HPV) 6 and 11. Symptoms include hoarseness, stridor, and airway obstruction. Spontaneous regression or progression may occur. With the latter the papilloma may extend into the trachea, bronchi, and lungs.

REFERENCES

Askin FB: Pulmonary interstitial air and pneumothorax in the neonate. In Stocker JT (ed): *Pediatric Pulmonary Disease*, New York, Hemisphere Publishing, 1989, p. 165.

Chen JC, Holinger LD: Congenital tracheal anomalies: Pathology study using serial macrosections and review of the literature. *Pediatr Pathol* 14:513, 1994.

Creasy G, Simon N. Sensitivity and specificity of the LS ratio in relation to gestational age. *Am J Perinatol* 1:302, 1984.

Cullinane C, Cox PN, Silver MM: Persistent pulmonary hypertension of the newborn due to alveolar capillary dysplasia. *Pediatr Pathol* 12:499, 1992.

Falciglia HS, Kosmetatos N. Brady K et al.: Intrauterine meconium aspiration in an extremely premature infant. *Am J Dis Child* 47:1035, 1993.

Floros J, guest editor. Special issue on structure, function, and expression of pulmonary surfactant proteins, *Ped Path Molec. Med.* 20:249, 2001.

Gale N. Poljak M, Kabic V, et al.: laryngeal papillomatosis: Molecular, histopathological, and clinical evaluations. *Virchows Arch* 425:291, 1994.

Gilbert-Barness E: The respiratory system. In Gilbert-Barness E (ed): *Potter's Pathology of the Fetus and Infant*, St. Louis, Mosby-Year Book, 1997, p. 712.

Gorenlfo M. Vogel M, Herbst L, et al.: Influence of clinical and ventilatory parameters on morphology of bronchopulmonary dysplasia. *Pediatr pathol* 19:214, 1995.

Husain AN, Hessell RG: Neonatal pulmonary hypoplasia: An autopsy study of 25 cases. *Pediatr Pathol* 13:475, 1993.

Katzenstein ALA, Gordon K, Oliphat M, Swender PT: Chronic pneumonitis of infancy. *Am J Surgical Pathol* 19(4):439, 1995.

Kulovich M Gluck L. The bioprofile II: the complicated pregnancy. *Am J Obstet Gynecol* 135:64, 1979.

Moerman PP, Vanderberghe K, Devlieger H, et al.: Congenital pulmonary lymphangiectasis with chylothorax: a heterogenous lymphatic vessel abnormality. *Am J Med Genet* 47:54, 1993.

Murphy JD, Vawles GF, Reid L: Pulmonary vascular disease in fetal meconium aspiration. *J Pediatr* 104:758, 1984.

Rodriguez RJ: Management of respiratory distress syndrome: an update. *Respiratory Care* 48:279, 2003.

Rosado-de-Christensen M, Frazier AA, Stocker JR: Extralobar sequestration: Radiologic-pathologic correlation. *Radiographics* 13:425, 1993.

Stocker JR: Congenital and developmental diseases. In Dail DH, Hammer SP (eds): *Pulmonary Pathology*, New York, Spring-Verlag, 1994, p. 212.

Stocker JT, Dehmer LP: Acquired neonatal and pediatric diseases. In Dail DH, Hammer SP (eds): *Pulmonary Pathology*, New York, Springer-Verlag, 1994, p. 212.

Stocker JT: The respiratory tract. In Dail DH, Hammer SP (eds): *Pulmonary Pathology*, New York, Springer-Verlag, 1994, p. 549.

Zuppan CW, Robinson CC, Langston C: Viral pneumonia in infants and children. *Perspect Pediatr Pathol* 18:111, 1995.

EIGHTEEN

Gastrointestinal Tract and Liver

ESOPHAGEAL ATRESIA (SEE ALSO CHAPTER 17)

Esophageal atresia results in a complete separation of the esophagus into upper and lower segments. This is often accompanied by communication of either segment or both with the trachea resulting in tracheoesophageal fistula (TEF). It is accompanied by polyhydramnios in which the fetus is unable to swallow amniotic fluid.

The incidence is from 1/800 to 1/5,000 live births.

Pathogenesis

At approximately 4 weeks of development, a diverticulum grows caudally from the ventral wall of the foregut to form the trachea and esophagus. Tracheoesophageal folds form a tracheoesophageal septum, which separates the trachea from the esophagus at the 5th week of embryonic development.

If there is failure of normal septum formation, it results in a TEF with two disconnected segments of the esophagus.

Esophageal atresia is usually sporadic, although there have been about 80 reports of familial atresia with TEF. It also may occur in trisomy 18 or 21.

In over 80% of cases, the upper esophageal segment ends blindly and the lower segment communicates with the trachea (TEF). In approximately 10%, there is isolated atresia of the esophagus; in 1–3%, the upper segment joins the trachea; in 5%, both segments join the trachea. In the region of the fistula, the trachea is often narrow, and tracheal cartilage may be hypoplastic or absent. (See Chapter 17.)

The most frequently associated malformations are gastrointestinal defects, with about one-half associated with an imperforate anus. Cardiovascular malformations, such as persistent ductus arteriosus, VSD, ASD, right-sided aortic arch, dextrocardia, and urogenital defects, such as renal agenesis and hydronephrosis may be associated. Vertebral defects, radial upper limb defects, rib defects, and skeletal abnormalities may also occur.

Atresia of the duodenum or colon or an imperforate anus may occur in familial cases.

Tracheoesophageal fistula with esophageal atresia is a component of the VATER association, which is a combination of vertebral defects (V), anal atresia (A), TE fistula (TEF), and radial and renal dysplasia (R).

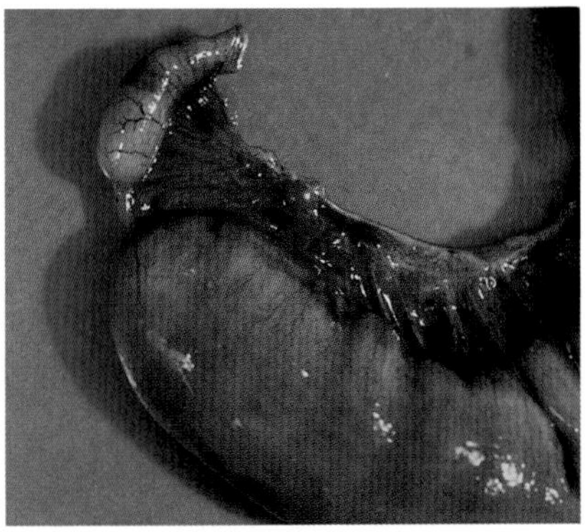

18.1. Jejunal atresia.

ATRESIA AND STENOSIS OF THE SMALL INTESTINE

Small bowel atresias occur in approximately 1/5,000 live births. The duodenum is the most common location for atresia in previable fetuses. It is an associated malformation in approximately 20% of trisomy 21 cases. Multiple atresias and stenoses occur in up to 20%. Most jejunal and ileal atresias result from intrauterine vascular disruptions (Figures 18.1 to 18.4).

Embryology

Embryologically, the lumen of the gastrointestinal tract becomes reestablished by the 11th week. The failure of normal recanalization is a cause of duodenal atresia.

In malrotation, volvulus, intussusception, and omphalocele, jejunal and ileal atresia by vascular disruption may produce infarction and atrophy. In cystic fibrosis, meconium in the intestinal lumen can produce obstruction with rupture, inflammation, granulation tissue, and scarring, which may lead to atresia and stenosis.

Intestinal atresia usually is sporadic. An autosomal recessive inheritance has been described in pyloroduodenal atresia, which is characterized by a septum between the stomach and the duodenum. Multiple bowel atresias, in which numerous atresias extend from the duodenum to the colon, are caused by an autosomal recessive gene. Jejunal atresia may also be an autosomal recessive disorder.

There are four types of intestinal atresia:

Type I – A transverse septum (diaphragm) obstructs the lumen.
Type II – Blind loops of gut are connected by a fibrous cord.
Type III – There is no connection between the two blind loops.

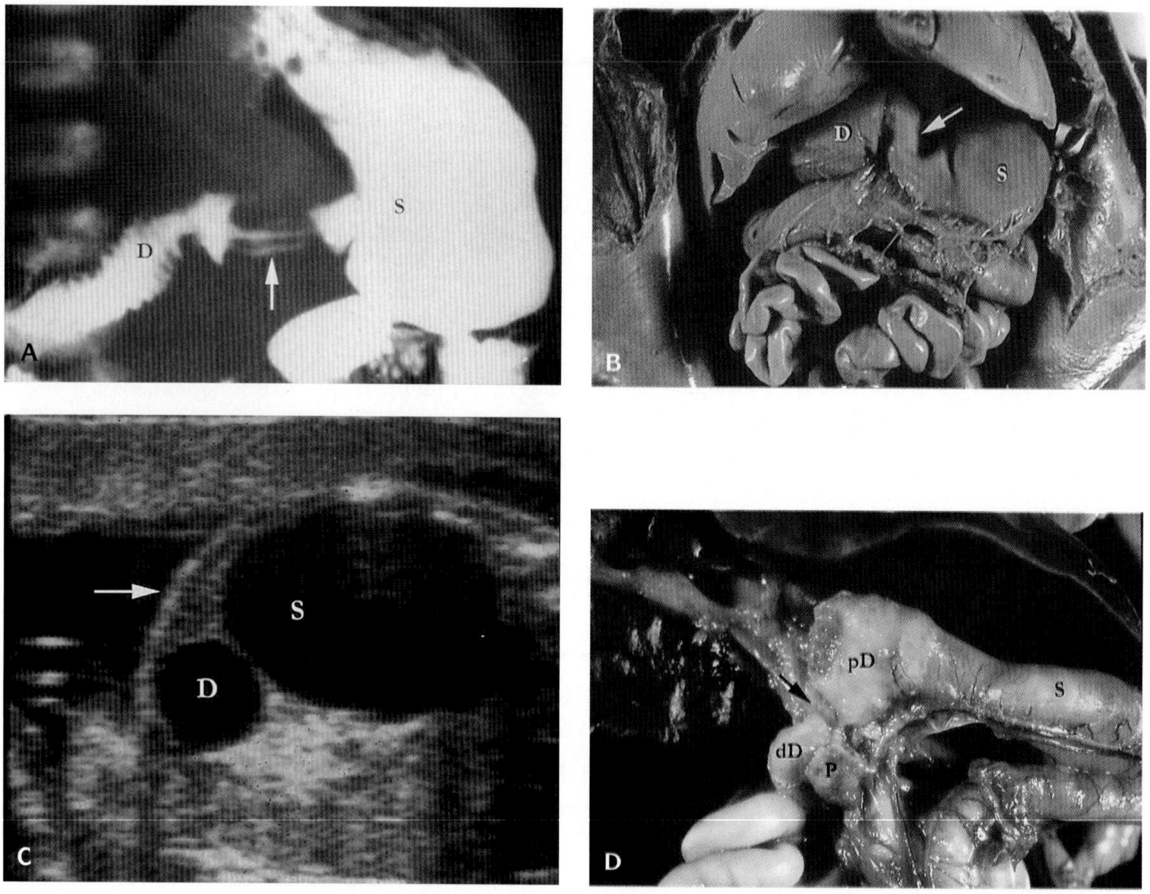

18.2. **(A)** Barium swallow x-ray shows pyloric stenosis (arrow). The stomach (S) is greatly dilated (D, duodenum). **(B)** Gross appearance of pyloric stenosis (arrow) (S, stomach; D, duodenum). **(C)** Ultrasound of duodenal atresia showing double bubble sign (arrow, abdominal wall; D, duodenum; S, stomach). **(D)** Duodenal atresia (arrow) (S, stomach; pD, proximal duodenum; dD, distal duodenum; p, pancreas).

Type IV – The atretic duodenum or jejunum spirals around the vascular supply. In this apple-peel-type of atresia, there is agenesis of the dorsal mesentery and absence of branches of the superior mesenteric artery.

Fifty to 70% of patients with intestinal atresia have associated abnormalities. The most common associated abnormality in duodenal atresia is congenital heart disease, and the next most frequent is TEF. The proportion of gastrointestinal abnormalities is reportedly higher in jejunal-ileal atresias than in duodenal stenosis.

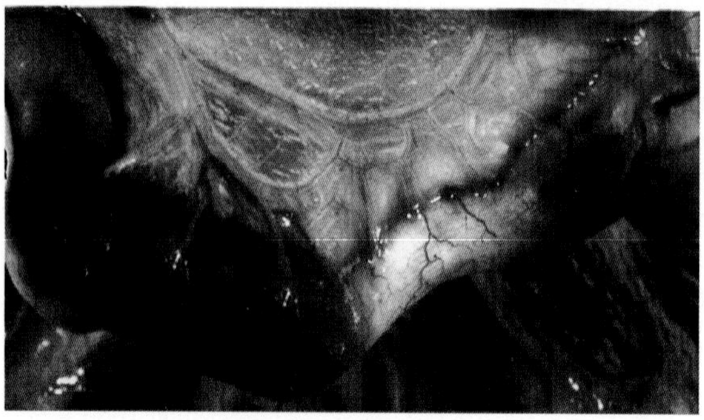

18.3. Stenosis of the terminal ileum.

Intestinal Duplications

Duplications are either tubular or cystic and are composed of mucosa and muscle that are closely adherent to the bowel on the mesenteric side (Figure 18.5). Only rarely is there a

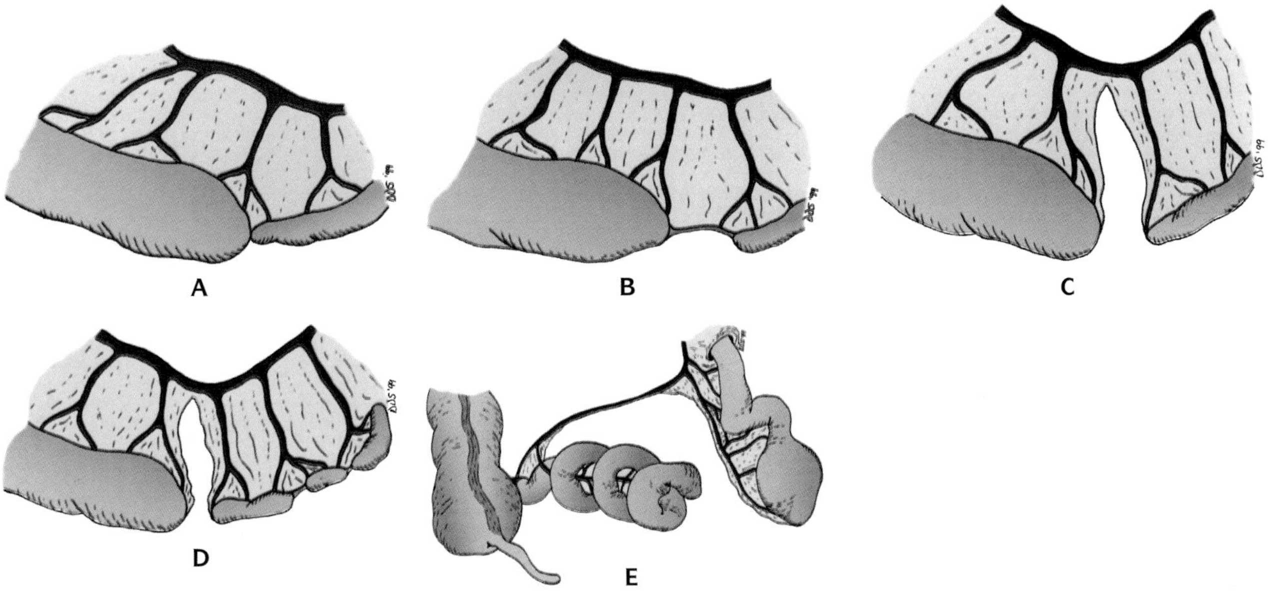

18.4. Illustrations of types of intestinal atresias. **(A)** Type I. **(B)** Type II. **(C)** Type III. **(D)** combination of Types I, II, and III. **(E)** Type IV.

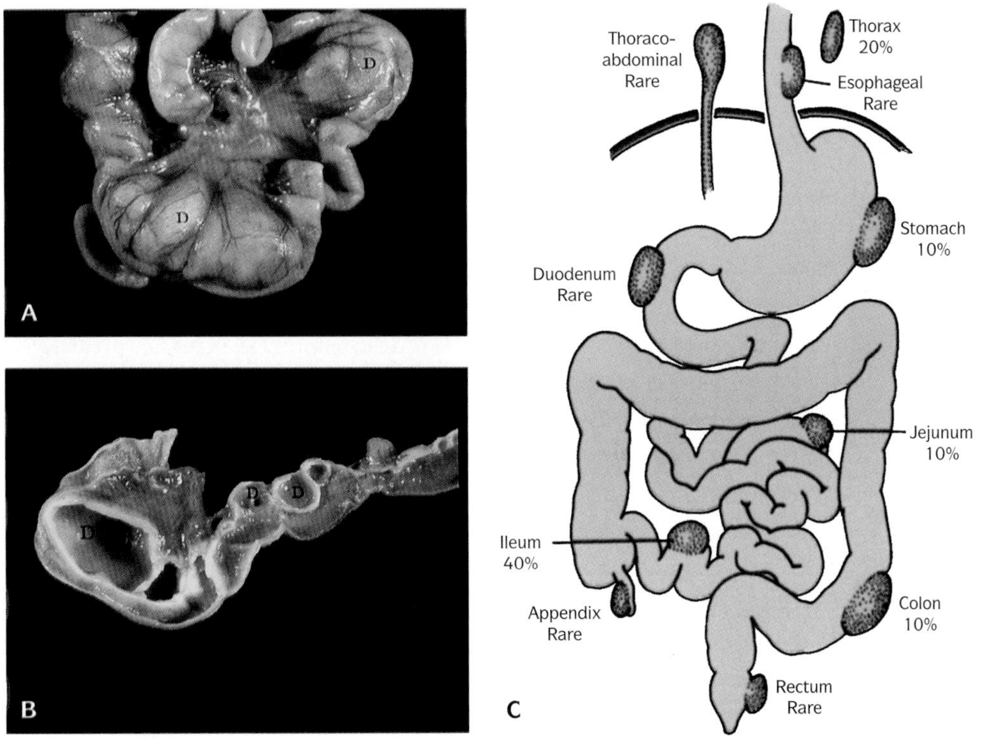

18.5. **(A)** Intestinal duplications. Unopened small bowel showing two duplication cysts (D). **(B)** Opened segment of bowel showing cystic duplications (D). **(C)** Sites of duplications.

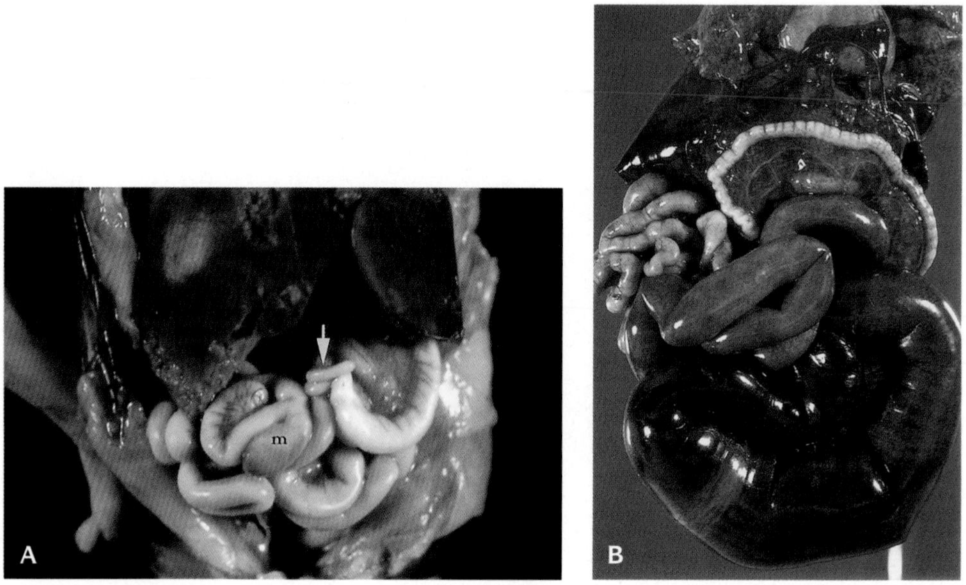

18.6. **(A)** Small intestinal malrotation. (Arrow on appendix in upper left abdomen; m, meckel diverticulum.) **(B)** Volvulus in malrotation.

communication with the lumen of the intestine. Duplications vary in length from a few to several centimeters. They are most common in the ileum and colon and they are filled with mucus.

MALROTATION OF THE BOWEL

Pathogenesis

At the 6th week of gestation, the growing midgut loop enters the umbilical cord where it rotates 180° in a counterclockwise direction. The cranial (prearterial) part of the loop elongates to form more intestinal loops. In the next stage, at 10 weeks, the intestines return to the abdomen. As they return, there is a further counterclockwise rotation of 90°, so the total rotation is 270°. Most of the prearterial part of the intestine enters the abdomen first, to the right of the superior mesenteric artery. Then the colon reenters, with the cecum, and, lastly, the terminal prearterial part of the small intestine. The third stage is fixation, which continues from 11–12 weeks until after birth. The mesenteries of the ascending and descending parts of the intestine fuse with the parietal peritoneum, and the cecum descends to the adult position.

In nonrotation, the colon reenters the abdomen first and lies on the left side; the cecum is in the middle and the small intestine is on the right. Vascular obstruction and volvulus may result if twisting occurs.

Malrotation may predispose to volvulus, vascular disturbances, abnormal adhesions, and, consequently, intestinal atresia or stenosis. Biliary obstruction, an annular pancreas, and mesenteric cysts have been associated with malrotation.

VITELLOINTESTINAL DUCT REMNANTS

The vitellointestinal (omphalomesenteric) duct connects the embryonic gut and the yolk sac. It is normally incorporated into the connecting stalk and later obliterated (Figures 18.7 and 18.8). The vitelline duct may persist as a diverticulum or as a fibrous cord connecting the ileum and the umbilical area or as a cyst(s) in the umbilical cord. The persistent diverticulum is called *Meckel diverticulum.* It is found at the terminal ileum in about 3% of normal individuals; it is more common in individuals with chromosome abnormalities. The

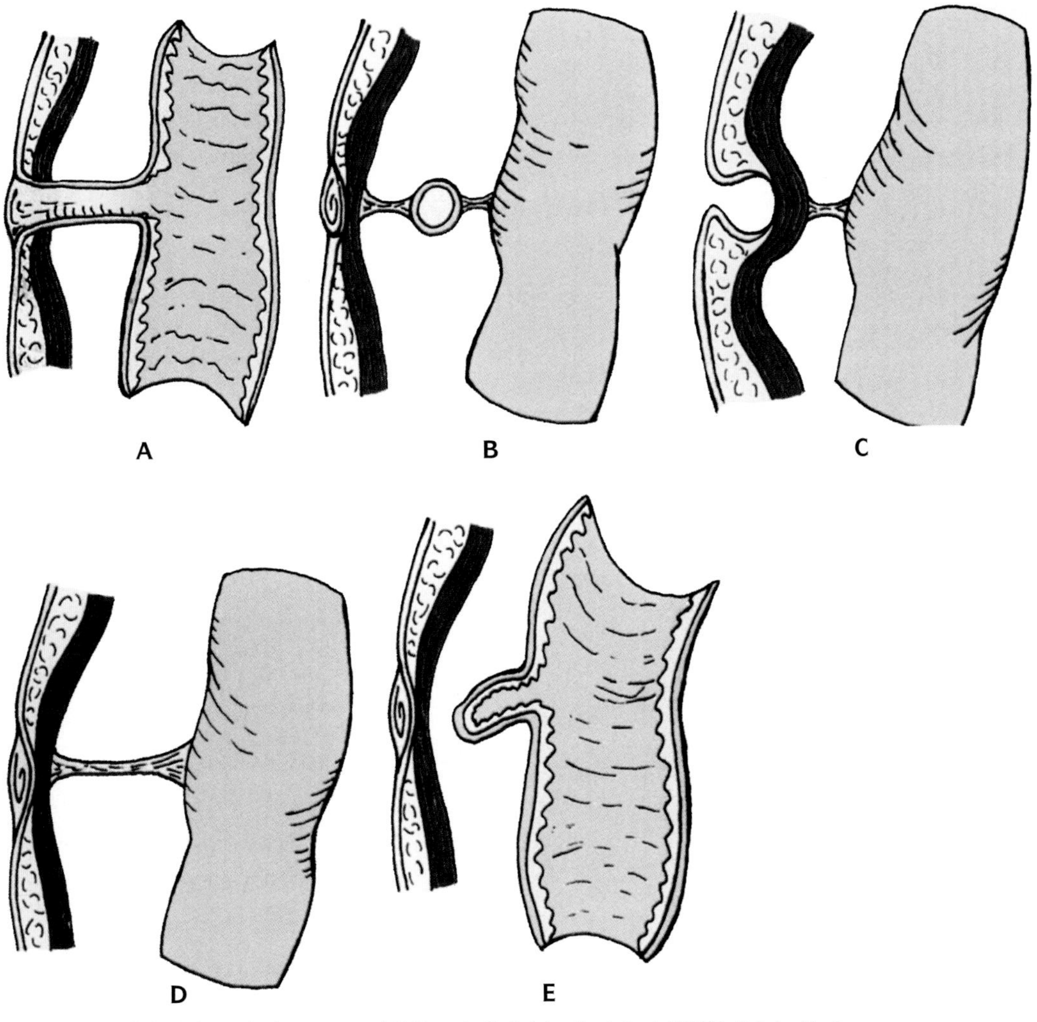

18.7. Types of vitellointestinal remnants. **(A)** Patent vitellointestinal duct. **(B)** Vitellointestinal cyst. **(C)** Fibrous cord with skin diverticulum. **(D)** Fibrous cord. **(E)** Meckel diverticulum.

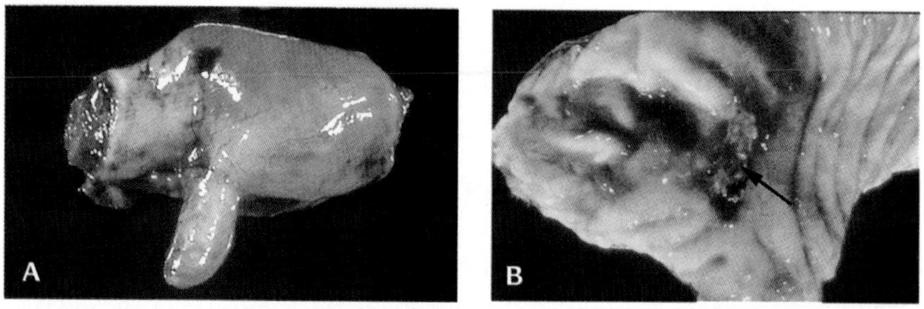

18.8. **(A)** Meckel diverticulum. **(B)** Opened Meckel diverticulum containing area of erosion due to the presence of gastric mucosa (arrow).

mucosal lining is usually small intestinal epithelium; however, gastric mucosa that may be the source of bleeding is seen in 25% of cases. Pancreatic tissue may also be present in a Meckel diverticulum.

SHORT BOWEL SYNDROME

The bowel may be shortened in omphalocele, gastroschisis, and jejunal and ileal atresia and in fetuses in whom swallowing movements are reduced as in oligohydramnios.

OMPHALOCELE

An omphalocele is a protrusion of the abdominal contents outside the abdominal wall (Figures 18.9 and 18.10). The defect is covered by a membrane consisting of amnion and peritoneum. The umbilical cord arises from the dome of the sac. A short umbilical cord may be etiologically related to the formation of an omphalocele. In 30–50% of cases it is associated with other congenital

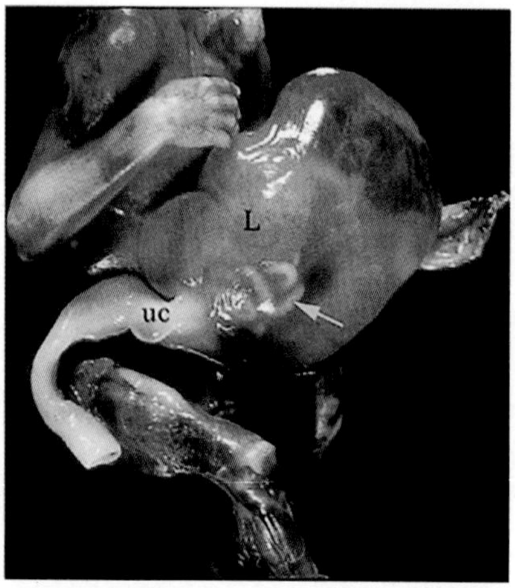

18.9. Omphalocele covered by peritoneum with short umbilical cord (UC). (L, liver; arrow, small bowel loops.)

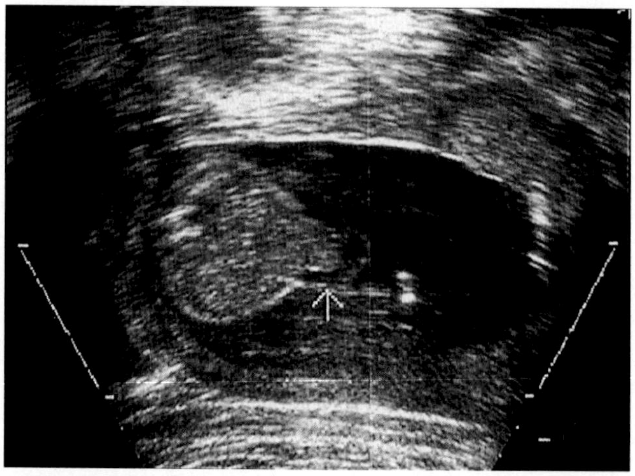

18.10. Ultrasound showing an omphalocele (arrow on cord insertion to omphalocele sac). The spine can be seen to the left as a white H-shaped structure.

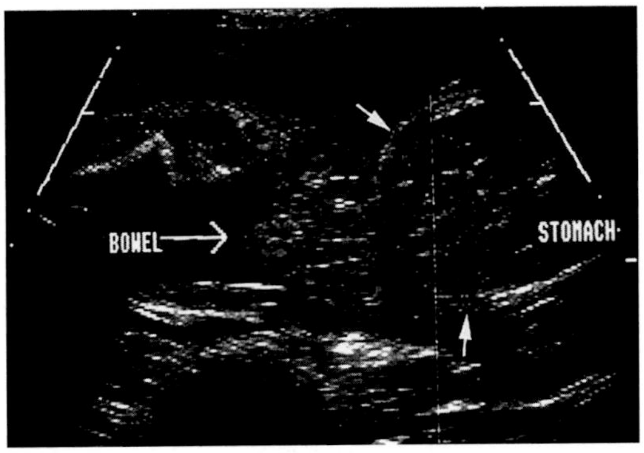

18.11. Ultrasound of gastroschisis (small arrows at abdominal wall).

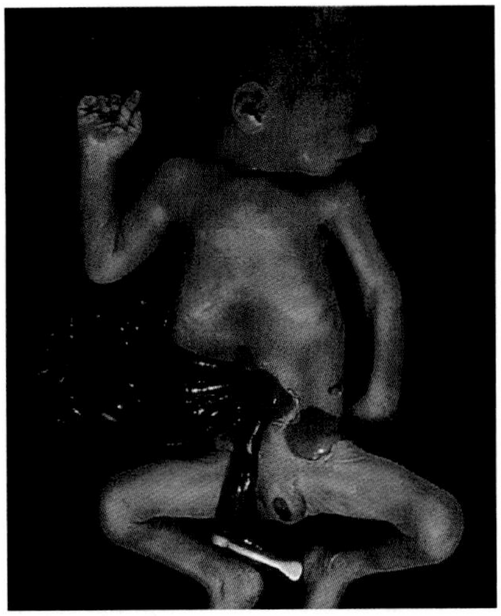

18.12. Gastroschisis. The intestinal contents are on the right side of the umbilical cord.

anomalies, including genitourinary anomalies, imperforate anus, intestinal malrotation, and congenital cardiac defects.

Gastroschisis

This is a paraumbilical defect of the anterior abdominal wall with evisceration of bowel through the defect (Figures 18.11 and 18.12). It is usually situated to the right of the umbilical cord. The total length of the intestine is greatly reduced. It is believed to be due to a vascular disruption of the right omphalomesenteric artery. It is usually an isolated defect unassociated with other malrotations.

ANORECTAL MALFORMATIONS

Anorectal malformations occur in 1/3,000 to 1/5,000 live births.

Anorectal abnormalities are associated with many syndromes and may be found in chromosomal abnormalities such as $13q^-$, trisomy 18, and cat-eye syndrome (Figures 18.13 to 18.16). These syndromes include dominant, recessive, and X-linked inheritances. Anal malformations are part of the VATER association and maternal diabetes predisposes a fetus to anorectal abnormalities.

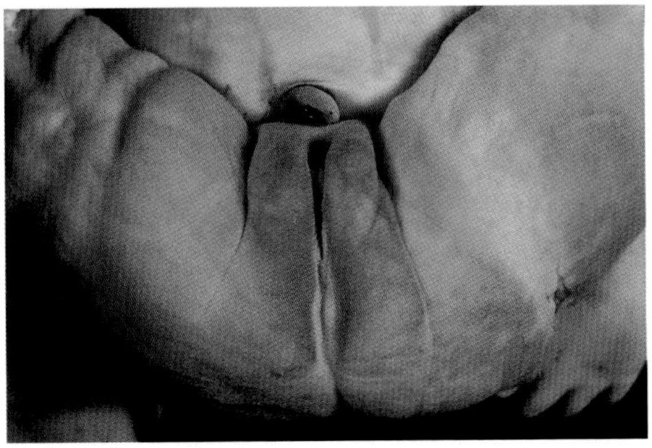

18.13. Anal atresia.

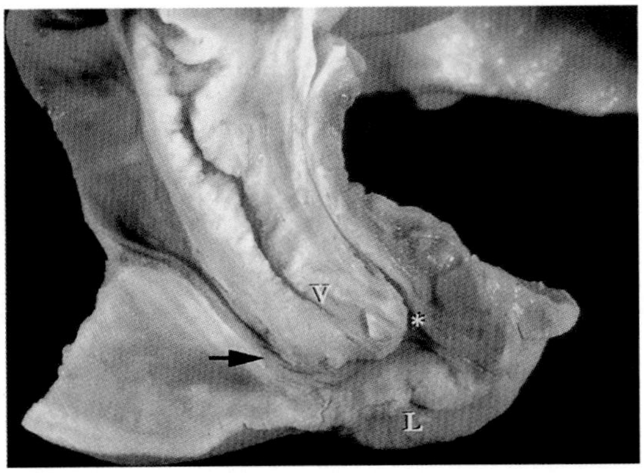

18.14. Imperforate anus with recto-perineal fistula (arrow). (*, urethra; L, labia; V, vagina.)

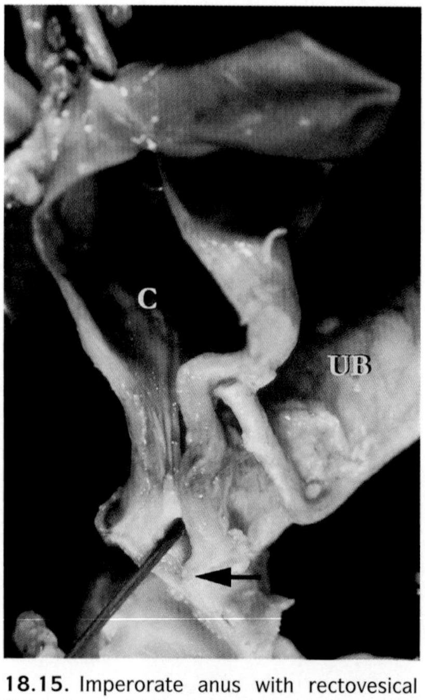

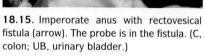

18.15. Imperorate anus with rectovesical fistula (arrow). The probe is in the fistula. (C, colon; UB, urinary bladder.)

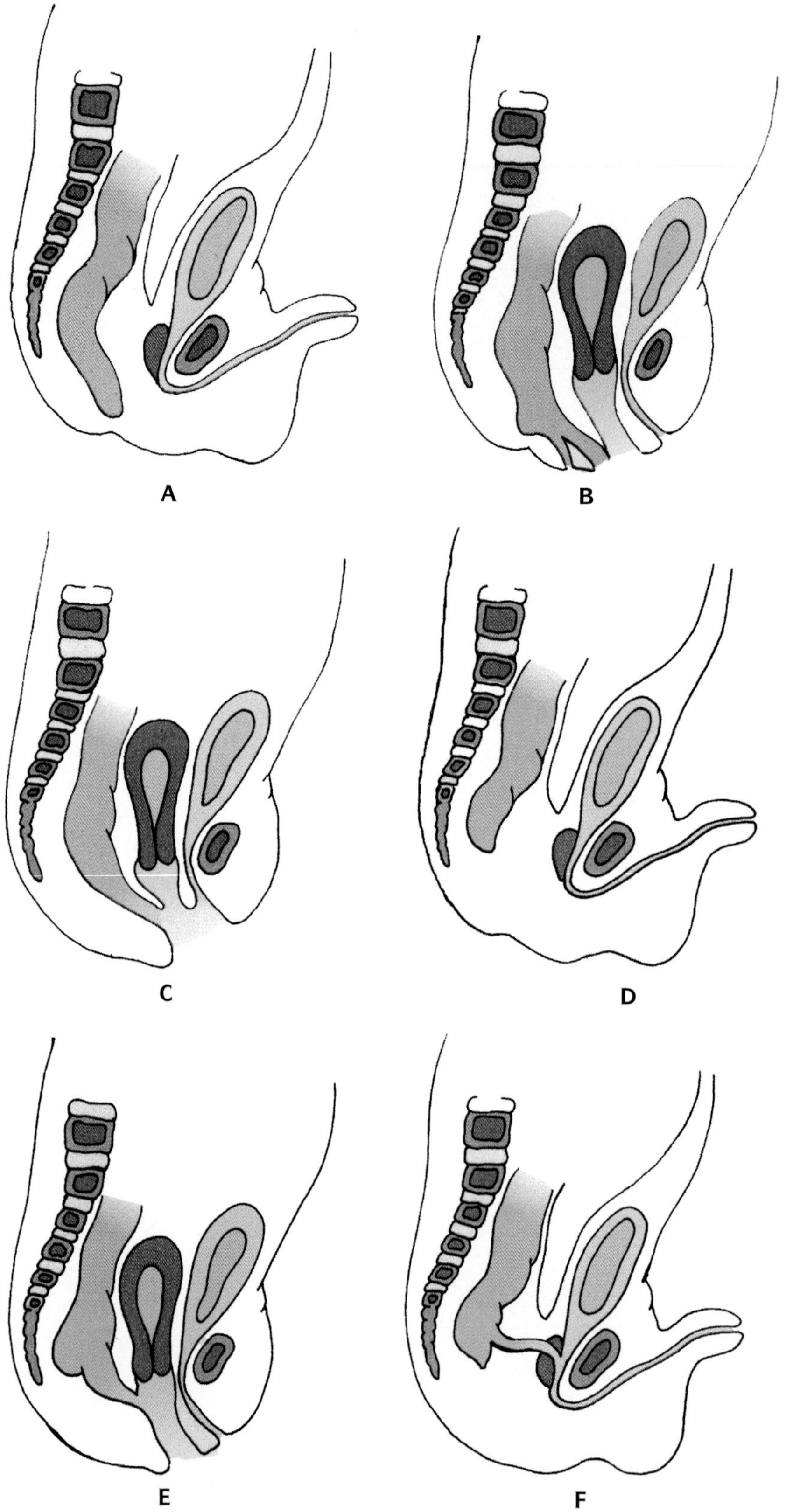

18.16. Types of imperforate anus. **(A)** Rectum ending blindly. **(B)** Rectoperineal fistula. **(C)** Rectovaginal vesicle fistula. **(D)** Sigmoid ending blindly. **(E)** Rectovaginal fistula. **(F)** Rectovesicle fistula.

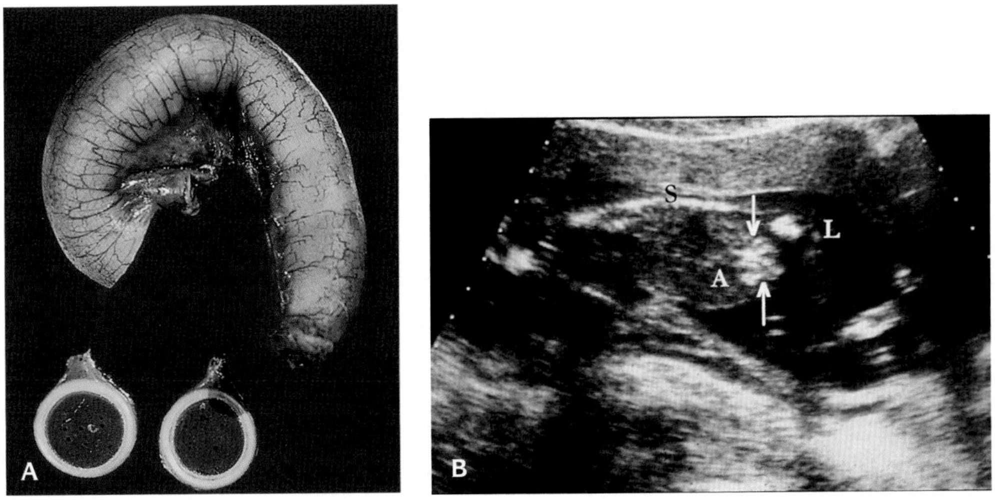

18.17. **(A)** Meconium ileus. The bowel is distended with viscid meconium. **(B)** Ultrasound of a fetus at 28 weeks gestation showing echogenic bowel (arrows) in the abdomen. (S, Spine; A, abdomen; L, leg.)

Pathogenesis

At 6 weeks gestation, the caudal end of the gastrointestinal tract communicates with the allantois through the urogenital sinus. The tissue in the angle between the gastrointestinal tract and the allantois is called the *urorectal septum*; it grows down until it reaches the surface ectoderm. The tissue separating the gut and urethra from the external surface degenerates to form the urethral and anal openings. In the female, an evagination from the urogenital sinus produces most of the vagina. Further growth completely separates the vagina and the urethra.

The most common defect of imperforate anus is a fistula between the gut and the vagina in the female and the gut and urethra in the male and results in the gut ending blindly.

Meconium Ileus

Meconium ileus is the most severe manifestation of cystic fibrosis (CF) and occurs in approximately 10% of newborns with CF (Figure 18.17). It is due to inspissation of thick, viscid meconium. On rare occasions it is due to abnormalities of the pancreas or pancreatic ducts not related to CF.

If the bowel perforates, meconium peritonitis occurs. This may become calcified and can readily be seen on x-ray examination.

Necrotizing Enterocolitis (See Also Stillbirth and Neonatal Death)

This usually occurs in premature infants during the first two weeks of life (Figure 18.18). The terminal ileum, cecum, and colon may be involved. The lesion may be continuous or

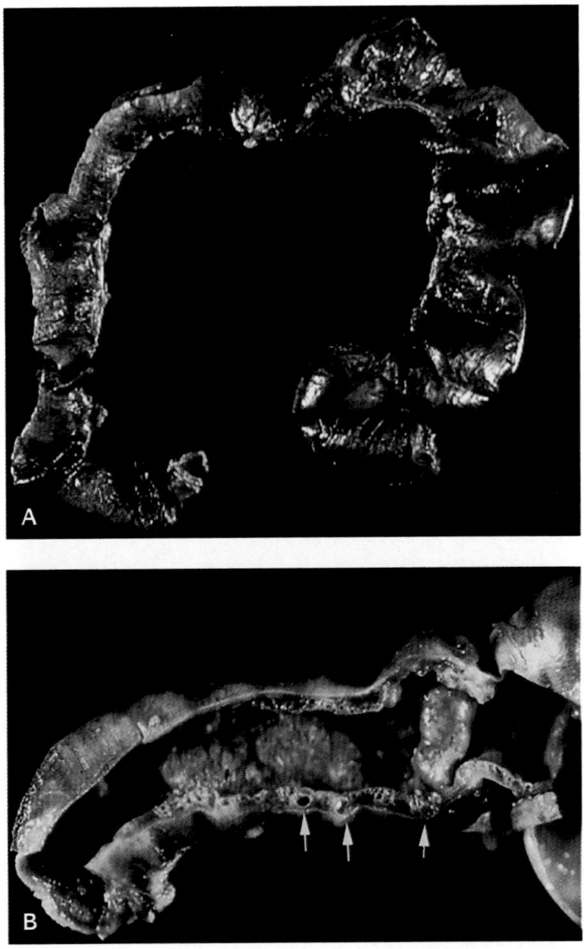

18.18. Necrotizing enterocolitis. **(A)** The small intestine is necrotic. **(B)** Necrotizing enterocolitis with pneumatosis intestinalis.

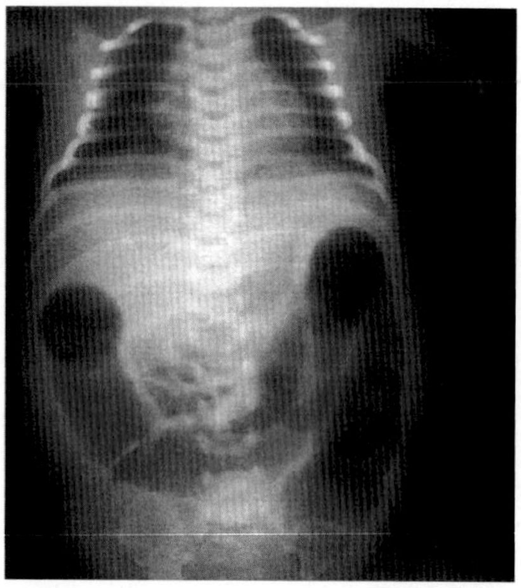

18.19. Hirschprung disease. X-ray showing distended loops of bowel above constriction site in rectosigmoid.

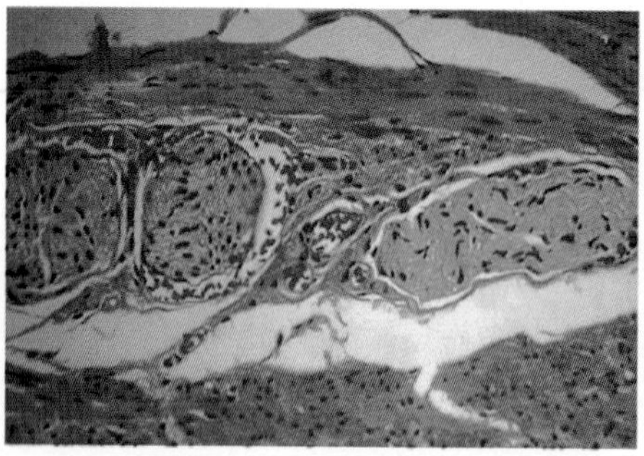

18.20. Hirschprung disease. The myenteric plexus is devoid of ganglion cells and the axons are hypertrophied.

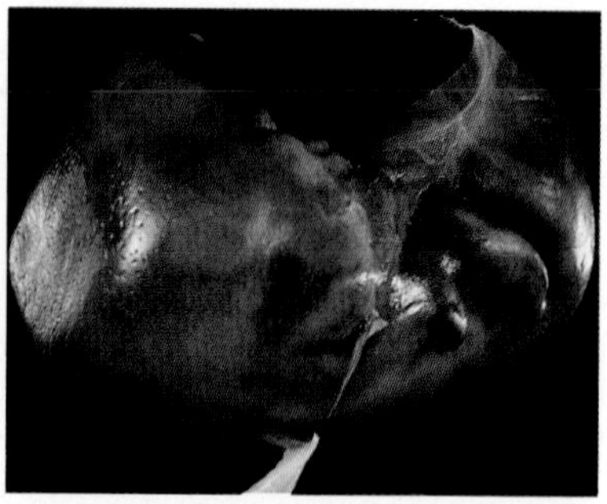

18.21. Abnormal lobation of the liver in a case of trisomy 18.

segmental. The bowel is friable hemorrhagic and necrotic. Intestinal perforation, necrosis, and pneumatosis intestinalis (air within the intestinal wall) develop. Prognosis is grave.

Hirschsprung Disease (Aganglionic Megacolon)

A constriction in the rectosigmoid results in distended loops of bowel above the constriction (Figure 18.19). In this disorder, there is a congenital absence of ganglion cells in the myenteric and submucous plexuses of the bowel wall (Figure 18.20). The axons are hypertrophied. The lesion is usually (75%) confined to the rectum and distal sigmoid colon. In 15% of cases, the aganglionosis extends to the transverse colon and in fewer than 10% there may be total aganglionosis. The incidence is 1/5,000 live births with a 3:1 male to female ratio. Five percent of cases are familial. It may be associated with trisomy 21, colonic and ileal atresias, congenital heart disease, genitourinary abnormalities, and neurofibromatosis type I.

DEVELOPMENTAL DEFECTS OF THE LIVER

Absence of the liver is extremely rare. Ectopic liver has been noted in the abdomen and thorax. Lobation is usually abnormal in trisomy 18 (Figure 18.21) and is not infrequent as a mild malformation in other chromosomal defects (Tables 18.1 to 18.3). Cysts are usually due to dilations of proliferating bile ducts (Figure 18.22). They may be solitary or multiple and unilocular. They are lined by cuboidal or columnar epithelium. Cystic disease of the liver usually occurs with renal cystic disease. The liver shows increased periportal fibrosis and an increased number of bile ducts that are serpiginous. This lesion is an accentuation of Meyenburg plexus and may progress to congenital hepatic fibrosis with portal hypertension. Caroli disease is a severe form in the spectrum of congenital hepatic fibrosis with cystic dilatation of extrabiliary ducts.

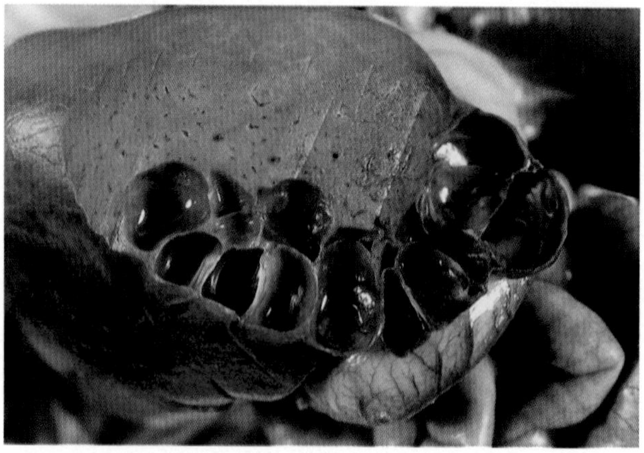

18.22. Multiple cysts in the liver.

Table 18.1 Special investigations in metabolic liver disorders

Histology	Ancillary investigations: Stain	EM	Other
Diagnostic			
α_1-antitrypsin deficiency*	PAS with diastase	+	Serum α_1-antitrypsin electrophoresis
Niemann-Pick disease type C*	Filippin	+	Skin fibroblast culture
Wolman disease (+ cholesterol ester storage disease)	Oil red O		Cholesterol crystal
	Sudan black		Birefringence (frozen tissue), skin fibroblast culture
Glycogen storage disease, type IV	Lugol's iodine	+	Pectinase digestion, liver −70°C
Cystic fibrosis*			Sweat test, molecular genetics
Cerebrohepatorenal syndrome of Zellweger*	Catalase activity	+	Serum VLCFA, fibroblast culture
Suggestive			
Bile acid synthesis or transport disorders (familial intrahepatic cholestatic syndromes)*		+	Serum, urine, bile, duodenal fluid for bile acid analysis, molecular genetics
Neonatal hemochromatosis*	Iron	+	Liver iron determination
Acute tyrosinemia			Urine succinyl acetone
Alagille syndrome			Bile duct determination
Hereditary fructose intolerance			Liver fructose-1, 6-diphospate aldolase
Galactosemia			Galactose-1-phosphate uridyl transferase
Mitochondrial respiratory chain disorders†	Various	+	Skeletal muscle −70°C

* May have pathologic changes of neonatal hepatitis
† Multiple enzymologies
EM, electron microscopy; VLCFA, very long chain fatty acids

Table 18.2 Assessment of infantile cholestasis

- Initial laboratory tests
  - Complete blood count
  - Bilirubin (direct/indirect)
  - Liver function tests including gamma glutamyl transferase (GGT)
  - Fasting glucose
  - Prothrombin time/partial
- Prothrombin time
  - Urinalysis
- Microbiology (as directed)
  - Viral serology
  - Cultures (blood, urine, cerebrospinal fluid)
- Metabolic (as indicated)
  - Blood gases
  - α_1-antitrypsin level ± phenotype
  - Urine-reducing substances
  - Sweat chloride/nasal potentiometry
  - Urine organic acids (succinylacetone)
  - Plasma amino acids
  - Red cell galactose-1-P uridyltransferase (GALT)
  - Thyroid function tests
  - Molecular genetics
  - Review neonatal metabolic screen
- Radiology
  - Ultrasound
  - Hepatobiliary scintography
- Procedures
  - Percutaneous liver biopsy
  - Transjugular liver biopsy
  - Endoscopic retrograde cholangiopancreatography
  - Exploratory laparotomy and intraoperative cholangiogram

Source: Ostry A et al.: *Pathol Case Rev* 4:134, 1999.

EXTRAHEPATIC BILIARY ATRESIA

The extrahepatic biliary ducts are atretic and represented by fibrous cord-like structures that may be completely obliterated (Figure 18.23). The gallbladder is absent, small, or cord-like. The bile ducts in the porta hepatis may have lumina of sufficient diameter (300 μm) to surgically attempt reestablishment of bile flow by portoenterostomy. Initially, the lesion in the liver appears to be a neonatal giant cell hepatitis that progresses to fibrosis and ultimately to biliary cirrhosis.

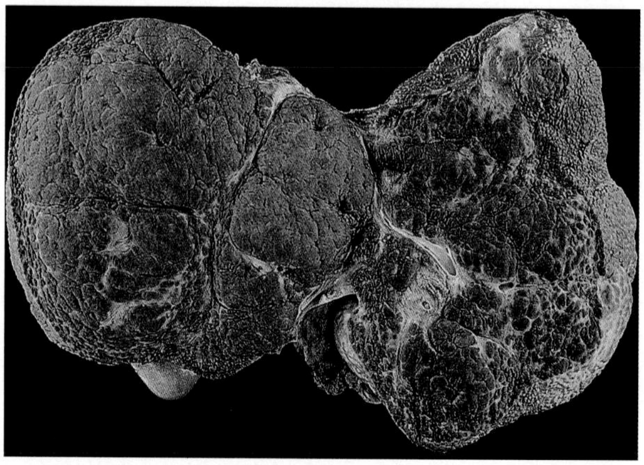

18.23. Biliary atresia with biliary cirrhosis after formalin fixation

α_1-ANTITRYPSIN (α_1-AT) DEFICIENCY

α_1-AT deficiency is an autosomal recessive disorder. The heterozygous state occurs in 10–15% of the general population, who have serum levels of ~60% of normal; the homozygous state occurs in 1/2,000 persons, who have serum levels of α_1-AT ~ 10% of normal. There are many alleles of the α_1-AT gene. An infant with α_1-AT deficiency may present at birth with neonatal cirrhosis. Cholestasis is present in hepatocytes and canaliculi. The portal areas may show fibrosis and bile duct proliferation. PAS-positive globules of α_1-AT positivity accumulate in the periportal hepatocytes and can be demonstrated by immunostaining with antibodies for α_1-AT (Figure 18.24). Patients with this disorder usually have the P_1ZZ phenotype. Liver transplantation is successful in the treatment of this disorder.

DEVELOPMENTAL DEFECTS OF THE GALLBLADDER

Absence of the gallbladder (Figures 18.25A and 18.25B) is usually associated with other malformations and is a common finding in fetal triploidy. The

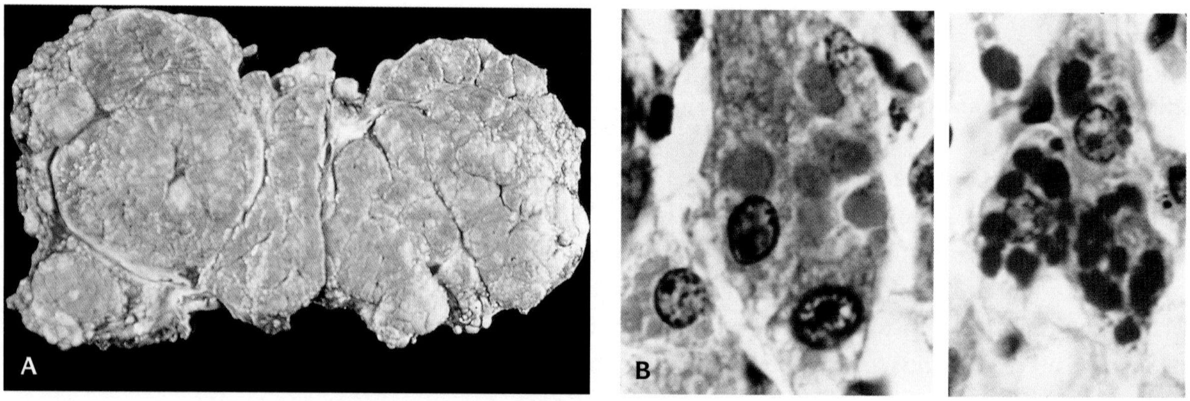

18.24. (A) α_1-antitrypsin congenital cirrhosis of liver. **(B)** α_1-antitrypsin globules in hepatocytes (left). PAS and stain for α_1-antitrypsin (right).

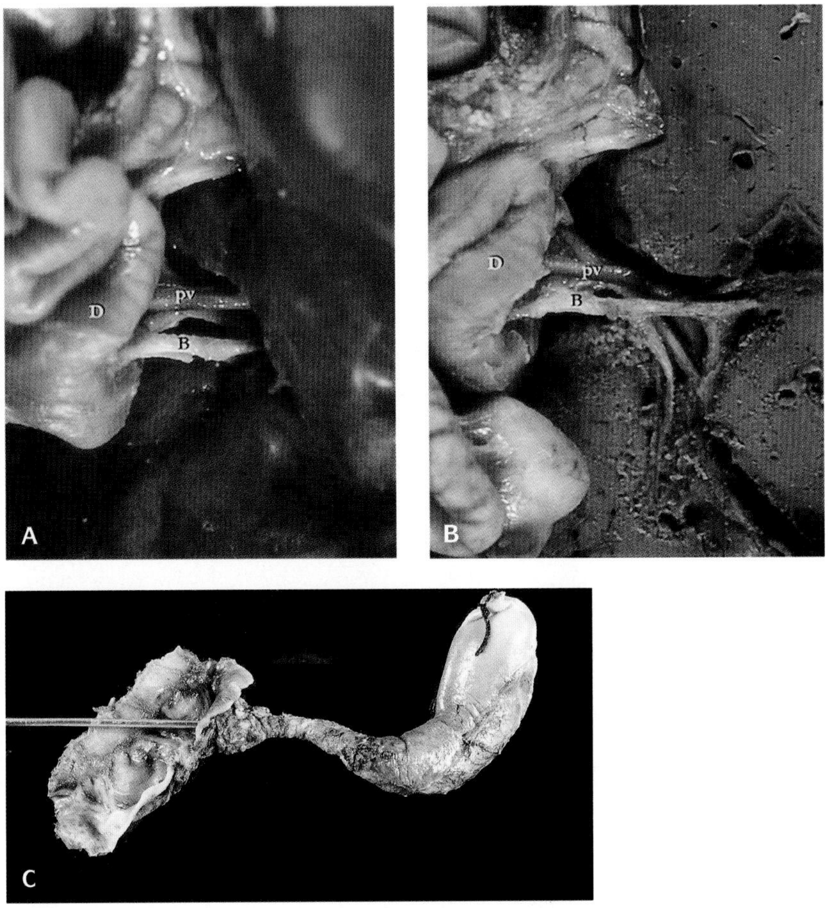

18.25. (A) Absence of gallbladder, external appearance. (D, duodenum; B, bile duct; pv, portal vein.) **(B)** Dissection of biliary ducts showing extension of bile ducts directly from the hepatic parenchyma into the duodenum. (B, bile duct; D, duodenum; pv, portal vein.) **(C)** Choledochal cyst of the gallbladder.

gallbladder may be embedded in the liver parenchyma. Double gallbladders and a floating gallbladder are rare defects (Figure 18.22).

CHOLEDOCHAL CYST

Dilatation of bile ducts is of five types (Figure 18.25C).

1. Choledochal cyst, a localized cystic dilatation of the extrahepatic bile duct.
2. Diverticulum of the common bile duct or gallbladder.
3. Choledochocele, a lesion that extends into the wall of the duodenum.
4. Multiple dilatations of extra- and intrahepatic ducts (Caroli disease).
5. Fusiform extra- and intrahepatic dilatation.

Jaundice and right upper quadrant pain is a triad seen in about 40% of cases. It may progress to cirrhosis of the liver with associated atresia or stenosis of the biliary tree. Radiological studies include isotope scan, ultrasonography, computed tomography, and cholangiography, which are used to diagnose the presence of a choledochal cyst. Prenatal diagnosis with early surgery has been curative. The cyst wall is 1–2 mm thick and bile stained and is composed of dense fibrous tissue containing a few inflammatory cells. The epithelial lining may be absent or have foci of residual columnar cells.

PAUCITY OF INTRAHEPATIC BILE DUCTS

The portal areas should contain at least six bile ducts. Paucity of bile ducts is present when fewer than 40% of the portal areas contain sufficient numbers of bile ducts. This condition may be syndromic (Alagille syndrome) or nonsyndromic. In Alagille syndrome, the facies are characteristic with a broad forehead, deep-seated eyes, and a saddle nose. The thoracic vertebrae have a butterfly appearance and the portal areas show a deficiency of bile ducts. Cholestasis and jaundice occur.

CHOLESTATIC SYNDROMES

A number of syndromes in the newborn may result in cholestasis in the liver and jaundice.

Table 18.3 Causes of cholestasis in infancy

Idiopathic neonatal hepatitis (INH)	Peroxisomal disorders, Zellweger syndrome
Extrahepatic biliary atresia (EHBA)	Familial intrahepatic cholestasis (FIC), including bile acid synthesis and transporter defects
Infectious	a. Progressive familial intrahepatic cholestasis, Byler disease (FIC 1 gene)
Bacterial	b. Bile salt export pump defect (FIC 2 gene)
Sepsis (Gram negative)	c. North American Indian cholestasis (FIC 1 gene)
Viral	d. Alagille syndrome (JAG 1 gene)
Hepatitis A, B, C	e. (4)-3-oxosteroid reductase 5β-reductase deficiency
Coxsackie	Mitochondrial respiratory chain disorders
Echo	Cystic fibrosis
Parvovirus B19	Neonatal hemochromatosis
HIV	Familial hemochromatosis
CMV	Total parenteral nutrition (TPN) associated cholestasis
Other	Dubin-Johnson syndrome
Toxoplasma	Gilbert syndrome
Syphilis	Others
Metabolic	Congenital hepatic fibrosis
Tyrosinemia type I	Drugs
Galactosemia	Neonatal lupus erythematosus
α_1-antitrypsin deficiency	
Fructose intolerance	
Glycogen storage type IV	
Niemann-Pick disease type II	
Wolman disease	
Gaucher disease	

Source: Ostry A et al.: *Pathol Case Rev* 4:133, 1999.

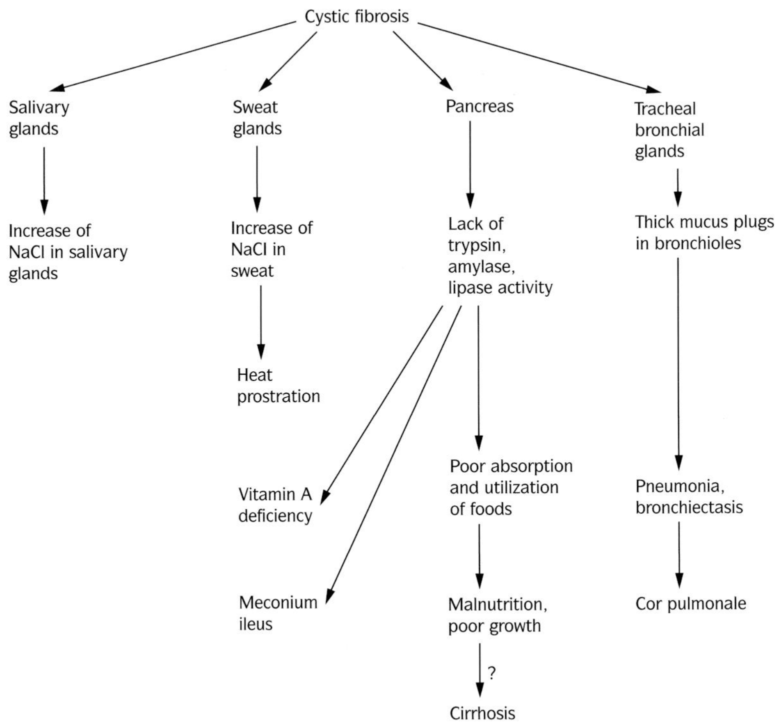

18.26. Cystic fibrosis.

DEVELOPMENTAL DEFECTS OF THE PANCREAS

Cysts

Multiple cysts of the pancreas may be a feature of von Hippel-Lindau syndrome, infantile polycystic disease of kidney and liver, Meckel syndrome, trisomy 13, and cystic fibrosis.

Cystic Fibrosis (CF)

CF is an autosomal recessive condition and is the leading cause of pancreatic insufficiency and malabsorption in infants and children (Figure 18.26 and Tables 18.4 and 18.5). The incidence is 1/2,500.

In the pancreas (Figure 18.27) there is widespread obstruction of exocrine gland ducts and acini by unusually viscid and dehydrated secretions. This

Table 18.4 Abnormalities in the gastrointestinal system in cystic fibrosis

Gastroesophageal reflux	Barrett esophagus
Malabsorption from pancreatic insufficiency	Hyperplasia and dilation of Brunner glands
Mucosis of the appendix	Meconium ileus, meconium peritonitis, meconium ileus equivalent
Lactase deficiency	Rectal prolapse
Volvulus	Small intestinal atresia
Peptic ulcer disease	Intussusception
Pneumatosis coli	

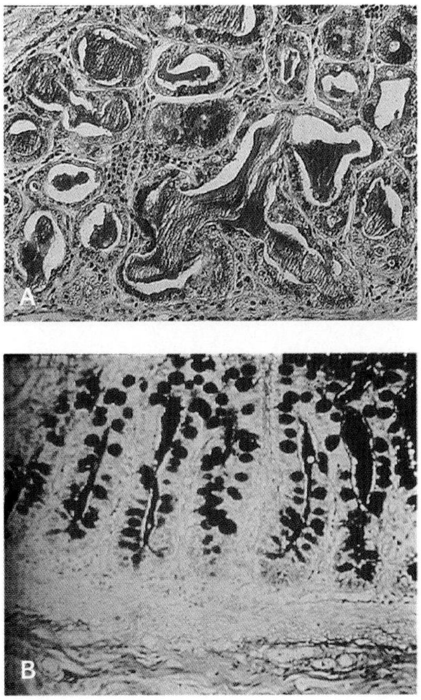

18.27. Cystic fibrosis. **(A)** The pancreatic ducts and acini are filled with mucus. **(B)** Small intestine showing mucus in intestinal mucosa.

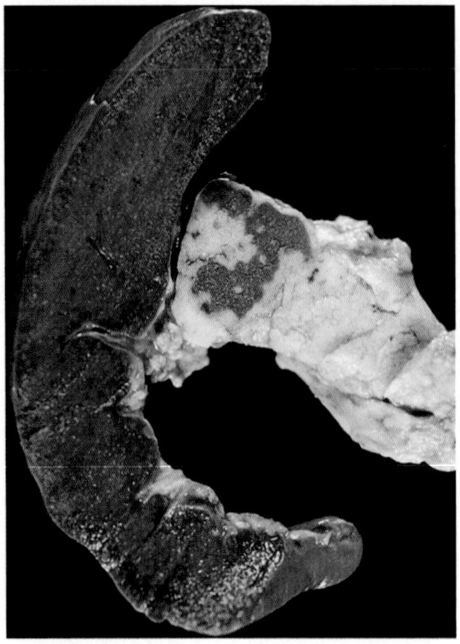

18.28. Heterotopic spleen in the pancreas in a case of CHARGE association.

Table 18.5 Cystic fibrosis of pancreas

Primary abnormality – altered secretion of exocrine glands
Mucous glands – secretion precipitated to form casts
Pancreas
Intestinal glands
Intrahepatic bile ducts
Gallbladder
Mucous salivary glands
Mucous glands – hypersecretion of histologically normal mucous
Mucous glands of respiratory tract
Brunner glands of duodenum
Serous glands – histologically normal but produce secretion of abnormally high electrolyte content
Sweat glands
Lacrimal glands
Serous salivary glands

results from abnormal chloride and sodium transport across cell membranes. Viscous secretions obstruct acini and ducts, and high luminal pressure from obstructing secretions in turn causes flattening and atrophy of epithelial cells and progressive dilatation of acini and ducts. Cyst formation results from ductular dilatation. Eventually acinar destruction and leakage of proteolytic enzymes into the parenchyma result in fibrosis.

Heterotopic Pancreas

Nodules of grossly apparent pancreatic tissue isolated from the main body of the pancreas are common incidental findings, usually in the wall of the stomach or proximal small intestine (Figure 18.28). Most commonly, they appear as small tan nodules on the serosal surface, but they may be intramural and, if so, are usually sessile submucosal masses projecting into the lumen. Heterotopic pancreatic tissue also is seen in Meckel diverticulum, liver, spleen, gastric wall, mesentery, umbilicus, and other remote sites.

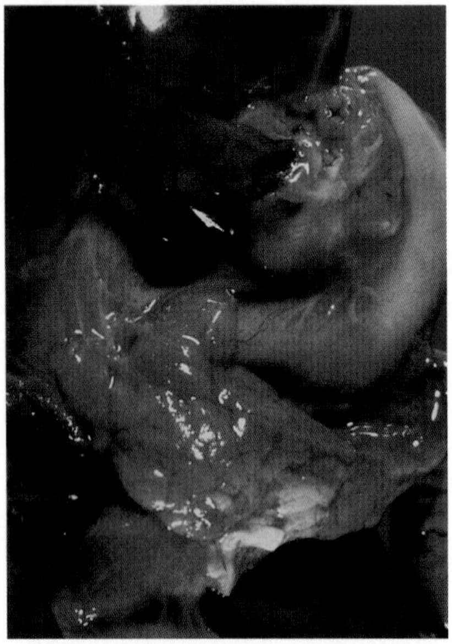

18.29. Annular pancreas.

Annular Pancreas

Annular pancreas is due to abnormalities in the migration of the embryonic ventral pancreas, which may result in a ring of pancreatic tissue completely encircling the duodenum (Figure 18.29).

Schwachman-Diamond Syndrome

Schwachman-Diamond syndrome is an autosomal recessive condition that occurs in early infancy and is characterized by growth retardation, steatorrhea, and frequent foul-smelling stools. Duodenal fluid analysis shows absent or low trypsin amylase and lipase activity. The pancreas is normal in size but largely replaced by fat.

INFANT OF DIABETIC MOTHER (IDM)

The pancreas in IDM responds to maternal hyperglycemia by marked increase in size and number of pancreatic islets with increased numbers of beta (insulin-secreting) cells (Figure 18.30).

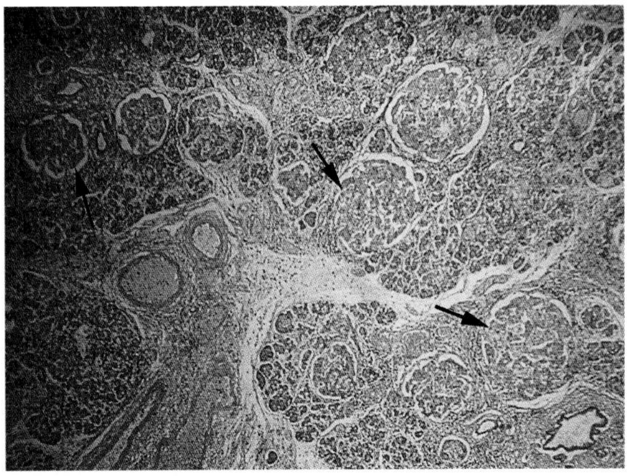

18.30. Pancreas in an infant of a diabetic mother. The pancreatic islets are increased in size and number and contain predominantely insulin-secreting cells. (Arrows, islets of Langerhans.)

ULTRASOUND OF GASTROINTESTINAL TRACT

Abdominal imaging and characteristics include:

A. The image should be obtained in a plane perpendicular to the major axis of the spine and should include the stomach bubble and hepatic vein in an area close to its insertion with the umbilical cord insertion site.
   1. The image *should not* include cross sections of the heart, kidneys, bladder, or umbilical cord insertion into the abdomen.
   2. The image is best localized by aligning the transducer with the spinal column, rotating the transducer 90° and sliding the transducer cephalad or caudad to obtain a scanning plane inferior to the heart and superior to the renal poles.
B. Is the stomach bubble present, normal in size, and situated on the left of the abdomen?
   1. Absent stomach bubble suggests tracheo-esophageal abnormalities and an abnormal swallowing mechanism
      a. Esophageal atresia is associated with trisomy 21; trisomy 18; and cardiac, gastrointestinal, and genito-urinary abnormalities
   2. Right-sided stomach bubble suggests possible situs inversus or complete transposition (depending on cardiac situs)
   3. The size of the stomach increases with gestational age

	16–18 wk 2 SD range	22–24 wk 2 SD range	28–20 wk 2 SD range	34–36 wk 2 SD range
Longitudinal	9–17 mm	13–25 mm	18–28 mm	19–37 mm
A-P diameter	4–8 mm	6–12 mm	9–15 mm	10–18 mm
Transverse	6–10 mm	15–21 mm	12–20 mm	12–20 mm

(From Goldstein et al.: *Obstet Gynecol*, 70:641, 1987)

   4. A double bubble sign suggests duodenal atresia and is strongly associated with trisomy 21
   5. Is the internal stomach bubble homogenous?
      a. Swallowed particulate material suggests possible meconium passage in utero

C. Absent stomach bubble
  1. Suggests esophageal atresia, congenital diaphragmatic hernia, situs inversus, and neurologic or musculoskeletal conditions that might affect swallowing
  2. Esophageal atresia
    a. Found in 1/1,000 to 1/5,000 deliveries
    b. Results from abnormal division of the primitive foregut into the trachea and esophagus during the 3rd through 8th weeks of embryonic life
    c. Should be suspected if polyhydramnios develops and the stomach bubble cannot be identified. In 10% of cases, an associated tracheoesophageal fistula may allow filling of the stomach, or gastric secretions may be present in sufficient quantity to distend the stomach and allow its visualization.
    d. Other structural congenital anomalies are present in 50–70% of cases
      i. Tracheal abnormalities in 90% of cases
      ii. Cardiac abnormalities in approximately 30%
      iii. Gastrointestinal abnormalities in 28%
      iv. Musculoskeletal abnormalities in 11%
      v. Central nervous system abnormalities in 7%
      vi. Facial abnormalities in 6%
    e. Associated with increased risk for aneuploidy
      i. Increased risk for trisomy 21 and trisomy 18
      ii. Associated with aneuploidy in 3–4% of live borns

D. Increased echogenicity of bowel or abdominal structures
  1. Bowel echogenicity – a subjective sonographic finding occasionally associated with karyotypic abnormalities
    a. It is important to avoid the combination of high ultrasound and low dynamic range when evaluating possibly echogenic bowel
    b. If the echo density of the structures in question approximate the brightness of local pelvic bone and sonographic "gain" and "dynamic range" are judged appropriate, hyperechogenicity is judged present.
    c. Differential diagnosis:
      i. Chromosomal aberrations
      ii. Infections, such as toxoplasmosis
      iii. Meconium ileus (cystic fibrosis)
      iv. Prior intra-amniotic hemorrhage with ingestion of red blood cells
      v. Placental insufficiency
      vi. Normal fetal development variation
      vii. Ultrasonic artifact related to high sonographic gain and low dynamic range

d. Echogenic bowel is associated with aneuploidy in 20% of cases
   i. 2–7% aneuploidy in fetuses with isolated abnormalities
   ii. 36–42% aneuploidy fetuses with one or more other structural abnormalities noted on sonography
e. Echogenic bowel in association with growth retardation is not associated with chromosomal abnormalities.

E. Abdominal calcifications
1. Bright specular intra-abdominal echos are often noted on sonography
2. If they shadow posteriorly, they are likely to represent calcifications
3. A wide variety of conditions are associated with such calcifications
   a. Meconium peritonitis – may be focal or diffuse and at times a meconium pseudo-cyst may develop
   b. Meconium plugging – can be associated with anorectal atresia (very distal lesions may not show dilated loops of bowel), small bowel atresia, or meconium ileus
   c. Infections – toxoplasmosis, cytomegalovirus
   d. Neoplasms – neuroblastoma, teratoma, hemangioma, hepatoblastoma
   e. Cholelithiasis

F. Do the bowel segments appear abnormally dilated?
1. The colon can be visualized by 28 weeks in most fetuses
2. Normal colonic diameter increases with gestational age

26wk	30 wk	35 wk	40 wk
10–90%	10–90%	10–90%	10–90%
1–9 mm	4–11 mm	8–15 mm	13–20 mm

(From Goldstein et al.: *Obstet Gynecol*, 70:682, 1987)

3. Abnormal dilation suggests distal obstruction
   a. Duodenal atresia
      i. Occurs in 1/5,000 to 1/10,000 live births. At 5 weeks of embryonic life, proliferating bowel epithelium obliterates the duodenal lumen, with subsequent restoration of patency within 6 weeks. Failures of vacuolation, vascular accidents, and interruption of the bowel lumen by a diaphragm or membrane may interrupt the recanulation of the duodenum. In the presence of atresia, amniotic fluid swallowed by the fetus does not transit further than the stomach or proximal duodenum, and these structures fill with amniotic fluid. As the pylorus is relatively nondistensible, the dilated stomach and proximal duodenum connected by the pylorus give a characteristic double-bubble appearance.
      ii. Atresia is often noted near the ampulla of VATER

            iii. Common bile duct obstruction may also be present
            iv. Often not noted until after 24 weeks
            v. Rarely, a central web within the stomach may obstruct flow out of the stomach, leaving a single bubble
    4. Associated with increased risk of aneuploidy
        a. 57% aneuploidy in antenatal cases of duodenal atresia
            i. 38% aneuploidy cases of isolated atresia
            ii. 64% of aneuploidy if other sonographic anomalies present
        b. Trisomy 21 is present in 8–30% of live-born infants with duodenal atresia
        c. Trisomy 13 present in approximately 2% of affected infants
    5. Historically, occurred often after exposure to thalidomide at 30–40 days of gestation
    6. Skeletal anomalies are present in 50%
        a. Skeletal defects – vertebral and rib abnormalities, sacral agenesis, radial abnormalities, talipes equinovarus
        b. Gastrointestinal anomalies – esophageal atresia, tracheo-esophageal fistula, intestinal malrotation, Meckel diverticulum, and anal-rectal atresia
        c. Renal abnormalities
    7. Mortality is 36%, primarily in infants with multiple anomalies
    8. Imperforate anus
    9. Volvulus
    10. Perforation/meconium ileus
    11. Hirschsprung disease
    12. May be confused with hydroureter
G. Most abnormalities are located near the umbilical cord insertion into the abdomen
H. Gastroschisis is usually situated to the right of the umbilicus and does not involve the umbilical cord directly.
    1. Occurs in 1/10,000 to 1/15,000 live births
    2. Elevated maternal serum α-fetoprotein is often present
    3. May form vascular compromise of either the umbilical vein or the omphalomesenteric artery. Premature involution of the right umbilical vein, before 28–32 conceptual days, may lead to ischemia and resultant mesodermal and ectodermal defects. Ischemic injury to the region of the superior mesenteric artery may explain high rates of jejunal atresia found in association with gastroschisis
    4. Defects are generally small, less than 4 cm in diameter, and bowel loops are often covered by an inflammatory exudate
        a. Defects are usually situated in the right paraumbilical area, free-floating bowel is noted in the peritoneal cavity, the liver is rarely involved, bowel obstruction is common, associated syndromes and anomalies are generally rare

   b. Be careful in evaluation for omphalocele, as the sac may have ruptured and no longer be evident (obscuring the diagnosis of omphalocele)
5. Risk for aneuploidy is 1% or less
   a. Many believe that gastroschisis has no apparent association with chromosomal abnormalities
   b. As previously noted, an omphalocele sac (see below) may no longer be evident because of rupture. In such cases, reliance on the diagnosis of gastroschisis in determining the need for antenatal karyotypic evaluation may yield inaccurate analysis of the likelihood of aneuploidy.
   c. If amniocentesis is not elected, care should be taken to ensure that the observed defect conforms closely to the preceding description. If defects are situated to the left of the midline, are moderate or large in size, involve the liver or other abdominal structures, or if other sonographic findings are present, the possibility of ruptured omphalocele should be considered and appropriate evaluation considered.
6. Omphalocele
   a. Occurs in 1/300 live births
   b. Ventral wall abnormalities that involve herniations of the peritoneal sac and its contents outside the abdominal wall. The anterior abdominal wall is formed by fusion of the cephalic fold with the lateral folds; failure of this fusion yields omphalocele with ectopia cordis, diaphragmatic, and sternal defects. Defective fusion of the lateral folds (between the 2nd and 4th conceptual weeks) leads to isolated omphalocele. Failed fusion of the caudal and lateral folds results in bladder exstrophy and cloacal exstrophy.
   c. Presentation – usually situated in the midline. Intra-abdominal contents herniate within the peritoneal sac into the amniotic cavity through the base of the umbilical cord. Bowel loops, stomach, and liver are commonly involved, and the size of the defect ranges from small to sacs containing most of the abdominal contents. The sac consists of peritoneum and amnion.
   d. Survival as an isolated structural abnormality in infants with normal karyotypes is approximately 95%.
   e. Omphaloceles should be categorized as either:
      i. herniation limited to bowel, possibly associated with persistence of the primitive body stalk
      ii. bowel, liver, and other organs herniated, possibly due to failure of body wall closure
   f. Additional structural abnormalities are commonly observed
   g. Aneuploidy is present in 35% of cases (trisomy 13, trisomy 18, trisomy 21, others)

i. 13% aneuploidy in isolated cases of omphalocele
ii. 46% aneuploidy in cases where other structural abnormalities are noted
iii. Trisomy 13 – cardiac anomalies, midline facial anomalies, microcephaly, holoprosencephaly, polydactyly, rocker-bottom feet, single umbilical artery
iv. Trisomy 18 – cardiac anomalies, growth retardation, cleft lip, single umbilical artery, cystic hygroma, hydrocephaly, overlapping fingers, rocker-bottom feet
v. Polyploidy – severe early onset asymmetric growth retardation, molar degeneration of the placenta, cardiac anomalies, central nervous system defects, oligohydramnios

REFERENCES

D' Aqata ID, Jonas MM, Pevez-Atayde AR, et al.: Combined cystic disease of the liver and kidney. *Semin Liver Dis*, 14:215, 1994.

Dahms BB: Gastrointestinal tract and pancreas. In Gilbert-Barness E. (ed): *Potter's Pathology of the Fetus and Infant*, St. Louis, Mosby-Year Book, 1997.

Dahms BB: The gastrointestinal tract. In Stocker JT, Dehner LP (eds): *Pediatric Pathology*, Philadelphia, JB Lippincott, 1992.

Dahms BB, Qualman SJ, Rosenberg HS, Bernstein J, eds: *Pediatric Gastrointestinal Pathology, Perspectives in Pediatric Pathology*, vol 20, Basel, Karger, 1997.

DeSa D: The alimentary tract. In Wigglesworth JC, Singer DB (eds): *Textbook of Fetal and Perinatal Pathology*, 2nd ed, Boston, Blackwell Scientific Publications, 1997, p. 799.

Manivel JC, Petinato G, Reinberg Y, et al.: Prune belly syndrome: clinicopathologic study of 29 cases. *Ped Path* 9:691, 1989.

Walker WA, Durie PR, Hamilton JR, Walker-Smith JA, Watkins JB: *Pediatric Gastrointestinal Disease*, 2nd ed. St. Louis, Mosby-Year Book, 1996.

Wyllie R, Hyams JS: *Pediatric Gastroinstinal Disease: Pathophysiology, Diagnosis, Management.* Philadelphia, WB Saunders, 1993.

NINETEEN

Genito-Urinary System

MALFORMATIONS

Horseshoe Kidney

A horseshoe kidney is a single, midline, horseshoe-shaped kidney.

The kidney is formed by an interaction between the ureteric bud and the metanephric blastema (Figures 19.1 to 19.3). If the ureteric buds are located more medially than normal or if the inducible metanephric blastema is continuous at the lower pole, then a fused horseshoe kidney may develop.

The horseshoe kidney is usually at a lower level than normal kidneys. Its renal pelves are displaced anteriorly and its ureters usually course across the anterior surfaces of the kidney. Dysplastic development may occur in the fused portion of the kidney.

The ureters may be duplicated or angulated, so that obstruction, which leads to hydronephrosis, occurs.

Ectopic Kidney

A kidney is **ectopic** when it is in the pelvis and not in its usual location. **Ureter duplication** is a double ureter that can be unilateral or bilateral. Ectopic kidney and ureter duplication usually are not functionally important in the prenatal period. Their frequency is increased in chromosome aneuploidies.

Renal Agenesis

In bilateral renal agenesis, both kidneys and ureters are absent (Table 19.1).

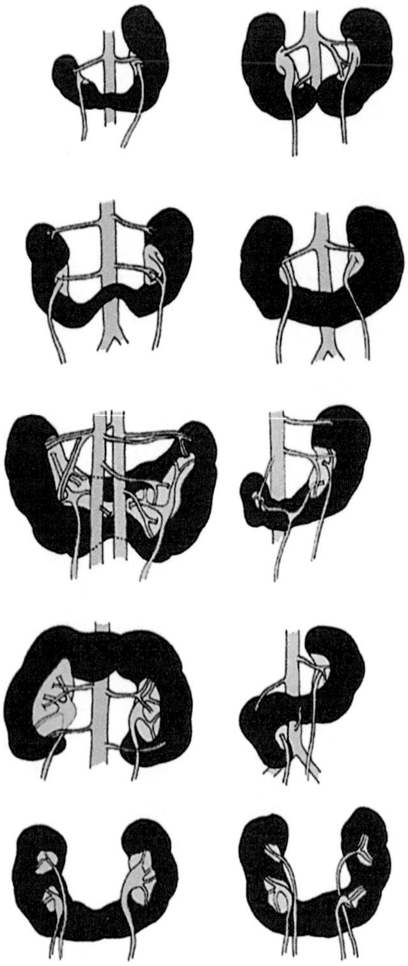

19.1. Types of horseshoe kidneys.

Table 19.1 Conditions associated with unilateral renal agenesis

Disorder	Associated features	Causation
Acrorenal field defect syndromes	Pectoral and nipple hypoplasia, limb defects	Heterogeneous
Brachio-oto-renal syndrome	Hearing loss, ear anomalies, branchial cleft fistula, or cyst	AD
Caudal regression syndrome	Lower limb defects, sacral agenesis, or hypoplasia	Heterogeneous
Cerebro-renal-digital field defect syndromes	Cerebral and cerebellar hypoplasia, lissencephaly, limb defects	Heterogeneous
Chromosomal defects	Multiple congenital anomalies, mental retardation	Structural and numerical aberrations
Diabetes, maternal	Limb defects, caudal regression, cardiac defects	Environmental
Fanconi pancytopenia	Hematologic, limb, and cardiac defects; increased risk of malignancy	AR
Fraser syndrome	Cryptophthalmos; nose, limb, and genital defects; mental retardation	AR
Kallmann syndrome	Anosmia, hypothalamic hypogonadism	AD, AR, XLR
Kousseff syndrome	Sacral meningocele, conotruncal heart defects	AR
MURCS association	Müllerian duct aplasia, vertebral and genitourinary defects	Unknown
Oculorenal syndromes	Optic nerve coloboma, aniridia, mental retardation	Heterogeneous
Smith-Lemli-Opitz syndrome	Microcephaly, mental retardation, ambiguous genitalia, polydactyly, syndactyly	AR
Urogenital adysplasia	Uterine anomalies, vaginal atresia, absence of the vas deferens	AD
VACTERL association	Vertebral, anal, cardiovascular, tracheoesophageal fistula, and limb defects	Sporadic

*AD, autosomal dominant; AR, autosomal recessive; XLR, X-linked recessive; MURCS, Müllerian duct aplasia, renal aplasia, and cervicothoracic somite dysplasia; VACTERL, vertebral anomalies, anal atresia, cardiac abnormalities, tracheoesophageal fistula and/or esophageal atresia, renal agenesis or dysplasia, and limb defects.

Source: Robson WL, Leung AKC, Rogers RC: Unilateral renal agenesis. *Adv Pediatr* 42:575, 1995.

Table 19.2 Renal aplasia

- May occur with dysplasia as a hereditary syndrome
- May be isolated
- Syndromatic
  - Brachio-oto-renal syndrome
  - Goldenhar syndrome, DiGeorge syndrome
  - Aplasia of female genital tract
  - Fraser-cryptophthalmos, syndactyly syndrome
  - Kallmann syndrome
  - Thymic-renal-anal-lung syndrome

Bilateral renal agenesis is rare, occurring in 1/3,000 to 1/4,000 live borns (Figure 19.4). Unilateral agenesis occurs in 1/1,000 newborns; it is more common in males.

It is postulated that renal agenesis is caused by the failure of the ureteric bud to develop. The ureteric bud normally induces the metanephric blastema to become a kidney. In some cases, however, it is possible that the mesenchyme is unable to respond to the ureteric bud, which would then degenerate.

Renal Aplasia

Extreme renal hypoplasia is referred to as renal aplasia where there are only tiny remnants of renal tissue (Table 19.2).

Oligohydramnios

Oligohydramnios is the most serious intrauterine consequence of bilateral renal agenesis. The lack of amniotic fluid interferes with normal lung development even before 20 weeks gestation and results in pulmonary hypoplasia (Figures 19.5 to 19.7).

Tracheoesophageal fistula, including the VATER association, duodenal atresia, and other gastrointestinal abnormalities and cardiovascular, skeletal, and CNS anomalies have been described also in association with renal agenesis.

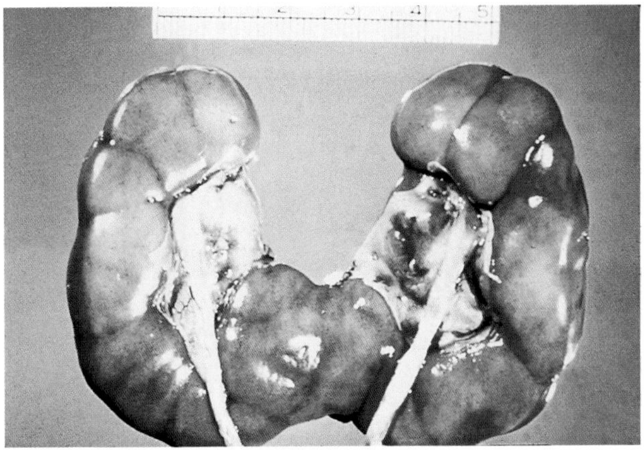

19.2. Horseshoe kidney.

RENAL CYSTIC MALFORMATIONS

Infantile Polycystic Kidneys

This autosomal recessive disease is characterized by bilaterally enlarged cystic kidneys (Tables 19.3 to 19.6). The renal lesion is usually accompanied by congenital hepatic fibrosis, with dilated intrahepatic bile ducts (Figures 19.8 to 19.11). Variation within an individual family occurs with variation in the severity of renal and hepatic involvement.

Hyperplasia and cystic dilation of the renal collecting ducts are attributed to an abnormal differentiation of the interstitial portion of the ureteric bud branches; the nephrons, ampulla, and pelvis are not affected.

Table 19.3 Classification of cystic renal diseases

Polycystic disease
Autosomal recessive polycystic kidney disease (ARPKD)
Classic infantile polycystic disease
ARPKD and congenital hepatic fibrosis in older individuals
Autosomal dominant polycystic kidney disease (ADPKD)
Classic adult polycystic disease
ADPKD in infants (glomerulocystic disease)
Glomerular cystic disease
Localized cystic disease
Renal cysts associated with syndromes of multiple malformations
Medullary cystic disease
Medullary sponge kidney
Familial nephronophthisis-medullary cystic disease (FNMCD) complex
Multilocular renal cysts
Renal dysplasia with cysts
Simple renal cysts
Acquired renal cystic disease
Miscellaneous extrarenal cysts

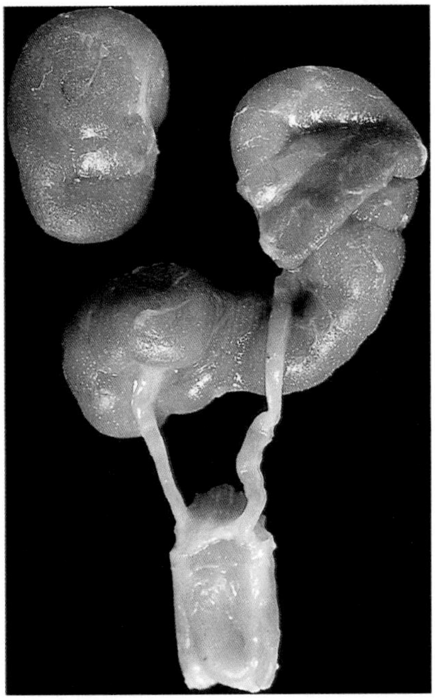

19.3. Fusion of kidneys forming partial horseshoe with S-shaped curve in a 17-week gestation fetus. The lower right kidney is pelvic. Note large misshapen adrenal on right.

Table 19.4 Recessive PKD (infantile)

Many presentations from in utero renal failure to childhood portal hypertension, inconsistent in families.
Reniform, sponge-like kidneys
Collecting tubule lesion
Linked to chromosome 6
Mouse model: mislocation of EGFR, other defects with cyclin-like function.

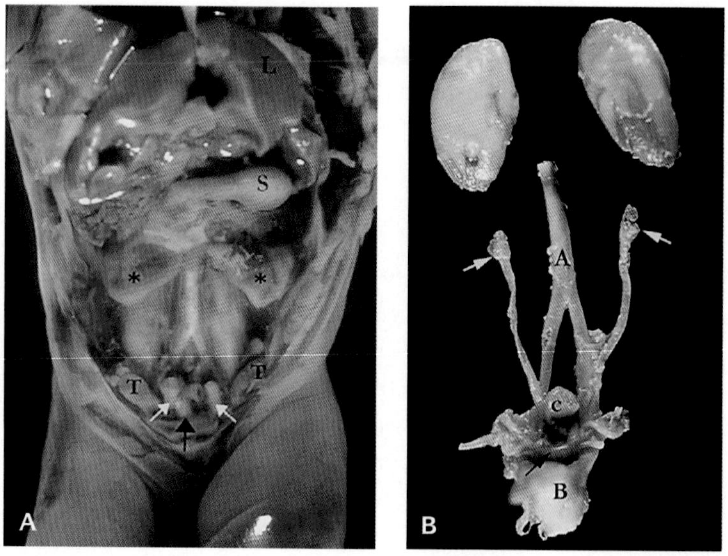

19.4. **(A)** Renal agenesis in a 17-week gestation fetus. The kidneys are absent. The adrenal glands are discoid (asterisks). (L, liver; T, testes; S, stomach; yellow arrow, umbilical arteries; black arrow, urinary bladder.) **(B)** Bilateral renal aplasia. Both kidneys (yellow arrows) are extremely small nubbins of dysplastic renal tissue. Note large discoid adrenals (A, aorta; C, colon; B, urinary bladder; black arrow, uterus).

The kidneys retain their usual shape but are diffusely spongy and grossly enlarged. The collecting ducts and tubules are dilated, and there is a medullary ductal ectasia with a radial arrangement of the elongated cysts. In the liver, there is a portal bile ductule proliferation, sometimes accompanied by periportal

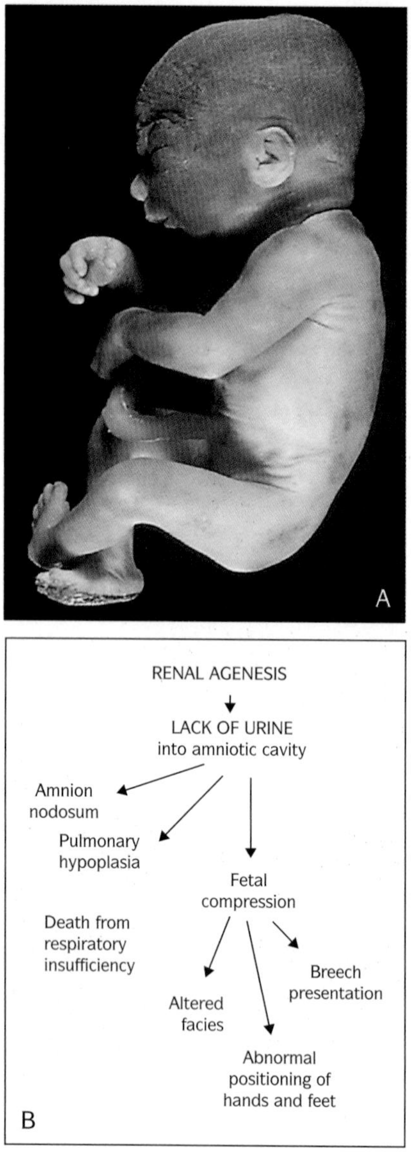

19.5. **(A)** Infant with Potter facies and arthrogryposis due to oligohydramnios. **(B)** Sequence of events in renal agenesis (left).

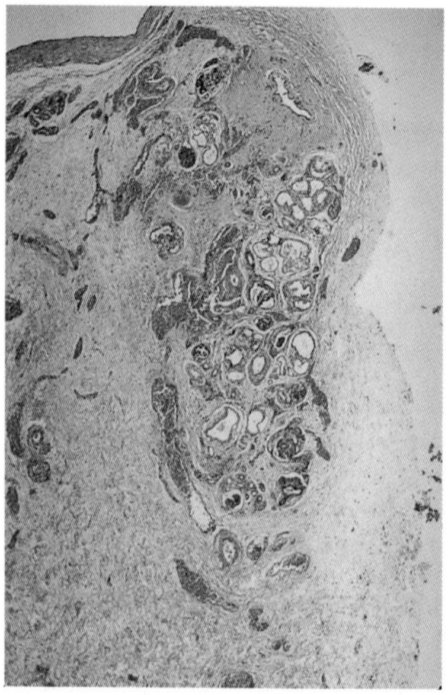

19.6. Microscopic section of kidney from a case of hereditary renal adysplasia. The kidney is aplastic with a small island of dysplastic renal tissue.

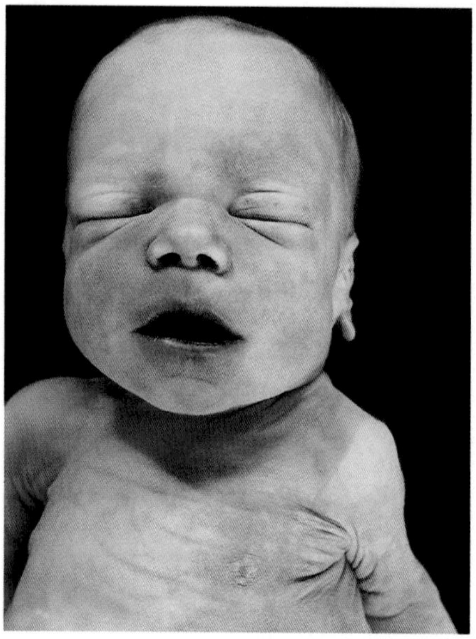

19.7. Thirty-four-week gestation infant with Potter facies due to renal agenesis.

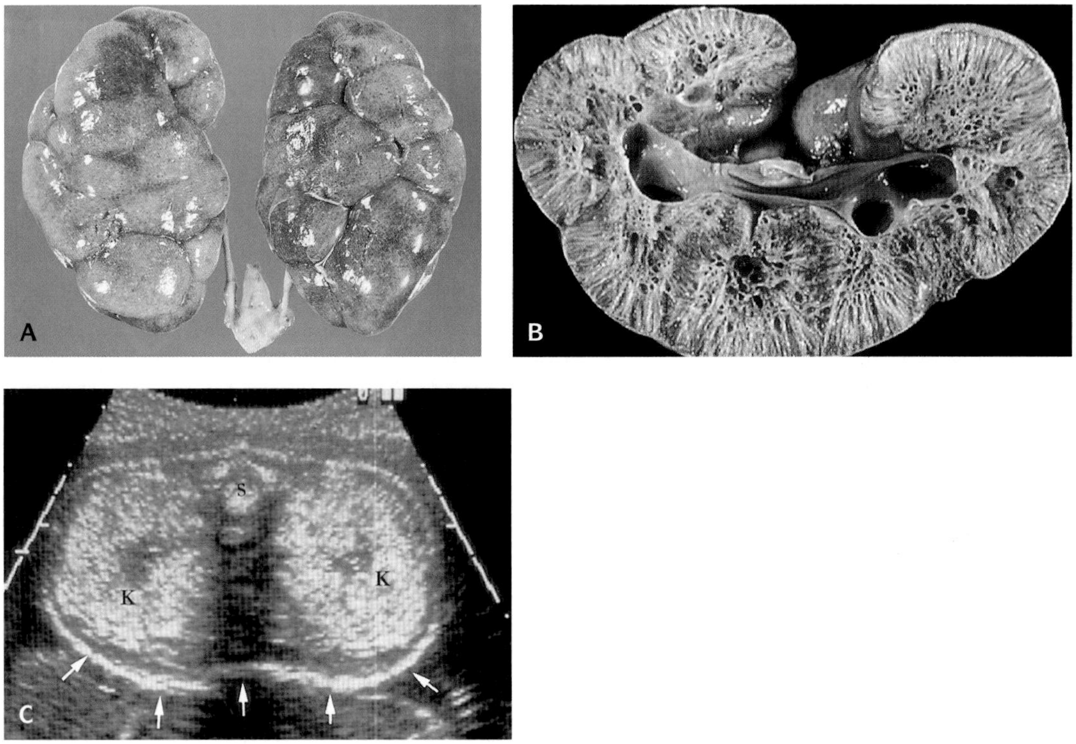

19.8. Gross appearance of infantile recessive polycystic kidneys. **(A)** External appearance. **(B)** Cut surface. **(C)** Ultrasound. (S, spine; K, kidneys; arrows, abdominal wall.)

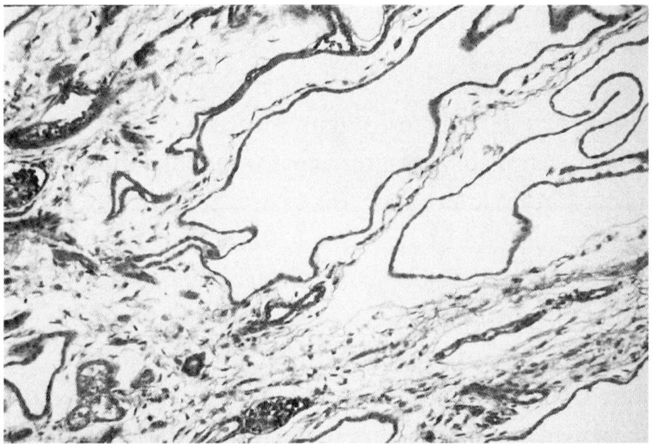

19.9. Microscopic appearance of infantile polycystic kidneys showing the cysts that are fusiform, dilated collecting ducts with interspersed normal glomeruli.

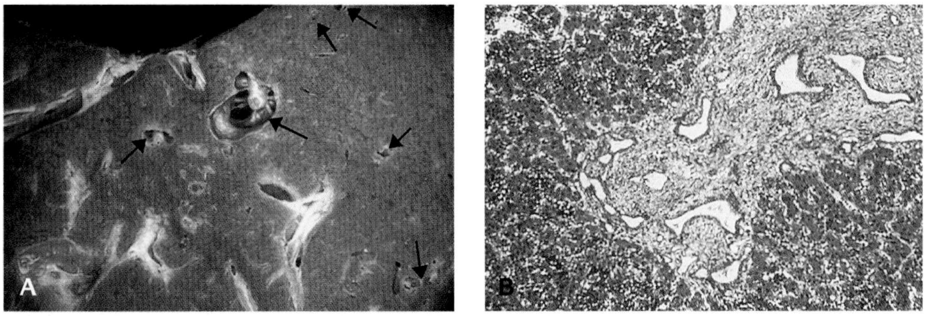

19.10. **(A)** Liver in infantile recessive polycystic kidneys showing small cystic spaces (arrows). **(B)** Microscopic appearance showing dilated serpiginous bile ducts in fibrotic stroma (congenital hepatic fibrosis).

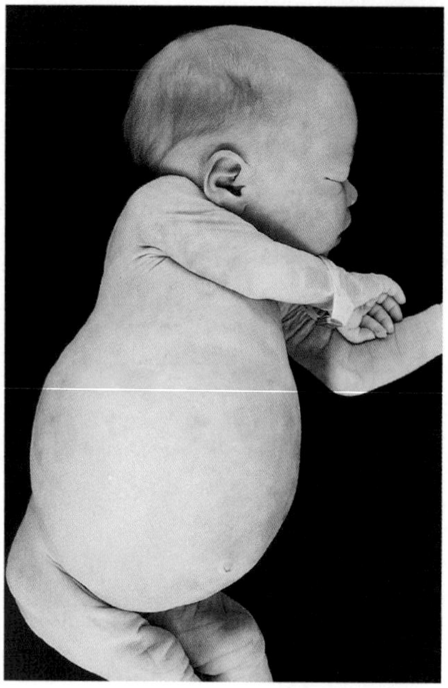

19.11. Newborn infant with markedly distended abdomen due to infantile recessive polycystic kidneys.

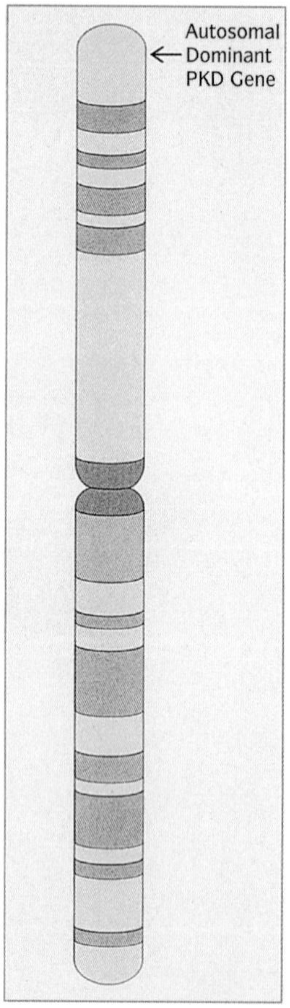

19.12. Location of gene for adult polycystic kidneys on chromosome 16.

Table 19.5 Presence of hepatic fibrosis in renal cystic disease

Congenital hepatic fibrosis: ARPKD, alone, tuberous sclerosis, MCA.
ARPKD: microscopic, like CHF, worse with age, constant
Caroli's: pure duct ectasia (macroscopic) or CHF like, may be local
ADPKD: autosomal dominant polycystic kidney disease, 30% adults to 75% increases with age, macroscopic, dilatation of interlobular ducts, 40% in autopsy
ARPKD: autosomal recessive polycystic renal disease
CHF: congenital hepatic fibrosis

Table 19.6 Dominant-polycystic kidney disease genetics

PKD1 (polycystin): 85% chromosome 16p next to TSC2 (tuberous sclerosis), neighboring duplicated genes? Ion channeling, multiple mutations, high germ line? Tissue somatic mutations, normal allele over expression, truncated transcript.
PKD2: chromosome 4 but homologous, Ca and Na channel proteins, same clinically. Gene interaction 1 and 2.

fibrosis. Cysts may also be present in the lungs, pancreas, spleen, and ovary. The gene locus is on chromosome 6p.

Adult Polycystic Kidney Disease

Adult polycystic disease is characterized by bilaterally enlarged kidneys. There is great variation in the severity of the disease (Figures 19.12 and 19.13). It may be present in the newborn or remain asymptomatic through the individual's life span. Symptoms usually begin around the fourth decade of life.

One in 1,000 people have this disease.

Cyst size varies from millimeters to several centimeters. They may be anywhere along the nephron but are usually due to dilation of the collecting tubules.

There may be cysts in other organs, such as the liver, lung, or pancreas.

A highly polymorphic DNA probe is available for prenatal diagnosis of the mutant gene on the short arm of chromosome 16 that causes dominant polycystic kidney disease. An affected fetus diagnosed by DNA studies and aborted at 12 weeks of gestation showed macroscopically normal kidneys. Microscopically, however, multiple glomerular and tubular cysts were seen in the renal cortex. The liver was macroscopically normal.

Renal Dysplasia

In renal dysplasia, the nephrons and ducts are immature and reduced in number (Figures 19.14 to 19.16 and Tables 19.7 to 19.9). The ducts are often cystic and the number of branches of the ureter is reduced.

The primitive appearance of the nephrons and ducts and the reduction in nephron number and in the amount of ureter branching suggest that differentiation of the renal mesenchyme and ureter is arrested early in development. The poorly differentiated glomeruli and collecting tubules often develop cystic dilations.

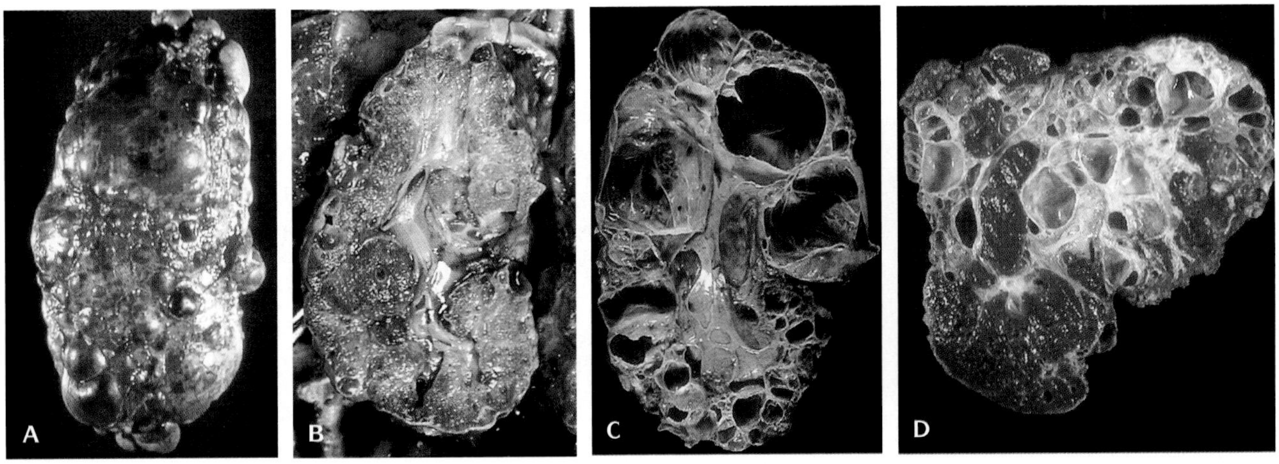

19.13. Adult dominant polycystic kidneys in a newborn showing large variably sized cysts. **(A)** External appearance. **(B)** Cut surface. **(C)** Adult dominant polycystic kidney in an adult, cut surface. **(D)** Cut surface of the liver in an adult.

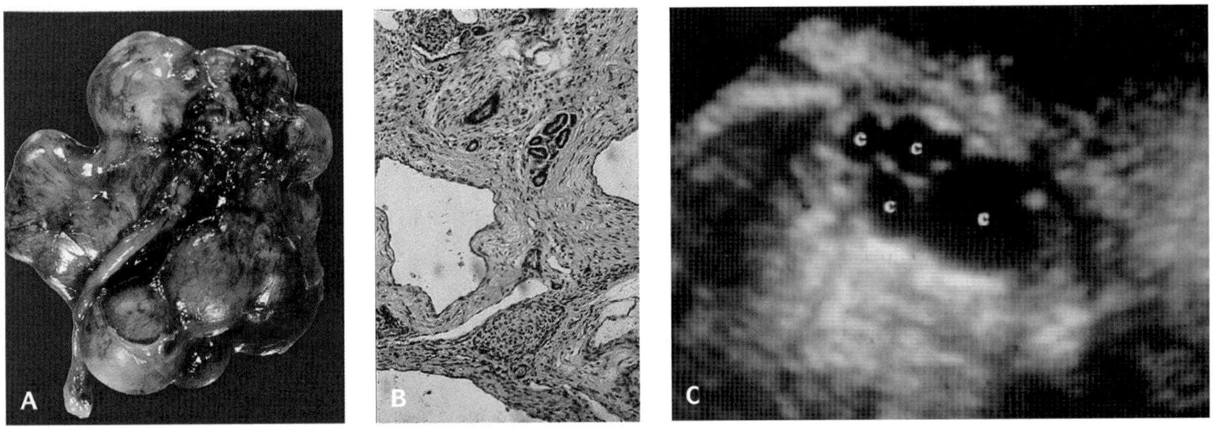

19.14. Multicystic renal dysplasia. **(A)** Gross appearance with cysts of varying size. **(B)** Microscopic appearance with cysts of varying size, a small island of cartilage and small clusters of primitive metaplastic ducts surrounded by a collar of fibroconnective tissue. **(C)** Ultrasound of a multicystic kidney (C, cysts).

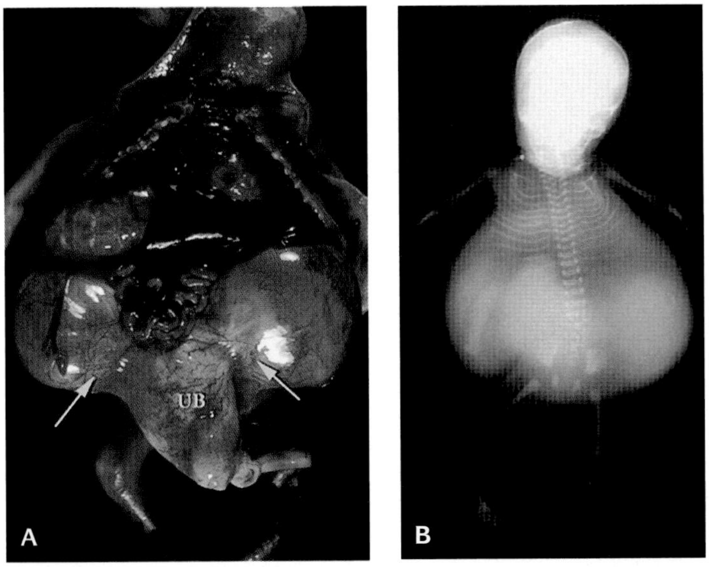

19.15. **(A)** Urethral agenesis with megacystis and huge bilateral urethral diverticula (arrows) in fetus of 27 weeks gestation (UB, urinary bladder). **(B)** X-ray of **(A)** showing massively distended bladder and bilateral ureteral diverticula.

Table 19.7 Incidence of renal dysplasia in GU anomalies

Anomaly	Incidence of renal dysplasia
Ectopic ureter	90%
Ureterocele	100%
Reflux megaureter	75%
Megaloureter	40%
Uteropelvic junction obstruction (UPJ)	23%
Ureteral atresia	100%

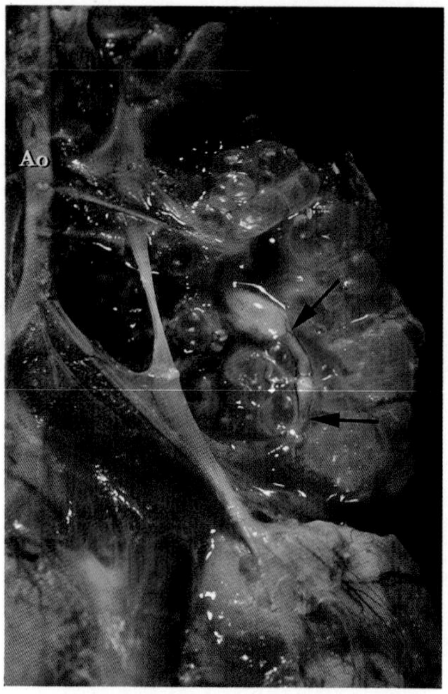

19.16. Multicystic renal dysplasia with atretic ureter (arrows). (Ao, aorta.)

Table 19.8 Variants of renal dysplasia

Dysplasia, dyshistogenesis not preneoplastic
Failure to undergo normal development. Abnormal development of renal parenchyma. Branches of ureteric bud (collecting ducts) with concentric fibroplasia.
Disorganization variable
Bilateral, multicystic
Hypoplastic, no cysts
Segmental-ureteral obstruction
Obstruction usual
Micromulticystic trisomy 13, 18, VATER polytopic field defect

Table 19.9 Syndromes with diffuse renal dysplasia

- Meckel syndrome, Goldston syndrome, Simopoulos syndrome, Miranda syndrome
- Short-rib polydactyly syndromes:
  - Jeune syndrome
  - Ellis-van Creveld syndrome
  - Elejalde syndrome
- Roberts syndrome
- Zellweger syndrome
- Trisomy syndromes 9 and 13
- Glutaric aciduria type 2
- Renal-hepatic-pancreatic dysplasia

Renal dysplasia is usually sporadic and frequently is caused by a urinary outflow tract obstruction, but a few cases of familial dysplasia have been reported. Renal dysplasia may be a component of many syndromes, such as the Meckel syndrome.

Dysplastic renal development may affect the whole kidney or it may be focal or segmental. Dysplasia can be multicystic or aplastic. The multicystic dysplastic kidney is grossly cystic and enlarged. The aplastic kidney is much smaller than a normal kidney and consists of dysplastic renal tissue or small cysts.

Bilateral renal dyplasia occurs in the oligohydramnios sequence. Unilateral renal dysplasia may be associated with other major developmental defects such as isolated ventricular septal defect, aortic coarctation, intestinal atresia, and meningomyelocele.

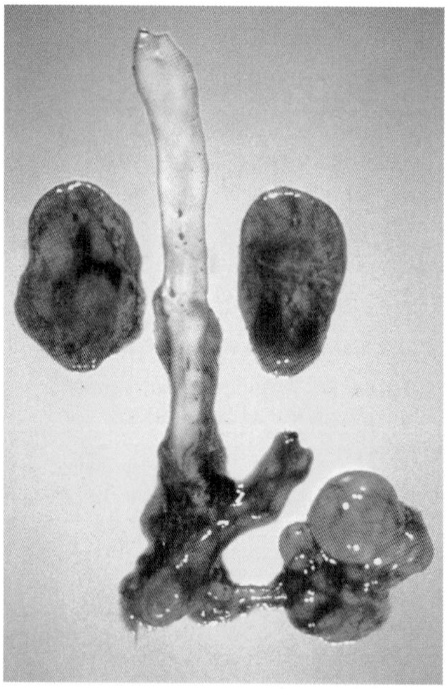

19.17. Hereditary renal adysplasia. There is renal agenesis of the right and a dysplastic cystic pelvic kidney on the left.

Hereditary Renal Adysplasia

Hereditary renal adysplasia (HRA) comprises unilateral dysplasia, unilateral agenesis, and lethal bilateral agenesis usually in a dominant mode of inheritance (Figures 19.17 and 19.18).

Hydronephrosis

In this condition, the renal pelvis is dilated and some of the renal parenchyma may be atrophied because of obstruction of the ureters or urethra, resulting in subsequent dysplastic development.

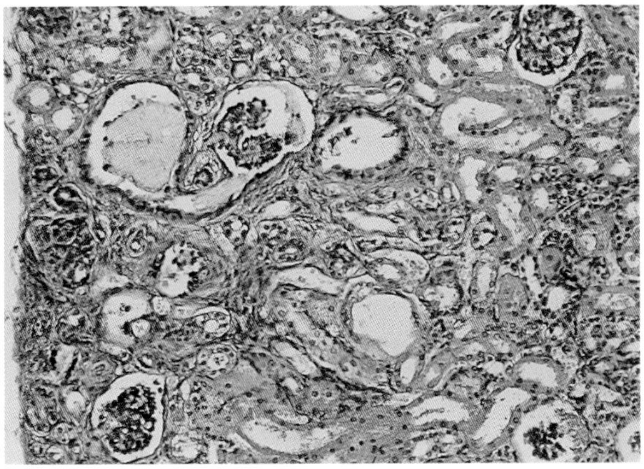

19.18. Micromulticystic kidney in a fetus with trisomy 13. The cysts are small, microscopic in size and are both tubular and glomerular.

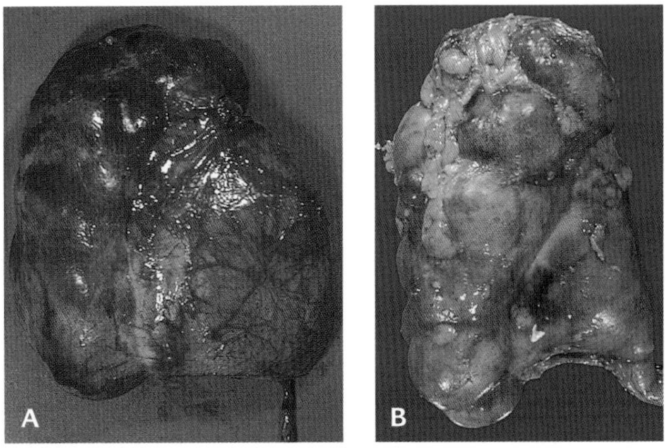

19.19. (A) Pelviectases. The pelvis of the kidney is greatly dilated and the ureter is atretic. **(B)** Hydronephrotic kidney with distension of the pelvis due to ureteral stenosis.

Obstruction to the outflow of urine is the cause of hydronephrosis, although it is not always possible to determine the location or to identify the cause of obstruction (Figures 19.19 to 19.21). Ureteropelvic obstruction is the most common cause of fetal hydronephrosis. Causes are:

1. Ureteropelvic junction obstruction
2. Pressure on the ureter by an aberrant blood vessel
3. Ureter muscle abnormalities, such as sparseness and fibrosis
4. Bladder diverticula adjacent to the ureter orifice
5. Posterior urethral valves and urethral maldevelopment.

The pelvicaliceal area is dilated and the renal parenchyma is atrophied depending on the degree of obstruction and the length of time it has been present. Other abnormalities of the urinary tract may cause hydronephrosis. Hydronephrosis is part of the **prune belly sequence** and the

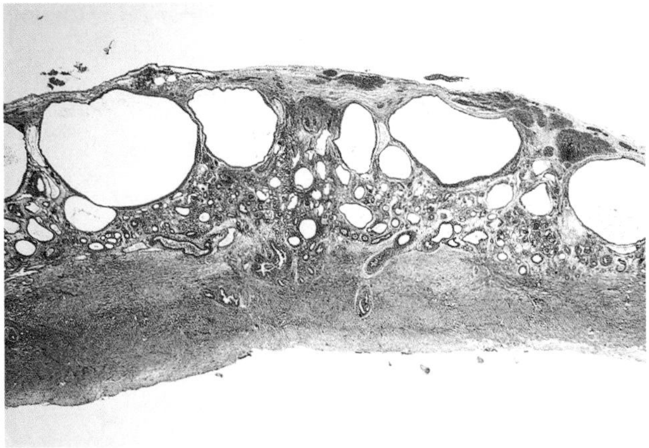

19.20. Microscopic appearance of congenital obstructive hydronephrosis with cysts located beneath the capsule.

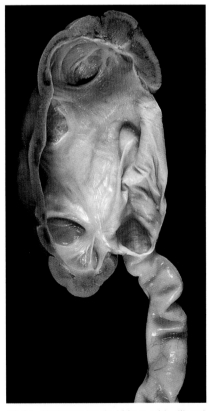

19.21. Hydronephrotic kidney with dilated tortuous ureters due to lower ureteral stenosis.

Table 19.10 Posterior urethral valve sequence

Males, bladder dilated
Oligohydramnios and its tetrad, crypto-orchidism, prune belly from megacystis, malrotation
VATER polytopic field defect

Table 19.11 Consequences of obstructive uropathy

Dilatation of renal outlet structures
Renal dysplasia and obstruction
Oligohydramnios
Fetal constraint: club feet, flat face
Amnion nodosum
Pulmonary hypoplasia pneumothorax

Table 19.12 Prostate in obstructive uropathy

Prune belly: No gross gland, few simplified glands, no acini, less muscle, loss of peripheral zone utricle, no junction with bladder
Posterior urethral valves: Gland small, hypertrophied junction with bladder, acini at periphery but small and dilated, loss of acini in periurethral zone, fibrosis.

megacystis-microcolon-intestinal hypoperistalsis syndrome, which is characterized by a large thin bladder, hydroureters, and hydronephrosis, with usually dysplastic kidneys. About 30% of cases of campomelic dysplasia have hydronephrosis, and it is occasionally present in thanatophoric dysplasia and dyssegmental dysplasia.

Posterior Urethral Valves

Valvular folds of the urethral mucous membrane occur only in the male. There are three types of valvular folds, but only types I and III can cause obstruction (Figures 19.22 and 19.23 and Tables 19.10 to 19.12):

1. Type I – The two folds that are normally present and extend from the verumontanum into the lateral wall of the urethra are enlarged and block urine outflow.
2. Type II – The folds extend posteriorly from the upper edge of the verumontanum without causing obstruction.
3. Type III – A transverse diaphragm blocks the urethra distal to the verumontanum.

Folds are normally present in the male urethra, but they are not large enough to cause obstruction. In type I, there seems to be an overgrowth of the folds, with a possible abnormal insertion of the distal end of the Wolffian duct. The transverse diaphragm seen in type III folds may be related to a defect of the urogenital membrane. Posterior urethral valves are almost always sporadic.

Obstruction of the urethra can produce enlargement and hypertrophy of the bladder and hydroureters and bilateral hydronephrosis. Renal dysplasia due to renal damage may be observed if the obstruction occurs early in development but more commonly cysts occur beneath the renal capsule due to the obstructive uropathy, originally described by Potter as type IV cystic kidneys.

Other abnormalities of the genitourinary tract, such as duplication of the urethra, hypospadias, and cryptorchidism, are commonly seen in obstructive uropathies due to posterior urethral valves. Abnormalities of other organs reported are imperforate anus, skeletal anomalies, and heart and blood vessel abnormalities. Posterior urethral valves may occur in the prune belly sequence.

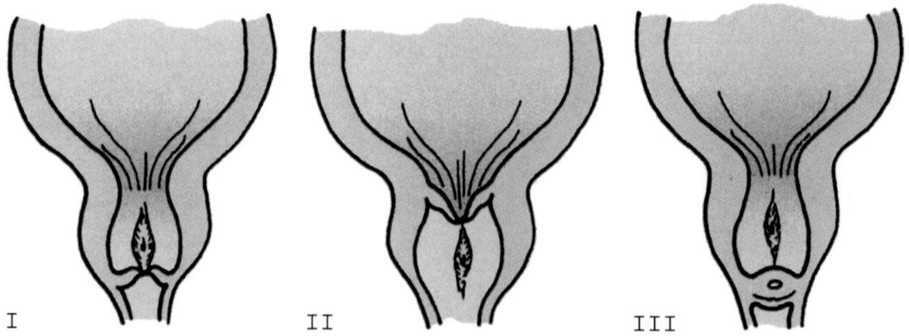

19.22. Types of posterior urethral valves.

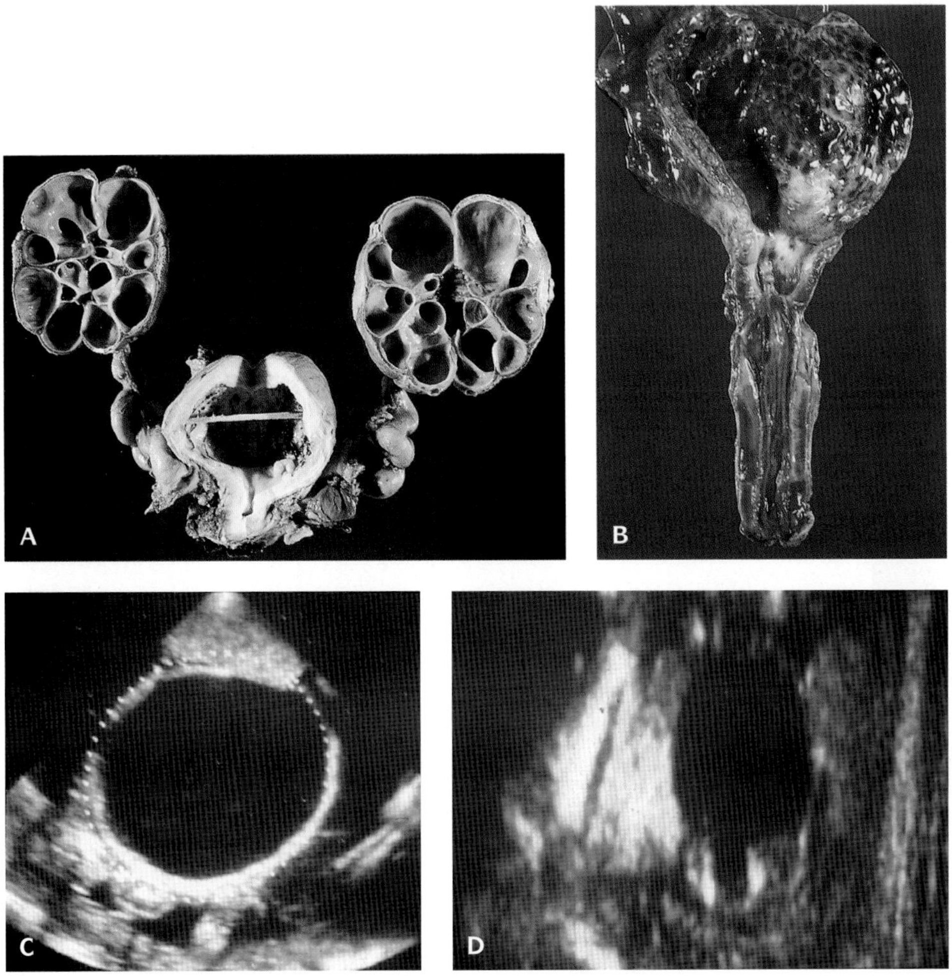

19.23. Posterior urethral valves. **(A)** Huge distended ureters and hydronephrotic kidney. **(B)** Gross appearance of posterior urethral valves. **(C)** Ultrasound showing large dilated bladder. **(D)** Ultrasound showing the keyhole urethral orifice with dilated bladder.

Prune Belly Sequence

The prune belly sequence consists of urinary tract abnormalities, cryptorchidism, and an abdominal muscle deficiency. Almost all cases are male.

The prune belly sequence occurs in 1/3,500 to 1/5,000 live-born infants. Prune belly sequence is usually sporadic (Figures 19.24 and 19.25). It has been reported in trisomy 13 and 18 and in 45,X.

Anterior abdominal wall muscle deficiency may occasionally be a primary muscle defect, but in most cases it is secondary to abdominal distension caused by a dilated hypertrophic urinary bladder. Abnormalities of the urethra may be the principal cause.

There may be atresia, posterior urethral valves, stenosis, or even urethral absence. The prostate may be hypoplastic. In some cases, no cause of urethral obstruction can be determined. The bladder is usually dilated and may be hypertrophic, the ureters are dilated, and the kidneys may be hydronephrotic and/or dysplastic.

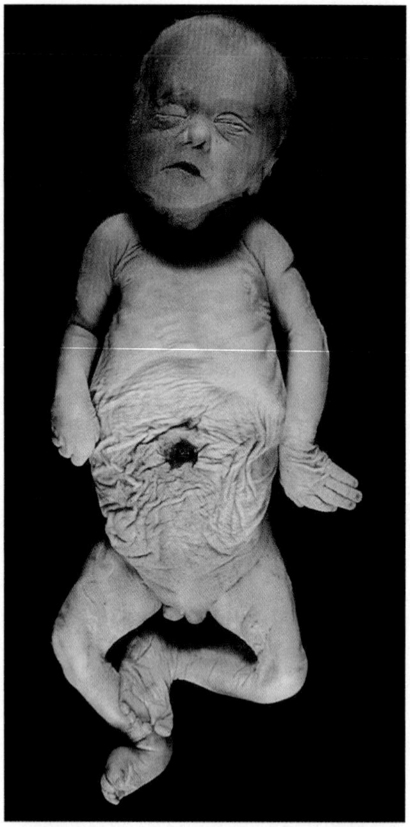

19.24. Prune belly sequence.

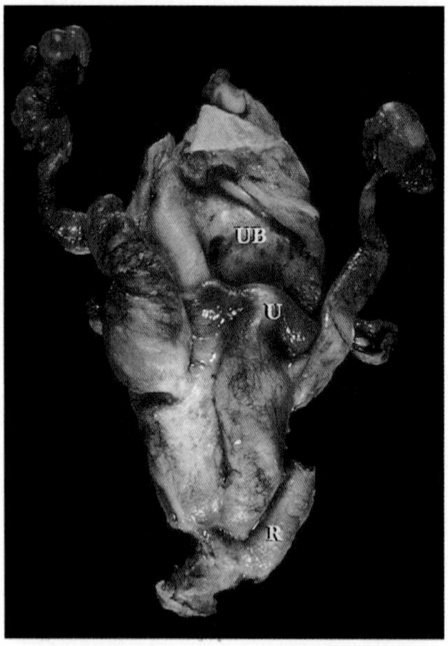

19.25. Posterior view of dilated urinary bladder with dilated distal ureters and small cystic dysplastic kidneys in a fetus at 32 weeks gestation with prune belly sequence. (UB, urinary bladder; U, uterus; R, rectum.) There was a rectovaginal vesicle fistula.

Table 19.13 Medullary cysts

ARPKD
Medullary sponge kidney
Medullary cystic-juvenile nephronophthisis
Beckwith-Wiedemann syndrome
Bardet-Biedl, Jeune, retinal dysplasia
Medullary necrosis
Pyelogenic cyst

Table 19.14 Medullary cyst disease

Often sporadic, but otherwise dominant
Small kidneys; corticomedullary and intramedullary low cuboidal epithelial lined cysts
Late childhood to adult onset
Diagnosis by IVP

Skeletal anomalies, especially of the rib cage, are common and cardiovascular abnormalities, cleft palate, and unilateral renal agenesis have also been reported. Intestinal malrotation and cryptorchidism are often present.

Medullary Cystic Kidneys

Ectasia of the intrapapillary ducts affecting the pyramids results in medullary cysts usually with calcific concretions (Figure 19.26). It is usually sporadic. Urolithiasis, hematuria and infection may occur (Tables 19.13 to 19.15).

Glomerulocystic Kidney Disease

This may occur in inherited or sporadic conditions including early onset ADPKD, Zellweger (cerebrohepatorenal) syndrome, tuberous sclerosis, short-rib polydactyly syndrome, and sometimes with renal dysplasia (Figure 19.27 and Tables 19.16 and 19.17).

Renal Cysts Associated with Multiple Malformation Syndromes

These include some hereditary syndromes, autosomal trisomies, short-rib polydactyly syndromes, Jeune asphyxiating thoracic dystrophy, Meckel syndrome, Zellweger syndrome, and von Hippel-Lindau syndrome.

Meckel Syndrome

This is an autosomal recessive trait and has been localized to chromosome region 17q21–q24 and has an incidence of 1/10,000. It consists of the triad of occipital encephalocele, large cystic dysplastic kidneys, and postaxial polydactyly, which is tetramelic (Figure 19.28). Hepatic involvement is histologically similar to that in ARPKD. Almost all males have underdevelopment of the external genitalia. The kidneys are bilaterally enlarged, causing extreme

Table 19.15 Medullary sponge kidney

Nephronophthisis, progresses to end-stage kidney
Thin cortex with no cysts to 2 cm, but 25% may have no or rare cysts.
Associated: hepatic fibrosis, retinal dysplasia
Tubular basal lamina disruption, inflammation, corticomedullary cysts, tubulointerstitial disease, periglomerular sclerosis
Cysts connect to collecting ducts
Large deletions in 2q (NPH1) in recessive type, 20% with no family history.

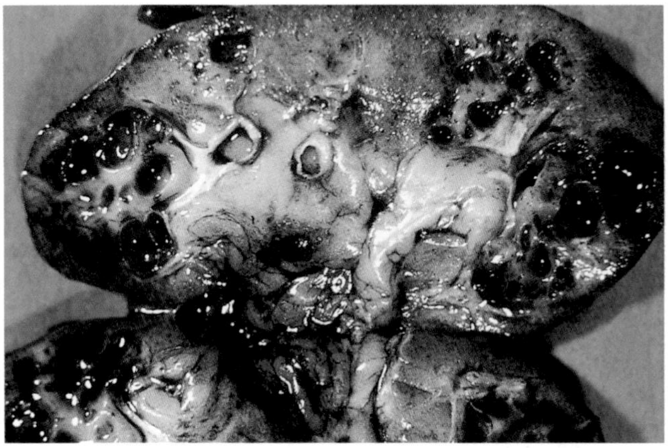

19.26. Medullary cystic kidney (medullary sponge kidney). Multiple medullary cysts with hemorrhage and calcification.

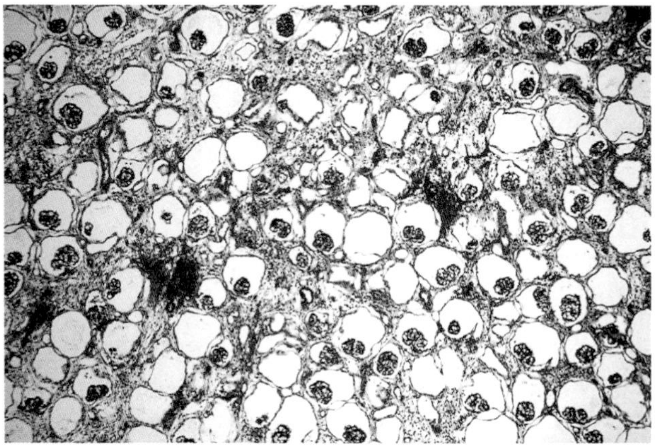

19.27. Glomerulocystic kidney.

abdominal bulging. The cysts vary in size up to several centimeters. The cysts may be seen as early as 10 weeks gestation. The cysts are tubular but may also be glomerular.

Tuberous Sclerosis (See Also Dysplasia Chapter)

This is a neurocutaneous autosomal dominant disorder characterized by epilepsy, mental retardation, and visceral hamartomas of the skin, kidney, brain, eye, bone, lung, and liver (Figure 19.29 and Table 19.18). Cutaneous lesions include angiofibromas. Renal lesions are present in most cases as angiomyolipomas and cysts. Cysts may be present in early infancy while angiomyolipomas are usually not discovered until adulthood.

The renal cysts appear to arise from proximal tubules as well as glomeruli. The cysts are lined by hyperplastic plump pale eosinophilic epithelial cells that may form polypoid projections into the lumina of the cysts.

Table 19.16 Types of glomerulocystic kidneys

- Glomerulocystic kidney disease
  - Autosomal dominant polycystic kidney disease in young infants
  - Dominant glomerulocystic kidney disease in older patients
  - Sporadic nonsyndromal glomerulocystic kidney disease
  - Familial hypoplastic glomerulocystic kidney disease
- Glomerulocystic kidneys in heritable malformation syndromes
  - Tuberous sclerosis
  - Orofaciodigital syndrome, type 1
  - Brachymesomelia-renal syndrome
  - Trisomy 13
  - Short rib-polydactyly syndromes
  - Jeune asphyxiating thoracic dystrophy syndrome
  - Zellweger cerebrohepatorenal syndrome
  - Familial juvenile nephronophthisis
- Glomerular cysts in dysplastic kidneys
  - Diffuse cystic dysplasia
  - Renal-hepatic-pancreatic dysplasia

Table 19.17 Glomerulocystic disease

- Cystic dilatation of Bowman space, diffuse
- ADPKD
- Dysplasia
- Obstruction
- Dominant/familial forms or sporadic
- Malformations: TS, trisomy, asphyxiating thoracic dystrophy, short rib polydactyly syndromes, nephronophthisis, Zellweger syndrome

Table 19.18 Tuberous sclerosis

Cysts like ADPKD, hyperplastic epithelium causes obstruction
Cysts, angiomyolipoma, renal cell carcinomas (2–3%)
20% children have cysts, 5% major cysts like ADPKD, newborns with small sponge-like cysts
Hyperplasia of lining and glomerular podocytes

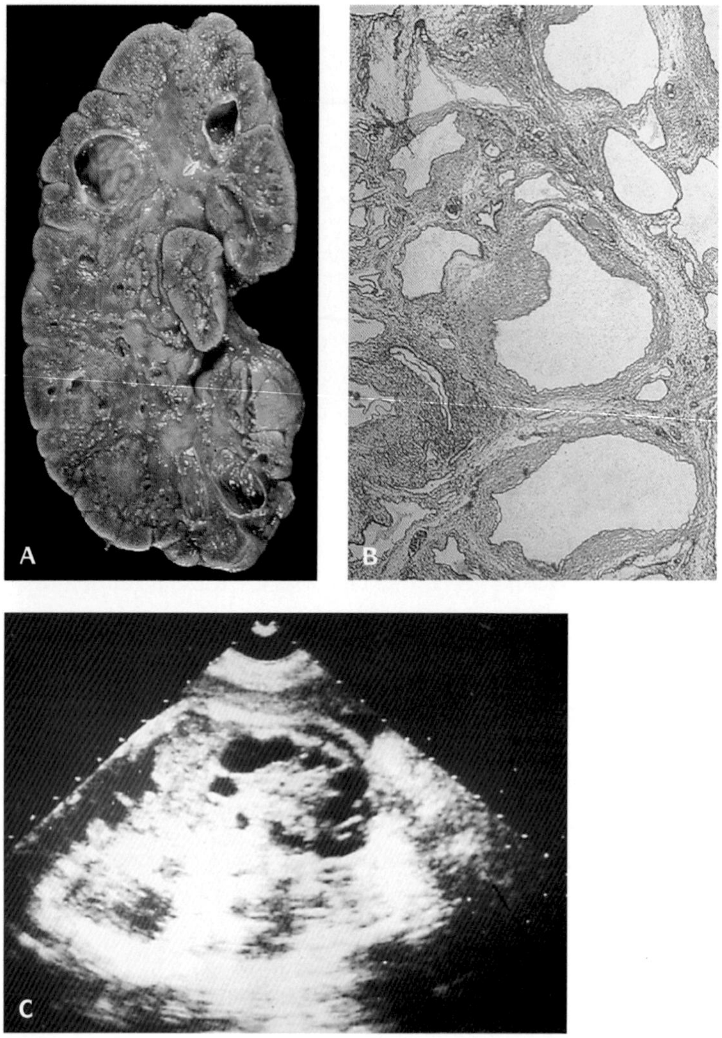

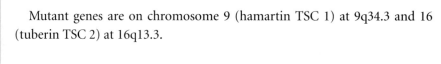

19.28. Meckel syndrome in a newborn infant. Gross appearance of large kidney with variable-sized cysts. **(A)** Cut surface. **(B)** Microscopic appearance showing cysts of variable size lined by tubular epithelium with dysplastic stroma and very little nephrotic tissue that is almost entirely cystic primitive ducts. **(C)** Ultrasound showing large cysts.

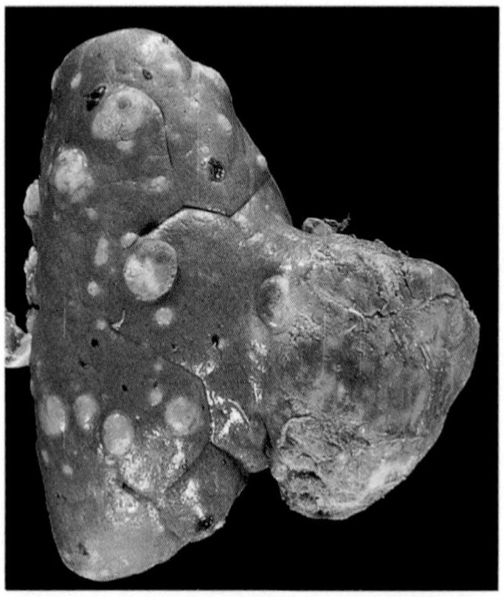

19.29. Tuberous sclerosis. Gross appearance of kidney with multiple angiomyolipomas.

Mutant genes are on chromosome 9 (hamartin TSC 1) at 9q34.3 and 16 (tuberin TSC 2) at 16q13.3.

Zellweger Syndrome (Cerebrohepatorenal Syndrome) (See Also Malformations Syndromes)

This is an autosomal recessive disorder characterized by dysmorphic features, mental retardation, malformations of the CNS, joint calcifications, hepatic fibrosis and siderosis, and renal cysts (Figure 19.30). The defect is a mutation of the gene responsible for peroxisomal assembly located on chromosome 8q21.1 The cortical cysts vary in size up to 1 cm in diameter and are both tubular and glomerular and are associated with increased stroma. By electron microscopy

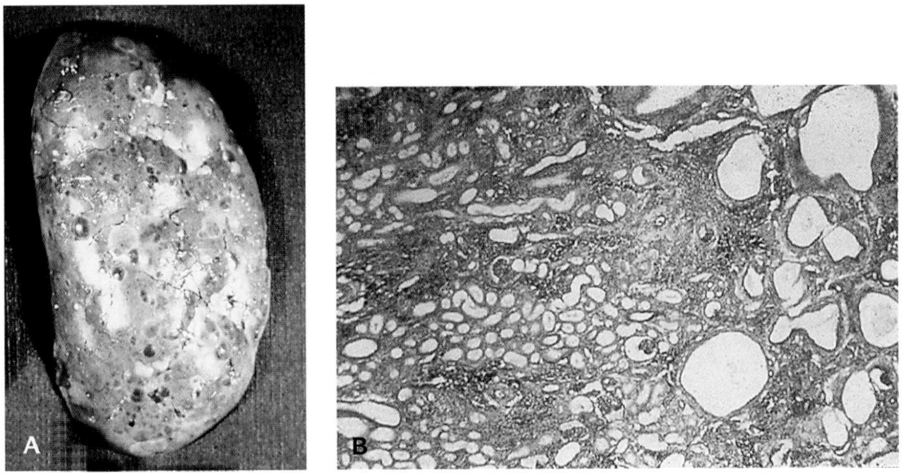

19.30. Zellweger syndrome. **(A)** Gross appearance of multiple cortical cysts in a newborn infant. **(B)** Microscopic section showing multiple tubular cysts.

peroxisomes are not present in the liver and the cells accumulate very long chain fatty acids and are deficient in plasmalogens. Prenatal diagnosis is made by demonstrations of fatty acid abnormalities from cultured amniotic cells or from chorionic villus sampling.

Von-Hippel-Lindau Syndrome (See Also Dysplasia Chapter)

This condition is inherited as an autosomal dominant trait characterized by retinal angiomatosis, cerebellar angiomas, and cysts of abdominal organs particularly pancreas and kidneys (Figure 19.31). The renal cysts vary in size and are lined by plump clear cells that may proliferate and result in renal cell carcinoma in 25% of cases. The gene locus is on chromosome 10 and is the same locus as renal cell carcinoma.

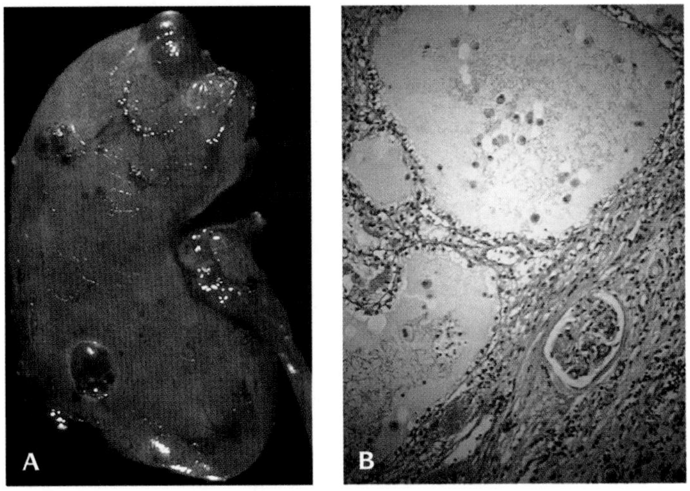

19.31. Von Hippel-Lindau. **(A)** Gross appearance of cystic kidney. The cysts are of variable size. **(B)** Microscopic appearance of renal cysts lined by prominent clear cells.

Smith-Lemli-Opitz Syndrome (See Also Dysplasia Chapter)

This condition is autosomal recessive and due to a deficiency of 7-dehydrocholesterol reductase that results in greatly reduced plasma cholesterol concentration (Figure 19.32). Distinct craniofacial appearance is present with microcephaly, ptosis of eyelids, inner epicanthal folds, strabismus, micrognathia, syndactyly of second and third toes, hypospadias, cryptorchidism, and mental retardation. Cystic renal disease, hypoplasia, hydronephrosis, and abnormalities of the ureters are frequent.

Congenital Renal Tubular Dysgenesis

This condition is characterized by absence of the proximal convoluted tubules that results in the oligohydramnios sequence with Potter facies (Figure 19.33). The kidneys are of normal size, with absence of proximal convoluted tubules and crowding of normal-appearing glomeruli. Atrophy of medullary pyramids and collecting ducts and squamous metaplasia of the pelvic transitional epithelium may be seen. Extrarenal manifestations may include large cranial fontanels and sutures, hypoplasia of calvarial bones, and severe neonatal liver disease with hemochromatosis. Autosomal recessive inheritance is suggested in some cases; however, the lesion has also been related to maternal administration of indomethacin and ACE inhibitors.

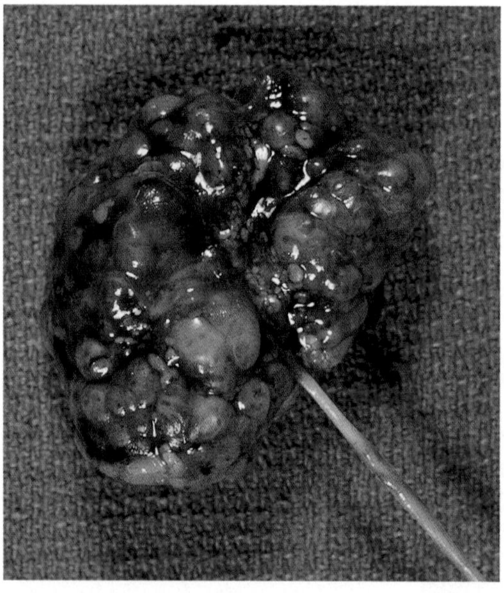

19.32. Smith-Lemli-Opitz syndrome. Gross appearance of a large cystic dysplastic kidney.

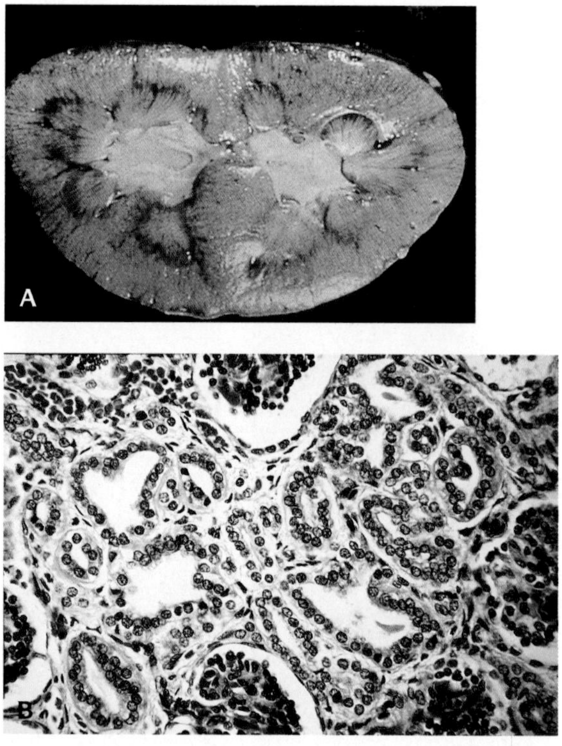

19.33. Congenital renal tubular dysgenesis. **(A)** Gross appearance of normal-appearing kidney. **(B)** Microscopic section shows no recognizable proximal tubules and the glomeruli are crowded.

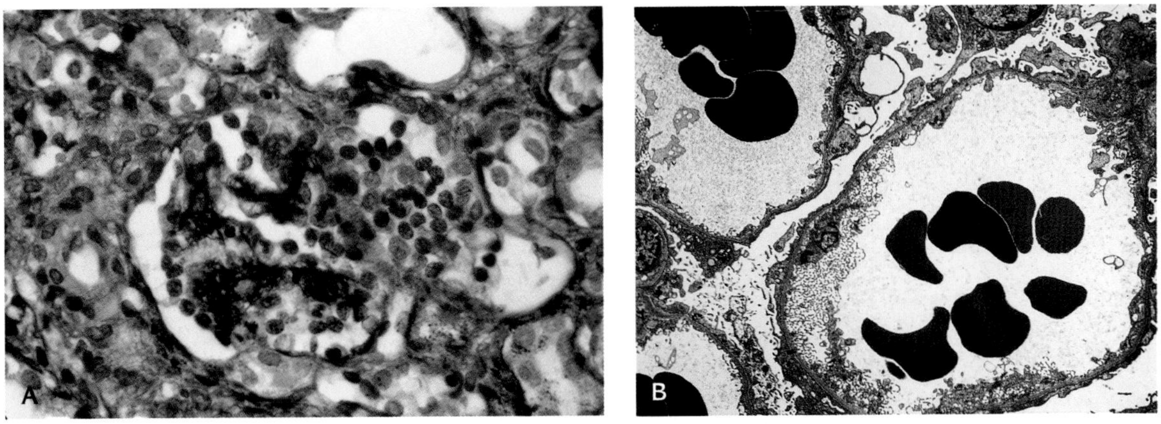

19.34. Congenital nephrotic syndrome. **(A)** Microscopic section of kidney. The glomerulus is enlarged with mesangial hypercellularity and increased matrix with adjacent tubular microcyst. **(B)** Electronmicroscopy shows extremely thin lamina densa with fusion of foot processes.

Congenital Nephrotic Syndrome

This condition, first described in Finland (congenital nephrosis of Finnish type) is inherited as an autosomal recessive trait. The gene locus is on chromosome 19q12–q13.1. At birth the placenta is large; there are deformities including talipes calcaneovalgus and contractures of the extremities (Figure 19.34 and Table 19.19). Proteinuria and edema are usually apparent at birth and the disorder is fatal within the first 2 years of life unless renal transplantation is performed.

The kidneys are large and pale, and the number of nephrons is increased. The characteristic renal lesion is tubular dilatation primarily of the proximal convoluted tubules. It is initially limited to the deep cortex but spreads radially

Table 19.19 Congenital nephrotic syndrome: differential diagnosis

- Congenital nephrotic syndrome, Finnish type
- Diffuse mesangial sclerosis, isolated
- Postinfectious glomerulonephritis
  - Congenital syphilis
  - Congenital toxoplasmosis
- Hemolytic-uremic syndrome
- C1q glomerulonephritis
- Congenital lupus nephritis
- Mercury (teething powder) toxicity
- Idiopathic nephrotic syndrome
  - Minimal change nephrotic syndrome
  - Diffuse mesangial hypercellularity
  - Focal segmental glomerular sclerosis
- Syndromal nephrosis
  - Drash syndrome of chronic renal disease, Wilms tumor, and gonadal dysgenesis
  - Nail-patella syndrome
  - Lowe oculocerebrorenal syndrome
  - Galloway-Mowat syndrome with cerebral maldevelopment and ocular abnormalities

Table 19.20 Cystic renal tumors

Benign cystic nephroma: part of spectrum of Wilms, myofibroblastic septae, flat epithelium, rare sarcomas, no treatment

Partially differentiated Wilms: septae have immature stroma and/or epithelium, good outcome, <2 years old.

Cystic Wilms: nephroblastoma with many cysts, solid tumor present.

Multilocular cystic renal cell carcinoma: adult female, 90% cystic, low-grade nuclear pleomorphism, epithelial cells may be clear cells.

Cystic hamartoma pelvis: adult females, present in pyramids

Table 19.21 Sexual identification

Type	Method	Time of recognition
1. Chromosomal		Fertilization
X positive	X chromatin	
Y positive	Y chromatin	
Morphology	Karyotype	
2. Gonadal	Histology	
Testis		$5\frac{1}{2}$ weeks
Ovary		6 weeks
3. Hormonal		
Androgen	Steroid assay	10–12 weeks
4. Duct differentiation	Visual	
Wolffian regression (female)		10–16 weeks
Mullerian regression (male)		10 weeks
Mullerian complete (female)		$24\frac{1}{2}$ weeks
5. External genitalia	Visual	
Phallus length and shape		11 weeks
Male type complete		16 weeks
6. Sex of rearing	Visual	After birth
7. Secondary sexual Differentiation	Visual	Puberty

to the peripheral cortex. Interstitial fibrosis and mesangial hypercellularity with wide and ectatic capillaries are present progressing to glomerular fibrosis and sclerosis. By electron microscopy the glomerular basement membrane is thin, visceral epithelial cells are edematous, and foot processes are lost. Fetal proteinuria results in an increase of amniotic α-fetoprotein.

Cystic Renal Tumors

A number of renal tumors are associated with cystic changes (Table 19.20).

GENITAL SYSTEM

The embryonic gonad is intrinsically programmed to become an ovary. If a gene(s) that produces testis-determining factor (TDF) is present, the gonad will start to develop into a testis between 6 and 8 weeks. Leydig cells and Sertoli cells begin to differentiate within the testes. The Leydig cells produce testosterone, which stimulates further development of the seminal vesicle, vas deferens, and epididymis. A derivative of testosterone, dihydrotestosterone, induces differentiation of the penis, scrotum, and prostate. The Sertoli cells produce the Müllerian inhibiting factor, which causes the Müllerian ducts to regress. The Sertoli cells begin to secrete at 45–50 days; the Leydig cells at about 60 days. If the indifferent gonad has not been exposed to TDF by 8–9 weeks, the gonad can no longer respond by becoming a testis.

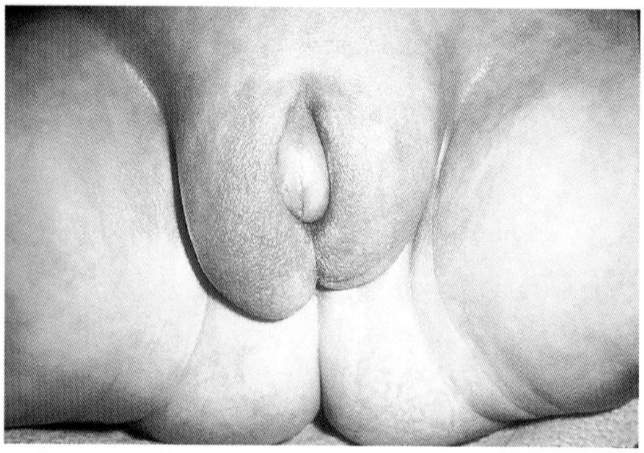

19.35. Ambiguous genitalia in infant with congenital adrenal hyperplasia due to 21-hydroxylase deficiency.

In the female, germ cells are found in primordial ovarian follicles, which develop at the epithelial side of the gonad that has become an ovary by the 7th week of development. The female external genitalia begin to develop at the 8th week.

Abnormalities of the genital system are divided into those with external manifestations and those with internal abnormalities.

Abnormal External Genitalia

The most common male abnormalities are hypospadias and small penis. Females with an enlarged clitoris are included in ambiguous genitalia (Figures 19.35 to 19.37 and Tables 19.21 to 19.31).

Ambiguous genitalia are rarely found in the previable period.

ABNORMAL INTERNAL REPRODUCTIVE TRACTS

Defects in the internal reproductive tracts are rare as isolated findings. They are usually found as a component of a complex malformation syndrome, such as sirenomelia (Figures 19.38 to 19.47). In female fetuses with a normal female karyotype, abnormalities of the internal reproductive tract include absent ovary, ovary showing gonadal dysgenesis, and Müllerian aplasia consisting of atresias, fistulas, and abnormal septa.

In male fetuses with a normal male karyotype, anorchia and Wolffian aplasia can be seen.

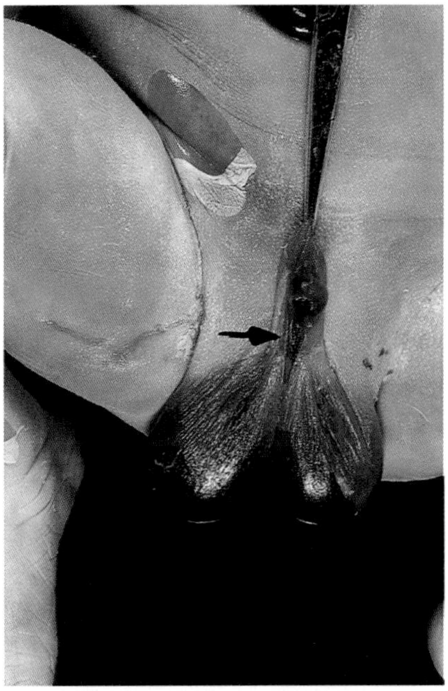

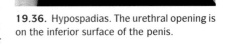

19.36. Hypospadias. The urethral opening is on the inferior surface of the penis.

Table 19.22 Evaluation of the neonate with ambiguous genitalia

History:
Family history, maternal exposure to toxic agents, endogenous androgen production

Physical examination:
Associated congenital anomalies, perineal orifices, phallic size, gonads palpable/not palpable

Imaging/laboratory studies:
Pelvic, adrenal, and renal ultrasonography
Vaginography
Karyotype
17α-Hydroxyprogesterone

Gonads not palpable/Müllerian structures present/46XX:
17α-Hydroxyprogesterone increased: 21-hydroxylase deficient congenital adrenal hyperplasia; measure sodium, potassium, plasma renin activity
17α-Hydroxyprogesterone normal or slightly increased, 17α-hydroxypregnenolone (low-deficiency or StAR; elevated deficiency of 3β-hydroxysteroid dehydrogenase), 11-deoxycortisol (elevated deficiency of 11α-hydroxylase)

Gonads palpable/Müllerian structures present/46XY or variant:
Measure AMH, intermediates of testosterone and dihydrotestosterone synthesis in basal specimens and after hCG administration

Gonads palpable/Müllerian Duct structures absent/46XY or variant:
Measure intermediates of testosterone and dihydrotestosterone synthesis in gonad Specimens and after hCG administration; assess androgen receptor

No diagnosis:
Gonadal biopsy for true hermaphroditism

StAR, steroidogenic acute regulatory protein.

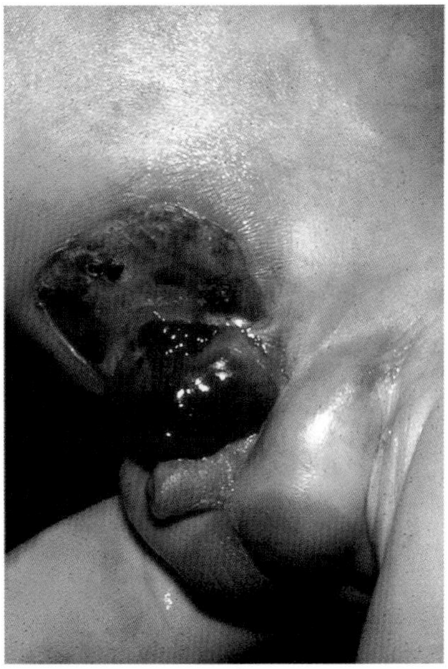

19.37. Extrophy of the bladder.

Table 19.23 Characteristics and diagnosis of the types of congenital adrenal hyperplasia (CAH)

Enzymatic defect	21α-Hydroxylase (virilizing CAH)		11β-Hydroxylase (virilizing CAH)		17α-Hydroxylase (nonvirilizing CAH)		Cholesterol desmolase system (nonvirilizing CAH)		3β-Hydroxysteroid dehydrogenase, $\Delta^5-\Delta^4$-isomerase (mixed CAH)	
Incidence	Classic: 1/5,000 births; approximately 90% of all CAH cases Late-onset: common		Classic: approximately 5% of all CAH cases Late-onset: rare		Rare		Rare		Classic: rare Late-onset: may be common	
Genotype	XX	XY	XX	XY	XX	XY	XX	XY	XX	XY
Phenotype	Female to ambiguous genitalia	Male	Female to ambiguous genitalia	Male	Female lack of secondary sex characteristics	Female to ambiguous genitalia	Female	Female to ambiguous genitalia	Ambiguous genitalia	Ambiguous genitalia
Chromosome location	6p	6p	8q	8q	10	10	15	15		
Hormones										
Adrenal										
Glucocorticoids	Deficiency	Deficiency	Deficiency	Deficiency	Deficiency	Deficiency	Deficiency	Deficiency	Deficiency	Deficiency
Mineralocorticoids	Deficiency	Deficiency	Excess (DOC)	Excess (DOC)	Excess (DOC)	Excess (DOC)	Deficiency	Deficiency	Deficiency	Deficiency
Androgens	Excess	Excess	Excess	Excess	Deficiency	Deficiency	Deficiency	Deficiency	Excess	Excess
Gonadal										
Androgens	–	–	–	–		Deficiency	–	Deficiency		Deficiency
Estrogens	–	–	–	–	Deficiency		Deficiency			
Addison's	infancy	infancy	infancy	infancy	infancy	infancy	+	+	+	+
Hypertension	–	–	+	+	+	+	–	–	–	–
Acid-base/ electrolytes	Hyperkalemic acidosis	Hyperkalemic acidosis	Hypokalemic alkalosis	Hypokalemic alkalosis	Hypokalemic alkalosis	Hypokalemic alkalosis	Hyperkalemic acidosis	Hyperkalemic acidosis	Hyperkalemic acidosis	Hyperkalemic acidosis
puberty-	prepubertal	isosexual	prepubertal	isosexual	hypergona-dotropic hypogonadism	hypergona-dotropic hypogonadism	hypergona-dotropic hypogonadism (?)	hypergona-dotropic hypogonadism (?)	prepubertal virilization hirsutism; menstrual irregularities; infertility	
Gynecomastia Postnatal	(heterosexual precocious puberty); premature adrenarche or prepubertal virilization; hirsutism; menstrual irregularities; infertility	precocious puberty; adrenal rest tumors in testes	(heterosexual precocious puberty); premature adrenarche or prepubertal virilization; hirsutism; menstrual irregularities; infertility	precocious puberty						

Diagnosis					
Homozygotes (or compound heterozygotes)	Increased urinary 17-ketosteroids and pregnanetriol excretion Plasma 17-hydroxy-progesterone Plasma renin activity	Increased 17-ketosteroids Plasma 11-deoxycortisol Urinary 170-HS excretion Urinary THS, THDOC excretion Plasma renin activity	Plasma pregnenolone/17-hydroxypregnenolone Plasma progesterone/17-hydroxypregnenolone Plasma renin activity		Increased 17-ketosteroids Plasma pregnenolone/progesterone 17-hydroxypregnenolone/17-hydroxyprogesterone
Prenatal	Amniotic fluid 17-hydroxyprogesterone HLA typing of amniotic cell	Amniotic fluid 11-deoxycortisol			Amniotic fluid DHEA/Δ^4-androstenedione
Heterozygotes (carriers)	Plasma 17-hydroxy-progesterone after ACTH stimulation HLA typing in family members	Not detectable biochemically			
Management	Karyotype Genitogram ultrasound Gender assignment Replacement Salt, hydration Glucocorticoid Mineralocorticoid (±) LHRH analogues Prenatal therapy with dexamethasone (wk 9–16) Surgery Clitoroplasty	Karyotype Genitogram ultrasound Gender assignment Replacement Hydration LHRH analogues Surgery Clitoroplasty	Karyotype Genitogram ultrasound Gender assignment Replacement Hydration Glucocorticoid Sex steroids Surgery	Karyotype Genitogram ultrasound Gender assignment Replacement Salt, hydration Glucocorticoid Mineralocorticoid Sex steroids Surgery	Karyotype Genitogram ultrasound Gender assignment Replacement Salt, hydration Glucocorticoid Mineralocorticoid Surgery Clitoroplasty

DOC, deoxycorticoid; DHEA, dehydroepiandrosterone; LHRH, luteinizing releasing hormone.

Table 19.24 Syndromes with ambiguous external genitalia

McKusick no.	Syndrome	Features	Inheritance
200110	Ablepharon-macrostomia	Absent eyelids, eyebrows, eyelashes, external ears; fusion defects of mouth; ambiguous genitalia; absent or rudimentary nipples; parchment skin; delayed development of expressive language	?AR
	Wilms tumor-aniridia, genital anomalies, mental retardation (WAGR syndrome)	Moderate to severe mental deficiency, growth deficiency, microcephaly, aniridia, nystagmus, ptosis, blindness, Wilms tumor, ambiguous genitalia, gonadoblastoma	Deletion at 11p13
205530	Asplenia, cardiovascular anomalies, caudal deficiency	Hypoplasia or aplasia of spleen, complex cardiac malformation, abnormal lung lobulation, anomalous position and development of abdominal organs, agenesis of corpus callosum, imperforate anus, ambiguous genitalia, contracture of lower limb	AR
209970	Beemer	Hydrocephalus, dense bones, cardiac malformation, bulbous nose, broad nasal bridge, ambiguous genitalia	AR
	Deletion 11q	Trigonocephaly, flat and broad nasal bridge, micrognathia, carp mouth, hypertelorism, low-set ears, severe congenital heart disease, anomalies of limbs, external genitalia	AR
194080	Drash	Wilms tumor, nephropathy, ambiguous genitalia with 46,XY karyotype	Unknown
219000	Fraser	Cryptophthalmia, defect of auricle, hair growth on lateral forehead to lateral eyebrow, hypoplastic nares, mental deficiency, partial cutaneous syndactyly, urogenital malformations	AR
	Lethal acrodysgenital dysplasia	Failure to thrive, facial dysmorphism, ambiguous genitalia, syndactyly, postaxial polydactyly, Hirschsprung disease, cardiac and renal malformation	AR
26870	Rutledge	Joint contractures, cerebellar hypoplasia, renal hypoplasia, ambiguous genitalia, urologic anomalies, tongue cysts, shortness of limbs, eye abnormalities, heart defects, gallbladder agenesis, ear malformations	AR
312830	SCARF	Skeletal abnormalities, cutis laxa, craniosynostosis, ambiguous genitalia, psychomotor retardation, facial abnormalities	Uncertain
263520	Short rib-polydactyly (type 2) Majewski	Short stature; short limbs; cleft lip and palate, ear anomalies; limb anomalies, including pre- and postaxial polysyndactyly; narrow thorax; short horizontal ribs; high clavicles; ambiguous genitalia	AR
207400	Smith-Lemli-Opitz	Microcephaly, mental retardation, hypotonia, ambiguous genitalia, abnormal facies, metabolic defect of 7-dehydrocholesterol reductase	AR
	Trimethadione, prenatal exposure	Mental deficiency, speech disorders, prenatal-onset growth deficiency, brachycephaly, midfacial hypoplasia, broad and upturned nose, prominent forehead, eye anomalies, cleft lip and palate, cardiac defects, ambiguous genitalia	Prenatal drug exposure
192350	VATER association	Vertebral, anal, tracheoesophageal, and renal anomalies; subjects with ambiguous genitalia as part of cloacal anomalies	Unknown

Modified from Simpson JL, Verp MS, Plouffe L Jr: Female genital system. In *Human Malformations and Related Anomalies*, Stevenson RE, Hall JG, Goodman RM, eds. New York, Oxford University, 1993, p. 584.

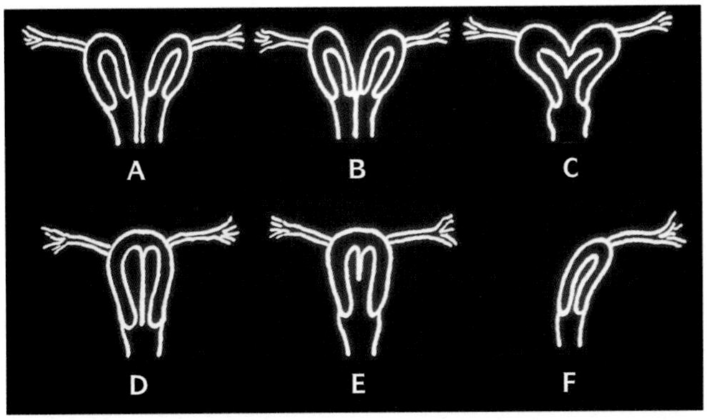

19.38. Abnormalities of the uterine fusion. **(A)** Double reproductive organs. **(B)** Bicornate uterus with septate vagina. **(C)** High bicornuate uterus. **(D)** Septate uterus with septate vagina. **(E)** Septate uterus. **(F)** Unicornuate uterus.

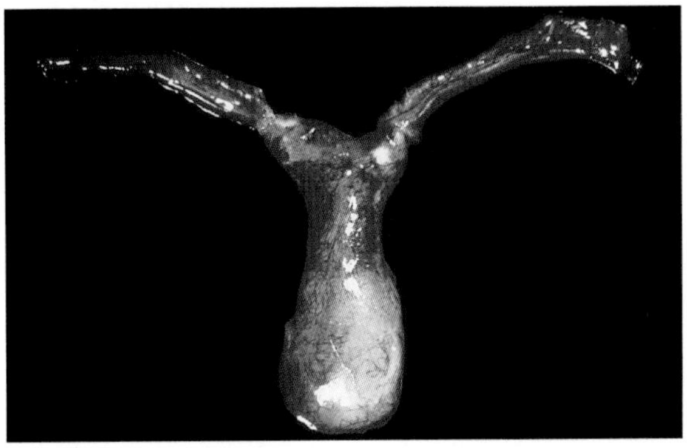

19.39. Atresia of the vagina with imperforate hymen.

Table 19.25 Congenital adrenal hyperplasia

Form	Genitalia	Androgens	Other
21-OH deficiency	Virilized female	↑	Salt losing, most common
11-OH deficiency	Virilized female	↑	Hypertension
Cholesterol desmolase	Ambiguous male	N	Lethal salt wasting
3β-OH	Virilized female or ambiguous male	↑	Lethal
17-OH deficiency	Ambiguous male	↓	Hypertension
17,20-lyase	Ambiguous male	↓	Isolated defect

Table 19.26 Genes involved in differentiation of the bipotential gonadal ridge

Gene	Chromosome	Function	Deficiency state
SF1	9q33	Regulates steroid synthesis, LH, FSH, GnRH, gonadal and adrenal differentiation	None identified
WT1	11p13	Regulates renal and gonadal differentiation	Denys-Drash, Frazier syndromes, WAGR
DAX1	Xp21.3–p21.2	Regulates adrenocortical differentiation; may influence ovarian differentiation	Loss-of-function: congenital adrenal hypoplasia, hypogonadotropism Gain-of-function: 46,XY sex reversal
SRY	Yp11.3	Regulates testicular differentiation	46,XY sex reversal
SOX9	17q24.3–q25.1	Influences testicular differentiation	46,XY sex reversal, campomelic dysplasia
AMH	19p13.3	Suppresses mullerian duct differentiation	Persistence of mullerian duct derivatives
LHCGR	2p21	Transmits effect of LH on androgen synthesis	46,XY sex reversal

LH, luteinizing hormone; FSH, follicle stimulating hormone; GnRH, gonadotropic releasing hormone.

Table 19.27 Discordance between external genitalia and karyotype

Female external genitalia with XY karyotype
- Androgen insufficiency syndromes
- XY gonadal dysgenesis (some)
- Leydig cell agenesis

Male external genitalia with XX karyotype
- XX males
- True hermaphrodites (some)

Table 19.28 Genes and gene products involved in glucocorticoid, mineralocorticoid, and sex hormone biosynthesis and action

Gene	Chromosome	Product	Function	Deficiency state
SLOS	7q32.1	7-Dehydrocholesterol reductase	7-Dehydrocholesterol→ Cholesterol	Smith-Lemli-Opitz syndrome
StAR	8p11.2	StAR	Transporter	Lipoid congenital adrenal hyperplasia (CAH); 46,XY sex reversal
CYP11A	15q23–q24	P450scc	Cholesterol→PREG	–
HSD3B2	1p13.1	3βHSD	PREG→PROG 17PREG→17PROG DHEA→A'DIONE	Male and female pseudohermaphroditism
CYP17	10q24.3	17α-Hydroxylase 17, 20-Lyase	PREG→17PREG PROG→17PROG 17PREG→DHEA 17PROG-A'DIONE	Male pseudohermaphroditism Female infantilism Hypertension
CYP21	6p21.3	P450c21	PROG→DOC 17PROG→deoxycortisol	CAH, classical and nonclassical
CYP11B1	8q21	P450c11	Deoxycortisol→cortisol	CAH, hypertensive form
CYP11B2	8q21	18-Hydroxylase (CMO I) Aldosterone reductase (CMO II)	Corticosterone→18-OH-Corticosterone→Aldosterone	Isolated aldosterone deficiency
HSD17B3	9q22	17βHSD	A'DIONE→Testosterone	Male pseudohermaphroditism
SRD5A2	2p23	Steroid 5α-reductase type 2	Testosterone→DHT	Pseudovaginal perineal hypospadias
AR	Xq11–q12	Transcription factor	Transmit effect of androgens on gene expression	Androgen insensitivity: complete, partial, mild
CYP19	15q21.1	P450arom	Aromatizes androgens to estrogens	Female pseudohermaphroditism
ESR	6q25.1	Transcription factor	Transmits effects of estrogens on gene expression	Male: osteopenia, delayed skeletal maturation

SLOS, Smith-Lemli-Opitz syndrome; StAR, steroidogenic acute regulatory protein; PREG, pregnenolone; 3βHSD, 3β-hydroxysteroid dehydrogenase; PROG, progesterone; 17PREG, 17α-hydroxypregnenolone; 17PROG, 17α-hydroxyprogesterone; DHEA, dehydroepiandrosterone; A'DIONE, androstenedione; DOC, desoxycorticosterone; DHT, dihydrotestosterone.

Table 19.29 Causes of female pseudohermaphroditism

Deficiencies of enzyme activity
- 3β-Hydroxysteroid dehydrogenase-type 2 (chromosome 1p13.1)
- 21-Hydroxylase (chromosome 6p21.3)

Deficiency of placental or germline aromatase

Maternal androgen excess
- Virilizing luteoma
- Congenital adrenal hyperplasia
- Ingestion of androgens/synthetic estrogens

Eponymic syndromes
- Fraser syndrome (cryptophthalmos, ambiguous internal and external genitalia)
- VACTERL association (vertebral-anal-cardiac-tracheoesophageal fistula-radial-renal-limb anomalies)

Table 19.30 Definitions of intersex abnormalities

Ambiguous genitalia – All genitalia that are not completely phenotypically normal are ambiguous, no matter how minor the apparent defect. In any infant with atypical genitalia, consideration must be given to the cause of the ambiguity before assigning the sex of rearing.

XX sex reversal – These phenotypically normal males with 46,XX karyotype are characterized often by short stature, small testes, primary hypogonadism, and the presence of translocated SRY to the distal portion of Xp.

XY sex reversal – These phenotypically normal females with 46,XY karyotype have "pure gonadal dysgenesis" associated with delayed puberty, tall stature, ovarian stroma without oogonia, increased risk for development of gonadoblastoma, and, in some patients, a mutation in SRY. Other examples of 46,XY sex reversal with normal female phenotype include complete androgen insensitivity syndrome and complete deficiency of 17α-hydroxylase.

XY gonadal dysgenesis – This disorder is also termed "mixed" gonadal dysgenesis and is associated with the 45X/46XY karyotype and a phenotype that may vary from that of Turner syndrome to that of a male with short stature and hypoplastic testes. Ambiguous genitalia, one dysgenetic testis, and a streak gonad are most commonly present in these patients.

True hermaphroditism – These patients have ambiguity of external genitalia or internal genitalia, or both, as well as histologic evidence of both ovarian and testicular tissue (either as separate structures or as an ovotestis). The karyotype of these patients is most frequently 46,XX, sometimes with SRY translocated to one of the X chromosomes.

Male pseudohermaphroditism – In these patients, the external and internal genitalia are ambiguous (incompletely masculinized), but the gonads are recognizable as testes, albeit often primitive; the karyotype is 46,XY.

"Vanishing testes" syndrome – Congenital anorchia occurs in phenotypic males with 46,XY karyotype, normal Wolffian duct structures but absent or rudimentary testes; it is likely that the testes were normally functional in the first trimester but then deteriorated, either because of a transplacentally transmitted environmental toxic agent or because of a genetic error (as yet unidentified) in factors necessary to maintain testicular integrity.

Female pseudohermaphroditism – In the female pseudohermaphrodite, the external genitalia are masculinized; the internal genitalia are feminine in the majority of individuals and ambiguous in a few patients.

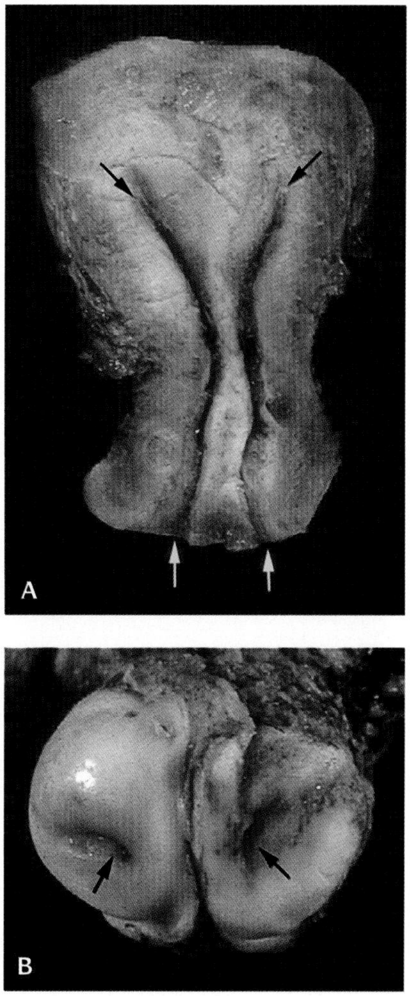

19.40. (A) Bicornuate uterus (black arrows) with septate cervix (yellow arrow) and vagina. **(B)** Septate cervices with vaginal resection margin between them (arrows indicate the os).

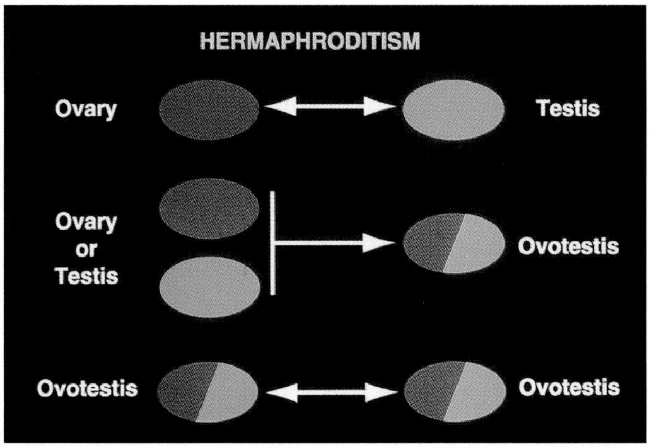

19.41. Types of hermaphroditism.

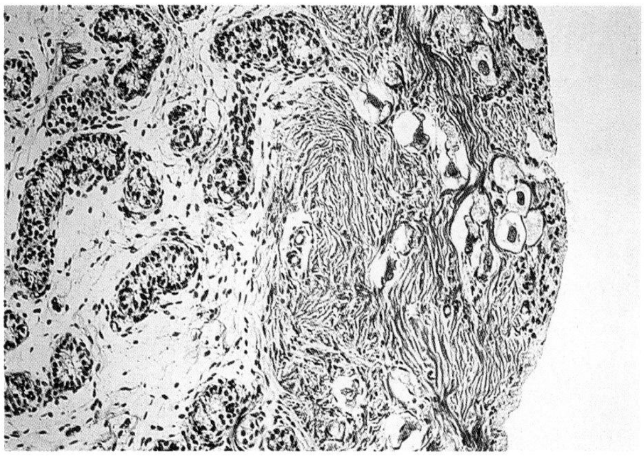

19.42. Microscopic section of ovotestis. Testicular tubules on left, ova on right.

Table 19.31 Types of gonadal dygenesis

	Karyotype	Gonad	Internal organs	External genitalia	Puberty	Fertility	Gonadal malignancy assignment	Sex
Gonadal dysgenesis (Turner syndrome)	XO, etc.	Streak	Immature Müllerian	Female	Eunuchoid	No (one exception)	Usually no	Female
Pure gonadal dysgenesis XX type	XX	Streak	Immature Müllerian	Female	Eunuchoid	No	Usually no	Female
Pure gonadal dysgenesis XY type	XY	Streak	Immature Müllerian	Female	Eunuchoid	No	Yes	Female
Mixed gonadal dysgenesis	XO/XY, etc.	Testis and streak	Wolffian and Müllerian	Ambiguous	Usually virilization	No	Yes	Variable
Reifenstein syndrome	XY	Testis	Wolffian	Hypospadiac male	Virilization with gynecomastia	No	No	Usually male
Testicular feminization syndrome	XY	Testis	Wolffian	Female	Feminization	No	Yes	Female
5α-reductase deficiency	XY	Testis	Wolffian	Female	Virilization	No	No	Female
Dysgenetic testes	XO/XY, etc.	Testis	Wolffian and Müllerian	Ambiguous	Virilization	No	Yes	Variable
	XXY, XX, etc.	Testis	Wolffian	Variable	Partial virilization	No	No	Variable

In previable female fetuses with an abnormal X, or monosomy X, there are usually no morphologic defects. The Müllerian ducts are well differentiated and the ovaries are appropriately developed for the gestational age. Loss of ova and an increase in fibrous tissue usually occur after 20 weeks gestation.

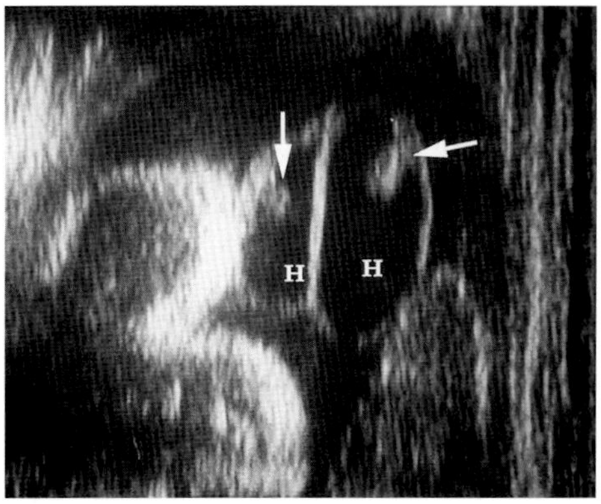

19.43. Ultrasound of bilateral hydroceles (H), testes (arrows) in hydrocele sac.

INTERSEX ABNORMALITIES: (FIGURES 19.48 AND 19.49)

ULTRASONOGRAPHY

A. Renal abnormalities are present in 2–3/100 pregnancies
B. In oligohydramnios due to renal agenesis, adrenals may be mistaken for kidneys
C. Renal dimensions by gestational age

	21–25 wk	26–30 wk	31–35 wk	≥36 wk
	2 SD	2 SD	2 SD	2 SD
AP Diameter	8–22 mm	16–23 mm	16–28 mm	17–30 mm
Transverse	8–24 mm	14–26 mm	15–32 mm	16–36 mm
Circumference	40–68 mm	52–79 mm	61–96 mm	56–112 mm
Kid Circ/Abd Circ	0.26–0.34	0.25–0.33	0.22–0.34	0.19–0.35

(From Grannum: *Am J Obstet Gynecol* 136:253, 1980)

D. Pyelectasis is associated with postnatal congenital hydronephrosis
E. Frequency of postnatal renal compromise or requiring corrective surgery

Renal Pelvis	14–23 wk	24–32 wk	33–42 wk
<3 mm	0	0	0
4–6 mm	19%	13%	0
7–9 mm	40%	6%	50%
>10 mm	73%	72%	59%

(From Corteville JE, Gray DL, Crane JP: Congenital hydronephrosis: correlation of fetal ultrasonographic findings with infant outcome. *Am J Obstet Gynecol* 165:384, 1991)

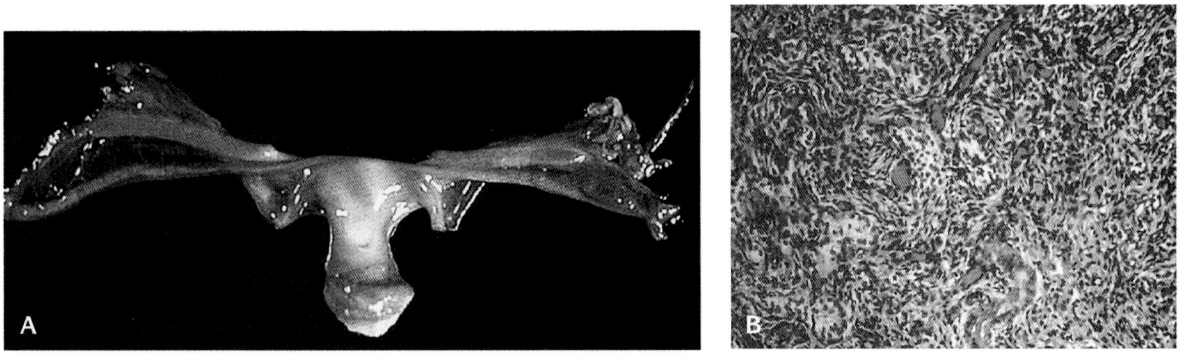

19.44. (A) Streak ovaries in a case monosomy X (Turner Syndrome). **(B)** Microscopic appearance of a streak ovary showing dense ovarian stroma lacking ova.

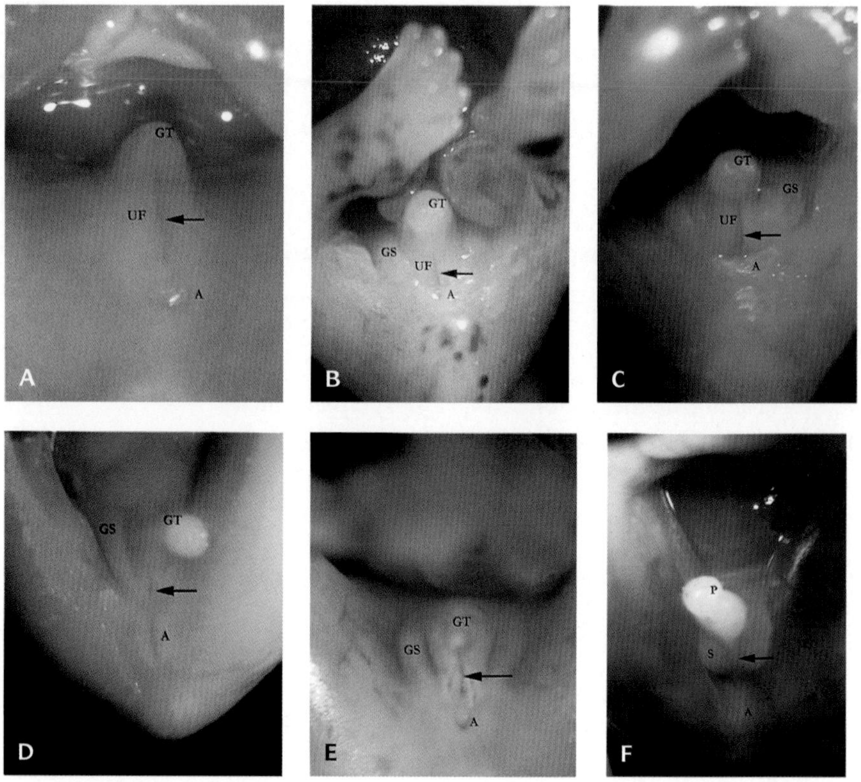

19.45. Normal development of external genitalia. **(A)** 7 weeks. **(B)** 8 weeks. **(C)** 9 weeks. **(D)** 10 weeks. **(E)** Female, 12 weeks (arrow, vaginal opening). **(F)** Male, 12 weeks (P, phallus; S, scrotum; arrow, scrotal septum). (GT, genital tubercle; UF, urethral fold; A, anus; GS, genital swelling; arrow, urethral groove.)

F. Recommendations for a follow-up evaluation if renal pelvic dilation (pyelectasis) is noted on initial sonography

>4 mm at 15–20 weeks gestation
>8 mm at 20–30 weeks gestation
>10 mm at >30 weeks gestation
(From Mandel J: *Radiology* 178:193, 1991)

G. Dilation of the renal pelvis is associated with:
   1. Aneuploidy present in 11% of cases (usually trisomy 21, trisomy 18, or trisomy 13)
      a. 3% aneuploidy in cases of isolated renal aberrations
      b. 24% aneuploidy if other abnormalities are present
      c. Risk of aneuploidy increases if other abnormalities are noted on sonogram
   2. Mild pyelectasis
      a. 3-fold increased risk for aneuploidy
      b. 30-fold increased risk for aneuploidy if additional abnormalities are present

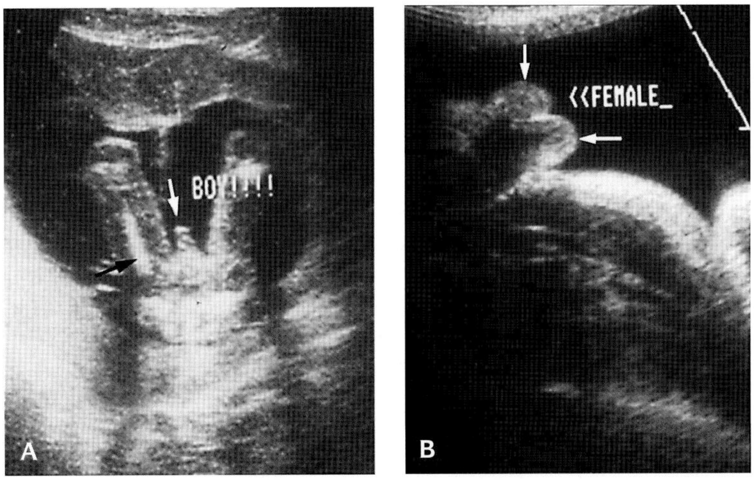

19.46. **(A)** Ultrasound of normal male at 16 weeks. **(B)** Ultrasound of female at 16 weeks.

3. Distal urinary tract obstruction or malformation
4. Uretero-pelvic junction (UPJ) abnormality
5. Ureteral atresia
6. Duplicated ureters
7. Posterior urethral valves (usually with megacystis and hydroureter)

H. Renal function can be evaluated antenatally:

	Prognosis	
	Poor	**Good**
Findings:		
Amniotic fluid volume	Moderate to severely decreased	Normal or moderately decreased
Appearance	Echogenic or cystic	Normal or echogenic
Urinary electrolytes		
Na	>100	<100
C1	>90	<90
Osmolarity	>210	<210
Urine output	<2mL/h	>2mL/h

(From Glick J: *Pediatr Surg* 20:376, 1985)

I. Cystic kidneys
  1. Adult polycystic kidney disease
     a. Multiple cysts of varying size replace the renal parenchyma. It is usually present in adulthood, but neonatal cases may occur
     b. One of the most common genetic disorders
     c. Usually bilateral, although only one kidney may initially appear abnormal
     d. Often does not manifest until the third trimester

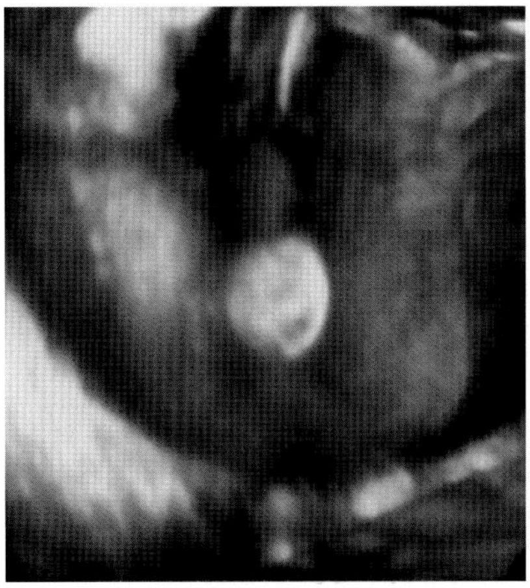

19.47. Three-dimensional ultrasound of a 26-week gestation male. The white area at midphotograph is the scrotum.

2. Infantile polycystic kidney disease
   a. Multiple cysts of varying size replace the renal parenchyma, with bilateral disease always present. It is not related to obstruction of the urinary system
   b. Similar to adult polycystic disease in appearance, but family history will usually provide ability to distinguish the two
   c. Autosomal recessive inheritance
   d. Four common presentations:
      i. Perinatal – In utero renal failure with massively dilated kidneys, 90% renal involvement, and high rates of neonatal demise

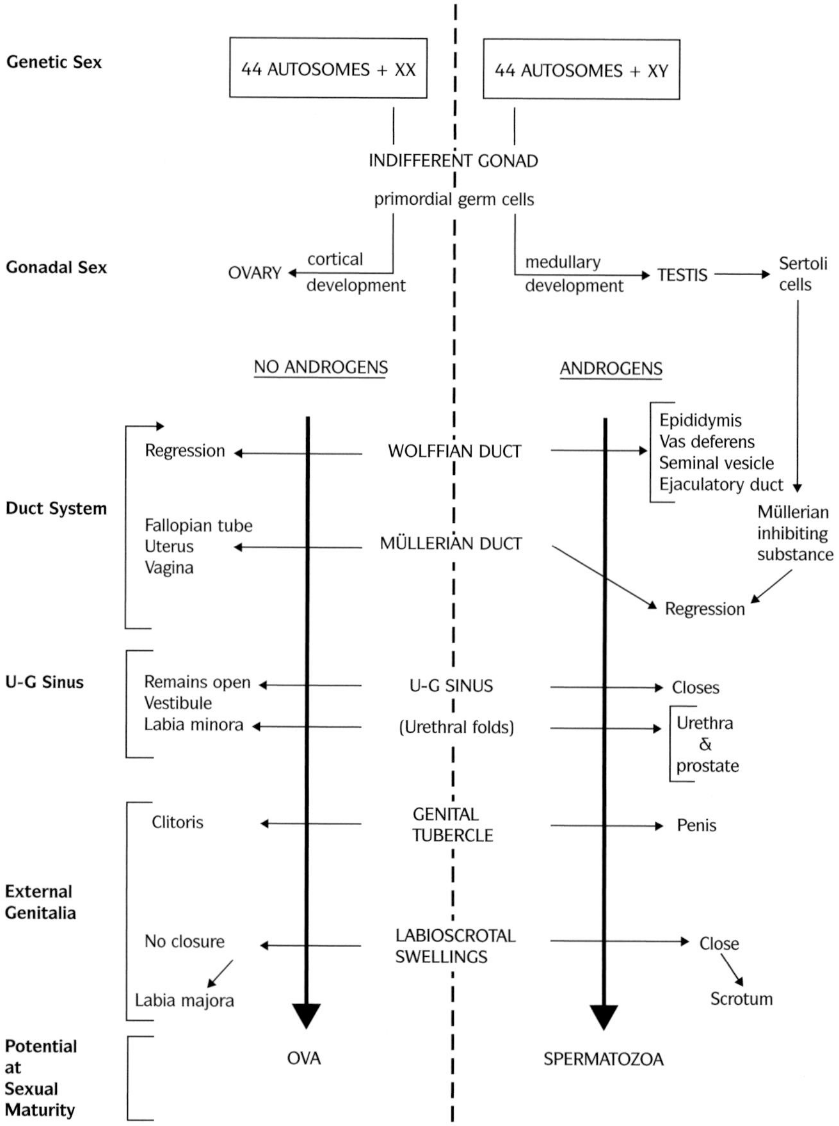

19.48. Flow sheet of sex differentiation and morphogenesis. U-G, urogenital. (From Gilbert-Barness E. *Potter's Pathology of the Fetus and Infant*. Philadelphia, Mosby, 1997.)

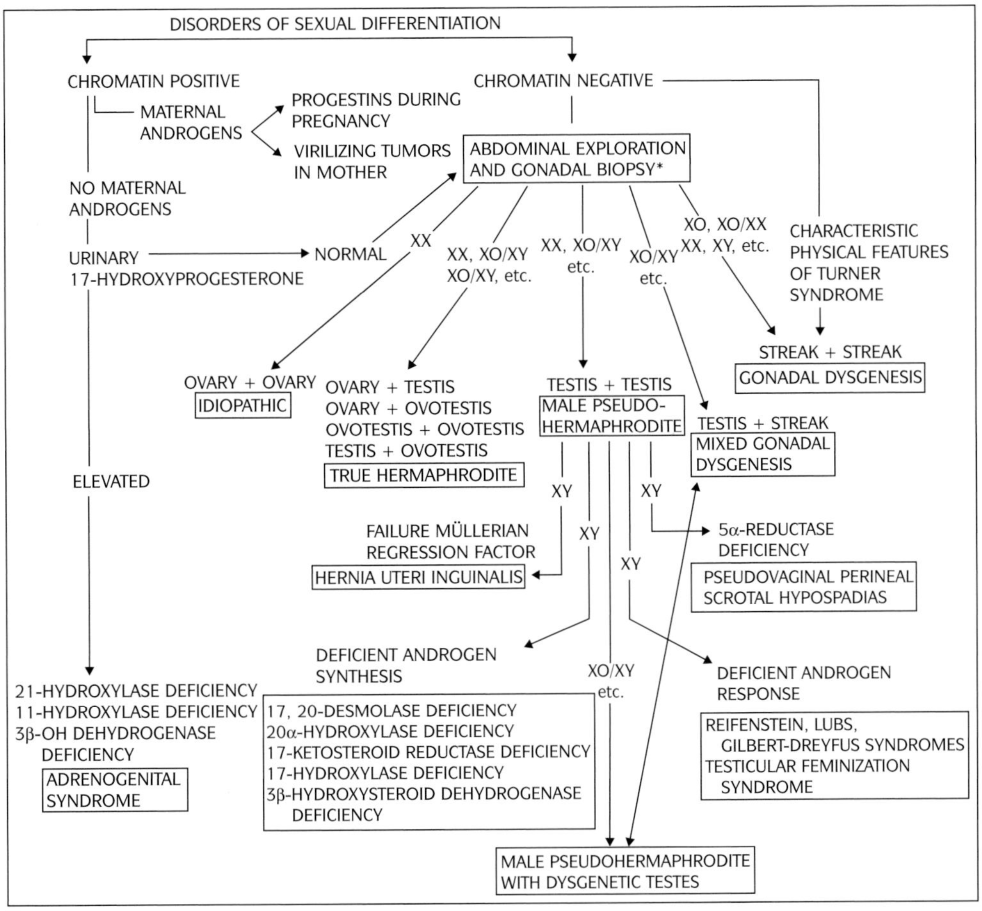

19.49. Schematic diagram of disorders of sexual differentiation. (Data from Allen TD: *Urology* 7 (Suppl 1): 1, 1976.)

ii. Neonatal – Onset occurring after 1 month of life with less significant renal enlargement, 60% renal involvement, mild hepatic fibrosis, and death occurs within 1 year of life

iii. Infantile – Disease presents at 3–6 months of age, with less renal involvement and a disease course similar to the infantile form.

e. Multicystic kidney disease

f. Bilateral, unilateral, or segmental dysplasia of the renal parenchyma corresponding to dilation of the collecting tubules which have a characteristic ultrasonic appearance. Multiple, round, peripheral cysts of variable size, enlarged kidneys (usually) with the appearance of grape-like clusters of cysts which do not communicate and obliterate the renal parenchyma. With bilateral disease, the fetal bladder does not fill over time, or with administration of furosemide. Oligohydramnios is usually present.

g. May result from either early obstructive uropathy or from developmental failure of the mesonephric blastema

h. Usually occurs sporadically or within families, and occasionally reported with maternal diabetes
i. Often occurs in association with autosomal recessive (Meckel, Dandy-Walker, Zellweger, Roberts, Fryns, Smith-Lemli-Opitz, others) and dominant (Apert) syndromes, and with aneuploidy (trisomy 9)
j. The differential diagnosis includes infantile polycystic kidney disease and ureteropelvic junction obstruction
k. Bilateral disease is a fatal condition, while those with unilateral disease are at increased risk for hypertension

Determine the presence of a bladder

- Presence of the bladder (and amniotic fluid after 16 weeks gestation) indicates some degree of renal function was present in the past
- Emptying and filling of the bladder can be quantitated
- An absent bladder indicates either poor fetal status (resulting in anuria), or genitourinary disease in proximal structures

Determine presence of a single umbilical artery

- Higher frequencies note in autopsy series
- More common in white fetuses
- More common in placentas with marginal or velamentous insertion
- More common in twins
  - Monozygotic twin fetuses are usually discordant for single umbilical artery
- May result from primary agenesis of one of the arteries, secondary atrophy of an umbilical artery, or persistence of the original single allantoic artery of the body stalk
- Umbilical artery evaluation should be performed near the abdominal cord insertion in the fetal abdomen.
  - Isolated single artery at the placental insertion site does not appear to have the same negative association as this same finding more proximally in the cord.
- Additional structural abnormalities are found in 20–50% of cases
  - Multiple anomalies noted in 20% of fetuses
  - Associated anomalies in single umbilical artery include:
    - Musculo-skeletal abnormalities – 23%
    - Genito-urinary abnormalities – 20%
    - Cardiovascular abnormalities – 19%
    - Gastrointestinal abnormalities – 10%
    - Central nervous system anomalies – 8%
- Single umbilical artery is associated with aneuploidy
  - Trisomy 18 (most often)
  - Trisomy 13
  - Turner syndrome
  - Triploidy

- The risk of aneuploidy is proportional to the presence of other anomalies. If present the rate of aneuploidy is 40%
- Rate of 33–43% aneuploidy reported if other anomalies are present
  - The combination of CNS abnormalities and single umbilical artery is associated with 50% aneuploidy.

REFERENCES

Bernstein, J, Risdon RA: Renal system. I. Kidneys and urinary tract. In Gilbert-Barness E (ed): *Potter's Pathology of the Fetus and Infant.* St. Louis, Mosby, 1997, p. 863.

Bernstein J, Risdon RA, Joshi VV: Renal System. In Gilbert-Barness E (ed): *Potter's Atlas of Fetal and Infant Pathology.* St. Louis, Mosby, 1998.

Bernstein J: Renal cystic disease in the tuberous sclerosis complex. *Pediatr Nephrol* 7:490, 1993.

Bernstein J: A classification of renal cysts. In Gardner KD Jr, Bernstein J (eds): *The Cystic Kidney.* Kluwer Academic Publishers, 147:70, 1990.

Bernstein J: Glomerulocystic disease: Nosological considerations. *Pediatr Nephrol* 7:464, 1993.

Bernstein J: Renal cystic disease in the tuberous sclerosis complex. *Pediatr Nephrol* 7:490, 1993.

Dedeoglu IO, Fisher JE, Springate JE, et al.: Spectrum of glomerulocystic kidneys: a case report and review of the literature. *Ped Path Lab Med* 16:941, 1996.

Dodd S: The pathogenesis of tubulointerstitial diseases and mechanisms of fibrosis. *Curr Top Pathol* 88:51, 1995.

Gagnadoux MF, Bacri JL, Broyer M, Hasbib H: Infantile chronic tubulointerstitial nephritis with cortical microcysts: variant of nephronophthisis or new disease entity. *Pediatr Nephrol* 3:50, 1989.

Griffin MD, Torres BE, Kumar R: Cystic kidney disease. *Current Opinion Neph & Hypertension* 6:276, 1997.

Habib R: Nephrotic syndrome in the first year of life. *Pediatr Nephrol* 7:347, 1993.

Kaplan BS, Restaino I, Raval D, et al.: Renal failure in the neonate associated with in utero exposure to non-steroidal anti-inflammatory agents. *Pediatr Nephrol* 8:700, 1994.

Kissane JM: Renal cysts in pediatric patients. A classification and overview. *Ped Nephro* 4:69, 1990.

Manivel JC, Pettinato G, Reinberg Y, et al.: Prune belly syndrome: clinicopathologic study of 29 cases. *Pediatr Pathol* 9:691, 1989.

Murugasu B, Cole BR, Hawkins EP, et al.: Familial renal adysplasia. *Am J Kidney Dis* 18:490, 1991.

Rapola J, Kaariaimen H: Morphologic diagnosis of recessive and dominant polycystic kidney disease in infancy and childhood. *Acta Pathol Microbiol Scand* 96:68, 1988.

Risdon RA: Renal dysplasia. 1. A clinico-pathologic study of 76 cases. II: A necropsy study of 41 cases. *J Clin Pathol* 24:57, 1971.

Risdon RA: Pyelonephritis and reflux nephropathy. In Tisher CC, Brenner BM (eds): *Renal Pathology with Clinical and Functional Correlations*, 2nd ed. Philadelphia, JB Lippincott, 1994, p. 832.

Root AW: Genetics errors of sexual differentiation. *Adv Pediatr* 46:67, 1998.

Shokeir MHK: Expression of "adult" polycystic renal disease in the fetus and newborn. *Am J Clin Pathol* 55:391, 1971.

TWENTY

Congenital Tumors

Congenital tumors are often composed of persistent embryonal or fetal tissues, suggesting a failure of proper cytodifferentiation or maturation during early life. Neuroblastoma develops from neural crest cells that migrate into the gland during embryonic and fetal life. Normally, these cells mature to ganglion cells.

Morphologic features of embryonic neoplasms include retinoblastoma, peripheral primitive neuroectodermal tumor (PNET), hepatoblastoma, yolk sac tumor of the testis, and embryonal rhabdomyosarcoma. Some teratomas show proliferation of embryonic tissues that fail to mature. A number of tumors in the young are associated with congenital malformations and growth disturbances.

Some embryonic tumors have a benign course despite a malignant microscopic appearance such as stage IV-S neuroblastoma, congenital fibrosarcoma, and nephroblastomatosis. These tumors may undergo cytodifferentiation and spontaneous regression. Malignant neoplasms are seldom seen in the newborn and only infrequently are responsible for neonatal death or spontaneous abortion. Chromosomal abnormalities associated with childhood tumors are shown in Table 20.1.

VASCULAR TUMORS

Hemangiomas are the most common tumors of the skin and soft tissues in infants (Figure 20.1).

Table 20.1 Chromosomal abnormalities associated with childhood tumors

Chromosomal defect	Childhood tumor
1p deletion	Neuoblastoma Melanoma Thyroid medullary carcinoma
3p deletion	Wilms tumor Hepatoblastoma Embryonal rhabdomyosarcoma Adrenal adenoma
11p13 deletion	Wilms tumor
13q14 deletion	Retinoblastoma Osteosarcoma
22q deletion	Neurofibroma
p32p36 deletion	Neuroblastoma
Monosomy 7	Leukemia
t(1:22)	Acute megakaryoblastic leukemia
Trisomy 18	Wilms tumor
Trisomy 21 (Down syndrome)	Leukemia
Gonadal dysgenesis (45,X/46XY)	Gonadoblastoma Germinoma
Klinefelter syndrome (XXY)	Teratoma Breast carcinoma

Data from Isaacs H Jr: *Tumors of the Fetus and Infant.* WB Saunders Co., Philadelphia, 1997.

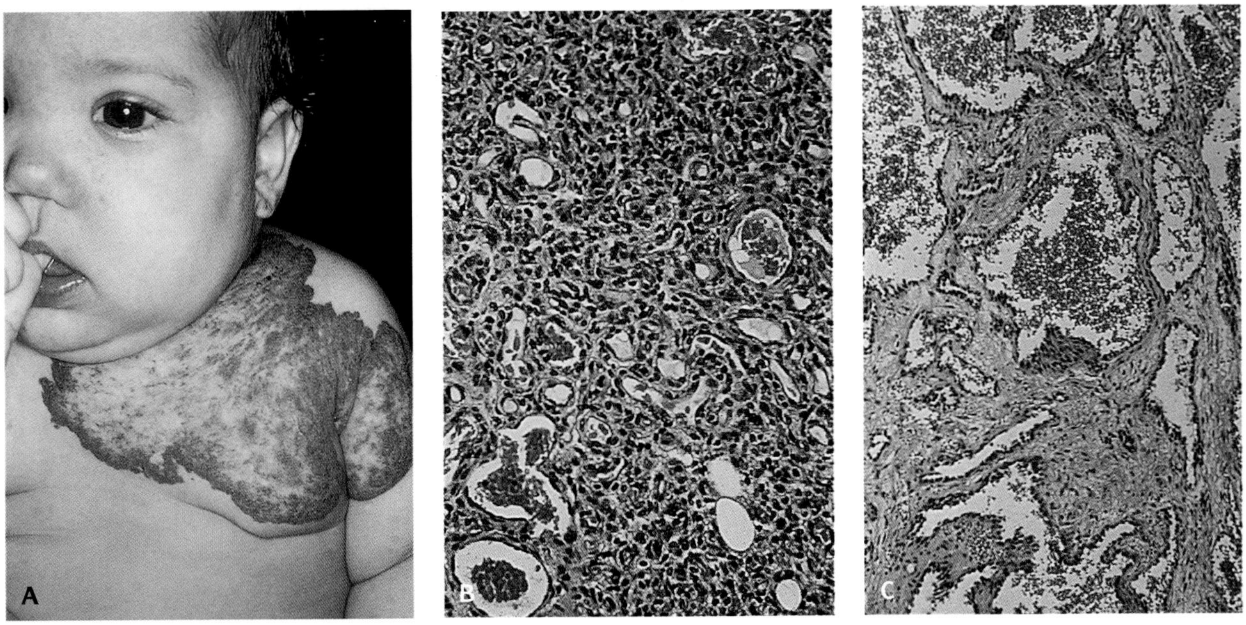

20.1. **(A)** Hemangioma of the neck and shoulder in a newborn. **(B)** Microscopic appearance of a capillary hemangioma. **(C)** Microscopic appearance of a cavernous hemangioma.

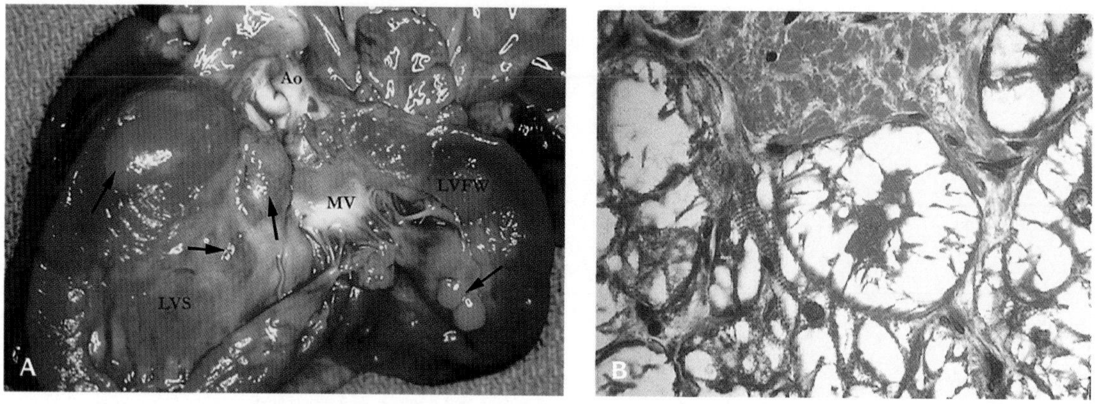

20.2. **(A)** Multiple rhabdomyomas of the heart in a newborn with tuberous sclerosis (arrows, tumor; AO, aorta; LVFW, left ventricular free wall; LVS, left side of ventricular septum). **(B)** Microscopic appearance of rhabdomyoma showing typical spider cells.

Benign Hemangiomas

Capillary hemangioma usually manifests at birth, grows steadily for 6–8 months, then stabilizes, and eventually regresses, although complete disappearance may take several years. It is composed of capillaries separated by stroma. It may present as a raised subcutaneous nodule that blanches under pressure. Because childhood hemangiomas are tumors that evolve in time, a capillary hemangioma is thought to originate from a more primitive form.

In a **cellular angioma** (infantile hemangioendothelioma), the number of tumor cells greatly exceeds the number of vascular lumina present.

Cavernous hemangioma is formed by vessels larger than capillary size.

Pyogenic granuloma is similar to capillary hemangioma but occurs at mucosal sites, is pedunculated, and has an epithelial collarette at the stalk.

Benign hemangiomas, both superficial and deep, may be part of numerous malformation syndromes:

- *Klippel-Trenaunay* (angio-osteohypertrophy)
- *Castleman disease* (angiofollicular hyperplasia of lymph nodes, may have a glomeruloid angiomatous pattern)
- *Takayasu* disease
- *Sturge-Weber* (encephalo-trigeminal angiomatosis)
- *Fabry disease* (angiokeratomas of the skin)
- *POEMS* (polyneuropathy, organomegaly, endocrinopathy, monoclonal protein, and skin changes)

TUMORS OF STRIATED MUSCLE

The benign rhabdomyoma, *fetal rhabdomyoma*, shows a marked propensity to arise in the head and neck and presents as a subcutaneous or submucosal polypoid mass at birth (Figure 20.2). It is composed of benign spindle cells interspersed with striated muscle cells. Fetal rhabdomyomas are benign tumors.

Rhabdomyosarcoma

Rhabdomyosarcoma is seldom noted at birth (Figure 20.3). Half the neonatal tumors arise caudally: buttock/sacrococcygeal, perirectal, bladder, and vagina. Other locations are neck, thorax, oropharynx, chest wall, and thigh.

Embryonal rhabdomyosarcoma – the most common type – has a >60% 5-year survival (Figure 20.4). It is composed of primitive mesenchymal cells. The nuclei are smaller than those of alveolar rhabdomyosarcoma cells, and the nucleoli are inconspicuous.

The sites of the botryoid, embryonal, and unspecified rhabdomyosarcoma types include the vagina, axilla, tongue, and paraspinal area.

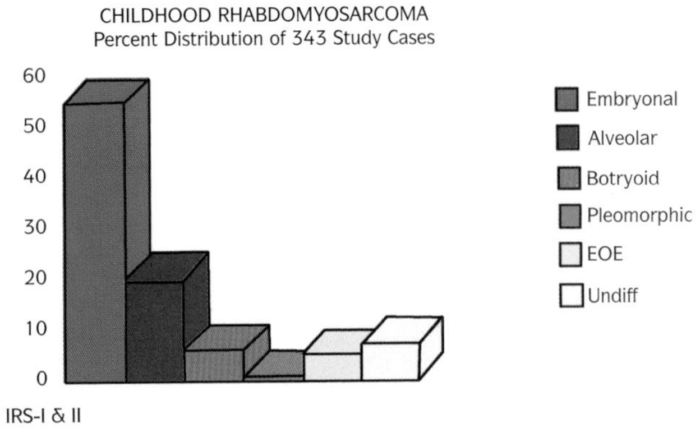

20.3. Childhood rhabdomyosarcoma. (Courtesy of Dr. Gonzales-Crussi.)

Subtypes of embryonal rhabdomyosarcoma with favorable prognosis (95% survival at 5 years) include the following:

1. *Spindle cell rhabdomyosarcoma* – occurs predominantly in the paratesticular region; it is composed of spindle-shaped cells reminiscent of smooth muscle cells.
2. *Botryoid rhabdomyosarcoma* – a polypoid growth projects into a mucosa-lined body cavity (Figure 20.5). It grossly resembles a bunch of grapes. Microscopic features are (1) presence of an intact epithelium at the surface, a feature required to evaluate the superficial condensation of cells; (2) presence of a well preserved, pluricellular layer of tumor cells under the surface epithelium (*cambium layer*).

Alveolar rhabdomyosarcoma usually arises in the neck area and foot regions. NMYC oncogene is amplified in alveolar but not in embryonal rhabdomyosarcoma (Figure 20.6). Fifty percent survive 5 years after diagnosis. It frequently involves the extremities. The cells are arranged against fibrous septa that partition the tumor into an alveolar pattern. The nuclei are round or oval with distinct nuclear membranes; the number of nucleoli is variable.

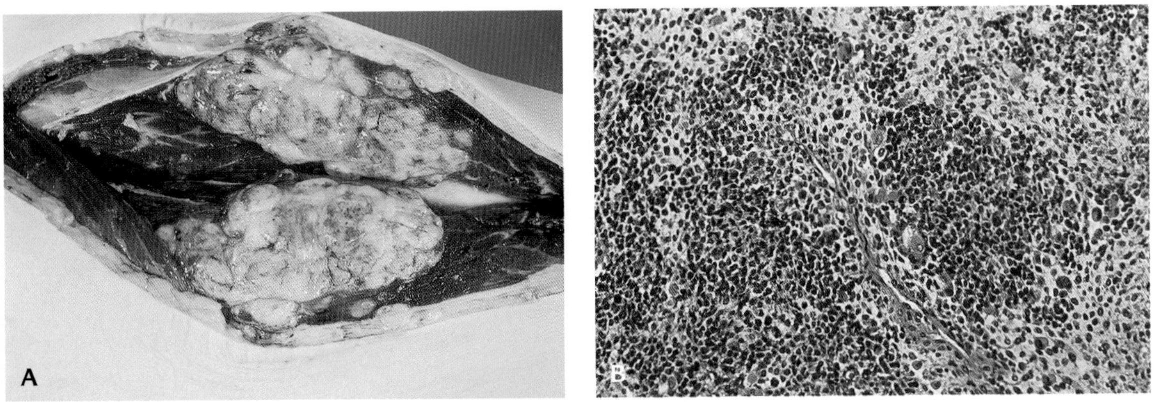

20.4. (A) Surgically excised rhabdomyosarcoma from the thigh. **(B)** Microscopic appearance of an embryonal rhabdomyosarcoma composed of small, dark blue cells.

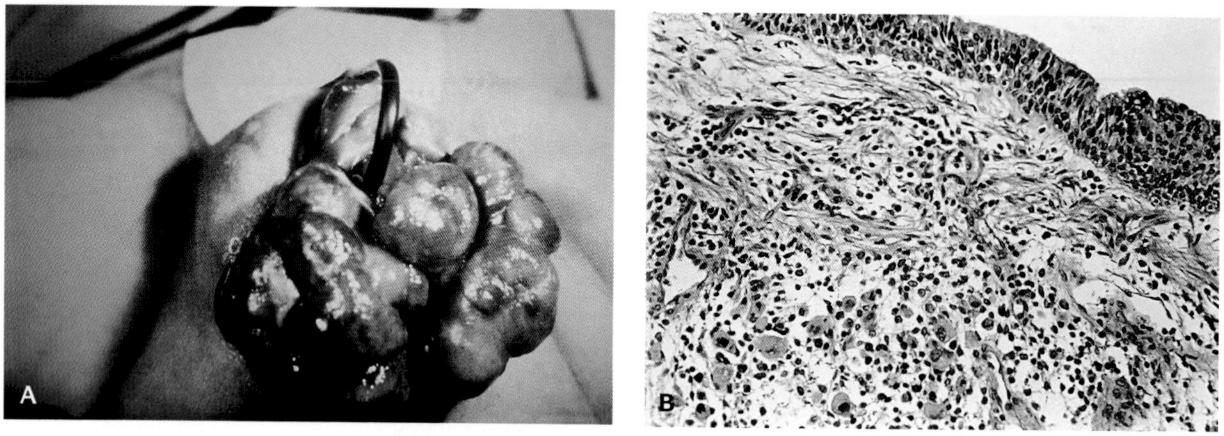

20.5. **(A)** Sarcoma botryoides with grape-like clusters emerging from the vaginal orifice in a newborn infant. **(B)** Microscopic appearance of sarcoma botryoides. Beneath the cambium layer are tumor cells.

Undifferentiated sarcomas are composed of closely packed, round cells with a scant to moderate amount of cytoplasm. The nuclei are irregular in contour, vesicular, with a single or a few prominent nucleoli.

Pleomorphic form of rhabdomyosarcoma is unusual in children. Foci of large cells with hyperchromatic, polyploid, "monstrous" nuclei are seen.

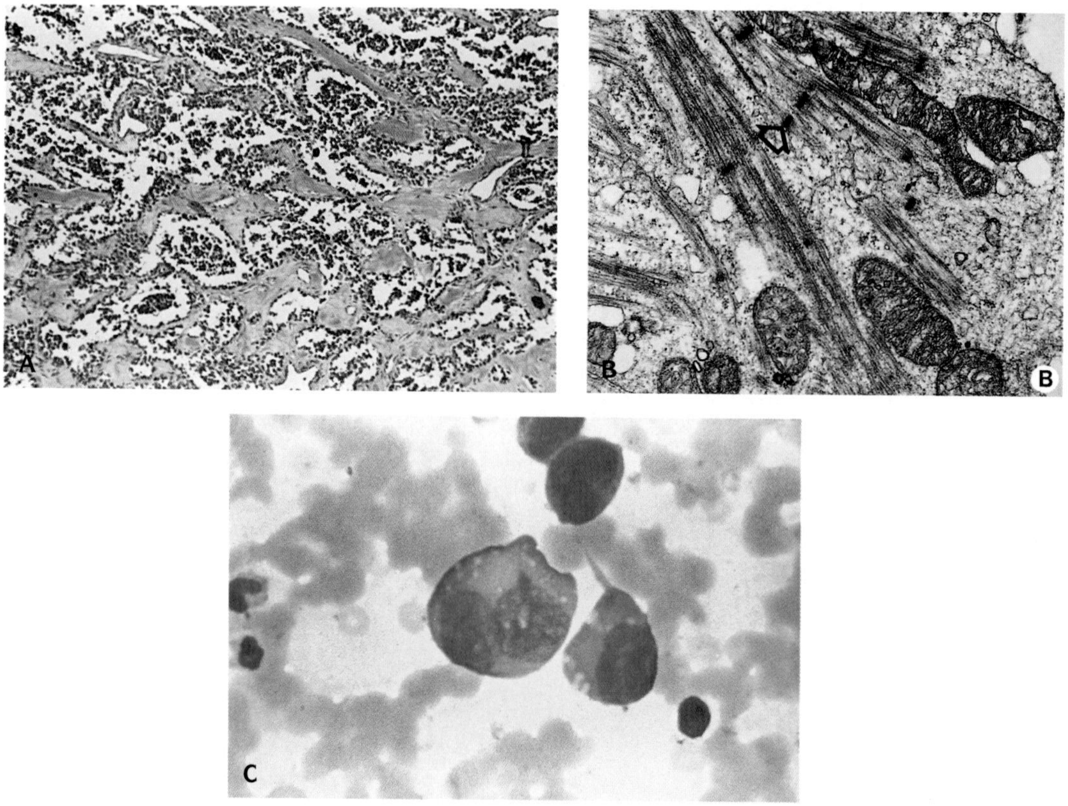

20.6. **(A)** Microscopic appearance of alveolar rhabdomyosarcoma. The tumor cells form an alveolar pattern separated by fibrous tissue septa. **(B)** Electron micrograph of alveolar rhabdomyosarcoma with myofilaments and z bands (arrow). **(C)** Bone marrow aspirate with rhabdomyosarcoma cells showing typical tails.

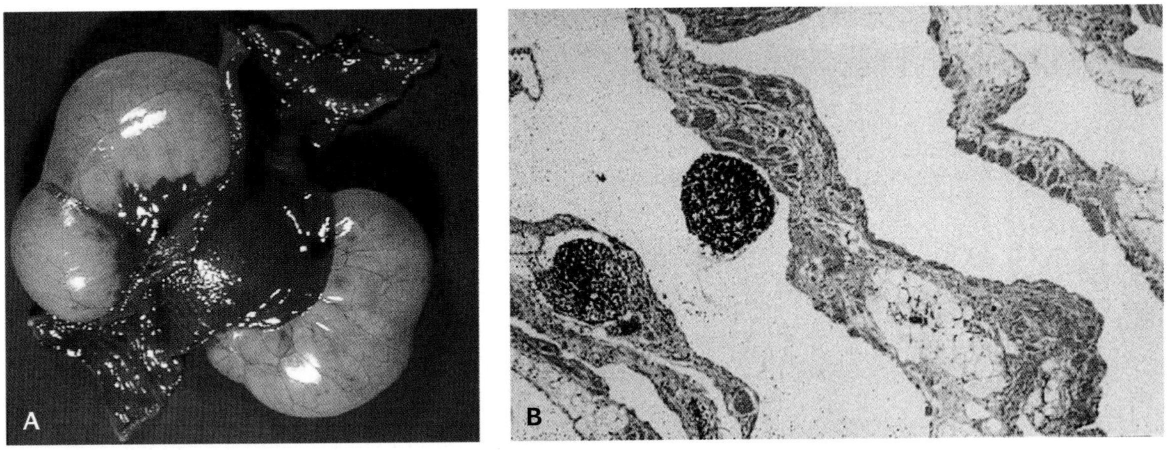

20.7. **(A)** Lymphangioma of the mesentery in a newborn. **(B)** Microscopic appearance showing dilated lymphatic spaces and clusters of lymphocytes.

Lymphangiomas

The usual location of cystic lymphangioma is the neck (cystic hygroma), axilla, inguinal region, or retroperitoneum (Figure 20.7). *Cystic lymphangioma of the mesentery* arises from the mesentery of the ileocecal region and terminal ileum, the jejunal mesentery, omentum, mesocolon, and retroperitoneum.

Table 20.2 WHO classification of germ cell tumors

Classification	Description
1. Dysgerminoma ("germinoma")	Variant – with syncytiotrophoblast cells
2. Yolk sac tumor (endodermal sinus tumor)	Variants – Polyvesicular vitelline tumor – hepatoid – glandular ("endometroid")
3. Embryonal carcinoma	
4. Polyembryoma	
5. Choriocarcinoma	
6. Teratomas	1. Immature 2. Mature Solid Cystic (dermoid cyst) With secondary tumor (specify type) Fetiform (homunculus) 3. Monodermal Stroma ovarii Carcinoid Mucinous carcinoid Neuroectodermal tumors (specify type) Sebaceous tumors Others 4. Mixed (specify types*)
7. Gonadoblastoma	Variant – with dysgerminoma or other germ cell tumor
8. Germ cell sex cord, stromal tumor	Variant – with dysgerminoma or other germ cell tumor

* For example, immature teratoma + yolk sac tumor

Adapted from Scully RE in Gilbert-Barness E (ed): *Potter's Pathology of the Fetus and Infant.* St. Louis, Mosby, 1997.

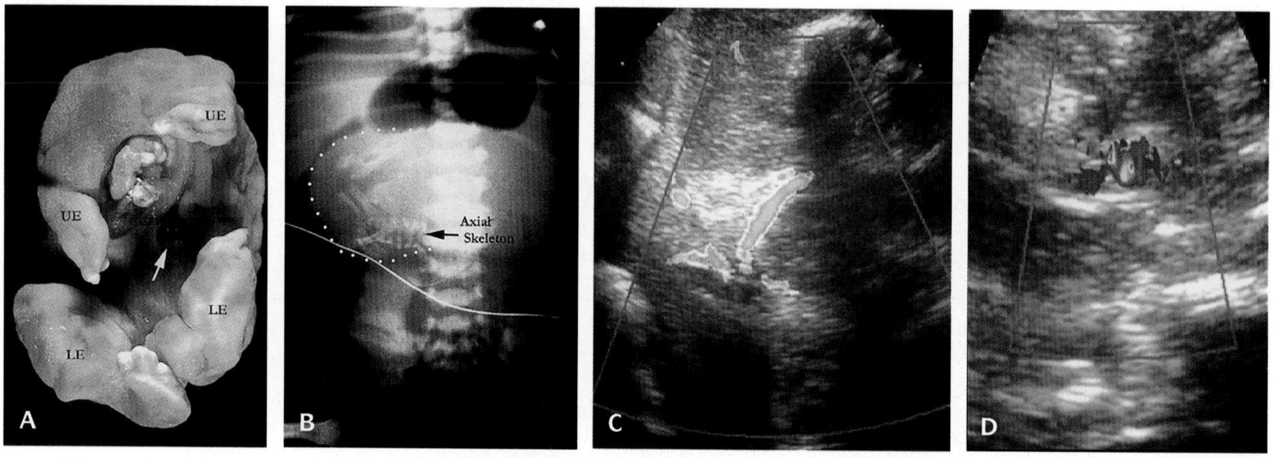

20.8. **(A)** Fetus in fetu from the retroperitoneum of a newborn infant. (LE, lower extremity; UE, upper extremity arrow-vascular attachment). **(B)** X-rays of fetus in fetu (outlined with white dots) showing axial skeleton and bony structures. **(C)** Doppler flow ultrasound of fetus in fetu showing a beating vessel from aorta. **(D)** Doppler flow ultrasound showing a beating heart.

GERM CELL TUMORS

Teratomas

A *teratoma* is defined as a true tumor composed of multiple tissues foreign to, and capable of growth in excess of, those characteristic of the part from which it is derived (Table 20.2). By definition, teratomas are composed of tissues representing each of the three layers of the embryonic disk.

The immature teratoma consists primarily of embryonic-appearing neuroglial or neuroepithelial components, which may coexist along with mature tissues.

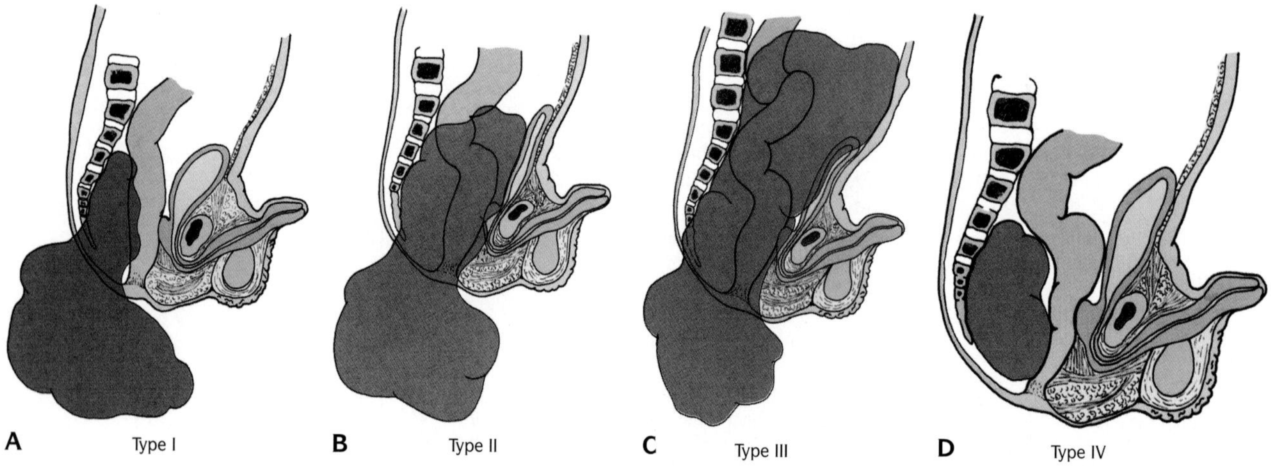

20.9. Types of sacrococcygeal teratomas. **(A)** Type I – The tumor presents externally without a significant intrapelvic extension. **(B)** Type II – The tumor is predominately external (sacrococcygeal) with only a minimal presacral component. **(C)** Type III – The tumor is apparent externally but the predominant mass is pelvic and extends into the abdomen. **(D)** Type IV – Presacral tumor with no external presentation.

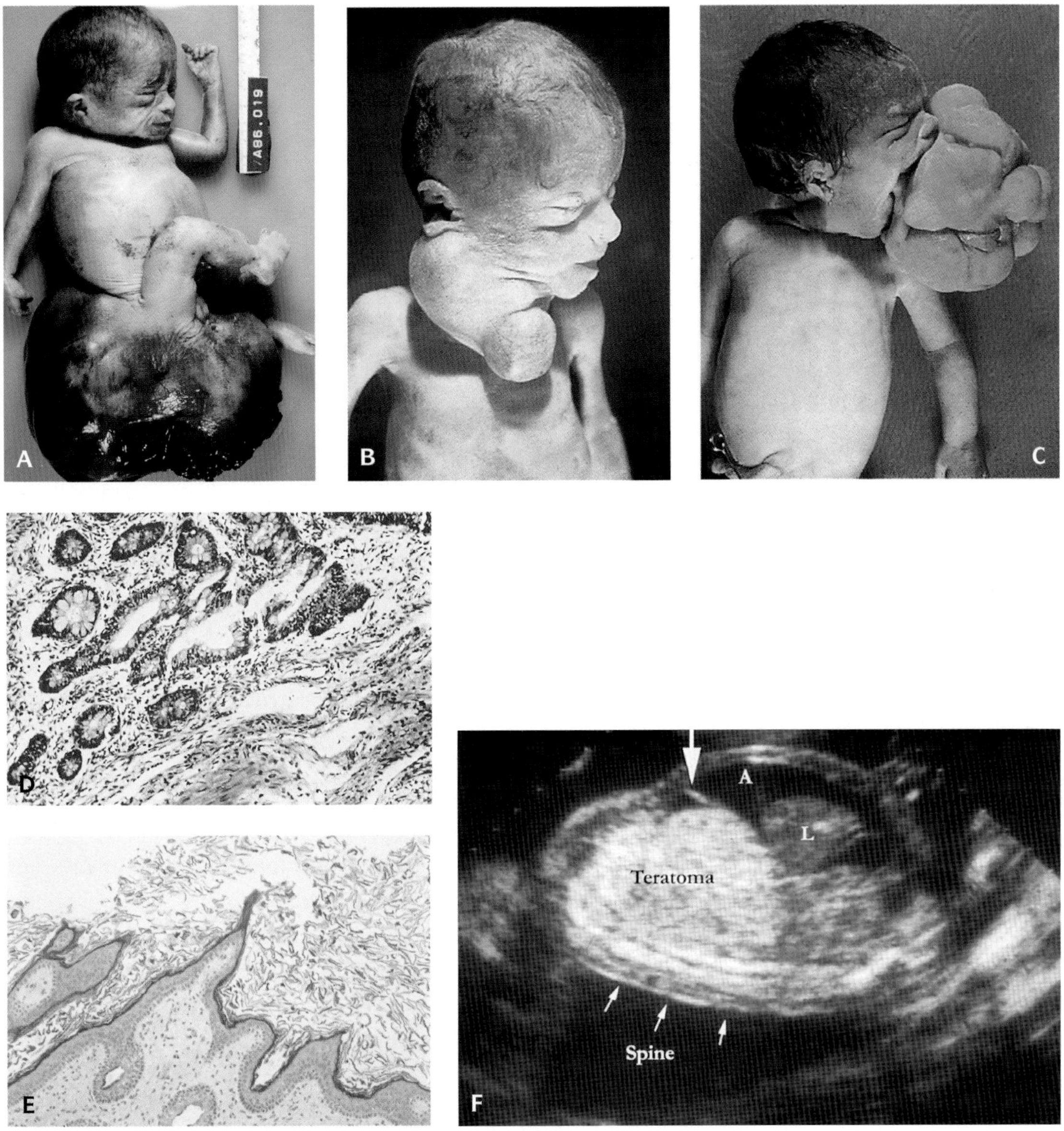

20.10. **(A)** Sacrococcygeal teratoma. **(B)** Thyrocervical teratoma. **(C)** Maxillary teratoma (epignathus). **(D)** Microscopic appearance of benign teratoma containing squamous mature glands and mesenchymal elements. **(E)** Squamous elements with keratin. **(F)** Ultrasound of a mediastinal teratoma. (Arrow, diaphragm; A, ascites; L, liver.)

Fetus in Fetu

The relationship between fetus in fetu and teratoma remains controversial (Figure 20.8). *Fetus in fetu* has vertebrae or notochord and a structural organization that exceeds that of a teratoma. An abdominal retroperitoneal mass is the most common clinical finding but may be found in other locations.

Sacrococcygeal Teratoma

Sacrococcygeal teratoma is the most common neoplasm in the fetus and newborn with an estimated incidence of 1/20,000 to 1/40,000 births, with a female predominance (Figures 20.9 and 20.10).

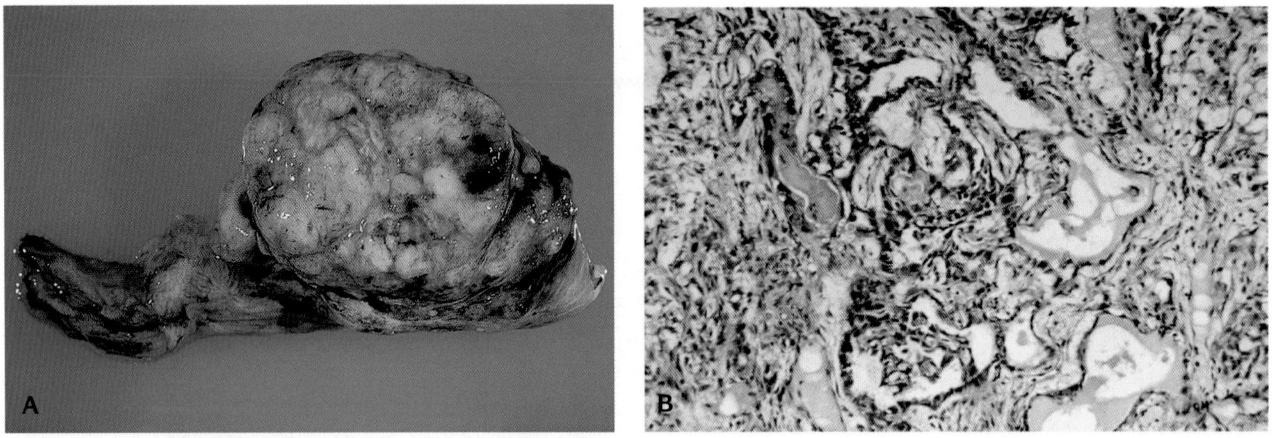

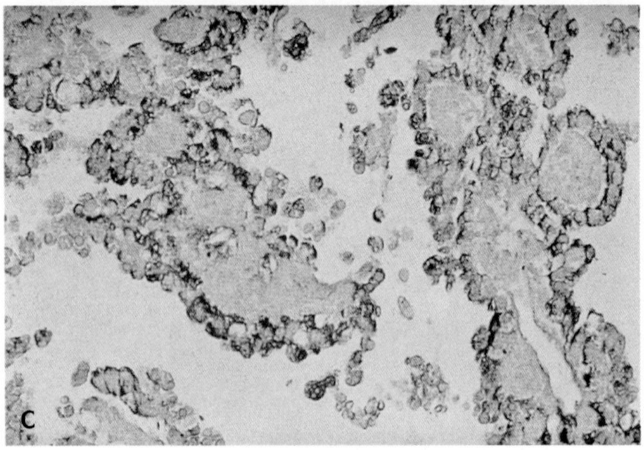

20.11. Yolk sac tumor. **(A)** A testicular tumor showing cystic and solid components. **(B)** Microscopic appearance with polyvesicular pattern. **(C)** Positive immunoperoxidase stain for AFP.

Eighteen percent of patients with sacrococcygeal teratomas have associated congenital defects, such as tracheoesophageal fistula, imperforate anus, anorectal stenosis, spina bifida, genitourinary malformations, meningomyelocele, and anencephaly.

Teratomas may also occur in other sites (Tables 20.3 and 20.4) including the cervico thyroidal region, maxillary area (epignathus), and in midline structures as well as the ovary and testis.

Yolk Sac Tumor

Yolk sac tumor (endodermal sinus tumor) is the leading malignant germ cell tumor affecting infants and children (Figures 20.11 and 20.12 and Tables 20.5 and 20.6). More arise from the sacrococcygeal area than from any other location during the first year of life. The head and neck, testis, pelvic retroperitoneum, vagina, and, seldom, the ovary are other sites. Childhood yolk sac tumors have deletions in chromosomes 1 (Ip) and 6 (6q) but no evidence of i(12p) deletion, which is described in adult germ cell tumors. It may involve the testis.

Table 20.3 Sites of perinatal teratomas

Spinal canal	Maxillary (epignathus)
Sacrococcygeal	Nasopharynx
Neck	Mediastinum
Head (face)	Pharynx
Occiput	Pericardium
Orbit	Liver
Retroperitoneum	Abdominal wall

Table 20.4 Sites of teratomas in children

	Percent
Mediastinal	10
Gonads – ovary	10
testis	
Sacrococcygeal and presacral	65
Cervical	10
Other sites	5
– Base of skull (epignathus)	
– Pineal gland	
– Viscera – stomach, kidney, lung, liver, heart	
– Paravertebral and vertebral canal	
– Intrapericardial	

Vaginal yolk sac tumor is a distinctive lesion. It is a polypoid mass projecting into the vaginal lumen. It is positive for α-fetoprotein (AFP) immunoperoxidase staining. Neonatal ovarian yolk sac tumor has not been reported.

Yolk sac tumors have a slimy, pale tan-yellow appearance with foci of necrosis and small cyst formations. Several histologic patterns include papillary, vesicular, and glandular, including the endometroid-like pattern.

Intracellular and extracellular hyaline droplets are present in most yolk sac tumors. The droplets stain with periodic acid-Schiff (PAS), are diatase-resistant, and are variably reactive to AFP.

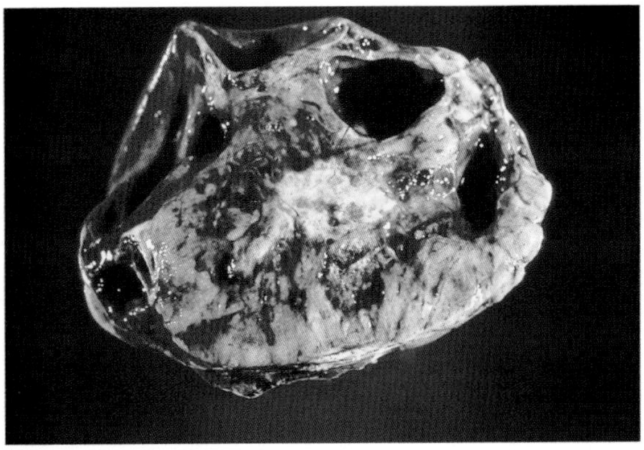

20.12. Gross appearance of yolk sac tumor of ovary.

Embryonal Carcinoma

Embryonal carcinoma is a malignant germ cell tumor that may be found in the first year of life. Embryonal carcinoma is a poorly differentiated malignant lesion composed of embryonal-appearing epithelial cells with characteristic large nucleoli (Figure 20.13). Human chorionic gonadotropin (hCG) and AFP immunoperoxidase staining are variable, but cytokeratin is positive.

Ovarian Tumors of Childhood

Ovarian tumors of childhood include: teratoma, yolk sac tumor, granuloma (theca cell tumor), Sertoli-Leydig cell tumor, dysgerminoma, and gonadoblastoma.

Gonadoblastoma

Gonadoblastoma typically arises from an abnormal gonad (Figure 20.14). Most patients with this tumor have a 46,XY or a 45,X/46,XY mosaic karyotype. It is composed of germ cells and characteristic calcifications.

Juvenile Granulosa Cell Tumor

Juvenile granulosa cell tumor is the most common ovarian tumor, overall, occurring in the perinatal period (Figure 20.15). It may also occur in the testis. Over 50% are diagnosed in the neonate, and 90% by 6 months of age.

Granulosa cell tumors of the ovary may occur in the newborn. It has both solid and cysts components.

Table 20.5 Testicular tumors of the newborn

Germ cell tumors	Sex cord, stromal tumors	Other tumors
Yolk sac tumor	Gonadal stromal tumor	Granular cell tumor
Gonadoblastoma	Juvenile granulosa cell tumor	Hamartoma
Teratoma		

Data from Kay R: Prepubetal testicular tumor registry. *Urol Clin Norm Am* 20:2, 1993.

Table 20.6 Testicular tumors of childhood

	Percent
Yolk sac tumor	60
Teratoma Embryonal carcinoma Choriocarcinoma	35
Interstitial cell tumor (Leydig cell tumor) Sertoli cell tumor Paratesticular rhabdomyosarcoma Retinal anlage tumor (melanotic progonoma)	5

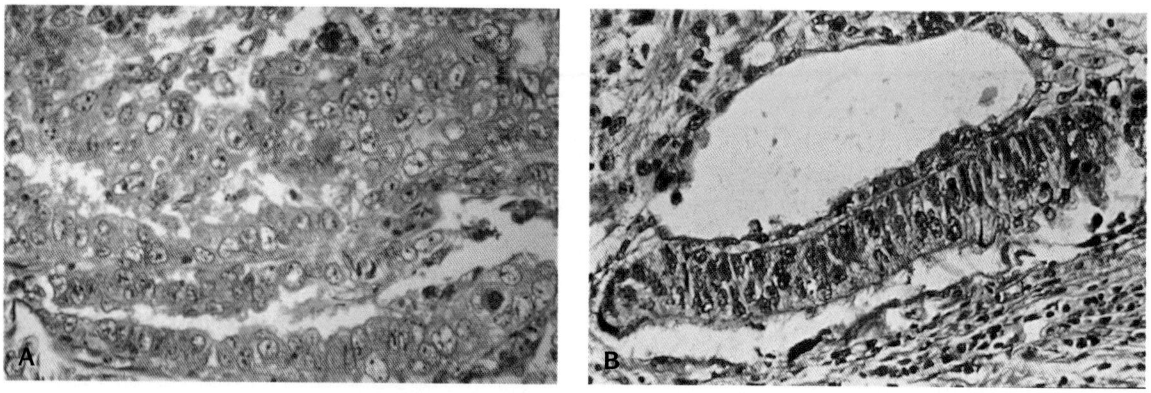

20.13. **(A)** Microscopic appearance of an embryonal carcinoma. **(B)** Higher magnification showing embryoid body.

Neurofibroma

Arising from a peripheral nerve, neurofibroma occurs as either a single lesion or as multiple tumors in association with café-au-lait spots and neurofibromatosis type I, an autosomal dominant disorder (von Recklinghausen's disease) (Figure 20.16). In neurofibromatosis, 50% have manifestations of the disease at birth. Microscopically, the tumor is composed of myxoid nerve trunks with waxy bundles of spindle-shaped cells.

Fibromatosis/Myofibromatosis

Fibromatosis (juvenile or infantile desmoid fibromatosis) is a benign, fibrous, connective tissue tumor that presents as a palpable mass in the fascia, skeletal muscle, or periosteum (Figure 20.17 and Table 20.7). In the newborn, the extremities and the head and neck region are the most frequent sites. Fibromatosis and fibrosarcoma are locally aggressive and often recur.

Fibromatosis consists of a firm, light gray or white mass with a rubbery, whorled, cut surface. Fibromatoses tend to be smaller than fibrosarcomas, averaging 2 cm in greatest dimension. Fibromatoses are spindle cell neoplasms with moderate variation in cellularity and the amount of intercellular collagen. The tumors stain positively with vimentin but do not react with desmin, S-100 protein, actin, or cytokeratin. The tumor cells are both fibroblasts and myofibroblasts. Thus, more appropriately they are called myofibromatoses.

Early, wide excision with adequate surgical margins is the treatment of choice.

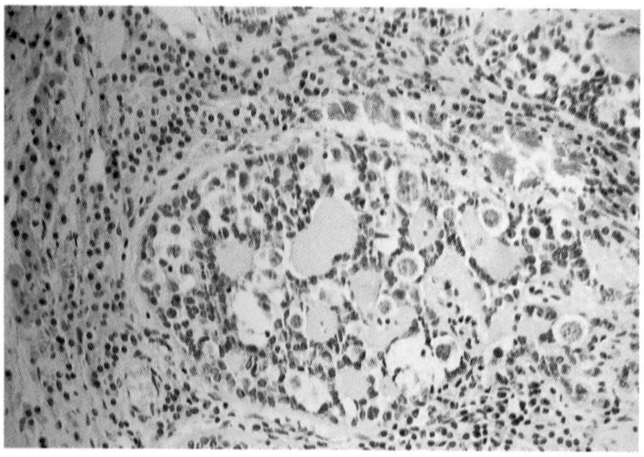

20.14. Gonadoblastoma showing tumor composed of nests of large germ cells with smaller, dark round to oval granulosa cells.

Infantile Digital Fibromatosis

This tumor involves the dorsolateral aspect of the distal phalanges of the fingers and toes (Figure 20.18). Inclusion bodies are characteristic. Almost 50% of these tumors are discovered within the first month of life. They are composed of white, firm nodules with a broad base and shiny surface and are composed of

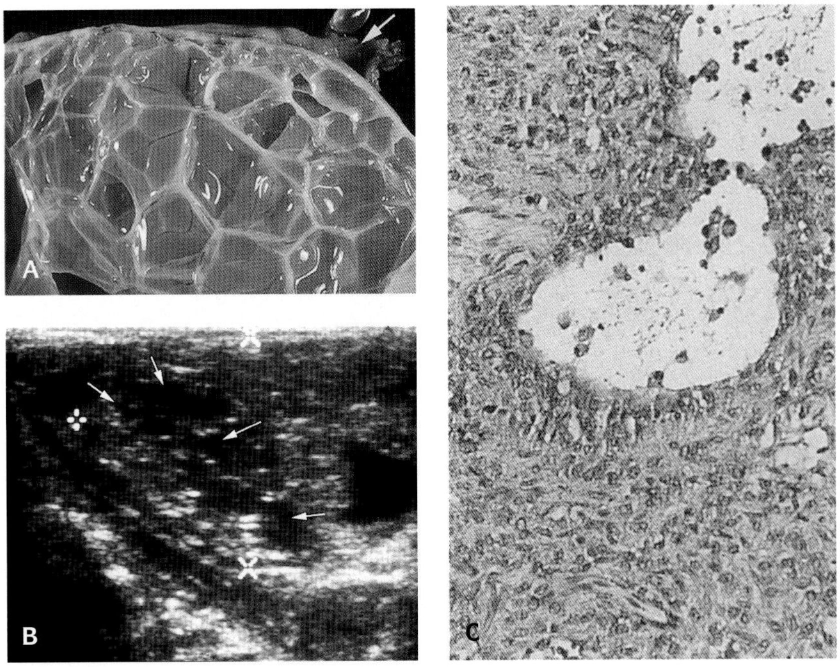

20.15. **(A)** Cystic juvenile granulosa cell tumor (note the arrow on the fallopian tube). **(B)** Ultrasound of a cystic juvenile granulosa cell tumor. **(C)** Microscopic appearance showing cystic spaces separating granulosa cells.

Table 20.7 Fibrous tumors of infancy and childhood benign entities
• Fibrous hamartoma of infancy
• Congenital/infantile myofibromatosis
• Fibromatosis colli
• Infantile fibromatosis (*)
• Calcifying aponeurotic fibroma (*)
• Digital fibromatosis (*)
• Hyalin fibromatosis
(*) Lesions that commonly recur
Adapted from Enzinger & Weiss, *Soft Tissue Tumors*, 3rd. ed. St. Louis, Mosby, 1995.

small, regular, spindle-shaped cells arranged in interlacing bundles or herringbone growth pattern with little or no mitotic activity, invading the dermis and subcutaneous tissue. A trichrome stain variably displays round or oval, red, paranuclear, intracytoplasmic inclusions, which, by electron microscopy, consist of packets of actin filaments.

Fibrous Hamartoma of Infancy

Ten to 20% of cases present at birth (Figure 20.19). It is a slowly growing, painless, palpable mass most often involving the axilla and shoulder and, less

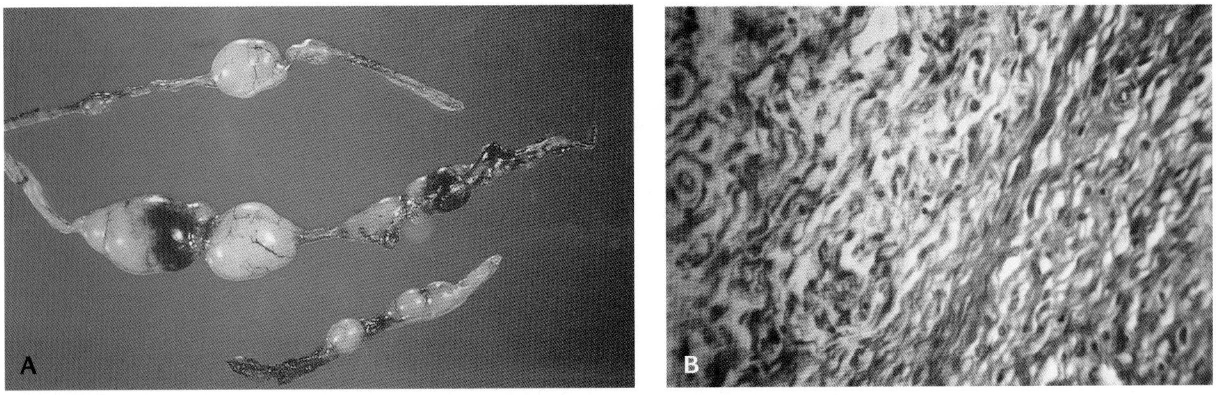

20.16. Neurofibroma. **(A)** Gross appearance showing tumor arising from a hypertrophied peripheral nerve. **(B)** Microscopic appearance showing wavy bundles of spindle cells.

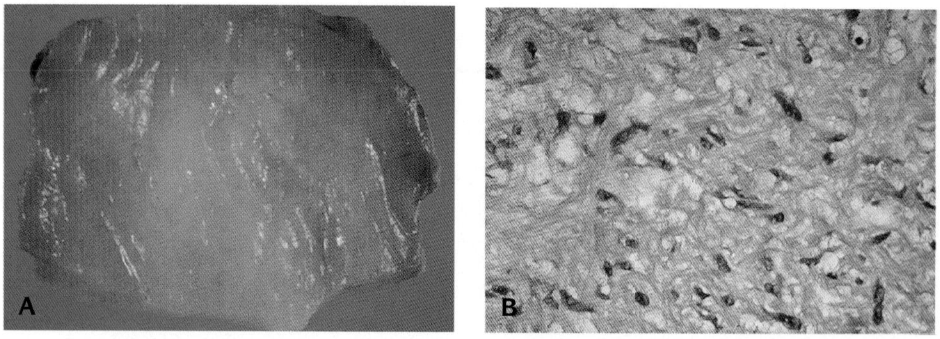

20.17. **(A)** Dense fibrous lesion of myofibromatosis. **(B)** Microscopic appearance of benign myofibroblasts.

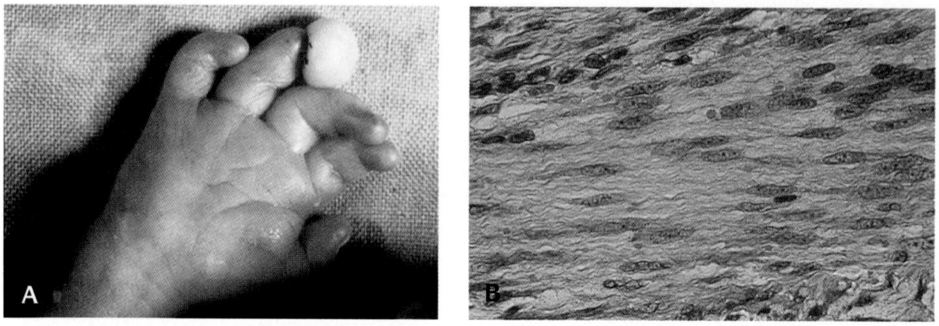

20.18. **(A)** Digital fibroma. **(B)** Microscopic appearance showing spindle cells with eosinophilic inclusions.

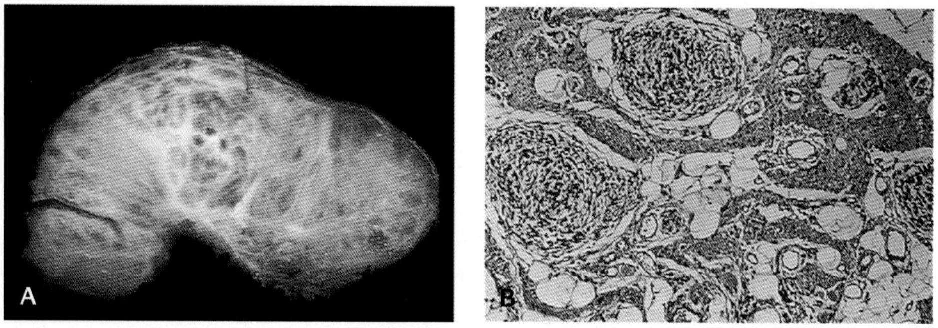

20.19. **(A)** Fibrous hamartoma of infancy from shoulder of infant. **(B)** Microscopic appearance showing adipose tissue, fibrous tissue and immature mesenchymal tissue.

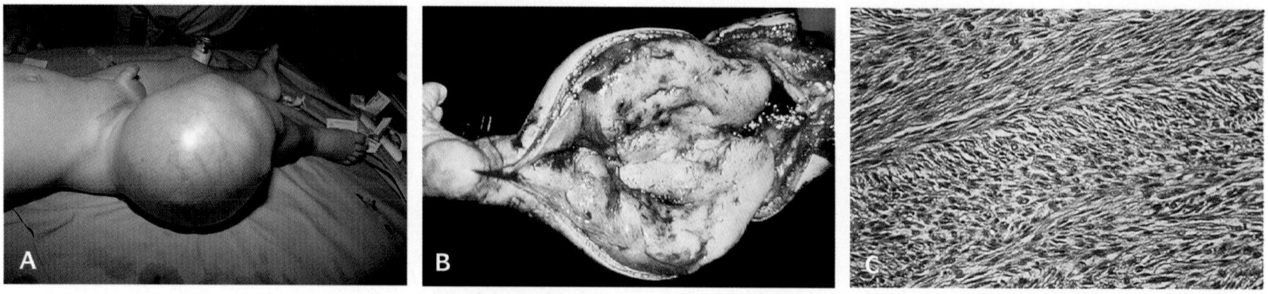

20.20. **(A)** Infantile fibrosarcoma involving lower extremity. **(B)** Cut surface of excised tumor. **(C)** Microscopic appearance showing spindle cells arranged in a herringbone pattern.

frequently, the chest wall, upper arm, neck, and inguinal region arising from the lower dermis or subcutaneous tissue.

It is composed of firm, glistening, gray-white fibrous tissue and yellow nodules of fat.

There are three main components: nests of immature spindle-shaped cells embedded in a myxoid background; interlacing, dense, fibrous trabeculae or cords resembling tendon; and lobules of mature adipose tissue situated between the other two components. It is a benign tumor that usually does not recur if completely excised.

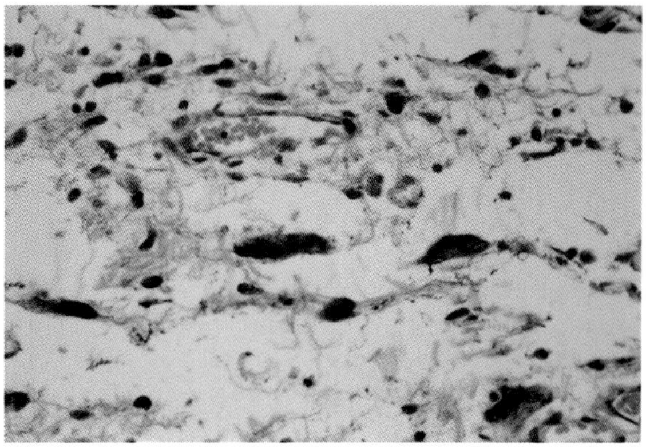

20.21. Giant cell fibroblastoma microscopic appearance showing giant fibroblast cells in a fibrous stroma.

GIANT CELL FIBROBLASTOMA

Congenital Fibrosarcoma

Although congenital (infantile) fibrosarcoma is relatively uncommon, it is the most common sarcoma of the newborn and presents as a bulky rapidly growing mass (Figures 20.20 and 20.21). The tumor has been described in stillborn infants. Local recurrence is as high as 50%; metastases seldom occur. There is a male/female ratio of 5:1. It is composed of plump spindle-shaped fibroblastic cells with moderate nuclear atypia.

Lipoblastoma

Lipoblastomas tend to grow slightly more rapidly than lipomas, have a much firmer consistency, and are paler and more myxoid or grayish in appearance than a typical lipoma on cross section (Figure 20.22). The tumor is composed of immature fat cells with varying degrees of differentiation that are separated by connective tissue septa and loose, grayish, myxoid areas. The presence of lipoblasts with a bubbly, vacuolated cytoplasm is a requisite for diagnosis.

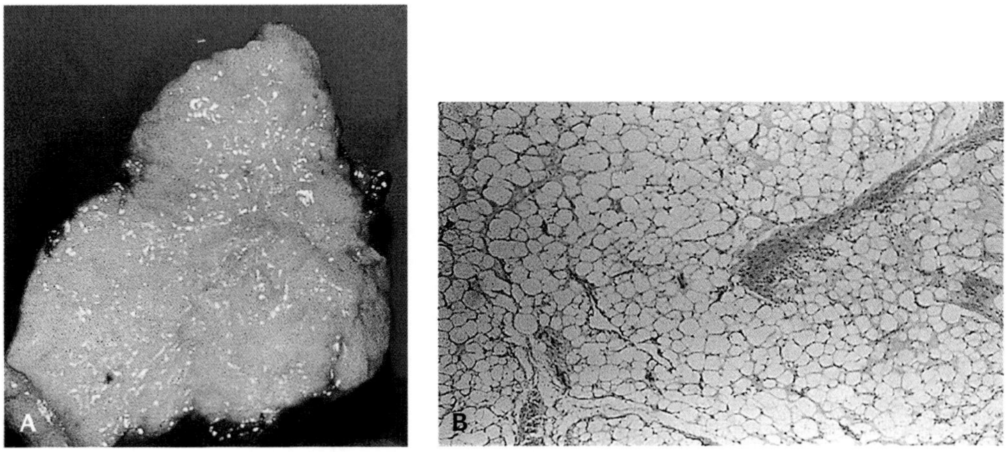

20.22. Lipoblastoma. **(A)** Gross appearance. **(B)** Tumor composed of benign lipoblasts.

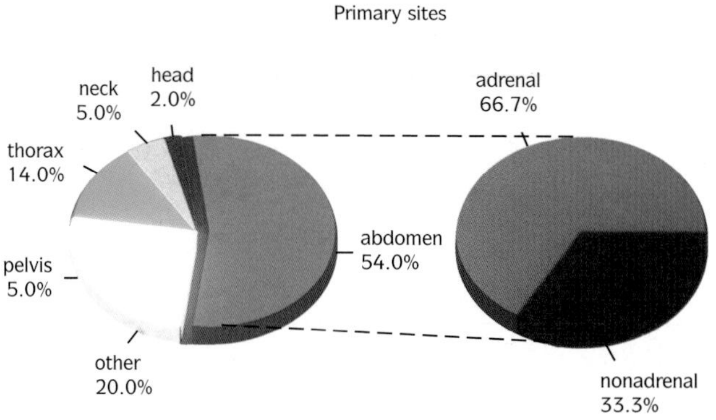

20.23. Primary sites of neuroblastoma. (Courtesy of Dr. Gonzalez-Crussi.)

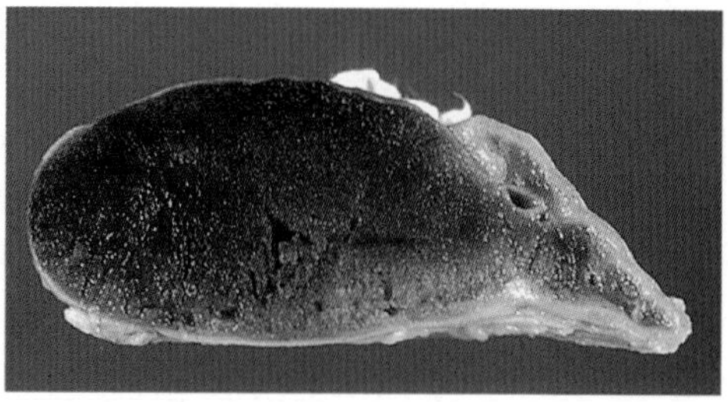

20.24. In situ tumor in the adrenal gland.

Mitoses are not seen. The tumor cells react positively to S-100 protein but are nonreactive to vimentin, actin, Leu-7, and factor VIII.

Treatment is complete excision of the mass; they have a favorable outcome.

NEUROECTODERMAL TUMORS

These tumors are included in the small blue cell tumors (Tables 20.8). Childhood blue cell tumors include the following:

- Embryonal rhabdomyosarcoma
- Ewing tumor and primitive neuroectodermal tumor (PNET)
- Lymphoma
- Neuroblastoma
- Wilms tumor
- Monophasic synovial sarcoma
- Germ cell tumors
- Thoracopulmonary tumor (Askin tumor)

Neuroblastoma

This tumor originates from neural crest cells (Figures 20.23 to 20.29). Typical primary sites are the adrenal gland, posterior mediastinum, or neck along the paraspinal region, in association with the distribution of sympathetic ganglia. It is usually found in patients under 2 years of age. Radiographically, there are calcific flakes in the mass. Catecholamines are excreted in the urine, and neuron-specific enolase is present in the serum.

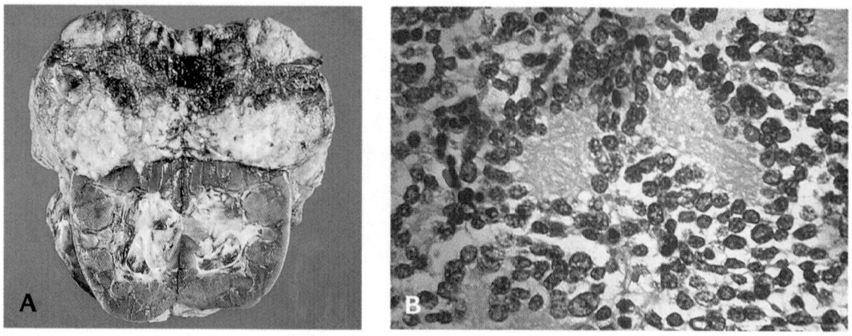

20.25. Neuroblastoma. **(A)** Tumor is hemorrhagic and necrotic in the adrenal gland. **(B)** Microscopic appearance of neuroblastoma showing small, dark blue cells with rosettes.

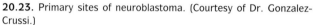

Table 20.8 **Histopathologic differential diagnosis of the small blue cell malignant tumors of the newborn**

Tumor	Light microscopy	Immunohistochemistry	Ultrastructure
Neuroblastoma	Small, round cells; rosettes; neurofilaments; nuclei with a peppery chromatin pattern	NSE+, NFP+, VIM+, DES−, MSA−, LCA−, CK−, HBA71−, β_2MG-M N1C2−, NB84+	Neurosecretory granules, microtubules, neurofilaments
Rhabdomyosarcoma	Spindle cells, eosinophilic cytoplasms, cross-striations, embryonal and alveolar patterns	DES+, MSA+, VIM+, NSE±, NFP−, HBA71−, CK−, LCA−	Spindle cells, primitive attachments, Z-bands, thick and thin filaments, basement membranes, glycogen ±
Leukemia	Diffuse infiltrates of small, round cells; granules ±	LCA+, VIM+, NFP±, MSA−, NFP−, CK−, HBA71−	Round cells, no attachments, no matrix, granules ±
Primitive neuroectodermal tumor (PNET)*	Small, round cells; rosettes; lobular pattern	NSE+, VIM+, NFP±, HBA71+, $\beta_2$mg+, LCA−, DES−, MSA−, CK−, M1C2+	Primitive cells, few organelles, rare neurosecretory granules, few intermediate filaments, primitive attachments ±
Rhabdoid tumor	Polygonal cells with eosinophilic cytoplasms; intermediate filament inclusions; round, vesicular nucleus with one large nucleolus	VIM+, CK+, DES−, MSA−, NFP−, LCA−	Bundles of cytoplasmic intermediate filaments

NSE, neuron specific enolase; NFP, neural fibullary protein; VIM, vimentin; LCA, leucolyte common antigen; DES, desmen; MSA, muscle specific antigen; CK, cytohexatin; B_2MG, B_2 microglobulin

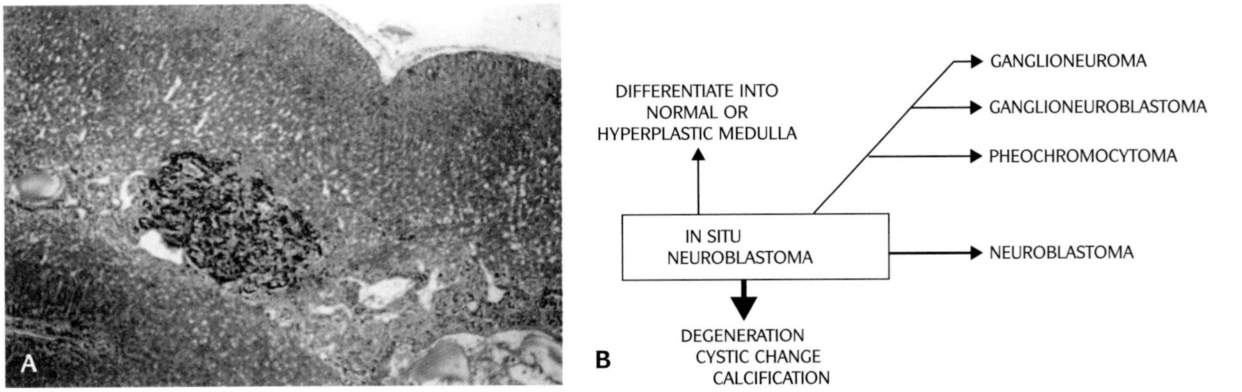

20.26. **(A)** Microscopic appearance of in situ neuroblastoma. **(B)** Fate of neuroblastoma in situ.

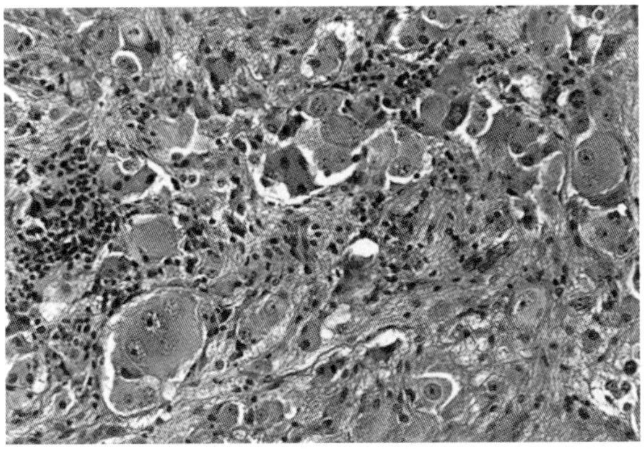

20.27. Microscopic appearance of a ganglioneuroblastoma from the mediastinum.

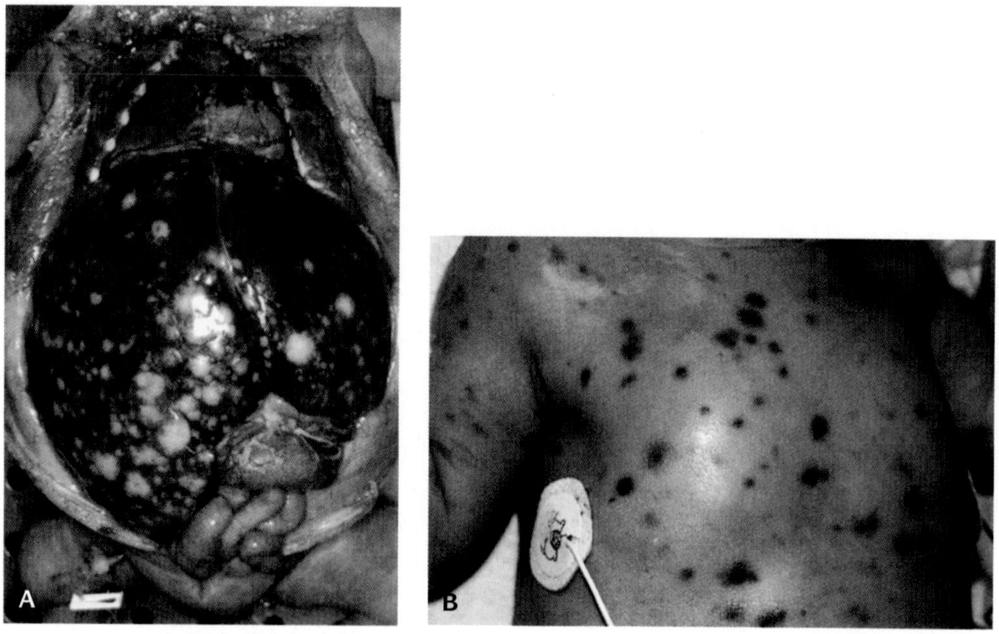

20.28. IV-S neuroblastoma. (A) Liver is studded with tumor nodules. (B) Skin lesions with "blueberry muffin" appearance.

Rosettes, neuronal differentiation, and a neurofibrillary background characterize the microscopic appearance. Expression of the neurotrophin receptor TRK-A, deletion or loss of heterozygosity of the short arm of chromosome 1, or amplification of NMYC indicate a poor prognosis.

Stage IVS is a specific pattern of metastatic neuroblastoma unique to the newborn with metastases to one or more of the following sites: liver, skin, and bone marrow (not bone). The adrenal is the most common primary site. Stage IVS neuroblastoma has a favorable prognosis.

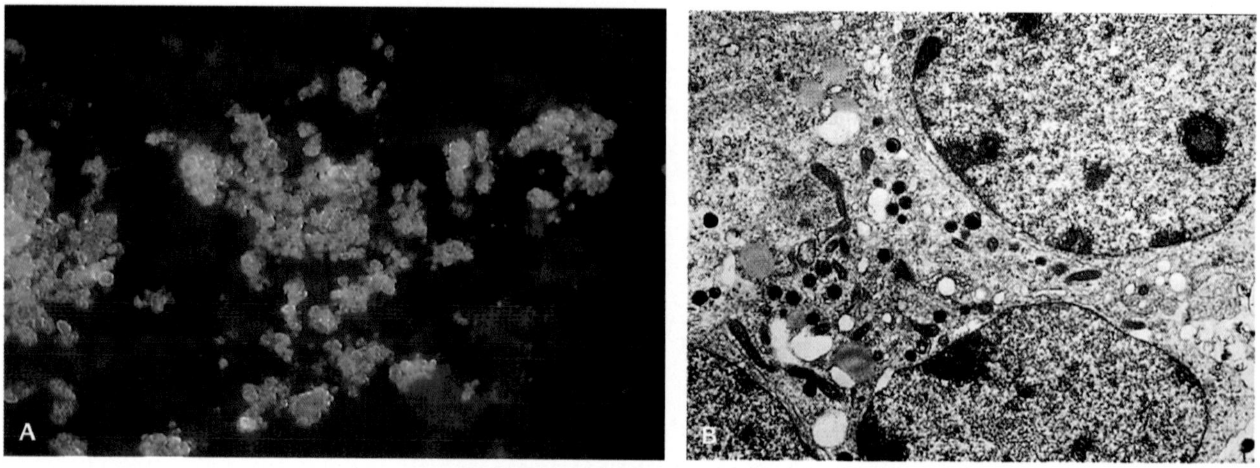

20.29. (A) Immunofluorescence of neuroblastoma. (B) Electronmicrograph showing neurosecretory granules.

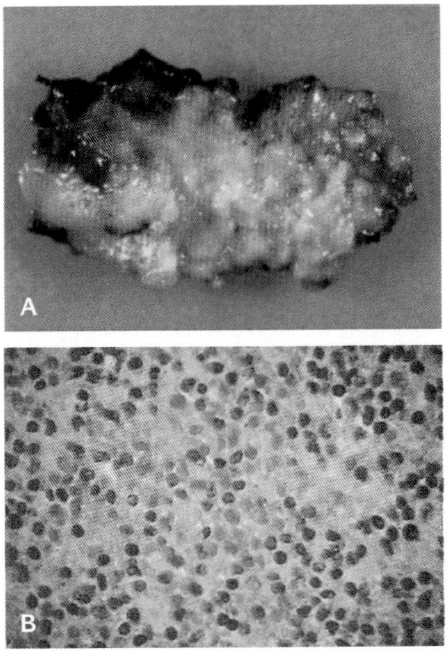

20.30. (A) Gross appearance of neuroectodermal tumor (PNET) of the forearm in a newborn infant. **(B)** Microscopic appearance showing small undifferentiated blue cells.

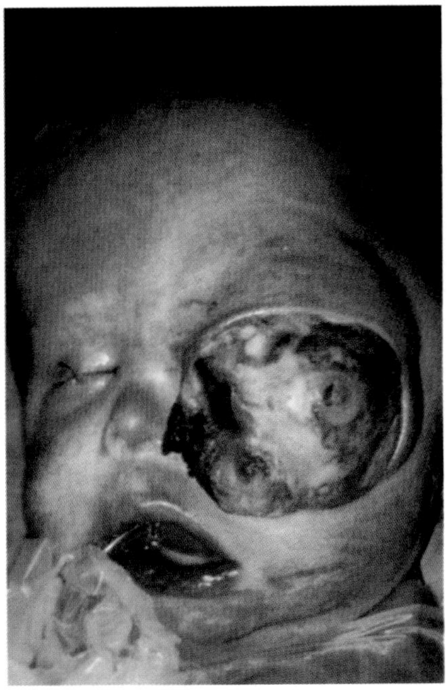

20.31. Polyphenotypic tumor of orbit in a newborn infant.

Primitive Neuroectodermal Tumor

The primitive neuroectodermal tumor (PNET) originates from cholinergic elements and the biologic characteristics are distinct from neuroblastoma (Figure 20.30). *Malignant small cell tumor of the thoracopulmonary region* accounts for about one-third of all PNETs. It is highly malignant, and pulmonary and skeletal metastases are common. Cells express β^2-microglobulin and share cytogenetic and immunocytochemical characteristics with PNET.

The PNET is a small blue cell malignant neoplasm that occurs in the central and peripheral nervous systems and soft tissues. The category of PNET comprises a wide variety of neoplasms, including entities such as meduloblastoma, retinoblastoma, Askin thoracopulmonary tumor, melanotic PNET of the jaws and peripheral neuroepithelioma of the soft tissues.

PNETs are sometimes the cause of death in fetuses and infants. The chest wall, extremities, and face are the primary sites.

Polyphenotypic Tumor

This primitive neoplasm is characterized by small dark-blue cells with a variety of positive immunostains (Figure 20.31) usually present in the newborn. It is aggressive and highly malignant.

Ewing sarcoma of bone and soft tissue occurs in childhood at a later age and constitutes the least differentiated part of a biologic spectrum of which PNET represents a better differentiated expression.

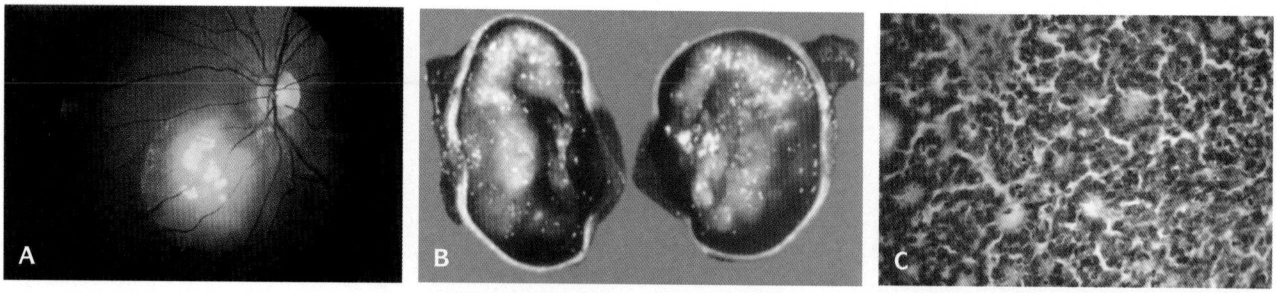

20.32. Retinoblastoma. **(A)** Ophthalmoscopic appearance. **(B)** Enucleated eye containing large tumor in a newborn. **(C)** Microscopic appearance of retinoblastoma showing Flexner-Winterstein rosettes.

Both PNET and Ewing sarcoma express a cell surface glycoprotein, p30/32, which is coded by the *MIC2* gene. Both tumors bear the translocation t(11;22)(q24;q12).

Retinoblastoma

This tumor may occur in the fetus or newborn and occurs with an incidence of 1/30,000 live births (Figure 20.32). The tumor may be bilateral (40%) or unilateral (60%). The gene, a suppressor gene, is located on chromosome 13q14 and deletions or mutations may occur at this locus.

The tumor may be hereditary (40%) or sporadic (60%). Bilateral cases are usually hereditary and the trait is dominant. Spontaneous regression has been documented as in neuroblastoma. The tumor is composed of a gray-white mass frequently with calcification involving the retina. It may disseminate into the cerebrospinal fluid with seeding of the leptomeninges. It is composed of small, dark blue cells presumably of neural crest origin with typical Flexner Winterstein rosettes.

Melanotic Neuroectodermal Tumor of Infancy

Typically, the melanotic neuroectodermal tumor is seen at birth or during the first year of life as a rapidly growing mass, usually arising from the anterior maxilla and less often from the brain, skull, and mandible, also the oropharynx and epididymis (Figure 20.33). Serum AFP and urinary VMA levels are elevated.

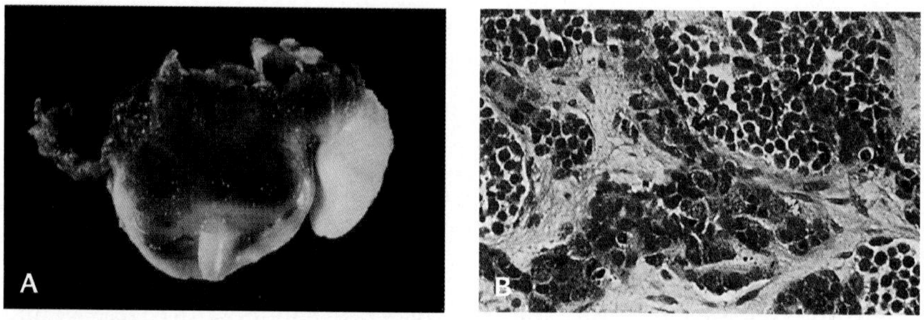

20.33. Pigmented neuroectodermal tumor (retinal anlage tumor, progonoma). **(A)** Gross appearance showing pigmented mass. **(B)** Microscopic appearance. The tumor is composed of pigmented epithelial cells and small, dark neuroectodermal cells resembling neuroblasts.

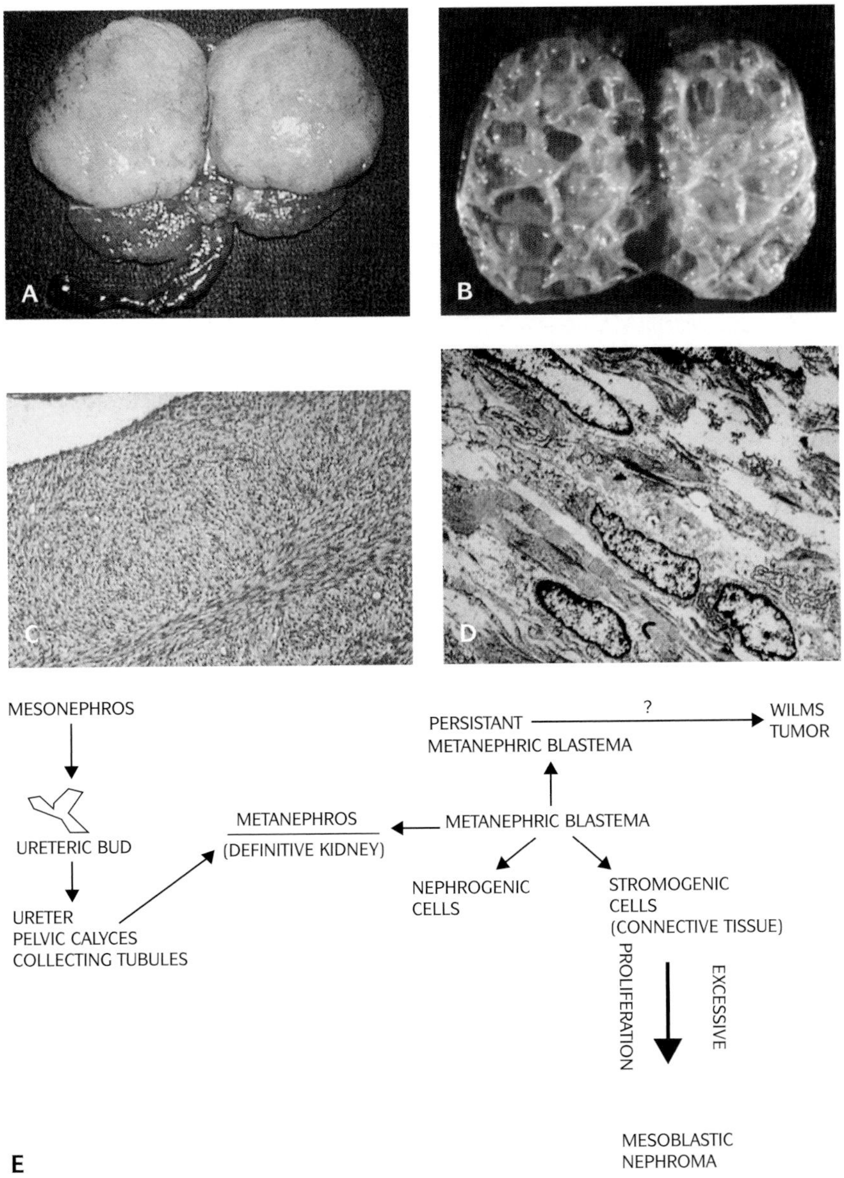

20.34. Mesoblastic nephroma of the kidney in a newborn. **(A)** The tumor is firm, nodular and sharply circumscribed. **(B)** A cystic mesoblastic nephroma. **(C)** Microscopic appearance of tumor showing spindle-shaped cells. **(D)** Electronmicrograph showing uniform spindle cells. **(E)** Mesoblastic nephroma flow chart.

KIDNEY TUMORS

Congenital mesoblastic nephroma (CMN) (fetal renal hamartoma) is a benign mesenchymal tumor of the kidney (Figure 20.34 and Table 20.9). It is the leading renal tumor of the fetus and newborn. It arises from the metanephric blastema.

Microscopically, there is a proliferation of uniform, spindle-shaped cells, demonstrated by electron microscopy to be myofibroblasts and fibroblasts.

Table 20.9 Classification of fetal and newborn renal tumors

Congenital mesoblastic nephroma	Cystic renal tumors
Classic mesoblastic nephroma	Cystic nephroma (multilocular cyst)*
Cellular mesoblastic nephroma	Cystic partially differentiated nephroblastoma
Wilms tumor*	Cystic Wilms' tumor
Classic triphasic	Rhabdoid tumor of kidney
Blastemal	Clear cell sarcoma of kidney
Epithelial (monomorphous)	Ossifying renal tumor of infancy
Fetal rhabdomyomatous	Renal cell carcinoma*
Wilms tumor with anaplasia*	Clear cell tumor
Nephroblastomatosis complex	

* Usually does not occur in newborns.

Adapted from Isaacs H Jr: *Tumors of the Fetus and Infant*. Philadelphia, WB Saunders Co., 1997.

Mitotic figures and small islands of cartilage are noted. Vimentin and actin staining are positive. The lesion is nonreactive to desmin or desmin may be focally expressed. A cellular histologic variant of CMN may occur. Nephroblastomatosis (Figure 20.35 and Table 20.9) is persistence of immature metanephric tissue beneath the capsule of the kidney.

RHABDOID TUMOR

Rhabdoid tumor is a rare highly malignant tumor with 6% occurring in the first year of life and some in the newborn with a 1–5:1 male/female ratio (Figure 20.36). Extrarenal rhabdoid tumor may also occur. Hypercalcemia is common. It is associated with apparently separate primary tumors of the central nervous system that have been diagnosed as medulloblastomas or PNET. There is a specific chromosomal translocation of chromosome 22q11 and 11p15.5. Rhabdoid tumor is a pale soft tumor that may be a single mass or have satellite nodules. It is composed of uniform, relatively large cells with prominent large nuclei and a single central nucleolus. Some cells contain prominent eosinophilic inclusions. Ultrastructurally there is an abundance of intermediate filaments. These tumors are vimentin positive and frequently have a polyphenotypic array of markers including epithelial and neural markers.

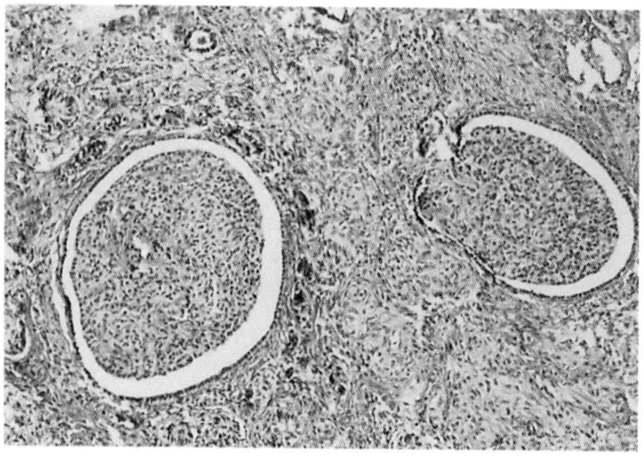

20.35. Nephroblastomatosis. Immature metanephric tissue present beneath the capsule of the kidney.

LIVER TUMORS

Hemangioma of the Liver

Most hemangiomas are diagnosed before 6 months of age and 50% are diagnosed within the first year of life (Figure 20.37). They may be small and regress, others are large and may rupture

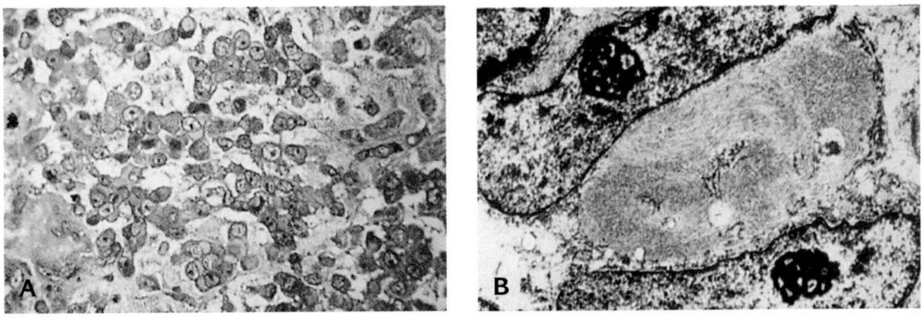

20.36. Rhabdoid tumor. (A) The cells are large, round or oval with prominent nucleoli with eosinophilic inclusions. (B) Electronmicrograph shows whorls of intermediate filaments.

in the perinatal period. Consumptive coagulopathy from disseminated intravascular coagulation, sequestration of platelets, and high-output cardiac failure are possible complications. About half of hepatic hemangiomas have hemangiomas in skin and other organs as well as chorangiomas in the placenta. These lesions can be detected prenatally and may be single or multiple. The cut surface reveals a dark, reddish-brown mass composed of blood vessels that may be capillary or cavernous. Capillary hemangiomas frequently become cavernous and thrombosis, necrosis, and fibrosis may result in regression. After surgical resection, the prognosis is favorable.

Mesenchymal Hamartoma

More than 50% of these tumors occur in infants, and 25% are found in the newborn (Figure 20.38). It is a tumor of developmental origin and may result from an anomalous blood supply to a liver lobule leading to ischemia and subsequent cystic change and fibrosis. It is sometimes attached to the liver by a pedicle. The lesion can be detected prenatally by ultrasonography. Most mesangial hamartomas occur in the right lobe of the liver and are cured by surgical resection. It is a well-demarcated multiloculated cystic mass. The cysts are lined by endothelium, sometimes cuboidal bile duct epithelium or by no epithelium, and are surrounded by dense, pale myxoid fibrous connective tissue septa containing blood vessels and small bile ducts.

Hepatoblastoma

More than 50% of hepatoblastomas are diagnosed in infants and 10% are diagnosed in the newborn (Figure 20.39 and Table 20.10). The tumor can be detected by ultrasonography. A number of clinical conditions may be associated with hepatoblastoma, including congenital anomalies, malformation syndromes, and Beckwith-Wiedemann syndrome. Hepatoblastoma has been described in siblings in association with fetal alcohol syndrome and maternal use of contraceptives. There is an increase in serum AFP levels as well as high serum cholesterol

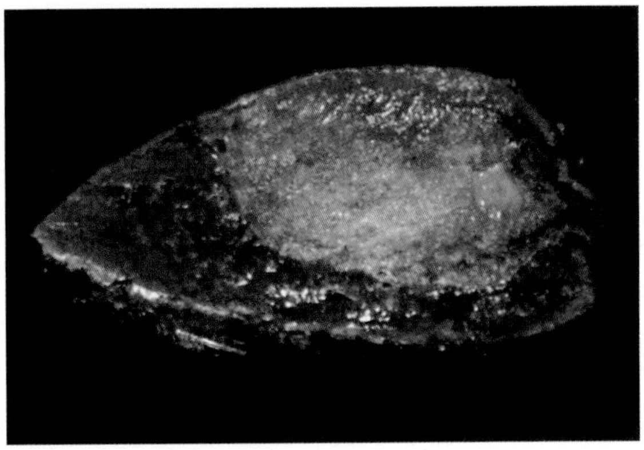

20.37. Hemangioma of liver in a newborn.

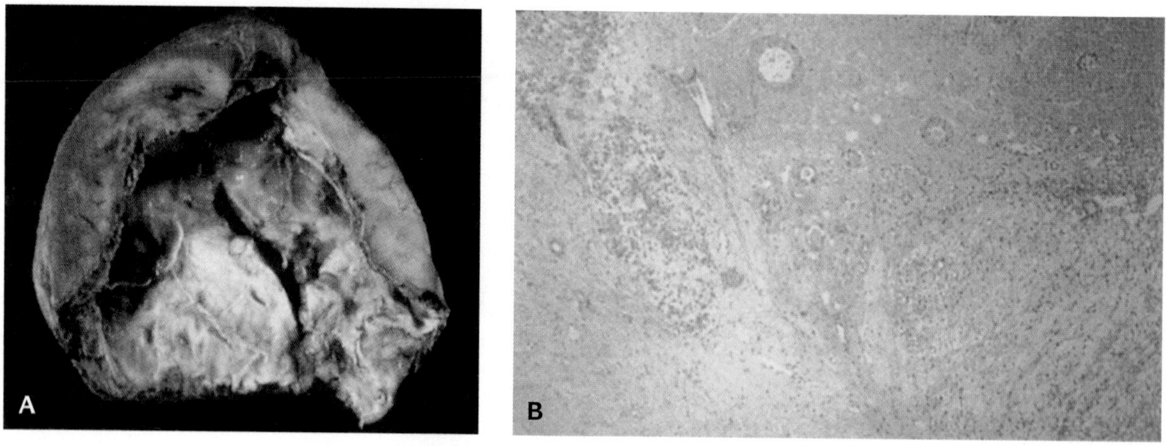

20.38. Mesenchymal hamartoma of liver in a newborn. **(A)** Gross appearance of the resected tumor from the right lobe of the liver. **(B)** Microscopic appearance showing scattered bile ducts and hepatocytes in a mesenchymal stroma.

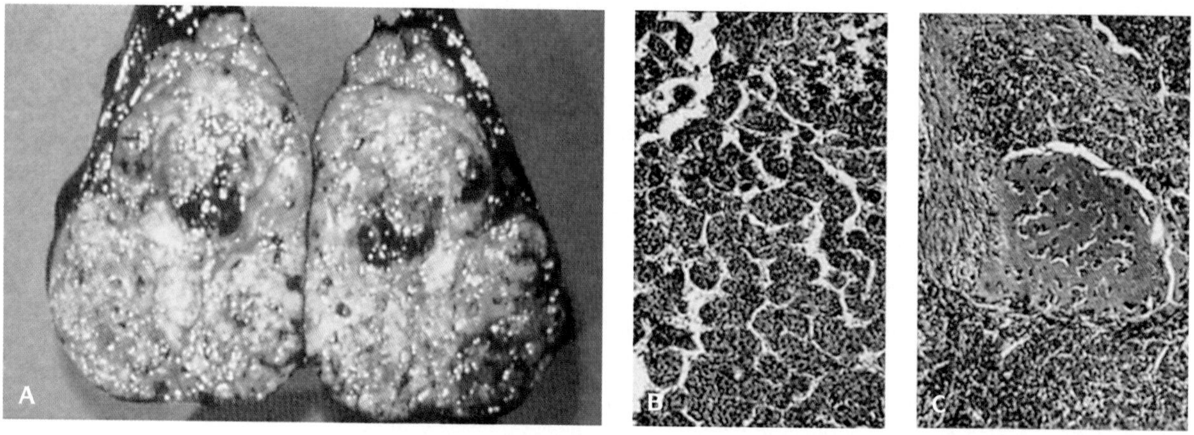

20.39. **(A)** Cut surface from a hepatoblastoma in the liver. **(B)** Microscopic appearance of fetal pattern in hepatoblastoma. **(C)** Island of cartilage in hepatoblastoma.

Table 20.10 Clinical conditions associated with hepatoblastoma

Hydrops fetalis	Stillbirth
Aicardi syndrome	Hemihypertrophy
α-antitrypsin deficiency	Beckwith-Wiedemann syndrome
Fetal alcohol syndrome	Cystathioninuria
Adenomatoid transformation of the renal epithelium	Isosexual precocity
	Polyhydramnios
Umbilical hernia	Maternal contraceptive use
Trisomy 18	Osteoporosis
Wilms tumor	Intestinal adenomatous polyposis

Adapted from Stocker JT, Ishak KG: Hepatoblastoma. In *Neoplasms of the Liver*, Okuda K, Ishak KG, eds. New York: Springer-Verlag, 1987.

values that correspond to a poor prognosis. The tumor is usually a single round mass that may measure up to 20 cm in diameter. It has a soft consistency and is pale yellow, frequently with necrotic areas. A variety of histologic patterns are described and there are prominent foci of hematopoiesis. Mitoses are frequent and both embryonal and fetal patterns may coexist and areas of osteoid formation may be present. On electron microscopy the cells contain abundant glycogen, prominent in the endoplasmic reticulum, tonofilaments, desmosomes, and canalicular microvilli. The cells are cytokeratin positive but stain negatively for vimentin desmin, S-100 protein, and neuron-specific enolase (NSE). Metastases occur in the lungs, abdomen, brain, lymphoid system, and vena cava. A teratoid variant contains tissue from all three germ layers. Survival depends on complete resection of the tumor, absence of metastases, and absence of embryonal or undifferentiated cell types.

THYROID TUMORS

A teratoma may involve the thyroid. Newborns with this tumor often have a maternal history of polyhydramnios and the tumor may cause airway compression, respiratory symptoms, and sometimes stillbirth. Histologically they are composed of mature tissues of various types as well as immature neuroglial elements.

Thyroglossal Duct Cyst

These cysts occur from the base of the tongue to the neck, inferior to the hyoid bone, usually in the midline. The cysts may enlarge and often rupture. The epithelial lining consists of columnar respiratory or squamous epithelium or a mixture of both. It may become infected and clusters of thyroid follicles may be found adjacent to the cysts.

SALIVARY GLAND TUMORS

Sialoblastoma

This tumor usually presents as a facial or submandibular mass that may be present at birth. It varies from 1 to 15 cm in diameter and has a lobulated surface. Microscopically it is characterized by solid nests of epithelial cells with small duct-like structures separated by thin septa; glycogen deposits are seen. The tumor is locally aggressive and may occur after surgical resection. The tumor cells are positive for vimentin. The myoepithelial cells are positive for smooth muscle actin, myosin, and S-100 protein, and the ductal cells stain for cytokeratin.

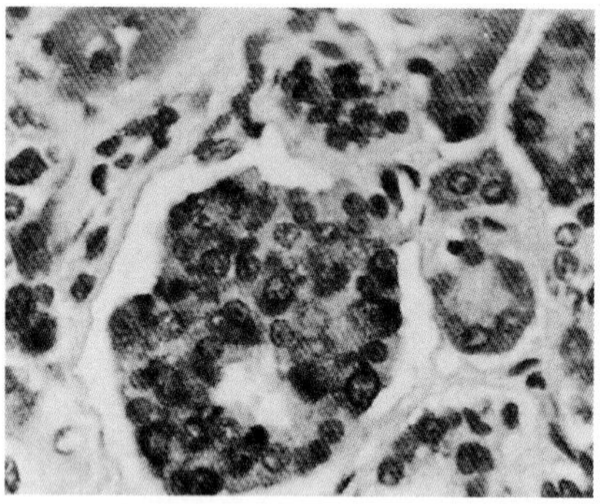

20.40. Nesidioblastosis. Microscopic appearance showing islet cell transformation of acini and ducts (immunoperoxidase stain for insulin).

CARDIAC TUMORS

Cardiac tumors seldom occur in the perinatal period. *Rhabdomyomas* are the most common and are usually associated with tuberous sclerosis. *Fibromas* and *myxomas* may involve the myocardium and may result in arrhythmias or sudden death.

PANCREATIC TUMORS

Tumors arising from islet cells, nesidioblastosis, and islet cell adenoma arise from the endocrine pancreas. In nesidioblastosis (Figure 20.40) neoformation of islets from pancreatic epithelium occur in which single islet cells or clusters of two to six islet cells, separate from islets, are located in acini and small pancreatic ducts.

Pancreatic adenoma is usually of small size and may be single or multiple and varies in size between 0.1 and 1 cm in diameter. It is composed of nests of islet cells and is separated from acinar tissue by a thin fibrous capsule. Both nesidioblastosis and islet cell adenoma are associated with severe hypoglycemia in the newborn.

Pancreatoblastoma

This tumor may be detected prenatally and may occur in the newborn. Microscopically the tumor is composed of a lobular pattern of acinar and ductular elements and central nodules of squamous cells. More than 50% of patients have Beckwith-Wiedemann syndrome. The tumors are usually found in the head of the pancreas and may be cystic; α_1-antitrypsin staining is positive as well as keratin and epithelium membrane antigen. The prognosis is generally good after complete surgical resection.

ADRENAL GLANDS

Congenital Adrenal Hyperplasia (Adrenogenital Syndrome)

This is an autosomal recessive disease caused by one of five different enzymatic defects in cortisol biosynthesis from cholesterol. It is the most frequent cause for ambiguous genitalia in the newborn. Deficiency of 21-hydroxylase enzyme accounts for more than 90% of cases, followed by 11-hydroxylase deficiency. The gene has been localized to 6p for 21-hydroxylase and to 8q for the 11-hydroxylase deficiency. Androgen levels are increased and manifested in the female by clitoral hypertrophy (a phallus-like clitoris), labial fusion, and sometimes scrotalization of the labia majora; in the male precocious puberty occurs. In one-half to two-thirds of patients with 21-hydroxylase deficiency, aldosterone synthesis is impaired and this results in the salt wasting-type of

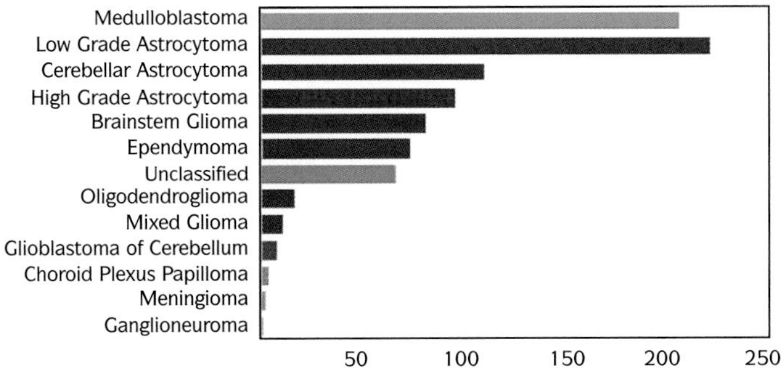

Duffner PK, Cohen ME, et al. *Neurology* 1986; 36:597, 1986.

20.41. Pediatric brain tumors distribution by tumor type.

congenital adrenal hyperplasia that principally occurs in males. The diagnosis of 21-hydroxylase deficiency in the newborn is established by determining the serum 17-hydroxyprogesterone level; prenatal diagnosis can be made by amniotic fluid analysis. The adrenal glands are enlarged and are frequently nodular with increased numbers of eosinophilic cells extending out toward the cortical surface.

Adrenal cortical hyperplasia may also be associated with Cushing syndrome. This may also occur in the newborn. It may be the result of adrenocortical carcinoma that occurs more frequently than adenomas in the newborn.

BRAIN TUMORS

Brain tumors are rare in the newborn (Figures 20.41 and 20.42 and Table 20.11). With the presence of a congenital brain tumor, there is an increased frequency of stillbirth; macrocephaly and hydrocephalus are the main presenting signs in the fetus and neonate. Brain tumors in the newborn may present as intracranial hemorrhage, chronic subdural hematoma, neurological deficits, unexplained hydrocephalus, or distortion of the cranium with bony defects.

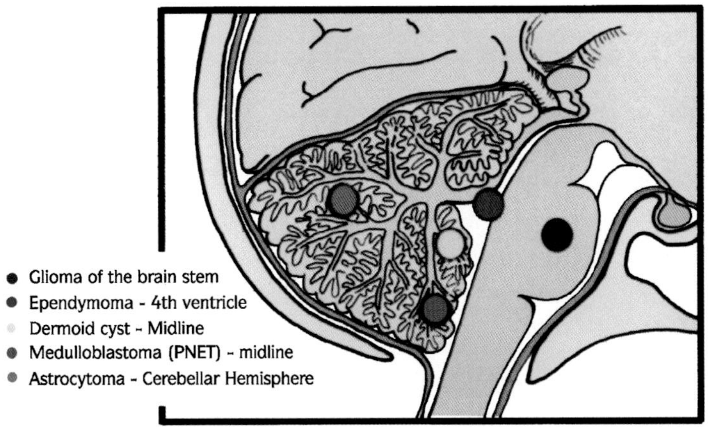

20.42. Brain tumors in the posterior fossa.

Table 20.11 Intracranial tumors of childhood

Posterior fossa	Pineal tumors – germinoma
Astrocytoma	teratoma
Medulloblastoma (PNET)	pinealoma
Ependymoma of the fourth ventricle	*Cerebral hemisphere* – rare
Glioma of the brain stem	Cerebral astrocytoma
Intracranial dermoids	Giant cell astrocytoma (tuberous sclerosis)
Hemangioblastoma of cerebellum	Supratentorial ependymoma
Region of third ventricle	Oligodendroglioma
Optic glioma	Papilloma of choroid plexus
Craniopharyngioma	Meningioma

Seizures may occur because of the ability of the skull to expand. *In utero* some brain tumors grow to an extremely large size and may result in fetal hydrops. The most common fetal and neonatal brain tumor is a teratoma. Other brain tumors that have been detected prenatally are choroid plexus papilloma, craniopharyngioma, and astrocytoma (Figures 20.43 to 20.45). Astrocytomas in the fetus and newborn usually are found outside the cerebellum and above the tentorium cerebelli. They are frequently large and may involve the cerebral hemisphere. They are usually pilocystic astrocytomas. Spontaneous intracerebral hemorrhage may occur. Subependymal giant cell astrocytoma is associated

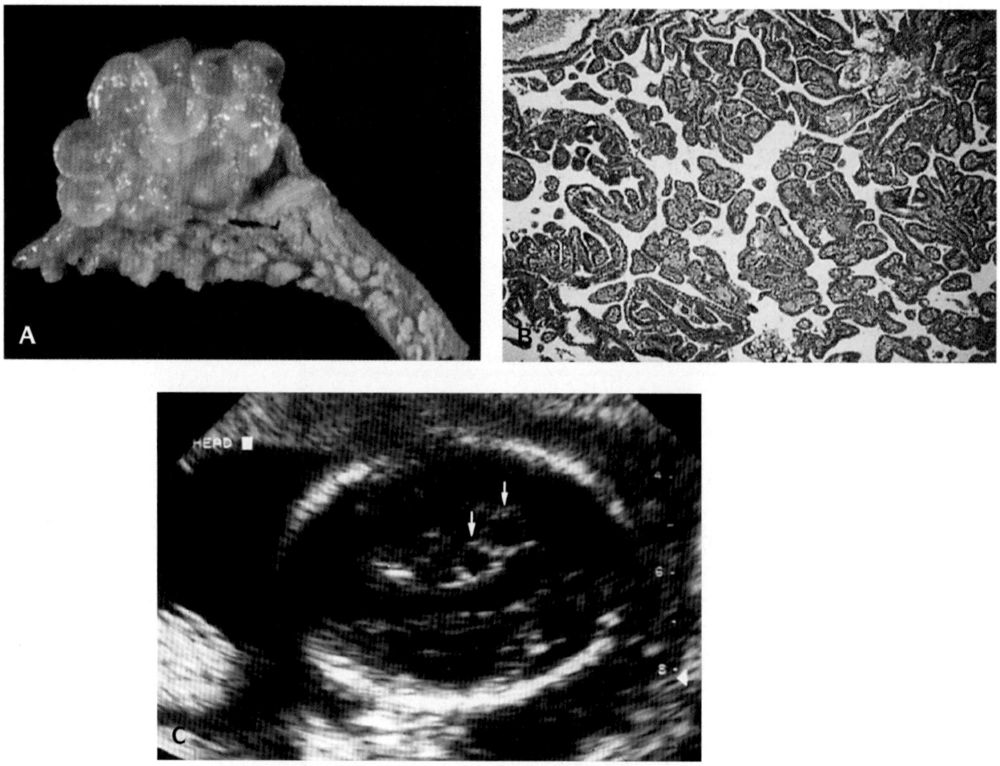

20.43. **(A)** Cystic choroid plexus papilloma. **(B)** Microscopic appearance of papillary choroid plexus papilloma. **(C)** Ultrasound of a choroid plexus papilloma.

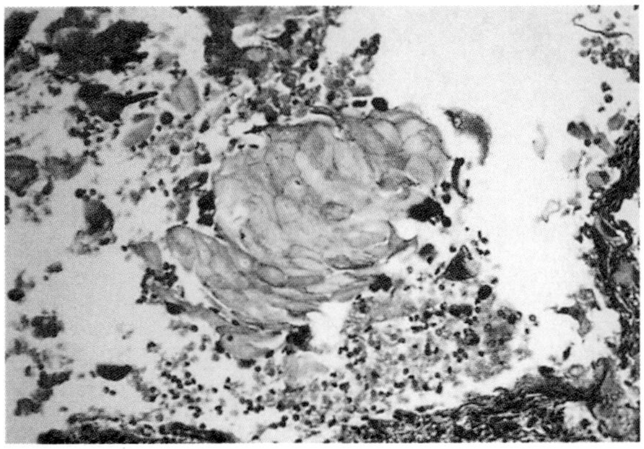

20.44. Craniopharyngioma. Microscopic appearance showing squamous cells and keratin.

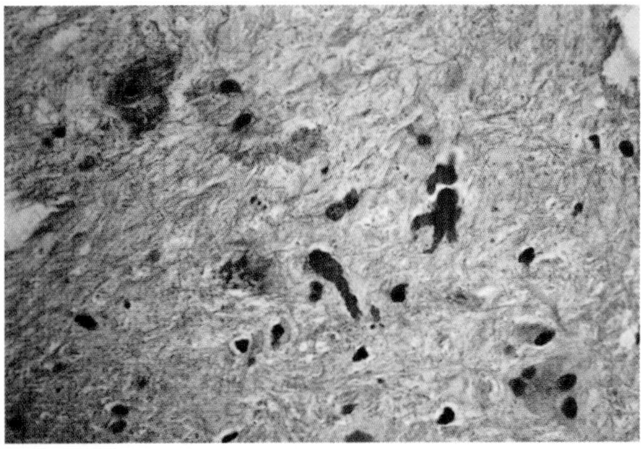

20.45. Pilocystic astrocytoma. Microscopic appearance showing astrocytic cells and Rosenthal fibers.

with tuberous sclerosis. Desmoplastic cerebrallar astrocytoma typically is found in infants and appears to be associated with a good prognosis. The prognosis for congenital brain tumors is poor. Hemangioblastomas (Figure 20.46) of the cerebellum occur in von Hippel-Lindau syndrome. Primitive neuroectodermal tumor (PNET) is a small blue cell malignant tumor occurring in the central and peripheral nervous systems and soft tissue (Figure 20.47). It is a very aggressive tumor and metastasizes widely within the cerebral spinal fluid pathways and may seed to the meninges and the spinal cord. It occurs predominantly in the midline of the cerebellum, the cerebellar hemispheres, pineal body, brainstem, spinal cord or olfactory nerve, and retina. It is composed of small or poorly differentiated dark staining cells.

Medulloblastoma (So-Called PNET of the Cerebellum)

This is a malignant tumor and is associated with a rather high frequency of stillbirth, hydrocephalus, and congenital defects, including cleft palate, malrotation of the intestine, imperfectness and imperforate anus, and exstrophy of the bladder (Figure 20.47). There is association of medulloblastoma and rhabdoid tumor of the kidney. The tumor originates from the roof of the fourth ventricle and causes obstruction of the cerebral aqueduct and hydrocephalus. The tumor may be detected prenatally by ultrasonography. Histologically the tumor consists of small darkly staining cells with variable amounts of intracellular pink-staining material. The cells have round, oval, or carrot-shaped nuclei with coarse chromatin and scant cystoplasm. Homer-Wright rosettes are present in fewer than 50% of cases. Immunostaining is positive for neuron-specific enclose (NSE) and synaptophysin as well as with vimentin. Medulloblastoma is a highly malignant tumor that is invariably fatal in the perinatal period.

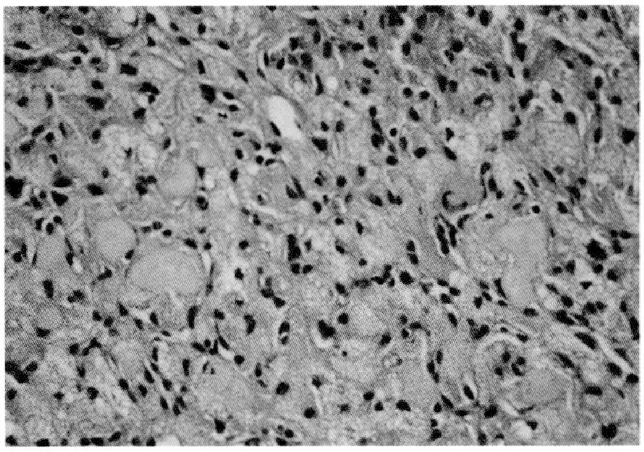

20.46. Hemangioblastoma. Microscopic appearance of a cerebellar tumor in a case of von Hippel-Lindau disease.

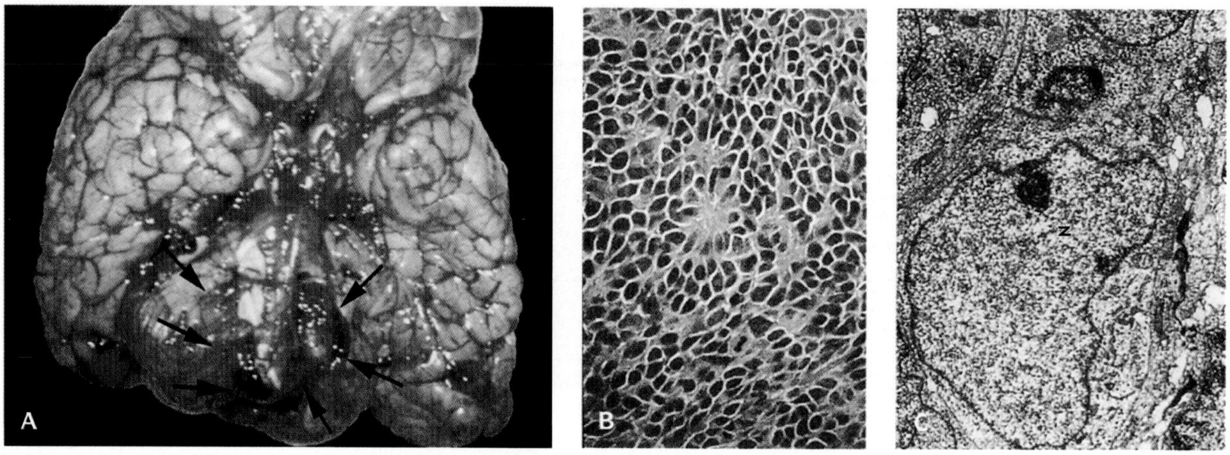

20.47. Medulloblastoma. **(A)** Gross appearance of midline cerebellar tumor (arrows). **(B)** Microscopic appearance of a midline cerebellar tumor composed of small, dark carrot-shaped cells with mitoses. **(C)** Electron micrograph showing large nuclei with prominent nucleolus and neurofilaments.

Ependymoma

Ependymomas may occur in the newborn and most arise from the wall of the fourth ventricle (Figure 20.48). Newborns present with hydrocephalus and signs of increased intracranial pressure. These tumors are responsible for dystocia, stillbirth, and spontaneous intracerebral hemorrhage. Congenital familial cases have been described. They consist of uniform, darkly staining cells with perivascular rosettes. Newborns with ependymomas have a poor prognosis; they may recur locally and may disseminate throughout the cerebrospinal fluid into the peritoneal cavity by ventricular peritoneal shunt catheters without filters.

Myxopapillary ependymoma occurs in the region of the chorda equina and has a distinctive papillary appearance. It is rarely seen in the newborn.

Choriocarcinoma may occur in the newborn from metastatic spread from a maternal choriocarcinoma. HCG levels are high. We have observed a male infant who died from massive intracranial hemorrhage secondary to metastatic choriocarcinoma to the brain, presumably from an unrecognized placental choriocarcinoma.

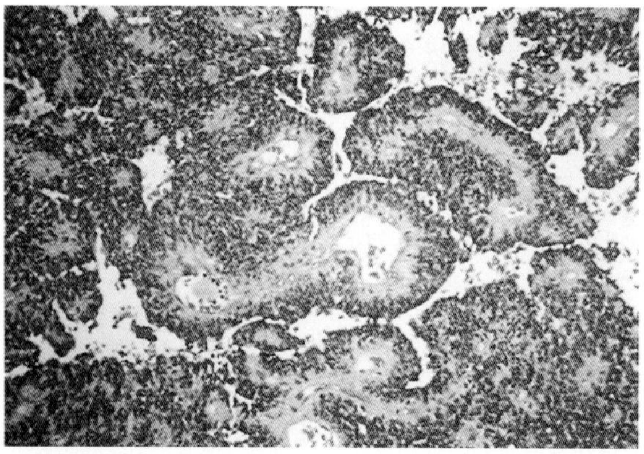

20.48. Microscopic appearance of ependymonas showing characteristic pseudorosette arrangement around blood vessels.

Craniopharyngioma

This tumor seldom occurs in the fetus and newborn (Table 20.12). It is intimally related to the pituitary gland and arises from Rathke's pouch, an ectodermal diverticulum or outgrowth developing from the roof of the mouth at about 24 days gestation. These tumors grow by expansion into the optic chiasm and into the floor of the fourth ventricle and posteriorly into the posterior fossa. Macrocephaly and hydrocephalus may result. These tumors are characterized by solid and cystic areas with

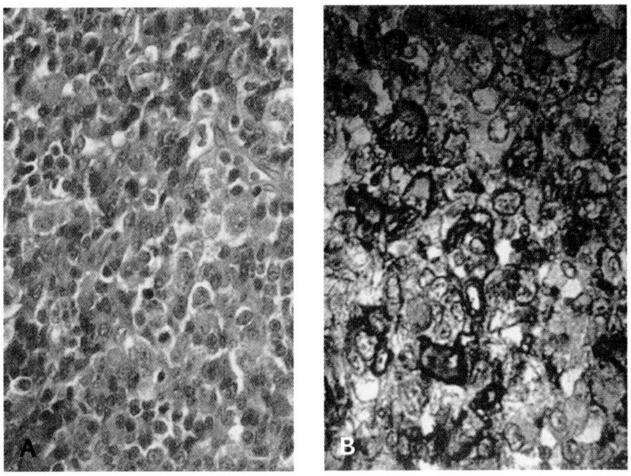

20.49. Atypical teratoma/rhabdoid tumor. **(A)** Microscopic appearance showing cells resembling rhabdoid tumor. **(B)** Positive for epithelial membrane antigen (EMA) immunostain.

Table 20.12 Craniopharyngioma

Arises from remnants of Rathke's pouch
Cystic and solid components
Microscopic
- Fibrous and glial tissue
- Giant cells
- Keratin
- Squamous epithelial nests
- Cords of columnar cells
- Loose myxoid stroma
- Calcification

squamous and adamantinomatous patterns with calcification and keratin pearls. This tumor has been detected by ultrasonography. Although it is a histologically benign tumor, the prognosis may be unfavorable because of its expansile growth.

Atypical teratoid/rhabdoid tumor is a highly malignant tumor that may occur in the newborn (Figure 20.49 and Table 20.13). It may arise in the cerebellum, the cerebrum, and the fourth ventricle. It may occur as a solitary tumor or concomitantly with rhabdoid tumor of the kidney or liver. It is characterized by aggressive growth, early metastases through the cerebrospinal fluid seeding the leptomeninges, and invasion of adjacent brain and spinal cord. The tumor is composed of cells with eosinophilic cytoplasm, round vesicular nuclei with a large nucleolus, and paranuclear cytoplasmic bodies composed of intermediate filaments and staining with epithelial membrane antigen (EMA), vimentin, and cytokeratin.

Table 20.13 Atypical teratoid/rhabdoid tumor

Patients are generally less than 2 years of age and most are boys
Clinical course is uncertain, although aggressive local recurrence and meningeal seeding are the rule
Pathology
- sheets of mitotically active, medium to large cells interrupted by fibrovascular septa;
- vacuolated cells give a "starry sky" appearance
- necrosis is common
- cells with rhabdoid features have round or reniform nuclei often displaced by hyaline,
- consistently vimentin positive,
- commonly positive for GFAP, EMA, cytokeratin

Monosomy 22 has been reported

OTHER NECK MASSES

- Cervical teratoma
  - Rarely identified prenatally
  - Usually unilateral and situated in the anterolateral portion of the neck
  - Cystic lesions that enlarge in pregnancy and become more complex over the course of pregnancy. Calcifications are present in 45%. Tumor sizes of 8–10 cm have been reported, and hydramnios is present in 30% of cases
  - Most (90%) are benign, but operative mortality is 9–15%
  - Untreated cervical teratomas have high (80–100%) mortality rates
  - Cesarean section has been recommended to facilitate prompt airway management
  - Other neck masses include branchial cleft cyst and thyroid enlargement, lipoma, fibroma, neuroblastoma, and (posterior mediastinum) thyroglossal duct cyst.

Goiter:

- Fetal goiter may present as a massive enlargement of the thyroid, often as a result of maternal thyroid blocking medications or ingestion of iodides, by transplacental passage of long-acting thyroid stimulant (LATS), or in association with congenital hypothyroidism (1/3,700 births).
- The enlarged thyroid usually presents as a solid, bilobed, homogenous mass in the anterior neck. The carotids may be displaced posteriorly, or the neck may be hyperextended. The common associated finding of hydramnios may be due to impaired fetal swallowing.
- Delivery at a high-risk neonatal facility is recommended because of the high risk of airway obstruction at birth.

Hemangioma:

- Localized proliferation of vascular tissue which rarely presents as fetal neck masses
- Complex sonographic appearance with many small vascular channels and an almost solid appearance. Color flow and pulsed Doppler will show heavy vascular flow patterns and make diagnosis highly likely
- High-output cardiac failure may develop, and close surveillance for hydrops, skin edema, ascites, and pleural effusion should be maintained
- Mode of delivery should be individualized, with consideration of cesarean section for large lesions

FAMILIAL TUMOR SYNDROMES

These are shown in Table 20.14. Progress in molecular and inherited cancer syndromes has led to the further understanding of carcinogenesis. Responsible genes have been identified and sequenced.

Table 20.14 Familial tumor syndromes

Syndrome	Gene	Chromosome	Nervous system	Skin	Other tissues
Neurofibromatosis 1	NF1	17q11	Neurofibromas, malignant peripheral nerve sheath tumors optic nerve gliomas, astrocytomas	Café-au-lait spots, axillary freckling	Iris hamartomas, osseous lesions, phaeochromocytoma, leukemia
Neurofibromatosis 2	NF2	22q12	Bilateral vestibular schwannomas, peripheral schwannomas, meningiomas, meningioangiomatosis, spinal ependymomas, astrocytomas, glial hamartomas, cerebral calcifications	–	Posterior lens opacities, retinal hamartoma
von Hippel-Lindau	VHL	3p25	Haemangioblastomas	–	Retinal haemangioblastomas, renal cell carcinoma, phaeochromocytoma, visceral cysts
Tuberous sclerosis	TSC1 TSC2	9q34 16p13	Subependymal giant cell astrocytoma, cortical tubers	Cutaneous angiofibroma ("adenoma sebaceum") peau chagrin, subungual fibromas	Cardiac rhabdomyomas, adenomatous polyps of the duodenum and the small intestine, cysts of the lung and kidney, lymphangio-leiomyomatosis, renal angiomyolipoma
Li-Fraumeni	TP53	17p13	Astrocytomas, PNET	–	Breast carcinoma, bone and soft tissue sarcomas, adrenocortical carcinoma, leukemia
Cowden	PTEN (MMAC1)	10q23	Dysplastic gangliocytoma of the cerebellum (Lhermitte-Duclos), megalencephaly	Multiple trichilemmomas, fibromas	Hamartomatous polyps of the colon, thyroid neoplasms, breast carcinoma
Turcot	APC hMLH1 hPSM2	5q21 3p21 7p22	Medulloblastoma Glioblastoma	– Café-au-lait spots	Colorectal polyps Colorectal polyps
Naevoid basal cell carcinoma syndrome (Gorlin)	PTCH	9q31	Medulloblastoma	Multiple basal cell carcinomas palmar and plantar	Jaw cysts, ovarian fibromas, skeletal abnormalities

Adapted from Kleihues P and Cavenee WK: *Pathology and Genetics. Tumours of the Nervous System*. International Agency for Research on Cancer, Lyon, 1997.

REFERENCES

Askin FB, Rosai J, Sibley RK, et al.: Malignant small cell tumor of the thoracopulmonary region in childhood: a distinctive clinicopathologic entity with uncertain histogenesis. *Cancer* 43:2438, 1979.

Coffin CM, Jaszcz W, O'Shea PA, Dehner LP: So-called congenital-infantile fibrosarcoma: does it exist and what is it? *Pediatr Pathol* 14:133, 1994.

Dehner LP: Primitive neuroectodermal tumor and Ewing's sarcoma. *Am J Surg Pathol* 17:1, 1993.

Enzinger FM, Weiss SW: *Soft Tissue Tumors*, 3rd ed. Philadelphia, Mosby Publishing, 1995.

Goldberg NS, Bauer BS, Kraus H, et al.: Infantile myofibromatosis: A review of clinicopathology with perspectives on new treatment choices. *Pediatr Dermatol* 5:37, 1988.

Isaacs H Jr: Tumors. In *Potter's Pathology of the Fetus and Infant*, Gilbert-Barness E, ed. Philadelphia, Mosby Publishing, 1997.

Isaacs H Jr: *Tumors of Fetus and Infant: An Atlas*, Springer-Verlag, New York, 2002.

Joshi VV, Cantor AB, Brodeur GM, et al.: Correlation between morphologic and other prognostic markers of neuroblastoma: a study of histologic grade, DNA index, n-myc gene copy number, and lactic dehydrogenase in patients in the Pediatric Oncology Group. *Cancer* 71:3173, 1993.

Leuschner I, Newton WA, Schmidt D, et al.: Spindle cell variants of embryonal rhabdomyosarcoma in the paratesticular region. A report of the Intergroup Rhabdomyosarcoma Study. *Am J Surg Pathol* 17:221, 19.

Panhan DM, ed: Pediatric Neoplasia; Morphology and Biology. Lippncott-Rowan, Phela, 1996.

Sotelo-Avila C, Bale PM: Subdermal fibrous hamartoma of infancy: pathology of 40 cases and differential diagnosis. *Pediatr Pathol* 14:39, 1994.

Sroeher and Dehner.

Weidner N, Tjoe J: Immunohistochemical profile of monoclonal antibody O13: Antibody that recognizes glycoprotein p30/32^{MIC2} and is useful in diagnosis Ewing's sarcoma and peripheral neuroepithelioma. *Am J Surg Pathol* 18:486, 1994.

TWENTY ONE

Fetal and Neonatal Skin Disorders

SEBORRHEA AND DRY DESQUAMATION

Miliaria

Secretion of sweat normally exudes from the glands but occasionally collects in the gland ducts, distending them so that they are visible at birth as discrete pinpoint elevations known as **milia crystallina** (Figure 21.1). They usually disappears during the first week of life. They are most often visible on the forehead, cheeks, and sides of the nose. Microscopically a keratinous plug and an intra- or subcorneal vesicle communicates with the underlying sweat duct, sometimes with a mild inflammatory infiltrate. When the process is deeper, prickly heat **(miliaria rubra)** occurs.

Milia are pearly yellow 1- to 3-mm papules on the face, chin, and forehead of 50% of newborns. Occasionally they erupt on the trunk and extremities. Although milia usually resolve without treatment during the first month of life, they may persist for several months. Microscopically they are miniature epidermal inclusion cysts, which arise from the pilosebaceous apparatus of vellus hairs.

Seborrheic Dermatitis

The scalp is most often affected in the newborn and is often associated with incomplete removal of the vernix caseosa. The lesions are poorly defined, yellow-red salmon-colored patches covered by waxy, greasy, easily removed scales.

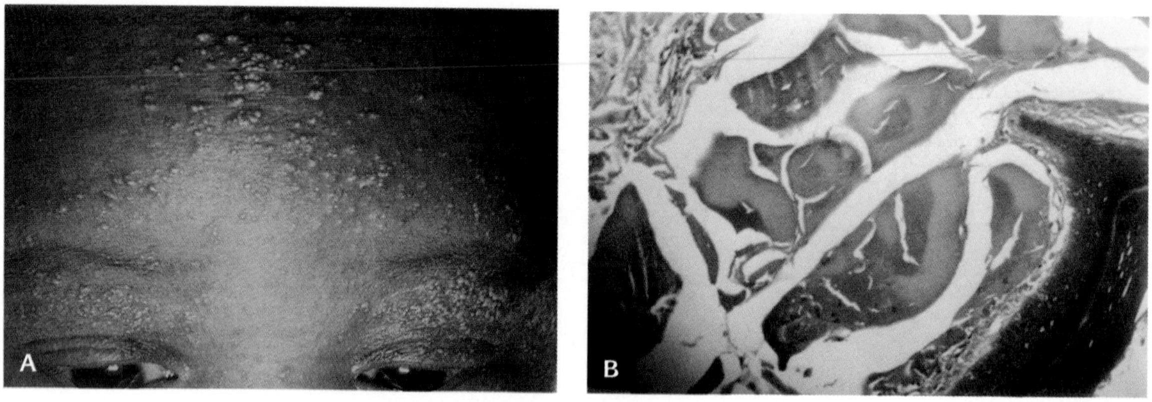

21.1. **(A)** Miliaria crystallina. Widespread milia were noted on the forehead and eyelids of this newborn. The white papules resolved spontaneously before 2-months. (Courtesy of Dr. Bernard Cohen.) **(B)** Milium. Section of skin of a newborn showing cyst containing keratinaceous and colloid material.

Acanthosis, edema, and occasional perivascular infiltration of leukocytes are present as well as spongiosis of the basal layer seen microscopically (Figure 21.2).

Leiner disease (desquamative erythroderma) is a more severe form of seborrheic dermatitis. This condition on the body is erythematous and covered by gray-white brawny or greasy scales. Intermittent fever, diarrhea, generalized lymphadenopathy, edema, and albuminuria may be present. The mortality rate is about 30%.

VESICULAR LESIONS IN THE FETUS AND NEWBORN

Vesicular lesions begin as blisters that may become pustules. They are characterized by a separation within the epidermis or between the epidermis and dermis with clefts that may be subcorneal, intraepidermal, suprabasal,

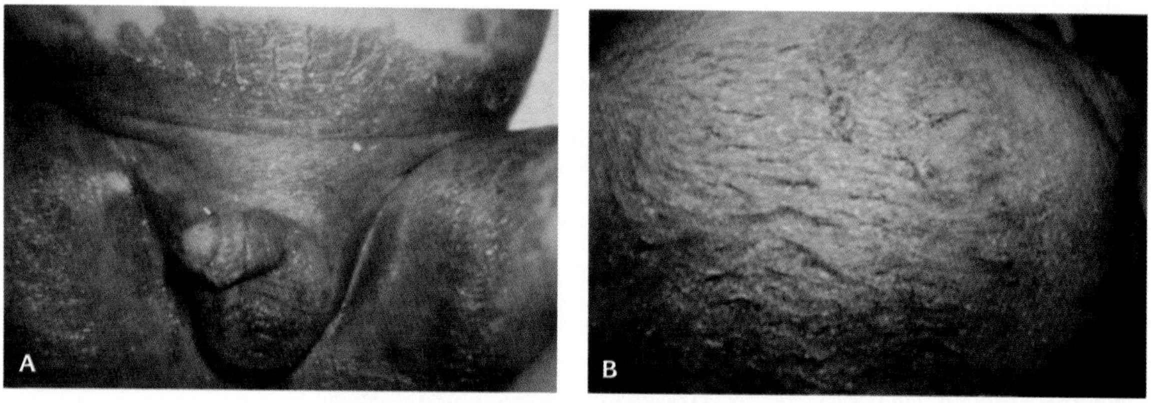

21.2. Seborrheic dermatitis. **(A)** The slightly greasy, red, scaling eruption typically begins in the groin creases and spreads throughout the diaper area. **(B)** "Cradle cap" consists of thick, tenacious scaling of the scalp. (Courtesy of Dr. Bernard Cohen.)

Table 21.1 Vesicular eruptions in the fetus or newborn

Genetic	Immunorelated	Infectious	Sporadic
Epidermolysis bullosa ectodermal dysplasia, incontinentia pigmenti, acrodermatitis enteropathica, hyperimmunoglobulinemia E syndrome	IgA dermatosis (chronic bullous disease of childhood) urticaria pigmentosa	Generalized sepsis (various organisms) 1. *herpes simplex infection* 2. *neonatal varicella congenital* 3. *neonatal candidiasis* 4. *staphylococcal pustulosis* 5. *streptococcal infections* 6. *Listeria monocytogenes*	Epidermal necrolysis Transient neonatal pustular melanosis Infantile acropustulosis Eosinophilic folliculitis Miliaria neonatal acne

or subepidermal (Table 21.1). The diagnosis is made by the location of this separation.

Epidermolysis Bullosa

Many types of epidermolysis bullosa (EB) have been described (Table 21.2 and Figure 21.3).

Table 21.2 Forms of epidermolysis bullosa (EB)

Name	Features	Genetics
1. Simplex EB (epidermolysis)	*Skin of skin cleavage: basal cells or suprabasal	AD
a. Localized EB, Weber-Cockayne	Bullae on hands and feet; presents in childhood; temperature dependent	
b. Generalized EB, Koebner	Generalized bullae; presents in infancy; heals without scarring	AD – K5, K14 keratin gene mutations
c. EB, herpetiformis, Dowling-Meara	Bullae with herpetiform pattern mainly on trunk	AD
d. EB with mottled pigmentation	Hyper- and hypopigmented spots on extremities	AD
e. EB simplex lethalis with neuromuscular disorder	Generalized bullae-presents at birth with associated neuromuscular disorder	AD (new mutation) or AR plectin gene mutation on chromosome 8
2. Junctional EB	*Site of cleavage is within lamina lucida of the epidermal–dermal junction but above the basement membrane	
a. Nonlethal	Bullae on neck, trunk, thighs, and legs; superficial bullae on extremities	AR
b. EB lethalis, Herlitz	Large bullae and skin erosions noted at birth; induced by friction and trauma; hemorrhage blisters; granulation tissue formation	AR – $\beta 3$ chain of laminin 5 bullous pemphigoid antigen, integrin $\beta 4$
3. Dystrophic (dermolytic) EB	*Site of cleavage below level of basement membrane	
a. Dominant dystrophic EB	Bullae present on hands, elbows, trunk and knees; scarring and atrophy	AD – Type VII (COL7A1) mutations
b. Recessive dermolytic EB	Bullae present at birth at sites of trauma; severe scarring, loss of nails, and fusion of digits; esophageal stricture; growth retardation	

EB, epidermolysis bullosa; AR, autosomal recessive, AD, autosomal dominant.
* Electron microscopy required to determine exact site of cleavage.

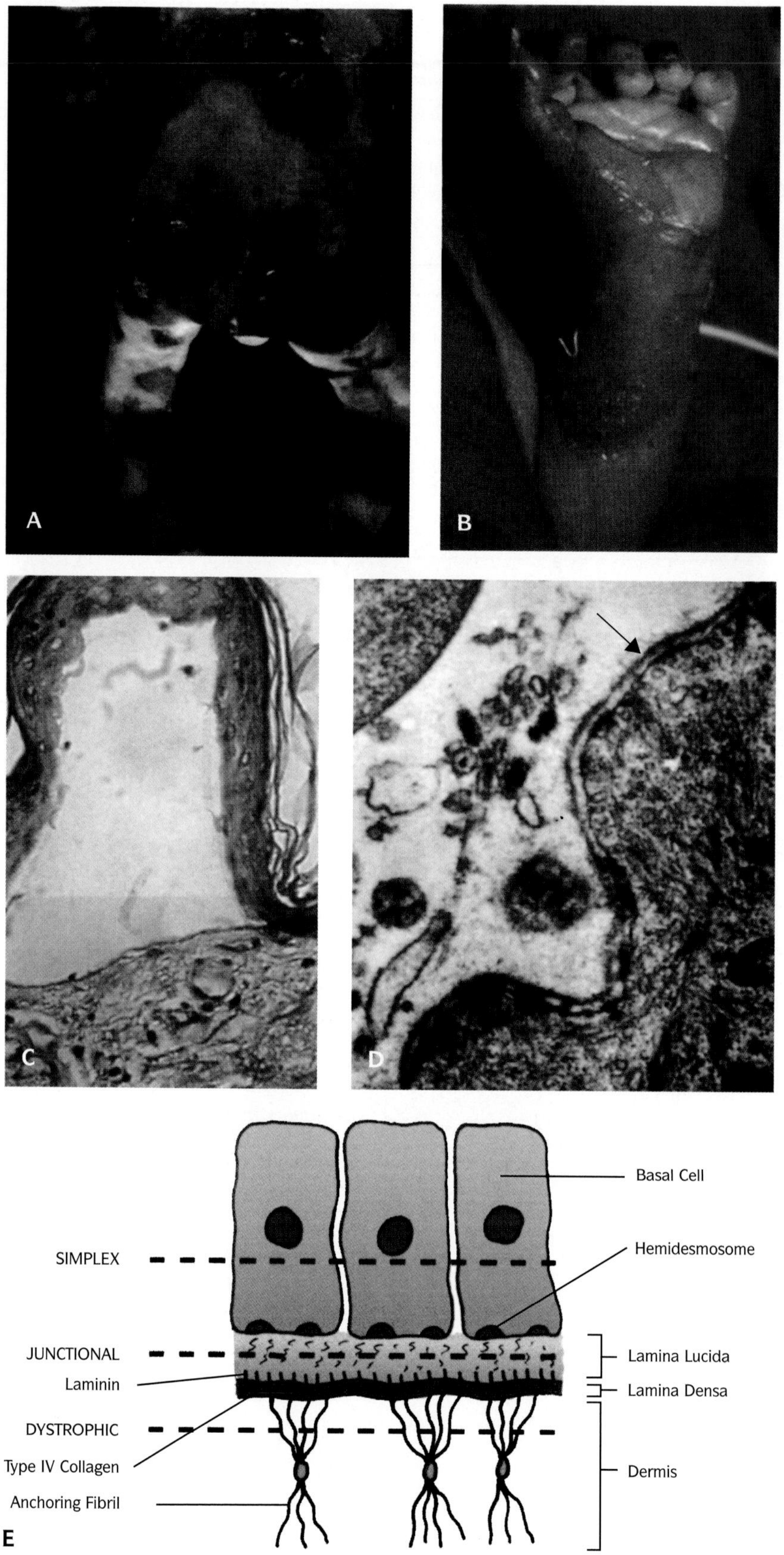

21.3. Epidermolysis bullosa (EB). **(A)** and **(B)** Widespread involvement in an infant at birth. The blisters break easily, leaving large denuded areas. **(C)** Microscopic appearance of dystrophic EB showing bullous lesion with clean separation below the level of the basement membrane. **(D)** Electron microscopy shows separation between the basal cells and the basement membrane (BM) due to degeneration and cytolytic changes of the basal cells. The anchoring fibrils of the BM are intact (arrow) and the plane of cleavage is in the basal epithelium. This occurs in EB simplex, EB of hands and feet (epidermolytic types), and EB lethalis and generalized atrophic benign EB (junctional forms). In dystrophic EB the separation occurs below the basement membrane (dermatolytic type). **(E)** Illustration of cleavage places in epidermolysis bullosa.

Toxic Epidermal Necrolysis (Lyell Type)

The disease may occur in the neonatal period. It begins with skin tenderness, erythema, a scalded appearance, and cleavage of the epidermis and is associated with skin and enteric infections. The lesion is an extensive necrosis and inflammation of epidermal cells and cleavage of most or the entire epidermis, which produces vesiculobullous lesions.

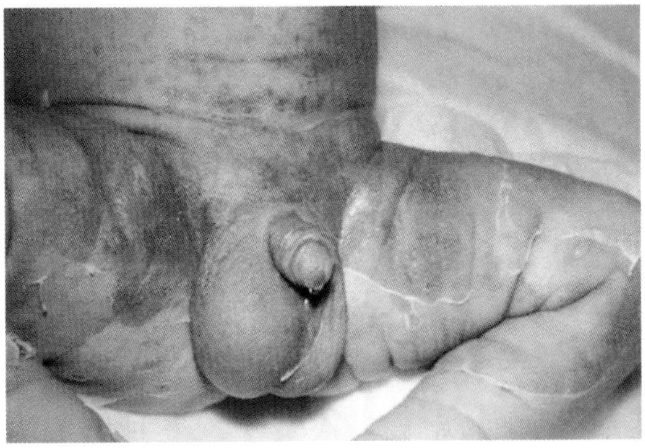

21.4. Staphylococcal scalded skin syndrome (toxic epidermal necrolysis) with desquamation of skin.

Staphylococcal Scalded Skin Syndrome (Ritter Disease)

This clinically resembles toxic epidermal necrolysis. Bullae form that, as they burst, leave a bright red, moist raw skin surface (Figure 21.4). Microscopically there are mild changes in the epidermal cells with separation of only the **superficial layers of the epidermis.**

Chronic Bullous Disease of Childhood (CBDC) (Linear IgA Dermatosis)

This lesion may occur in the newborn but more frequently occurs later in childhood (Figure 21.5). It presents with variably pruritic vesicles and bullae usually located on the perineum, thighs, buttocks, and lower abdomen, and less commonly on the arms, face, and legs. Blisters tend to cluster around the periphery of older, resolving lesions, giving it "a string of pearls" appearance. Oral mucosal erosions occur in up to 50% of patients.

The vesicles are caused by separation of the basal layer from the basement membrane with neutrophils and eosinophils. It has a characteristic immunofluorescence pattern with a linear IgA deposition in the basement membrane.

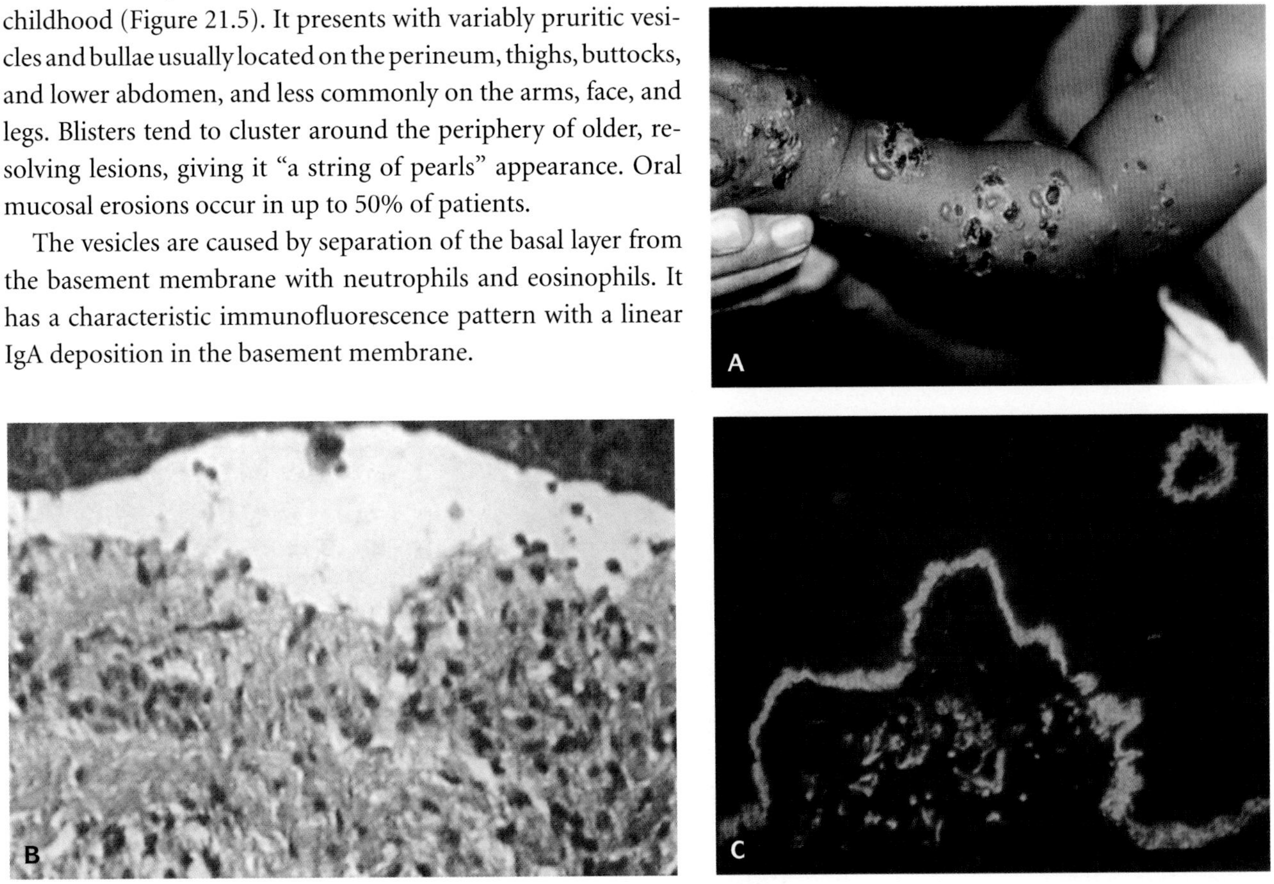

21.5. Chronic bullous disease of childhood. **(A)** Ruptured bullae have left annular and scalloped erosions. **(B)** Microscopic appearance of bullous lesion with epidermal-dermal separation. **(C)** IgA immunofluorescence at epidermal-dermal junction.

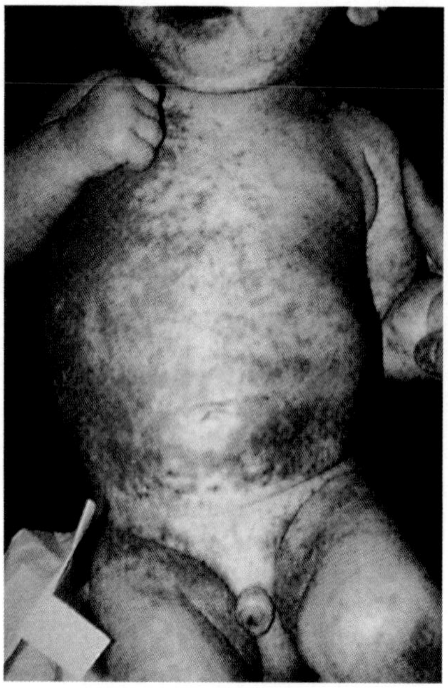

21.6. Acrodermatitis enteropathica. A bright-red scaling dermatitis that spread to the intertriginous areas, face and extremities of this four-week-old infant. (Courtesy of Dr. Cohen.)

Treatment with sulfonamides alone or in addition to prednisone may require 6 months or longer for improvement.

Acrodermatitis Enteropathica

This is an autosomal recessive vesiculobullous disease due to a zinc deficiency. The lesions are weeping, crusted erythematous patches affecting the diaper region, perioral, acral, and intertriginous areas (Figure 21.6). It may present in the neonatal period with diarrhea, anooral dermatitis, and alopecia. Affected infants have a defect in zinc binding protein in the gastrointestinal tract with resultant zinc malabsorption. Breast milk is protective because it contains a zinc binding ligand that facilitates zinc absorption. Acquired forms of this disease occur in infants receiving hyperalimentation with a low or absent zinc content and in malabsorption states (cystic fibrosis, chronic diarrhea, short bowel syndrome).

Incontinentia Pigmenti

Incontinentia pigmenti is an X-linked dominant trait and is lethal in males. The incidence in females is 1/40,000 (Figure 21.7).

Papules, vesicles, and pustules occur progressively on an erythematous base and are present at birth and may persist for months with peripheral eosinophilia. This is followed by verrucous pigmented hyperkeratosis and finally symmetrical hyperpigmentation. Dental anomalies and focal alopecia may be present.

Ichthyosis

The most severe form of ichthyosis occurs as the **harlequin fetus**, which is inherited as an autosomal recessive characteristic and is present at birth (Figure 21.8). The skin is extremely hyperkeratotic with large, rigid plaques between which are fissures imparting a grotesque appearance. The hands may appear moist and weeping with no apparent skin covering, and the nails may be

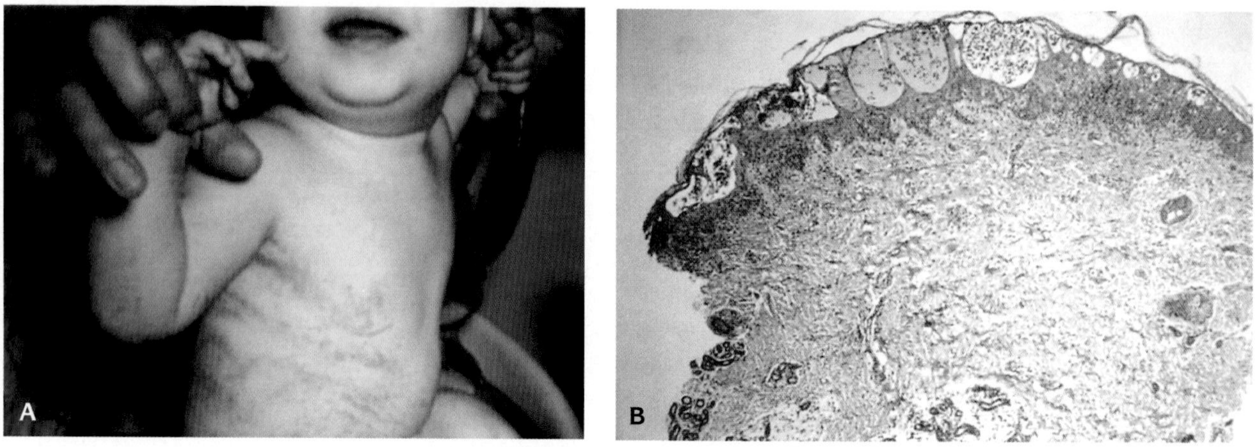

21.7. Incontinentia pigmenti. **(A)** Linear verrucous pigmented lesions on the trunk and arm present since birth. **(B)** A lesional biopsy specimen shows vesicular stage of incontinentia pigmenti with eosinophilic spongiosis and intraepidermal, eosinophil-containing vesicles.

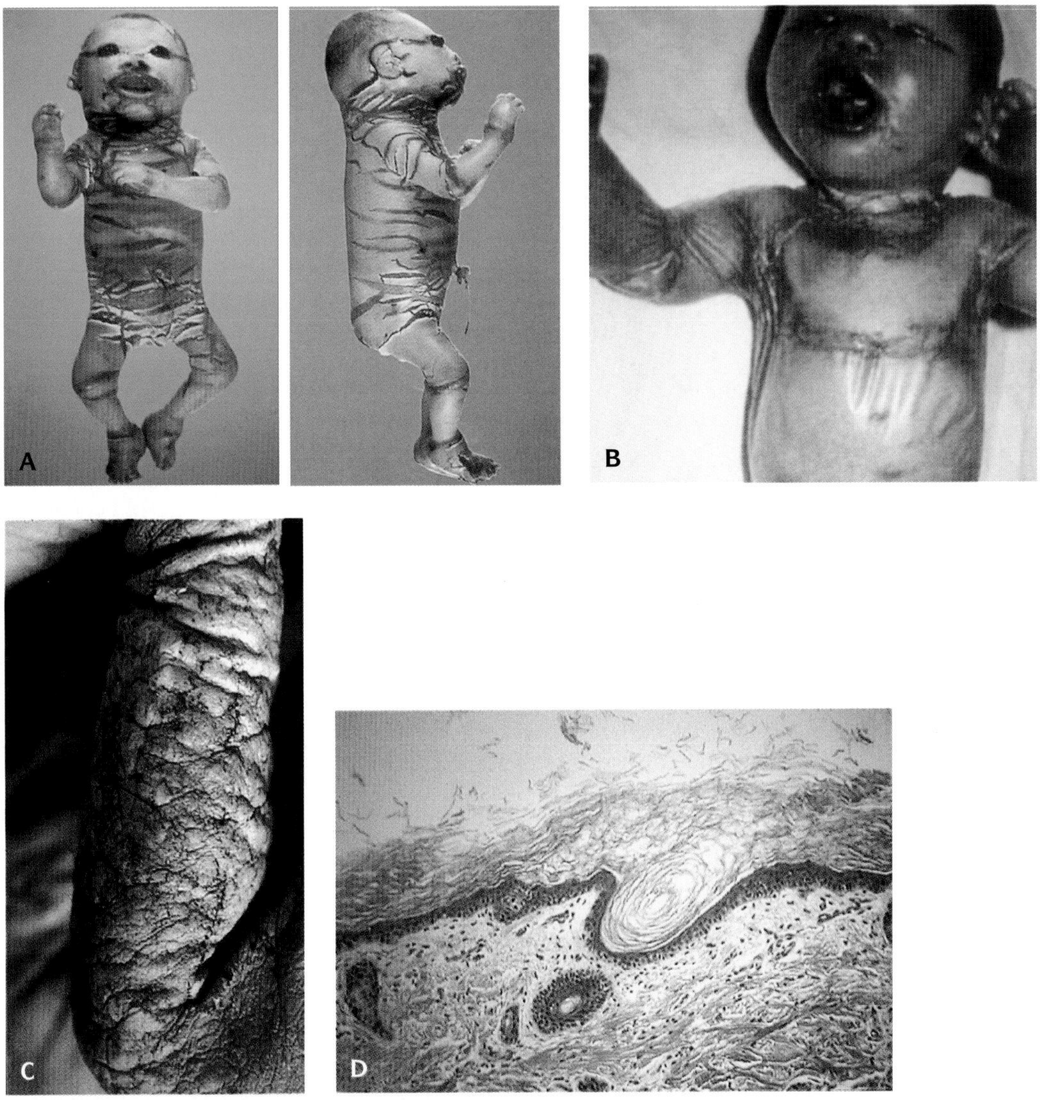

21.8. Ichthyosis. **(A)** Harlequin baby. This infant developed thick plate-like scales and ectropion immediately after birth followed by respiratory failure and death. **(B)** Collodion baby. A shiny transparent membrane covered the baby at birth. **(C)** Lamellar ichthyosis with thick brown scales covering the skin. **(D)** Microscopic appearance of hyperkeratotic skin in lamellar ichthyosis.

unrecognizable. The **collodion baby** (lamellar ichthyosis) is encased in a thick cellophane-like membrane with an incidence of 1/300,000 births. In about 30%, this may desquamate leaving normal skin. It is autosomal recessive. Ichthyosis simplex (vulgaris) is autosomal dominant with onset after birth. The skin is rough and scaly, and the lesion is most prominent on the extensor surfaces, especially elbows and knees. There is hyperkeratosis with decreased or absent granular layers. Incidence is 1/250 births.

X-linked ichthyosis is characterized by generalized large, dark scales with sparing of the palms and soles. In one-third, the lesions are present at birth; the incidence is 1/6,000 male births. There is hyperkeratosis and decreased steroid sulfatase C activity. Increased cholesterol sulfate in low density lipoproteins

Table 21.3 Major forms of ichthyosis

Form	Features	Age of onset	Genetics
Ichthyosis vulgaris	Atopy, mild scales, generalized	Childhood	AD
X-linked, ichthyosis	Corneal opacities, large trunk scales	Birth or infancy	XLR – most have steroid sulfatase deficiency
Lamellar ichthyosis	Ectropion, skin infections, collodion baby	Birth	AR and AD – most have mutations of transglutaminase 1
Epidermolytic hyperkeratosis (congenital ichthyosiform erythroderma)	Bullae, skin infections, offensive odor	Birth	AD – K1 and K10 keratin gene mutations
Ichthyosis congenita (ichthyosis gravis, harlequin fetus)	Thick plaques of stratum corneum, fissures, death in neonatal period	Birth	AR
Epidermolytic palmoplantar keratoderma	Diffuse thickening of epidermis on entire surfaces of palms and soles.	Infancy	AD – K9 keratin gene mutations
Nonepidermolytic palmoplantar keratoderma	Thick palms and soles	Birth	AD – K16 keratin gene mutations

result in increased mobility on lipoprotein electrophoresis. Steroid sulfatase locus is on the distal arm of the X chromosome.

Prenatal diagnosis by fetoscopic skin biopsy in all forms of ichthyosis is possible.

Trichothiodystrophy

Trichothiodystrophy is a term that describes ichthyosis with brittle hair, intellectual impairment, decreased fertility, and short stature (IBIDS) (Figure 21.9 and Table 21.4). There is a low concentration of cystine in an amino acid analysis of the hair.

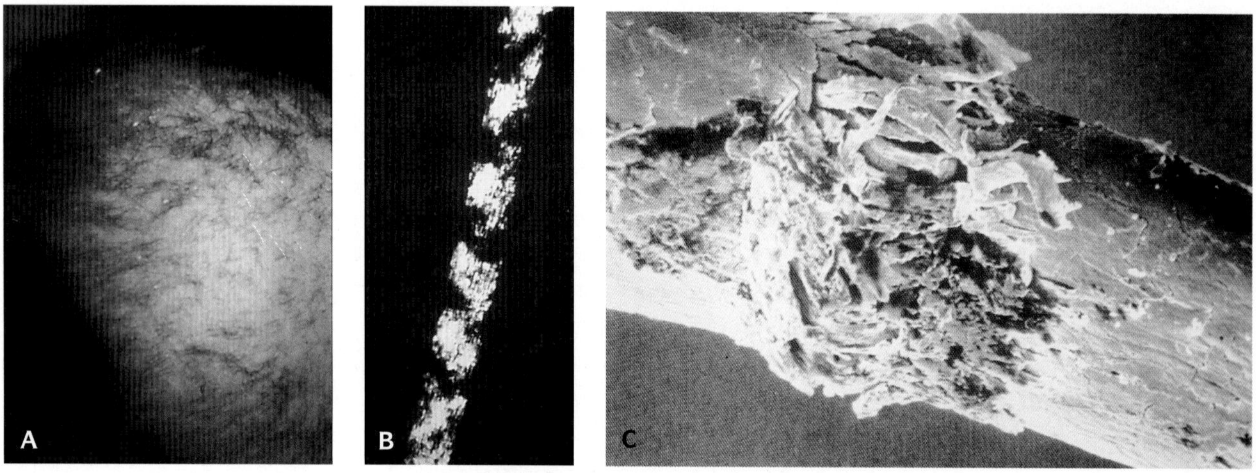

21.9. Trichothiodystrophy. **(A)** Sparse, brittle coarse hair of scalp. **(B)** Polarized light reveals alternating segments of light and dark bands with ribbon-like appearance. **(C)** Scanning electron microscopic appearance of hair shaft showing disruption.

Table 21.4 Signs and symptoms commonly associated with trichothiodystrophy

Skin	Ichthyosis, collodion baby, photosensitivity, eczema, erythroderma, xeroderma, pigmentosum
Nails	Dysplasia, splitting, koilonychia
Eyes	Cataracts, conjunctivitis, pale optic disc
Genital organs	Hypoplasia, cryptorchism
Morphologic changes and dysmorphic	Protruding ears, dental abnormalities, caries, thin-beaked nose, progeria, receding chin, growth retardation
Nervous system	Retardation, microcephaly, microdolichocephaly
Immune system	Recurrent infection
Amino acid	Low cystine content analysis

Modified from Itin and Pittelkow: Trichothiodystrophy update on the sulphur deficient brittle hair syndromes. *J Am Acad Dermatol* 44:891, 2001.

Menkes kinky hair syndrome is X-linked due to a defect in intestinal copper absorption resulting in a low serum copper level and low ceruloplasmin. All copper enzymes are deficient. Deficiency of the elastin leads to tortuosity of arteries. There is profound mental retardation.

An eyebrow hair biopsy by fetoscopy has confirmed the diagnosis in a 20-week fetus (Figure 21.10).

VESICULOPUSTULAR ERUPTIONS IN THE NEWBORN

Erythema Toxicum Neonatorum (ETN)

A common disorder, ETN affects as many as 70% of all newborns, in whom erythematous macules and pustules are simultaneously present (Table 21.5 and Figure 21.11). These lesions last 3 or 4 days and usually disappear with no sequelae, but in malnourished or compromised infants secondary infection may cause serious illness. Peripheral eosinophilia occurs in 20% of cases.

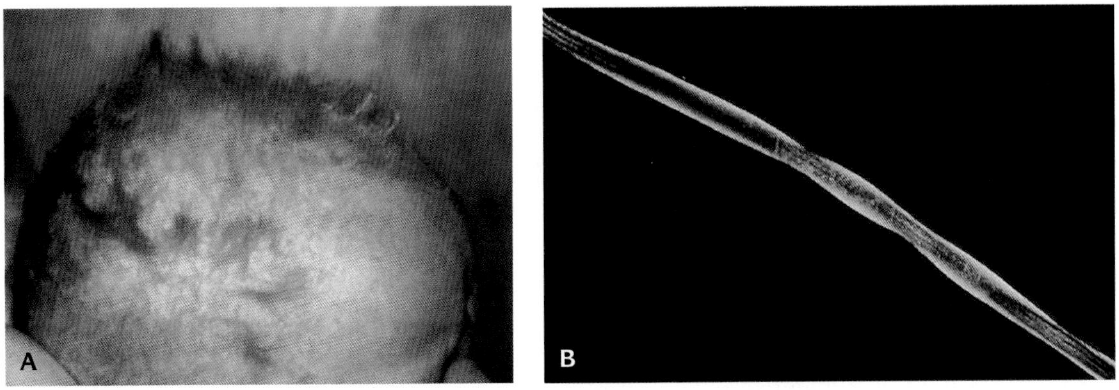

21.10. Menkes kinky hair syndrome. **(A)** The scalp hair is coarse, kinky, and brittle. **(B)** Hair under polarized light shows pili torti.

Table 21.5 Conditions with vesiculopustular and/or bullous lesions in the newborn

Vesicles and pustules	Bullae
*Acne vulgaris: neonatal	‡Acrodermatitis enteropathica
‡Acrodermatitis enteropathica	‡Aplasia cutis congenita
†Acropustulosis of infancy	*Bullous impetigo
‡Behcet disease: neonatal	‡Chronic bullous dermatosis of childhood
†Candidiasis: congenital cutaneous	‡Diffuse cutaneous mastocytosis
*Candidiasis: neonatal	‡Ectodermal dysplasias
‡Cytomegalovirus	‡Epidermolysis bullosa
‡Eosinophilic pustular folliculitis	†Epidermolytic hyperkeratosis
*Erythema toxicum neonatorum	‡Erythropoietic porphyria
†Herpes simplex: perinatal	‡Gangrene of buttock: perinatal
‡Histiocytosis: congenital self-healing	‡Maternal bullous disease
‡Histocytosis: Langerhans' cell	‡Protein C or S deficiency: congenital
‡Hyperimmunoglobulin E syndrome	‡*Pseudomonas* infection
†Incontinentia pigmenti	†Staphylococcal scalded skin syndrome
‡*Listeria monocytogenes*	*Sucking blisters
*Miliaria crystallina	‡Syphilis: congenital
*Miliaria rubra	‡Toxic epidermal necrolysis
†Scabies	‡Varicella: neonatal
†Sepsis	
*Staphylococcal pyoderma	
*Transient neonatal pustular melanosis	
‡Varicella: neonatal	

*Common cause; †uncommon causes; ‡rare causes.

Microscopically the dermis is edematous with intense eosinophilic infiltration with a few neutrophilic polymorphonuclear and mononuclear cells in a perivascular distribution.

Neonatal pustular melanosis (**NPM**) is a transient lesion characterized by pustules and pigmented macules appearing at birth that rupture easily leaving a collarette of fine white scales and a tiny central brown macule on the chin, forehead, nape, lower back, and skin.

Skin biopsy reveals hyperkeratosis, acanthosis, and intracorneal vesicles with small collections of neutrophils, eosinophils, and keratinous debris.

Acropustulosis of Infancy

Infantile acropustulosis may be present in the neonatal period. It is characterized by crops of very pruritic, recurrent vesiculopustules ranging from 1 to 3 mm in diameter. The lesions occur primarily on the palms and soles.

Microscopically, there is focal intraepidermal necrolysis followed by the formation of vesicles that become filled with neutrophils and eosinophils.

INFECTIOUS ERUPTIONS

Impetigo

The skin lesions of bullous impetigo, which frequently are noted at birth, usually are characterized initially by vesicles, rapidly progressing to large bullae

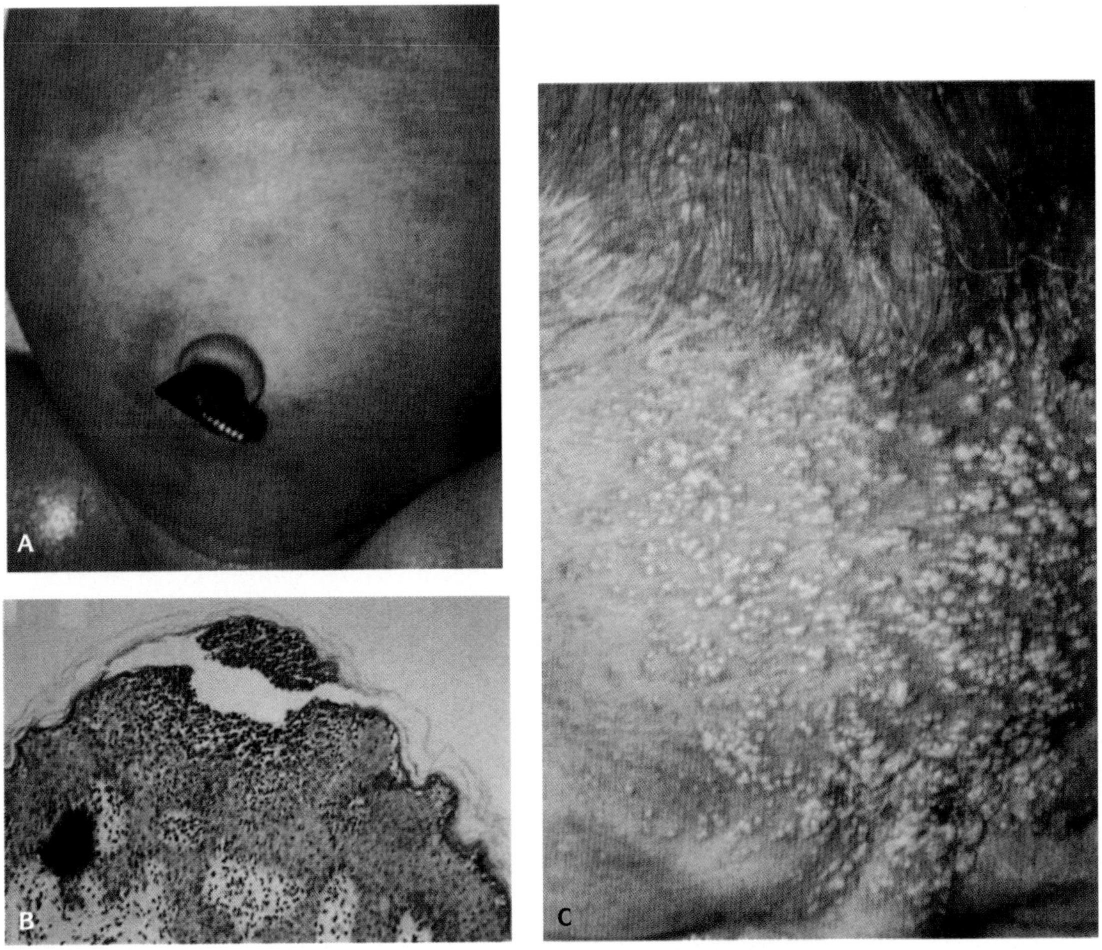

21.11. Erythema toxicum neonatorum. **(A)** Numerous yellow papules and pustules are surrounded by large, intensely erythematous rings on the trunk of this infant. **(B)** Microscopic appearance of intracorneal pustule containing polymorphonuclear leukocytes. **(C)** Transient neonatal pustular melanosis. Numerous tiny pustules dot the forehead and scalp of this neonate. (Courtesy of Dr. Bernard Cohen.)

filled with clear or cloudy fluid (Figure 21.12). The causative agent is usually *Staphylococcus aureus*, phage group II.

Candida Infection

Candida colonizes the gastrointestinal tract and skin shortly after birth and may produce both localized (thrush and diaper dermatitis) and disseminated cutaneous infection as well as systemic infection in the newborn (Figure 21.13). This lesion also should raise the suspicion of heritable or acquired immunodeficiency. Recurrent and persistent infection in infancy may be associated with the use of antibiotics.

Syphilis

The skin lesions of congenital syphilis are the result of an intrauterine syphilitic infection (Figure 21.14). The diffuse lesions have a special predilection for the

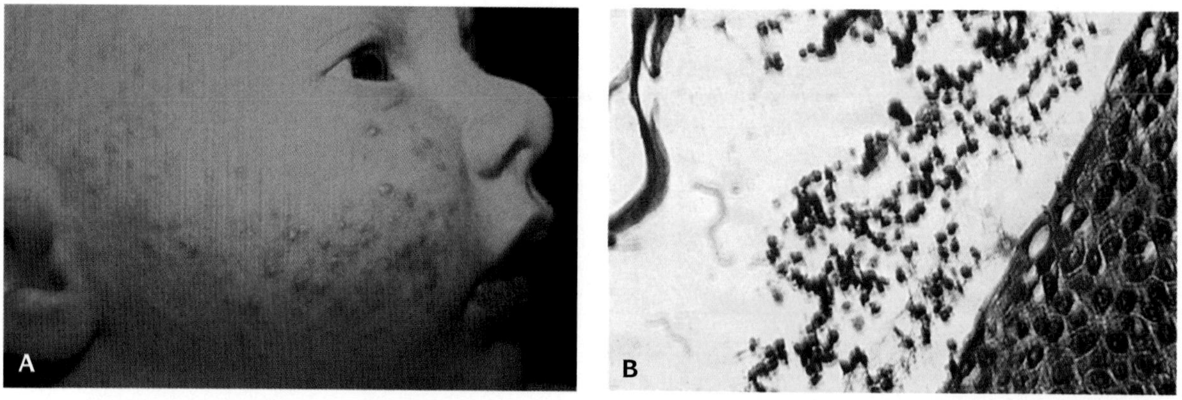

21.12. Impetigo in a newborn infant. **(A)** Child with pustules, erythema and crusts on the chin. **(B)** Microscopic examination shows a pustule beneath the keratin layer containing polymorphonuclear leukocytes. It progresses to involve the epidermis.

face, palms, and soles. Skin is brittle and shiny, often cracked and covered by large thick scales. In macerated stillborn fetuses, spirochetes can be detected, and there is hepatosplenomegaly, nucleated red blood cells in villous capillaries, and chorioamnionitis.

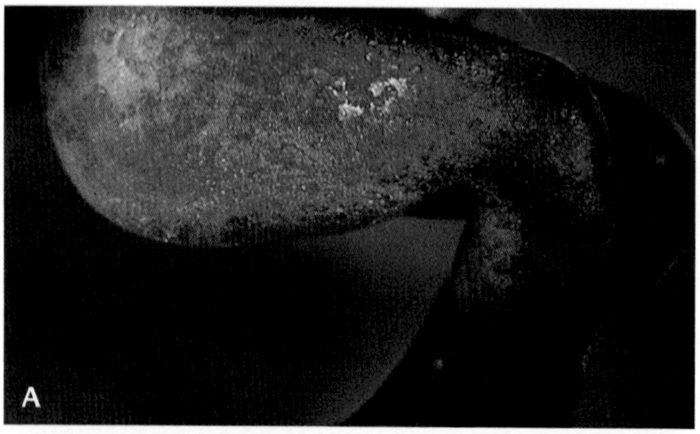

Rhagades develop in the first few days of life as moist, ulcerating lesions extending outward in a liner manner from the angles of the eyes, nose, and mouth.

Herpes Simplex

This infection results from inoculation from genital herpes in the mother. Infection in the neonate has a high risk of dissemination (Figure 21.15). It has an incidence of 1/3,500 deliveries. A skin rash occurs in 70%, and 90% of those infants develop systemic disease with lung, liver, gastrointestinal, and brain involvement with high mortality.

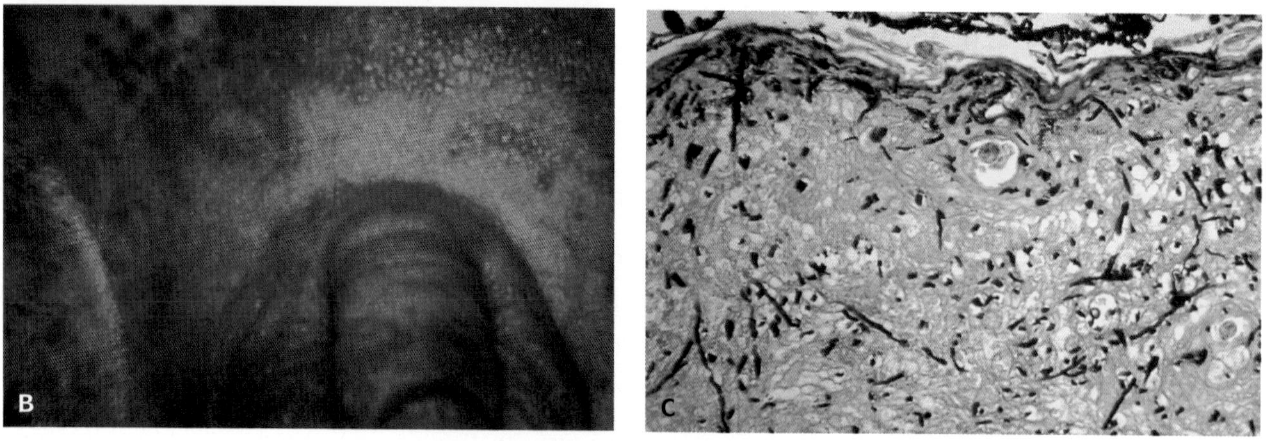

21.13. *Candida* infection. **(A** and **B)** The eruption is bright red with numerous pinpoint satellite papules and pustules. Intertriginous areas are prominently involved. [**(B)** is courtesy of Dr. Bernard Cohen.] **(C)** Microscopic appearance shows dermal infiltrate of predominantly plasma cells with candida hyphae (Gomori methenamine silver stain).

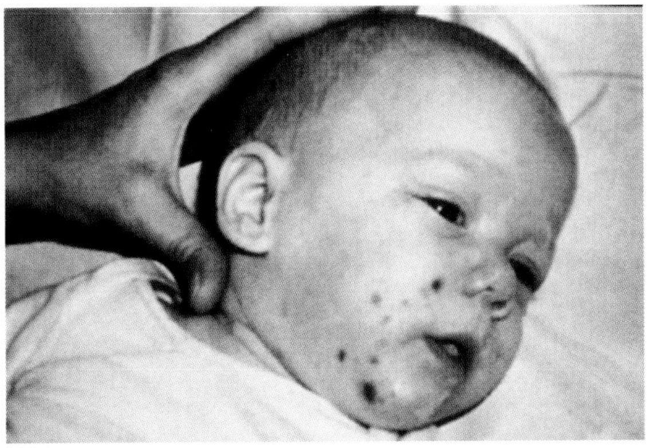

21.14. Congenital syphilis. Infant with a scaly eruption reminiscent of the lesions of secondary syphilis may appear on the face, trunk, and extremities. (Courtesy of Dr. Bernard Cohen.)

Varicella-Zoster

Perinatal infection with varicella has a high mortality risk and has been recorded in both stillborn and liveborn infants. It is a dermatomal cutaneous infection caused by reactivation of varicella-zoster virus in the mother. It is a generalized infection with involvement predominantly of the brain, liver, and spleen as well as the skin.

Subcutaneous Fat Necrosis (SFN)

Obstetric trauma in the form of extreme pressure against hard underlying structures has been implicated as a primary cause of this lesion (Figure 21.16).

It consists of sharply defined, nonelevated areas of subcutaneous induration that appear a few days after birth in large, well-developed, otherwise healthy infants, most commonly on the back, cheeks, arms, thighs, buttocks, calves, and shoulders. The lesions are woody in consistency and do not pit on pressure; the overlying skin is blue or violet. These lesions ordinarily disappear in 3 or 4 months.

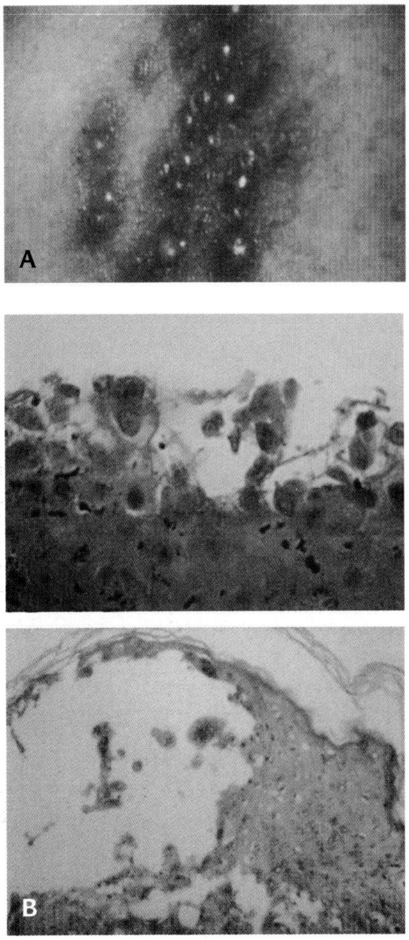

21.15. **(A)** Herpes simplex vesicular lesions of skin. **(B)** Microscopic appearance of skin showing intranuclear inclusion (top). Intraepidermal vesicle (bottom).

Sclerema Neonatorum

This lesion appears to be a complication of multisystem failure with cooling of the skin and subcutaneous adipose tissue from decreased cutaneous perfusion. It is characterized by a widespread induration of the skin that begins between the third and fourth day after birth. It appears first on the legs or face and in a short time may involve all the body surfaces except the palms, soles, and scrotum. The affected areas are smooth, hard, dry, cold to touch, and whitish or waxy in appearance. A skin biopsy shows edema of the fibrous septae without necrosis of fat cells. The prognosis is poor, with death occurring in 75% of cases in a short time. The condition is limited almost exclusively to premature infants.

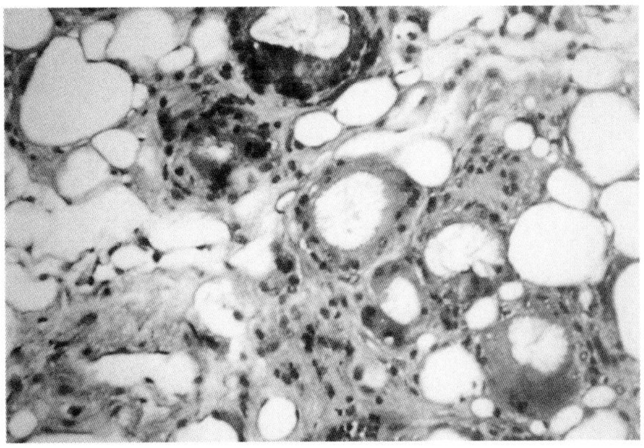

21.16. Subcutaneous fat necrosis with multinucleated giant cells and refractile crystals representing triglycerides are present.

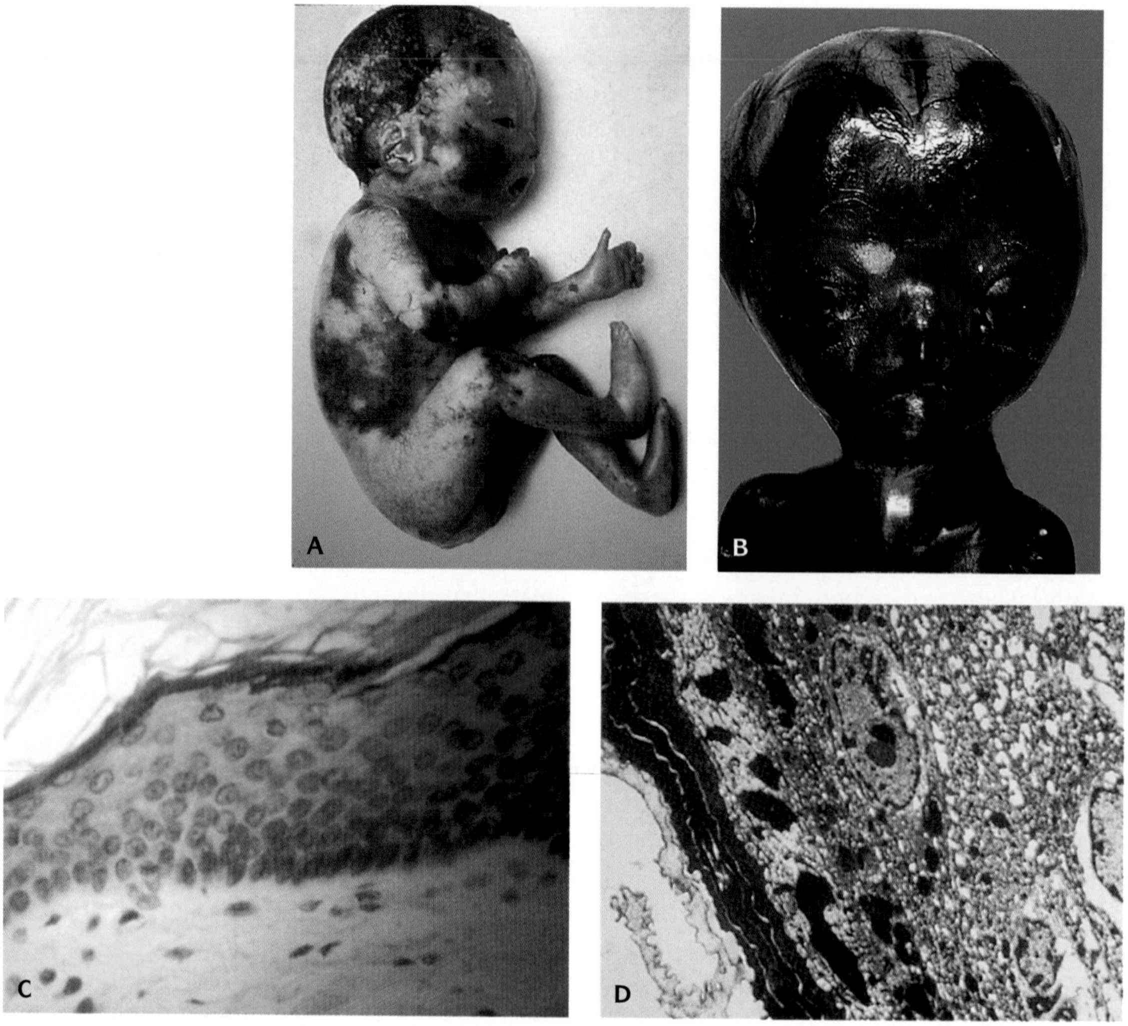

21.17. Restrictive dermopathy. **(A)** Term female infant. Absent nipples, elbow and hip contractions, skin thicker across buttocks, patulous everted anus, no gluteal crease. **(B)** A 29-week fetus weighed 760 g. The sagittal suture is 6 cm across, brain shows through dura, cataracts, membrane across nares, mouth, and ears. **(C)** Hyperkeratosis, parakeratosis, flat DE junction, dense dermis with atrophic glands, thick collagen bands parallel to epidermis, rare elastin fibrils. **(D)** Electron microscopy shows abnormal keratohyalin granules, decreased numbers of desmosomes, and epidermolysis. (Courtesy Dr. Karen Schmidt.)

Scleredema

This lesion is similar to sclerema except for edema; it most often begins in the legs. The affected areas are swollen and doughy in consistency and pit on pressure. Scleredema usually appears as a diffuse waxlike hardening of the skin in a severely ill newborn from the second to the fourth day after delivery.

Intense edema with mild nonspecific changes such as dilation of the vessels, edema, and minimal inflammation in the skin, the subcutaneous tissue, and sometimes the underlying muscle characterize the lesion.

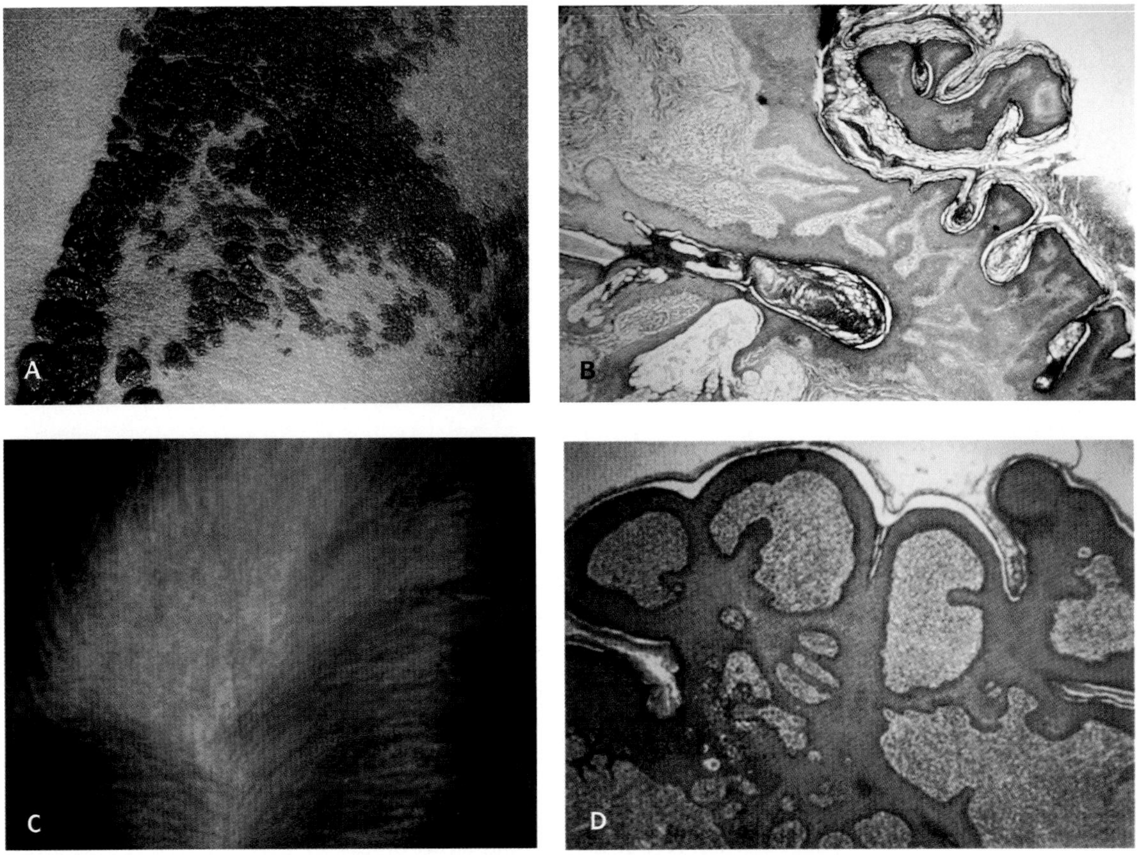

21.18. Epidermal nevus. **(A)** Child with multiple hyperpigmented verrucous epidermal nevi present on the face and trunk. **(B)** Microscopic appearance with epidermolytic hyperkeratosis. **(C)** Nevus sebaceous of Jadassohn. A yellow hairless patch was present since birth. **(D)** Microscopic appearance of nevus sebaceous of Jadassohn. (Courtesy of Dr. Bernard Cohen.)

Restrictive Dermopathy

Restrictive dermopathy is an autosomal recessive disorder in which the skin is thickened, scaly, and noncompliant with irregular shiny erythematous thin patches and hypoplastic nails (Figure 21.17). The eyebrows, eyelids, and scalp hair are sparse. The epidermis is hyperplastic, keratin proteins are quantitatively abnormal, and, ultrastructurally, keratin filaments are deficient and keratohyalin is abnormal. Prenatal fetal skin biopsy may be diagnostic. It is usually rapidly fatal.

MALFORMATION OF THE SKIN AND ITS APPENDAGES

Sebaceous Nevus of Jadassohn

Sebaceous nevus of Jadassohn is observed in the neonate as flat or slightly raised, yellow-brown to pink hairless plaques distributed over the scalp or forehead, face, and trunk (Figure 21.18). The nevus tends to regress after birth only to enlarge again at puberty. The skin appendages appear malformed and irregular and the sebaceous glands are increased in number. There is a predisposition to basal cell carcinoma and adnexal tumors arising from the lesion, and therefore removal is indicated.

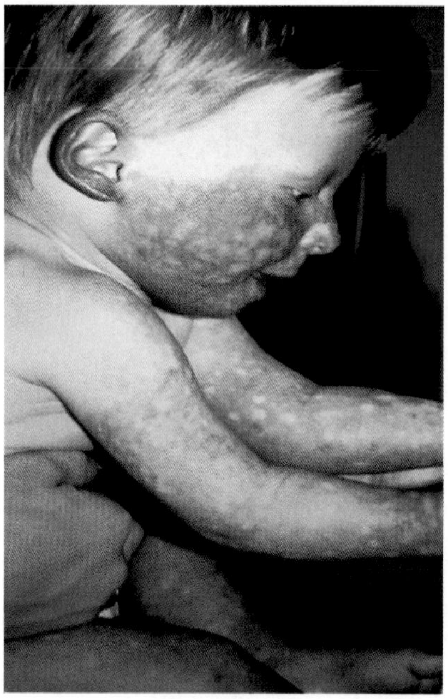

21.19. Congenital cutaneous dystrophy (Rothmund-Thomson syndrome). This infant has a diffuse erythematous rash involving the face, arms, and legs.

Linear Sebaceous Nevus Syndrome

This lesion is associated with visceral malformations, including meningeal hemangiomas, congenital heart disease, urinary tract anomalies, nephroblastomatosis, hydrocephalus, vitamin D-resistant rickets, colobomas, ocular desmoids, seizures, and mental retardation. It is usually sporadic but autosomal dominant inheritance has been reported.

Congenital Cutaneous Dystrophy (Rothmund-Thomson Syndrome, Poikiloderma Congenitale)

This autosomal recessive disease is characterized by skin lesions and congenital cataracts. The skin lesions that are light sensitive early in life begin as a network of fine red lines separating areas of normal skin over part or all of the body. The involved skin becomes irregularly atrophic, hyperkeratotic, and pigmented (Figure 21.19). Abnormalities of the teeth and dystrophic nails, minor skeletal malformations, dwarfism, and hypogonadism occur in more than one-third of patients.

Focal Dermal Hypoplasia (Goltz Syndrome)

In this condition there is thinning of the dermis, hypopigmentation and hyperpigmentation, telangiectasia, focal absence of the skin appendages, and

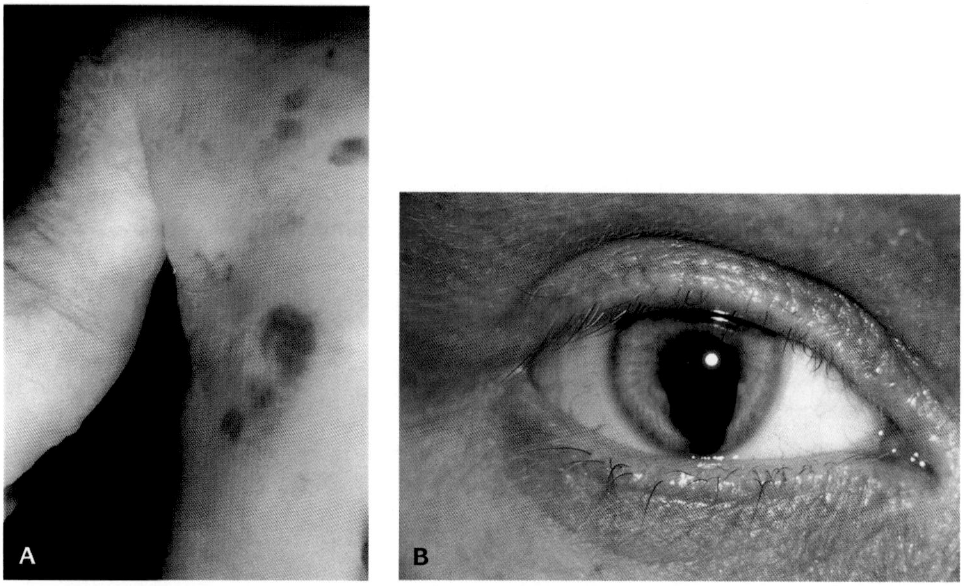

21.20. Focal dermal hypoplasia (Goltz syndrome). **(A)** Multiple lesions of aplasia and hypoplasia of the skin in this newborn infant. **(B)** Coloboma of iris.

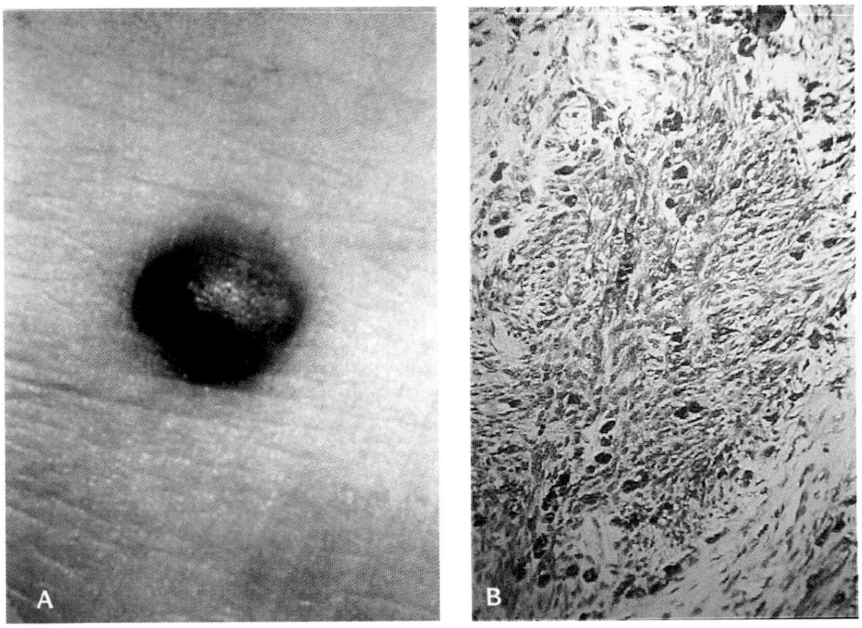

21.21. Blue nevus. **(A)** This firm blue nodule is composed of deep nevus cells. **(B)** Histiologic appearance with dendritic, oval, fusiform and spindle melanocytes deep within the dermis.

herniation of the subcutaneous adipose tissue into the skin due to thinning of the dermis and the absence of dermal elastic tissue (Figure 21.20). The nails are fissured, striated, and atrophic. Associated anomalies may include those of bone (e.g., spina bifida, fuse vertebral, syndactyly, and hypoplasia of the ribs) and eye (e.g., microphthalmia, strabismus, and coloboma). This is an X-linked abnormality with a variety of malformations of other parts of the body.

Melanocytic Lesions

One percent of melanocytic nevi are congenital. Nevi less than 2 cm in greatest dimension are by far more frequent than the giant pigmented nevi, which are noted in fewer than 1/20,000 newborns. Giant melanocytic nevi range from flat to nodular to rough and verrucous. The amounts of pigmentation and hair differ. The incidence of malignant melanoma arising from a giant pigmented nevus is approximately 6%.

An extra chromosome 7 (trisomy 7), reported in malignant melanomas, has been found in congenital pigmented nevi also. Giant hairy nevi may have leptomeningeal involvement (meningeal melanosis).

Microscopically nevus cells extend deep into the dermis and subcutaneous fat and connective tissue and surround skin appendages, blood, and lymphatic vessels in an infiltrative fashion. In addition to the melanocytic component, the congenital nevus may contain blue nevus and neural elements.

Blue Nevus is a small firm blue-purple lesion composed of dendritic melanocytes deep within the dermis. It is seldom recognized in the newborn.

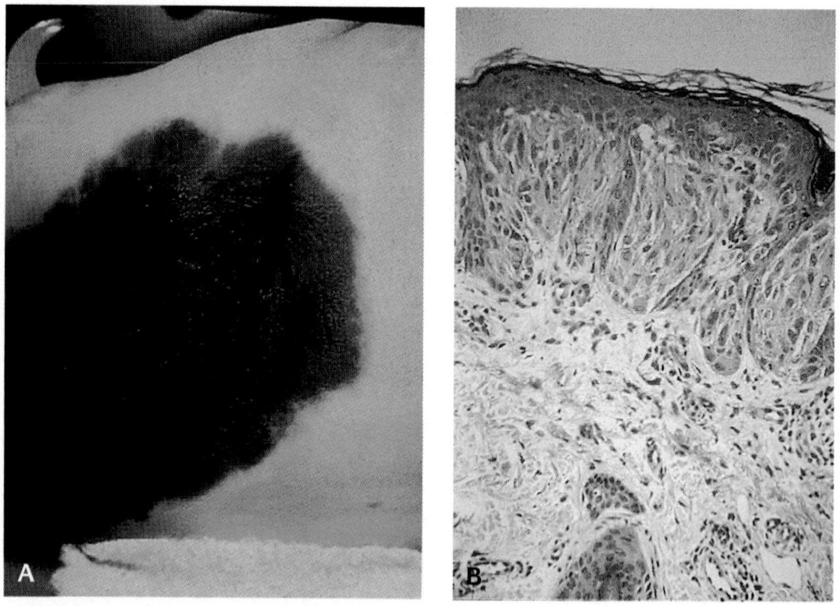

21.22. **(A)** Congenital giant hairy nevus on the trunk of a newborn infant. **(B)** Nevus cells in the papillary dermis with extension into the deep dermis.

LEOPARD (multiple lentigines) syndrome (**l**entigines, **e**lectrocardiographic changes, **o**cular hypertelorism, **p**ulmonary stenosis, **a**bnormal genitalia, **r**etarded growth, **d**eafness) is an autosomal dominant trait with numerous lentigines up to 5 mm in diameter present over the skin (Figures 21.21 to 21.23). Cardiac disorders, growth retardation, and conduction deafness are also present.

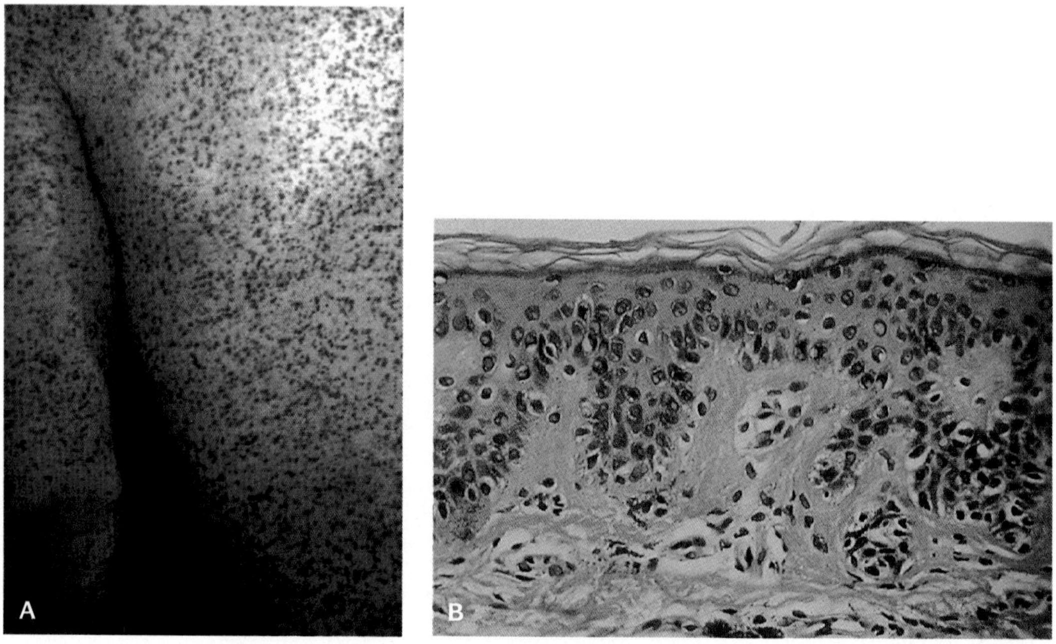

21.23. LEOPARD syndrome. **(A)** The skin is covered with sharply circumscribed lentiginous lesions. **(B)** The lentigo lesion shows elongation and melanin hyperpigmentation of the rete ridges.

Urticaria Pigmentosa

In this condition bullous or nodular lesions associated with focal or diffuse infiltration of mast cells in the skin appear in infants (Figure 21.24). They may be preceded by a pink macular rash and fever; later, plaques may develop in the dermis. The lesions consist of masses of mast cells located in the upper part of the dermis with the overlying dermis normal except for increased melanin in the basal layers. The cells are often spindle shaped, and their identity may not be appreciated without a Giemsa stain to demonstrate the presence of metachromatic granules. When discrete, the lesions usually disappear in childhood. When diffuse, they may persist throughout life; the disease may be generalized and the liver, spleen, and bone marrow may become involved. Leukemia may eventually develop. Mastocytoma arising as a separate nodule from within a congenital melanocytic nevus has been documented.

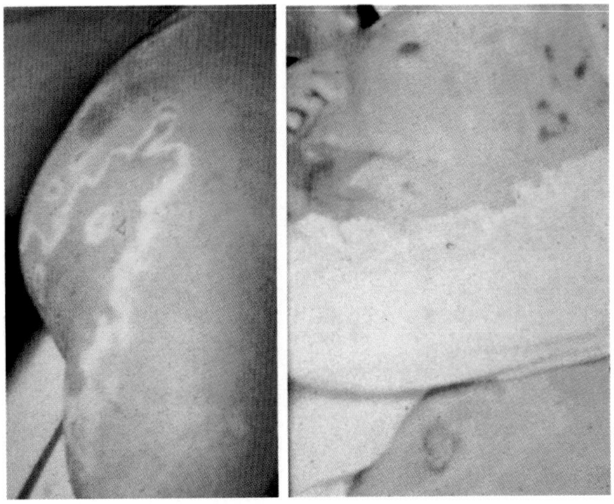

21.24. Urticaria pigmentosa. (Left) Lesion of the buttock. (Right) Lesions on the face and chest.

XERODERMA PIGMENTOSUM

This lesion belongs to a group of disorders due to abnormalities in DNA repair. It is an autosomal recessive disorder. Marked photosensitivity and ultraviolet skin damage predispose to malignancy (Figure 21.25). It consists of at least seven complementation groups (A to G) and additional variants. The skin becomes atrophic and punctate stellate telangiectasias appear. The lesions become hypo- or hyperpigmented and poikiloderma results. Ocular abnormalities occur in 40% of cases and mental deficiency and neurologic abnormalities occur in 20%. Prenatal diagnosis is possible by detecting impairment in DNA repair after irradiation of cultured amniotic fibroblasts with UV light.

Ectodermal Dysplasia

Ectodermal dysplasias are a complex heterogeneous group of congenital, nonprogressive, developmental disorders of structures derived from ectoderm – i.e., the epidermis, hair, nails, teeth, and sweat glands.

The **hidrotic form** (Clouston ectodermal dysplasia), in which the sweat glands are not affected, is inherited as an autosomal dominant characteristic (Figure 21.26). Sparse thin hair and scanty eyelashes and brows are characteristic findings.

In the **X-linked recessive anhidrotic** form (Christ-Siemens-Touraine syndrome), the sweat glands are absent or rudimentary, and both dermis and epidermis are abnormally thin. The scalp hair is soft and sparse, the eyebrows are absent, the eyelashes are few, the internal structures are dry, and ozena (foul smell) is present; the teeth are hypoplastic, the nails are absent,

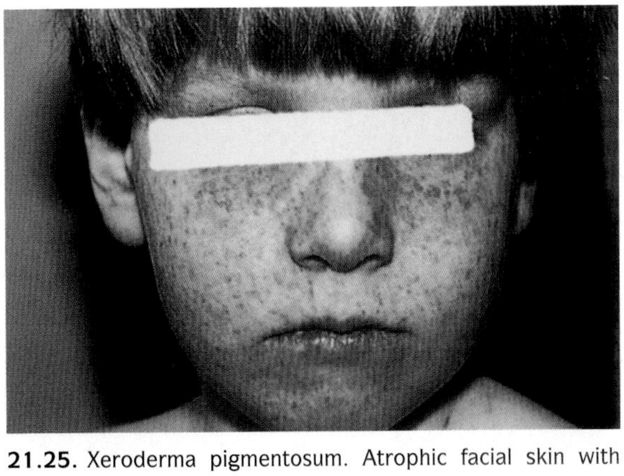

21.25. Xeroderma pigmentosum. Atrophic facial skin with multiple pigmented lesions. A nodule on the forehead was a squamous carcinoma.

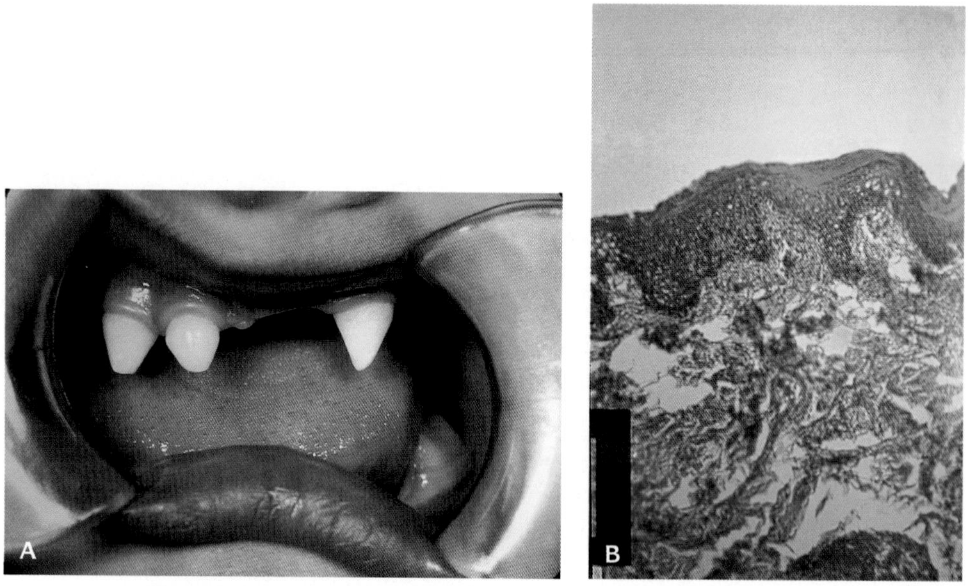

21.26. Ectodermal dysplasia. **(A)** Most of the teeth are missing but others are peg-shaped. **(B)** Microscopic section of skin shows absence of hair follicles and sebaceous glands.

and the subcutaneous tissue is so sparse that the skin is easily picked up and folded on itself.

Multiple Pterygia (Fetal Akinesia)

This may be multiple and familial. The condition restricts movement of the extremities and may result in arthrogryposis (Figure 21.27).

Langerhans Cell Histocytosis

Langerhans cell histiocytosis (LCH) is a group of disorders previously referred to as histiocytosis X, Letterer-Siwe, Hand-Schüller-Christian disease, or eosinophilic granuloma. LCH is a proliferative disorder of histiocytes in which the consistent pathologic finding is the presence of Langerhans cells, dendritic cells that originate in the bone marrow mononuclear-phagocytic system (Figure 21.28). LCH is defined as an abnormal proliferation of cells that express S100 and CD1a, a phenotype similar to the normal Langerhans cells of the epidermis, and demonstrate the presence of Birbeck granules by electron microscopy.

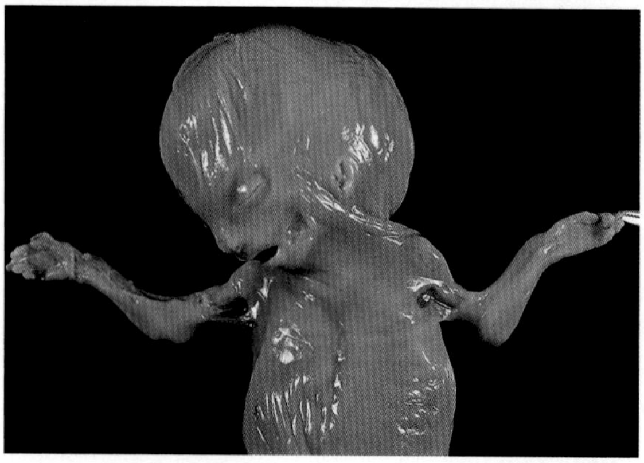

21.27. Multiple pterygia in a fetus. Note the pterygia at the neck, axilla, and antecubital fossa.

Skin lesions in LCH can present clinically as a generalized or focal disorder except in the newborn, in whom the disease is limited to the skin. The definitive diagnosis is based on ultrastructural demonstration of Birbeck granules and/or CD1a immuno positivity.

Microscopically the infiltration in the skin is histiocytes that have light pink eosinophilic cytoplasm, with oval or elongated grooved nuclei, fine chromatin, and a small nucleolus with multinucleated giant cells, lymphocytes, plasma cells, and eosinophils.

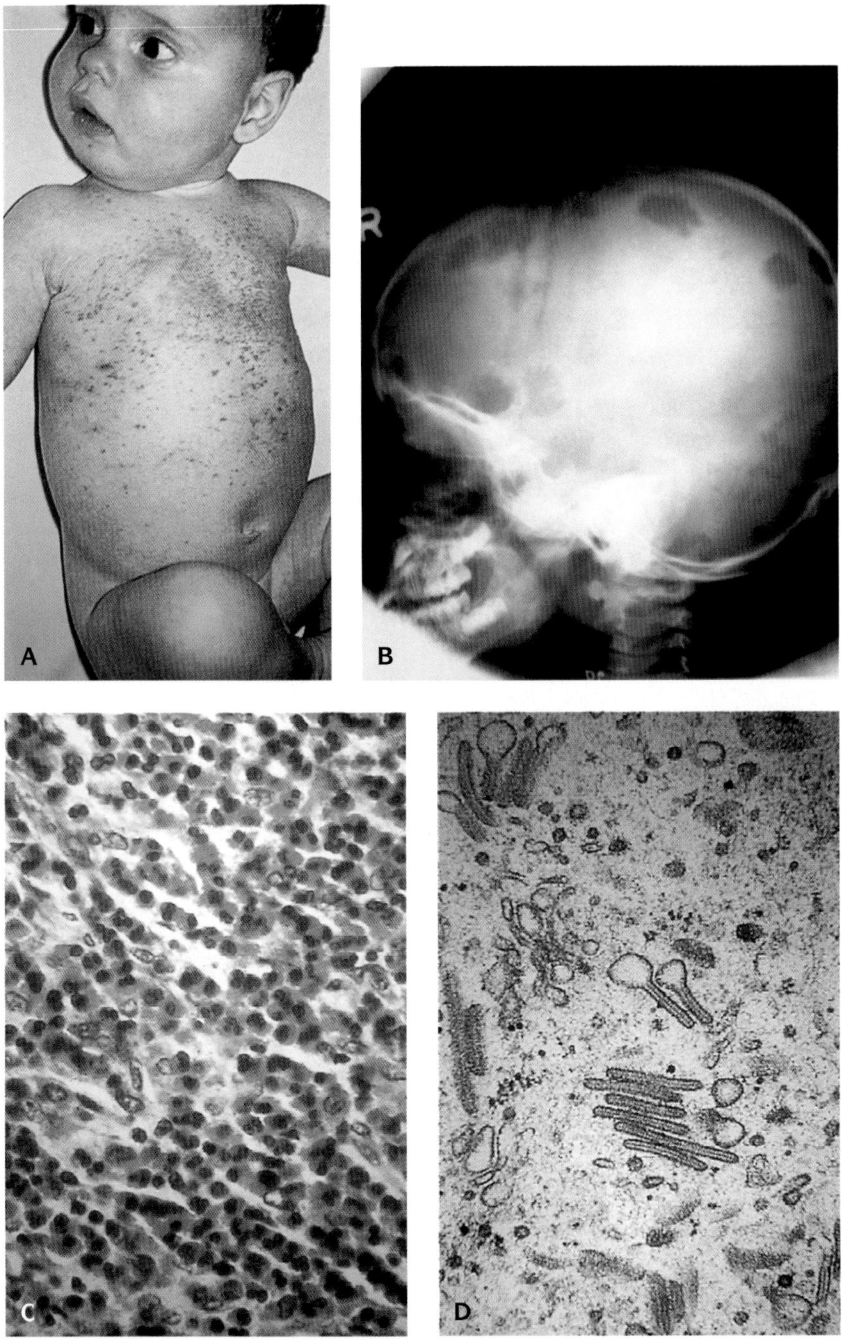

21.28. Histiocytosis. **(A)** Infant with generalized red papular rash. **(B)** X-ray of skull showing punched out lesions of skull. **(C)** Microscopic section showing infiltrate of histocytes and eosinophils. **(D)** Electron micrograph showing Birbeck bodies.

Monoclonal antibodies of choice are S100 neuroprotein and CD1a, both highly specific antibodies that recognize skin Langerhans cells, and LCH cells. CD1a is best demonstrated in smears, frozen sections, or flow-cytometric studies. CD68, a macrophage-associated antigen usually confined to the Golgi area, is usually present. Racquet-shaped Birbeck granules are seen by electron microscopy.

ACKNOWLEDGMENT

The authors gratefully acknowledge the illustrations kindly provided by Dr. Bernard Cohen, Dr. Robert Gorlin, Dr. Michael Morgan, and Dr. Jane Messina.

REFERENCES

Cohen, BA: *Atlas of Pediatric Dermatology.* St. Louis, Mosby, 1993.

Cohen BA: Pediatric Dermatology, 2nd ed., Mosby, 1999.

Harper J, Oranje AP, Prose NS, Esterly N: *Textbook of Pediatric Dermatology,* Blackwell Science Inc., 2000.

Infant with congenital erosions of the skin of several fingers and gastroschisis. *Am J Med Genet* Aug 15; 102(3):297, 2001.

Isaacs H, Jr: Skin Diseases. In Gilbert-Barness E (ed): *Potter's Pathology of the Fetus and Infant.* St. Louis, Mosby-Year Book, Inc., 1997.

Isaacs H, Jr: Skin Diseases. In Gilbert-Barness E (ed): *Potter's Pathology of the Fetus and Infant,* 2nd ed., St. Louis, Mosby-Year Book, 1997.

Johnson, BC, Honig PJ, Jaworsky C: *Pediatric Dermatopathology.* London, Butterworth-Heinemann Publishers, 1994.

Novice FM, Collison DW, Burgdorf WHC, Esterly NB: *Handbook of Genetic Skin Disorders.* Philadelphia, WB Saunders, 1994.

Quintero RA, Morales WJ, Gilbert-Barness E: In utero Diagnosis of Trichothiodystrophy by Endoscopically-Guided Fetal Eyebrow Biopsy. *Fetal Diagn Ther* 15:152, 2000.

Schachner LA, Hansen RC: *Pediatric Dermatology,* 2nd ed. New York, Churchill Livingstone, Inc., 1996.

Schachner LA, Hansen RC: *Pediatric Dermatology,* 3rd ed., Mosby, 2003.

Sybert VP: *Genetic Skin Disorders.* Oxford University Press, 1997.

Weinberg S, Kristal L, Prose NS: *Color Atlas of Pediatric Dermatology,* 3rd ed., MaGraw-Hill Companies, 1997.

TWENTY TWO

Intrauterine Infection

The symptoms and signs and laboratory findings in congenital infections are listed in Table 22.1.

BACTERIAL INFECTIONS

Bacterial infections in the fetus (Figure 22.1) are more frequently recognized than viral, parasitic, or fungal infections. In most cases acquisition of the organism is believed to be from the maternal genital tract by an ascending route. Premature rupture of membranes or a sudden spontaneous abortion may be the first indication of intrauterine infection.

Other routes of infection are:

1. Hematogenous spread of maternal infection
2. Iatrogenic infections introduced during prenatal procedures such as amniocentesis
3. Direct infection from the maternal peritoneal cavity.

In addition, bacteria can be carried asymptomatically in the male urogenital tract and can infect the conceptus by the ascending route after sexual intercourse in pregnancy.

Infection may occur by access secondary to rupture of membranes. Once bacteria are in the amniotic sac, they incite maternal leukocyte migration from the intervillous space toward the amniotic cavity (Tables 22.1 and 22.2). The

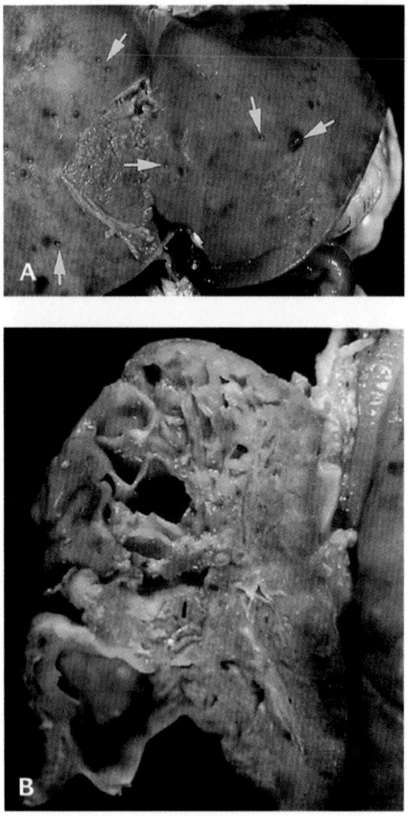

22.1. Staphylococcal septicemia in a neonate. **(A)** The liver shows multiple abscesses (arrows). **(B)** The lungs show multiple cavitary abscesses.

Table 22.1 Signs, symptoms, and laboratory findings commonly associated with congenital infections

- Intrauterine growth retardation
- Jaundice at birth
- Hepatosplenomegaly
- Hepatitis (elevated transaminases, direct and indirect hyperbilirubinemia)
- Skin lesions (petechiae, purpura, vesicles, maculopapular rash, scars)
- Hematologic abnormality (thrombocytopenia, anemia, lymphopenia, neutropenia)
- Generalized adenopathy
- Pneumonitis
- Cardiac lesions (myocarditis, congenital defects)
- Bone lesions
- Eye lesions (glaucoma, chorioretinitis, retinopathy, cataracts, optic atrophy)
- Microphthalmia, uveitis, keratoconjunctivitis
- Sensorineural hearing loss
- Central nervous system disease (microcephaly, meningoencephalitis, ventriculomegaly, hydrocephalus, intracranial calcifications)

accumulation of neutrophils leads to a loss of translucency of the membranes, which become creamy yellow. Most bacteria infect the membranes diffusely. Inhalation and ingestion of infected amniotic fluid by the fetus (amniotic infection syndrome) can be diagnosed microscopically by sectioning of the fetal lungs and stomach, which will contain neutrophils from the amniotic fluid. Infection of the amniotic fluid can result in intrauterine aspiration pneumonia in the fetus or the development of septicemia particularly if the organism is strongly virulent as with group B streptococci (Figures 22.2 and 22.3). Oranisms most frequently resulting in chorioamnionitis are shown in Table 22.2.

Acute chorioamnionitis frequently induces labor, presumably because the neutrophils and bacteria that are present release phospholipases, which in turn enzymatically release arachidonic acid from the fetal membranes. The

Table 22.2 Bacterial pathogens associated with chorioamnionitis

Gram positive	Gram negative	Other bacteria
Group B streptococci	*Bacteroides* sp.	*Ureaplasma urealyticum*
Listeria monocytogenes	Coliform bacteria	*Chlamydia*
Coagulase-negative staphylococci	*Hemophilus* sp.	*Mycoplasma hominis*
Viridans streptococci	Brucella sp.	*Treponema pallidum*
Group D streptococci	*Neisseria* gonorrhoeae	*Borrelia* sp.
Anaerobic Gram-positive cocci	Campylobacter sp.	*Mobiluncus* sp.
Lactobacilli	*Fusobacterium* sp. Miscellaneous non-fermentative bacteria (*Pseudomonas, Aeromonas*)	*Gardnerella vaginalis*

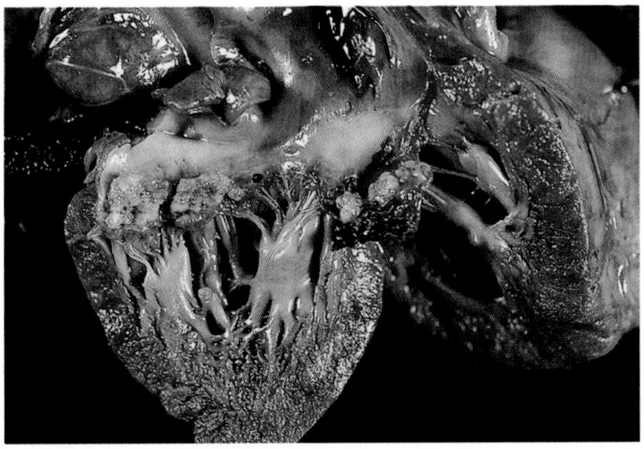

22.2. Infective endocarditis in a newborn where mother had hemolytic group B streptococcal chorioamnionitis. Note the vegetations on the valve.

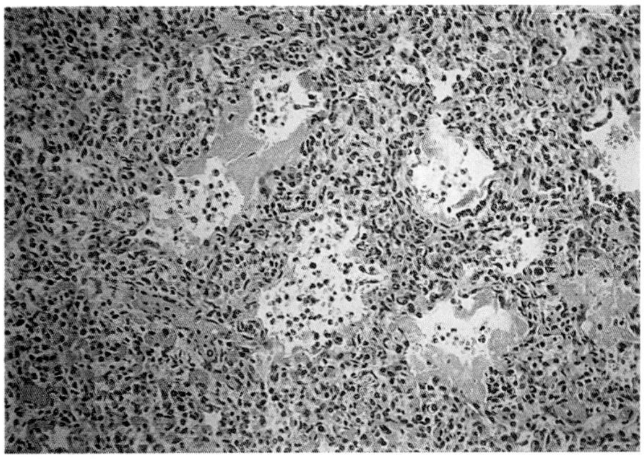

22.3. Intrauterine pneumonia in the infant due to hemolytic group B streptococcal chorioamnionitis. Note also hyaline membranes.

arachidonic acid rapidly converts to prostaglandin E_2 and to $F_{2\alpha}$. Prostaglandin E_2 causes the cervix to dilate and $F_{2\alpha}$ initiates uterine contractions.

Genital *Mycoplasma hominis* and *Ureaplasma urealyticum* were implicated in the cause of repeated spontaneous abortion after it was shown that the organisms were isolated more often from the cervix and endometrium of habitual aborters than from those of controls. Infection with *Chlamydia trachomatis* is uncommon as a cause for early pregnancy loss. In intrauterine bacterial infection, the infection extends into the decidua basalis from which bacteria may reach the fetus hematogenously by being shed into the intervillous blood. Infection usually occurs only by the ascending route.

Listeria monocytogenes a Gram-positive motile bacillus is a serious prenatal infection with a characteristic gross and histologic pattern of granulomatous lesions in the fetus and placenta (Figure 22.4). It may infect the fetus by the ascending or hematogenous route. Severely infected fetuses may be hydropic, showing typical granulomatous lesions and microabscesses affecting skin and multiple viscera including the leptomeninges, sometimes with calcification and placental lesions. Abortions, stillbirths, and IUGR are frequent. In congenital infection there is always meconium staining even in fetuses less than 32 weeks when it is very suggestion of listerosis. Diagnosis is by culture isolation and Brown-Hopps stain demonstrates in the lesions Gram-positive pleomorphic rods, 0.4–0.5 μm by 0.5–2.0 μm. The bacillius also can be revealed by Gomori methenamine-silver stain, Warthin-Starry, or other argentic methods. It is important to consider that the organisms sometimes may appear Gram-negative particularly in longstanding disease and when the patient has been treated with antibiotics. To confirm the histopathologic diagnosis, immunohistochemistry and DNA hybridization can be used.

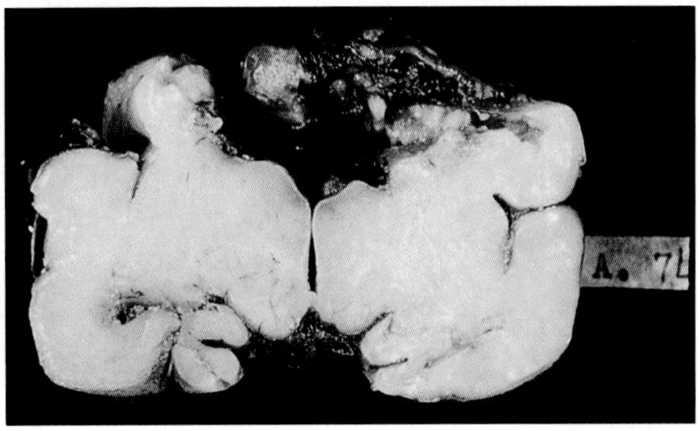

22.4. Early onset listeriosis. Extensive destruction of the cerebral tissue. (Picture courtesy of Dr. Achilea Bittencourt.)

Syphilis infects the fetus by hematogenous spread from the mother with primary or secondary disease; although organisms

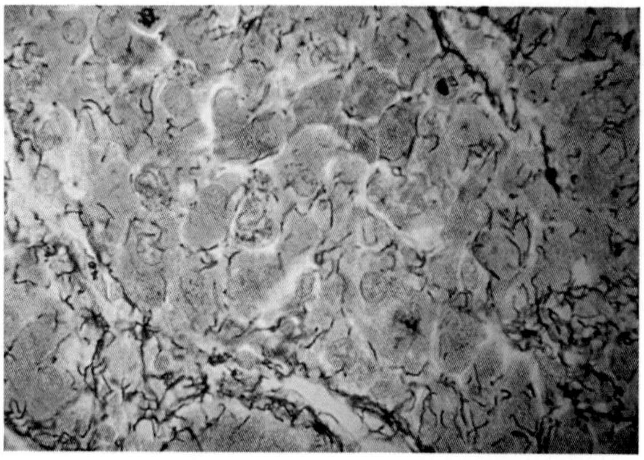

22.5. Congenital syphilis. Spirochetes are present in the placenta (Warthin-Starry stain).

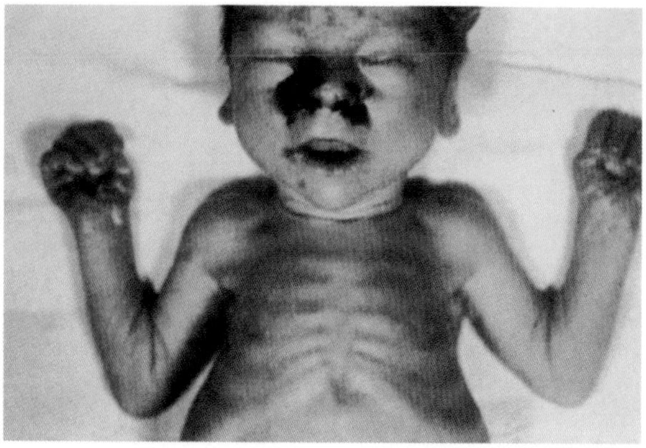

22.6. Congenital syphilis. Infant with hemorrhagic nasal discharge (snuffles).

have been recovered from first trimester abortuses, lesions in the fetus develop only with active infection after about 16 weeks gestation (Figures 22.5 to 22.7 and Tables 22.3 to 22.5). Infection with *Treponema pallidum* can present at autopsy in a fetus with profound changes or may be quite subtle, and even unconfirmable.

The great majority of infected fetuses are macerated. Hydrops and hepatosplenomegaly are most common. In Brazil syphilis represents one of the most common cause of nonimmune hydrops. The basilar meninges may appear thickened, especially around the brain stem and the optic chiasm.

In congenital syphilis besides macular, papular, and papulo-annular eruptions, an extensive vesicle-bullous lesion can be observed. In addition, a marked sloughing of the epidermis may be seen especially on the palms, soles, and around the mouth and anus. In cases of severe infection the lungs appear pale and heavy. For this reason the pulmonary lesions have been described as pneumonia alba. The pancreas may be increased in size and is firm due to

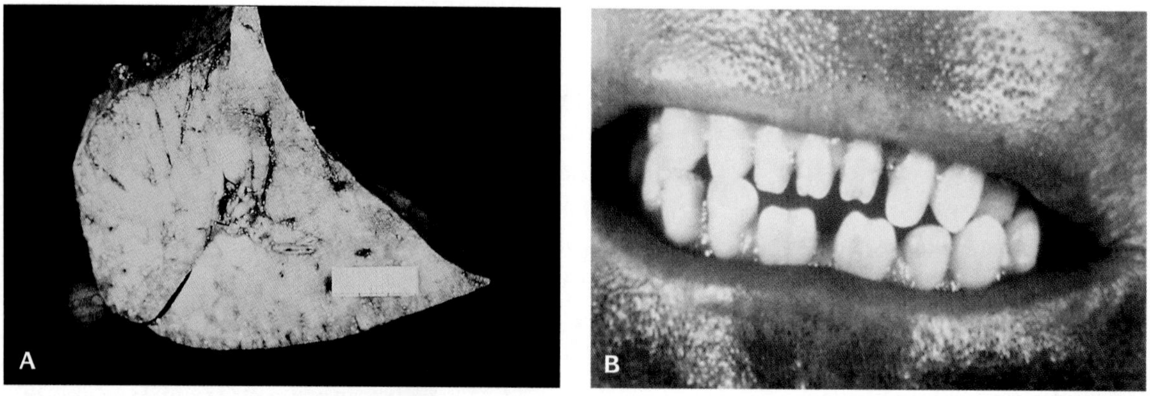

22.7. **(A)** Lung in congenital syphilis showing "pneumonia alba" due to fibrosis. **(B)** Hutchinson teeth (notching of the incisors) seen later after eruption of permanent teeth due to congenital syphilis.

Table 22.3 Serologic tests used in congenital syphilis

Nontreponemal	Treponemal
Standard tests	
Venereal Disease Research Laboratory (VDRL)	Fluorescent treponemal antibody (FTA)
Rapid plasma reagin (RPR)	Fluorescent treponemal antibody-absorbed (FTA-ABS)
	Microhemagglutination assay for antibody to *Treponema pallidum* (MHA-TP)
	Hemogglutination treponemal test for syphilis (HATTS)
Experimental tests	
VDRL ELISA for IgG and IgM	19S–IgM FTA-ABS*
	T. pallidum ELISA for IgG and IgM*
	T. pallidum Western blot
	Rabbit infectivity test (RIT)
	Polymerase chain reaction for *T. pallidum* (PCR)
	T. pallidum antigen-capture ELISA

* These tests are available through the Centers for Diseases Control or other reference laboratories.

fibrosis. The thymus is involuted and may present with abscesses of Dubois that constitute a pathognomonic sign of congenital syphilis.

The histologic hallmark of congenital syphilis is obliterative endarteritis. Virtually every organ may be involved in congenital syphilis but most frequently are the liver, kidney, bones, pancreas, spleen, eyes, bowel, skin and mucosa, testes and epididymus, hypophysis, lymph nodes, thymus, heart, lungs, and brain.

The lungs may be affected by a diffuse interstitial fibrosis. Intestinal lesions occur and may cause a heavy intestinal inflammation. Interstitial fibrosis in the kidneys may lead to tubular atrophy.

The lymph nodes present macrophage proliferation and the testes often have marked inflammation and interstitial fibrosis.

The CNS is frequently involved and 86% of infants with clinical manifestations of syphilis present spirochetes in the cerebrospinal fluid and there is a frequent mononuclear infiltration in the leptomeninges.

Syphilitic osteochondritis and periostitis may affect all bones, although lesions of the nose and lower legs are most distinctive. Destruction of the vomer

Table 22.4 Signs of late congenital syphilis

Frontal bossing	Sternoclavicular thickening
Small maxillae	Saber shins
Saddle nose	Flaring scapulas
Protruding mandible	Interstitial keratitis
High-arched palate	Neurologic abnormalities
Peg-shaped upper incisors	Mental retardation
Mulberry molars	Eighth cranial nerve deafness
Perioral fissures (rhagades)	Hydrocephalus
Bilateral knee effusions	

Table 22.5 Findings in symptomatic cases of congenital syphilis

Rash
Fever
Failure to thrive
Low birth weight
Rhinitis
Hepatosplenomegaly
Pseudoparalysis
Pneumonitis
Central nervous system involvement
Renal manifestations
Lymphadenopathy
Acites
Leukocytosis
Anemia
Thrombocytopenia
Radiologic changes
Metaphyseal involvement
Periostitis
Osteochondritis

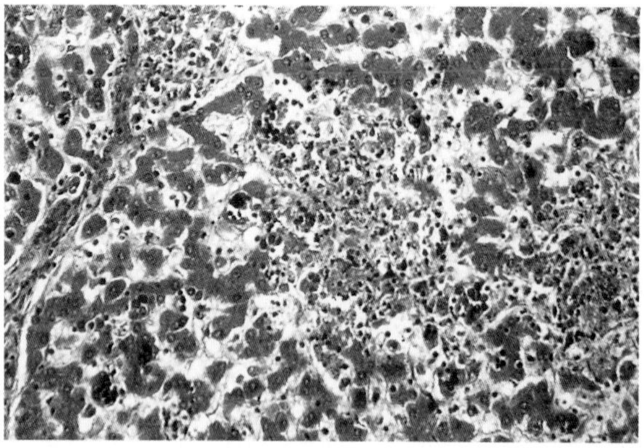

22.8. Liver in congenital tuberculosis. See two areas of caseous necrosis without granulomatous reaction. There is a mild infiltration of mononuclear cells around the necrotic areas. (Picture courtesy of Dr. Achilea Bittencourt.)

causes collapse of the bridge of the nose and, later on, the characteristic saddle nose deformity.

Through silver impregnation or immunohistochemistry the organisms may be demonstrated in many organs. They also can be detected in fresh imprints of the organs and umbilical cord in dark-field examination.

Mycobacterium tuberculosis as a congenital infection is rare. Spread from the mother is by the hematogenous route from the placenta or through the amniotic fluid (Figure 22.8).

TORCH Infections

TORCH infections include toxoplasmosis, other (congenital syphilis and other viruses), rubella, cytomegalovirus, and herpes simplex virus infections.

Toxoplasmosis (Figures 22.9 to 22.12) caused by *Toxoplasma gondii* affects cats, dogs, sheep, rabbits, guinea pigs, and other animals as well as humans. Because most pregnant women are infected during the third trimester, about two-thirds of newborns present the subclinical form of infection. This form has the potential of manifesting symptomatology later. Nonetheless, the severe sequelae of the encephalic form may be present at birth. Congenital toxoplasmosis (Table 22.6) includes the tetrad of hydrocephalus or microcephalus, chorioretinitis, convulsions, and cerebral calcification; skin rash, purpura, prolonged jaundice, hepatosplenomegaly, and extramedullary hematopoiesis are common. Multiple necrotic nodules in the brain may coalesce and result in massive destruction of brain tissue leading to hydranencephaly. Toxoplasma

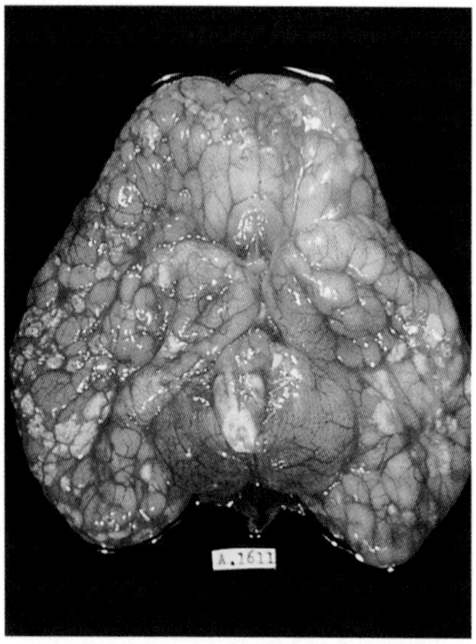

22.9. Congenital toxoplasmosis. The milky areas on the cerebral surface correspond to necrosis and calcification. (Picture courtesy of Dr. Achilea Bittencourt.)

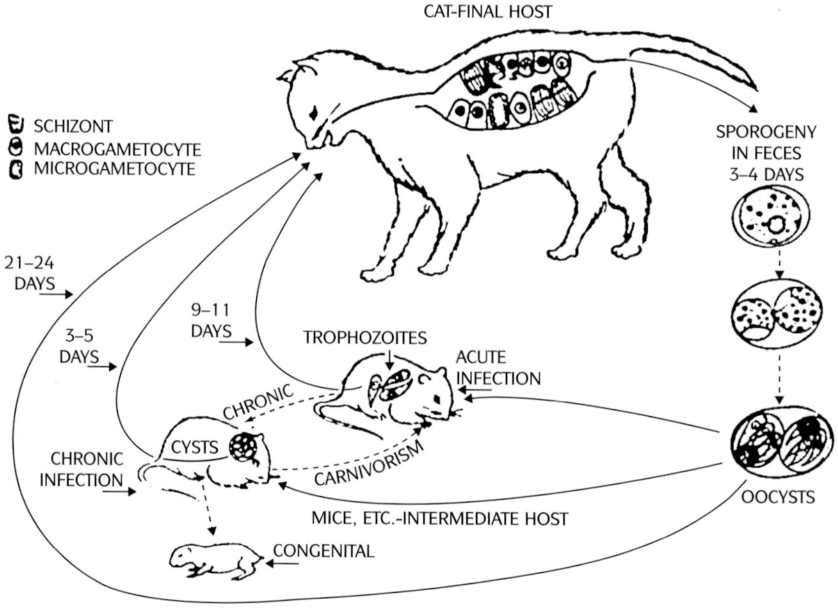

22.10. Congenital toxoplasmosis. Life cycle of *Toxoplasma gondii*.

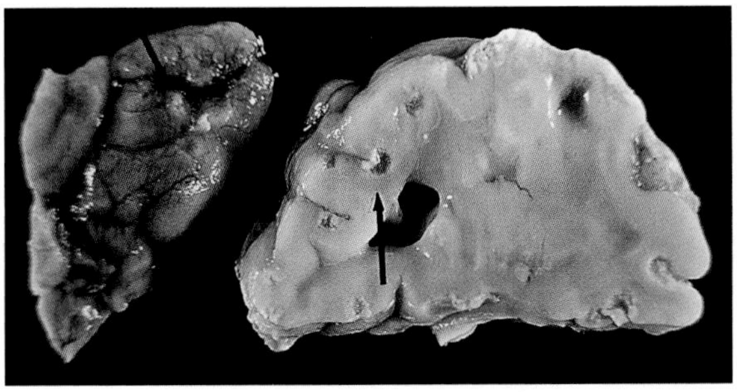

22.11. Congential toxoplasmosis. Multiple necrotizing lesions in the brain.

Table 22.6 Congenital toxoplasmosis

Prematurity	31%
Chorioretinitis	99%
Cerebral calcification	63%
Psychomotor retardation	56%
Hydrocephalus or microcephalus	50%

organisms may be found in the myocardium, adrenal glands, lungs, subcutaneous tissue, testes, ovaries, pancreas, stomach, liver, and kidneys (Figure 22.12). Placental infection is characterized by placentomegaly with hydropic changes.

Necrosis represents the most characteristic lesions in the CNS. The necrotic lesions are more marked in the cerebral cortex, basal ganglia, and periventricular areas. Later on the lesions became calcified or transform into cavities. By immunohistochemistry parasites are frequently identified in the lesions.

The presence of *T. gondii* (tachyzoites or cysts) in tissues confirms the histopathologic diagnosis of congenital toxoplasmosis. The cysts are strongly positive with PAS; however, the cyst wall stains weakly with PAS but it is strongly argyrophilic. To differentiate toxoplasma from *Histoplasma capsulatum*, a silver stain with the Grocott method must be used.

Diagnosis of congenital toxoplasmosis also may be made by in situ hybridization or polymerase chain reaction (PCR) with using formalin-fixed paraffin-embedded tissues. Isolation of the parasite from tissue or body fluid by means of cell culture or animal inoculation are other methods to detect toxoplasma in autopsy material. However, PCR assay produces more positive results than the other methods.

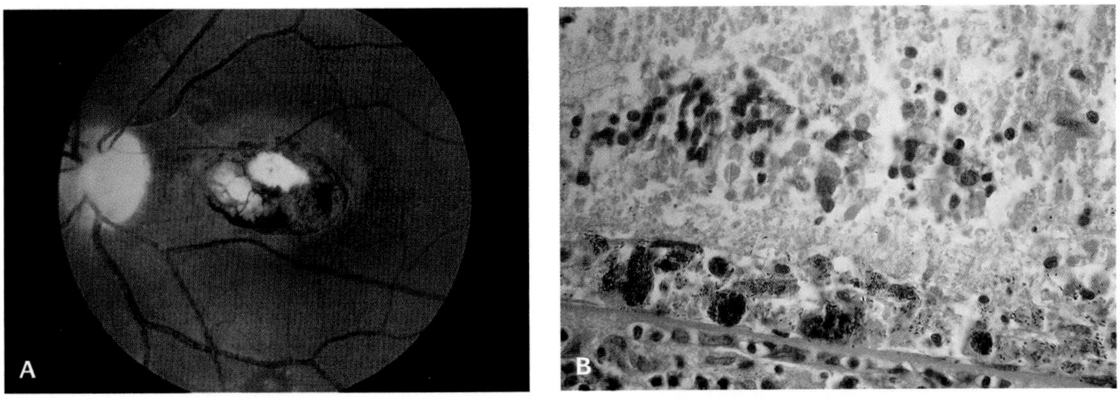

22.12. Chorioretinitis in congenital toxoplasmosis. **(A)** Macular scarring of the retina. **(B)** Necrosis and inflammation of the retina.

Table 22.7 Viruses that may cause congenital or perinatally acquired infection or disease

DNA viruses
Cytomegalovirus
Herpes simplex virus types 1 and 2
Varicella-zoster virus
Human parvovirus B19
Hepatitis B virus
Variola virus (smallpox virus)
Human papilloma viruses

RNA viruses
Rubella virus
Mumps virus
Measles virus
Enteroviruses (coxsackie virus, echo virus, polio viruses)
Hepatitis C virus
Lymphocytic choriomeningitis virus
HIV

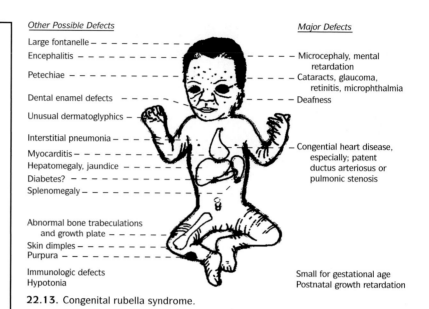

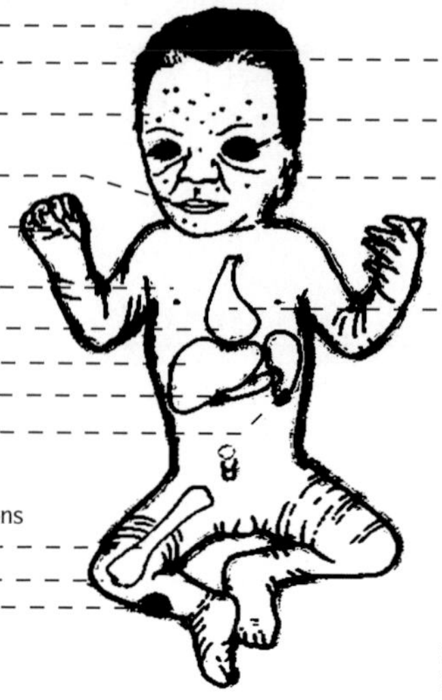

22.13. Congenital rubella syndrome.

VIRAL INFECTIONS

Spontaneous abortion is a rare complication of maternal viral disease; chronic fetal disease is the usual result of intrauterine viral infection. Growth retardation and destructive brain lesions are frequent findings including hepatomegaly, and splenomegaly with focal necrosis (Table 22.7).

Rubella Infection

Rubella is an RNA virus. Fetal infection can result from maternal rubella viremia. Spontaneous abortion is found in only 8% (Figures 22.13 to 22.15). Fetuses infected before 11 weeks gestation are always malformed, with heart defects, deafness and cataracts being present in about 85% of fetuses and infants (Table 22.8). Isolated deafness occurs in 35% of survivors who are infected between 13 and 16 weeks gestation. Fresh tissue from the heart, brain, liver, and placenta should be submitted for rubella culture, antigen detection, and nucleic acid hybridization.

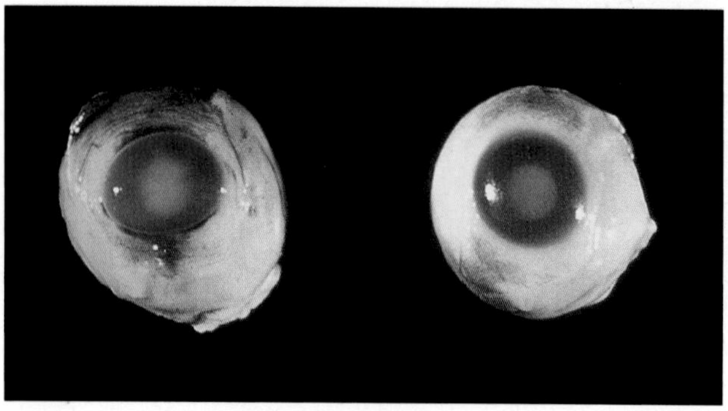

22.14. Cataracts in congenital rubella.

Resorption of the embryo may occur during the first 2 months of pregnancy. The fetus may be spared in cases of placental infection. Only one identical twin may be infected. The hallmark of rubella infection is its chronicity, with the tendency for virus to persist throughout fetal and postnatal life. More than 80% of newborns eliminate a great quantity of virus through nasopharyngeal secretions and urine, and 3% present persistent viral elimination up to 20 months of age.

Abortuses and stillborns show generalized involvement with hepatosplenomegaly, thickening of the intima of the aorta and other large elastic arteries, and hypoplasia of the

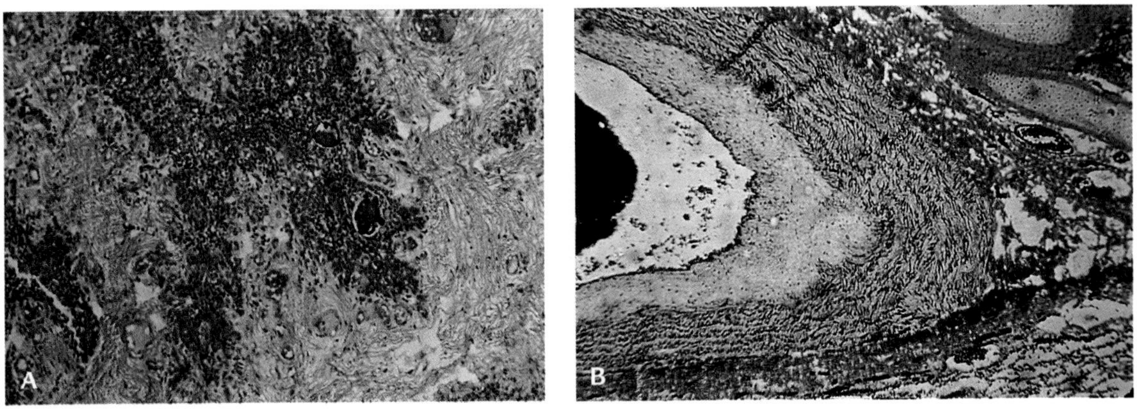

22.15. Congenital rubella. **(A)** Atrophy of the thymus lobules, depletion of lymphocytes, absence of Hassall corpuscles, and presence of foci of calcification. **(B)** Branch of the pulmonary artery showing intimal thickening and reduction of the lumen. (Courtesy of Dr. Achilea Bittencourt.)

thymus. Hassall corpuscles are absent, cystic, or calcified. Other changes include hepatocyte swelling, cholestasis, portal phlebitis, proliferation of biliary ducts, and a giant cell transformation of hepatocytes as well as periportal fibrosis by rubella virus in formalin-fixed or cryopreserved lens aspirates.

The diagnosis is generally made taking into account the history of recent maternal infection, the serologic reactions, and the pathologic observations in the autopsy. Confirmation can be achieved by isolation of the rubella virus from placental or fetal tissues or by reverse transcriptase-PCR with formalin-fixed paraffin-embedded fetal tissues.

Herpes Infection

The herpes viruses include:

- cytomegalovirus (CMV)
- herpes simplex virus (HSV)
- varicella-zoster virus (VZV)
- Epstein–Barr virus (EBV)

Table 22.8 Malformations in congenital rubella

Cardiac	Gastrointestinal tract
Patent ductus arteriosus	Isolated defects
isolated	Tracheoesophageal fistula
associated with ventricular septal defect, atrial septal defect or aortic coarctation	Duodenal atresia
Tetralogy of Fallot	Imperforate anus
Vascular malformations (persistence of the left superior vena cava, anomalies of the left subclavian artery, and the renal artery)	Persistent cloaca
Hypoplastic left heart	Malrotation of the small bowel
Ventricular septal defect	Multiple defects
Truncus arteriosus	Rectourethral fistula and imperforate anus
Transposition of the great vessels	Duodenal atresia and imperforate anus
Endocardial cushion defect	Ectopic anus, malrotation of the intestine

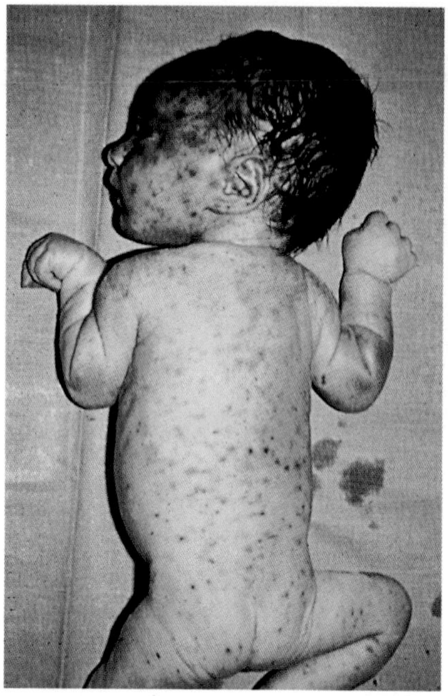

22.16. Newborn with multiple petechial hemorrhages in CMV infection.

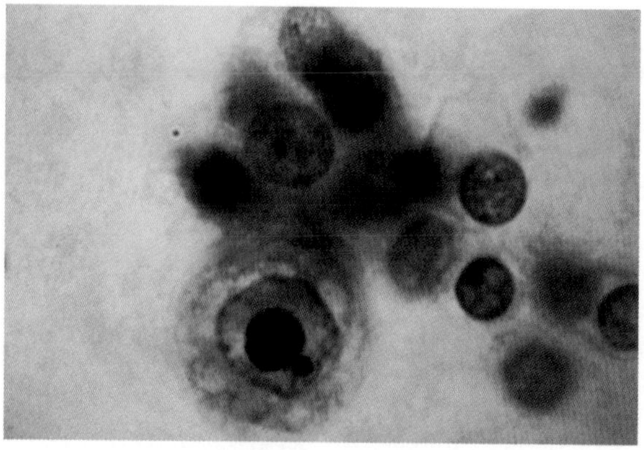

22.17. Congenital cytomegalovirus infection. Urinary sediment with large intranuclear inclusion.

Maternal antibody status IgG and IgM can be helpful in diagnosing and distinguishing primary and reactivated infections.

Cytomegalovirus Infection (CMV)

Intrauterine transmission of CMV infection occurs in 30–40% of pregnant women with primary infection but may also result from maternal reinfection (Figures 22.16 to 22.19). Fewer than 5% of congenitally infected infants develop symptoms during the newborn period.

The manifestations of fetal CMV infection include intrauterine growth retardation, hepatosplenomegaly, hepatitis with hyperbilirubinemia, pneumonitis, encephalitis, cerebral calcification, and microcephaly and chorioretinitis. Enterocolitis due to congenital CMV infection may cause multiple strictures, ulceration, and perforation. The intestinal involvement may constitute the only manifestation of congenital CMV.

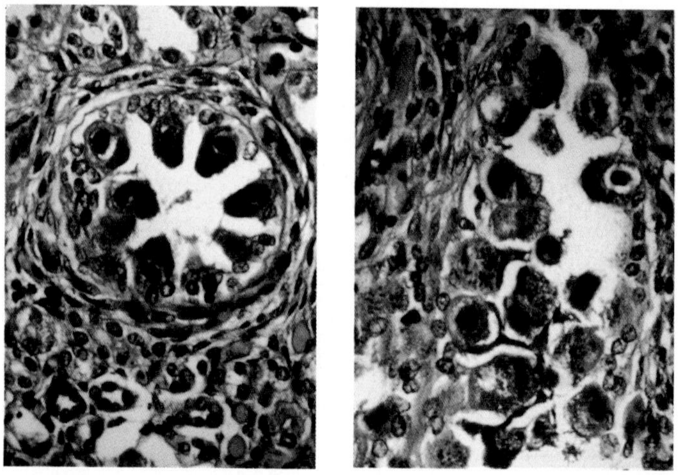

22.18. Cytomegaloviral infection in renal tubular epithelial cells (left) and alveolar lining cells in lung (right).

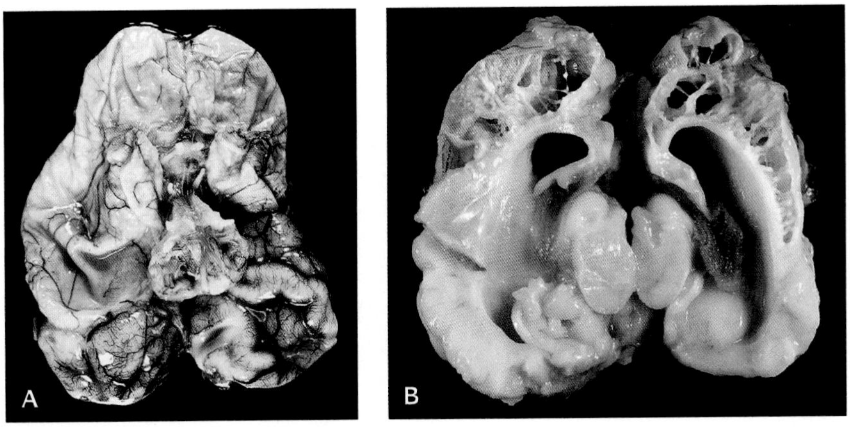

22.19. CMV. Brain showing **(A)** extensive necrosis **(B)** cut surface with destruction and necrosis of brain parenchyma.

Cytomegalic cells frequently are seen in the renal tubules, especially in the distal convoluted tubules and the collecting ducts, associated with an interstitial inflammatory infiltrate. Inclusions also may be detected in many other organs. Extramedullary hematopoiesis is also observed in the kidneys.

Placental changes include villitis, with prominent plasma cell infiltration, focal villus necrosis, and hemorrhage.

The diagnosis of CMV infection is made by identification of the typical inclusion as well as taking into account the maternal serologic data. In cases without the typical inclusions, the presence of the CMV can be demonstrated by immunohistochemistry or in situ hybridization with monoclonal antibodies or specific anti-CMV probes. These techniques can be performed in fresh and in paraffin-embedded tissues.

Herpes simplex virus type 2 may occur after rupture of membranes or during passage of the fetus through an infected birth canal. Developmental defects include microcephaly, intracranial calcifications, chorioretinitis, and microphthalmia (Figures 22.20 to 22.24).

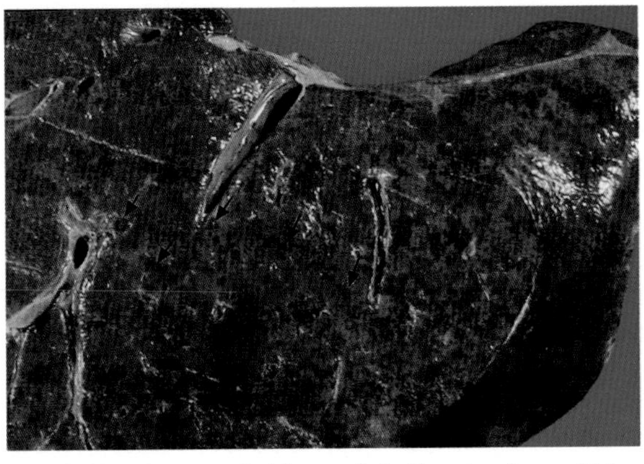

22.20. Liver in congenital herpes infection showing multiple abscesses (arrows).

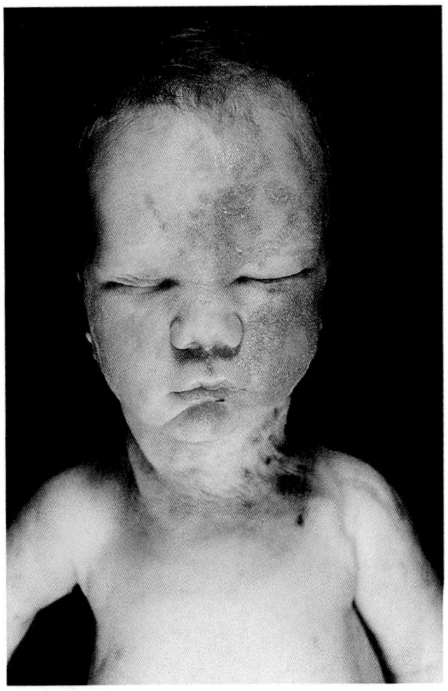

22.21. Newborn with congenital herpes viral infection. Vesicles are present on the skin of the face and neck.

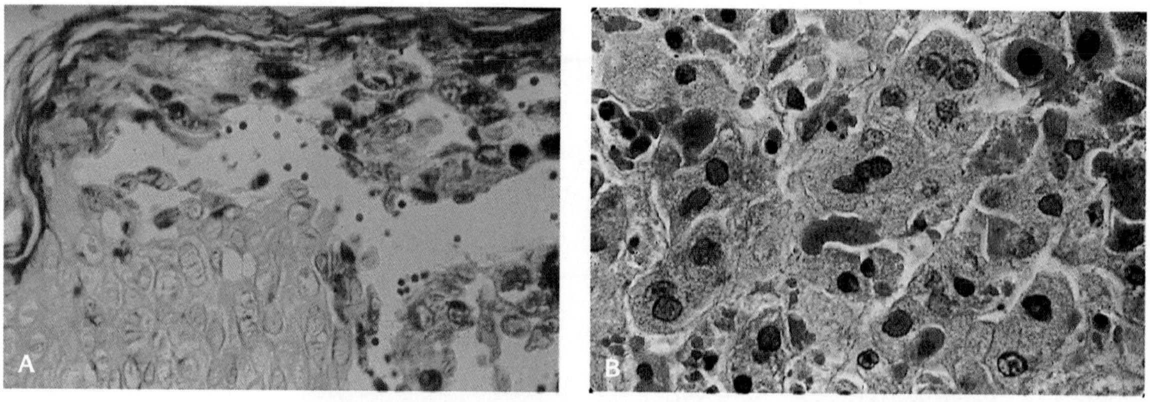

22.22. **(A)** Section of skin in congenital herpes infection showing vesicle and intranuclear inclusions in the epithelial cells. **(B)** Intranuclear inclusions in hepatocytes.

Most of infected newborns are born prematurely. Infection may also be a cause of abortion. The disseminated form of the infection generally involves liver, adrenals, lungs, brain, and heart. Hemorrhagic necrosis is the predominant aspect observed but lymphocytic infiltration can also be seen. These lesions cause extensive destruction. Secondary to necrosis, extensive areas of calcification can occur.

Intrauterine herpes simplex infection may appear as cutaneous vesicles or scars, eye lesions, and severe CNS abnormalities such as microcephaly and hydranencephaly. The main ocular changes are keratoconjunctivitis and chorioretinitis.

The diagnosis can be made through the finding of balloon cells with inclusions in tissues in hematoxylin and eosin-stained sections. Viral cultures or typing of HSV-1 and HSV-2 by immunohistochemistry techniques can be used to prove the diagnosis. Herpesvirus DNA may be detected in paraffin sections of formalin-fixed organs by PCR.

Women of childbearing age with congenital *varicella-zoster* virus infection in pregnancy may have fetal loss. If the mother's rash begins more than 4 days

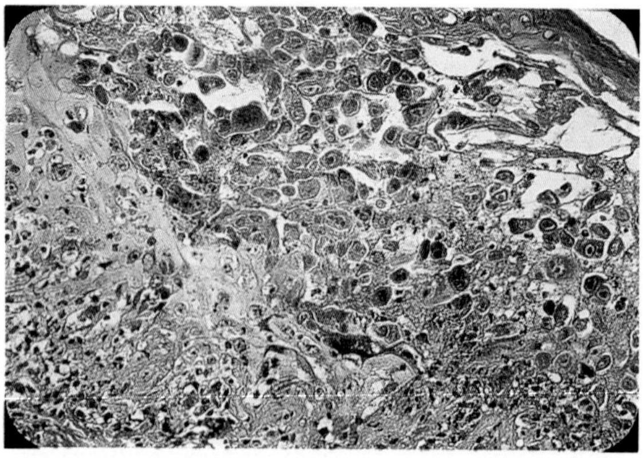

22.23. Congenital herpes simplex. A multiloculated intraepidermal vesicle with necrotic keratinocytes, some of them with intranuclear inclusions. (Courtesy of Dr. Achilea Bittencourt.)

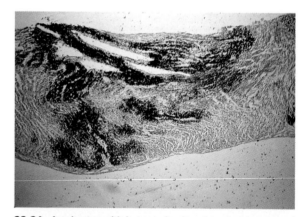

22.24. An abortus with herpes simplex. An extensive area of calcification is seen in the endocardium, myocardium, and epicardium. (Courtesy of Dr. Achilea Bittencourt.)

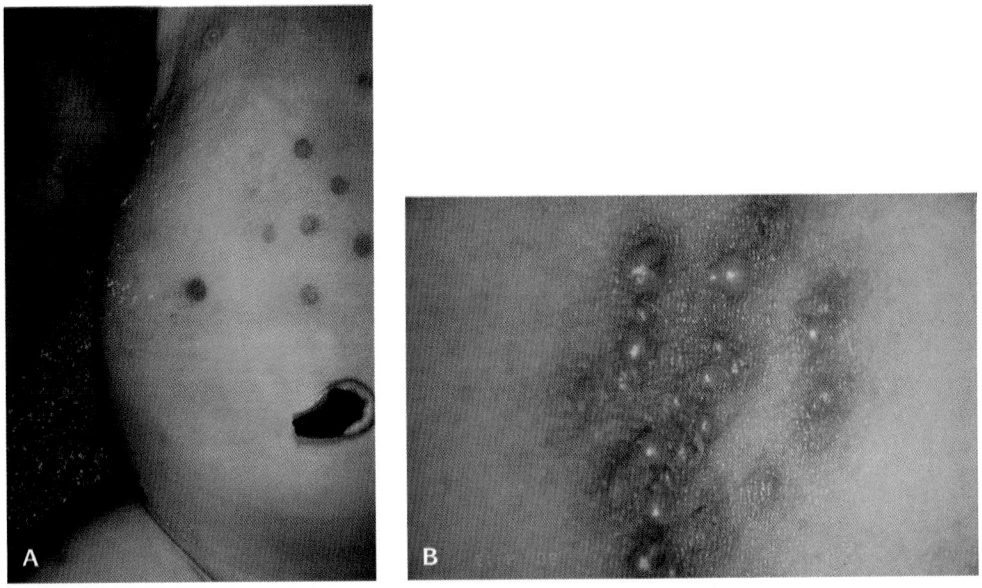

22.25. Congenital varicella infection. **(A)** Skin of newborn showing vesicles. **(B)** Close up view of varicella vesicles.

before delivery, the infant usually presents only skin lesions because of the transference of specific antibodies (Figure 22.25). Fetal infection may occur during maternal varicella or maternal herpes zoster; however, it is more frequent in the course of gestational varicella infection.

In the varicella syndrome widespread lesions can be observed as fibrotic areas or inflammatory changes in the heart, liver, lungs, adrenals, and pancreas.

The ocular abnormalities are chorioretinitis, anisocoria, microphthalmia, and cataract. In the limbs, hypoplasia, absence of digits, talipes equinovarus, and calcaneovalgus have been reported.

Ulcerations can be observed in the gastrointestinal tract and are the cause of intestinal fibrosis and strictures. Mucosal fibrosis of the trachea and bladder are the result of healed ulcerations.

Other aspects not frequently observed in the varicella syndrome are hydronephrosis and hydroureters.

When infection occurs early in gestation, the fetal effect may be catastrophic with the development of a constellation of anomalies known as congenital varicella syndrome. Newborns with acute disease may present with generalized lesions or only a varicelliform rash.

Bone abnormalities are caused by the direct viral invasion of the dorsal root ganglia and spinal cord.

Massive malformation of the cerebral hemisphere can constitute the only lesion in congenital varicella syndrome.

In the acute and generalized infection the skin, liver, and lungs are always involved. Varicella pneumonitis, fulminant hepatitis, and disseminated intravascular coagulation are causes of death of perinatal VZV infection.

The pathologic findings can be confirmed by viral culture or through the demonstration of VZV antigen in fetal organs. Besides detection of the VZV, DNA can be retrieved in fetal tissues by PCR.

Epstein–Barr Virus

Epstein–Barr virus infection does not appear to be associated with fetal loss.

Influenza Virus

A casual relationship between influenza virus and developmental defects remains unclear. High rates of fetal loss, however, were reported in the influenza pandemic of 1918–1919, especially when the disease was complicated by maternal pneumonia.

Enteroviruses

Enteroviruses include Coxsackie viruses A and B, ECHO virus, polio virus, and all the picorna virus group. These viral infections have not been associated with an increase in developmental defects.

Evidence of intrauterine infection has been shown for Coxsackie viruses A3, A9, and B2–B4 and B6 but these cases are rare. Transplacental passage of Coxsackie viruses is generally detected at term; however, this virus also may be responsible for abortion. Coxsackie virus B infection may cause myocarditis, meningoencephalitis, pneumonitis, and inflammatory foci with necrosis in the liver, pancreas, and adrenals. Pneumonitis and mild myocarditis have been found in A3 and A9 congenital Coxsackie virus infection.

ECHO virus (enteric cytopathogenic human orphan virus) is subdivided into 31 different serotypes. Abortion, stillbirth, and congenital infection may occur. Pneumonitis has been described as well as hepatic fibrosis with regenerative nodules, adrenal hemorrhagic necrosis, and foci of myocardial, hepatic, and adrenal calcification.

The histopathologic diagnosis of ECHO virus and Coxsackie viruses is accomplished by identification of the viral antigens by immunocytochemistry in paraffin-embedded tissue samples. Virus particles also can be visualized by electron microscopy. ECHO viruses also can be isolated from placental and fetal tissues.

Poliomyelitis is associated with an increased incidence of abortion.

Hepatitis Viruses

Hepatitis viruses have not been associated with an increase in fetal loss or in the frequency of developmental defects.

Transplacental transmission of hepatitis B virus (HBV) and hepatitis C virus (HCV) has been well documented; however, vertical transmission may also occur at the time of delivery or postnatally. Reports about transplacental transmission of hepatitis A virus (HAV), hepatitis E virus (HEV), and hepatitis G virus (HGV) are rare.

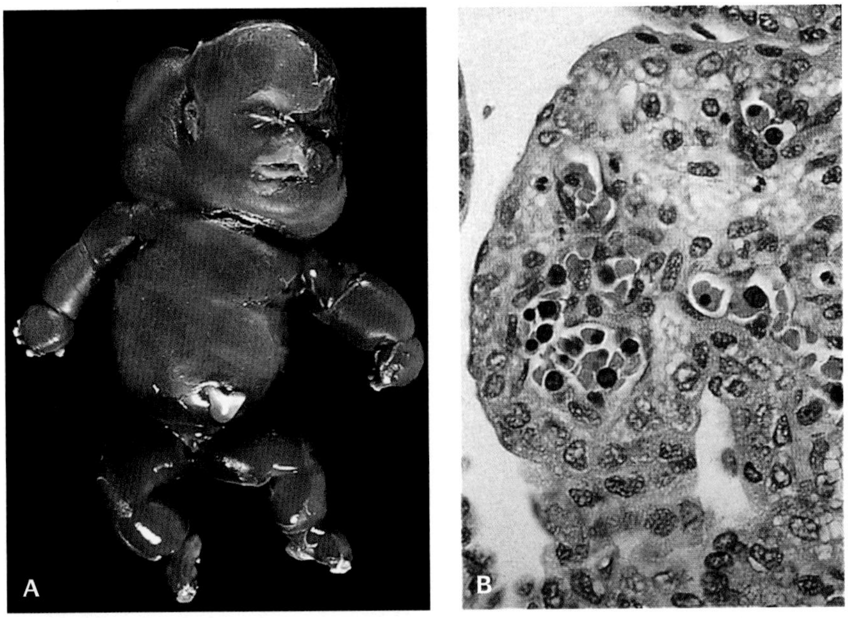

22.26. **(A)** Hydropic fetus with profound anemia due to parvovirus B19 infection. **(B)** Placenta of hydropic infant with parvoviral inclusions in nucleated red blood cells in chorionic villus capillaries.

Transplacental transmission of HBV is 50% of HbsAg-positive mothers. The frequency of vertical transmission of HBV is higher when acute hepatitis occurs in the third trimester. Once infected, infants usually remain HBsAg carriers indefinitely.

Vertical transmission is much lower in HBsAg-positive–HBeAg-negative mothers than in HBe-Ag-positive mothers.

The risk of vertical HCV transmission is higher in infants of HCV-positive–HIV-positive mothers.

Most infants vertically infected with HCV are asymptomatic but may develop severe liver disease by 6 months of age; fetal infection in HAV is rare.

Demonstration of HBsAg in liver biopsies either by specific immunohistochemical or by nonimmunologic methods such as orcein or Victoria blue stain serves to distinguish the ground-glass hepatocytes of chronic HBV infection. HBsAg is observed in chronic hepatitis and only rarely in the acute type of hepatitis. Molecular hybridization techniques also demonstrate the presence of HBV DNA in the hepatocytes.

Parvovirus

Parvovirus B19 a DNA virus is the cause of "fifth disease," also called erythema infectiosum (Figures 22.26 and 22.27). Transmission of the virus occurs in one-fourth to one-third of cases and it may occur at any time during gestation. Most of the B-19-associated fetal deaths occur during the second trimester of gestation. Visceral pallor and enlargement of the liver and the spleen are the most frequent internal abnormalities. A skin rash called blueberry muffin skin

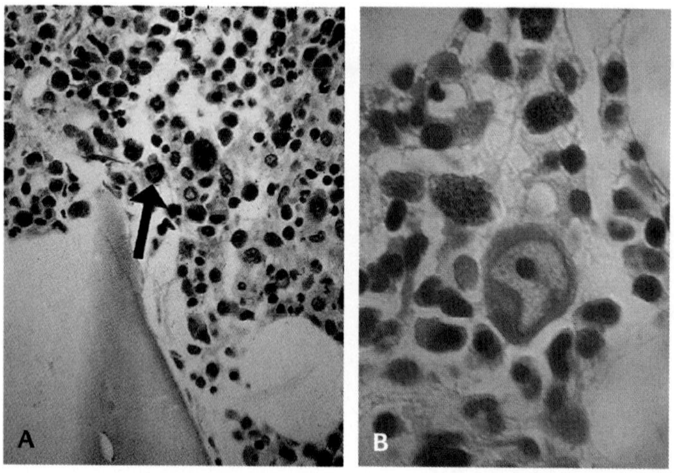

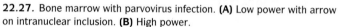

22.27. Bone marrow with parvovirus infection. **(A)** Low power with arrow on intranuclear inclusion. **(B)** High power.

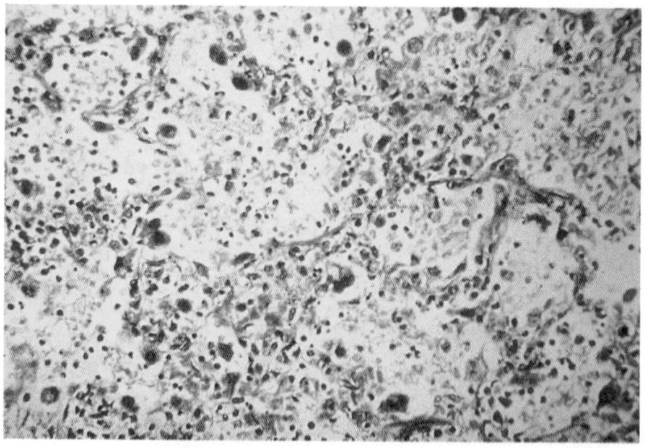

22.28. Adenovirus pneumonia in a newborn with multiple adenoviral inclusions in the alveolar cells.

rarely can be observed and represents foci of extramedullary hematopoiesis. The heart may be normal or symmetrically enlarged and the thymus is abnormally small. It may result in hydrops fetalis due to anemia caused by red blood cell destruction by the virus. Histologic features consist of intranuclear inclusions in erythroid precursors and excessive iron pigment in the liver, hepatitis, a leukoerythroblastic reaction, and eosinophilic nuclear inclusions in hematopoietic cell nuclei. In situ hybridization with labeled viral DNA is best for confirmation of the diagnosis.

Adenovirus

Adenoviral infections usually occur in immunocompromised infants (Figure 22.28).

Human Immunodeficiency Virus

Congenital human immunodeficiency virus (HIV) infections (AIDS) have been reported with an estimate of *in utero* transmission of 35% (Figure 22.29).

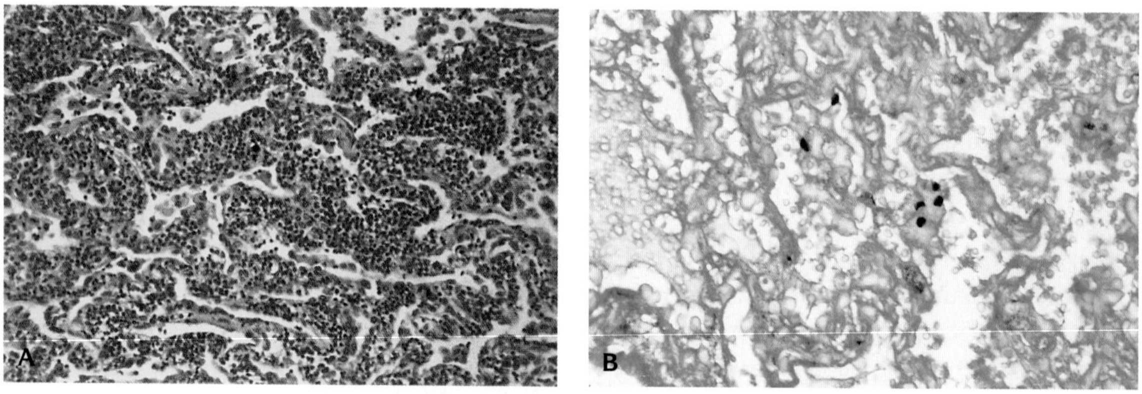

22.29. **(A)** Microscopic section of lung of newborn with HIV infection. There is a marked mononuclear interstitial infiltrate. **(B)** Pneumocystis carinii in lung (methenamine silver stain).

There are no well-documented cases of HIV infection causing specific dysmorphic features or malformations. The rate of pregnancy loss in healthy HIV-infected mothers is increased.

No manifestations of HIV-1 infection are observed at birth. Of infected children 80% develop acquired immunodeficiency syndrome (AIDS) at a median age of 5 months.

Chagas Disease (South American Trypanosomiasis)

T. cruzi presents in the mammalian host in two morphologically distinct forms: the trypomastigotes and the amastigotes (Figure 22.30). The trypomastigotes are motile, spindle-shaped, and nonmultiplying blood forms of the parasite. Intracellularly they are transformed into amastigotes, which multiply and are later released as a trypomastigotes upon lysis of infected cells. The trypomastigotes enter other cells, initiating a new cycle, or they penetrate the fetal bloodstream, disseminating the infection. The trypomastigotes are present in the blood during the acute phase of the disease but thereafter in the chronic phase of infection, parasitemia is intermittent.

Stillborns and newborns with severe disease may present with hydrops and hepatosplenomegaly. When the conceptus dies of cardiac insufficiency, cardiomegaly is observed. Parasites may be detected in most of the organs, but they predominate in the brain, heart, esophagus, intestines, skeletal muscles, and skin. The inflammatory infiltrate consists of mononuclear cells with some neutrophils; less commonly, small granulomas of epithelioid cells are seen.

The inflammatory infiltration in the myocardium is generally diffuse and is associated with edema and disruption of the myofibers.

Encephalitis may occur. The muscular layer and Auerbach's plexus of the esophagus and intestines show a marked focal inflammatory infiltration with parasitism of myofibers or macrophages. Degeneration or destruction of neurons is responsible for early digestive manifestations.

In the lungs, besides mononuclear infiltration in the interalveolar septa, parasitized cells can be observed in the alveolar wall or inside the alveolus. There is also frequent involvement of the skeletal muscles.

Miliary granulomas may be observed in the liver. The lymph nodes and spleen are enlarged.

The histopathologic diagnosis of congenital Chagas disease is made by finding amastigotes in hematoxylin and eosin-stained preparations. They are spherical or oval, are 2 μm in diameter, and present a nucleus and kinetoplast.

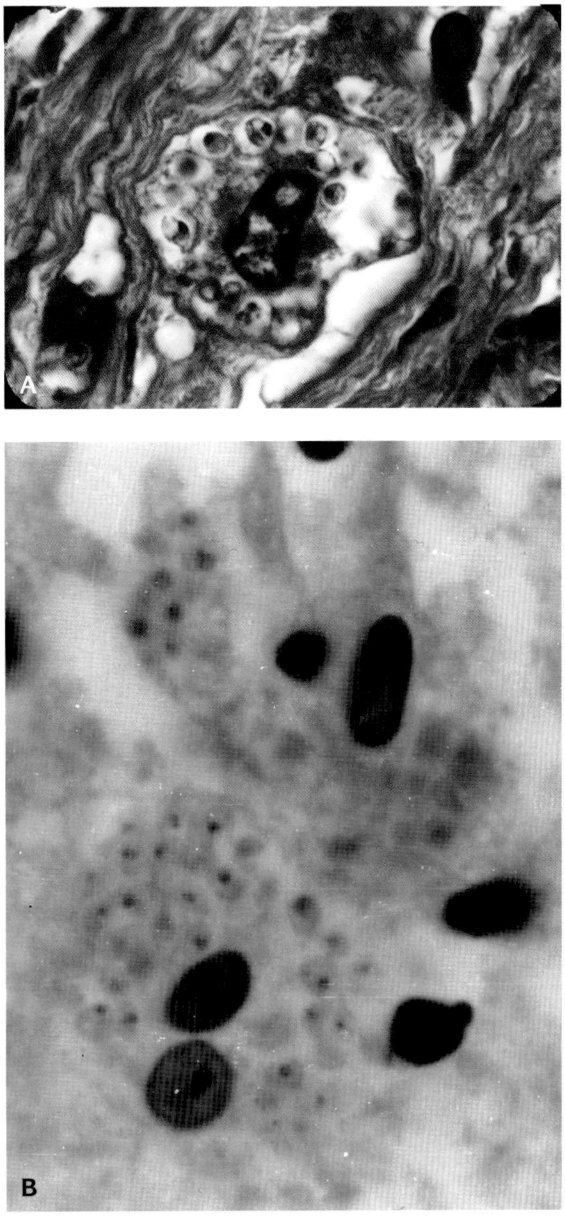

22.30. Congenital Chagas disease. Tissues from a fetus with marked maceration. **(A)** Skeletal muscle presenting mononuclear cells containing amastigotes dissociating the fibers. **(B)** Presence of parasitized microglial cells in the brain. (Courtesy of Dr. Achilea Bittencourt.)

Malaria

Congenital malaria may be caused by *Plasmodium vivax*, *Plasmodium malariae*, *Plasmodium ovale*, and *Plasmodium falciparum*; however, it is of rare occurrence. Even in infants born to mothers with low levels of immunity, symptoms of congenital malaria are usually delayed until 4–12 weeks after birth. It is believed that fetal hemoglobin protects the fetus against malarial infection, and infection is very low in the first 3 months of postnatal life when the level of fetal hemoglobin is high. Sporozoites introduced into the bloodstream mature in the liver and form the mature schizont, which contains a great number of merozoites. After the release of merozoites the ring stage appears within erythrocytes in the peripheral blood with a subsequent transformation into tachyzoites. The sexual form is called gametocyte. In infections with *P. vivax*, *P. malariae*, and *P. ovale* all forms are seen in the blood but in infections with *P. falciparum* only rings and gametocytes are found.

Although the parasite is rarely detected in umbilical cord blood, the placenta shows parasitism and sometimes is so affected that it affects the fetus. Maternal malaria is an important cause of IUGR due to placental lesions as well as maternal anemia. The mean birthweight of the fetus is lower if the placenta is infected with *P. falciparum*.

Congenital infection occurs mainly in malaria caused by *P. falciparum* and *P. vivax*. The reported congenital cases present in the first few months of life with splenomegaly and less frequently with hepatomegaly. Evidence for malaria causing stillbirths is sparse.

Q-Fever

Q-fever caused by *Coxiella burnetii* may cause abortion, prematurity, low birthweight, and fetal death. *C. burnetti* has been isolated from the placenta and fetal kidney.

African Trypanosomiasis

Most congenital cases of African trypanosomiasis are not well documented. Considering that the clinical manifestations of this infection generally are of late appearance, it is impossible in endemic areas to consider as congenital late manifestations of the disease. Two cases of congenital disease have been observed in Europe in infants born to infected mothers. One had hydrocephalus at birth and repeated convulsive episodes. The other was healthy until 18 months when the infant developed trypanosomal CNS infection.

Visceral Leishmaniasis (Kala-Azar)

Pregnant women with the generalized disease may infect the placenta and possibly the fetus. IUGR and placental parasitism have been described.

Borreliosis (Lyme Disease)

Fetal infection has been described in *Borrelia burgdorferi* infection. Spirochetes have been found in brain, spleen, myocardium, and bone marrow, but inflammatory changes are much less than in adult cases and sometimes are absent.

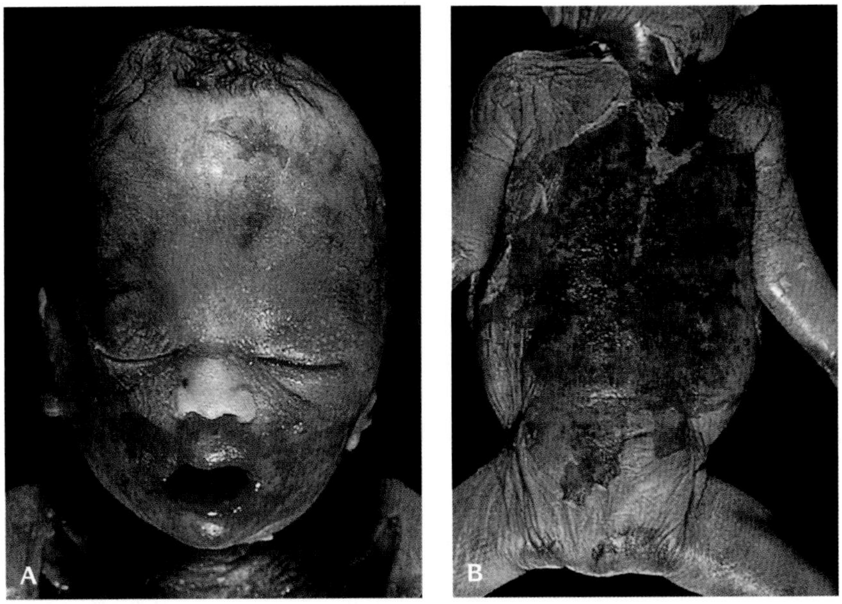

22.31. Candida septicemia in a newborn with hemorrhagic excoriation of the skin. **(A)** Face. **(B)** Body of infant.

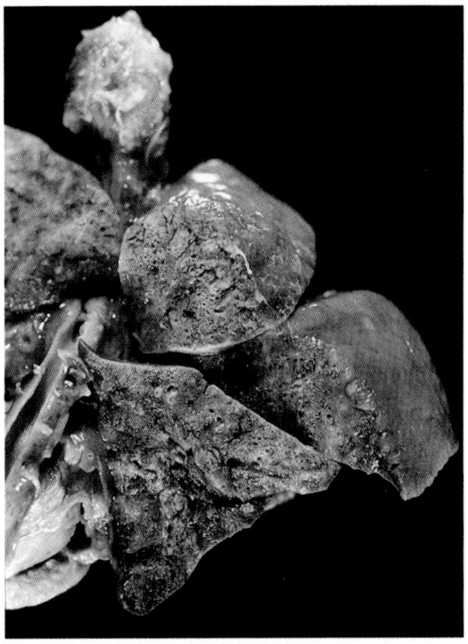

22.32. Candida septicemia with necrotizing lesions in the lung of a newborn.

The organisms can be demonstrated by silver impregnation by immunofluorescence with monoclonal antibodies.

Campylobacter (*Vibrio*) *fetus* Infection

Campylobacter fetus, a common enteric pathogen in humans, has been described as the cause of prematurity, fetal death, and acute villitis. It may

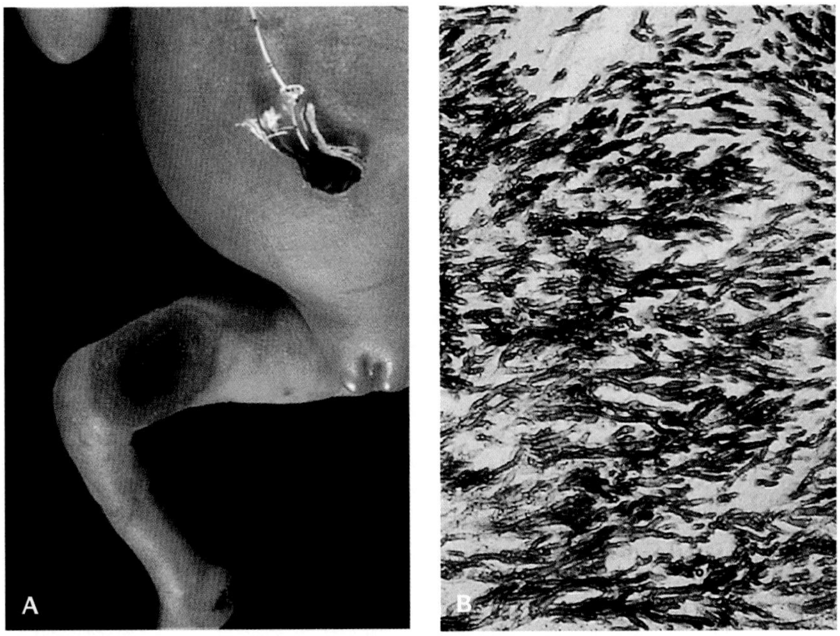

22.33. Aspergillus septicemia in a newborn. **(A)** A large necrotizing ulcer is present on the thigh. **(B)** Branching hyphae (methenamine silver stain).

Table 22.9 **Fungi and parasites and protozoa associated with congenital or perinatal infection**

Fungi
Candida albicans
Coccidioides immitis
Cryptococcus neoformans
Blastomyces dermatitidis
Mycoplasma and chlamydia
Mycoplasma hominis
Ureaplasma urealyticum
Chlamydia trachomatis
Parasites and protozoa
Toxoplasmosis gondii (toxoplasmosis)
Plasmodium vivax, P. falciparum, P. malariae, P. ovale (malaria)
Trypanosoma cruzi (Chagas disease)
Trypanosoma brucei (African sleeping sickness)
Ascaris lumbricoides
Trichinella spiralis (trichinosis)

cause meningitis and meningoencephalitis, and it has been isolated from fetal organs.

Fungal Infections

Candida results in rounded yellow plaques varying in size from 0.5 to 2 mm seen on the umbilical cord surface and in membranes with an intense cellular response by polymorphonuclear and mononuclear cells (Figures 22.31 and 22.32 and Table 22.9). This is usually an incidental finding in an otherwise normal pregnancy that has resulted in a normal newborn. Aspergillus infection (Figure 22.33) also may occur in a debilitated or immunocompromised infant.

REFERENCES

Agha S, Sherif LS, Allan MA, et al.: Transplacental transmission of hepatitis C virus in HIV-negative mothers. *Res Virol* 149:229, 1998.

Alter MJ, Gallagher M, Morris TT, et al.: Acute non-A-E hepatitis in the United States and the role of hepatitis G virus infection. Sentinel countries virus hepatitis study team. *N Engl J Med* 336:741, 1997.

Basso NG, Fonseca ME, Garcia A, et al.: Enterovirus isolation from foetal and placental tissues. *Acta Virol* 34:49, 1990.

Bates HR: Coxsackie virus B13 calcified pancarditis and hydrops fetalis. *Am J Obstet Gynecol* 106:629, 1970.

Bittencourt AL, Ashworth T: American trypanosomiasis (Chagas' disease). In Doerr W, Seifert G (eds): *Tropical Pathology.* Berlin, Springer Verlag, 1995, pp. 653–704.

Bittencourt AL, Garcia AGP: Pathogenesis of hematogenous infections of the fetus and newborn. *Ped Path Molec Med* 21:253, 2002.

Bittencourt AL, Garcia AGP: The placenta in hematogenous infections. *Ped Path Molec Med* 21:401, 2002.

Bortolussi R, Schlech WF: Listeriosis. In Remington JS, Klein JO (eds): *Infections Diseases of the Fetus and Newborn.* Philadelphia, WB Saunders, 1995, pp. 1055–1068.

Brown KE, Hibbs JR, Gallinella G, et al.: Resistance to parvovirus B19 infection due to lack of virus receptor (erythrocyte P antigen). *N Engl J Med* 330:1192, 1994.

Chouquet C, Burgard M, Richardson S, et al.: Timing of mother-to-child HIV-1 transmission and diagnosis of infection based on polymerase chain reaction in the neonatal period by a non-parametric method. *AIDS* 11:1183, 1997.

Cooper LZ, Preblud SR, Alford CA, Jr: Rubella. In Remington JS, Klein JO (eds): *Infectious Diseases of the Fetus and Newborn.* Philadelphia, WB Saunders, 1995, pp. 268–311.

Dimova PS, Karparov AA: Congenital varicella syndrome case with isolated brain damage. *J Child Neurol* 16:595, 2001.

Duray PH, Chandler FW: Lyme disease. In Connor DH, et al. (eds:) *Pathology of Infectious Disease.* Stamford, Appleton and Lange, 1997, pp. 635–646.

Esterly JR, Oppenheimer EH: Pathological lesions due to congenital rubella. *Arch Pathol* 87:380, 1969.

Greco MA, Zagzag D: Human immunodeficiency virus infection lesion in the pediatric age group. In Cannor DH, Chandler FW, Schwartz DA, et al. (eds): *Pathology of Infectious Disease.* Stamford, Appleton and Lange, 1997, pp. 169–181.

Guarner J, Greer P, Barlett J, et al.: Congenital syphilis in a newborn: an immunopathologic study. *Mod Pathol* 12:87, 1999.

Hartwig NG, Vermejj-Keers C, Van Elsacker-Niele AMW, et al.: Embryonic malformations in a case of intrauterine parvovirus B19 infection. *Teratology* 39:295, 1989.

Jones MJ, Kolb M, Votava HJ, et al.: Intrauterine echovirus type II infection. *Mayo Clin Proc* 55:509, 1980.

Jordan JA: Identification of human parvovirus B19 infection in idiopathic nonimmune hydrops fetalis. *Am J Obstet Gynecol* 174:37, 1996.
Lachaux A, Lapillonne A, Bouvier R, et al.: Transplacental transmission of hepatitis B virus: a familial case. *Pediatr Infect Dis J* 14:60, 1995.
Lack EE, Chandler FW, Pearson GR: Cytomegalovirus infection. In Connor DH, Chandler FW, Schwartz DA, et al. (eds): *Pathology of Infectious Diseases.* Stamford, Appleton & Lange, 1997, pp. 91–99.
Leikin E, Lysikiewicz A, Garry D, et al.: Intrauterine transmission of hepatitis A virus. *Obstet Gynecol* 88:690, 1996.
MacLeod CK: Malaria. In MacLeod CL (ed): *Parasitic Infections in Pregnancy and the Newborn.* New York, Oxford Medical Publication, 1988, pp. 8–42.
Magliocco AM, Demetrick DJ, Sarnat HB, et al.: Varicella embryopathy. *Arch Pathol Lab Med* 116:181, 1992.
Mayauz MJ, Teglas JP, Mandelbrot L, et al.: Acceptability and impact of zidovudine for prevention of mother-to-child human immunodeficiency virus-1 transmission in France. *J Pediatr* 131:857, 1997.
Nakamura Y, Yamamoto S, Tanaka S, et al.: Herpes simplex viral infection in human neonates: an immunohistochemical and electron microscopic study. *Hum Pathol* 16:1091, 1997.
Pham Duy L, LeVan N, Truong HNC: Congenital miliary tuberculosis. A propos of a case. *Rev Pneumol Clin* 54:207, 1998.
Quinn TC, Jacobs RF, Mertz GJ, et al.: Congenital malaria: a report of four cases and a review. *J Pediatr* 101:229, 1982.
Racult D, Stein A: Q-fever during pregnancy-a risk for women, fetuses and obstetricians. *N Engl J Med* 330:371, 1994.
Remington JS, McLeod R, Desmonts G: Toxoplasmosis. In Remington JS, Klein JO (eds): *Infectious Diseases of the Fetus and Newborn.* Philadelphia, WB Saunders, 1995, pp. 140–267.
Scharf A, Scherr O, Enders G, et al.: Virus detection in the fetal tissue of a premature delivery with a congenital varicella syndrome. A case report. *J Perinat Med* 18:317, 1990.
Schroter B, Chaoui R, Meisel H, et al.: Maternal hepatitis B infection as the cause of nonimmunologic hydrops fetalis. *Z Geburtshilfe Neonatol* 203:36, 1999.
Schweitzer IL, Dunn AEG, Peters RL, et al.: Viral hepatitis B in neonates and infants. *Am J Med* 55:762, 1973.
Sharma R, Malik A, Rattan A, et al.: Hepatitis B virus infection in pregnant women and its transmission to infants. *J Trop Pediatr* 42:352, 1996.
Signer DB: Infections of fetuses and neonates. In Wigglesworth JS, Singer DB (eds): *Textbook of Fetal and Perinatal Pathology.* Oxford, Blackwell Scientific Publications, 1991, pp. 525–591.
Stagno S: Cytomegalovirus. In Remington JS, Klein JO (eds): *Infectious Diseases of the Fetus and Newborn.* Philadelphia, WB Saunders, 1995, pp. 312–345.
Stiskal J, Jacquette M, Kaplan G, et al.: Congenital cytomegalovirus infection with gastrointestinal involvement. *J Pediatr* 131:168, 1997.
Toce SS, Keeman WJ: Congenital echovirus II pneumonia in association with pulmonary hypertension. *Pediatr Infect Dis J* 7:360, 1988.
Whitley RJ, Arvin AM: Herpes simplex virus infections. In Remington JS, Klein JO (eds): *Infectious Diseases of the Fetus and Newborn.* Philadelphia, WB Saunders, 1995, pp. 354–372.
Yeung LTF, King SM, Roberts EA: Mothers-to-infant transmission of hepatitis C virus. *Hepatology* 34:223, 2001.
Zanetti AR, Tanzi E, Paccagnini S, et al.: Mother-to-infant transmission of hepatitis C virus. *Lancet* 345:289, 1995.

TWENTY THREE

Multiple Gestations and Conjoined Twins

TYPES OF TWINS AND THEIR ORIGINS

For naturally conceived multiple pregnancy, about 70% are dizygotic (DZ) twins, resulting from double or multiple ovulations in the same cycle; this is attributed to higher levels of maternal follicle-stimulating hormone (FSH) or increased FSH receptor sensitivity. Monozygotic (MZ) twinning involves postzygotic splitting, resulting in two or more embryos. This can occur at any time up to about 14 days postconception.

A third type of twin, the "polar body" twin, is very rare.

DETERMINATION OF ZYGOSITY

Zygosity determination is best carried out by analysis of restriction fragment length polymorphisms in variable number tandem repeat sequences of DNA, extracted from chorionic villus samples, amniotic fluid cells, peripheral blood white cells, placenta, cord and membranes, and tissues sampled at autopsy, including macerated stillborn fetuses (Table 23.1).

PLACENTAL ANATOMY OF ZYGOSITY

Of MZ twins, about one-third have dichorionic (DC) placentas (separate or fused disks), while two-thirds have truly single monochorionic (MC) placentas

Table 23.1 Zygosity of naturally conceived triplets

	Monozygotic	Dizygotic	Trizygotic	Total
Monochorionic	100	0	0	15%
Dichorionic	30	70	0	45%
Trichorionic	5	20	75	40%

(Figure 23.1). Most MC placentas have two amniotic cavities (MC, DA), while a minority (about 1% of all twins) have a single amniotic cavity (MC, MA). Conjoined twins are MZ, and most are MC, MA.

Types of placentation in MZ twins reflect timing of MZ twinning events.

1. Unlike-sexed twin pairs are DZ (Figures 23.2 to 23.4).
2. MC pairs are MZ. With a very rare exception, MC twin placenta may be dizygotic due to fusion of separately fertilized embryos at late morula stage (Redline 2003).
3. Like-sexed DC twins are of unknown zygosity. It is incorrect to assume that like-sexed DC twins are DZ.

Risks for MZ twins:

1. Prenatal twin-twin transfusion (Figures 23.5 to 23.7).
2. Acute perinatal twin-twin transfusion (Tables 23.2 to 23.4 and Figures 23.5 to 23.9).
3. Twin reversed arterial perfusion (TRAP) (Figure 23.8).
   One twin actively perfuses the co-twin (acardiac twin) via large artery to artery and vein to vein anastomosis. Blood flows retrogradely in the arterial

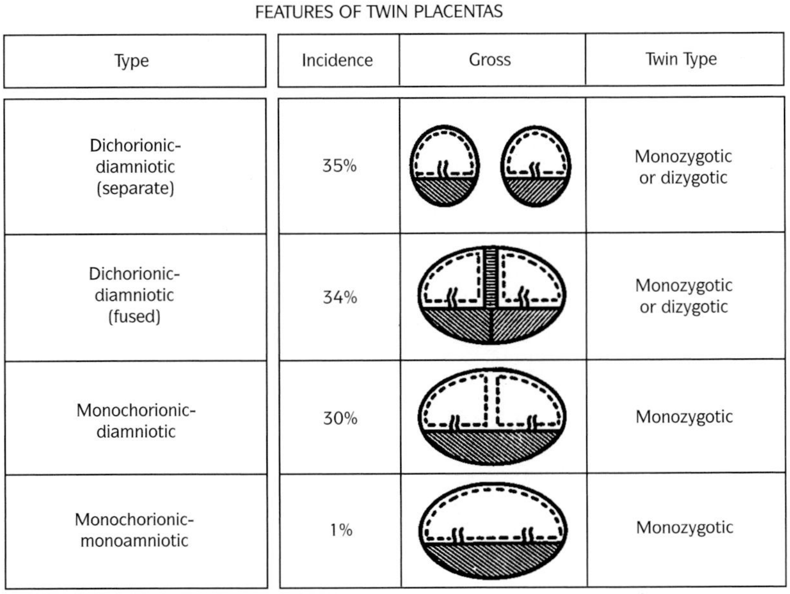

FEATURES OF TWIN PLACENTAS
Type
Incidence
Gross
Twin Type
Dichorionic-diamniotic (separate)
35%
Monozygotic or dizygotic
Dichorionic-diamniotic (fused)
34%
Monozygotic or dizygotic
Monochorionic-diamniotic
30%
Monozygotic
Monochorionic-monoamniotic
1%
Monozygotic

23.1. Types of placentas in twin gestation.

Table 23.2 Acardia-acephalus: Autopsy findings

Absence of cardiac remnants
  Hemiacardiacs have some tissue that is not functional
Absence of central nervous system
Most have no functional urinary system
Most have a single umbilical artery

Table 23.3 Vanishing twin phenomenon

Placental membranes may show yellow-white thickened areas
May find portions of a fetal sac or umbilical cord
Sectioning may reveal fetal remnants
Histology: fetal remnants
Cytogenetics should be attempted on remnants

Table 23.4 Fetus papyraceus

Histological findings
  Fetal remnants
  Increased amounts of perivillous fibrin
Radiographic findings
  Fetal skeleton on x-ray
  May see on ultrasound
Cytogenetics should be attempted

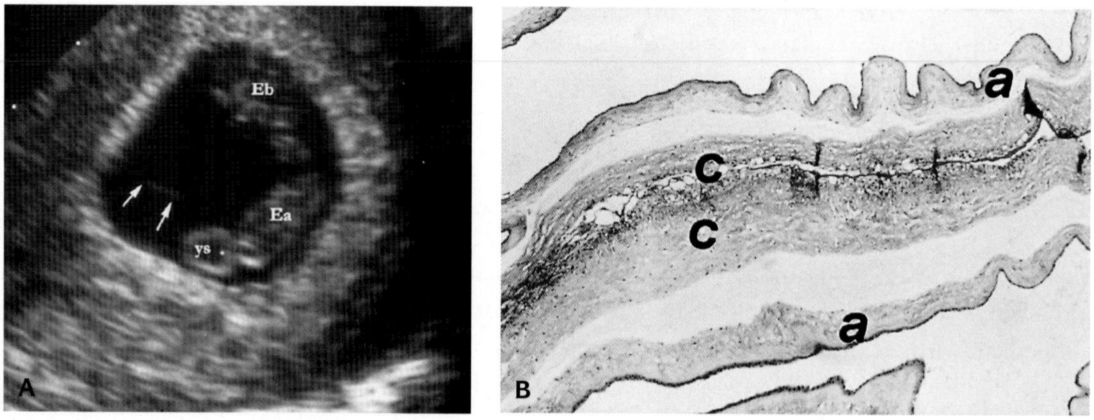

23.2. **(A)** Ultrasound showing twins with dividing membrane (arrows). (YS, yolk sac; Ea, embryo A; Eb, embryo B.) **(B)** Microscopic section of dividing membranes in DA DC twin placenta (a, amnion; c, chorion).

tree to the acardiac twin perfusing only the lower portion of the body while the brain, heart, and upper limbs undergo ischemic necrosis.

4. Unequal parenchymal sharing. The placental parenchyma may be unequally shared by the twins, particularly with respect to venous return. Marked growth discordance can occur in the absence of transfusion.
5. Fetal death of one twin. This is a perilous condition in MC twins, because the survivor is likely to suffer vasculogenic organ damage.
6. Cardiovascular flow lesions. There is an excess of flow-type cardiovascular lesions in MC twins. These are thought to result from transfusional events in MC twins.
7. Cord entanglement of both umbilical cords (Figure 23.9).
8. During delivery, the cord of the second twin may prolapse before the birth of the first twin, or it may be around the neck of the first-born twin.

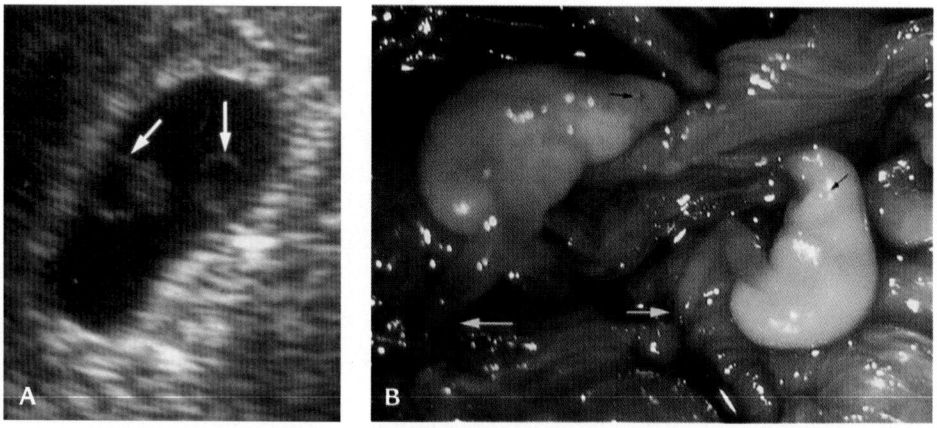

23.3. **(A)** Ultrasound of early twin gestation showing two yolk sacs (arrows). **(B)** MA MC twin embryos. Yellow arrows at umbilical cord insertions, black arrows indicate retinal pigment on the left twin and optic vesicle on the right twin. These twins are GD3.

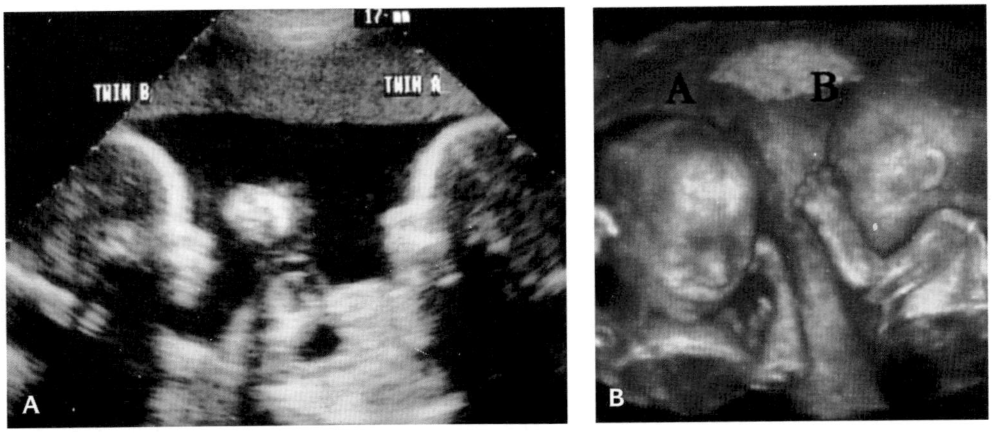

23.4. **(A)** Ultrasound of twins at 20 weeks gestation. **(B)** Three-dimensional ultrasound of twins at 28 weeks gestation.

Fetal death of one twin may occur in the first trimester, resulting in resorption of the dead fetus (vanishing twin) up to 30% of early twin pregnancies revert to single gestations (Figures 23.10 and 23.11).

In the second trimester, fetal death of one twin usually results in fetus papyraceous (Figure 23.12). Fetal death of a twin may cause tissue damage to the remaining twin with aplasia cutis and multiple bowel atresias.

In the third trimester, fetal death in a MC twin can result in a disseminated intravascular coagulopathy by resorption of the products of the dead twin by the surviving twin, resulting in hypoxic ischemia of the brain with multicystic encephalomalacia and porencephaly (Swiss-cheese brain) (Figure 23.13).

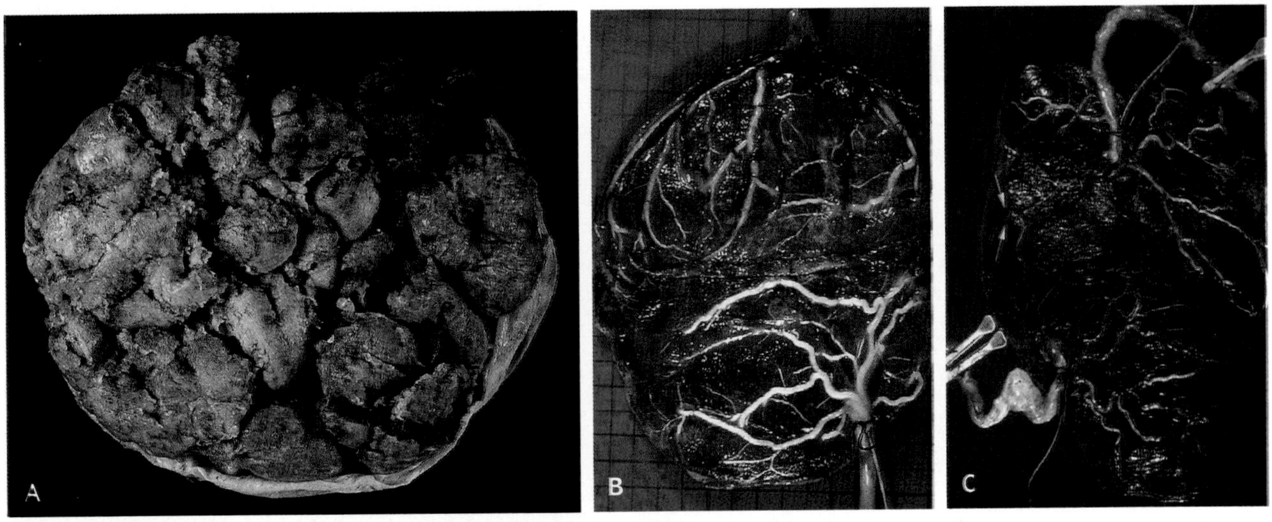

23.5. Twin-to-twin transfusion. **(A)** Diamniotic monochorionic (DA MC) placenta. Donor side on left; recipient side on the right. **(B)** Injection study in DA DC twin placenta with no vascular anastomosis. **(C)** Injection study in DA MC twin placenta showing feeding vessel (arrows).

Table 23.5 Placentation in triplets

Placentation	Incidence	
	Survivors	Deaths
Trichorionic triamniotic	54	36
Dichorionic triamniotic	34	32
Monochorionic triamniotic	10	26
Dichorionic diamniotic	2	6

Source: Baldwin VJ: *Pathology of Multiple Pregnancy*. New York, Springer-Verlag, 1994.

TRIPLETS

In the United States triplets (Figure 23.14) range from 1/1,300 in the southeastern area to 1/10,000 in Chicago (Table 23.5). One-third of spontaneous triplets actually deliver as singletons, 7.7% loss of all three, to 15% loss of two, and 43% loss of one conceptus by 20 weeks gestation. Up to 83% of triplet deliveries are the result of hormonal ovulation induction and many are the result of in vitro fertilization (IVF). The pattern of placentation in triplets ranges from one disk with a single inner layer of amnion (monoamniotic) to three separate disks and gestational sacs (trichorionic triamniotic). Umbilical cord anomalies are more common than with twins. Eighteen percent of triplets have velamentous insertions, abnormally long cords, and one single-artery cord.

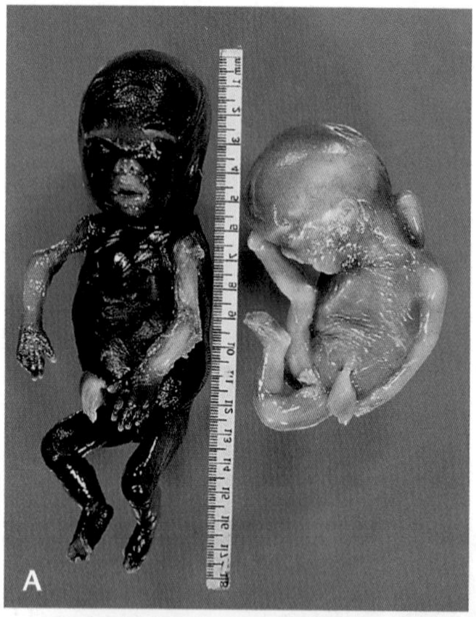

QUADRUPLETS AND HIGHER MULTIPLES

The zygosity combinations in natural multiples probably represent a random distribution, whereas induced multiples are more likely to be polyovulatory. Assisted reproduction technology has increased the incidence of quadruplets; fewer than 5% are spontaneous. Gestational complications reported with

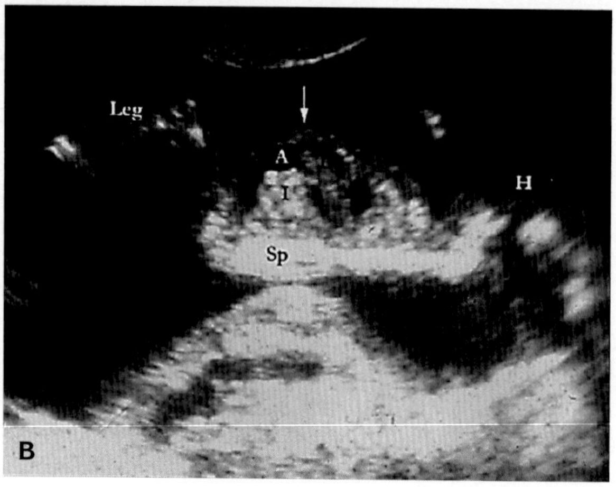

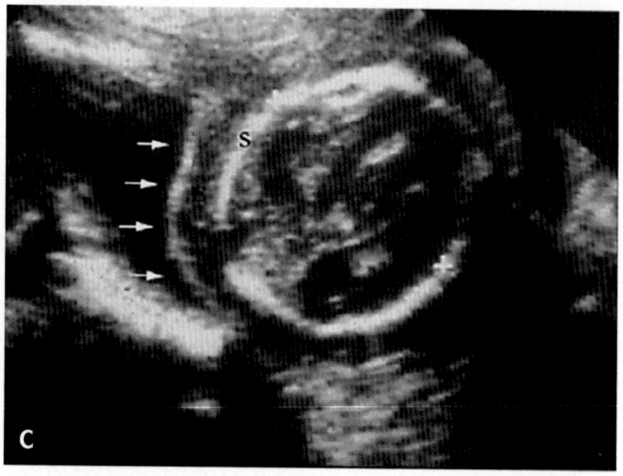

23.6. **(A)** Intrauterine death due to twin-to-twin transfusion, plethoric recipient on left, anemic donor on right. Note also inequality of fetal size. **(B)** Ultrasound of recipient twin with ascites (A). (H, head; I, intestine; L, liver; SP, spine; arrow, distended abdomen.) **(C)** Ultrasound of the recipient head showing scalp edema (E) (S, skull; arrows, scalp skin).

quadruplet pregnancies include gestational diabetes mellitus in 10–50%, pregnancy-induced hypertension in 17–90%, first trimester bleeding in 35%, anemia in 10–25%, and urinary tract infection in 14–17%. Tendency of preterm labor occurs earlier and is more resistant to tocolysis with increasing numbers of fetuses. The mean gestational age at delivery is 31.1 weeks. Mean birth weights have ranged from 1,000 g to 1,700 g. Neonatal morbidity is related to prematurity with hyaline membrane disease. There are four patterns of quadruplet zygosity (Figure 23.15), with the embryos originating from one, two, three, or four ova – monozygotic, dizygotic, trizygotic and quadrizygotic.

High orders with 6, 7, and 8 fetuses rarely have been described.

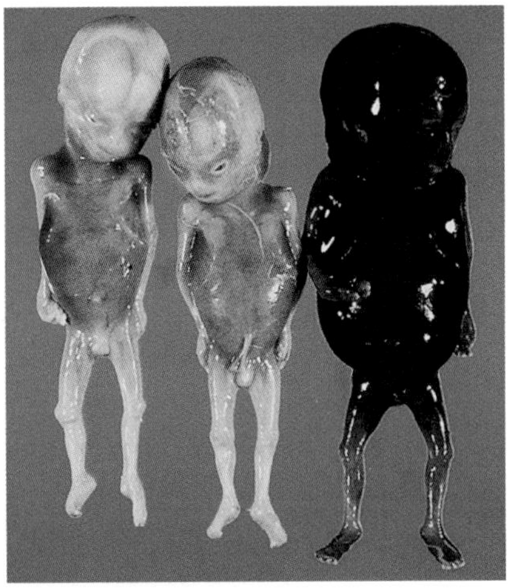

23.7. Triplet transfusion in triamniotic dichorionic (TA DC) placenta, two donors on left and center, recipient on right.

CONJOINED TWINS (CT)

Conjoined twins (CT) (Table 23.6) result from very late, partial twinning events at or about the time when the notochordal axes are being laid down – i.e., at

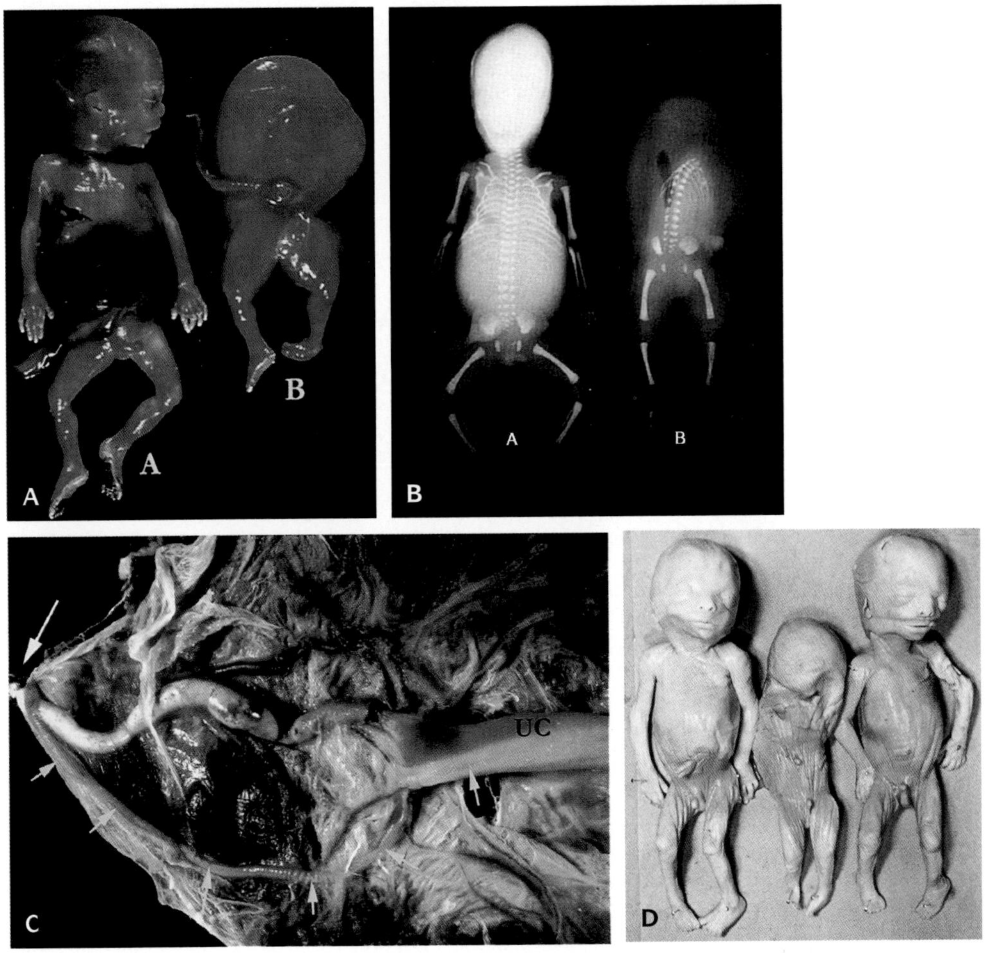

23.8. Twin reversed arterial perfusion (TRAP). **(A)** Normal twin on left. Acardiac acephalic twin on the right. **(B)** X-ray of TRAP. **(C)** Placenta of TRAP showing velamentous insertion (white arrow) of two vessel cord in acardiac twin. A placental artery (yellow arrows) communicates directly with umbilical cord of normal twin (UC). **(D)** Triplets. Center triplet is acardiac due to TRAP.

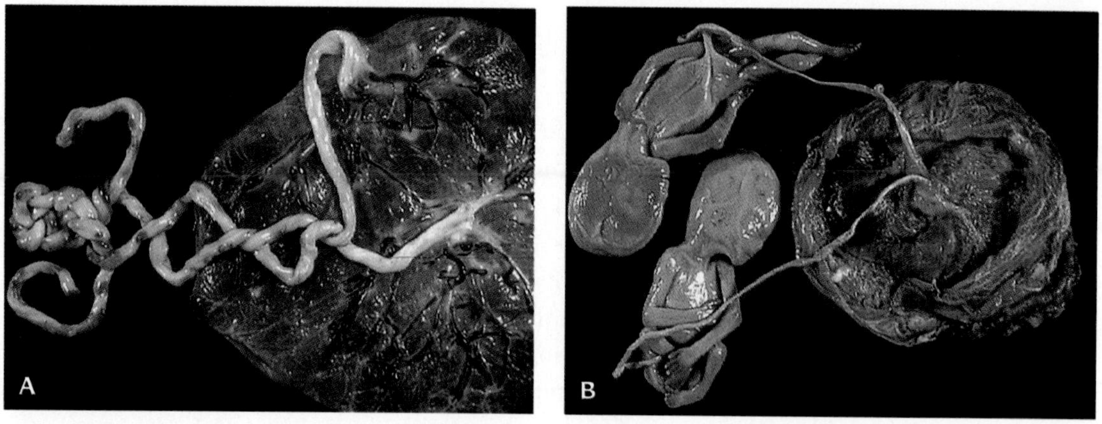

23.9. **(A)** Cord entanglement in twins with fetal death. **(B)** Cord insertion of monochorionic (MoA MoC) twin umbilical cords with vascular compromise and fetal death.

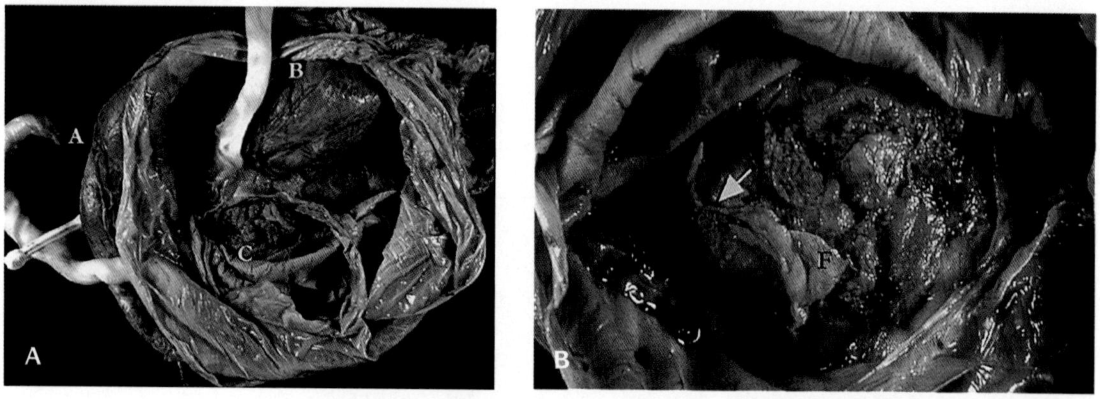

23.10. Vanishing triplet. **(A)** The placenta shows three amniotic sacs (A, B, C). **(B)** "C" contained an amorphous fetus (F) with attenuated umbilical cord (arrow).

Table 23.6 Anatomic classification of conjoined twins

I. Axis orientation:
  A. Notochordal axes in parallel:
    1. Dicephalus, with two spines and heads, two or more upper limbs, single pelvis, two lower limbs.
    2. Diprosopus, with single spine and head, but two faces.
  B. Notochordal axes as far apart as possible:
    1. Ventro-ventral, cranial end – i.e., cephalo-thoracopagus or janiceps, with expression of "new" faces and other organs out laterally.
    2. Ventro-ventral, mid-torso – i.e., thoracopagus, sternopagus, xiphopagus, omphalopagus.
    3. Dorso-dorsal, end-to-end, caudal end – i.e., pygopagus.
    4. End-to-end, cranial end – i.e., craniopagus.
    5. Ventro-ventral, caudal end – i.e., ischiopagus, with 'new' pelvic axes expressed out laterally.

II. Axis symmetry:
  For type IB, notochordal axes may be oriented perfectly dorsodorsally or ventroventrally (disymmetric) or obliquely (asymmetric), with reduced expression of one-half.

III. Axis expression:
  A. Each axis fully expressed (or nearly so) – i.e., diplopagus.
  B. One axis incompletely expressed (parasite) and attached to complete axis (autosite).
  Note that dipagus twins do not represent a side-by-side arrangement with splitting caudally, previously classified as a type of anadidymus CT; in fact they are attached ventroventrally and are best considered as a variant of ischiopagus in which one axis is parasitic.

Source: Baldwin VJ: *Pathology of Multiple Pregnancy*. New York, Springer-Verlag, 1994.

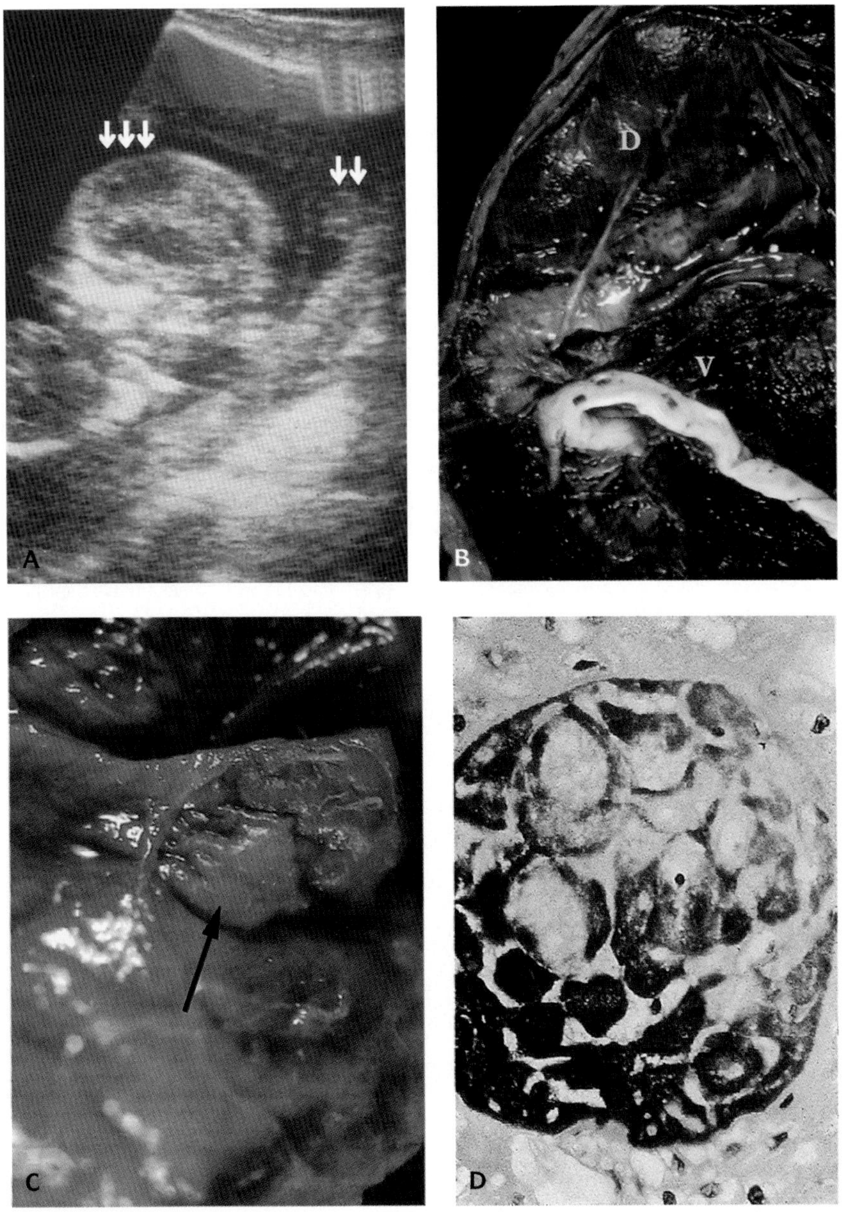

23.11. Vanishing twin. **(A)** Ultrasound showing normal twin (three arrows) and dead (vanishing) twin (two arrows). **(B)** Placenta showing viable twin placenta (V) and small placenta (D) on left. **(C)** Gross appearance of the amorphous calcified vanishing twin (arrow). **(D)** Microscopic appearance of **(C)**.

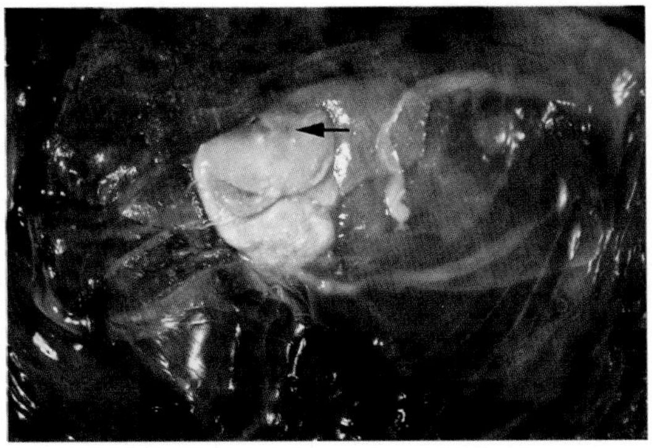

23.12. Fetus papyraceus. Retinal pigment of fetus (arrow). The fetus is compressed onto the placenta.

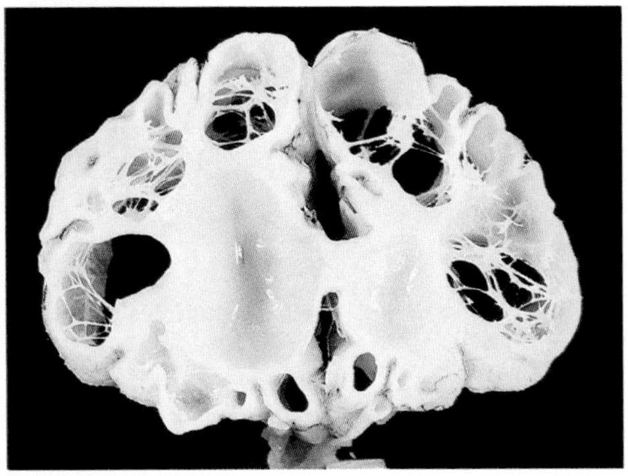

23.13. Swiss cheese brain in surviving twin after death of other twin.

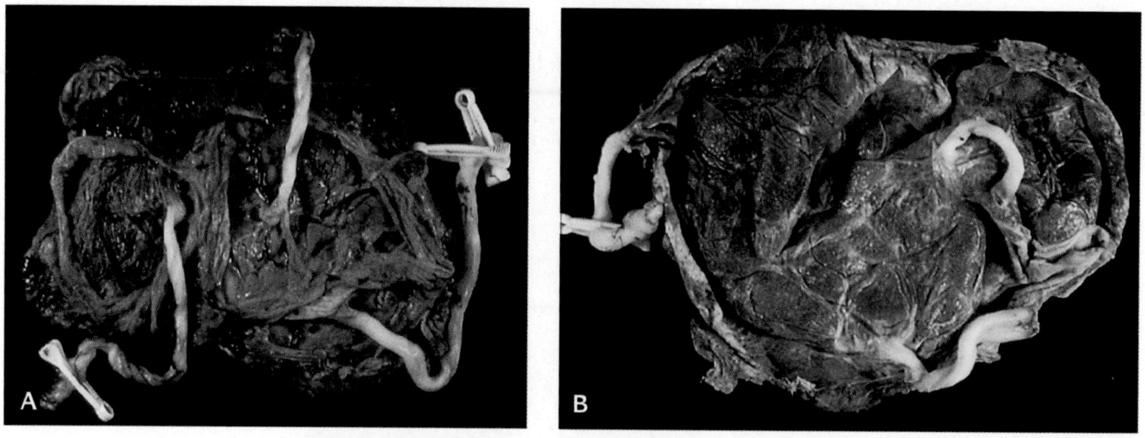

23.14. **(A)** Triamniotic trichorionic fused triplet placenta. Note thick membranes separating each placenta. **(B)** Monochorionic monoamniotic triplet placenta with single amniotic sac and no dividing membranes.

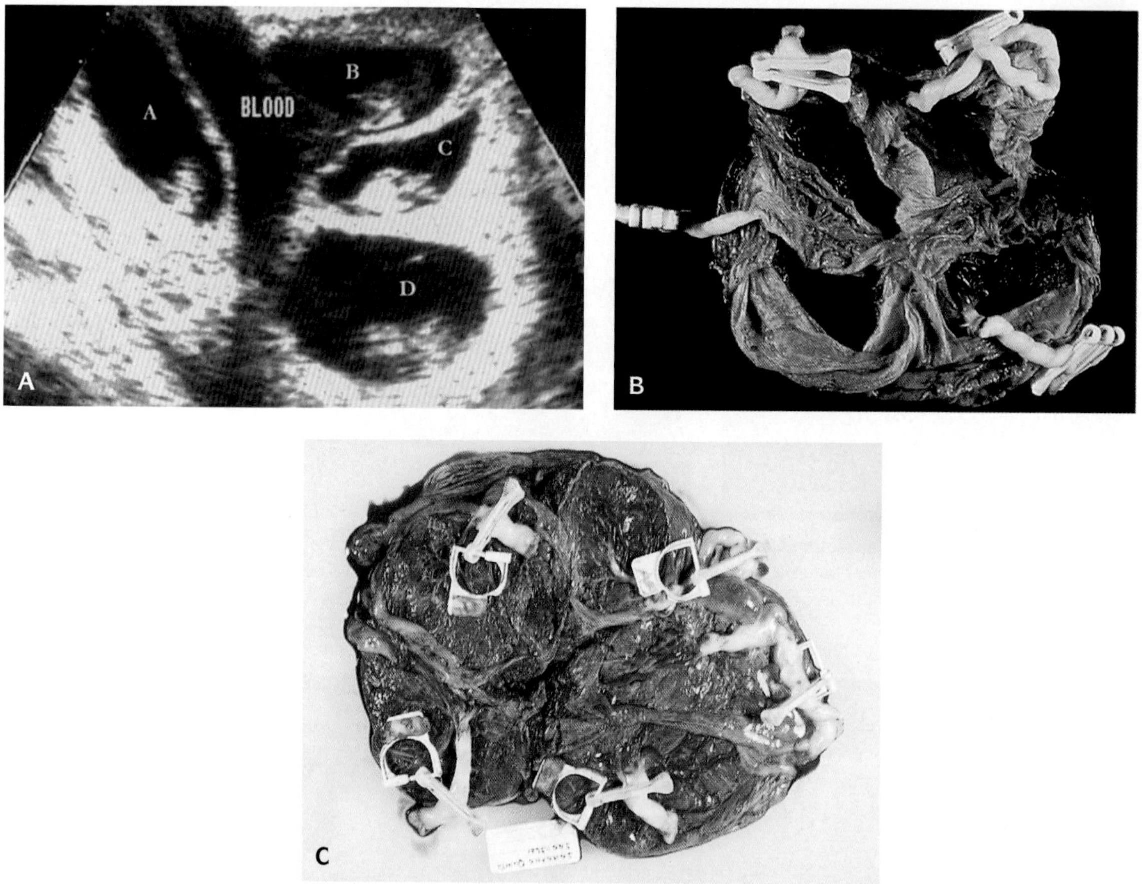

23.15. Quadruplet placenta. **(A)** Ultrasound showing four sacs (A, B, C, D) at 8–10 weeks gestation. **(B)** Four separate sacs in a fused quadraamniotic, quadrachorionic placenta. **(C)** Quintuplet placenta, quinta-amniotic, and qunitachorionic following *in vitro* fertilization. All infants survived. Born at 30 weeks gestation.

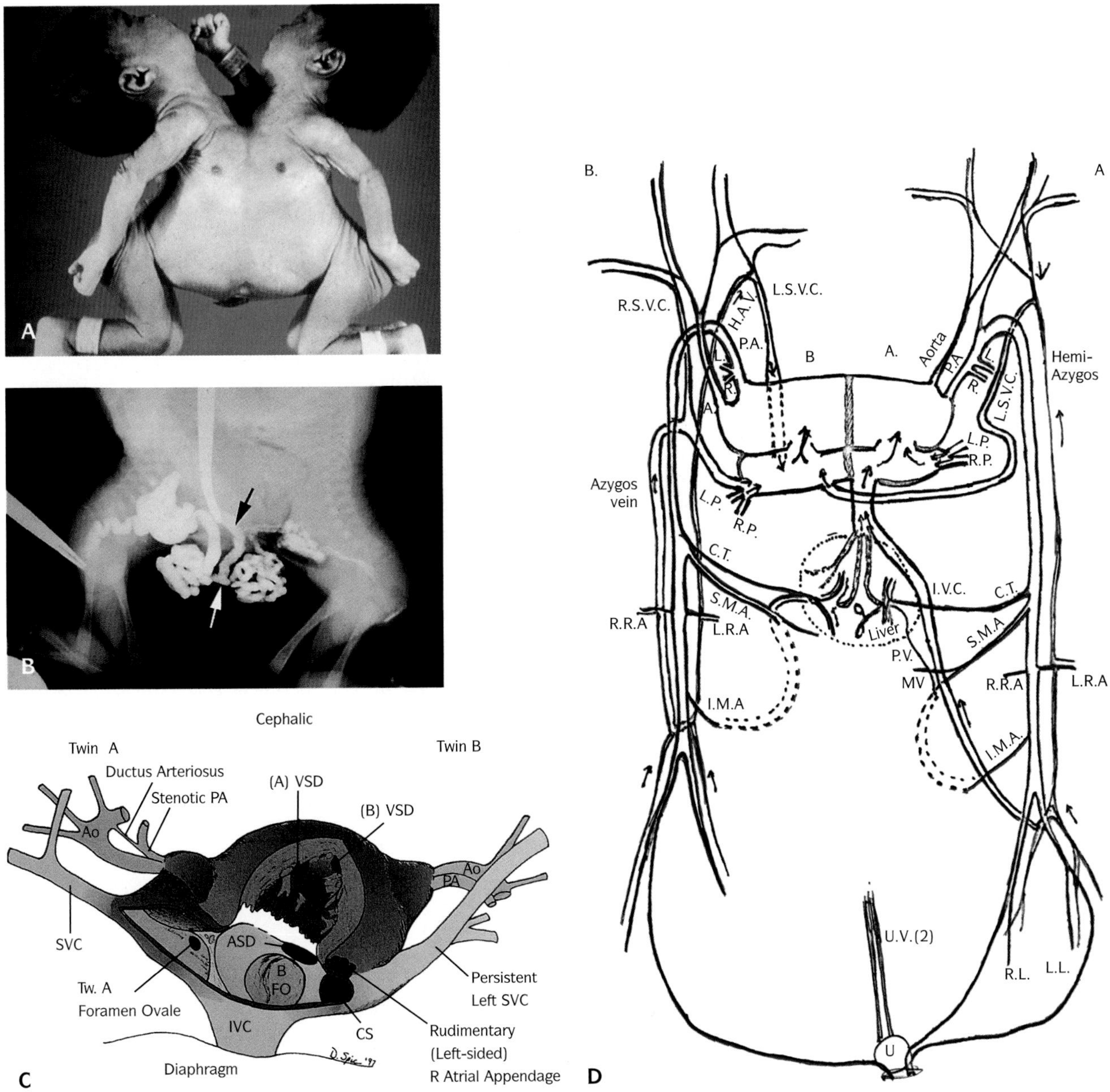

23.16. **(A)** Thoracopagus conjoined twins. **(B)** Barium injection of intestinal tract with shared small bowel (black arrow) and two separate colons (white arrow = separation point). **(C)** Diagram of a five chambered heart in thoracopagus conjoined twins. (PA, pulmonary artery; VSD, ventricular septal defect; SVC, superior vena cava; IVC, inferior vena cava; CS, coronary sinus; ASD, atrial septal defect; FO, foramen ovale; AO, aorta.) **(D)** Illustration of the flow of blood in thoracopagus conjoined twins. (RSVC, right superior vena cava; LSVC, left superior vena cava; HAV, hemiazygos vein; PA, pulmonary artery; AO, aorta; A, azygos vein; R, right; L, left; LP, left pulmonary vein; RP, right pulmonary vein; CT, celiac trunk; SMA, superior mesenteric artery; RRA, right renal artery; LRA, left renal artery; PV, portal vein; MV, mesenteric vein; IMA, inferior mesenteric artery; RL, right leg; LL, left leg; U, umbilicus.)

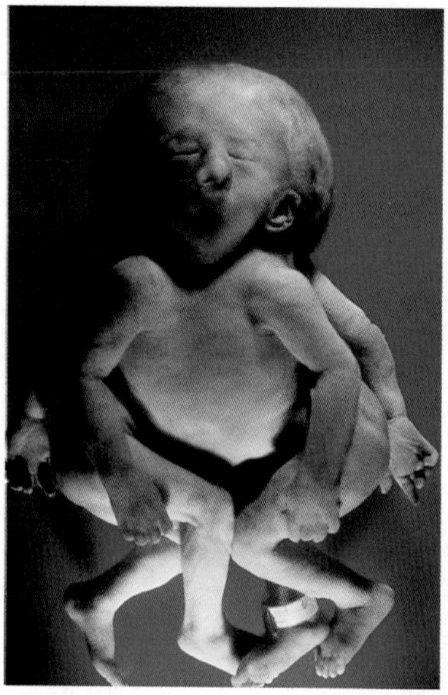

23.17. Cephalothoracopagus (janiceps) conjoined twins.

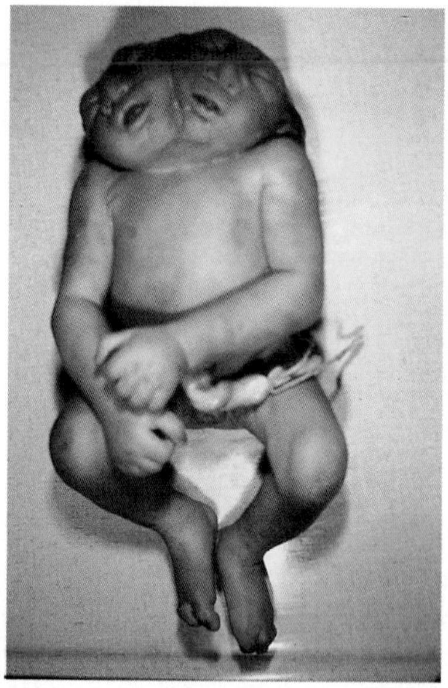

23.18. Diprosopus (one head, two faces).

about 12 days post conception (Table 23.6 and Figures 23.16 to 23.19). The two axes are contained within one ectodermal covering, and placentation is almost always MA, MC. It results from an incomplete separation between monozygotic twins. The incidence is approximately 1/150,000 births and represents fewer than 1% of monozygotic twins. In these there is sharing of viscera including fusion of multichambered hearts and a common midgut as far as the ileocecal valve. Conjoined twins frequently have other congenital anomalies including

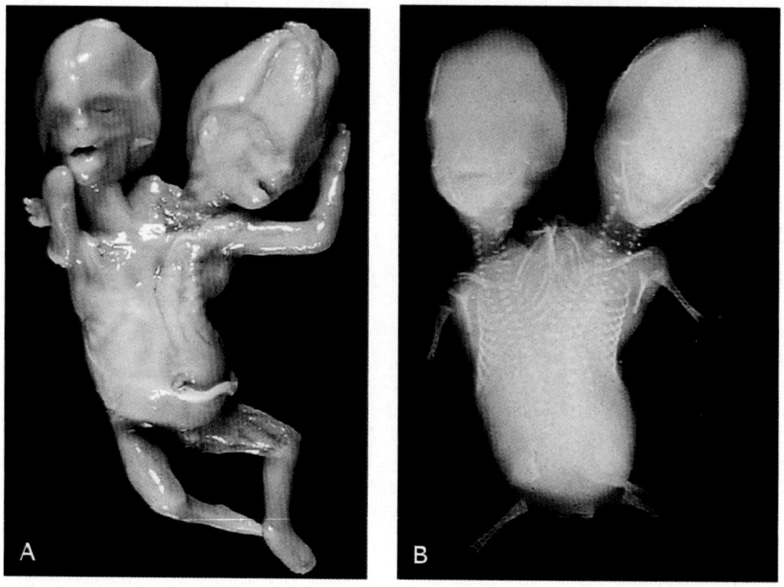

23.19. **(A)** Dicephalus dibrachus dipus (two heads, two arms, two legs). **(B)** X-ray of twins.

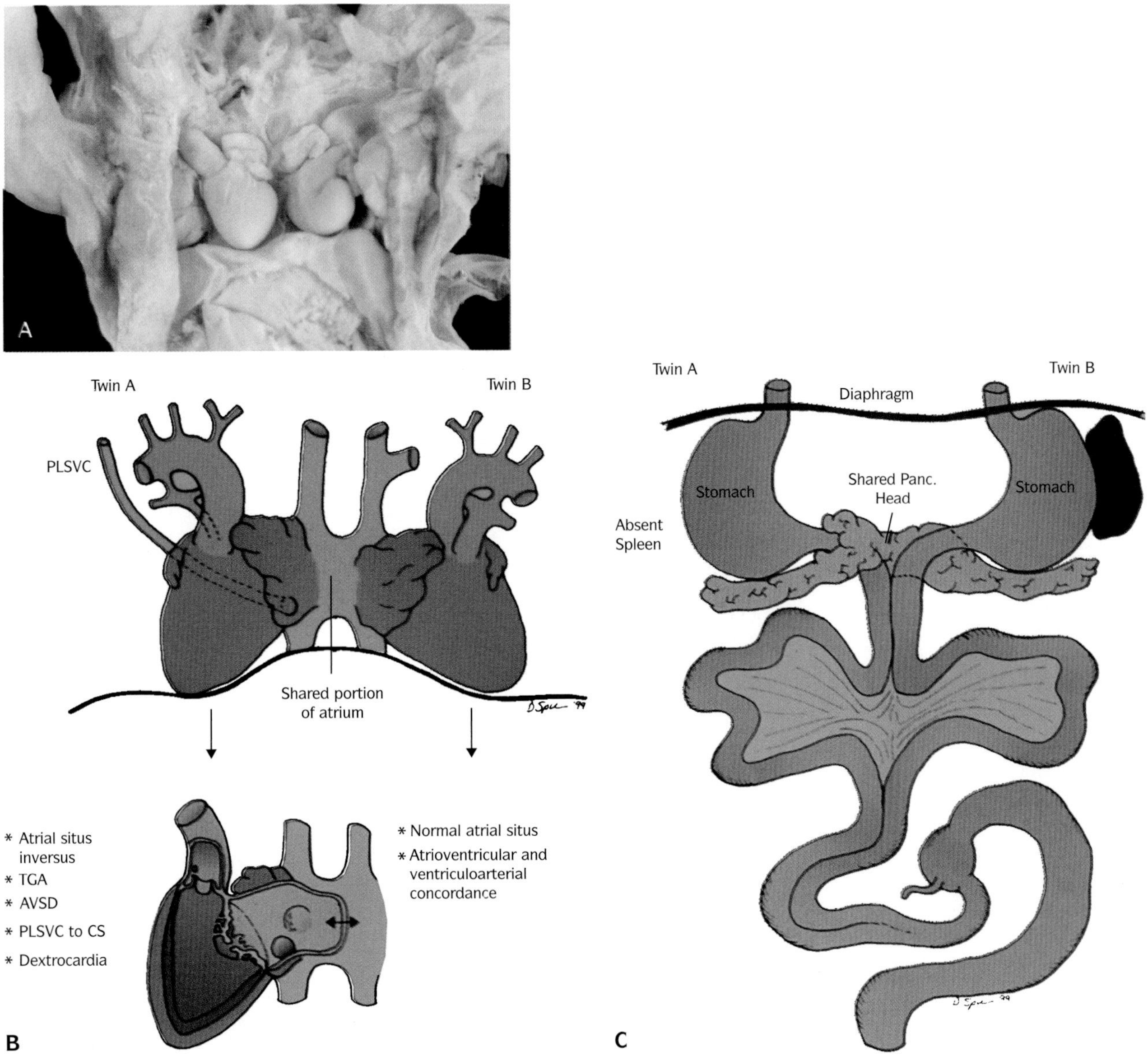

23.20. **(A)** Gross appearance of two separate hearts with shared right atrium in conjoined twins in Figure 23.19. **(B)** Diagram of disposition of the two hearts. **(C)** Diagram with two separate, small bowels and shared colon.

cleft palate, anencephaly, and complex cardiac defects. Seventy-five percent are thoracopagus. About one-third are stillborn. It is a sporadic occurrence. Polyhydramnios is frequent. They may be detected by ultrasound as early as 9 weeks. Color doppler studies are useful in viewing arterial circulation particularly in the heart and liver, and fetal echocardiography will determine the cardiac abnormalities. All conjoined twins with rare exceptions require surgical separation. A shared heart and/or shared brain (Figure 23.20 and 23.21) precludes survival for both twins.

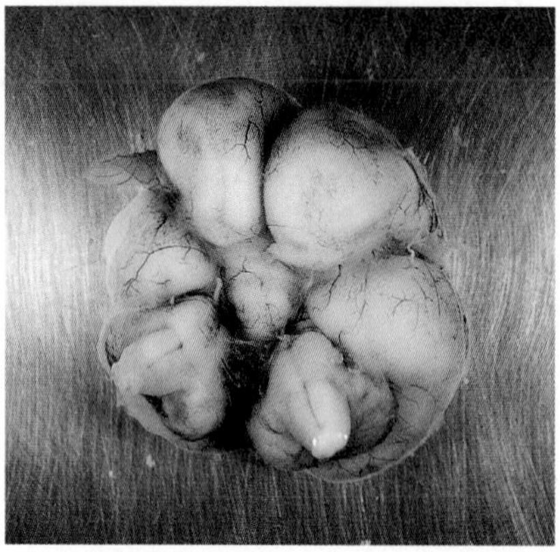

23.21. Diprosopus conjoined twin with one brain and two cerebelli and spinal cords with two spinal axes.

FETUS IN FETU

This refers to a reduced parasitic fetus. Such a fetus usually derives its blood supply from the superior mesenteric or renal vessels that are usually located in the upper retroperitoneum (Figure 23.21). There may be considerable overlap between sacrococcygeal teratoma and fetus in fetu. The distinguishing feature is the presence of an axial skeleton in fetus in fetu.

REFERENCES

Baldwin VJ: *Pathology of Multiple Pregnancy.* New York, Springer-Verlag, 1994.

Benirschke K, Kaufmann P: *Pathology of the Human Placenta,* 3rd ed. New York, Springer-Verlag, 1995.

Botting BJ, Davies IM, Macfarlane AJ: Recent trends in the incidence of multiple births and associated mortality. *Arch Dis Child* 62:941, 1987.

Gilbert-Barness E: Multiple pregnancies. In Gilbert-Barness E (ed): *Potter's Pathology of the Fetus and Infant.* St. Louis, Mosby-Year Book, 1997.

Machin GA, Bamforth F: Zygosity and placental anatomy in 15 consecutive sets of spontaneously conceived triplets. *Am J Med Genet* 61:247, 1996.

Machin GA: Conjoined twins: Implications for blastogenesis. In Opitz JM, Paul NW (eds): *Blastogenesis: Normal and Abnormal.* March of Dimes Birth Defects Foundation. Birth Defects: Original Article New York, March of Dimes, Series 29:141, 1993.

Machin GA, Keith LG: *An Atlas of Multiple Pregnancy.* London, U.K., Parthenon Publications, 1999.

Machin GA: Multiple pregnancies and conjoined twins. In Gilbert-Barness E (ed): *Potter's Pathology of the Fetus and Infant.* St. Louis, Mosby-Year Book, 1997, p. 281.

Machin GA, Still K, Lalani T: Correlations of placental vascular anatomy and clinical outcomes in 69 monochorionic twin pregnancies. *Am J Med Genet* 62:229, 1996.

Monteagudo A, Timor-Tritsch IE, Sharma S: Early and simple determination of chorionic an amniotic type in multifetal gestations in the first fourteen weeks by high-frequency transvaginal ultrasonography. *Am J Obstet Gynecol* 170:624, 1994.

Philips DIW: Twin studies in medical research: Can they tell us whether diseases are genetically determined? *Lancet* 341:1008, 1993.

Redline RW: Non identical twins with a single placenta – disproving dogma in perinatal pathology. *N Eng J Med* 349:111, 2003.

Strong SG, Corney G: *The Placenta in Twin Pregnancy.* Oxford, Pergamon Press, 1967.

TWENTY FOUR

Metabolic Diseases

Most metabolic disorders due to inborn errors of metabolism are inherited as autosomal recessive traits; some are X-linked. A few are dominant traits. Mitochondrial enzymes are coded by both the maternal nuclear genome and by the mitochondrial DNA. Some disorders can be detected by newborn screening (Table 24.1). Placental changes (Table 24.2) may be present and suggest a lysosomal storage disease. Skin fibroblasts, conjunctiva, intestinal biopsy, peripheral nerve, muscle, bone marrow and amniocytes may be used in the diagnoses of metabolic disease (Table 24.3). Vacuolated lymphocytes (Table 24.4) also may be seen in a number of storage diseases.

AMINO ACID DISORDERS

A number of disorders of amino acid metabolism have been described including phenylketonuria, tyrosinemia, alkaptonuria, homocystinuria, lysinemia, and cystinosis (Figures 24.1 and 24.2 and Tables 24.5 and 24.6). These disorders are rarely observed in the fetus or newborn infant.

MUCOPOLYSACCHARIDOSES

These disorders are distinguished by storage of glycosaminoglycans (GAG) (mucopolysaccharides) and glycolipids in the lysosomes of different cell types,

Table 24.1 Disorders detected by newborn screening

Cystic fibrosis	Immunoreactive tryptinogen test (IRT) (not valid after 3 months of age), sweat test, DNA probes
Galactosemia	Galactokinase deficiency Galactose-1-phosphate uridyl transferase deficiency Galactose-4-epimerase deficiency
Glycogen storage diseases	
Amino acid disorders	Maple syrup urine disease Tyrosinemia homocystinuria Arginase deficiency Acute neonatal citrullinemia Phenylketonuria Pyroglutamic aciduria
Congenital adrenal hyperplasia	Salt wasting 21-hydrolase deficiency Simple virilizing 21-hydroxylase deficiency
Biotinidase deficiency	
Adrenosine deaminase deficiency (SCID)	
Acylcarnitine disorders	Organic acid Methylmalonic acidemias Methylmalonyl-CoA mutase deficiencies (mut$^-$ and mut$^+$) Adrenosylcobamin synthesis defects (Cb1A and Cb1B) Combined adenosylcobalamin and methylcobalamin defects (Cb1C and Cb1D) Propionic acidemia Isovaleric acidemia Glutaric acidemia type I Multiple CoA carboxylase deficiency 3-Methylcrotonyl-CoA carboxylase deficiency 3-Ketothiolase deficiency 3-Hydroxy-3-methylglutaryl-CoA lyase deficiency 3-Methylglutaconyl-CoA hydratase deficiency 3-Hydroxyisobutyl-CoA hydrolase deficiency 2,4-Dienoyl-CoA reductase deficiency
Fatty acid oxidation defects	Medium-chain acyl-CoA dehydrogenase deficiency (MCAD) Short-chain acyl-CoA dehydrogenase deficiency (SCAD) Long-chain acyl-CoA dehydrogenase deficiency (LCAD) 3-Hydroxy acyl-CoA dehydrogenase deficiency Carnitine palmityl transferase deficiency type II Multiple Acyl-CoA dehydrogenase deficiency (glutaric acidemia type II)
Congenital hypothyroidism	
Sickle cell disease	

Table 24.2 Inherited metabolic disorders – placental pathology

Disease	Vacuolated trophoblast	Vacuolated stromal/ Hofbauer cells	Ultrastructural/histochemical pathology only
GM1 generalized gangliosidosis	+	+	
Mucopolysaccharidosis I	−	+	
Mucopolysaccharidosis III	+	+	
Mucopolysaccharidosis IV	−	+*	
Sialidosis	+	+	
Infantile free sialic acid storage disease	+	+	
Salla disease	+	+	
Mucolipidosis II	+	+	
Mucolipidosis IV	−	+	
Cholesteryl ester storage disease	+	?	
Niemann-Pick disease	+	+	
Gaucher disease**	−	−	
Ceroid lipofuscinosis	−	−	+
Glycogen storage disease II (Pompe)	−	−	+
Peroxisomal deficiencies	−	−	+

* Uncertain if villus edema or lysosomal storage ** Villus intravascular Gaucher cells only

Table 24.3 Tissues used for diagnosis of metabolic disorders

I. Skin
  A. Fibroblasts
    1. Lysosomes
    2. Enzymes
II. Conjunctiva
  A. Lysosomes
III. Intestinal – neurogenic plexus
  A. Gangliosides
  B. Neuronal ceroid lipofuscinosis
  C. Sphingolipidosis
  D. Niemann-Pick
IV. Peripheral nerve
  A. Fabry
  B. Niemann-Pick
  C. Metachromatic leukodystrophy
V. Muscle
  A. Carnitine
  B. Glycogen
  C. Enzyme histochemistry
VI. Bone marrow
  A. Cystinosis
  B. Gaucher
  C. Niemann-Pick
VII. Aminocytes
  A. Gaucher
  B. Mucopolysaccharides
  C. Gangliosidosis

Adapted from Barness LA, Gilbert-Barness E: Metabolic Diseases. In *Potter's Pathology of the Fetus and Infant*, Gilbert-Barness E, ed. Philadelphia, Mosby Publishing, 1997.

Table 24.4 Presence of vacuolated lymphocytes in storage disorders

Disease	Vacuolated lymphocytes
GM1-gangliosidosis, infantile	Frequent, large
Niemann-Pick A	Occasional, small
Niemann-Pick C	Occasional, small
Sialidosis	Frequent, large
Aspartylglycosaminuria	Frequent, large
Mannosidosis	Frequent, large
Fucosidosis	Occasional, small
Sialic acid storage disorders	Frequent, large
Mucolipidosis, type II and III	Frequent, large
Mucopolysaccharidoses, types 1–3	Occasional, variable
Glycogenosis, type II	Occasional, small
Wolman disease	Occasional, small
Juvenile neuronal ceroid lipofuscinosis	Frequent, large

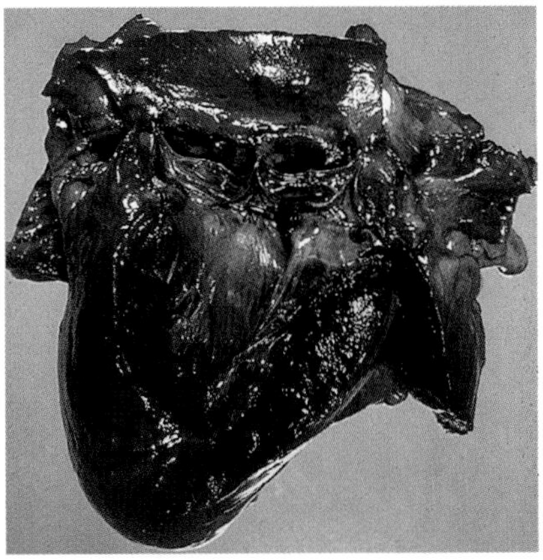

24.1. Alkaptonuria. Pigment is present in the endocardium and heart valves.

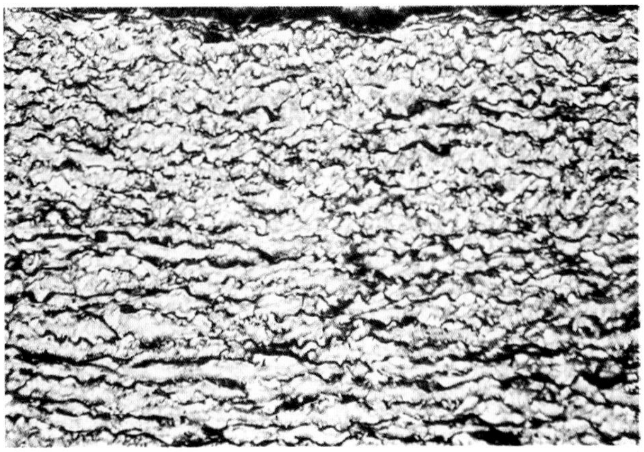

24.2. Homocystinuria. Basket weave pattern of elastic tissue in the aorta.

Table 24.5 Aminoaciduria

OMIM #	Disease	Enzyme defect	Diagnosis
261600	Phenylketonuria 12q22–q24.1 AR 1/10,000	Phenylalanine hydroxylase, pterins	Phenylalanine level blood; enzyme assay (liver) biopterin
276700	Tyrosinesmia I 15q23q25 AR 1/100,000	Fumarylacetoacetate	Enzyme assay (liver), blood and urine, tyrosine
276600	Tyrosinesmia II 16q22.1–22.3 AR	Tyrosine aminotransferase	Enzyme assay, liver, blood, and urine for tyrosine
*203500	Alkaptonuria 3q2 AR 1/100,000	Homogentisic acid oxidase	Homogentisic acid, urine, enzyme deficiency (tissues)
*238331	Hyperglysinemia, nonketotic 9q13 AR 1/250,000	Glycine cleavage enzyme	Glycine in blood, spinal fluid, enzyme deficiency (brain and liver)
#219800	Cystinosis, AR 1/100,000	Transport of cystine	Cystine crystals, bone marrow, cornea, amniocytes
219500	Homocystinemia AR 21q22.3 1/200,000	Cystothionine β-synthase	Cystine decreased in plasma, increased urinary homocysteine, absent cystothionine β-synthase in cultured fibroblasts, lymphocytes, or liver biopsy

including fibroblasts, macrophages, white blood cells, parenchymal cells of liver, kidneys, brain and other organs, and neurons, and by excretion of mucopolysaccharide in the urine (Table 24.7).

When the tissue is fixed in GAG-insoluble fixatives such as alcohol, the accumulated material shows intense metachromasia (purple-blue staining) with toluidine blue and stains with Alcian blue, weakly with periodic acid-Schiff (PAS), and is impregnated with colloidal iron. Lipid may be abundant.

Table 24.6 Homocystinuria

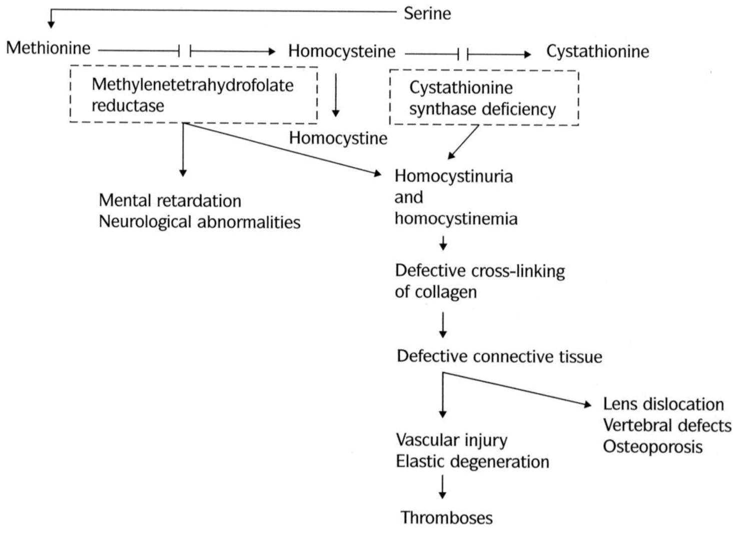

Table 24.7 Mucopolysaccharidoses (MPS)

Disorder	Inheritance	Defective enzyme	Clinical pathologic features
MPS 1H (Hurler)	AR	α-1-iduronidase	Abnormal facies, visceromegaly, skeletal changes, cardiovascular disease, mental retardation, corneal clouding
MPS 1S (Scheie)	AR	α-1-iduronidase (defect allelic with above)	Cardiac valve disease, corneal clouding, joint stiffness, normal intelligence
MPS 1H/1S genetic compound	AR	α-1-iduronidase	Intermediate between MPS 1H and MPS 1S
MPS 2A (Hunter, clinically severe subset)	XLR	Sulfoiduronate sulfatase	Abnormal facies, growth retardation, hepatosplenomegaly, cardiovascular disease, death by second decade
MPS 2B (Hunter, clinically milder subset)	XLR	Sulfoiduronate sulfatase (? defect allelic with 2A)	Features less severe than above with longer survival
MPS 3A (Sanfilippo A)	AR	Heparan sulfate sulfatase	Visceral/skeletal features slight; mental defect severe
MPS 3B (Sanfilippo B)	AR	*N*-acetyl-α-D-glucosaminidase	Similar to above
MPS 3C (Sanfilippo C)	AR	Acetyl CoA: α-glucosaminide *N*-acetyl transferase	Similar to above
MPS 3D (Sanfilippo D)	AR	*N*-acetylglucosamine 6-sulfate sulfatase	Similar to above
MPS 4A (Morquio A)	AR	β-Galactosamine-6-sulfate sulfatase	Thoracic skeletal deformity, aortic valve
MPS 4B (Morquio B)	AR	β-Galactosidase (presumably allelic with forms of generalized GM1 gangliosidosis)	Skeletal disease, corneal clouding mild, intellect normal
MPS 5 – now MPS 1S			
MPS 6 (Maroteaux-Lamy)	AR	Arylsulfatase B	Skeletal disease, corneal clouding severe, intellect normal until late in course
MPS 7 (Sly)	AR	β-Glucuronidases	Short stature, major feature
MPS 8	AR	Glucuronidases-6-sulfate sulfase	Short stature, hepatomegaly, mental retardation, normal corneas

AR, autosomal recessive; XLR, X-linked recessive.

Hurler disease is characterized by coarse features, prominent supraorbital ridges, depressed nasal bridge and dysostosis multiplex (Figures 24.3 to 24.5). Beaking of the vertebral bodies may be apparent in the fetus and newborn.

Mucolipidoses

All types have coarse facial features, mental retardation, and dysostosis multiplex and resemble the Hurler phenotype except for the lack of mucopolysacchariduria.

Mucolipidosis II (I-cell disease) is characterized by a Hurler phenotype.

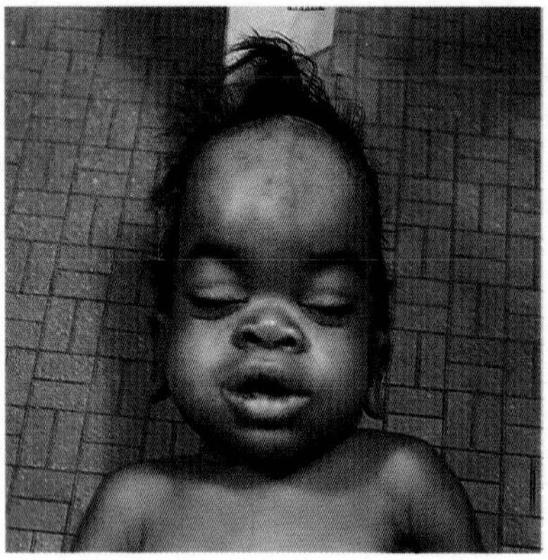

24.3. Hurler syndrome. Phenotypic appearance of child showing coarse features, prominent supraorbital ridges, and depressed nasal bridge.

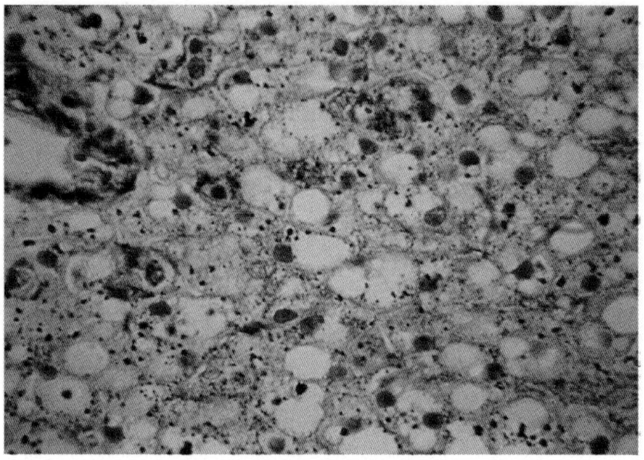

24.4. Microscopic section of liver in mucopolysaccharidosis I (Hurler syndrome) (collodial iron stain).

Hepatocytes, macrophages, hepatic and splenic sinusoidal lining cells, neurons, and renal glomerular and collecting tubular epithelial cells are most severely affected (Figures 24.6 to 24.10).

The accumulated cytoplasmic acid mucopolysaccharides exhibits histochemical characteristics of a weakly sulfated compound, producing a positive reaction with Hale's colloidal iron, Alcian blue at pH 2.5, and toluidine blue at pH 2.0, but a negative reaction with Alcian blue at pH 1.0.

LYSOSOMAL LIPID STORAGE DISEASE (TABLE 24.8)

Gaucher Disease

Gaucher disease is the most common of the lysosomal storage disorders. Three types represent different allelic disorders with different mutations in the

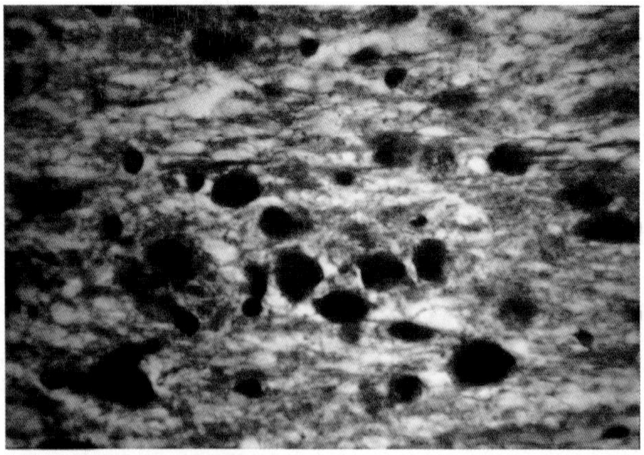

24.5. High magnification of greatly distended neurons of anterior horn cells in the spinal cord.

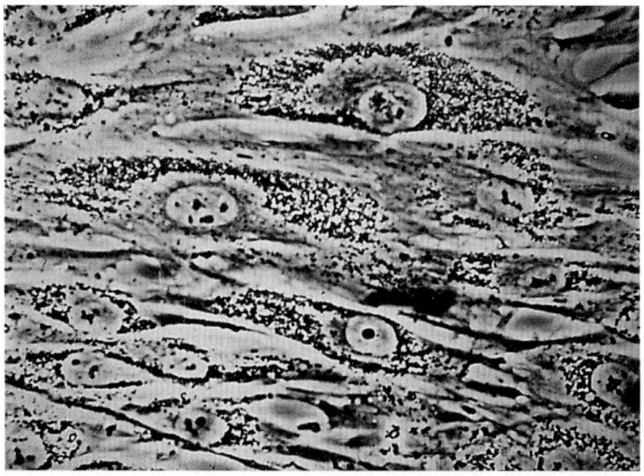

24.6. I cell disease (mucolipidosis II). Cultured fibroblasts viewed under phase microscopy showing coarse cytoplasmic granules.

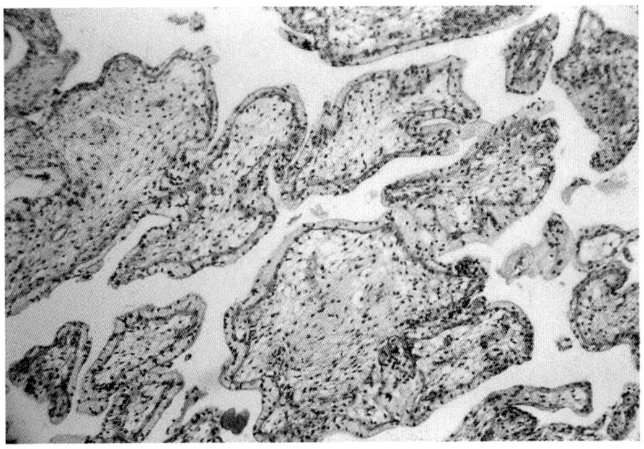

24.7. I cell disease. Microscopic section of the placenta. The stromal cells of the chronic villi are vacuolated and distended with storage material.

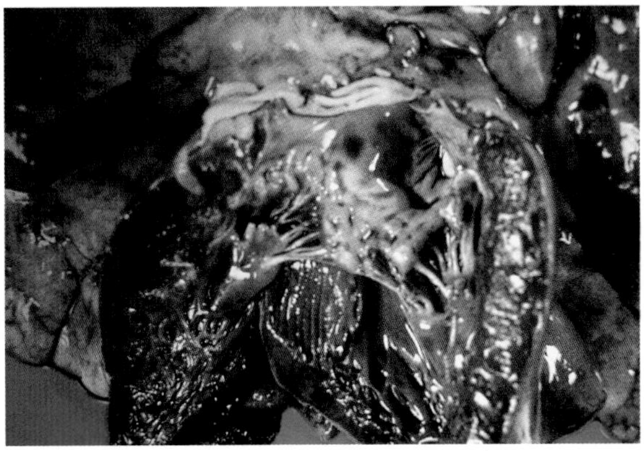

24.8. I cell disease. The heart valves are thickened and distorted.

structural gene of the deficient enzyme, β-glucocerebrosidase (Figure 24.11). In the absence of this enzyme, glucocerebroside cannot be catalytically converted into ceramide and glucose and thus accumulates in reticuloendothelial tissues.

Type 1 – Gaucher disease is characterized by marked hepatosplenomegaly, anemia, Erlenmeyer flask deformity of the femurs, and Gaucher cells in the bone marrow. It is nonneuronopathic.

Type 2 – This form is neuronopathic and results in severe neurologic symptoms soon after birth with death early in life.

Type 3 – This form (Norrbottnian type) is intermediate between type 1 and type 2.

Sphingolipid Storage Diseases

Sphingolipidosis (Niemann-Pick disease) is associated with deficiency of isoelectric forms of sphingomyelinase with the accumulation of sphingomyelin, cholesterol, glycolipid, and acylglyceropyrophosphate in various organs

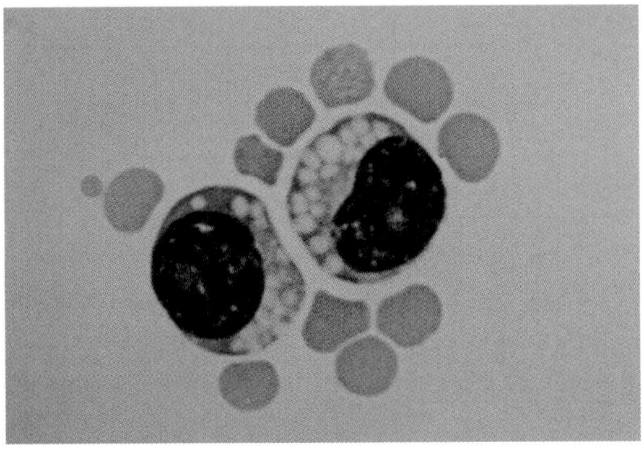

24.9. Vacuoles in peripheral blood lymphocytes in sialidosis.

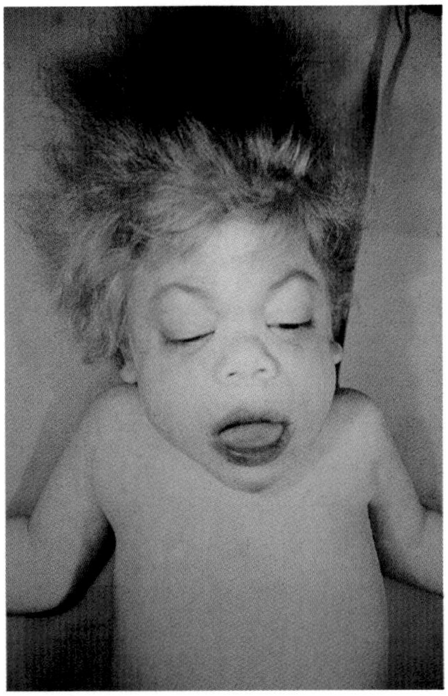

24.10. I cell disease. Child with Hurler-like features with brushed out hair.

Table 24.8 Lysosomal lipid storage diseases

McKusick no.	Disease	Inheritance	Deficient enzyme
Triglyceride/cholesteryl ester storage diseases			
27800	Wolman, infantile	AR	Acid lipase (cholesterol ester hydrolase)
21500	Cholesteryl ester storage diseases	AR	Acid lipase
Sphingomyelin storage diseases			
25720	Niemann-Pick A (infantile cerebral type)	AR	Sphingomyelinase
257200	Niemann-Pick B (juvenile noncerebral type)	AR	Sphingomyelinase
	Niemann-Pick (neonatal malignant cholestatic jaundice)	AR	Presumably sphingomyelinase, ? Subset of NP-A
257220	Niemann-Pick C (subacute juvenile neuropathic type)	AR	Same as above
257250	Niemann-Pick E (adult noncerebral type) (Primary sea-blue histiocyte syndrome)	AR	Not established, ? sphingomyelinase
Cerebroside storage diseases			
230800	Gaucher 1 (adult Gaucher disease)	AR	Glucocerebrosidase β-*o*–glucosyl-*N*-acyl sphingosine hydrolase
230900	Gaucher 2A (infantile cerebral type)	AR	Glucocerebrosidase
	Gaucher 2B (rapidly progressive with ichthyosis)	AR	Glucocerebrosidase
23100	Gaucher 3 (chronic neuropathic or Norrbottnian type)	AR	Glucocerebrosidase
245200	Krabbe, infantile type	AR	Galactocerebroside β-galactosidase
245200	Krabbe, late infantile/juvenile type	AR	Galactocerebroside β-galactosidase
301500	Farber lipogranulomatosis a. Early onset b. Infantile type	AR	Ceramidase
301500	Fabry (angiokeratoma corporis diffusum)	XLR	α-Galactosidase A (ceramide trihexosidase)
Gangliosidoses			
230500	GM1 type 1 gangliosidosis, infantile	AR	β-Galactosidase
230600	GM1 gangliosidosis type 2 infantile (Derry)	AR	As above, presumably allelic
272800	GM2 type 1 gangliosidosis, infantile (Tay-Sachs disease, B form)	AR	Hexoaminidases A (α-unit mutation)
268800	GM2 type 2 gangliosidosis, infantile generalized form (Sandhoff)	AR	Hexoaminidases A and B (β-unit mutation)
Sulfatide storage diseases			
250100	Metachromatic leukodystrophy, infantile	AR	Arylsulfase A (cerebroside sulfate sulfatase (allele 1 mutation)
27200	Multiple sulfatase deficiency (Austin mucosulfatidosis)	AR	Arylsulfatases A, B, and C; clinical type 1 – onset in first year, survival to 6–10 years; type 2 – onset in later infancy, survival into second decade; type 3 – onset in second decade, survival to third–fourth decades, probably due to continuous spectrum of severity rather than allelic differences

AR, autosomal recessive; XLR, X-linked recessive.

(Figures 24.12 and 24.13). Type A is the most common and most severe infantile form with hepatosplenomegaly and neurological deterioration in the first year of life. Type B is the nonneuronopathic form. Type C is the juvenile form with onset in childhood and severe neurological deterioration. Niemann-Pick cells may be found in the bone marrow in all forms.

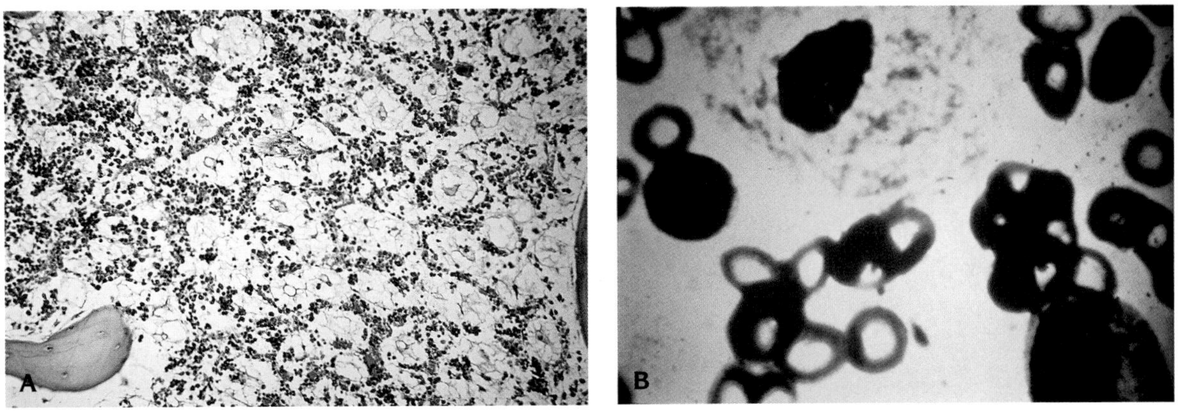

24.11. Gaucher disease. **(A)** Histiocytes in bone marrow aspiration. The cells are large and vacuolated. **(B)** High magnification of typical Gaucher cells showing cytoplasmic striations (wrinkled tissue paper appearance).

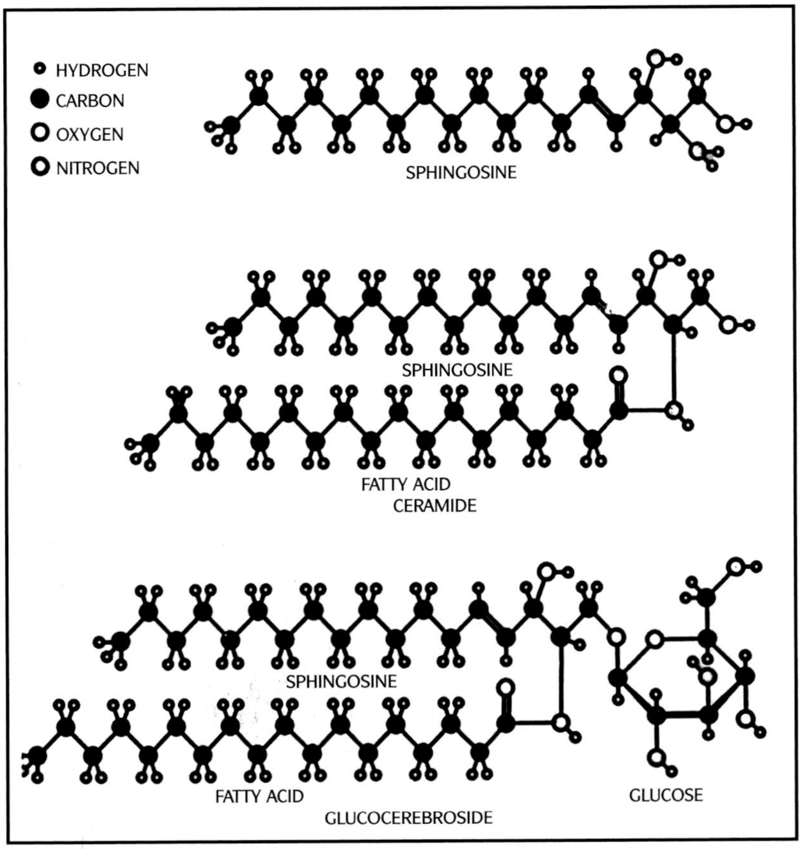

24.12. Structure of sphingolipids. Sphingosine (top) attached to a fatty acid ceramide (middle); ceramide attached to a single sugar forms a glucocerebroside (bottom); if ceramide is combined with polysaccharide (complex sugar) with one or more molecules of *N*-acetylneuraminic acid, the result is a ganglioside. (From Brady RO: Hereditary fat metabolism diseases. *Sci Am* 229:88, 1973.)

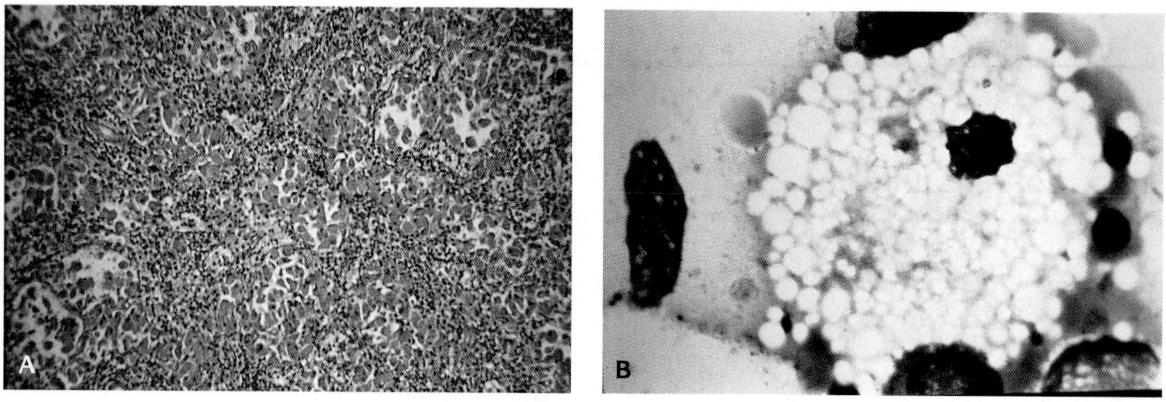

24.13. Niemann-Pick disease. **(A)** Spleen shows sinusoids filled with storage cells. **(B)** Niemann-Pick cell showing typical soap-bubble appearance.

Gangliosidoses

In these (autosomal recessive) disorders there is deficient activity of β-galactosidase with accumulation of ganglioside in neurons, and in other sites. GM1 type 1 generalized gangliosidosis presents in early infant with death by 2 years of age. GM2 type 1 (Tay Sach's disease) has a high incidence in the Jewish population. Infants develop rapid neurologic and psychomotor deterioration with seizures and blindness and death by 35 years of age.

Metachromatic-Leukodystrophy (Autosomal Recessive)

In this disorder, there is deficiency of arylsulfatase A, which hydrolyzes galactocerebroside sulfatide (GCS) to galactocerebroside.

Presence of urinary sulfatide excretion is detected by the presence of brown metachromasia on a filter paper urine spot test with cresyl violet (Figure 24.14). In the tissues brown metachromatsia is exhibited by special stains with cresyl violet. It is characterized by severe progressive neurological and psychomotor deterioration.

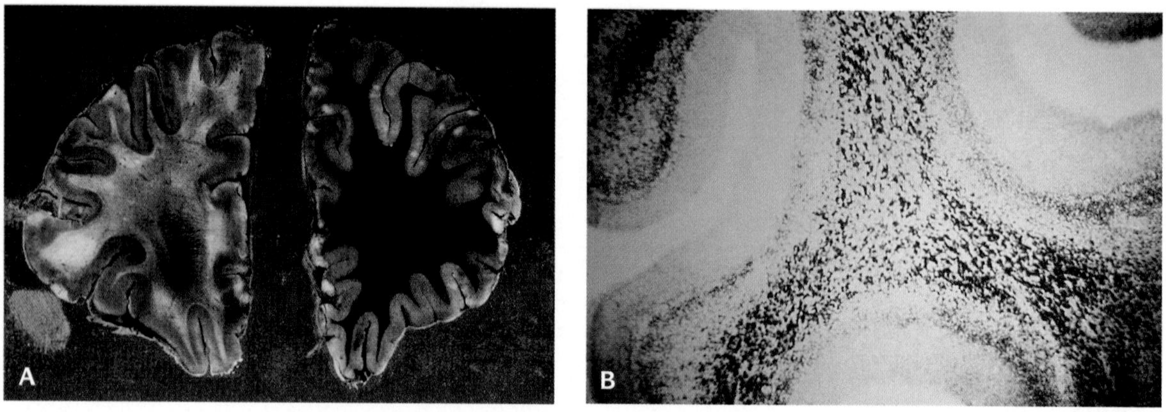

24.14. Metachromic leukodystrophy. **(A)** The white matter stains brown with cresyl violet. **(B)** Brown metachromasia due to sulfatide storage in neurons and astrocytes of cerebellum.

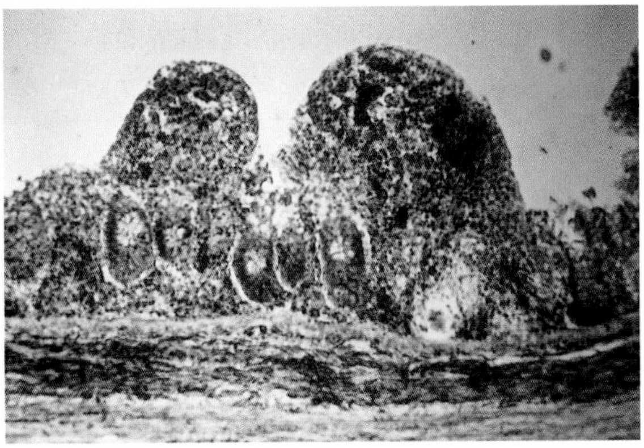

24.15. Wolman disease. Microscopic section of gastrointestinal mucosa showing an abundance of lipid laden histiocytes (Oil Red O stain).

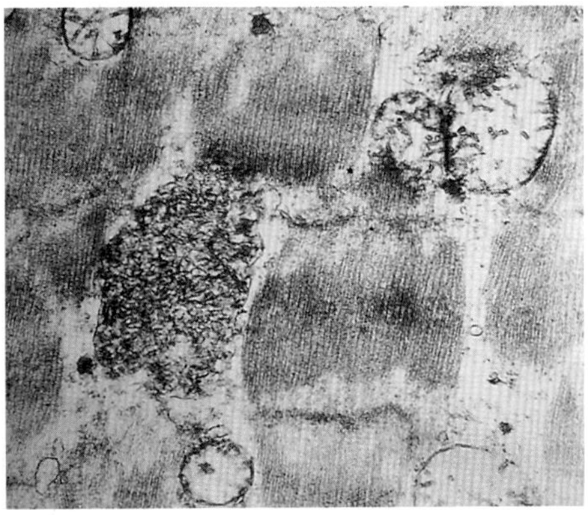

24.16. Neuronal ceroid lipofuscinosis (Batten disease). Electron micrograph of the heart showing curvilinear bodies.

Multiple Sulfatase Deficiency (Austin Disease)

A deficiency of arylsulfatase A, B, and C results in increased amounts of mucopolysaccharides (MPS) and sulfatide in the affected tissues and in the urine. Rapid psychomotor and mental deterioration occurs with death in the first decade of life.

WOLMAN DISEASE AND CHOLESTERYL ESTER STORAGE DISEASES

Deficiency of lysosomal acid lipase results in accumulation of cholesteryl esters and triglyceride.

Wolman disease (Figure 24.15) presents in early infancy. The liver is enlarged, yellow with foam cells, in the periportal areas in both hepatocytes and Kupffer cells, and cholesterol and triglycerides can be identified histochemically. The adrenal glands become calcified with necrotic cells and foam cells.

Cholesteryl ester storage disease is similar but milder than Wolman disease.

NEURONAL CEROID LIPOFUSCINOSIS (NCL) (BATTEN DISEASE)

This disease comprises a group of neurological disorders sharing features of progressive psychomotor retardation and accumulation of large amounts of lipopigments in neural and extraneural cells (Figure 24.16 and Table 24.9). The infantile form has its onset at 8–18 months of life with death by 8–14 years.

CARBOHYDRATE DISORDERS

Galactosemia

The pathological changes are similar to those in hereditary fructose intolerance and tyrosinemia and include marked steatosis of the hepatocytes with a progressive pseudoacinar change of hepatic architecture, ductular proliferation,

Table 24.9 Clinical and neurophysiological features of neuronal ceroid lipofuscinosis (NCL)

	INCL	LINCL	JNCL	Adult NCL
Age of onset	8–18 months	2–4 years	4–8 years	30 years
Mental retardation	early	late	late	late
Visual failure	relatively early	late	early, leading symptom	not present
Ataxia	moderate to marked	marked	marked	variable
Myoclonus	constant	constant	mild-marked	severe, symptom in some patients
Nonambulant	8–30 months	3–5 years	13–28 years	over 35 years
Retinal pigment aggregations	not present	rare	constant	not present
Vacuolated lymphocytes	negative	negative	positive	negative
Age at death	8–14 years	6–15 years	13–40 years	over 40 years

NCL, neuronal ceroid lipofuscinosis; I, infantile; L, late; J, juvenile.

cholestasis, focal giant cell transformation, focal necrosis and finally cirrhosis, pancreatic islet cell hyperplasia, and vacuolization of renal tubular epithelial cells (Figure 24.17). Brain edema, gliosis, and neuronal necrosis are attributed to hypoxic-ischemic damage. Girls develop ovarian failure. Hereditary fructose intolerance and tyrosinemia have similar pathological changes.

GLYCOGEN STORAGE DISEASES

There are many enzymatic steps in the synthesis of glycogen.

Type I (von Gierke disease) has predominant **liver** involvement with accumulation of glycogen and liver failure early in life, massive hepatomegaly, failure to thrive, ketosis, and hyperuricemia.

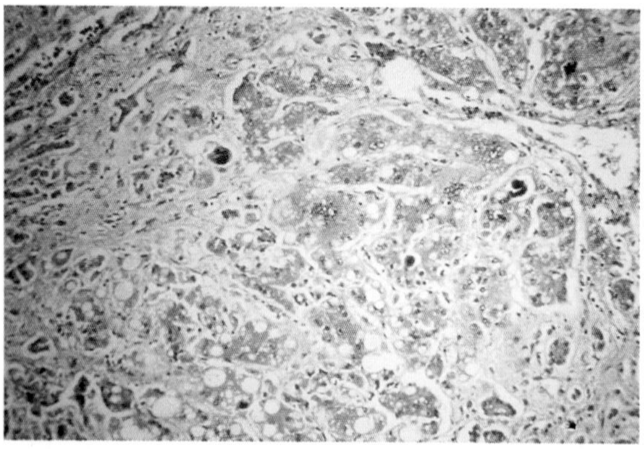

24.17. Galactosemia. Liver showing pseudoacinar arrangement of hepatocytes, giant cell transformation, fibrosis, cholestasis, and ductular proliferation.

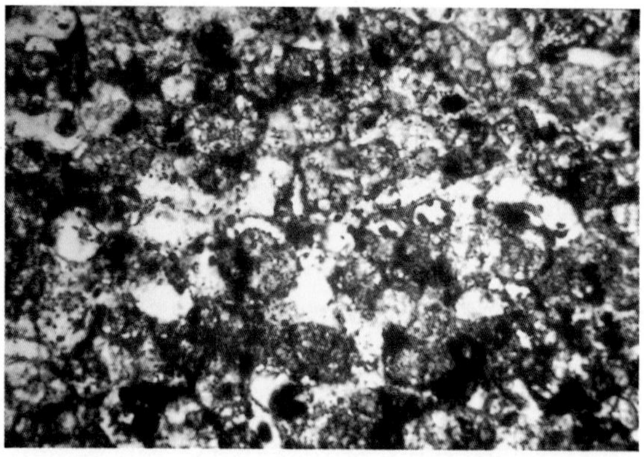

24.18. Glycogen storage disease type II (Pompe disease). Hepatocytes are distended with glycogen (PAS stain).

Table 24.10 Glycogen storage diseases

McKusick #	Type	Inheritance	Enzyme defect
24060	0	AR	Glycogen synthetase
23220	1A (von Gierke)	AR	Glucose-6-phosphatase
232230	2 (Pompe)	AR	α-1, 4-glucosidase (acid maltase)
23240	3 GSD (Forbes/Cori limit dextrinosis)	AR	Amylo-1, 6-glucosidase (Debrancher enzyme)
23250	4 (Anderson-amylopectinosis)	AR	amylo 1,4-1,6 transglucosidase (Brancher enzyme)
23260	5 (McArdle)	AR	Myophosphorylase; (1,4-α-D-glucan:orthophosphate-α-D-glucosyl transferase)-D-glucanotho-phosphatase-α-D-glucosyl transferase)
23270	6 (Hers)	AR	Hepatophosphorylase
23280	7 (Tarui)	AR	Muscle phosphofructokinase
26175 30600	8	AR XLR	Hepatic phosphorylase b kinase
	9	AR	Hepatic phosphorylase kinase
	10	AR	Cyclic 3′,5′-AMP-dependent kinase

AR, autosomal recessive; XLR, X-linked recessive; GSD, glycogen storage disease.

Type II (Pompe disease (Figure 24.18) generalized glycogenosis) predominantly involves heart, skeletal muscle, and CNS. Glycogen accumulates within lysosomes. It affects all tissues and is referred to as generalized glycogenosis. Death usually results from cardiac failure before two years of age (Table 24.10). Tissues should be fixed in alcohol to preserve the glycogen. After formalin fixation the hepatocytes appear empty and vacuolated. Other forms of glycogen storage diseases are rare.

UREA CYCLE DISORDERS

These disorders include 1. carbamyl phosphate synthase deficiency; 2. ornithine transcarbamylase deficiency; 3. citrullinemia; 4. argininosuccinic aciduria; 5. argininemia; 6. hyperornithinuria, hyperammonemia, homocitrullinuria (HHH disease) (Figure 24.19); and 7. lysinuric protein intolerance (Table 24.11). These disorders are characterized by hyperammonemia usually presenting in the neonatal period, convulsions, coma, and frequently death.

ORGANIC ACIDEMIAS

These disorders (Table 24.12) include 1. maple syrup urine disease; 2. isovaleric acidemia; 3. propionic acidemia; 4. methylmalonic acidemia; 5. glutaric acidemia type 1; 6. glutaric acidemia type II; and 7. biotinidase deficiency. These disorders are characterized by symptoms beginning in the neonatal

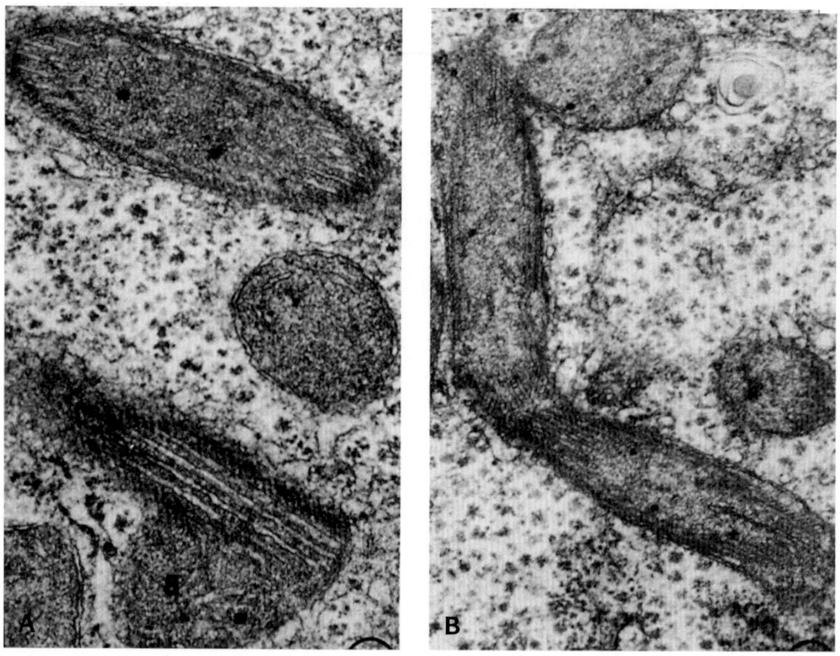

24.19. HHH disease (hyperornithinemia, hyperammonemia, and homocitrullinuria syndrome). Electron micrograph. **(A)** Showing large mitrochondria. **(B)** Bulbous end of a mitochondrium.

Table 24.11 Urea cycle disorders

Disease	Enzyme defect	Diagnosis
Carbamyl phosphate synthase, 2pAR	CP synthase	ammonemia, low citrulline, arginine: (blood); enzyme, (liver)
Ornithine transcarbamylase deficiency Xp21,1mXL 1/100,000	OTC	ammonemia, orotic acid (urine), low citrulline, (plasma); enzyme, (liver)
Citrullinemia, 9q34,AR, 1/100,000	argino–succinase	ammonemia; enzyme, (WBC, fibroblasts)
Arginino-succinic aciduria, 7cen-p 21, AR, 1/100,000	arginino–succinic lyase	high citrulline, argininosuccinate, (plasma), enzyme, (liver)
Argininemia, 6p23,AR, 1/100,000	arginase	ammonemia; enzyme (liver)
Hyperornithinuria, ammononemia, homocitrullinuria, AR		ammonemia, ornithinemia, homocitrullinura
Lysinuric protein intolerance	transport	transport dibasic acidemia acids, low serum lysine, arginine, ornithine, urea, urine: orotic acid

AR, autosomal recessive; CP, carbamyl phosphate; OTC, ornithine transcarbamylase; WBC, white blood cells; XL, X-linked recessive.

Table 24.12 Organic acidurias

Disease	Enzyme defect	Diagnosis
Maple syrup urine disease, 19q13,AR, 1/120,000	Ketoacid dehydrogenase	amino, organic acids (urine, serum) enzyme (WBC, fibroblasts)
Isovaleric acidemia, 15q14–q15,AR	Isovaleryl-CoA dehydrogenase	Organic acids (urine) enzyme (WBC, fibroblasts)
Propionic acidemia, 13q32,3q13.3–q22,AR	Propionyl CoA carboxylase	Organic acid (urine), enzyme (WBC, fibroblasts) glycine, serum
Methylmalonic acidemia, 6p12–p21.2,AR, 1/20,000	Methylmalonyl mutase, apoenzyme	Organic acid (urine), enzyme (WBC, fibroblasts)
Glutaric acidemia type I, 19?AR, 1/30,000	Glutaryl CoA dehydrogenase	Organic acid (urine)
Glutaric acidemia type II, AR	Electron transport defect	Organic acid, urine, electron transport, flavoproteins
Biotinidase deficiency, 3p25,AR, 1/60,000	Carboxylases deficient	dicarboxylic acids, (urine) enzyme: (serum) fibroblasts, (WBC) glycine

AR, autosomal recessive; WBC, white blood cells.

period, severe CNS dysfunction, coma, seizures, and death if these disorders are not diagnosed and promptly treated.

FATTY ACID β OXIDATION DEFECTS

Inherited defects in the β oxidation pathway include LCAD, MCAD (1q31), and SCAD deficiencies (Table 24.13). Symptoms of hypoglycemia develop especially after fasting. Coma may be a presenting sign. Ketosis does not occur. Fatty acid metabolites are excreted in the urine. Carnitine esters are increased and free carnitine levels are low in the plasma, skeletal muscle, and liver. Muscle cells, cardiac myocytes, and hepatocytes show fatty infiltration (Figure 24.20). MCAD has an incidence of 1/5,000 live births and may be a cause of sudden infant death.

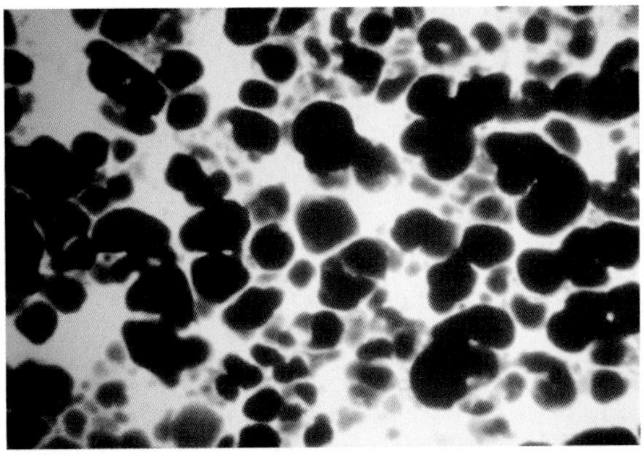

24.20. Medium-chain acyldehydrogenase deficiency (MCAD). Liver shows marked fatty change. (Oil Red O stain.)

Carnitine Deficiency

Carnitine deficiency results from a defect in fatty acid transport across the inner mitochondrial membrane (Figure 24.21). Primary carnitine deficiency (CPT II) (1,AR) occurs as a myopathic, a systemic, and a mixed form. The myopathic form manifests as progressive skeletal muscle weakness. Serum carnitine is normal but muscle carnitine is low. Systemic

Table 24.13 Characteristic features of fatty acid oxidation defects

MIM#	Disorder	Tissue distribution	Chromosome location	Symptoms and signs	Laboratory findings
212140	Carnitine deficiency	Kidney, heart, muscle, FB, liver		Cardiomyopathy, coma, muscle weakness, Reye-like syndrome, sudden infant death	Glucose (P) ↓, ammonia (B) ↑, acidosis + carnitine (P) ↑, long-chain acylcarnitine (P) n, cellular carnitine uptake ↓
255120	Carnitine palmitoyl transferase I	Liver, FB	11q22–q23	Coma, liver insufficiency, hepatomegaly	Glucose (P) ↓, ammonia (B) n-↑, acidosis +, carnitine (P) n-↑, long-chain acylcarnitine (P) n
212138	Acylcarnitine translocase	FB, liver, heart muscle		Coma, cardiac abnormalities, liver insufficiency, vomiting	Glucose (P) ↓, ammonia (B) ↑, acidosis ±, free carnitine (P) ↓, acylcarnitine (P) ↑, long-chain acylcarnitine (P) ↑, seizures ±
255110	Carnitine palmitoyl transferase II	Muscle, heart, liver, FB	1p32	Coma, Reye-like syndrome, hepatomegaly, exercise intolerance, myalgia, cardiomyopathy, developmental delay ±, sudden death	Glucose (B) ↓, ketosis, liver enzymes (P) ↑, creatine kinase (P) ↑, myoglobin (P,U), dicarboxylic acids (U) ±, carnitine (P) ↓, long-chain acylcarnitine (P) ↑
	Very-long chain acyl-CoA dehydrogenase			Cardiomyopathy, coma, respiratory arrest, Reye-like syndrome, muscle weakness, muscle pain	Glucose (B) ↓, acidosis +, CK (P) ↑, dicarboxylic acids (U) ↑, $C_{14:1}$ fatty acid (P) ↑, $C_{14:1}$ acylcarnitine (P) ↑, carnitine (P) ↓, long-chain acylcarnitine (P) ↑
201450	Medium-chain acyl-CoA dehydrogenase	Liver, muscle, FB, WBC	1p31	Coma/lethargy, hepatopathy, hypotonia, apnea/respiratory arrest, sudden death, seizures ±, mental retardation, attention deficit disorder	Glucose (B) ↓, ketosis ±, acidosis +, transamines (P) ↑, ammonia (B) ↑, uric acid (P) ↑, dicarboxylic acids (U) n-↑, glycine conjugates (U,P) ↑, decanoate (P) ↑, acylcarnitines (U) ↑, carnitine (P) n-↓, long-chain acylcarnitine (P) n
201470	Short-chain acyl-CoA dehydrogenase	Muscle, liver, FB, WBC	12q22-qter	Muscle weakness, lethargy, failure to thrive, mental retardation	Ketosis +, acidosis +, ethylmalonic acid (U) n-↑, carnitine (P) ↓ n
143450	Long-chain 3-hydroxyacyl-CoA dehydrogenase	Liver, muscle, heart, FB, WBC	7	Coma/lethargy, hepatopathy, cardiomyopathy, neuropathy, retinopathy, muscle weakness, sudden death	Glucose (B) ↓, acidosis, lactate (P) ↑, myoglobin (P,U), CK (P) ↑, dicarboxylic acids (U) ↑, hydroxy-dicarboxylic acids (U) ↑, long-chain 3-hydroxy-fatty acids (P) ↑, carnitine (P) ↓, long-chain acylcarnitine (P) ↑
600890	Short-chain 3-hydroxyacyl-CoA dehydrogenase deficiency	Muscle, FB	—	Cardiomyopathy, muscle weakness, lethargy	Glucose (B) ↓, myoglobinuria +, CK (P) ↑, AST/ALT (P) ↑, ketosis +, ketones (U) ↑, dicarboxylic acids (U) n-↑

MIM, Mendelian Inheritance in man number; B, blood; U, urine; P, plasma; FB, fibroblasts; WBC, white blood cells; AST, aspartate transferase; ALT, alanine transferase; n, normal.

Source: Gilbert-Barness E, Barness LA: *Metabolic Diseases: Foundations of Clinical Management, Genetics, and Pathology*, Vol. I, Natick, Massachusetts, Eaton Publishing, 2000.

Table 24.14 Classification of mitochondrial disorders

Disorder	Systemic lesions	CNS lesions
Luft disease	Ragged red fibers (muscle)	–
Leigh disease	–	Deep and periventricular gray matter: spongy change; vascular proliferation; cystic lesions
Pyruvate dehydrogenase complex		
Pyruvate decarboxylase	–	Cerebrum; deep and periventricular gray matter: cystic lesions in white > gray; Leigh disease
Pyruvate carboxylase	Hepatic steatosis	Cerebral white matter; neocortex: paucity of myelin; neuronal loss
Glioneuronal dystrophy (some Alper disease)	Hepatic fibrosis	Neocortex: spongy change and neuronal loss
Respiratory chain enzymes	Cardiomyopathy	
Biotin-dependent enzymes:		
Biotinidase	Skin rash; alopecia	Insufficient data
Carboxylases	Skin rash; alopecia	Insufficient data
Carnitine deficiency	Lipid myopathy	–
Carnitine palmitoyl-transferase	Rhabdomyolysis	–
Ragged red fiber-related diseases:		
Kearns-Sayre disease	Ragged red fibers	Brainstem, cerebellar white matter: spongy change
MERRF	Ragged red fibers	Dentate nucleus; brainstem: neuronal loss; tract degeneration
MELAS	Ragged red fibers	Neocortex: microinfarcts

–, nonreported; CNS, central nervous system; MELAS, mitochondrial encephalomyopathy, lactic acidosis, and stroke; MERRF, myoclonic epilepsy with ragged red fibers.

Adapted from Powers JM and Haroupian DS: Central nervous system. In Damijanov I and Linder J (eds): *Anderson's Pathology*. St. Louis, Mosby, 1996.

carnitine deficiency is characterized by low serum and tissue carnitine concentrations.

Pathologic changes include lipid accumulation in skeletal muscle (Figure 24.22) in type I myocytes, liver, and frequently in the cardiac muscle cells.

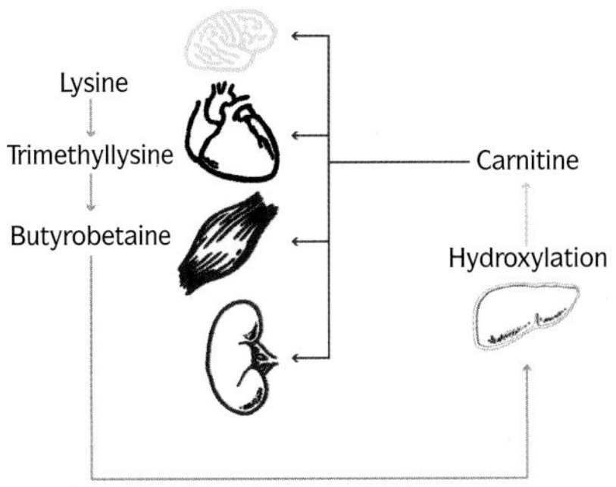

24.21. Carnitine deficiency. Metabolism and transport of carnitine.

ABNORMALITIES OF MITOCHONDRIA

Most mitochondrial disorders (Table 24.14) are inherited as autosomal recessive traits. All disorders caused by mitochondrial DNA defects and intergenomic signaling defects result in impaired respiratory chain and/or oxidative phosphorylation. Pathologic changes of mitochondrial disease are

1. abnormalities associated directly with altered number and structure of the mitochondria;

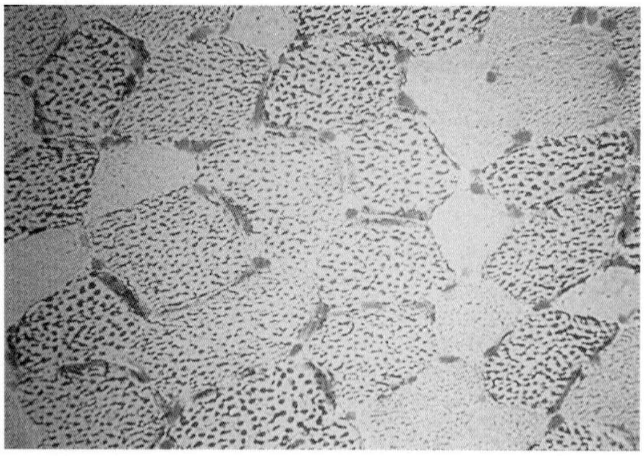

24.22. Carnitine deficiency. Lipid vacuoles of muscle biopsy in type I cells.

2. secondary degenerative and destructive changes due to impaired function of the mitochondria. These changes include status spongiosis in the brain, neuronal degeneration, astrogliosis, demyelinization, neuronal necrosis, and mineral deposits in the brain.

PEROXISOMAL DISORDERS

Peroxisomal diseases are genetically determined and caused by failure to form or to maintain the peroxisome or by impaired function of a single peroxisomal enzyme (Figures 24.23 to 24.25). These include

- Zellweger syndrome
- Neonatal adrenoleukodystrophy
- Hyperoxaluria type I
- Classic Refsum disease
- X-linked adrenoleukodystrophy
- Hyperpipecolic acidemia
- Acatalasemia and
- Rhizomelic chondrodysplasia punctata (RCDP).

DISORDERS OF METAL METABOLISM

Neonatal Iron Storage Disease (Neonatal Hemachromatosis) (6p21.3,AR)

Neonatal iron storage disease or perinatal hemachromatosis is clinically and pathologically defined by severe liver disease of intrauterine onset associated with extrahepatic siderosis that spares the reticuloendothelial system (Figure 24.26). Hemachromatotic siderosis in the perinate may be a sequel of

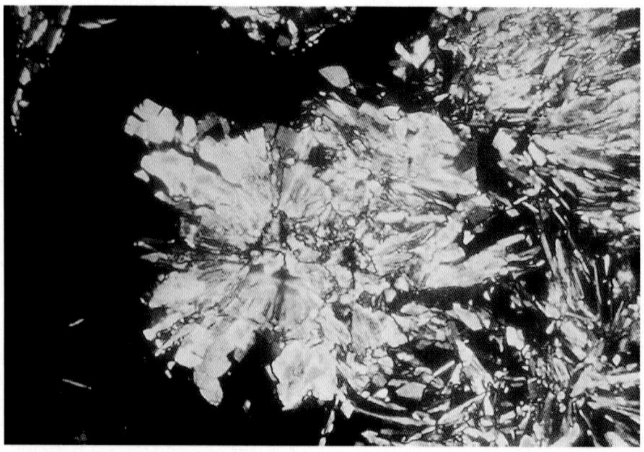

24.23. Primary oxalosis. Oxalate crystals of urinary sediment viewed under polarized light.

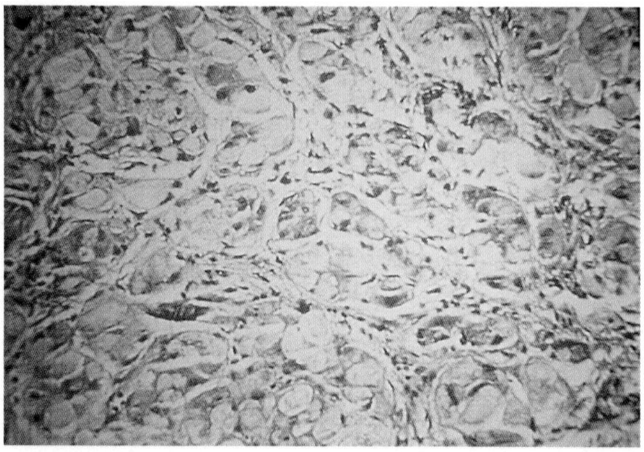

24.24. X-linked adenoleukodystrophy. Microscopic section of adenal gland. The cells are large with pink granular cytoplasm and striations.

intrauterine liver disease. Transaminase activities are usually low and serum concentrations of α-fetoprotein are high; hepatocellular injury results in low levels of clotting factors, hypotransferrinemia, or hypoerythropoietinemia. Hyperbilirubinemia and hyperferritinemia are present soon after birth.

The liver weighs less than normal, is fibrotic and cirrhotic, and may be bile stained. Cholestasis and giant cell transformation are characteristic. Iron accumulation is massive in liver cells with lesser quantities in biliary epithelium and Kupffer cells. Hyperplasia and hypertrophy of the islets of Langerhans are constant findings. Extrahepatic sites for iron accumulation include pancreatic acinar and islet cells, renal tubules, adrenal cortex, and thyroid follicular epithelium. The reticuloendothelial system is not involved.

Electron microscopy demonstrates hemosiderin in lysosomes within hepatocytes and to a lesser extent in Kupffer cells and in liver cytoplasm. Electron-dense masses and membranous arrays are observed in the lysosomes. Neonatal hemachromatosis has been associated with maternal autoantibodies against RO/SS-A and LA/SSB ribonucleoproteins.

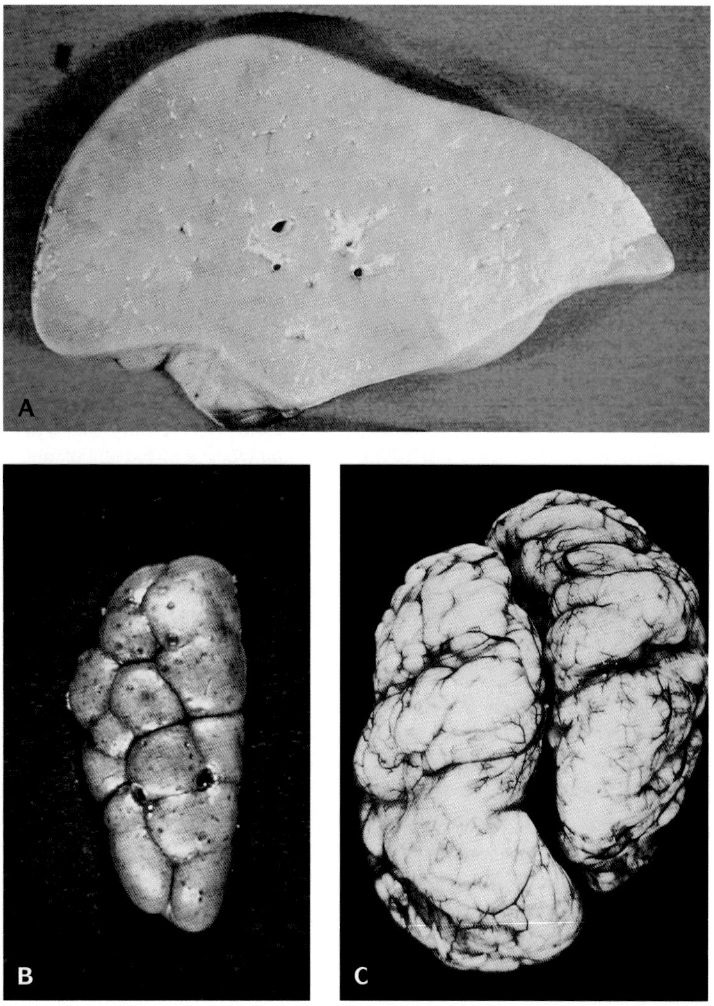

24.25. Zellweger syndrome. **(A)** Liver shows brown discoloration due to iron deposition. **(B)** Kidney with multiple cortical cysts. **(C)** Brain shows pachygyria.

DEFECTS IN COPPER METABOLISM

Wilson Disease (13q14,AR)

Wilson disease is an inborn error of copper metabolism (Figure 24.27). Hepatic copper is elevated, liver and serum ceruloplasmin are usually decreased,

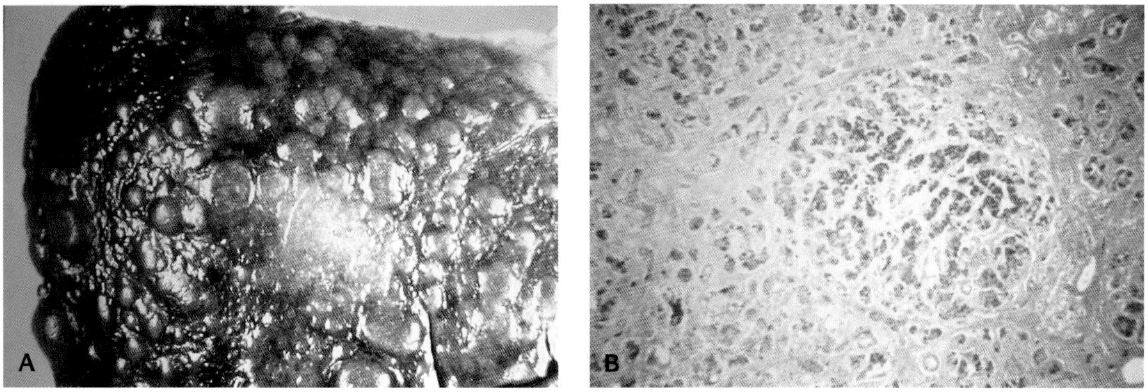

24.26. Neonatal iron storage disease. **(A)** Liver of a newborn shows advanced cirrhosis. **(B)** Iron stain of liver shows abundance of iron (Prussian blue stain).

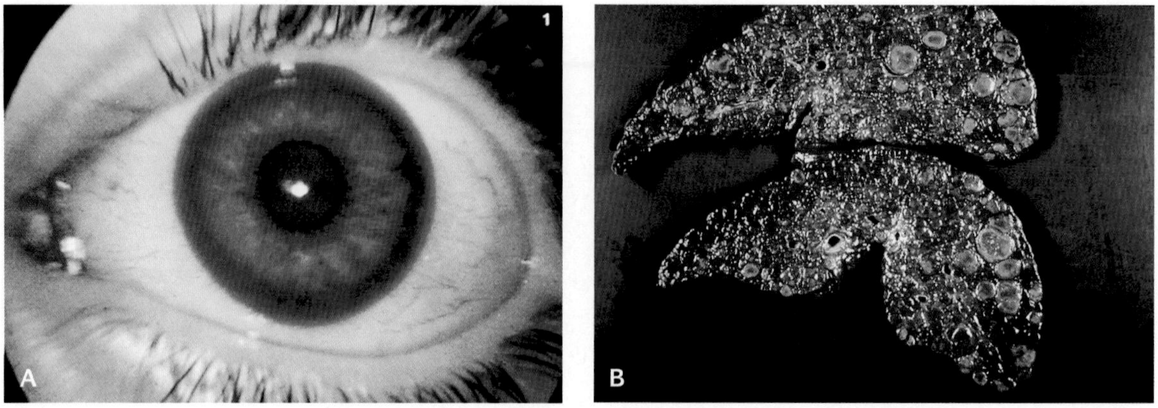

24.27. Wilson disease. **(A)** Eye with Kayser-Fleischer ring. A brown deposit on Descemet membrane of the limbus of the cornea. **(B)** Liver showing advanced cirrhosis.

serum copper levels are usually low, and copper excretion in the urine is increased.

The pathologic effects on the liver, kidneys, and brain are directly related to the accumulation of copper ions. In the precirrhotic stage, the changes resemble a chronic, active hepatitis with focal necrosis, scattered acidophilic bodies, and moderate to marked steatosis. Glycogenated nuclei in periportal hepatocytes is a typical finding. Kupffer cells are hypertrophied and may contain hemosiderin. Copper may not be cytochemically demonstrable in the precirrhotic stage. In later stages, periportal fibrosis, portal inflammation, cholangiolar proliferation and, finally, cirrhosis (macronodular or macro and micronodular) occur. In young, asymptomatic patients, the copper is diffusely distributed in the

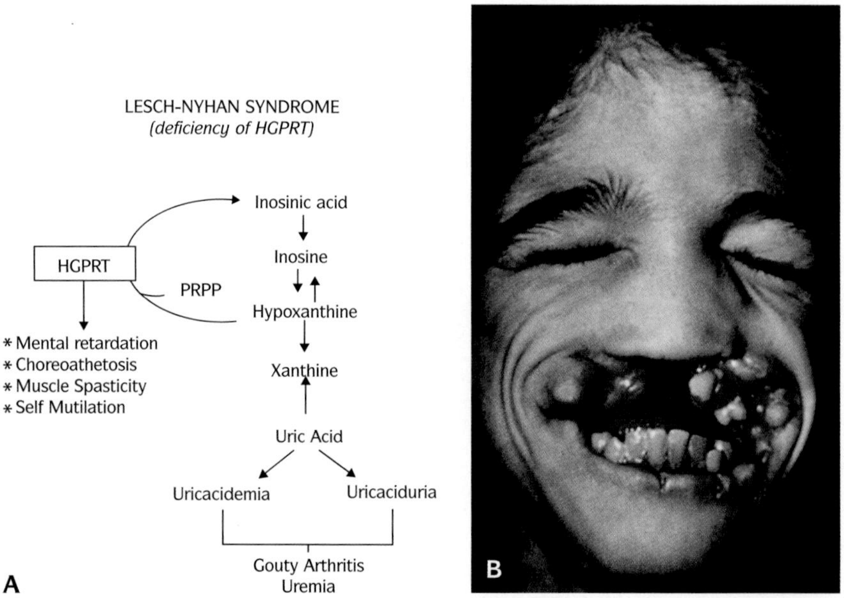

24.28. Lesch-Nyhan syndrome. **(A)** Metabolic pathway. **(B)** Self-mutilation in a child with Lesch-Nyhan syndrome.

cytoplasm but later accumulates in lysosomes. Rhodamine and rubeanic acid stains specifically detect the presence of copper. Copper-associated protein can be stained with orcein or aldehyde fuchsin. Electron microscopy changes are pathognomonic. The mitochondria show marked pleomorphism, intracristal spaces widen, and microcysts form at the tips of the cristae. Copper deposits are extremely electron dense.

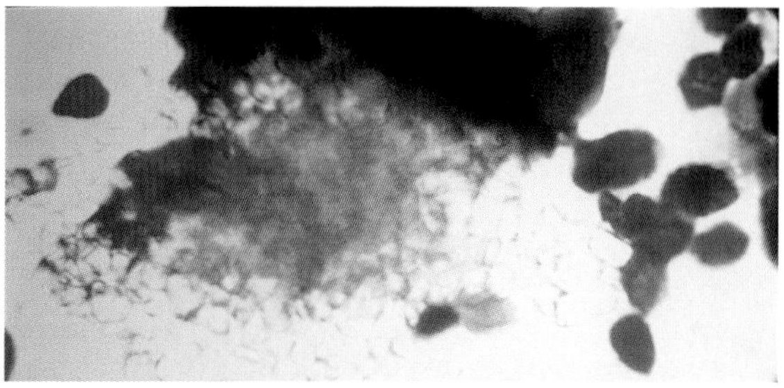

24.29. Cystinosis. Cystine crystals in the bone marrow.

Menkes Syndrome (Xq13)

Menkes syndrome is an X-linked disorder due to a defect in intestinal copper absorption resulting in a low serum level of copper and ceruloplasmin in affected male infants. All copper-containing enzymes – e.g., cytochrome oxidase, superoxide dismutase, tyrosinase, dopamine hydroxylase, and lysyl oxidase – are deficient. Arterial elongation and tortuosity are due to deficiency of copper-dependent cross-linking in the internal elastic membrane of the arterial wall. By histofluorescence peculiar torpedo-like swellings of catecholamine-containing axons are seen in the peripheral nerve tracts along with reduced numbers of adrenergic fibers in the mid-forebrain. (See chapter 21.)

α_1-Antritrypsin Deficiency (See Chapter 18)

ERRORS IN PURINE METABOLISM

Lesh-Nyhan Syndrome (Figure 24.28)

Hypoxanthine-guanine phosphoribosyltransferase deficiency is an X-linked recessive disorder characterized by delay in mental development, choreoathetoid movements, self-mutilation, hyperuricemia, gouty tophi, and arthritis. Absence of the enzyme can be found in erythrocytes, fibroblasts, and other tissues.

Defects in Renal Transport (Cystinosis)

This condition – an autosomal recessive disorder – is due to a defect in the gene for lysosomal cystine transport (CTNS). Three phenotypes are identified. The most severe form is nephrepathic cystinosis that becomes manifest in the first year of life. Benign and intermediate forms exist. The major abnormal manifestation is Fanconi syndrome with renal failure. Cystine crystals are formed in the kidneys, organs of the reticulo-endothelial system, and in the cornea and bone marrow (Figure 24.29). These can be seen in polymorphonuclear leukocytes and cultured fibroblasts, and predominantly in amniotic fluid or chorionic villus sampling that can be used for prenatal diagnosis.

REFERENCES

Applegarth DA, Dimmick JE, Toone JR: Laboratory detection of metabolic disease. *Pediatr Clin North Am* 36:49, 1989.

Barness L, Gilbert-Barness E: Metabolic diseases. In Gilbert-Barness E (ed): *Potter's Pathology of the Fetus and Infant.* St. Louis, Mosby-Year Book, 1997, p. 571.

Dimmick JE, Applegarth DA: Inherited metabolic disease. In Stocker JT, Dehner LP (eds): *Pediatric Pathology.* Philadelphia, JB Lippincott, 1992, p. 161.

Fernandez J, Saudubray J-M, Tada K, eds: *Inborn Metabolic Diseases: Diagnosis and Treatment.* Berlin, Springer-Verlag, 1990.

Gilbert-Barness E, Barness L: Metabolic disorders. In Gilbert-Barness E (ed): *Atlas of Fetal and Infant Pathology.* Philadelphia, Mosby-Year Book, 1998.

Gilbert-Barness E, Barness L, eds: *Metabolic Diseases*, Natick, Massachusetts, Eaton Publishing Co., 2000.

Ishak KG: Pathology of inherited metabolic disorders. In Balistreri WF, Stocker JT (eds): *Pediatric Hepatology.* Washington, DC, Hemisphere Publishing, 1990.

Kaler SG: Menkes disease. In Barness LA (ed): *Advances in Pediatrics*, Vol 41, St. Louis, Mosby-Year Book, 1994.

McAdams AJ, Hug G, Bove KE: Glycogen storage diseases types I-X, *Hum Pathol* 5:463, 1974.

Roberts DJ, Ampola MG, Lage JM: Diagnosis of unsuspected fetal metabolic storage disease by routine placental examination. *Pediatr Pathol* 11:647, 1991.

Scheinberg IH, Sternlieb I: *Wilson's Disease*, Philadelphia, WB Saunders, 1984.

Scriver CR, Beaudet AL, Sly WS, Valle D, eds: *The Metabolic and Molecular Bases of Inherited Disease*, 7th ed, New York, McGraw-Hill, 1995.

Appendices

APPENDIX 1. CYTOGENETIC TERMINOLOGY

Aneuploid. An unbalanced state that arises through loss or addition of whole or pieces of chromosomes; always considered deleterious.

Chromosome. The location of hereditary (genetic) material within the cell. This hereditary material is packaged in the form of a very long, double-stranded molecule of DNA surrounded by and complexed with several different forms of protein. Genes are found arranged in a linear sequence along chromosomes, as is also a large amount of DNA of unknown function.

Confined placental mosaicism. A viable mutation in trophoblast or extraembryonic progenitor cells of the inner cell mass resulting in dichotomy between the chromosomal constitution of the placenta and the embryo or fetus.

Deletion. Pieces of chromosomes are missing in persons having 46 chromosomes.

Diploid (2n). The whole set of 46 chromosomes in a somatic cell.

Duplications. Extra pieces of chromosomes occur in individuals with 46 chromosomes.

Endomitosis. Duplication of the chromosomes without accompanying spindle formation or cytokinesis, resulting in a polyploid nucleus.

Fluorescence in situ hybridization (FISH). This technique can use nondividing cells from smears or sections. By use of commercially available, chromosome-specific fluorescent probes that can hybridize to complementary *DNA* sequences, the number of fluorescent signals in interphase cells can be counted to determine the number of copies of the target chromosomes present in those cells.

Fragile X. The most frequent mental retardation syndrome caused by a mutant gene. The syndrome is due to an altered gene on the X chromosome characterized by too many copies of a trinucleotide repeat that compromises the function of a gene thought to specify a brain protein (FMR-1). Since it is sex linked, it is more frequent in males, but it also occurs in heterozygous females who have extensive amplification of the Xq27.3 region.

Genotype. The total of the genetic information contained in the chromosomes of an organism; the genetic make-up of an organism.

Haploid (n). One-half set (23 chromosomes) of a gamete.

Homologue. The individual members of a pair of chromosomes.

Inversion. Inversions require two breaks. Both breaks on one side of the centromere produce a paracentric inversion; breaks in both arms produce a pericentric inversion.

Isochromosomes. Chromosomes that arise from several different mechanisms, principally transverse rather than longitudinal division of the centromere during mitosis or meiosis.

Monosomy. Lack of one whole chromosome.

Mosaicism. Two or more chromosomally different cell lines in the same person.

Nondisjunction. Failure of paired chromosomes or sister chromatids to disjoin at anaphase during mitotic division or in the first or second meiotic division.

Oncogenes. Normal growth-related genes that become activated and/or amplified in somatic cells, thereby causing increased cell proliferation and abnormal growth.

Phenotype. The observable properties of an organism resulting from the interaction between its genotype and the environment.

Polymorphisms. Chromosomes or chromosome regions that may vary in size without effect because they contain heterochromatin (nontranscribing DNA) versus euchromatin, which cannot be deleted or amplified without significant phenotypic effect. The most common human polymorphisms involve 1q, 9q, 13p, 14p, 15p, 16q, 21p, 22p, and Yq.

Polyploidy. More than two complete sets of chromosomes (i.e., 69 is triploidy, 92 is tetraploidy).

Ring chromosomes. Formed after at least two chromosomal breaks and can be mitotically unstable; they rarely survive meiosis to be transmitted from one generation to the next.

Southern blotting. Can be used to assess gene or DNA sequence copy number by using specific endonucleases to cut the DNA into fragments. Using gel electrophoresis to separate the fragments on the basis of size, followed by use of specific radioactive DNA probes that hybridize to the target sequence, the presence of abnormal DNA sequences can be detected. This is the basis of molecular testing for the fragile X in which the band hybridizing to the probe can be demonstrated by autoradiography.

Tetraploidy. Four copies of haploid set (92,XXXX or 92,XXYY). This occurs in many tumors and also occurs at conception or shortly thereafter, resulting in spontaneous abortion or (rarely) in term delivery of a malformed infant.

Tetrasomy. Two extra chromosomes (of one pair); if they belong to two different pairs, the state is called double trisomy.

Translocation. Reciprocal exchange of material between two chromosomes in which the unbalanced state of one or the other altered chromosome in offspring represents a duplication or deficiency, which also can arise through crossing over in a pericentric inversion. Robertsonian translocation involves the acrocentric chromosomes only. The breakpoints are in the short arms, and the translocation arises from end-to-end pairing.

Triploidy. Three copies of haploid set (69,XXX, 69,XXY, or 69,XYY) due to an accident at fertilization, dispermy, or failure to extrude the second polar body. Triploidy is not viable and results in spontaneous abortion or premature delivery of a nonviable infant with multiple malformations. The finding most diagnostic of a triploid abortus is molar degeneration of the placenta.

Trisomy. One whole extra chromosome.

APPENDIX 2. TIME PERIODS OF EMBRYONIC AND FETAL DEVELOPMENT IN HUMANS

Developmental event	Developmental age (days)
Somites first appear	20
Rostral neuropore closes	24
Caudal neuropore closes	26
Upper limb bud appears*	26–27
Lower limb bud appears*	28–30
Crown rump length, 5 mm	29–30
Paddle-shaped hand plate	31–32
Paddle-shaped foot plate	33–36
Spiral septum begins	34
Herniation of gut	34
Eye pigment*	34–35
Crown-rump length, 10 mm	37
Ossification begins	40–43
Müllerian duct appears	40
Digital rays, upper extremity*	41–43
Cloaca divided by urorectal septum	43
Testes, histologic differentiation	43
Notches between finger rays	44–46
Digital rays, lower extremity*	44–46
Heart septation complete	46–47
Webbed fingers	49–51
Notches between toe rays	49–51
Free fingers*	52–53
Webbed toes	52–53
Eyelids closed	56–58
Palate closed completely	56–58
Herniation of gut reduced*	60
Urethral groove closed in male	90

**Important landmarks.*

APPENDIX 3. SUMMARY OF EMBRYONIC DEVELOPMENT

Crown-rump length (mm)	Days after ovulation	Carnegie stage	Main external features
0.1	0–2	1	Fertilized oocyte
	2–4	2	Morula
	4–6	3	Blastocyst
		4	Bilaminar embryo
0.2–0.4	6–15	5	Bilaminar embryo with primary yolk sac
		6	Trilaminar embryo with primitive streak
0.4–1.0	15–17	7	Trilaminar embryo with notochordal process
1.0–1.5	18–20	8	Primitive pit and notochordal canal formed
1.5–2.0	20–22	9	Deep neural groove; first somites present; heart tubes begin to fuse
2.0–3.0	22–24	10	Neural folds begin to fuse; heart begins to beat; embryo straight; 4–12 pairs of somites
3.0–4.0	24–26	11	Rostral neuropore closing, embryo slightly curved; 13–20 pairs of somites
4.0–5.0	26–30	12	Upper limb buds appear; caudal neuropore closed; tail appearing; 21–29 pairs of somites
5.0–6.0	28–32	13	Four pairs of branchial arches; lower limb buds appear; tail present; 30 or more somites
6.0–7.0	31–35	14	Lens pits and nasal pits visible; optic cups present
7.0–10.0	35–38	15	Hand plates formed; lens vesicles and nasal pits prominent
10.0–12.0	37–42	16	Foot plates formed; nasal pits face ventrally; pigment visible in retina
12.0–14.0	42–44	17	Finger rays appear; auricular hillocks developed; upper lip formed
14.0–17.0	44–48	18	Toe rays and elbow region appear; eyelids are forming; ambiguous genital tubercle seen
16.0–20.0	48–51	19	Trunk elongating and straightening; midgut herniation to umbilical cord
20.0–22.0	51–53	20	Fingers distinct but webbed; scalp vascular plexus appears
22.0–24.0	53–54	21	Fingers free and longer; toes still webbed
24.0–28.0	54–56	22	Toes free and longer; eyelids and external ear more developed
28.0–30.0	56–60	23	Head more rounded; fusing eyelids

Data from Jirasek JE: *Atlas of Human Prenatal Morphogenesis*, Boston, Martinus Nijhoff, 1983. Moore KL, Persaud TVN: *The Developing Human: Clinically Oriented Embryology*, 5th ed. Philadelphia, WB Saunders, 1993. O'Rahilly R, Muller F: *Developmental Stages in Human Embryos*, Washington, DC, Carnegie Institution, Publication 637, 1987. Streeter GL: *Developmental Horizons in Human Embryos*, Washington, DC, Carnegie Institute of Embryology, 1951.

APPENDIX 4. CROWN-RUMP LENGTH AND DEVELOPMENTAL AGE IN PREVIABLE FETUSES

Crown-rump length (mm)	Days after ovulation		Crown-rump length (mm)	Days after ovulation	
30–31	56	9th week	98–99	92	14th week
32–34	57		100–101	93	
35–36	58		102–103	94	
37	59		101	95	
38–39	60		105–106	96	
40–41	61		107–108	97	
42	62		109–110	98	
43–44	63				
45–46	64	10th week	111–112	99	15th week
47–48	65		113–114	100	
49	66		115–116	101	
50–51	67		117–118	102	
52–53	68		119–120	103	
54	69		121–122	104	
55–56	70		123–124	105	
57–58	71	11th week	125–126	106	16th week
59–60	72		127–128	107	
61–62	73		129	108	
63–64	74		130–131	109	
65	75		132–134	110	
66–67	76		135–136	111	
68–69	77		137–138	112	
70–71	78	12th week	139	113	17th week
72–73	79		140–141	114	
74	80		142–143	115	
75	81		144–145	116	
76–78	82		146–147	117	
79–80	83		148–149	118	
81	84		150	119	
82	85	13th week	151–152	120	18th week
83–86	86		153	121	
87–89	87		154–155	122	
90–91	88		156–157	123	
92–93	89		158	124	
94	90		159–160	125	
95–97	91		161–162	126	
			163–164	127	20th week
			165	128	

Modified from McBride ML, Baillie J. Poland BJ: Growth parameters in normal fetuses. *Teratology* 29:185, 1984.

APPENDIX 5. HAND AND FOOT LENGTHS CORRELATED WITH DEVELOPMENTAL AGE IN PREVIABLE FETUSES

Developmental age (wk)	Hand length (mm)	Foot length (mm)
11	10 ±2	12 ±2
12	15 ±2	17 ±3
13	18 ±1	19 ±1
14	19 ±1	22 ±2
15	20 ±3	25 ±3
16	26 ±2	28 ±2
17	27 ±3	29 ±4
18	29 ±2	33 ±2

Modified from McBride ML, Baillie J, Poland BJ: Growth parameters in normal fetuses. *Teratology* 29:185, 1984.

APPENDIX 6. WEIGHTS AND MEASUREMENTS OF FETUSES OF 8 TO 26 WEEKS GESTATION (MEAN VALUES)

Gestation (wk)	Weight (g)*	Crown-heel length (cm)*	Crown-rump length (cm)	Foot length (cm)
8	10	2		
9	11	3		
10	14	4		
11	18	6	4	0.9
12	25	7	6	1.1
13	27	9	7	1.4
14	38	10	8	1.7
15	53	13	9	2.1
16	73	14	10	2.2
17	122	17	12	2.4
18	161	19	13	2.6
19	188	20	14	2.9
20	227	21	15	3.2
21	303	24	16	3.4
22	384	26	18	3.8
24	389	27	19	4.1
26	394	28	20	4.5

* Modified from Potter EL, Craig JM: *Pathology of the Fetus and Infant*, 3rd ed. Chicago, Mosby-Year Book, 1975.

APPENDIX 7. ORGAN WEIGHTS IN FETUSES FROM 9 TO 20 WEEKS OF DEVELOPMENT

Developmental age (days)	Weight (g)	Crown-rump length (cm)	Brain (g)	Heart (g)	Lungs (g)	Liver (g)	Adrenals (g)	Kidneys (g)	No. of cases
63	11	3	1.2	0.1	0.1	0.2	0.1	0.1	30
67	13	4	1.5	0.2	0.3	0.7	0.1	0.1	27
71	15	6	2.6	0.2	0.4	0.8	0.1	0.1	15
73	20	7	4.3	0.3	0.4	1.1	0.1	0.2	21
76	25	7	4.8	0.4	0.7	1.1	0.2	0.2	14
79	30	8	5.4	0.4	1.0	1.3	0.2	0.2	15
84	35	9	6.2	0.5	1.4	2.0	0.2	0.3	14
89	45	9	7.4	0.5	1.9	2.5	0.4	0.4	22
90	50	10	8.5	0.5	1.9	3.0	0.5	0.5	23
91	60	10	10	0.5	2.5	3.4	0.6	0.6	21
92	70	11	11	0.6	3.0	3.6	0.6	0.8	24
96	80	11	12	0.7	3.0	4.3	0.6	0.8	7
100	90	12	14	0.9	3.0	4.7	0.7	0.9	15
105	100	12	17	1.1	3.9	5.6	0.7	1.4	28
109	125	13	23	1.3	4.1	7.4	0.7	1.4	21
115	150	14	23	1.4	5.3	9.2	0.8	1.4	20
117	175	14	23	1.4	5.6	11	0.8	1.8	27
118	200	15	33	1.7	7.2	12	1.1	2.2	39
124	250	16	39	2.2	9.1	15	1.2	2.7	37
130	300	17	46	2.4	10	17	1.5	3.1	43
133	350	18	54	2.9	11	21	2.0	3.8	31
143	400	18	61	3.4	11	23	2.2	4.2	32

APPENDIX 8A. MEANS AND STANDARD DEVIATIONS OF WEIGHTS AND MEASUREMENTS OF STILLBORN INFANTS

Gestation (wk)	Body weight (g)	Crown-rump (cm)	Crown-heel (cm)	Toe-heel (cm)	Brain (g)	Thymus (g)	Heart (g)	Lungs (g)	Spleen (g)	Liver (g)	Kidneys (g)	Adrenals (g)	Pancreas (g)
20	313	18.0	24.9	3.3	41	0.4	2.4	7.1	0.3	17	2.7	1.3	0.5
	±139	±2.0	±2.3	±0.6	±24	±0.3	±1.0	±3.0	±1.0	±9	±2.9	±0.6	±0.1
21	353	18.9	26.2	3.5	48	0.5	2.6	7.9	0.4	18	3.1	1.4	0.5
	±125	±4.8	±3.6	±0.6	±18	±0.3	±0.9	±3.8	±0.6	±7	±1.3	±0.7	±0.4
22	398	19.8	27.4	3.8	55	0.6	2.8	8.7	0.5	19	3.5	1.4	0.6
	±117	±9.6	±2.5	±0.4	±15	±0.4	±0.9	±3.1	±0.4	±10	±0.8	±0.6	±0.5
23	450	20.6	28.7	4	64	0.8	3	9.5	0.7	21	4.1	1.5	0.7
	±118	±2.3	±3.3	±0.5	±18	±0.5	±1.4	±5.7	±0.5	±7	±1.7	±0.8	±0.3
24	510	21.5	29.9	4.2	74	0.9	3.3	10.5	0.9	22	4.6	1.5	0.7
	±179	±3.1	±4.3	±0.8	±25	±0.7	±1.8	±5.6	±0.7	±8	±2.4	±0.8	±0.3
25	581	22.3	31.1	4.4	85	1.1	3.7	11.6	1.2	24	5.3	1.6	0.8
	±178	±4.0	±6.5	±0.8	±31	±0.8	±1.3	±4.9	±0.4	±35	±2.4	±0.8	±0.7
26	663	23.2	32.4	4.7	98	1.4	4.2	12.9	1.5	26	6.1	1.7	0.8
	±227	±4.1	±5.3	±0.9	±37	±1.4	±2.2	±8.7	±1.1	±16	±3.6	±0.9	±0.7
27	758	24.1	33.6	4.9	112	1.7	4.8	14.4	1.9	29	7	1.9	0.9
	±227	±2.9	±3.2	±1.4	±37	±1.1	±3.6	±9.7	±1.0	±24	±3.1	±1.5	±0.3
28	864	24.9	34.9	5.1	127	2	5.4	16.1	2.3	32	7.9	2.1	1
	±247	±2.2	±5.6	±1.2	±39	±2.1	±2.6	±7.0	±1.1	±32	±2.5	±1.6	±0.3
29	984	25.8	36.1	5.3	143	2.4	6.2	18	2.7	36	9	2.4	1.1
	±511	±4.1	±5.9	±1.2	±57	±2.6	±2.4	±13.6	±2.0	±23	±4.5	±1.2	±1.2
30	1115	26.6	37.3	5.6	160	2.8	7	20.1	3.1	40	10.1	2.7	1.2
	±329	±2.4	±3.6	±0.7	±72	±4.1	±2.8	±8.6	±1.5	±22	±6.0	±1.3	±0.2
31	1259	27.5	38.6	5.8	178	3.2	8	22.5	3.6	46	11.3	3	1.4
	±588	±3.0	±2.7	±0.7	±32	±1.9	±3.1	±10.1	±4.0	±38	±4.1	±1.8	±1.4
32	1413	28.4	39.8	6	196	3.7	9.1	25	4.2	52	12.6	3.5	1.6
	±623	±2.8	±5.4	±0.6	±92	±2.2	±4.1	±10.7	±2.4	±32	±8.0	±1.8	±0.6
33	1578	29.2	41.1	6.2	216	4.3	10.2	27.8	4.7	58	13.9	3.9	1.8
	±254	±3.5	±3.1	±0.4	±51	±1.5	±2.0	±5.8	±2.3	±17	±3.5	±1.4	±0.8
34	1750	30.1	42.3	6.5	236	4.8	11.4	30.7	5.3	66	15.3	4.4	2
	±494	±3.5	±4.3	±0.8	±42	±5.6	±3.2	±15.2	±2.5	±22	±5.1	±1.3	±0.5
35	1930	30.9	43.5	6.7	256	5.4	12.6	33.7	5.9	74	16.7	4.9	2.3
	±865	±3.9	±5.8	±0.9	±70	±3.4	±5.3	±14.3	±6.8	±46	±7.1	±1.9	±0.7
36	2114	31.8	44.8	6.9	277	6.1	13.9	36.7	6.5	82	18.1	5.4	2.6
	±616	±4.0	±7.2	±0.8	±94	±4.1	±5.8	±16.8	±2.9	±36	±6.3	±2.4	±2.6
37	2300	32.7	46	7.2	297	6.7	15.1	39.8	7.2	91	19.4	5.8	2.9
	±647	±5.1	±7.9	±0.9	±69	±3.9	±9.9	±11.1	±6.3	±57	±9.7	±6.2	±3.1
38	2485	33.5	47.3	7.4	317	7.4	16.4	42.9	7.8	100	20.8	6.3	3.2
	±579	±2.6	±3.9	±0.8	±83	±6.1	±4.4	±15.7	±5.9	±44	±6.0	±2.1	±1.6
39	2667	34.4	48.5	7.6	337	8.1	17.5	45.8	8.5	109	22	6.7	3.5
	±596	±3.7	±4.9	±0.5	±132	±4.7	±3.9	±15.2	±4.5	±53	±5.8	±5.3	±1.9
40	2842	35.2	49.7	7.8	355	8.9	18.6	48.6	9.2	118	23.1	7	3.9
	±482	±6.4	±3.2	±0.7	±57	±4.3	±12.9	±19.4	±4.1	±49	±8.6	±2.9	±1.7
41	3006	36.1	51	8.1	373	9.6	19.5	51.1	9.9	126	24.1	7.1	4.2
	±761	±3.7	±5.4	±0.8	±141	±5.6	±4.9	±17.0	±4.5	±53	±10.5	±3.0	
42	3156	36.9	52.2	8.3	389	10.4	20.3	53.2	10.6	135	24.9	7.2	4.5
	±678	±2.0	±3.0	±0.5	±36	±5.0	±4.5	±10.1	±3.7	±54	±8.1	±2.9	±2.3

Data from Women & Infants Hospital, Providence, RI. From Jones Kl., Harrison JW, Smith DW: Palpebral fissure size in newborn infants, *J Pediatr* 92:787, 1978; with permission.

APPENDIX 8B. MEANS AND STANDARD DEVIATIONS OF WEIGHTS AND MEASUREMENTS OF LIVE-BORN INFANTS

Gestation (wk)	Body weight (g)	Crown-rump (cm)	Crown-heel (cm)	Toe-heel (cm)	Brain (g)	Thymus (g)	Heart (g)	Lungs (g)	Spleen (g)	Liver (g)	Kidneys (g)	Adrenals (g)	Pancreas (g)
20	381 ±104	18.3 ±2.2	25.6 ±2.2	3.6 ±0.7	49 ±15	0.8 ±2.3	2.8 ±1.0	11.5 ±2.9	0.7 ±0.3	22.4 ±8.0	3.7 ±1.3	1.8 ±1.0	0.5 ±0.5
21	426 ±66	19.1 ±1.2	26.7 ±1.7	3.8 ±0.1	57 ±8	1 ±0.3	3.2 ±0.4	12.9 ±2.8	0.7 ±0.2	24.1 ±4.2	4.2 ±0.7	2 ±0.5	0.5
22	473 ±63	20 ±1.3	27.8 ±1.6	4 ±0.4	65 ±13	1.2 ±0.3	3.5 ±0.6	14.4 ±4.3	0.8 ±0.4	25.4 ±5.2	4.7 ±1.5	2 ±0.6	0.6 ±0.3
23	524 ±116	20.8 ±1.9	28.9 ±3.0	4.2 ±0.5	74 ±11	1.4 ±0.7	3.9 ±1.3	15.9 ±4.9	0.8 ±0.4	26.6 ±8.0	5.3 ±1.8	2.1 ±0.8	0.7 ±0.4
24	584 ±92	21.6 ±1.4	30 ±1.7	4.4 ±0.3	83 ±15	1.5 ±0.7	4.2 ±1.0	17.4 ±5.9	0.9 ±0.5	28 ±7.1	6 ±1.8	2.2 ±0.8	0.8 ±0.5
25	655 ±106	22.5 ±1.6	31.1 ±2.0	4.6 ±0.4	94 ±25	1.8 ±1.2	4.7 ±1.2	19 ±5.3	1.1 ±1.6	29.7 ±9.8	6.8 ±1.9	2.2 ±1.4	0.9 ±0.3
26	739 ±181	23.3 ±1.9	32.2 ±2.4	4.8 ±0.7	105 ±21	2 ±1.1	5.2 ±1.3	20.6 ±6.3	1.3 ±0.7	32.1 ±10.9	7.6 ±2.5	2.4 ±1.1	1 ±0.5
27	836 ±197	24.2 ±2.5	33.4 ±3.5	5 ±0.5	118 ±21	2.3 ±1.2	5.8 ±1.9	22.1 ±9.7	1.7 ±1.0	35.1 ±13.3	8.6 ±3.0	2.5 ±1.1	1.2 ±0.5
28	949 ±190	25 ±1.7	34.5 ±2.3	5.2 ±0.6	132 ±29	2.6 ±1.5	6.5 ±1.9	23.7 ±10.0	2.1 ±0.8	38.9 ±12.6	9.7 ±12.0	2.7 ±1.2	1.4 ±0.5
29	1077 ±449	25.9 ±2.8	35.6 ±4.4	5.4 ±0.8	147 ±49	3 ±1.9	7.2 ±2.7	25.3 ±12.6	2.6 ±0.9	43.5 ±15.8	10.9 ±4.4	3 ±1.2	1.5 ±1.0
30	1219 ±431	26.7 ±3.3	36.7 ±4.2	5.7 ±0.7	163 ±38	3.5 ±2.6	8.1 ±2.6	26.9 ±20.3	3.3 ±2.0	49.1 ±18.8	12.3 ±8.5	3.3 ±2.7	1.7 ±1.0
31	1375 ±281	27.6 ±3.8	37.8 ±3.1	5.9 ±0.7	180 ±34	4 ±3.4	9 ±2.8	28.5 ±13.2	4 ±1.2	55.4 ±17.3	13.7 ±5.2	3.7 ±1.3	1.8 ±0.6
32	1543 ±519	28.4 ±9.5	38.9 ±5.7	6.1 ±1.1	198 ±48	4.7 ±3.6	10.1 ±4.4	30.2 ±19.0	4.7 ±5.4	62.5 ±30.0	15.2 ±7.4	4.1 ±1.7	2 ±0.8
33	1720 ±580	29.3 ±3.3	40 ±3.5	6.3 ±0.7	217 ±49	5.4 ±3.2	11.2 ±4.0	31.8 ±13.5	5.5 ±3.5	70.3 ±25.4	16.8 ±7.7	4.6 ±1.5	2.1 ±0.8
34	1905 ±625	30.1 ±4.3	41.1 ±4.0	6.5 ±0.6	237 ±53	6.1 ±3.8	12.4 ±2.8	33.5 ±16.5	6.4 ±3.0	78.7 ±30.2	18.5 ±9.3	5.1 ±2.2	2.3 ±1.1
35	2093 ±309	30.9 ±2.0	42.3 ±2.9	6.7 ±0.4	257 ±45	6.9 ±4.5	13.7 ±3.6	35.2 ±20.5	7.2 ±5.2	87.4 ±30.6	20.1 ±10.9	5.6 ±2.8	2.5 ±0.6
36	2280 ±615	31.8 ±3.9	43.4 ±5.9	6.9 ±1.1	278 ±96	7.7 ±5.0	15 ±5.1	36.9 ±17.5	8.1 ±3.1	96.3 ±33.7	21.7 ±6.8	6.1 ±3.1	2.6 ±0.7
37	2462 ±821	32.6 ±5.0	44.5 ±7.0	7.1 ±1.2	298 ±70	8.4 ±5.6	16.4 ±5.7	38.7 ±22.9	8.8 ±6.4	105.1 ±33.7	23.3 ±9.9	6.6 ±3.3	2.8 ±0.9
38	2634 ±534	33.5 ±3.2	45.6 ±5.1	7.3 ±0.8	318 ±106	9 ±2.8	17.7 ±5.4	40.6 ±17.1	9.5 ±3.5	113.5 ±34.7	24.8 ±7.2	7.1 ±2.9	3 ±1.1
39	2789 ±520	34.3 ±1.9	46.7 ±4.4	7.5 ±0.5	337 ±91	9.4 ±2.5	19.1 ±2.8	42.6 ±14.9	10.1 ±3.5	121.3 ±39.2	26.1 ±4.9	7.4 ±2.5	3.3 ±0.5
40	2922 ±450	35.2 ±2.8	47.8 ±4.2	7.7 ±0.8	356 ±79	9.5 ±5.0	20.4 ±5.6	44.6 ±22.7	10.4 ±3.3	127.9 ±35.8	27.3 ±11.5	7.7 ±3.0	3.6 ±1.3
41	3025 ±600	36 ±3.1	48.9 ±5.4	7.9 ±0.8	372 ±65	9.1 ±4.8	21.7 ±10.9	46.8 ±26.2	10.5 ±4.5	133.1 ±55.7	28.1 ±12.7	7.8 ±2.8	3.9 ±1.5
42	3091 ±617	36.9 ±2.4	50 ±3.8	8.1 ±1.1	387 ±61	8.1 ±3.8	22.9 ±6.2	49.1 ±14.6	10.3 ±3.6	136.4 ±38.9	28.7 ±9.7	7.8 ±3.2	4.3 ±1.9

Data from Women & Infants Hospital, Providence, RI. From Jones KL, Harrison JW, Smith DW: Palpebral fissure size in newborn infants. *J Pediatr* 92:787, 1978; with permission.

APPENDIX 9. THE FETOPLACENTAL EXAMINATION AND THE PATH TO PRIMARY CAUSE

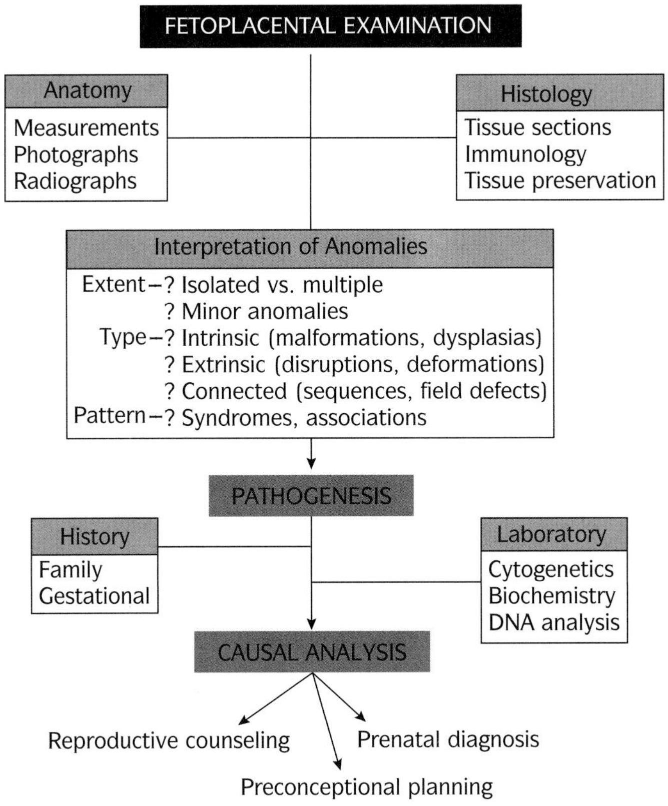

Source: Gilbert-Barness E, ed: *Potter's Pathology of Fetus and Infant*, Philadelphia, CV Mosby Co, 1997.

APPENDIX 10. ORGAN WEIGHTS OF CHILDREN

			Lungs				Kidneys		
Age	Body length (cm)	Heart (g)	Right (g)	Left (g)	Spleen (g)	Liver (g)	Right (g)	Left (g)	Brain (g)
Birth-3 days	49	17	21	18	8	78	13	14	335
3–7 days	49	18	24	22	9	96	14	14	358
1–3 wk	52	19	29	26	10	123	15	15	382
3–5 wk	52	20	31	27	12	127	16	16	413
5–7 wk	53	21	32	28	13	133	19	18	422
7–9 wk	55	23	32	29	13	136	19	18	489
9–3 mo	56	23	35	30	14	140	20	19	516
4 mo	59	27	37	33	16	160	22	21	540
5 mo	61	29	38	35	16	188	25	25	644
6 mo	62	31	42	39	17	200	26	25	660
7 mo	65	34	49	41	19	227	30	30	691
8 mo	65	37	52	45	20	254	31	30	714
9 mo	67	37	53	47	20	260	31	30	750
10 mo	69	39	54	51	22	274	32	31	809
11 mo	70	40	59	53	25	277	34	33	852
12 mo	73	44	64	57	26	288	36	35	925
14 mo	74	45	66	60	26	304	36	35	944
16 mo	77	48	72	64	28	331	39	39	1,010
18 mo	78	52	72	65	30	345	40	43	1,042
20 mo	79	56	83	74	30	370	43	44	1,050
22 mo	82	56	80	75	33	380	44	44	1,059
24 mo	84	56	88	76	33	394	47	46	1,064
3 yr	88	59	89	77	37	418	48	49	1,141
4 yr	99	73	90	85	39	516	58	56	1,191
5 yr	106	85	107	104	47	596	65	64	1,237
6 yr	109	94	121	122	58	642	68	67	1,243
7 yr	113	100	130	123	66	680	69	70	1,263
8 yr	119	110	150	140	69	736	74	75	1,273
9 yr	125	115	174	152	73	756	82	83	1,275
10 yr	130	116	177	166	85	852	92	95	1,290
11 yr	135	122	201	190	87	909	94	95	1,320
12 yr	139	124	–	–	93	936	95	96	1,351

APPENDIX 11. CALCULATED VALUES OF LENGTH OF THE EXTREMITIES AT THE CLOSE OF EACH FETAL MONTH (mm)

Portion of extremity measured	3 mo	4 mo	5 mo	6 mo	7 mo	8 mo	9 mo	10 mo
Length of lower extremity	23.4	59.8	91.0	118.6	143.7	166.8	188.5	208.9
Thigh length (trochanter to knee)	11.5	27.5	41.3	53.5	64.6	74.8	84.4	93.4
Leg length (knee to lateral malleolus)	9.7	26.6	41.1	53.9	65.6	76.4	86.4	95.9
Foot length	4.8	18.4	30.0	40.2	49.6	58.2	66.3	73.8
Length of upper extremity	24.3	58.2	87.2	112.8	136.2	157.7	177.9	196.8
Arm length (acromion to elbow)	10.2	23.6	34.8	44.8	53.8	62.2	70.0	77.3
Forearm length	7.7	18.7	28.1	36.5	44.1	51.1	57.6	63.8
Hand length	3.5	15.6	24.3	32.0	39.1	45.5	51.6	57.2

Data from Scammon RE, Calkins LA: *The Development and Growth of the External Dimensions of the Human Body in the Fetal Period*, Minneapolis, University of Minnesota Press, 1929, with permission.

APPENDIX 12. CALCULATED VALUES OF EXTERNAL DIMENSIONS OF THE HEAD AT THE CLOSE OF EACH FETAL MONTH (mm)

Dimensions of head	3 mo	4 mo	5 mo	6 mo	7 mo	8 mo	9 mo	10 mo
Occipitofrontal circumference	60.8	117.9	166.8	210.1	249.6	285.9	319.9	351.9
Occipitofrontal diameter	20.6	40.5	57.6	72.6	86.4	99.0	110.9	122.0
Suboccipitobregmatic circumference	60.3	113.1	158.4	198.5	235.1	268.7	300.2	329.8
Suboccipitobregmatic diameter	20.2	37.1	51.6	64.4	76.1	86.9	96.9	106.4
Suboccipitofrontal circumference	61.0	116.0	163.1	204.8	242.8	277.8	310.6	341.3
Suboccipitofrontal diameter	22.2	40.4	56.0	69.8	82.4	93.9	104.8	114.9
Occipitomental circumference	53.6	106.9	152.6	193.0	229.8	263.7	295.5	325.3
Occipitomental diameter	18.6	38.5	55.6	70.6	84.4	97.0	108.9	120.0
Biparietal diameter	15.5	31.5	45.3	57.5	68.6	78.8	88.4	97.4

Data from Scammon RE, Calkins LA: *The Development and Growth of the External Dimensions of the Human Body in the Fetal Period.* Minneapolis, University of Minnesota Press, 1929, with permission.

APPENDIX 13. ORGAN WEIGHT (g) IN RELATION TO TOTAL BODY WEIGHT (g)

	Total body weight								
Organ	500–999	1,000–1,499	1,500–1,999	2,000–2,499	2,500–2,999	3,000–3,499	3,500–3,999	4,000–4,499	≥4,500
Thyroid	0.8	0.8	0.9	1.1	1.3	1.6	1.7	1.9	2.4
Thymus	2.1	4.3	6.6	8.2	9.3	11.0	12.6	14.3	17.3
Both lungs	18.2	27.1	37.9	43.6	48.9	54.9	58.0	65.8	74.0
Heart	5.8	9.4	12.7	15.5	19.0	21.2	23.4	28.0	36.0
Spleen	1.7	3.4	4.9	7.0	9.1	10.4	12.0	13.6	16.7
Pancreas	1.0	1.4	2.0	2.3	3.0	3.5	4.0	4.6	6.2
Both kidneys	7.1	12.2	16.2	19.9	23.0	25.3	28.5	31.0	33.2
Both adrenals	3.1	3.9	5.0	6.3	8.2	9.8	10.7	12.5	15.1
Brain	108.7	179.5	255.6	307.6	358.7	403.3	420.6	424.1	406.2
Liver	38.8	59.8	76.3	98.1	127.4	155.1	178.1	215.2	275.6

APPENDIX 14. AUTOPSY PROTOCOL

Autopsy protocol

Autopsy # ____________

Hospital Chart # ________

Birthweight: __________

Name: ______________________________

Age: ______________________________

Gestational age: ______________________________

Sex: ______________________________

Race: ______________________________

Date and time of admission: ______________________________

Date and time of death: ______________________________

Date and time of autopsy: ______________________________

Autopsy performed by: ______________________________

Protocol:

The body is that of a ______ infant weighing ___ gm. The crown-rump length is ___ cm; the rump-heel, ____ cm. The occipitofrontal circumference is ____ cm, that of the chest is ___ cm, and that of the abdomen is ___ cm. Rigor ____________

Hypostasis ____________. Icterus ____________

Cyanosis; ____________. Edema ____________

The pupils are ______________________________

The sclerae are ______________________________

The ears ______________________________

The nose ______________________________

The mouth ______________________________

There is/are ____________ needle puncture mark(s) ____________

____

The umbilical cord is ______________________________

The anus is ______________________________

The external genitalia are ______________________________

The skin is ______________________________

____

____

Peritoneal cavity:

The peritoneal surfaces are ______________________________

____

The peritoneal cavity contains ______________________________

____

The diaphragm arches to the ________ on the right and to the ________ on the left.

APPENDIX 14. (CONTINUED)

The umbilical vein ______________________________

There are __________ umbilical arteries.

The measurements of the liver are as follows: ______________________________

The spleen ______________________________

____

The appendix is in the right lower quadrant. The stomach is ______________________________

____

The small intestine is ______________________________

The large intestine is ______________________________

The mesenteric lymph nodes are ______________________________

The root of the mesentery ______________________________

____

Pleural cavities:

The pleural surfaces are ______________________________

____

The right pleural cavity contains ______________________________

____

The left pleural cavity contains ______________________________

____

The lungs occupy ____________ of their respective pleural cavities.

Each lung has a normal number of lobes.

Pericardial cavity:

The pericardial surfaces are ______________________________

____

The cavity is free from adhesions and contains ______________________________

____

Cardiovascular system:

Heart: The heart weighs ____ g (normal is ____ g).

The foramen ovale is ______________________________

The ductus arteriosus is ______________________________

The mural and valvular endocardium is ______________________________

The myocardium is ______________________________

The coronary ostia and coronary sinus are in normal position. The great vesels arising from the heart and those arising from the aortic arch do so in normal position.
The measurements of the heart are as follows:

TV ____, PV ____, MV ____, AV ____, RVM ____, LVM ____ cm.

The thoracic and abdominal arota ______________________________

____

(*continued*)

APPENDIX 14. (CONTINUED)

Respiratory system:

Lungs: The combined weight of the lungs is ____ g (normal is ____ g).

On section ____

____

The trachea and major bronchi are lined by ______ mucosa; their lumina contain ______

Hematopoietic system:

Spleen: The spleen weighs ____ g (normal is ____ g). The capsule is ______________

On section the parenchyma is ____

The malpighian corpuscles are ____

The lymph nodes are ____

Bone marrow is ____

Gastrointestinal system:

The mucosa of the esophagus is ____

and its lumen contains ____

The mucosa of the stomach is ____

and its lumen contains ____

The mucosa of the small intestine is ____

and its lumen contains ____

The length of the small bowel is ____ cm; the large bowel, ____ cm.

The mucosa of the large intestine is ____

and its lumen contains ____

Liver: The liver weighs ____ g (normal is ____ g).

The capsule is ____

On section the parenchyma is ____

____

The sinus intermedius and ductus venosus are ____

____

The bile, which is ______________________, is freely expressed from the gallbladder into the duodenum.

Pancreas: The pancreas is tan and coarsely lobulated. On section______________

____

____

Endocrine system:

Adrenals: The combined weight of the adrenals is ____ g. They are ______________

____

The cut surfaces reveal ____

peripheral zones and ______________________ central zones.

APPENDIX 14. (CONTINUED)

Genitourinary system:

Kidneys: The combined weight of the kidneys is ___ g (normal is ___ g).

The renal arteries and veins are free from thrombi. The capsules strip easily from ___ surfaces ______________________________

____

On section the cortex and medulla are ______________________________ demarcated. The renal pelves and ureters are lined by ______________

Bladder: The mucosa of the bladder is ______________________________

____

The relations at the trigone are normal.

Genitalia: The prostate is small and firm and reveals no gross abnormalities. The vaginal mucosa is ______________________________

The uterus, tubes, and ovaries reveal no gross abnormalities. The uterus and ovaries are of normal size.

Organs of the Neck: The thymus weighs ___ g. The surface is ______________

____

The cut surfaces ______________________________

The thyroid and larynx reveal no gross abnormalities. The larynx is lined by ______________ mucosa and is empty. The submaxillary glands ______________

____

______________ parathyroids are identified. Positions: ______________

____

Head: The soft tissues of the scalp are ______________________________ . The anterior fontanelle measures ___ cm.

The posterior fontanelle is ______________________________

The sutures ______________________________

The dura mater is ______________________________

The falx cerebri and the tentorium cerebelli are intact. The pia arachnoid is ______________

____

There is no subarachnoid hemorrhage nor exudate. The convolutions and sulci are ___
The brain is fixed in toto. The dural sinuses are free from thrombi.

The middle ears are ______________________________

A segment of the ______________ spinal cord is removed by the anterior approach and reveals no gross abnormalities.

The pituitary ______________________________

Musculoskeletal system:

Bones: The manubrium sternum contains ______________ center of ossification. The ______________, ______________, ______________ sternbrae each contain ______________ centers of ossification. There are ______________ pairs of ribs. Two lower costochondral junctions are removed from each side.

APPENDIX 15. NOMOGRAM FOR EVALUATION OF GROWTH OF OCCIPITOFRONTAL DIAMETER

	Occipitofrontal diameter (mm)		
Age (weeks)	5th	50th	95th
11	11	18	25
12	16	23	30
13	20	27	34
14	24	31	38
15	29	36	43
16	33	40	47
17	37	44	51
18	41	48	55
19	46	53	60
20	50	57	64
21	54	61	68
22	58	65	72
23	62	69	76
24	65	72	79
25	69	76	83
26	73	80	87
27	76	83	90
28	80	87	94
29	83	90	97
30	86	93	100
31	89	96	103
32	92	99	106
33	95	102	108
34	97	104	111
35	99	106	113
36	102	109	116
37	104	111	118
38	105	112	119
39	107	114	121
40	108	115	122
41	109	116	123
42	110	117	124

APPENDIX 16. RELATIONSHIP BETWEEN GESTATIONAL AGE AND BIPARIETAL DIAMETER

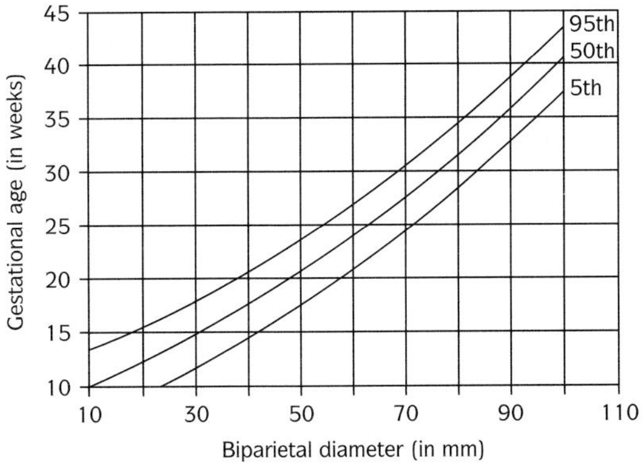

APPENDIX 17. CORTICAL MANTLE THICKNESS

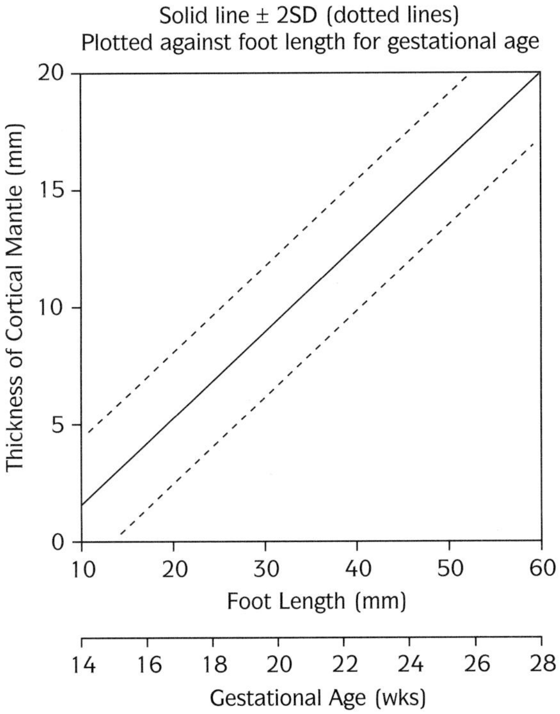

Index